Radiology of the Heart

Cardiac Imaging in Infants, Children, and Adults

Hugo Spindola-Franco
Bernard G. Fish

Radiology
of the
Heart

*Cardiac Imaging in Infants,
Children, and Adults*

With Contributions by
Robert Eisenberg, Charles B. Higgins,
Richard M. Steingart, and John P. Wexler

With over 552 halftone illustrations in 1202 parts
and 62 line illustrations

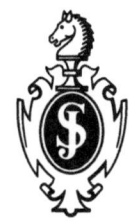

Springer-Verlag
New York Berlin Heidelberg Tokyo

Hugo Spindola-Franco, M.D., F.A.C.C., F.A.C.R., Professor of Radiology, Albert Einstein College of Medicine, Yeshiva University; Attending Radiologist, Montefiore Medical Center; Director of Cardiovascular Radiology, Montefiore Medical Center; Consultant in Radiology and Medicine (Cardiology), Bronx Veterans Administration Hospital, New York. Address correspondence to Department of Radiology, Montefiore Medical Center, Moses Division, 111 East 210th Street, Bronx, New York, U.S.A. 10467.

Bernard G. Fish, M.D., F.A.A.P., Assistant Professor of Pediatrics and Assistant Professor of Radiology, Albert Einstein College of Medicine, Yeshiva University; Associate Attending in Pediatrics (Pediatric Cardiology), Montefiore Medical Center. Address correspondence to Department of Pediatrics, Montefiore Medical Center, Moses Division, 111 East 210th Street, Bronx, New York, U.S.A. 10467

Library of Congress Cataloging in Publication Data
Spindola-Franco, Hugo.
    Radiology of the heart.
  Includes bibliographies and index.
    1. Heart—Radiography. 2. Heart—Diseases—
Diagnosis. I. Fish, Bernard G. II. Title.
[DNLM: 1. Heart—radiography. 2. Heart Diseases—
diagnosis.   WG 141.5.R2 S757r]
RC683.5.R3S65 1985   616.1'20757   84–23631

© 1985 by Springer-Verlag New York, Inc.
Softcover reprint of the hardcover 1st edition 1985

X-ray reproductions by Carlin Medical Photography, New York City.
Line drawings by Stanley R. Waine, Medical Multimedia Corp., 211 East 43rd Street, New York, New York.
Text and cover design by Robert Hollander.
Typeset by Kingsport Press, Kingsport Tennessee.

9 8 7 6 5 4 3 2 1

ISBN-13:978-1-4613-8207-2   e-ISBN-13:978-1-4613-8205-8
DOI: 10.1007/978-1-4613-8205-8

Dedicated to
HAROLD G. JACOBSON, M.D.
The teacher, the scholar, the scientific father

and to our wives
EDITH BALDERAS DE SPINDOLA, JUDITH NAOMI OPHIR FISH
and our children, who patiently awaited completion of this book.

Foreword

In this unprecedented era of revolutionary developments in clinical imaging, in no area of the body are dramatic breakthroughs better exemplified than in imaging of the heart.

It is difficult for this writer to be objective about this work because he has watched its development in the exceptionally capable hands of a cardiovascular radiologist and a cardiovascular internist, functioning as an ideal amalgam in its preparation. In the process, the author of this Foreword has developed an unbounded enthusiasm for the content of the work.

At the outset it must be stressed that the dramatic gains in the development of new imaging modalities and the improvements in the old [e.g., ultrasonography, echocardiography, radionuclides, computerized tomography (CT), cineradiography, magnetic resonance (MR)] have changed our concepts about the anatomy of a number of organ systems. Anatomy and even physiology virtually are being rewritten. These changes apply particularly to the chest (mediastinum), biliary tract, central nervous system (brain), heart and great vessels and the hemodynamics of the cardiovascular system. The authors have demonstrated in this exhaustive treatise how far our understanding of the many cardiac abnormalities has progressed, made possible by the application of the new modalities and further advances in those already established, particularly echocardiography and radioisotope scanning. These developments have altered and added significantly to our body of information, particularly in the many complex congenital anomalies and in coronary artery disease.

This work is presented in ten chapters. Chapter 1 consists of an updated delineation of normal anatomy of the heart and great vessels; Chapter 2 constitutes an introductory but thorough discussion of the clinical application of echocardiography (including Doppler echocardiography); Chapter 3 deals with the almost startling newly discovered efficacy of cardiovascular nuclear medicine (contributed by Drs. Richard Steingart and John Wexler); Chapter 4 discusses an increasingly important subject—ischemic heart disease; Chapter 5 describes in detail the various forms of valvular heart disease; Chapter 6 evaluates the various cardiomyopathies in depth; Chapter 7, by far the largest of the book, is divided into six sections describing both the commonplace and the esoteric congenital abnormalities of the heart and great vessels. This chapter constitutes a monograph unto itself, discussing a very complex subject in superb detail and with great clarity; Chapter 8 details the various neoplasms of the heart; the number of neoplasms considered is extraordinary; Chapter 9 discusses diseases of the pericardium; and finally, Chapter 10 is a contribution from Dr.

Charles B. Higgins of the University of California at San Francisco on imaging of the heart by magnetic resonance.

This work is encyclopedic in its scope and yet brilliantly organized and written with admirable lucidity. The authors go into the most minute detail regarding even the most obscure of lesions. The tome is a thoroughly scholarly effort. The reproductions are of superior quality lending to the enhancement of an impressive array of descriptive illustrations of an unusually large volume of material—both commonplace and esoteric. A very considerable, very thorough, yet relevant bibliography is appended to each chapter, promising to be of inestimable value to the scholar in the field.

In all instances, the authors diligently correlate the interrelationship of the anatomical features, the clinical data, the findings on echocardiography, the hemodynamics, the application of radionuclides where appropriate. In addition, a description in depth of the imaging (radiological) features with plain films, cine radiography for opacification studies, and other "state of the art" imaging techniques is presented. Even a concise but pragmatic discussion of treatment in each disorder is provided.

It is very difficult to write an objective Foreword for this work. This enthusiastic evaluation of the treatise probably overcomes any degree of objectivity in evaluating the tome and yet the author of this Foreword has no compunction about being biased in this instance. In a sense this Foreword constitutes a review of the book—a review that appears to sing constant paeans of praise for the quality and scope of the work. If the impression is gained that this writer is prejudiced, *so be it*. Calling it "like you think it is" is still fundamentally a sound aphorism, even if the judgment of the "caller" is suspect.

This important work is an unusual example of a cooperative effort by a clinical cardiovascular radiologist and a clinical cardiovascular internist in the production of a treatise of great scope and significance. In this writer's judgment, an outstanding contribution has been prepared on a highly complex but fundamentally important subject—a contribution badly needed in the discipline of cardiac radiology. This treatise should prove to be of inestimable value to a whole array of different groups of physicians: the general radiologist, the primary care physician in all areas, the residents in training, all medical students and, of course, the cardiac radiologist and cardiac internist. The work, with its deftly organized presentation of inexhaustible details, promises to become a landmark on the subject.

The authors are to be congratulated on the preparation of an important contribution on a complex but overwhelmingly vital subject.

HAROLD G. JACOBSON, M.D.

Preface

The purpose of this book is to provide comprehensive coverage of all aspects of cardiovascular disease. Each topic is presented systematically and concisely leading the reader to correlate clinical findings and non-invasive studies with invasive studies and treatment modalities.

A detailed description of the patterns of pulmonary vasculature and a new classification of congenital heart disease based on radiological findings should facilitate an accurate diagnosis in simple as well as complex cardiac defects.

The stepwise approach used in this book is used by the authors in the evaluation of patients and in the instruction of trainees as well as colleagues.

We are confident that by using this approach others will become proficient in a field which has been, even for sophisticated professionals, an impenetrable enigma.

Acknowledgments

We are grateful to many people who contributed to this work, including members of the Departments of Radiology, Medicine, Pediatrics, and Cardiothoracic Surgery at Montefiore Medical Center and the Albert Einstein College of Medicine. Among those who cooperated extensively in performing hemodynamic and angiographic studies and in providing an atmosphere of learning were Drs. Doris Escher, Richard Grose, and Norman Solomon. Drs. Grose and Solomon, through their friendship, their understanding, and their willingness to assume extra responsibility, provided an atmosphere conducive to the development and completion of this work. Dr. Mark Greenberg reviewed the chapter on Valvular Heart Disease and made many helpful suggestions. Other members of the Division of Cardiology who contributed were Drs. Janet Strain, Robert Rosenblum, and Thasana Nivatpumin.

We acknowledge the faculty and staff of the Bronx Veterans Administration Hospital, especially the late Dr. Kam F. Chan and Dr. Howard Friedman, who provided acccess to material from that institution and invited the senior author to provide teaching conferences. The material for this book stems from a collection gathered in preparation for conferences at Montefiore Medical Center and at the Bronx VA.

Drs. Michael V. Cohen, Maxine Rosoff, and Naftali Neuberger were especially helpful in contributing echocardiograms on adults. Dr. Robert Eisenberg with Drs. Rajamma Mathew and Henry Issenberg performed the pediatric cardiac catheterizations at Montefiore Medical Center.

Special thanks are due to Drs. George Robinson, Lari Attai, Robert Frater, Abraham Merav, and Richard Brodman, who not only contributed material, but more importantly provided surgical correlation with the angiocardiographic studies.

Dr. James Scheuer had maintained a standard of excellence within his division and has encouraged close cooperation between the Divisions of Cardiology and the Department of Radiology.

Dr. Spindola-Franco has been particularly fortunate to be able to work and develop under giants in the field of Radiology: Dr. Harold G. Jacobson, Dr. Herbert L. Abrams, and Dr. Douglass F. Adams in the United States and the late Jorge Ceballos Labat in Mexico, who taught discipline and uncompromising excellence.

Dr. Jacobson noted the abundance of material being collected and insisted that it be brought together into a book. He also diligently reviewed and meticulously edited the entire manuscript and made innumerable helpful changes. Dr. Jacobson deserves full credit for the existence of this book.

Drs. Sven Paulin, Richard Gorlin, and Michael V. Herman at Harvard Medical School and Drs. Seymour Sprayregen and Thomas C. Beneventano at Montefiore Medical Center also taught special skills required, and served as models for excellence in teaching.

Dr. Spindola-Franco's former associates in Cardiac Radiology, Enrico Cappiello, Robert Greenbaum and Elliot Wein, and his present associate, Ayodeji Fayemi, have contributed material and have enabled Dr. Spindola-Franco to spend the time required to write this book.

Zina Zilo, Chief Technologist in the Cardiac Catheterization Laboratory, in cooperation with Lilly Sharaz and Kevin Early, photographed innumerable cineangiographic studies, from which many of the illustrations were selected.

The late Dr. Dennison Young, former Director of Pediatric Cardiology at Montefiore Medical Center and a pioneer in the field of congenital heart disease, was most influential in Dr. Fish's training and continued as his mentor until his recent death. Dr. Fish also trained with Dr. Norman Talner at Yale University, who encouraged excellence in academic pursuits.

Mr. Michael Carlin deserves credit for the superb work he did in converting all of the roentgenographic studies into photographic prints. The excellent drawings were produced by Mr. Stanley Waine.

The staff of Springer-Verlag have been enthusiastic in their cooperation in the production of this book. In addition to their meticulous attention to technical details, the production staff coordinated the process in such a way as to make an overwhelming and complex task manageable.

Mrs. Eleanor Schultz deserves special mention. Her patience and diligence in preparing the manuscript contributed in a major way to the quality of this book. She functioned as a research and editorial assistant, checking innumerable details, proofreading text and bibliography, and communicating with the publisher.

Contents

Contributors

Robert Eisenberg, M.D., Assistant Professor of Pediatrics and Attending in Pediatrics (Pediatric Cardiology), Albert Einstein College of Medicine, Yeshiva University, and Montefiore Medical Center, Bronx, New York, U.S.A.

Charles B. Higgins, M.D., Professor of Radiology and Chief, Magnetic Resonance Imaging, University of California San Francisco Medical Center, San Francisco, California, U.S.A.

Richard M. Steingart, M.D., Assistant Professor of Medicine, Division of Cardiology, Albert Einstein College of Medicine, Yeshiva University, and Montefiore Medical Center, Bronx, New York, U.S.A.

John P. Wexler, M.D., PH.D., Assistant Professor of Radiology, Albert Einstein College of Medicine, Yeshiva University, and Montefiore Medical Center, Bronx, New York, U.S.A.

1 Normal Heart and Great Vessels

The radiological appearance of the heart and great vessels has a wide variation. The configuration of the cardiovascular silhouette varies according to the body build (chest shape) or habitus, respiratory cycle, the age and sex of the individual, and position (effects of gravity) at the time of examination (supine, erect), changes in intrathoracic pressure (Valsalva and Mueller maneuvers), and the like.

The heart is situated in the middle mediastinum and casts a homogeneous shadow (water density). Approximately two thirds of the heart project to the left of the midline and one third projects to the right. The cardiac borders are clearly outlined by the radiolucent lungs. The inferior heart border may blend with the diaphragm, making its differentiation difficult. The shadows of the heart and pericardium cannot often be separated. When optimal roentgenograms are obtained, however, the epicardial fat allows these structures to be distinguished in the frontal and lateral projections and especially over the apex. Pericardial fat, however, may obscure the cardiophrenic angles. Fat in obese patients and in those taking steroids (fat redistribution) and the thymus in children may obscure the vascular structures in the superior mediastinum. Evaluation of heart size and chamber enlargement requires intimate knowledge of the position of the chambers and their contribution to the formation of the cardiac outline.

Heart Size. Many methods and innumerable tables are available for determination of normal heart size. However, most of these are cumbersome and inaccurate. Although the cardiothoracic ratio (the ratio of the transverse cardiac diameter to the maximum internal diameter of the thorax) and the absolute transverse cardiac diameter (Ungerleider method) are grossly inaccurate, they are useful guidelines for the unsophisticated. A cardiothoracic ratio of 55%–60% is considered normal. The measurement of the transverse cardiac diameter alone is a useful baseline for future comparison and gross determination of cardiac enlargement.

Determination of cardiac volumes on plain films pro-

vides a more accurate index of overall cardiac size. It is cumbersome, however, and seldom used.

Normal Heart

The Posteroanterior (PA) Projection (Fig. 1–1A)

The right heart border is composed of two segments. The inferior segment is smooth and convex, being formed by the lateral wall of the right atrium. The superior segment is usually straight and is formed by the superior vena cava and right innominate vein. The ascending aorta may cause a gentle convexity of the lower part of the superior segment. The junction of the superior and inferior segments is often delineated by a shallow notch.

The left heart border is made up of three segments: The upper segment is usually round and convex laterally and is formed by the aortic arch (aortic knob). The middle segment is variable in shape, usually slightly convex but on occasion straight or even concave, depending on the age and habitus of the patient. This segment is formed by the main pulmonary artery. The lower and longest segment is convex, being formed by the left ventricle. The degree of convexity of the lower segment is variable, depending on the age and habitus of the patient. The junction of the middle and lower segments usually demarcates the region of the left atrioventricular groove. The left circumflex artery generally runs in that plane. The edge of the left atrial appendage may contribute to this small segment. The left cardiophrenic angle may be obliterated by pericardial fat, which may simulate cardiomegaly.

Lateral Projection (Fig. 1–1B)

From above downward the anterior border of the cardiovascular silhouette is formed by the ascending aorta, the pulmonary artery and the right ventricle (outflow tract superiorly and sinus portion inferiorly). Between the sternum and the outflow tract of the right ventricle is a clear

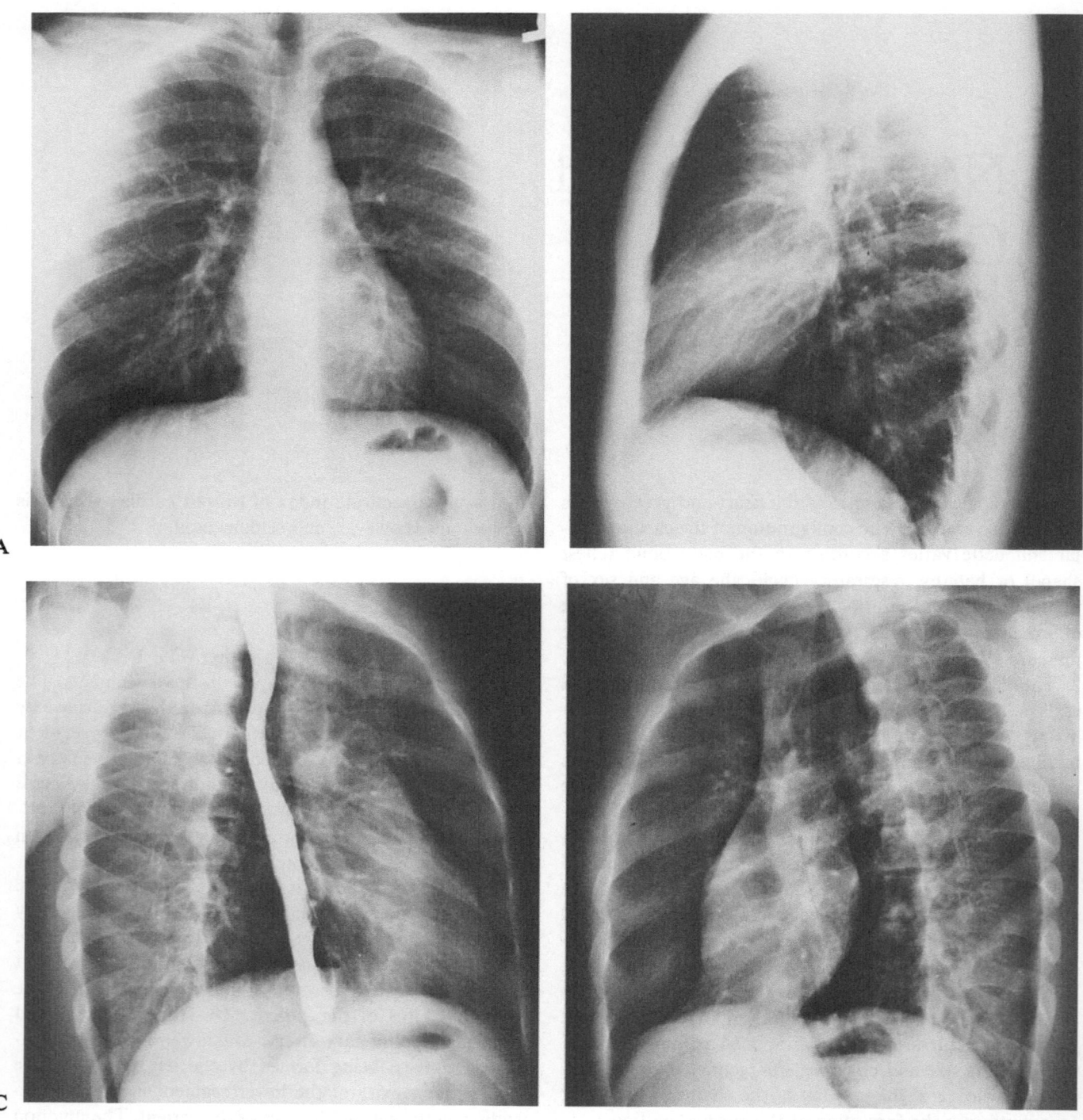

Fig. 1–1, A–D. *Normal cardiac configuration, normal pulmonary vascularity.* **A** PA view. Comprising the right heart border are the outlines of the superior vena cava, right atrium, and inferior vena cava. The outer contour of the left heart border consists of the aortic arch, main pulmonary artery (MPA) and left ventricle. The pulmonary vessels to the upper segments of the lungs are of smaller caliber than are those to the lower segments. Gradual tapering of the vessels is apparent. **B** Lateral view. The anterior heart border is formed by the ascending aorta, MPA and right ventricle. The posterior cardiac border is formed by the left atrium, left ventricle and inferior vena cava. The right pulmonary artery appears as a spheroid density. The left pulmonary artery arches posteriorly and inferiorly above the left main bronchus. **C** Right anterior oblique (RAO) view. The anterior (left) heart border is formed by the ascending aorta, pulmonary artery, right ventricular outflow tract and right ventricular sinus (body of the right ventricle). The posterior (right) heart border is formed by the aorta, left atrium, right atrium and inferior vena cava. The barium-filled esophagus is indented by the aorta above. **D** Left anterior oblique (LAO) view. The anterior (right) heart border is formed by the superior vena cava, ascending aorta, right atrial appendage and right ventricle. The posterior (left) heart border is formed by the left atrium and the left ventricle. A radiolucent space (the aortic window) is present below the aortic arch.

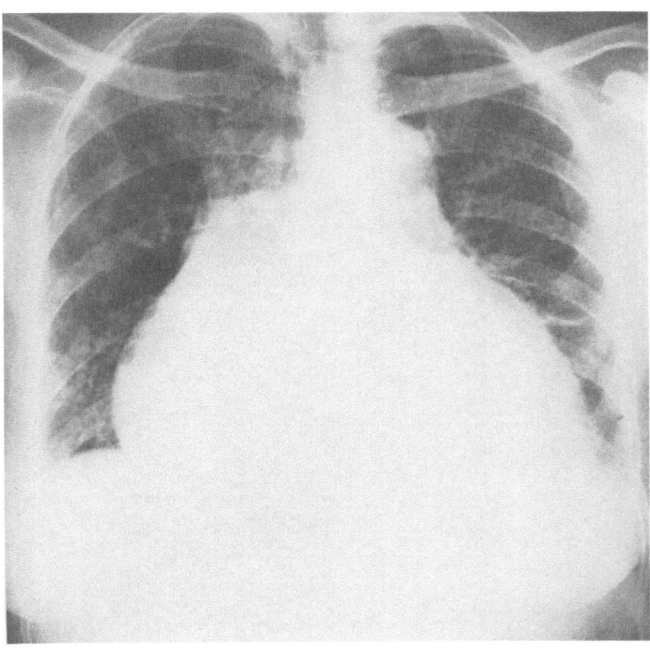
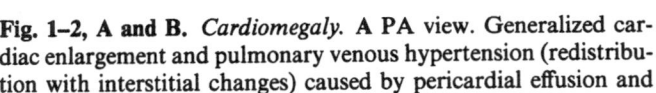

A

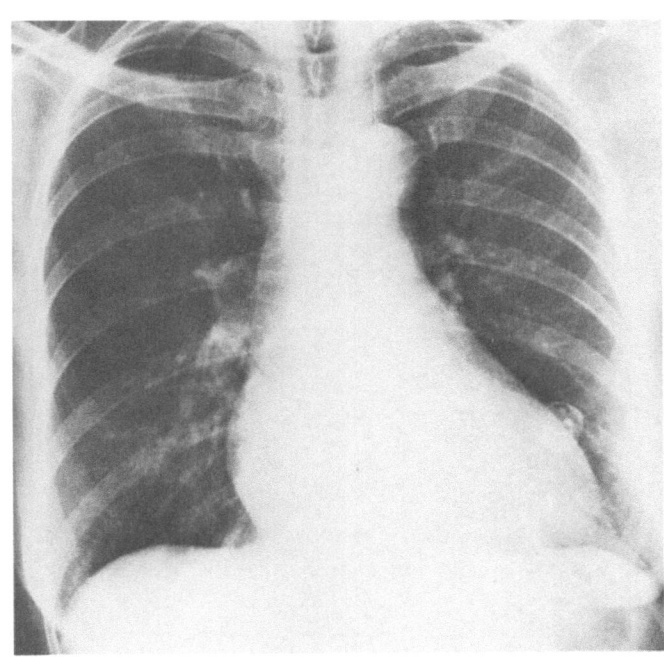

B

Fig. 1–2, A and B. *Cardiomegaly.* A PA view. Generalized cardiac enlargement and pulmonary venous hypertension (redistribution with interstitial changes) caused by pericardial effusion and cardiac tamponade. B After resolution of pericardial effusion. An incidental large granuloma is noted overlying the left heart border.

space (retrosternal clear space) that is important in the analysis of chamber enlargement. The posterior border is formed by the left atrium superiorly and the left ventricle inferiorly. The inferior vena cava casts a slightly concave linear density as it enters the right atrium from below. The aortic arch is usually well outlined, as is the ascending aorta and proximal portion of the descending aorta. The right pulmonary artery is visualized as a spheroid or ovoid density in front of the lucency cast by the opening of the eparterial bronchus. This first branch of the right bronchus is called eparterial because it lies above the right pulmonary artery. The left pulmonary artery is represented by a tubular density that arches in a posterior direction above the left main pulmonary bronchus (the hyparterial bronchus).

Right Anterior Oblique (RAO) Projection (Fig. 1–1C)

The anterior cardiovascular border is formed from above downward by the ascending aorta, pulmonary artery and outflow tract of the right ventricle and the sinus portion of the right ventricle. The posterior border is formed again from above downward by the aorta, left atrium, right atrium and the inferior vena cava as it enters the right atrium.

Left Anterior Oblique (LAO) Projection (Fig. 1–1D)

The anterior (right) border is formed from above downward by the ascending aorta, the right atrial appendage, and the right ventricle. Above the outline of the ascending aorta the virtually straight density of the superior vena cava can be appreciated. The posterior border is formed by the left atrium and the left ventricle, which are below the pulmonary artery. The aortic arch is outlined virtually in its entirety, and, depending on the degree of inspiration, a radiolucent clear space (aortic window) may be noted below it. The aortic window is thus outlined by the undersurface of the aorta and the superior surface of the left pulmonary artery.

Cardiomegaly

Enlargement of the heart may be generalized, or it may involve one or more chambers. Generalized cardiac enlargement may be difficult to distinguish from pericardial effusion (Fig. 1–2). However, if one or more chambers are enlarged the cardiac silhouette usually shows characteristic changes recognizable on plain films.

Left Ventricular Hypertrophy

In most cases left ventricular hypertrophy does not alter the left heart border. However, in some instances rounding and elevation of the cardiac apex on the frontal roentgenograms are noted. Right ventricular hypertrophy also causes rounding and elevation of the cardiac apex but is usually associated with abnormalities of the main pulmonary artery (concavity or dilatation).

Left Ventricular Enlargement (LVE) (Fig. 1–3)

On the PA projection dilatation of the left ventricle (LV) causes an increase in the transverse cardiac diameter and in the length of the left heart border with the apex pointing downward. The apex projects below the left hemidiaphragm, and the prominence of the left heart border may be pronounced in contrast to the adjacent concavity of the pulmonary artery segment.

On the lateral projection LV dilatation increases the

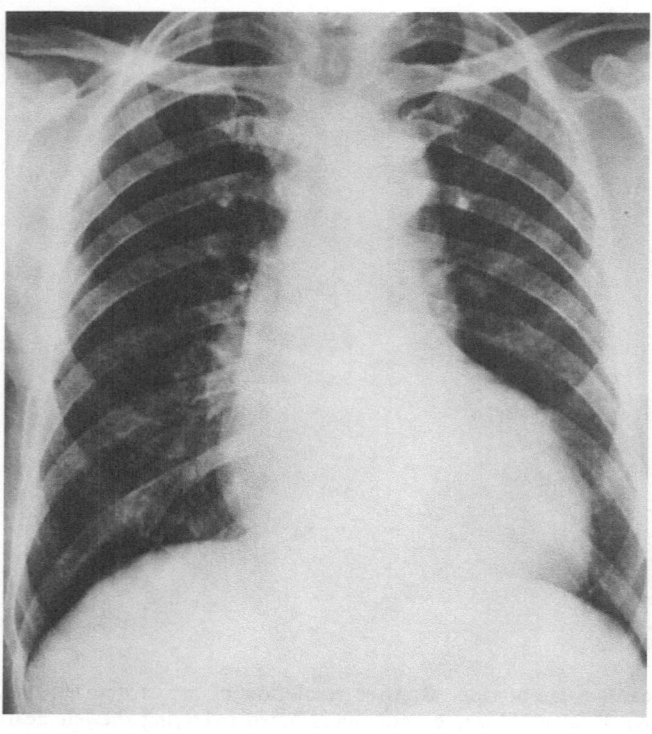

A

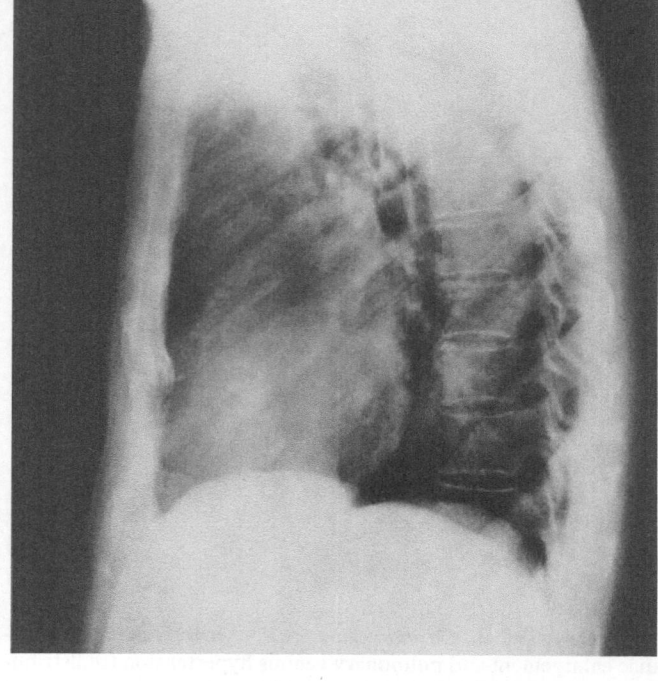

B

Fig. 1–3, A and B. *Left ventricular enlargement in a hypertensive male.* A PA view. An increase in the transverse cardiac diameter with rounding and elongation of the left heart border is observed. The apex points downward. The dilated ascending aorta can be identified as a convexity along the right heart border between the superior vena cava and right atrium. The aortic arch and descending aorta are also dilated. **B** Lateral view. The enlarged left ventricle presents as a convexity along the lower segment of the posterior heart border, extending more than 1.8 cm behind the inferior vena cava.

convexity of the lower posterior contour. The LV should not extend more than 1.8 cm behind the posterior border of the inferior vena cava at a level 2 cm cephalad to their crossing (the Rigler sign). The sharp angle between the heart and the diaphragm disappears. The left ventricle may also extend behind the barium-filled esophagus with reduction of the retrocardiac space. Depending on the extent of the dilatation, the left ventricle may become border forming anteriorly.

On the RAO projection the enlarged LV may displace and indent the esophagus, and on the LAO projection the LV may project over the spine.

The LV is enlarged in patients with hypertension, aortic valvular disease (insufficiency), coarctation of the aorta, myocardial disease (including ischemic myopathy), mitral valvular disease (insufficiency) and shunt lesions (e.g., ventricular septal defect, patent ductus arteriosus).

Left Atrial Enlargement (LAE) (Fig. 1–4)

On the PA projection the enlarged left atrium (LA) usually produces a double density within the cardiac silhouette. A double density also may be observed in some individuals with a normal LA. In these individuals the double density is the size of a normal LA and is not as radiopaque as that of an enlarged LA. In LAE, however, the density of the right atrium is considerably less than that of the left atrium, and it tends to be more lateral and inferior. When the LA is markedly enlarged (giant LA) it may bulge just

superiorly to the right atrium or it may form the right heart border. Other signs of LAE include elevation of the left main bronchus and splaying of the carina, which on occasion is associated with collapse of the left lower lobe (LLL). The esophagus is generally displaced to the right, but displacement may also occur to the left. The descending thoracic aorta may also be displaced to the left. Enlargement of the left atrial appendage produces straightening of the left heart border or a convexity (bulge, third mogul) below the pulmonary artery segment in the frontal view.

Indentation of the barium-filled esophagus by the LA is observed optimally in the RAO and left lateral projections. It should be noted that in some individuals with marked enlargement of the LA the barium-filled esophagus tends to remain in a relatively normal position with minimal or no displacement. This is because the LA dilates laterally. On the RAO projection the enlarged LA projects posterior to the esophagus. In some older individuals with uncoiling of the aorta the esophagus tends to follow the aorta and may on occasion simulate LAE, particularly on the lateral projection.

On the LAO projection the contour corresponding to the LA is prominent, and the elevation of the left main bronchus can be best appreciated. The left main bronchus may be narrow and associated with LLL collapse.

The left atrium is enlarged in rheumatic heart disease (mitral valvular disease), shunt lesions (ventricular septal defect, patent ductus arteriosus, aorticopulmonary win-

Fig. 1–4, A–C. *Left atrial enlargement* (LAE) in a patient with mitral stenosis. **A** PA view. The enlarged left atrium produces a double density within the cardiac contour. The left atrial appendage produces a slight convexity in the region of the AV groove along the left heart border (*arrows*). In instances in which this convexity is more pronounced it is called the third mogul. Another sign of LAE observed in this film is mild elevation of the left main stem bronchus. **B** Lateral view. A bulge in the region of the left atrium displaces the left main bronchus posteriorly and superiorly. **C** RAO view. Characteristic indentation of the barium-filled esophagus by the enlarged left atrium is present.

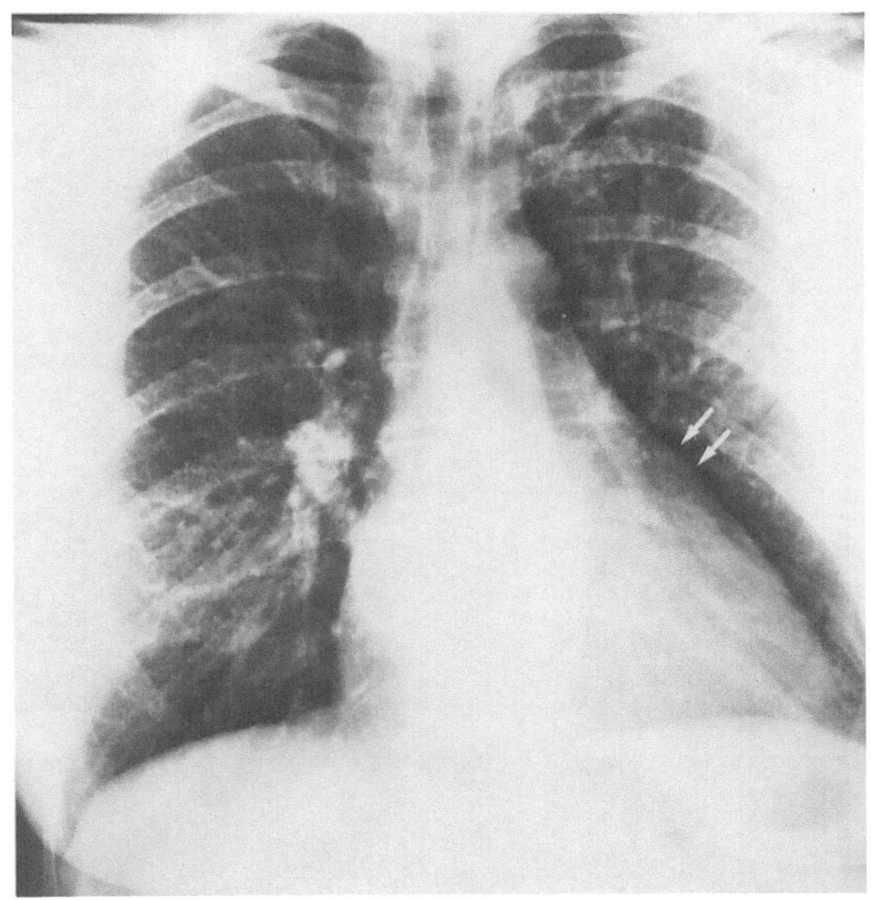

A

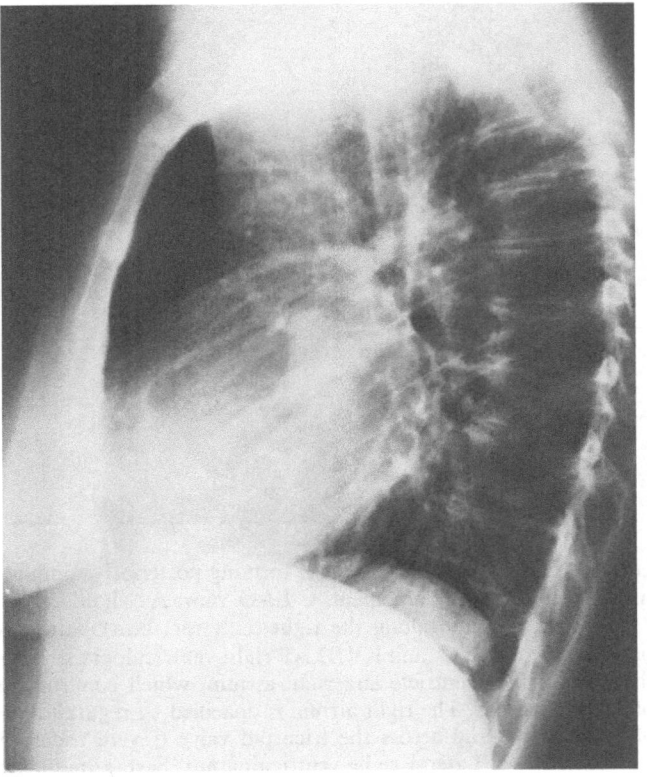

B

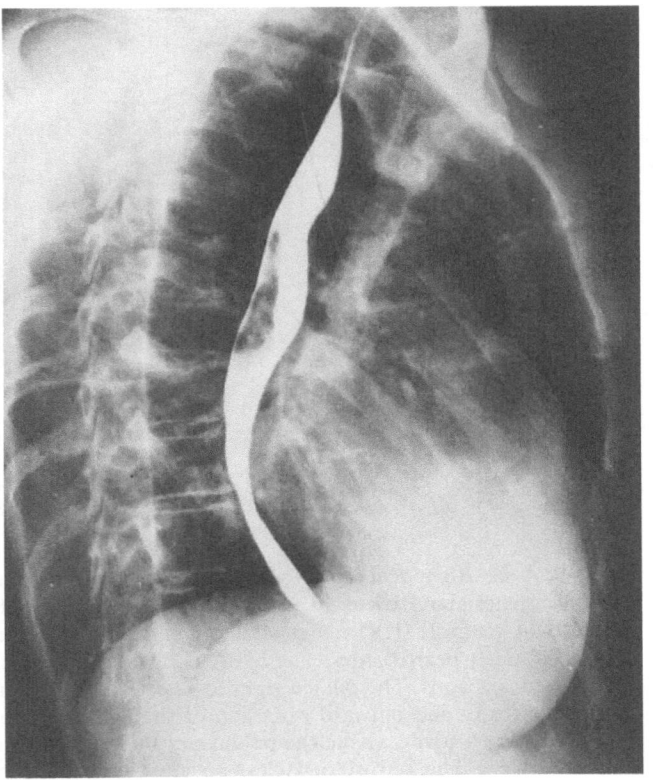

C

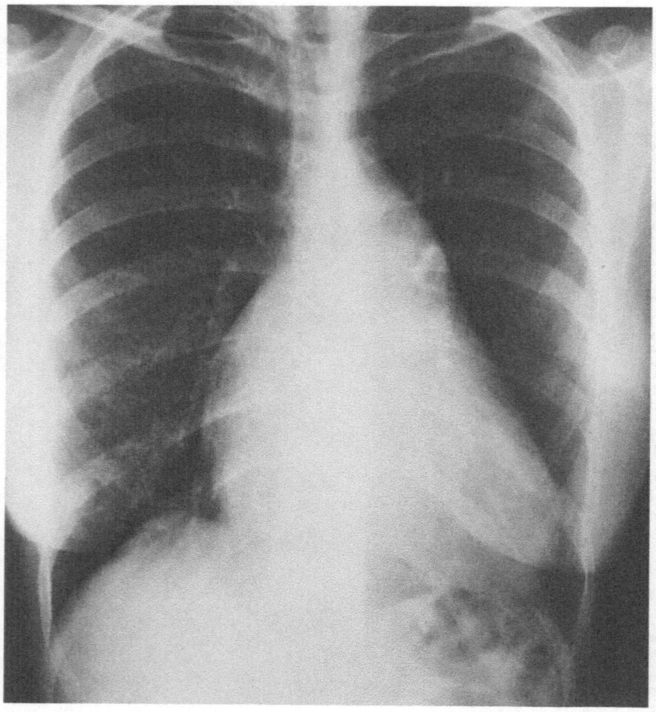

Fig. 1-5, A-E. *Right ventricular enlargement* in a patient with pulmonic stenosis and tricuspid insufficiency. **A** PA view. The dilated right ventricle (RV) causes straightening and slight convexity of the left heart border. The MPA is dilated. The aortic arch is inconspicuous. The dilated right atrium (RA) causes increased convexity and outward extension of the lower segment of the right heart border. Note the pulmonary undercirculation. **B** Lateral view. The retrosternal clear space is obliterated by the dilated RV and RA. Specifically the dilated right atrial appendage (RAA) is elevated so that it becomes the major contributor to obliteration of the retrosternal clear space. The markedly enlarged right atrium is also border forming posteriorly, simulating left ventricular enlargement. **C** LAO view. A "shoulder" or "shelf" configuration along the right (anterior) heart border is produced by the RAA and RV. **D** AP right ventriculogram. Note the dilated right ventricle and right atrium, which confirm the plain film findings. The right atrium is opacified by regurgitation of contrast material across the tricuspid valve (severe tricuspid insufficiency). **E** Lateral right ventriculogram. Severe pulmonic valve stenosis is present, with doming of the pulmonary valve and a narrow jet emptying into a markedly dilated main pulmonary artery (poststenotic dilatation).

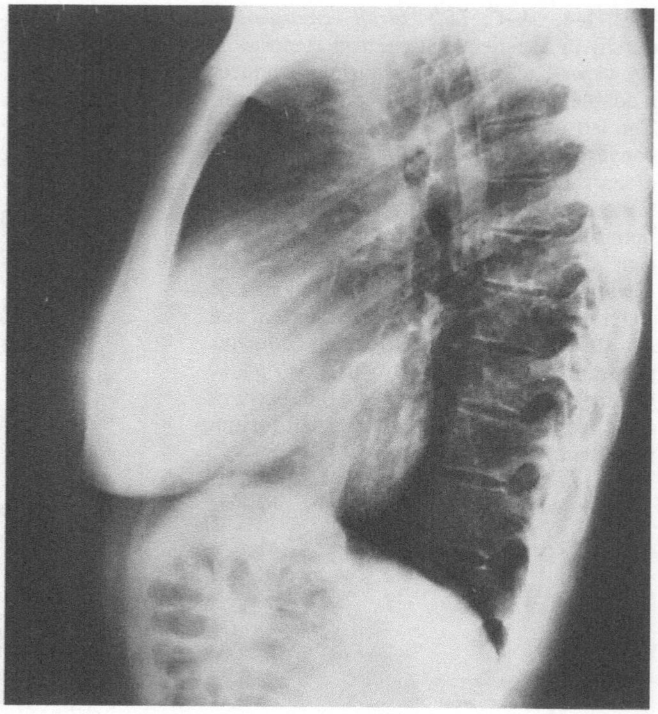

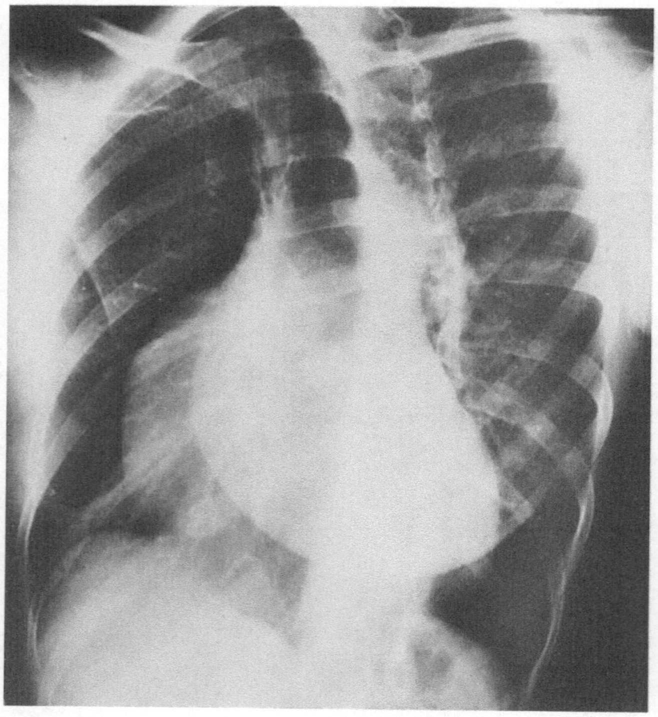

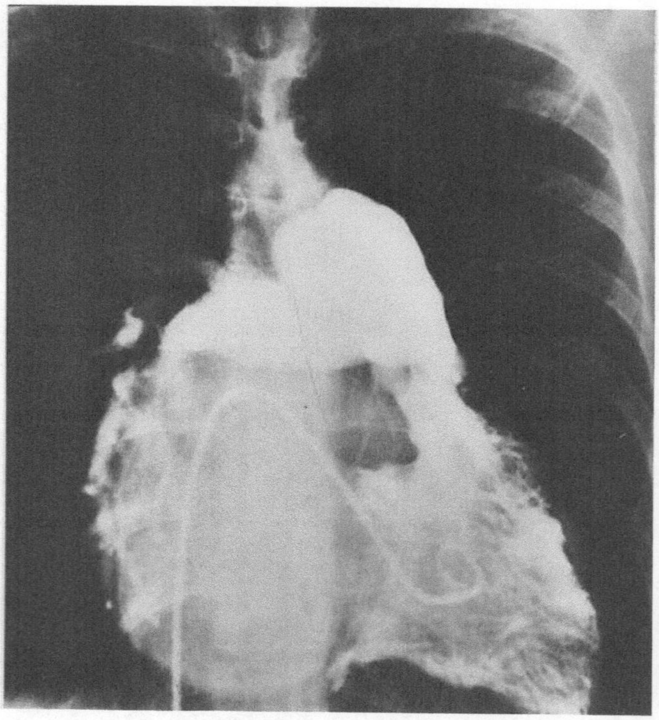

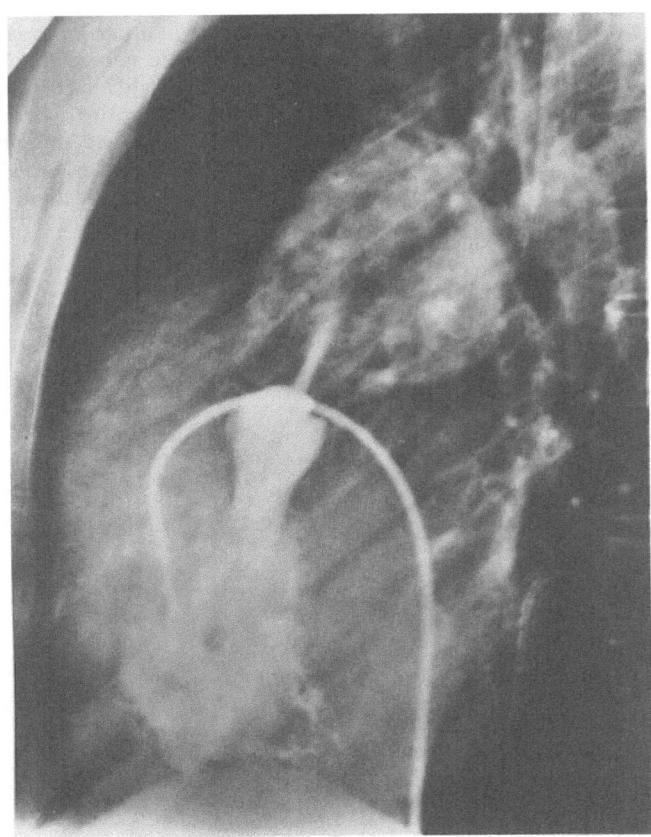

E

configuration) results from elevation of the right atrial appendage by an enlarged RV. In the RAO projection, RVE causes an abnormal convexity or rounding of the anterior heart border. The lateral projection is very useful in the evaluation of RVE, demonstrating obliteration (increase in density) of the retrosternal clear space caused by dilatation of the outflow tract of the RV as shown by right ventriculography. Elevation of the right atrial appendage by an enlarged RV also contributes to obliteration of the retrosternal clear space. The LV is usually retrodisplaced by an enlarged RV. Thus the lower segment of the posterior heart border may project behind the esophagus, or it may project far behind the posterior border of the inferior vena cava at its entrance to the RA, simulating LV enlargement. Analysis of the other projections and the presence of obliteration of the retrosternal clear space (lateral view) will clarify the situation.

On occasion, RVE will also displace the LA, causing an exaggerated convexity of the superior segment of the posterior heart border that simulates LAE. In such instances, the signs of LA enlargement will be lacking in other projections.

Right Atrial Enlargement (Figs. 1–5, 1–6)
Dilatation of the right atrium (RA) causes increased rounding of the lower segment of the right heart border and a prominence or bulge in the region of the right atrial appendage (RAA) in the LAO projection. In the RAO projection RA dilatation is reflected in increased convexity or rounding of the posterior heart border above the diaphragm and below the contour of the left atrium. A dilated RA may displace the LA, simulating LA enlargement in the lateral and LAO projections; however, a double density is not present in the frontal view. RA enlargement may be accompanied by dilatation of the superior vena cava (SVC), which causes widening or fullness of the right upper mediastinum. In extreme forms of RA dilatation (e.g., Ebstein anomaly) the RA becomes border forming in the lateral projection (Fig. 1–6).

A bulge in the upper segment of the anterior (right) heart border (shelf or shoulder configuration) in the LAO projection may be due to enlargement of the RA, RV or both. Dilatation of the intracardiac portion of the aorta (aortic root) (e.g., cystic medial necrosis) will displace the RAA in the LAO projection, producing the shoulder configuration and mimicking right heart enlargement (Fig. 1–7). Review of the PA and lateral projections will show the lack of signs of RV and RA enlargement.

If the RA and RV are both enlarged the frontal and lateral views will show signs of combined enlargement. It should be noted that a dilated RAA also causes obliteration of the retrosternal clear space.

In addition to alterations in the size of the cardiac chambers, the size and shape of the SVC and supradiaphragmatic portion of the inferior vena cava (IVC) may change in response to abnormal pressure or volume overload. The dilated SVC will cause widening of the superior mediasti-

dow), in some instances of left ventricular failure (from any cause), tumors (myxoma), and in other unusual causes (e.g., idiopathic left atriomegaly).

Enlargement of the left atrial appendage is usually associated with mitral valvular disease and to a lesser extent with shunt lesions. Idiopathic dilatation of the left atrial appendage is rare (noted above).

Right Ventricular Hypertrophy
Right ventricular hypertrophy usually does not result in cardiac enlargement on plain films. When it does, the cardiac apex is uplifted and rounded, particularly on the frontal projection.

Right Ventricular Enlargement (RVE) (Fig. 1–5)
When the right ventricle dilates it becomes border forming, producing an abnormal convexity of the left heart border on the frontal view. The degree of rounding of the left heart border depends on the extent of RV dilatation. In mild RV dilatation, straightening of the left heart border may mimic enlargement of the left atrial appendage. In moderate RV dilatation, rounding of the junction of the middle and lower segments of the left heart border occurs. This rounding or abnormal convexity may encompass most of the left heart border when the RV is markedly enlarged.

In the LAO projection, RV dilatation causes abnormal convexity of the right (anterior) heart border, which may be accentuated superiorly in the region of the right atrial appendage. This abnormal upper convexity ("shoulder"

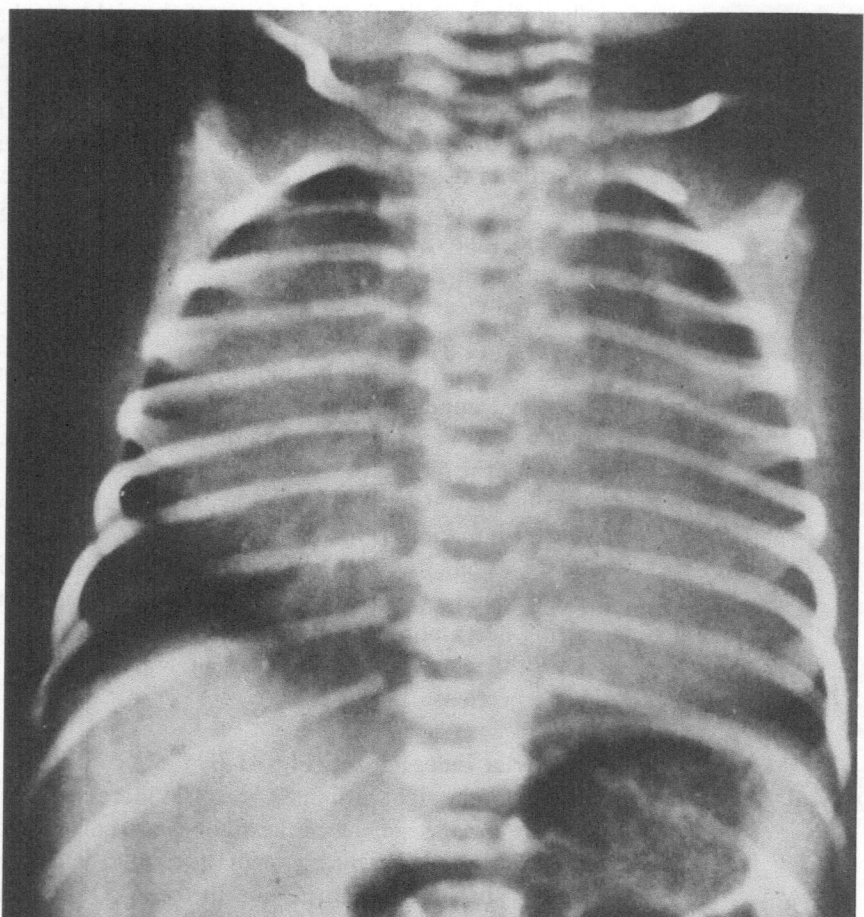

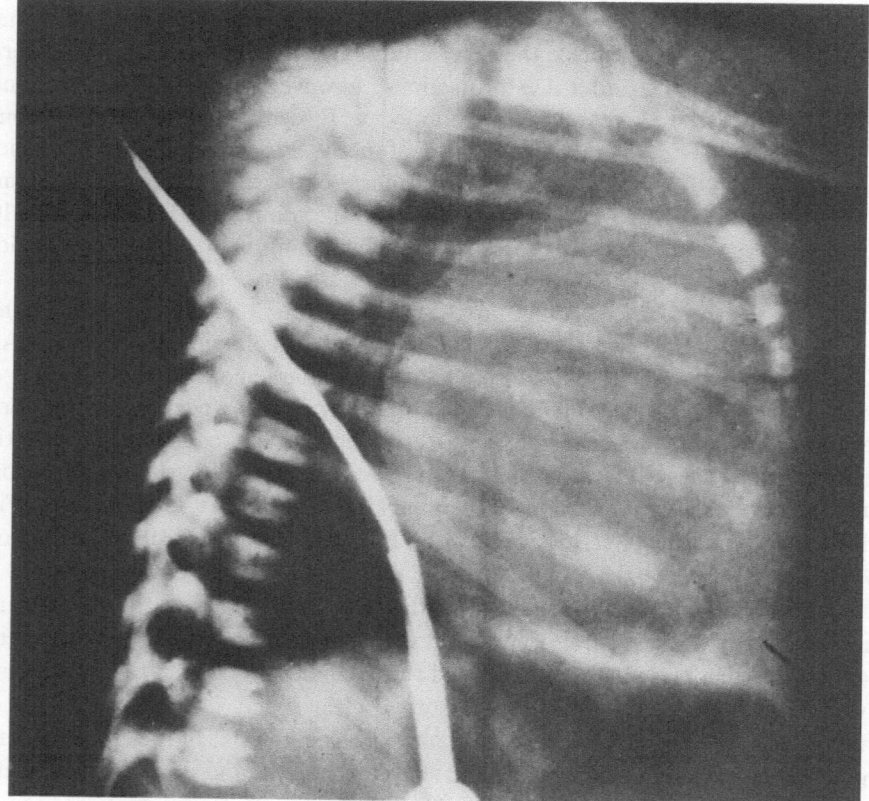

Fig. 1–6, A and B. *Right atrial enlargement* in an infant with Ebstein anomaly. **A** PA view, **B** lateral view. The right atrium is massively enlarged, forming the entire right heart border on the frontal view and the entire posterior border on the lateral view. Note the severe pulmonary undercirculation.

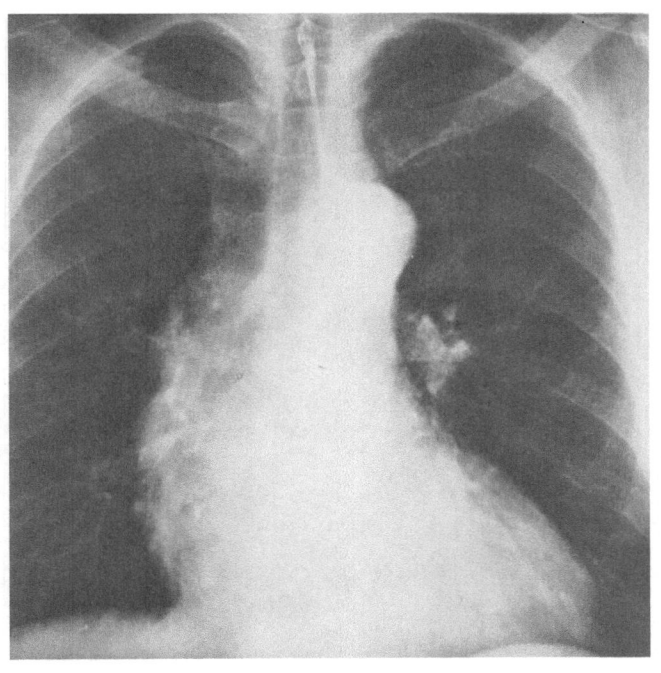

A

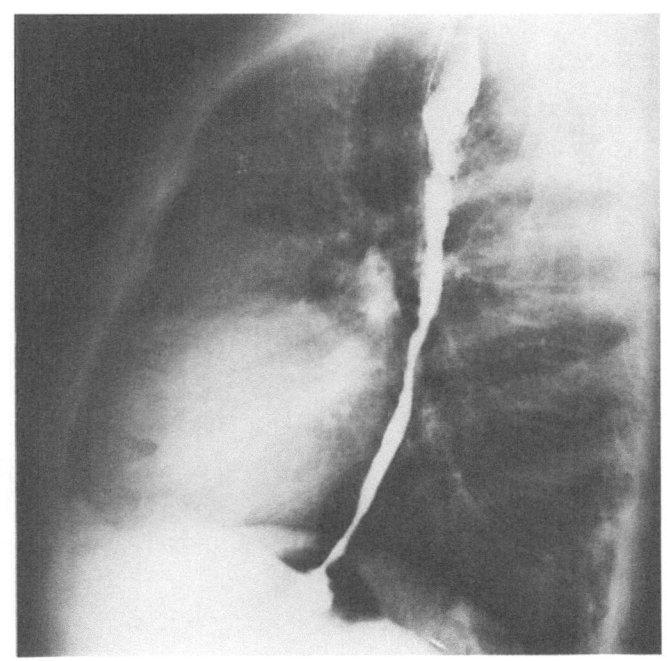

B

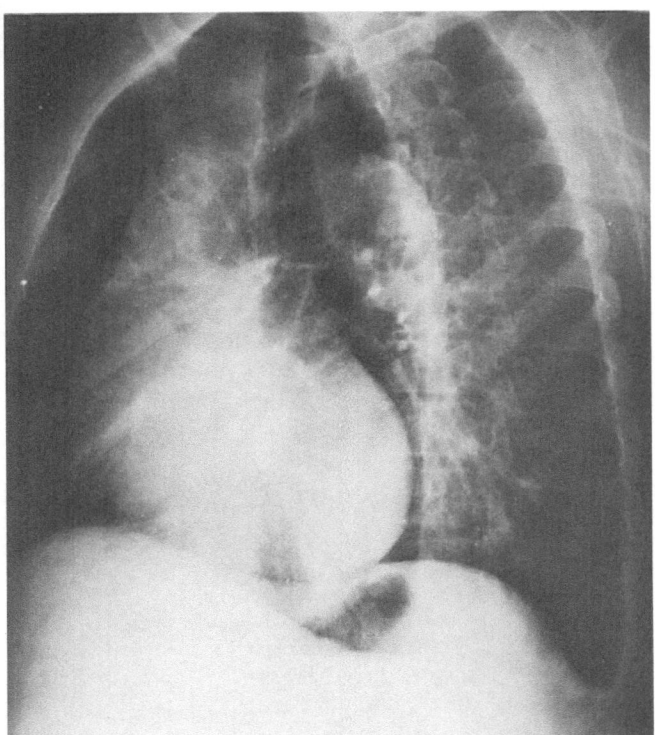

C

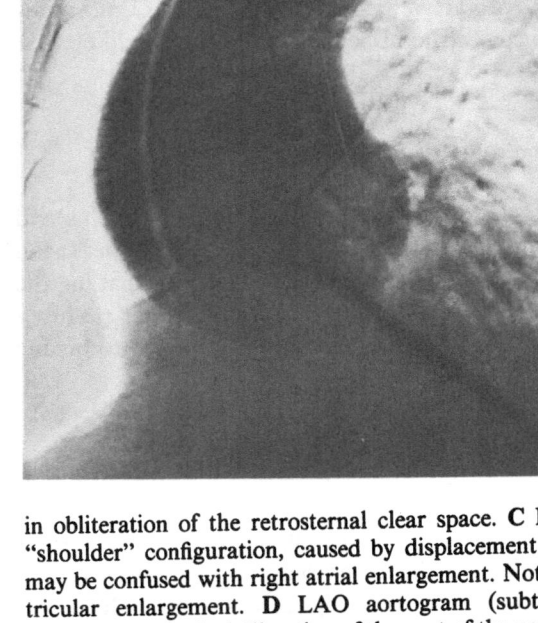

D

Fig. 1–7, A–D. *Enlargement of the aortic root* (intracardiac segment of the aorta) in a man with cystic medial necrosis. **A** PA view. The dilated aortic root and dilated ascending aorta form a convexity along the upper segment of the right heart border. The aortic arch is also enlarged but to a lesser extent than the root of the aorta. Left ventricular enlargement is also present. **B** Lateral view. Enlargement of the root of the aorta is responsible for displacement of the right atrial appendage (RAA), resulting in obliteration of the retrosternal clear space. **C** LAO view. A "shoulder" configuration, caused by displacement of the RAA, may be confused with right atrial enlargement. Note the left ventricular enlargement. **D** LAO aortogram (subtraction film). Marked symmetrical dilatation of the root of the aorta and effacement of the sinuses of Valsalva are apparent. The aortic arch is relatively spared.

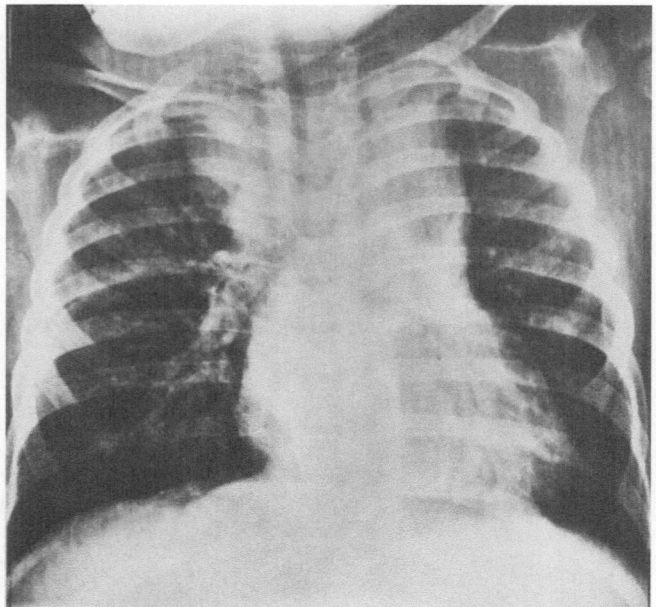

A

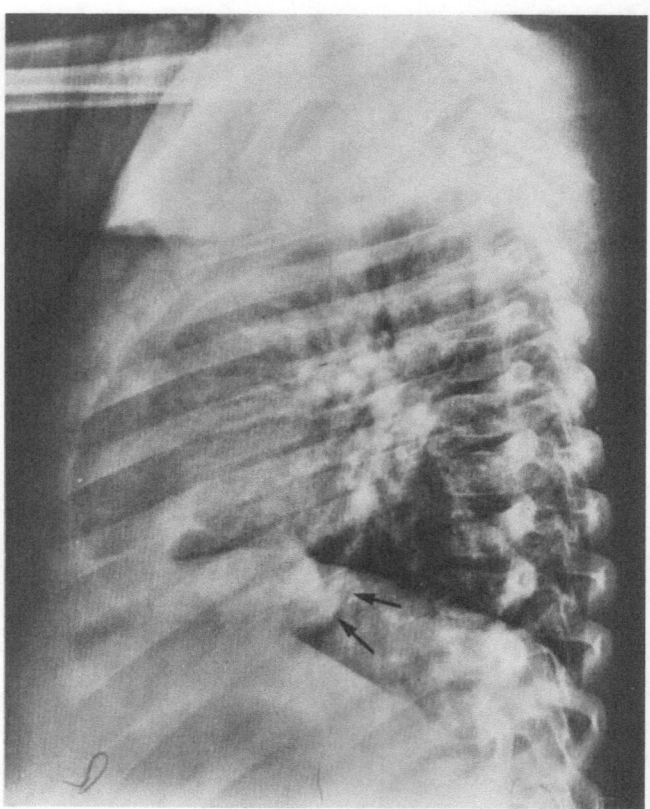

B

Fig. 1–8, A–C. *Dilatation of the superior vena cava* in a child with venous obstruction after Mustard procedure (intraatrial baffle) for dextrotransposition of the great vessels. **A** Frontal view. Marked widening of the superior mediastinum is caused by the superior vena cava and azygos vein on the right and by the left innominate vein on the left. **B** Lateral view. The dilated IVC forms a convex density (*arrows*) as it enters the right atrium. **C** Superior vena cava injection. Obstruction (*arrow*) at the entrance to the superior limb of the baffle is present. Note the retrograde flow from the SVC into the dilated azygos vein and from there to the anterior spinal veins. The left innominate vein is not opacified.

num on the frontal view (Fig. 1–8). The IVC, normally a slightly concave structure on the lateral view, will become convex.

Pulmonary Vasculature

Even though the distribution of the pulmonary veins and arteries is uniform throughout the lungs, their perfusion differs. Bjure and Laurell in 1927 observed that in the erect position the bases of the lungs were better perfused than the apices. They believed this phenomenon to be due to gravity.

Normal Pulmonary Vasculature (Figs. 1–1A, 1–9)
Because of the gravitational dependence of the distribution of pulmonary flow, the vessels to the lower lobes are significantly larger than those to the upper lobes (the normal ratio of the caliber of the lower to upper pulmonary vessels is approximately 4:1). Radiologically, the lower lobe vessels, particularly near the hilum and the left atrium, are clearly visualized, whereas those in the upper lobes may be difficult to identify because of their smallness. The pulmonary vessels taper gradually from center to periphery, becoming imperceptible in the outer third of the lungs. At no point does any abrupt change in caliber occur. Arteries and veins cannot be differentiated by their radiodensity,

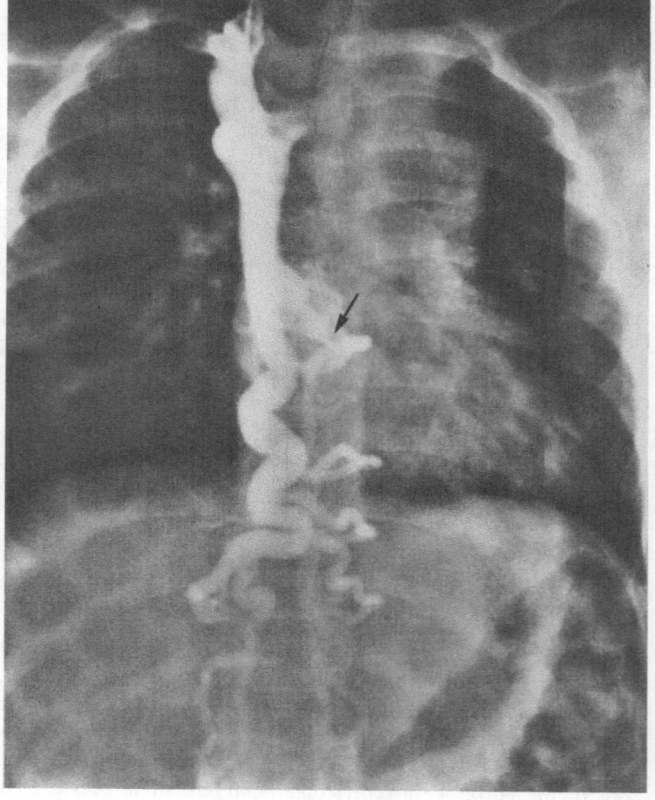

C

size, or numerical quantity; however, they can be distinguished by their characteristic directional arrangement. The pulmonary arteries originate from the hilus at about the level of the seventh posterior rib, approximately 3 cm

Fig. 1–9, A and B. *Normal pulmonary angiogram.* **A** arterial phase; **B** venous phase. Pulmonary arteries and veins can be differentiated by the direction of their courses and by the location of their attachments to the heart. In the upper lobes the arteries and veins have an approximately parallel course. The veins are lateral to their corresponding arteries and enter the heart at a lower level. In the lower lobes the arteries descend in a vertical course, whereas the veins pass horizontally to join the left atrium lower down.

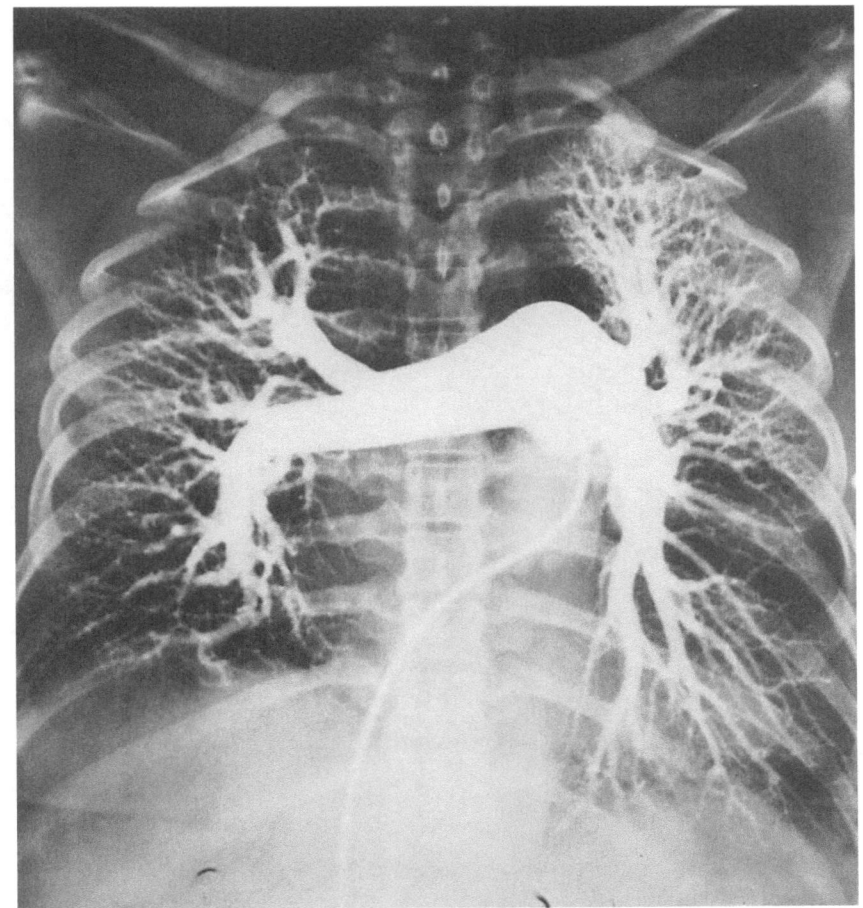

A

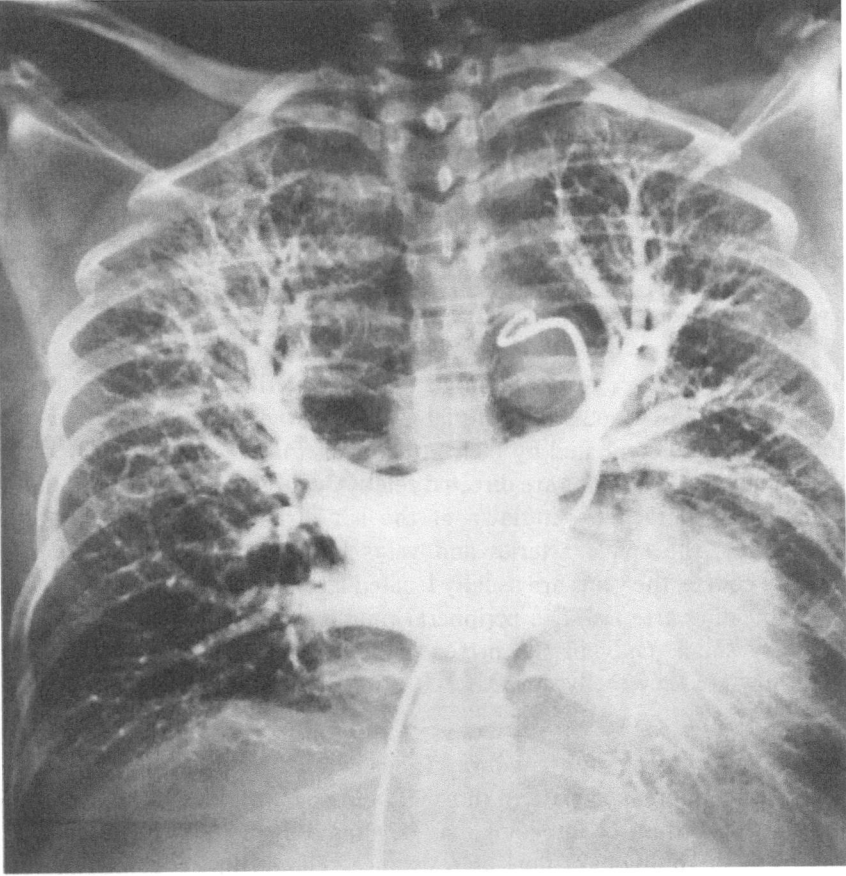

B

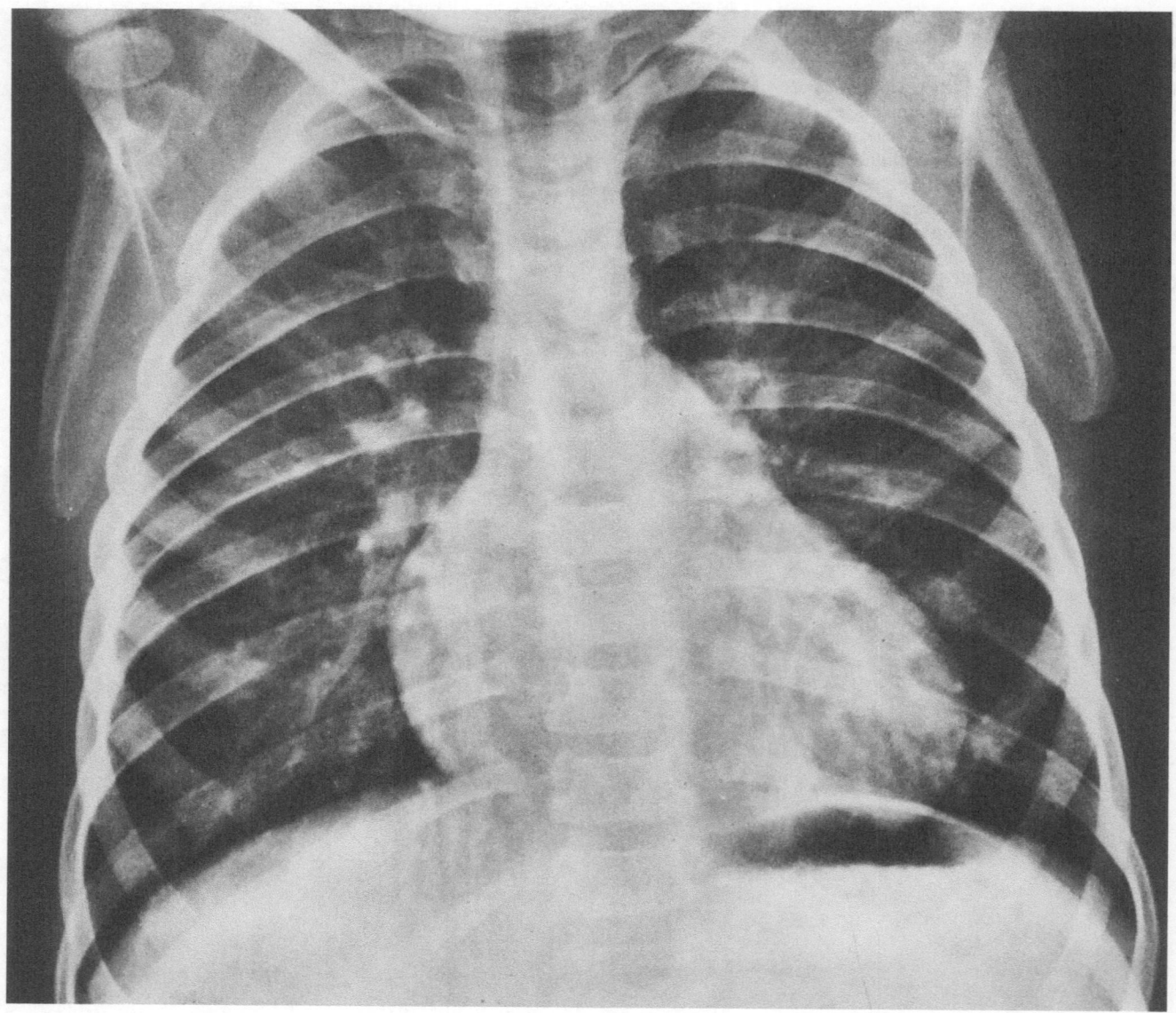

A

Fig. 1–10, A–C. *Bilateral (generalized) pulmonary overcircula-tion.* **A** A frontal plain film in a child with coronary aneurysm and coronary arteriovenous fistula shows mild enlargement of the pulmonary vessels. **B** Marked pulmonary overcirculation in a woman with endocardial cushion defect. The pulmonary arteries are markedly dilated all the way to the periphery. **C** An aortogram from the patient in A demonstrates an aneurysm of the sinoatrial node artery, associated with a fistula emptying into the right atrium.

above the confluence of the pulmonary veins entering the left atrium. The venous and arterial vessels in the lower lobes can be differentiated by their attachment to the car-diac silhouette. The veins are directed relatively more hori-zontally and attach lower down at the left atrial level. Conversely, the apical arteries and veins have a nearly parallel course; the veins are usually located lateral to their corresponding arteries. The peripheral pulmonary vessels are very small. Only in the presence of an abnormally high flow are they easily defined.

Abnormal Pulmonary Vasculature (Table 1–1)

The normal pulmonary pattern (normal pulmonary vascu-larity) described in the foregoing may be altered by distur-bances in the pulmonary flow or resistance. The changes in pressure are secondary manifestations of abnormal flow or resistance or both. Accordingly, the abnormal radiologi-cal patterns can be categorized in three groups: (1) in-creased pulmonary blood flow (pulmonary overcircula-tion); (2) increased pulmonary resistance; and (3) decreased pulmonary blood flow (pulmonary undercirculation). A fourth group, called the variegated pattern, consists of a combination of (1) and (2).

Increased Pulmonary Blood Flow (Pulmonary Overcirculation)

Increased pulmonary blood flow (overcirculation pattern) may be bilateral (generalized), unilateral or segmental. Bi-lateral or generalized overcirculation (Fig. 1–10) may be observed in (1) high output states (e.g., anemia, hyperthy-roidism, fever, exercise, pregnancy); (2) left-to-right shunts

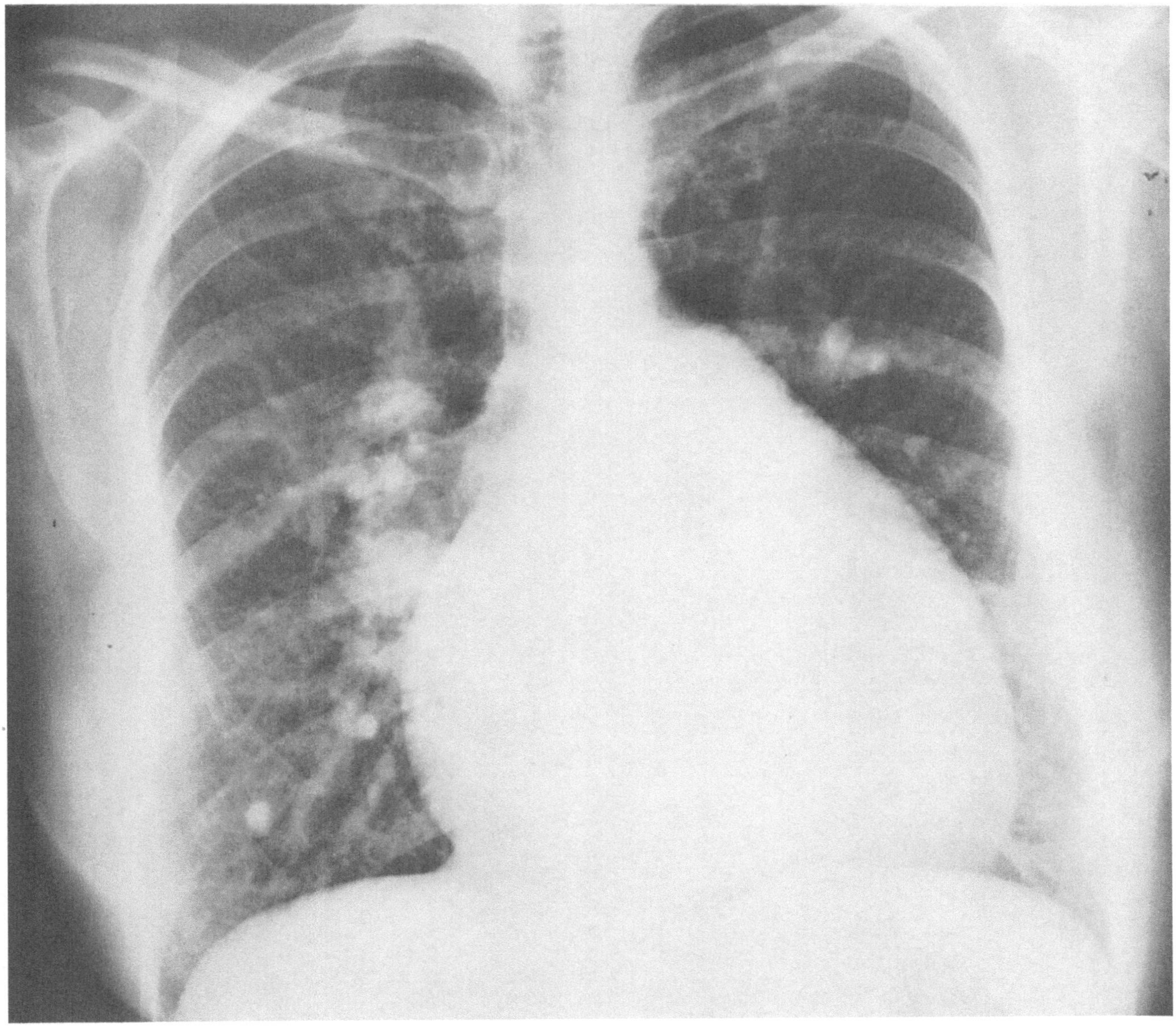

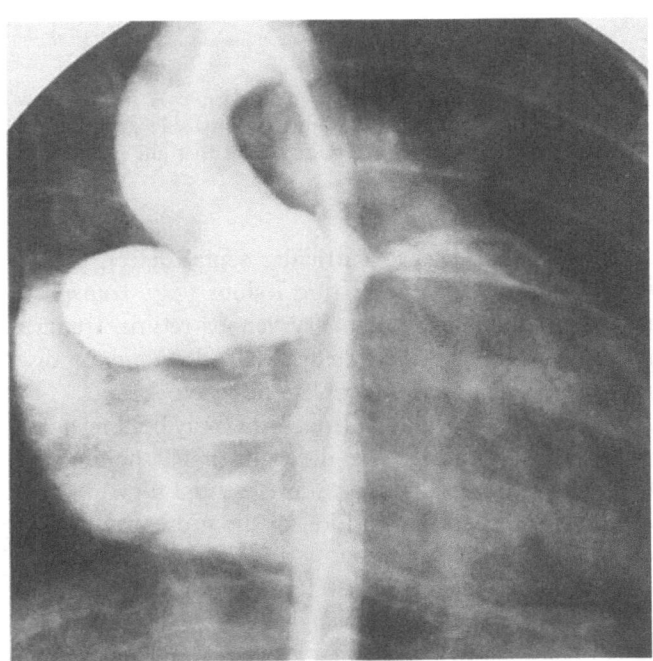

B

C

Table 1–1. Radiological Patterns of Abnormal Pulmonary Vasculature

Increased pulmonary blood flow (pulmonary overcirculation)
  Bilateral (generalized)
  Unilateral
  Segmental

Decreased pulmonary blood flow (pulmonary undercirculation)
  Bilateral (generalized)
  Unilateral
  Segmental
  Unilateral undercirculation and contralateral overcirculation

Variegated pattern of pulmonary blood flow

Increased pulmonary resistance
  Postcapillary (pulmonary venous hypertension)
  Precapillary (pulmonary arterial hypertension)

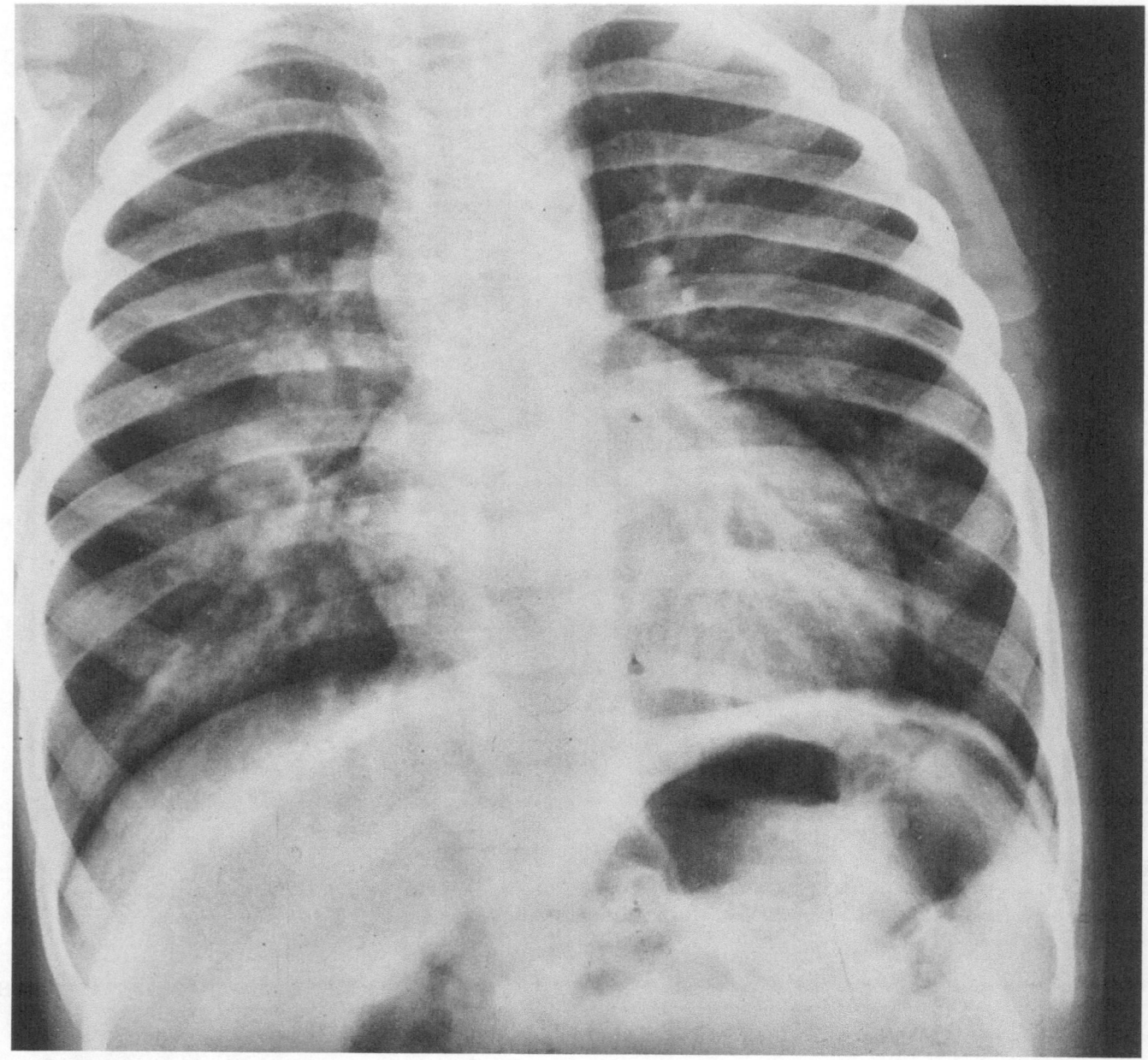

Fig. 1–11. *Unilateral pulmonary overcirculation.* A frontal view in an infant with a Waterston shunt (side-to-side anastomosis of the posterior wall of the ascending aorta to right pulmonary artery). Marked dilatation of the right pulmonary artery and branches is present. In contrast, the left lung shows undercirculation.

(e.g., atrial septal defect, ventricular septal defect, patent ductus arteriosus); (3) admixture lesions (e.g., transpositions, total anomalous pulmonary venous return, truncus arteriosus communis, single ventricle); (4) conduction disturbance (e.g., congenital complete heart block).

Unilateral overcirculation (Fig. 1–11) may be congenital (e.g., ectopic origin of either the right or left pulmonary artery from the ascending aorta, preferential flow in some patients with dextrotransposition of the great arteries) or acquired (Waterston anastomosis for cyanotic congenital heart disease). Segmental overcirculation (Figs. 1–12, 1–13) may be congenital (e.g., single or multiple pulmonary arteriovenous fistulas, pulmonary steal syndrome) or ac-

quired (faulty Waterston anastomosis causing tenting or kinking of the right pulmonary artery).

Decreased Pulmonary Blood Flow (Pulmonary Undercirculation)

Decreased pulmonary blood flow may be bilateral (generalized), unilateral or segmental. Unilateral undercirculation may be associated with contralateral overcirculation. Bilateral or generalized undercirculation (Fig. 1–14) is observed in obstructing lesions such as pulmonic stenosis (valvar, supravalvar and infravalvar), double-chambered right ventricle, RV tumors (e.g., rhabdomyoma, rhabdomyosarcoma), cystic lesions of the pulmonary valve, multiple pul-

Fig. 1–12, A and B. *Segmental pulmonary overcirculation* in a woman with a pulmonary arteriovenous (A-V) fistula. **A** PA view. A mass density in the right base (*F*) is associated with dilatation of an artery (*A*) and vein (*V*). **B** AP pulmonary angiogram. The pulmonary A-V fistula is opacified.

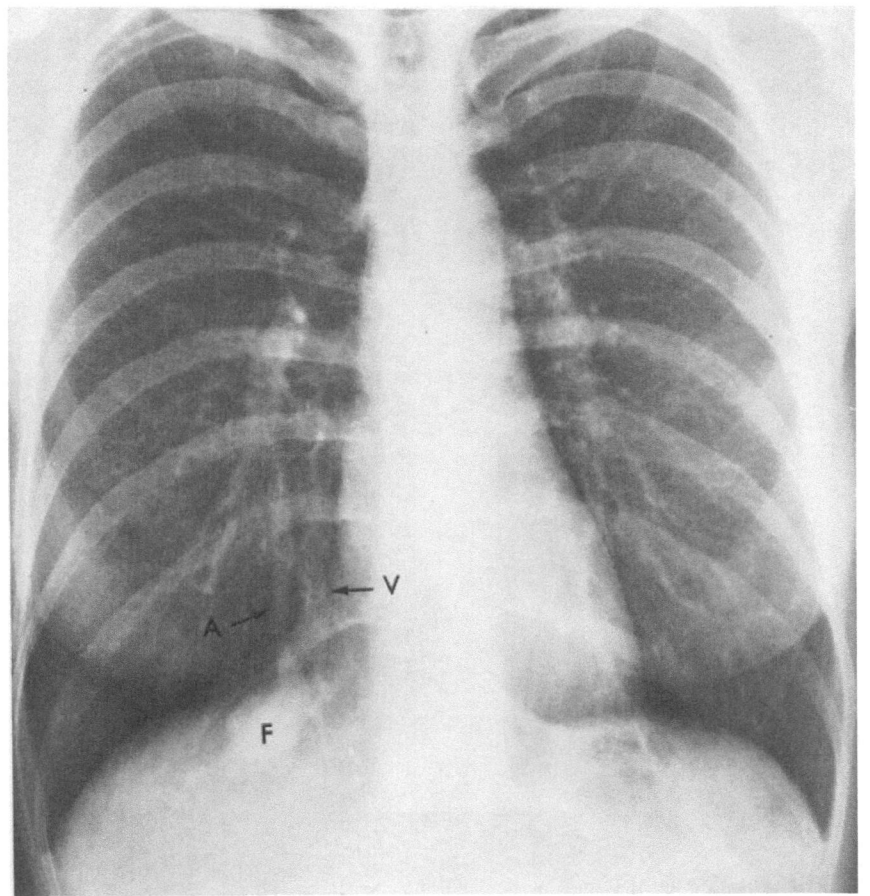

A

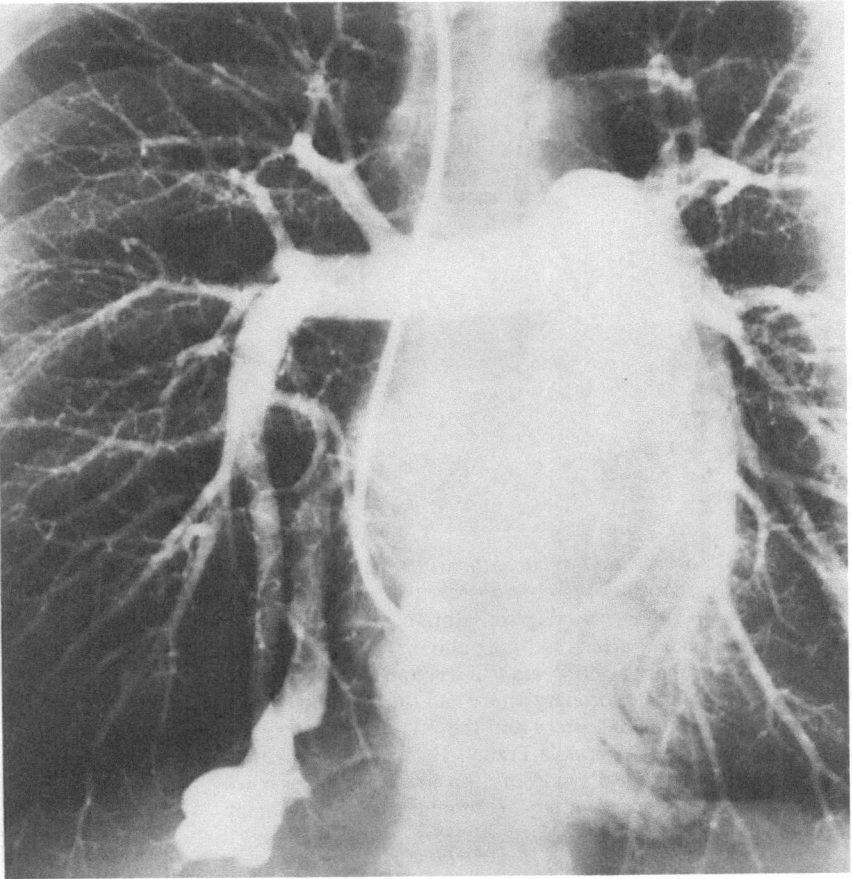

B

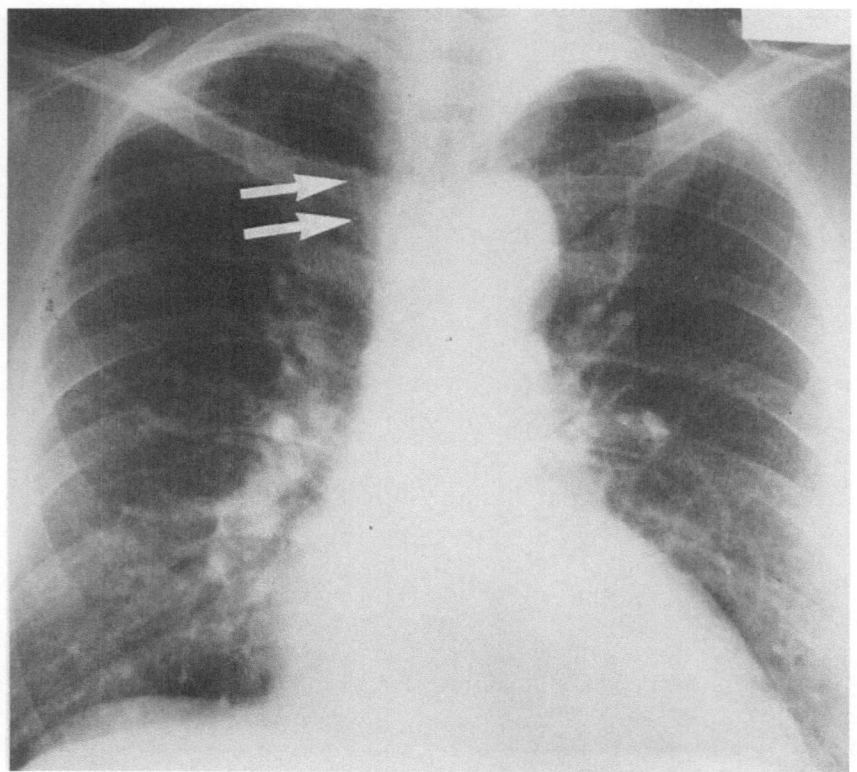

A

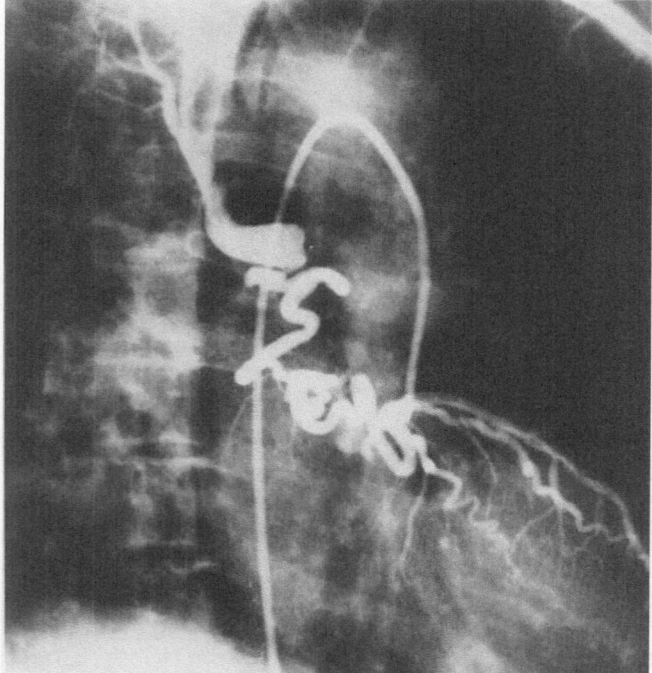

B

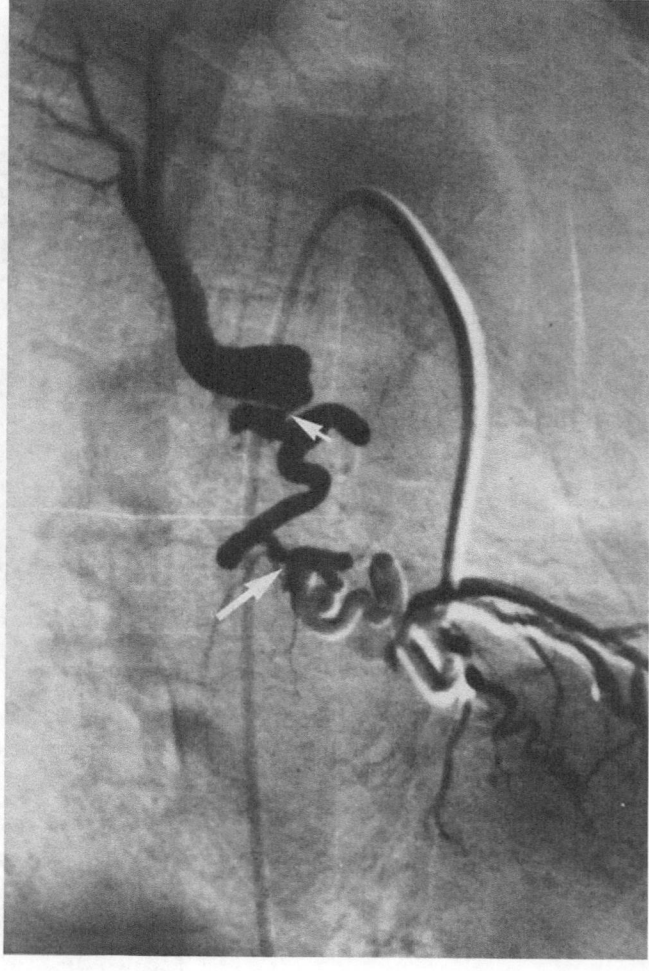

C

Fig. 1–13, A–C. *Segmental overcirculation* in a man with angina. **A** PA view. An abnormal vessel is observed in the right upper lobe (*arrows*). **B** Coronary angiogram. Note communication between the left coronary artery and the pulmonary artery (pulmonary steal). **C** Coronary arteriogram (subtraction film). The anastomoses between the left coronary artery and the bronchial artery and between the bronchial artery and the pulmonary artery are demonstrated (*arrows*). Spindola-Franco H, Weisel A, Delman AJ (1978) Pulmonary steal syndrome: An unusual case of coronary-bronchial pulmonary artery communication. Radiology 126:25–27

Fig. 1–14, A and B. *Generalized pulmonary undercirculation* in an infant with rhabdomyoma of the right ventricular outflow tract. **A** Frontal view. The lungs show marked undercirculation. **B** Lateral view of right ventriculogram. A large mass nearly fills the RV outflow tract.

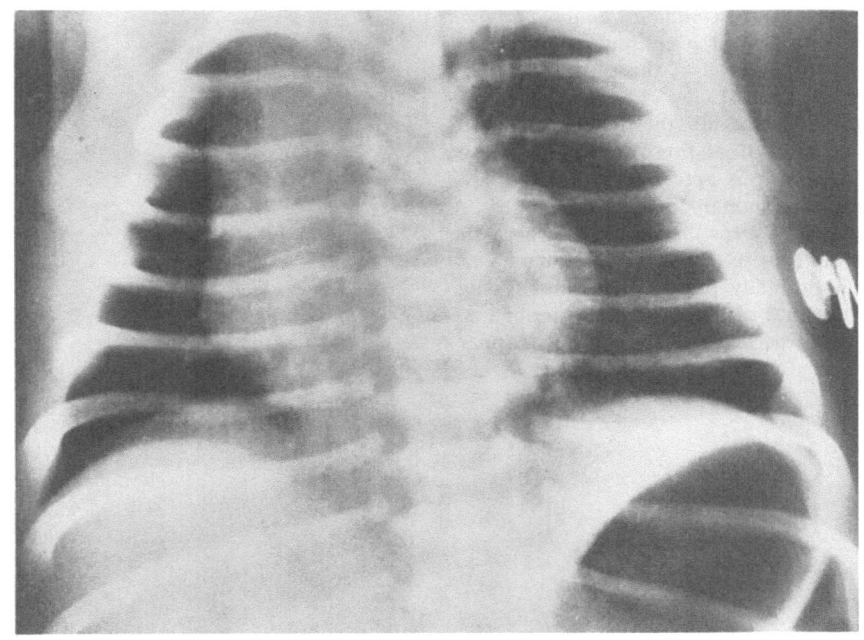

A

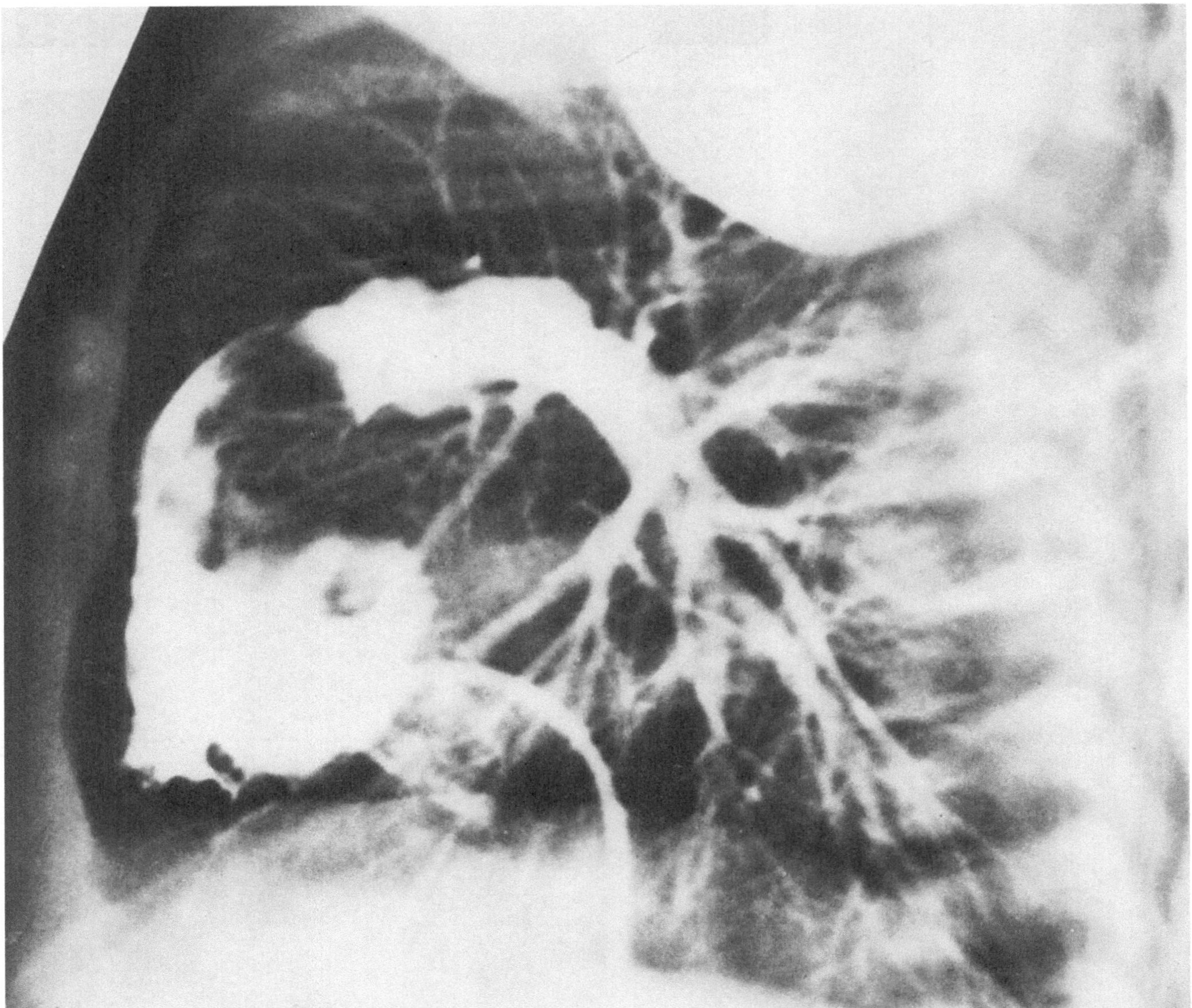

B

Fig. 1–15, A–C. *Unilateral undercirculation* with contralateral overcirculation in a patient with agenesis of the right pulmonary artery. **A** Frontal view. The left lung shows overcirculation while the right lung demonstrates undercirculation. Loss of volume of the right lung is apparent. **B** Lateral view. The left pulmonary artery is enlarged. A clear space (*arrow*) is observed where the spheroid density of the right pulmonary artery is normally present. This finding suggests absence of the RPA. **C** Posterior lung scan. Only perfusion of the left lung is apparent.

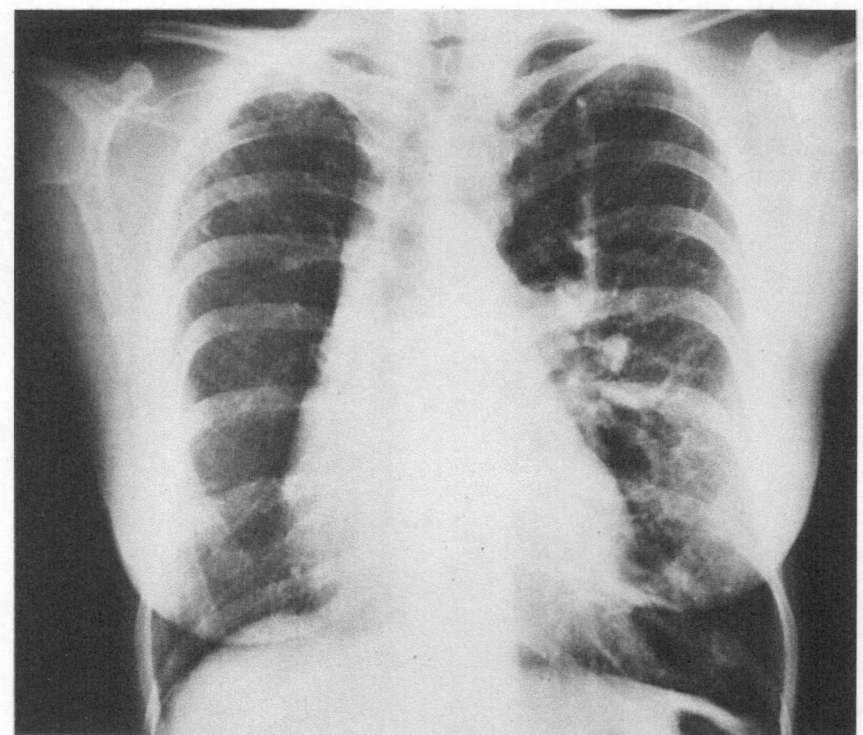

A

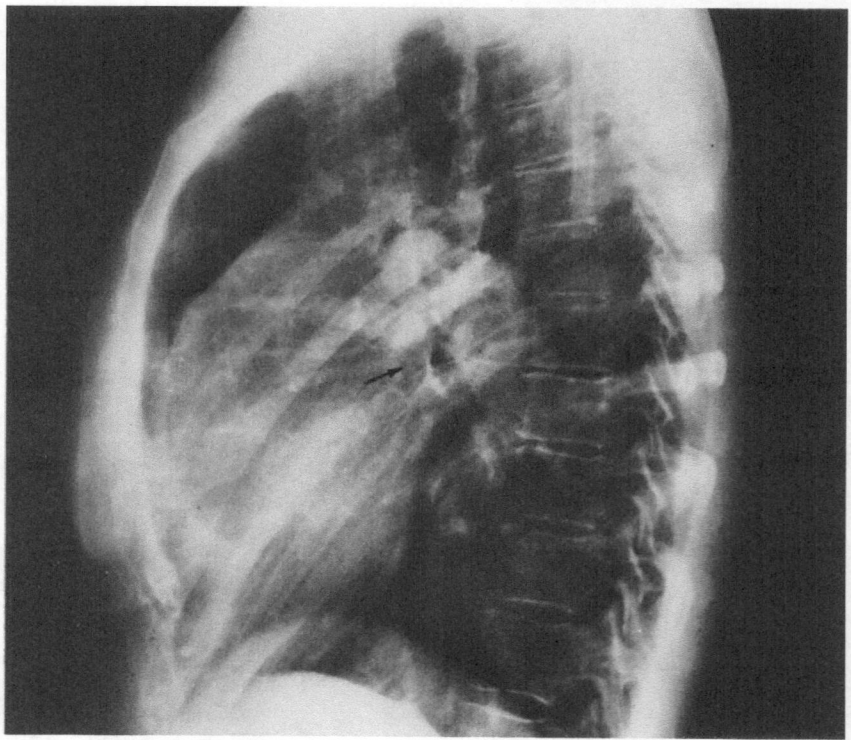

B

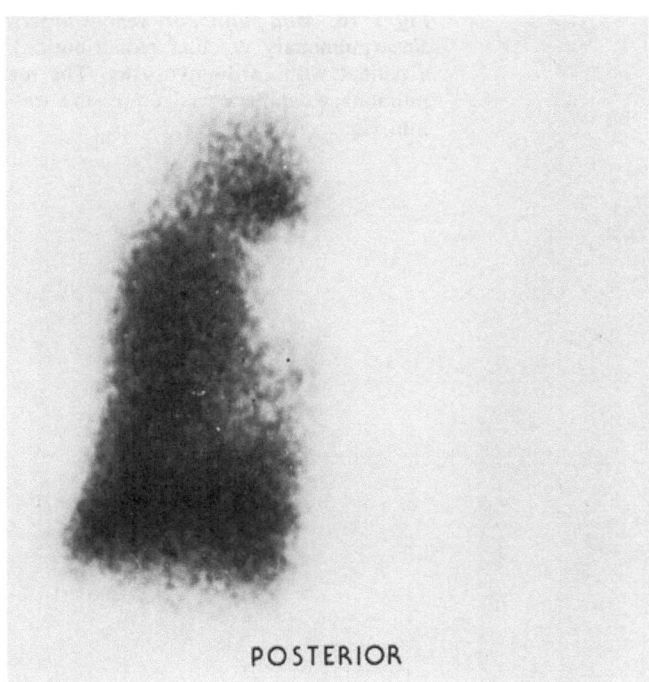

POSTERIOR

C

monary branch stenosis, and persistence of fetal circulation in neonates. Unilateral undercirculation may be noted in such disorders as stenosis of one pulmonary artery and pulmonary embolism. Segmental undercirculation is observed in isolated stenosis of interlobar branches and bronchial atresia and other disorders. Unilateral undercirculation with contralateral overcirculation may be noted in patients with agenesis or severe stenosis of one pulmonary artery (Fig. 1–15).

Variegated Pattern of Pulmonary Vasculature

A variegated pattern of pulmonary vasculature consists of a mixture of overcirculation and undercirculation patterns. Some areas appear overcirculated, and some are normal or undercirculated, producing a nonhomogeneous or patchy appearance of one or both lungs. A variegated pattern of pulmonary vasculature occurs in pulmonary atresia with ventricular septal defect, in which the pulmonary circulation is supplied by multiple systemic (or bronchial) collateral vessels. These vessels join the pulmonary arteries directly, some of them being stenotic at their anastomotic sites and some having no stenosis. The result is that the areas of lung supplied by nonstenotic collaterals carry systemic blood pressure and are overcirculated, while the areas supplied by stenotic vessels carry low blood pressure and are normally perfused or undercirculated. The radiological appearance reflects the pathophysiology. (See section on pulmonary atresia with VSD, Chapter 7.)

Increased Pulmonary Resistance

The appearance of the pulmonary vasculature on plain films varies with the location (precapillary or postcapillary) and degree of the increased resistance.

Table 1–2. Causes of Increased Pulmonary Resistance

Postcapillary (pulmonary venous hypertension)
  LV failure (from any cause)
  Mitral valvular disease (acquired)
  Congenital obstructive lesions (Table 1–3)

Precapillary (pulmonary arterial hypertension)
  Obstructive (pulmonary vascular disease)
    Thromboembolism
    Arteritis
    Schistosomiasis
    Idiopathic (primary) pulmonary hypertension
  Obliterative (pulmonary parenchymal disease)
    Emphysema
    Pulmonary fibrosis (from any cause)
  Constrictive (hyperkinetic)
    Hypoxia (from any cause)
    Left-to-right shunts (chronic and large)

Combined (postcapillary + Precapillary)
  Severe mitral stenosis

Table 1–3. Congenital Lesions Causing Pulmonary Venous Hypertension

Pulmonary venous obstruction
  With normal pulmonary venous return
    Pulmonary vein stenosis
    Pulmonary vein atresia
    Intimal fibrosis (focal, diffuse)
    Pulmonary vein diaphragm
    Pulmonary veno-occlusive disease
  With total anomalous pulmonary venous connection
    Usually subdiaphragmatic

Left Atrial Obstruction
  Cor triatriatum
  Supravalvular left atrial ring

Mitral Valve Disease
  Atresia
  Hypoplasia
  Stenosis
  Insufficiency

Left Ventricular and/or Aortic Obstruction
  Subaortic stenosis
  Aortic valve stenosis or atresia
  Hypoplastic left heart syndrome
  Coarctation of aorta
  Shone Syndrome

Pulmonary venous hypertension (PVH), also known as postcapillary hypertension, results from increased pressure beyond the capillary bed. Left ventricular failure (from any cause) and mitral valvular disease are the most common causes, (Table 1–2). Uncommon causes are cor triatriatum and abnormalities of the pulmonary veins (e.g., stenosis, thrombosis) (Table 1–3). Radiologically, PVH may manifest as pulmonary vascular redistribution, pulmonary edema (interstitial or alveolar) and pleural effusion. Pulmonary hemosiderosis and ossification are secondary late manifestations. The degree of pulmonary venous hypertension

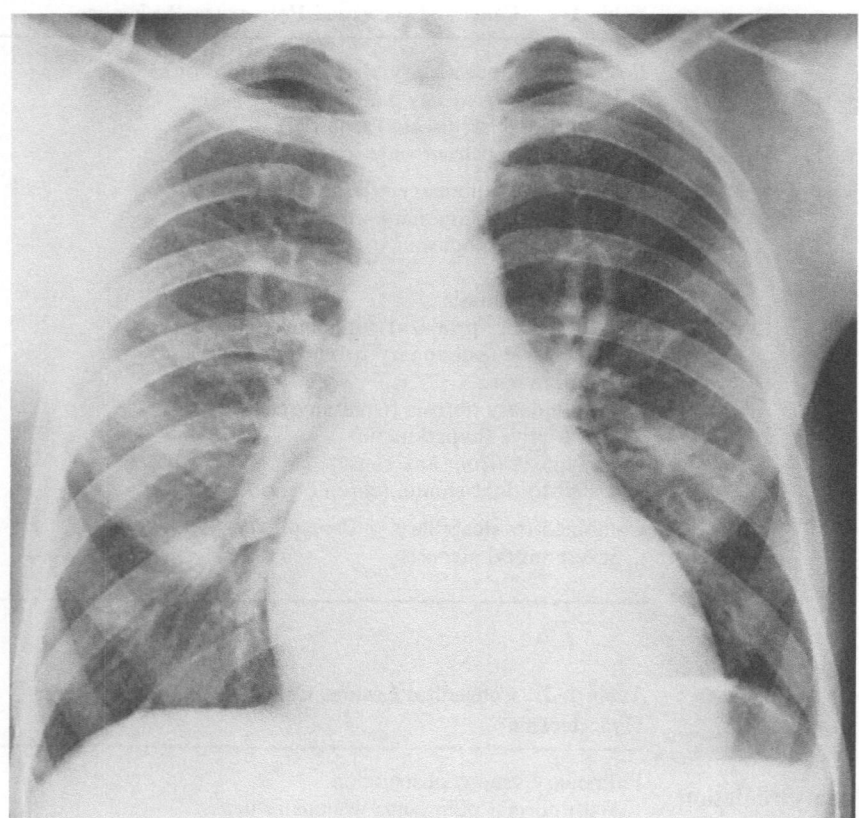

Fig. 1–16. *Mild pulmonary venous hypertension* (pulmonary vascular redistribution) in a patient with cardiomyopathy. The mean pulmonary capillary wedge pressure was 18 mm Hg.

Table 1–4.   Radiological Findings with Pulmonary Venous Hypertension

Mild pulmonary venous hypertension (12–20 mm Hg)*
  Equal perfusion
  Pulmonary vascular redistribution

Moderate pulmonary venous hypertension (20–30 mm Hg)*
  Interstitial edema (Kerley lines)
  Pulmonary "interstitial veiling"
  Subpleural edema
  Perihilar, perivascular, peribronchial haziness
  Small pleural effusions

Severe pulmonary venous hypertension (>30 mm Hg)*
  Alveolar and/or interstitial edema
  Large pleural effusions

* Correlates with mean pulmonary capillary wedge pressure or left atrial mean pressure in older children and adults. In infants the corresponding pressures are much lower.

(pulmonary venous pressure) and its response to therapy can be estimated by careful analysis of plain films (Table 1–4).

Mild PVH (12–20 mm Hg) is characterized by pulmo-

nary vascular redistribution (dilatation of the upper lobe vessels). The vessels of the lower lobes are constricted (Fig. 1–16). This reversal of the normal relationship is secondary to an elevation of the pulmonary venous pressure, causing interstitial and perivascular edema. The perivascular edema causes compression of the pulmonary capillaries in the lower lobes. Consequently an increase in the pulmonary vascular resistance in the lung bases occurs, and blood flow is diverted to the upper lobes, which have a lower resistance. Friedman and Braunwald showed by radionuclide studies that a linear relationship exists between left atrial pressure and the upper/lower lobe flow ratio.

Equal distribution of pulmonary blood flow to the upper and lower lobes (same vessel caliber of upper and lower lung zones on chest roentgenograms) may precede pulmonary vascular redistribution. This equalization of the caliber of the vessels should be differentiated from a left-to-right shunt. In left-to-right shunts the peripheral pulmonary vessels which are usually not visualized are dilated and thus become visible because of the increased blood flow.

Moderate PVH (20–30 mm Hg) is characterized by the

Fig. 1–17. *Severe pulmonary venous hypertension* in a patient with congestive heart failure. Interstitial pulmonary edema with hilar haze and a large right pleural effusion are noted. The left ventricular end-diastolic pressure was 36 mm Hg.

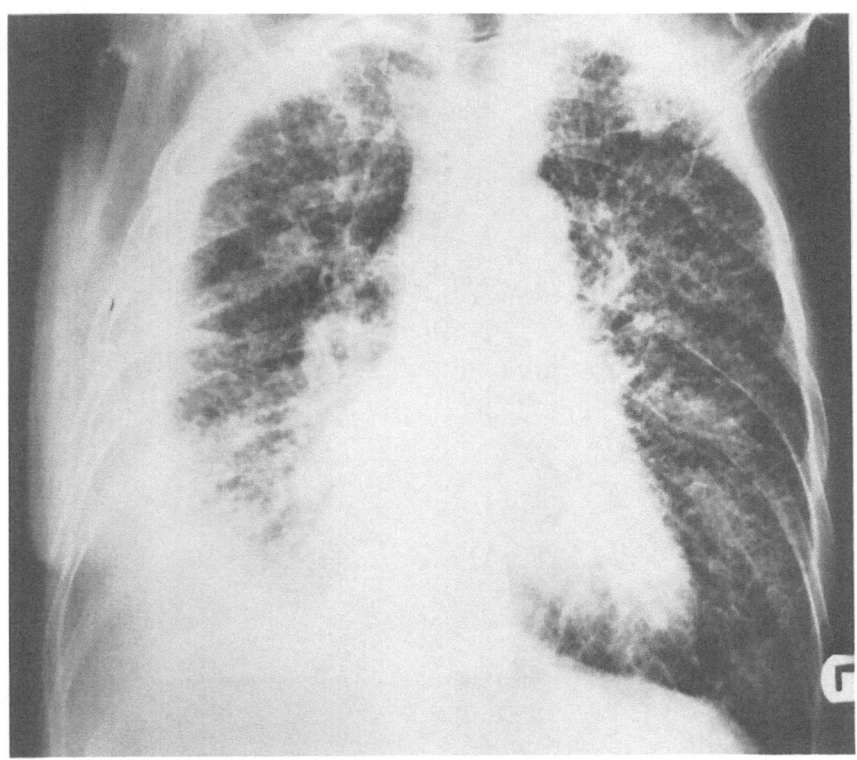

presence of interstitial edema. Interstitial pulmonary edema may be septal (Kerley lines), subpleural or perivascular. Septal lines are distended interlobular septa. Septal lines may also be due to interstitial fibrosis, hemosiderosis, lymphangitic metastatic spread and lymphatic obstruction. Septal lines are therefore nonspecific. They are sharp, linear densities about 1 mm in width and 2–3 cm in length extending from the pleural surface toward the center of the thorax. They usually run transversely in the frontal projection and are more common in the costophrenic angles. Perivascular edema produces "interstitial veiling" and unsharpness of both the central and peripheral vessels (perivascular cuffing). Loss of definition of the clear space between the right hilum and the heart (perihilar haziness) occurs (Fig. 1–17). Subpleural edema represents the accumulation of fluid between the lung and the adjacent pleural surface (visceral pleura) (Fig. 1–18) and should be differentiated from encapsulated interlobar effusion (pseudotumor or vanishing tumor) and middle lobe collapse. An interlobar effusion has biconvex margins (spindle shaped) (Fig. 1–19).

Severe PVH (> 30 mm Hg) is characterized by pulmonary edema and pleural effusions. Acute pulmonary edema (alveolar pulmonary edema) usually occurs in patients with acute left heart failure. Rapid transudation of fluid from the capillary bed into the alveoli takes place beyond the capacity of the pulmonary lymphatics to resorb it. The pulmonary capillary pressure is usually greater than 30 to 35 mm Hg. The radiological appearance of pulmonary edema consists of fluffy densities more prominent in the hilar areas of the lungs and fading toward the periphery ("butterfly" configuration) (Fig. 1–20). On occasion, a miliary or nodular pattern may be observed. The distribution of pulmonary edema is variable. It may be central (hilar) or peripheral, symmetrical or asymmetrical, bilateral or unilateral (Fig. 1–21) or combinations thereof.

Uremic alveolar edema that occurs in patients with renal failure may be differentiated on occasion from the acute pulmonary edema of heart failure. Uremic edema tends to be less basal in distribution than in cardiac failure. Often, evidence of narrowing of the basal vessels is lacking. The upper lobe vessels are dilated, resulting in an upper lobe/lower lobe flow ratio of approximately 1. Thus a 1/1 flow distribution should lead one to suspect renal failure rather than cardiac failure.

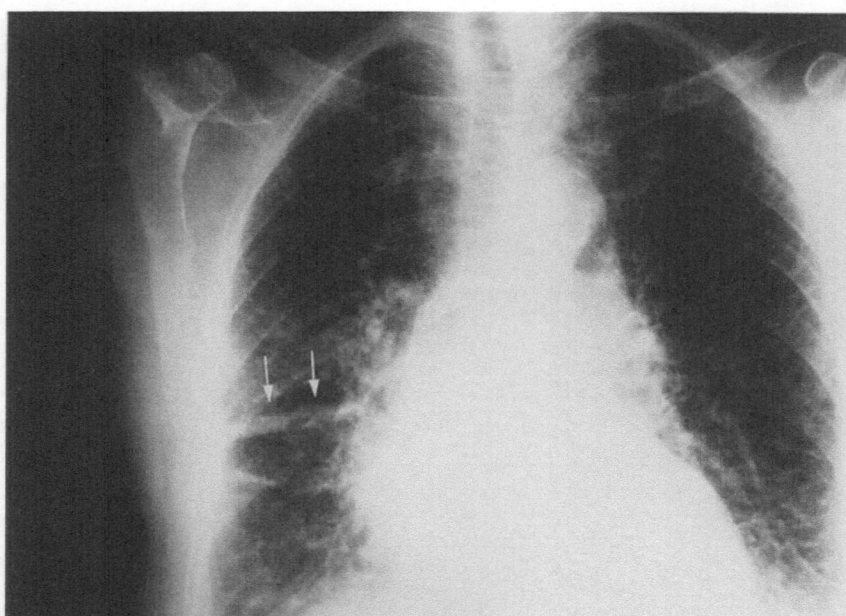

A

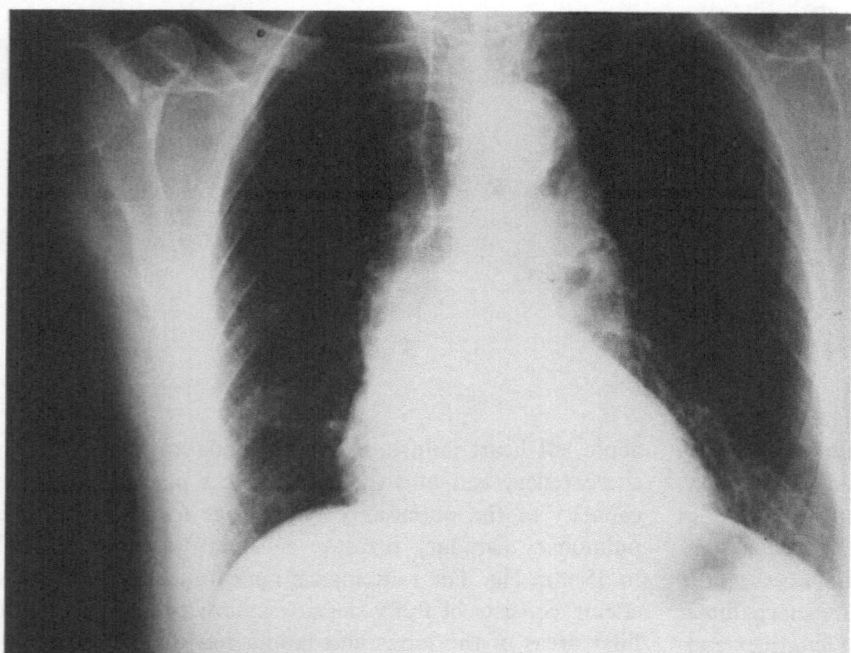

B

Fig. 1–18, A and B. *Subpleural edema* in a patient with ischemic cardiomyopathy. **A** before treatment; **B** after treatment. The linear density in **A** (*arrows*) represents a collection of fluid between the lung and the visceral surface of the pleura. The lower margin is sharp because it is delineated by the pleural surface. The upper margin is indistinct because it is in contact with the pulmonary surface. Subpleural edema may be the only clue to distinguish interstitial edema from interstitial fibrosis.

Pulmonary Arterial Hypertension

Numerous disorders (Table 1–2) that cause an increase in the pulmonary artery resistance (increased precapillary resistance) result in pulmonary arterial hypertension. Under normal circumstances the pulmonary artery pressure does not exceed 30/10 mm Hg., with a mean pressure of 20. Mild pulmonary hypertension is defined as systolic pressure of 35–50 mm Hg; moderate, from 50–75 mm Hg; and severe, from 75 mm Hg to systemic level or greater.

In chronic moderate to severe pulmonary arterial hypertension, dilatation of the pulmonary trunk (pulmonary artery segment) and both pulmonary arteries is present, and the intrapulmonary arterial (lobar and segmental) branches are uniformly constricted, producing the "pruned-tree" appearance (Fig. 1–22). Because of the diminished blood flow through the capillary bed, the caliber of the pulmonary veins is also decreased. Calcification of the main pulmonary artery (trunk) and branches may be observed. Angiocardiography is generally contraindicated in patients with severely elevated pulmonary resistance. If a pulmonary angiogram is obtained a slow washout of contrast material from the lungs occurs.

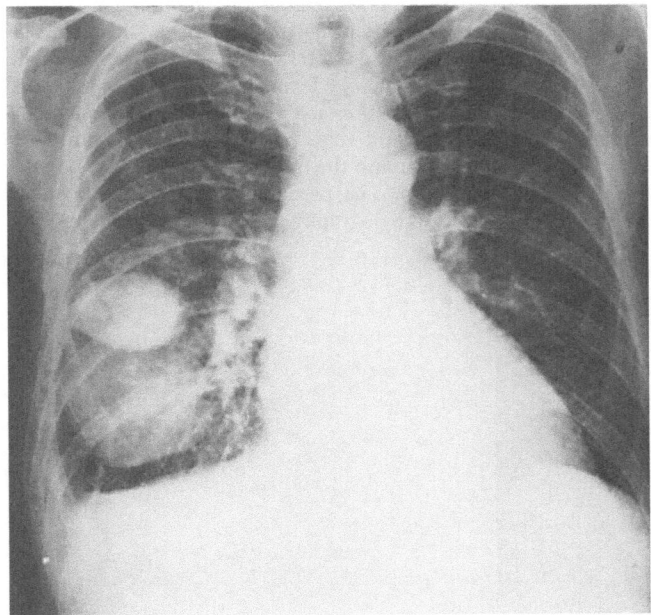 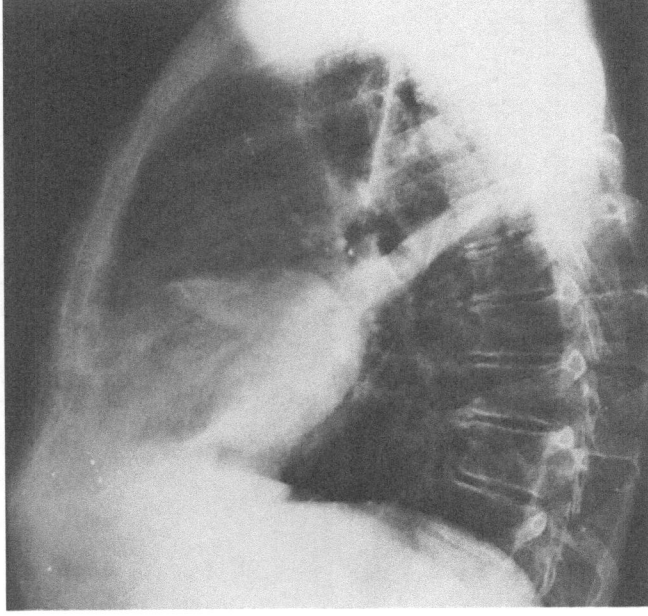

A   B

Fig. 1–19, A and B. *Interlobar effusion.* **A** PA view. Compare the fusiform appearance of the pseudotumor with subpleural edema present in Fig. 1–18. The haziness projecting below the pseudotumor proved on the lateral view (**B**) to be a second pseudo- tumor. The fusiform appearance of both pseudotumors is demon- strated on the lateral view. In addition, fluid is observed in a major fissure.

Fig. 1–20. *Bilateral alveolar pulmonary edema.* Note the Swan-Ganz catheter in the right pulmonary artery. Injection of contrast medium through the second catheter demon- strates opacification of the pericardiophrenic vein. The position of the catheter may simu- late perforation. A nasogastric tube is also noted.

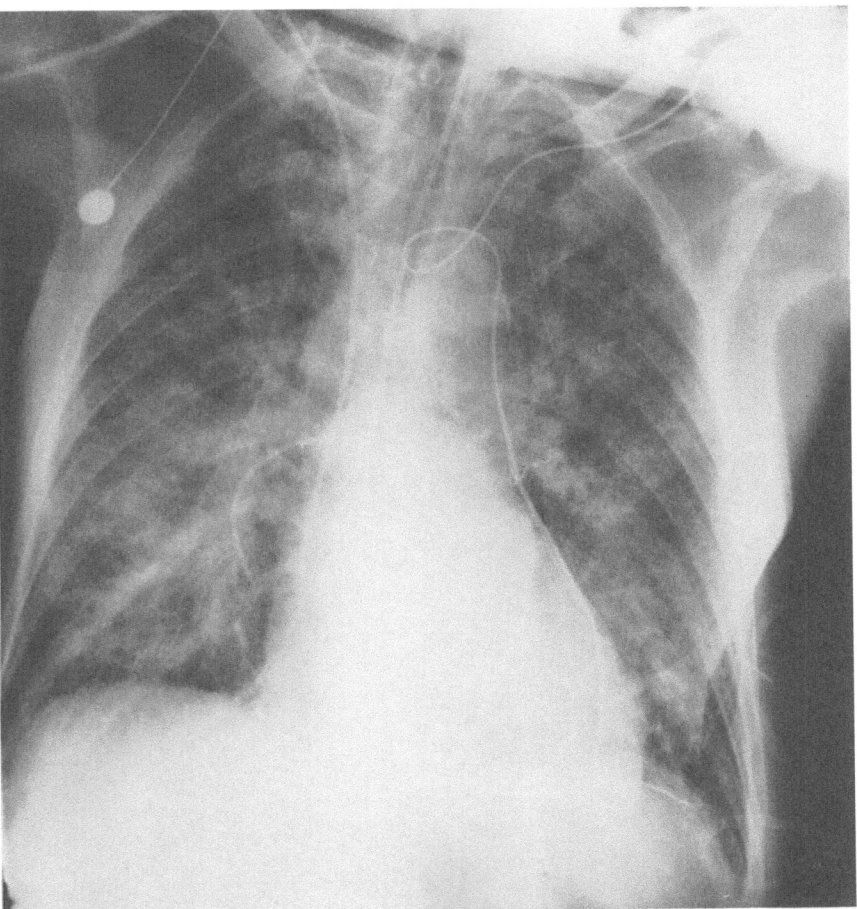

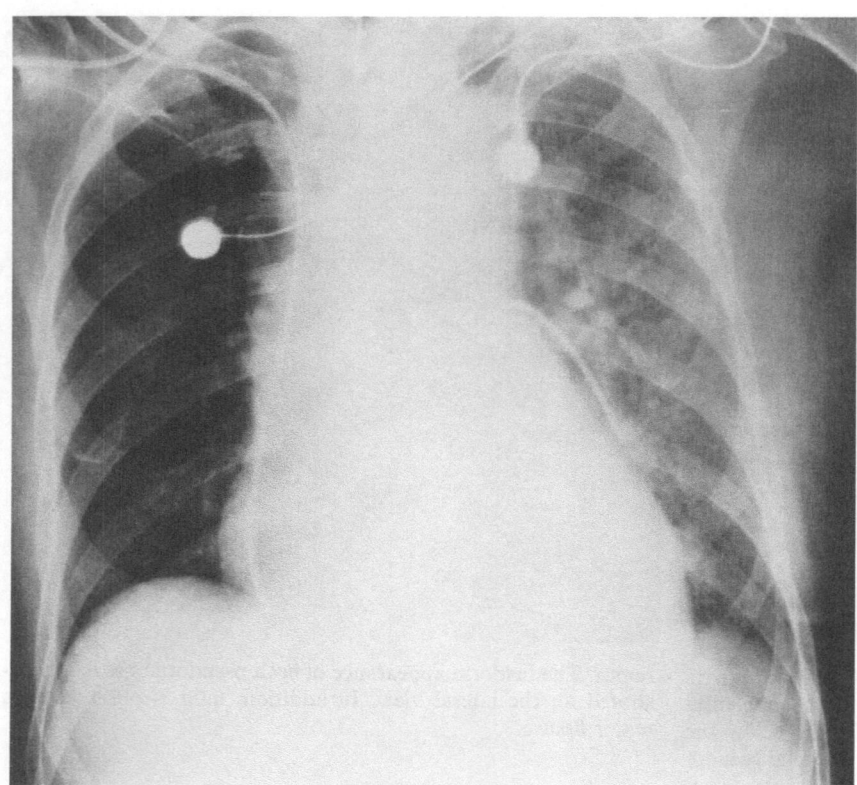

Fig. 1–21. *Unilateral pulmonary edema.* The patient had severe aortic and mitral insufficiency after aortic valve replacement. Pulmonary edema on the right was prevented by compression of the right pulmonary artery and veins by a pseudoaneurysm of the aorta into the transverse sinus of the pericardium. The pseudoaneurysm was diagnosed by angiography and confirmed at surgery.

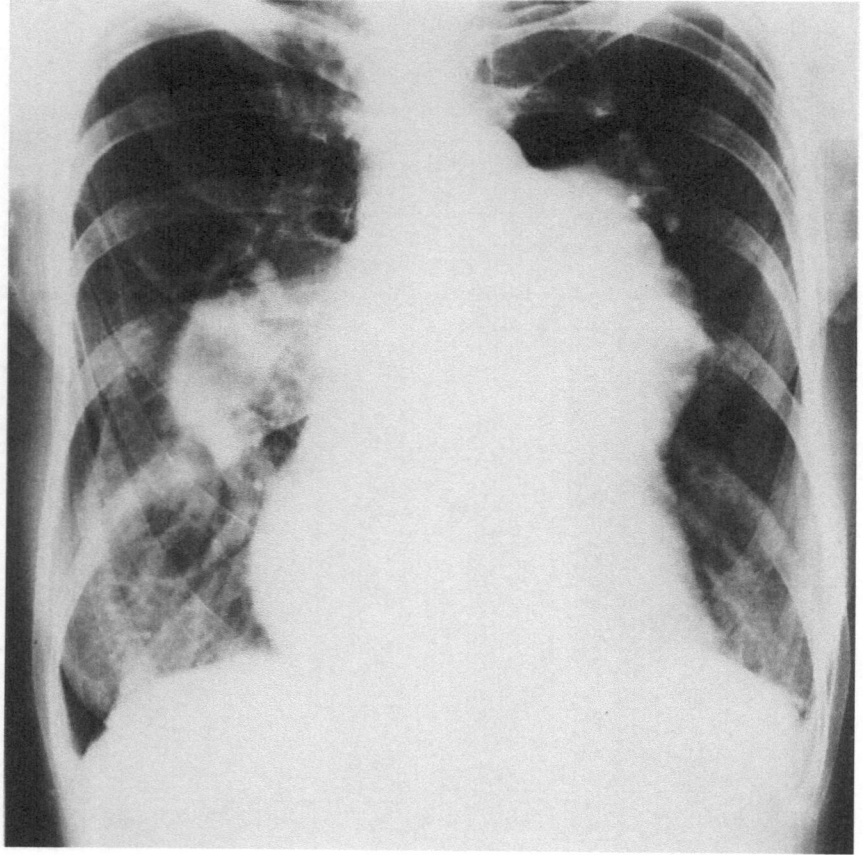

Fig. 1–22. *Pulmonary arterial hypertension due to markedly elevated pulmonary resistance (precapillary).* The central pulmonary arteries are massively dilated. The interlobar vessels taper abruptly ("pruned-tree" appearance).

Bibliography

General References

Amundsen P (1959) The diagnostic value of conventional radiological examination of the heart in adults. Acta Radiol 181:1–87

Elliot LP, Taylor WJ, Schiebler GL (1963) Combined ventricular hypertrophy in infancy. Vectocardiographic observations with special reference to the Katz-Wachtel phenomenon. Am J Cardiol 11:164–172

Eyler WR, Wayne DL, Rhodenbaugh JE (1959) The importance of the lateral view in the evaluation of left ventricular enlargement in rheumatic heart disease. Radiology 73:56–61

Hansen JF, Rygg I, Efsen F (1974) Intrapericardial left atrial aneurysm. Am Heart J 87:113–116

Higgins CB, Reinke RT, Jones NE, Broderick T (1978) Left atrial dimension on the frontal thoracic radiograph: A method for assessing left atrial enlargement. Am J Roentgenol 130:251–255

Holt JF (1947) Epicardial fat shadows in differential diagnosis. Radiology 48:472–479

Jacobson HG, Poppel MH, Hanenson IB, Dewing SB (1952) Left atrial enlargement. The optimum roentgen method for its demonstration. Am Heart J 43:423–436

Keats TE, Rudhe U, Foo GW (1964) Inferior vena caval position in the differential diagnosis of atrial and ventricular septal defects. Radiology 83:616–621

Klatte EC, Tampas JP, Campbell JA (1963) Evaluation of right atrial size. Radiology 81:48–56

Toombs BD, Miller SW (1979) Clinical implications of the convex supradiaphragmatic inferior vena cava. Radiology 132:577–581

Ungerleider HE, Gubner R (1942) Evaluation of heart size measurements. Am Heart J 24:494–510

Pulmonary Vasculature

Bjure A, Laurell H (1927) Abnormal static circulatory phenomena and their symptoms; arterial orthostatic anaemia as neglected clinical picture. Ups Lakaref Forh 33:1–23

Case Records of the Massachusetts General Hospital (1979) Bronchial atresia of the left upper lobe, with emphysema and hyperlucent lung. N Engl J Med 301:829–835

Chen JTT, Robinson AE, Goodrich JK, Lester RG (1969) Uneven distribution of pulmonary blood flow between left and right lungs in isolated valvular pulmonary stenosis. Am J Roentgenol 107:343–350

Davies H, Dow J (1971) Differential pulmonary vascularity and the orientation of the right ventricular outflow tract with special reference to corrected transposition. Br J Radiol 44:258–264

Felson B (1960) Fundamentals of chest roentgenology. Saunders, Philadelphia, pp 193

Friedman WF, Braunwald E (1966) Alterations in regional pulmonary blood flow in mitral valve disease studied by radioisotope scanning. A simple nontraumatic technique for estimation of left atrial pressure. Circulation 34:363–376

Glancy DL, Roberts WC (1976) Congenital obstructive lesions involving the major pulmonary veins, left atrium, or mitral valve: A clinical, laboratory, and morphologic survey. Cathet Cardiovasc Diagn 2:215–252

Lucas RV Jr, Anderson RC, Amplatz K, Adams P, Jr, Edwards JE (1963) Congenital causes of pulmonary venous obstruction. Pediatr Clin N Am 10:781–836

Milne ENC (1973) Correlation of physiologic findings with chest roentgenology. Radiol Clin North Am 11:17–47

Muster AJ, Paul MH, Van Grondelle A, Conway JJ (1976) Abnormal distribution of the pulmonary blood flow between the two lungs in transposition of the great arteries. In: The child with congenital heart disease after surgery. Langford Kidd BS, Rowe RD (eds) Futura Publ, Mount Kisco, N.Y., pp 165–178

Ovenfors C, Ounjian ZJ (1977) Aberrant position of central venous catheter introduced via internal jugular vein. Am J Roentgenol 128:483–484

Race GA, Scheifley CH, Edwards JE (1957) Hydrothorax in congestive heart failure. Am J Med 22:83–89

Shone JD, Sellers RD, Anderson RC, Adams P Jr, Lillehei CW, Edwards JE (1963) The developmental complex of "parachute mitral valve," supravalvular ring of left atrium, subaortic stenosis, and coarctation of the aorta. Am J Cardiol 11:714–725

Spindola-Franco H (1978) Plain film diagnosis of congestive heart failure. J Med Soc N J 75:783–784

Spindola-Franco H, Weisel A, Delman AJ (1978) Pulmonary steal syndrome: An unusual case of coronary bronchial pulmonary artery communication. Radiology 126:25–27

Turner AF, Lau FY, Jacobson G (1972) A method for the estimation of pulmonary venous and arterial pressures from the routine chest roentgenogram. Am J Roentgenol 116:97–106

West JB, Dollery CT, Heard BE (1965) Increased pulmonary vascular resistance in the dependent zone of the isolated dog lung caused by perivascular edema. Circ Res 17:191–206

West JB, Dollery CT, Naimark A (1964) Distribution of blood flow in the isolated lung: Relation to vascular and alveolar pressure. J Appl Physiol 19:713–724

Wilson WJ, Amplatz K (1967) Unequal vascularity in tetralogy of Fallot. Am J Roentgenol 100:318–321

2 Introduction to Echocardiography

Physical Principle

The principle upon which ultrasound imaging is based is similar to that used in sonar depth finders. Sound waves are produced by a piezoelectric crystal that vibrates within a known frequency range when excited by an electric current. Such crystals also act as receivers, transforming acoustic energy back into electrical energy with extreme efficiency. Some naturally occurring crystals such as quartz and Rochelle salt have piezoelectric properties. Ultrasound transducers are usually made of ceramics such as barium titanate and lead zirconate.

The piezoelectric crystal is excited by a short burst of electrical energy so that it vibrates at its intrinsic frequency for a very short period. The sound is directed in a straight line, with some dispersion beyond the focal depth of the transducer. In a liquid medium and in most body tissues the sound travels with a known velocity (1540 m/sec). It is reflected by any interface between substances of differing acoustic impedance. Each interface reflects a greater or lesser fraction of the signal, depending on the difference between the ultrasound impedances. Bone and air reflect all of the signal because their ultrasound impedances are markedly different from that of soft tissues. Heart valves and heart muscle have acoustic impedances close to that of blood. Therefore many layers of heart tissue can be imaged without total attenuation of the transmitted signal. As the reflected sound reaches the transducer the crystal transforms the acoustic energy back into electrical energy and transmits electrical impulses to the receiving amplifier. *A-mode* or amplitude mode is the simplest method of display of the returning signals. In this mode the echocardiograph displays a spike on the baseline to represent each returning echo. The spike is closer to the origin if the returning echo is relatively early and further from the origin if the echo returns later. The amplitude of the spike is proportional to the intensity of the returning echo (Fig. 2–1).

B-mode (brightness mode) is made up of an array of points of light along a line, each representing a returning echo. The distance of each point from the origin is proportional to the distance the sound has traveled before returning to the transducer (i.e., the depth of the structure). The intensity or brightness of each point is proportional to the intensity of the returning echo reaching the transducer (Fig. 2–2).

TM-mode (time-motion mode) or *M-mode* (Figs. 2–3 to 2–6) is made by sweeping the dots of the B-mode across a persistence screen or photographic paper so that the changing depth (motion) of the structure is displayed versus time. Use of M-mode for imaging motion of cardiac structures was described by Hertz and Edler in 1954. Even with the advent of two-dimensional echocardiography (2-DE), M-mode remains an important method of imaging cardiac structures. M-mode is especially useful when timing of events is crucial. M-mode allows precise measurements of thickness, leaflet velocity, chamber diameter, and mean velocity of circumferential fiber shortening (mean VCF). Subtle abnormalities of leaflet motion (e.g., fine flutter) are also better identified on M-mode than on 2-DE. M-mode echocardiography is particularly useful as an aid in recognition of noncalcified bicuspid aortic valve, aortic insufficiency (mitral flutter), mitral prolapse, flail mitral leaflet, pedunculated vegetations and pedunculated intracardiac tumors.

The following are descriptions of the M-mode images of the cardiac valves and chambers. The patient is supine or in left lateral decubitus position. The transducer is generally placed in the third or fourth (or occasionally in the second or fifth) left intercostal space.

Aortic valve motion (Figs. 2–3, 2–4, and 2–7) is characterized by a rapid opening motion anteriorly and posteriorly, probably representing the right (anterior) and noncoronary cusps within the aortic root. Sometimes a third leaflet can be seen fluttering in the middle of the aortic root during systole (Fig. 2–7B). The opening is sustained

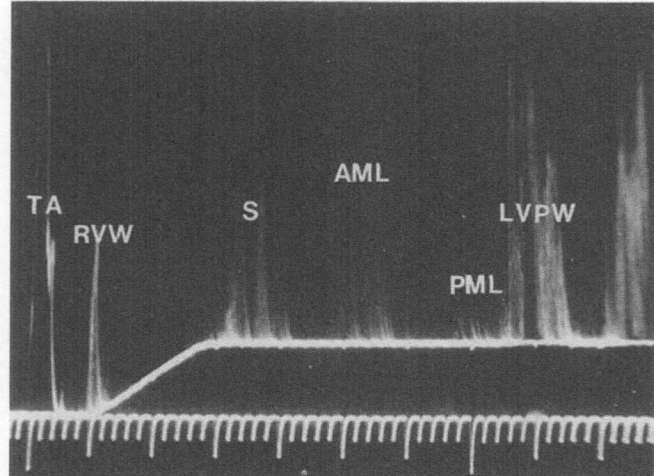

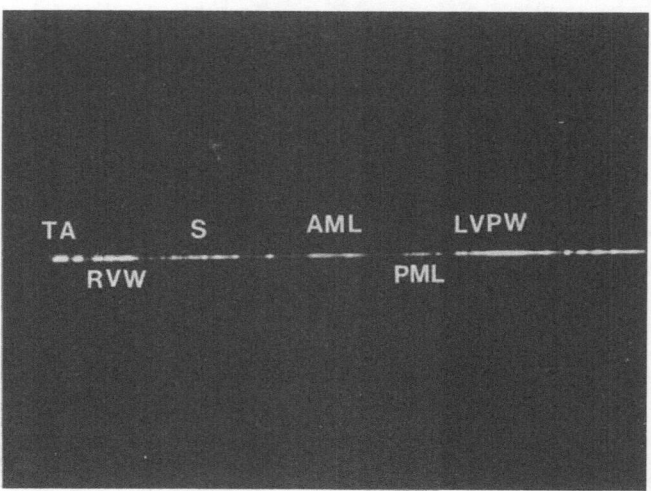

Fig. 2–1. *A-mode (amplitude mode).* The height of the spikes is proportional to the intensity of the returning echoes. The distance from the origin is proportional to the depth of the reflecting interface. The centimeter scale indicates the depth. *TA* = transducer artifact; *RVW* = right ventricular wall; *S* = septum; *AML* = anterior mitral leaflet; *PML* = posterior mitral leaflet; *LVPW* = left ventricular posterior wall.

Fig. 2–2. *B-mode (brightness mode).* The intensity of the dots is proportional to the intensity of the returning echo. The distance from the origin indicates the depth of the reflecting interface. This representation is swept across a persistence screen or polaroid film or along photographic paper to produce the T-M mode (Fig. 2–3 to 2–5). Abbreviations same as Fig. 2–1.

throughout systole. The leaflets then fall together, completing a parallelogram. The leaflets coapt in the middle of the aortic root throughout diastole. The entire aortic root is moved anteriorly during ventricular systole and then falls posteriorly as the left ventricle fills. The atrial kick can usually be seen as a posterior dip of the aortic walls and the coapted valve just before systole. The *right ventricular outflow tract* is anterior to the aortic valve. The *left atrium* is behind the aorta. The left atrium is generally measured at the end of ventricular systole from the initial echoes of the posterior aortic root to the initial echoes of the left atrial free wall. The aortic root is measured during diastole, from the initial echoes of its anterior wall to the initial echoes of its posterior wall. Normal measurements are found in Table 2–1.

The *pulmonary valve* (Figs. 2–4 and 2–8) is encountered as the transducer is angled superiorly and to the left of the aortic valve. In infants a parallelogram can be identified if the transducer is moved to the second intercostal space to transect the valve perpendicular to its opening motion. In older children and adults the transducer is positioned in the left third or fourth interspace, so that the valve is imaged from below. Therefore the opening motion of the valve is away from the transducer and its closing motion is toward the transducer. During systole coarse flutter is normally observed. During diastole the coapted valve tends to move slowly away from the transducer. The atrial kick is observed just prior to the opening of the valve.

Semilunar Valves in Complex Congenital Defects In congenital heart defects it is not possible to differentiate the aortic from the pulmonic valve by motion. Usually the semilunar valves can be differentiated by use of systolic time intervals. In infants beyond a few hours of age, pulmonary pressure should be less than systemic. The preejection

period (PEP) of the pulmonary valve should therefore be shorter than that of the aortic valve. The ventricular ejection time (VET) of the pulmonic valve tends to be longer than that of the aortic valve. With normally related great vessels the aortic valve (long PEP, short VET) should be posterior, to the right and inferior relative to the position of the pulmonary valve (short PEP, long VET) (Figs. 2–7, 2–8). If the aorta is anterior and to the right, D-transposition is likely (Fig. 2–9). If the aorta is anterior and to the left, L-transposition should be suspected (Fig. 2–10).

The *mitral valve* (Fig. 2–11) is identified as the transducer is angled caudally and laterally from the fourth left intercostal space. The normal motion of the anterior leaflet during diastole is like the letter M. The initial rapid opening motion of the anterior leaflet is anterior (toward the transducer). The posterior leaflet moves posteriorly (away from the transducer) but to a lesser extent than the anterior leaflet. During the slow filling phase the mitral leaflets tend to fall together. The atrial kick again spreads the leaflets before they close with onset of ventricular systole. The

Fig. 2–3. *Cardiac anatomy as observed on M-mode echocardiography.* The upper part of the diagram is a cross section along the long axis of the left ventricle. M-mode can only image one position at a time. By angling the transducer through positions, 1,2 and 3, all structures can be imaged in sequence. The characteristic motions of the structures are observed in the lower part of the drawing. At position 1 the left ventricle (*LV*) and chordae tendineae (*CH.T*) are imaged (Figs. 2–5, 2–6). At position 2 the mitral valve is demonstrated (see also Fig. 2–11). At position 3 the aortic root (*Ao*) is noted (Fig. 2–7) with the right ventricular outflow tract (*RVOT*) anterior to it and the left atrium (*LA*) behind it. *Ao.V* = aortic valve; *AML* = anterior mitral leaflet; *PML* = posterior mitral leaflet; *PM* = papillary muscle; *RVW* = right ventricular free wall; *LVPW* = LV posterior wall.

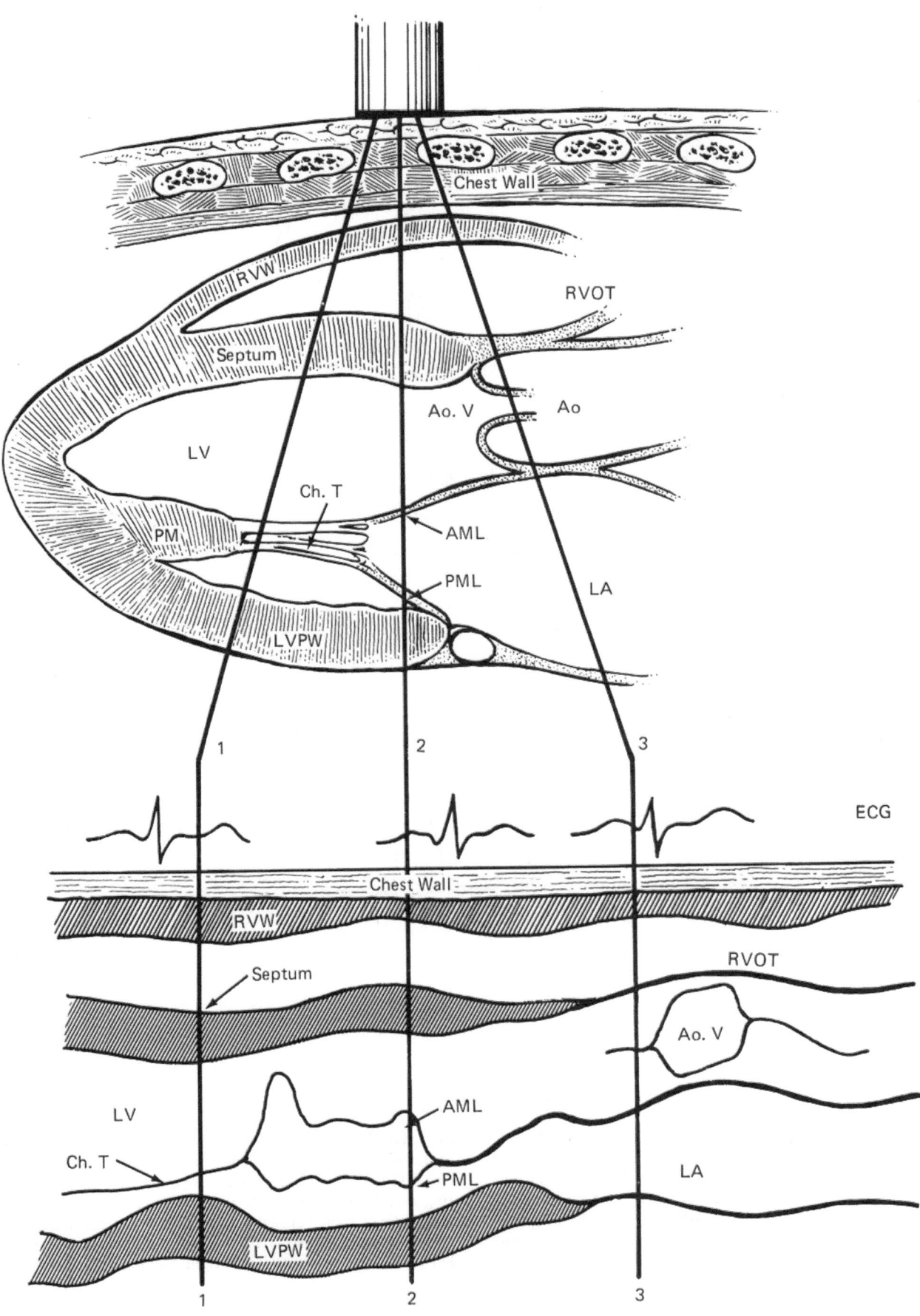

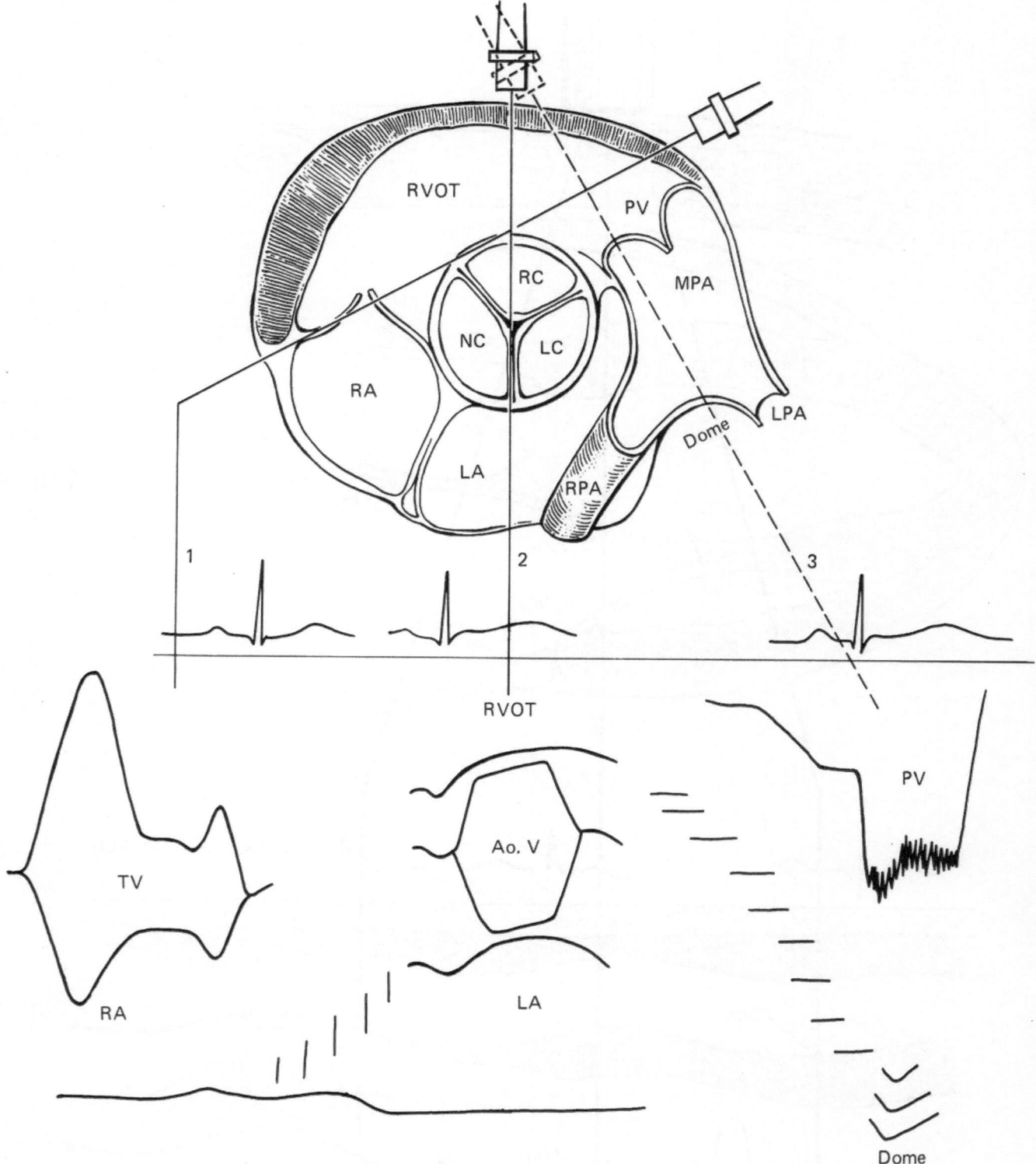

Fig. 2–4. *Cardiac anatomy as defined on M-mode echocardiography.* The upper image represents a horizontal cross section of the heart at the level of the aortic valve (*Ao.V*). The tricuspid valve (*TV*) is to the right of the aortic valve (position 1) (see also Fig. 2–12). The right ventricular outflow tract (*RVOT*) (position 2) is wrapped around the front of the aortic root. The pulmonary valve (*PV*) (position 3) is superior and to the left of the aortic valve. When the transducer is held in the third or fourth left intercostal space the pulmonary valve is imaged from within the RVOT. Therefore both leaflets move away from the transducer during systole (see Fig. 2–8). *LA* = left atrium; *RA* = right atrium; *RC* = right coronary cusp; *LC* = left coronary cusp; *NC* = noncoronary cusp; *MPA* = main pulmonary artery; *LPA* = left pulmonary artery; *RPA* = right pulmonary artery.

Table 2-1. Normal Measurements Using M-Mode Echocardiography

Age, weight	Ao (cm)	LA (cm)	LVIDd (cm)	SF	mVCF (circ/sec)	LVW and septal thickness (cm)	Mitral E-to-F slope (mm/sec)	RVID (cm)
Premature newborn								
1–1.2 kg	0.66 ± 0.09[J]	0.76 ± 0.15[J]	1.23 ± 0.17[J]	31.2 ± 7.2[J]	1.8 ± 0.49[J]			
2.3 kg	0.93–1.13[Sol] (1.03)	0.68–1.05[Sol] (0.87)	1.61–2.17[Sol] (1.89)			0.20–0.34[Sol] (0.27)		
Term newborn								
2.7–4.5 kg	0.8–1.2[H]	0.5–1.0[H]	1.2–2.3[H]		0.9–2.2[S] (1.51)	0.2–0.4[H] (0.3)		0.8–1.9[H] (1.4)
4–12 mo 7.77 ± 1.8 kg	1.21 ± 0.14[M]	1.59 ± 0.33[M]	2.28 ± 0.36[M]		1.34 ± 0.30[G]	0.38 ± 0.08[M]		1.12 ± 0.18[M]
1–2 yr 10.86 kg ± 2.15 kg	1.38 ± 0.15[M]	1.82 ± 0.30[M]	2.82 ± 0.26[M]		1.34 ± 0.30[G]	0.45 ± 0.09[M]		1.12 ± 0.22[M]
26–50 lb	1.3–2.2[F] (1.7)	1.7–2.7[F] (2.2)	2.4–3.8[F] (3.4)		1.34 ± 0.30[G]	0.5–0.7[F] (0.6)		0.4–1.5[F] (1.0)
51–75 lb	1.7–2.3[F] (2.0)	1.9–2.8[7] (2.3)	3.3–4.5[F] (3.8)		1.34 ± 0.30[G]	0.6–0.7[F] (0.7)		0.7–1.8[F] (1.1)
76–100 lb	1.9–2.7[F] (2.2)	2.0–3.0[F] (2.4)	3.5–4.7[F] (4.1)		1.34 ± 0.30[G]	0.7–0.8[F] (0.7)		0.7–1.6[F] (1.2)
101–125	1.7–2.7[F] (2.3)	2.1–3.0[F] (2.7)	3.7–4.9[F] (4.3)		1.34 ± 0.30[G]	0.7–0.8[F] (0.7)		0.8–1.7[F] (1.3)
Adult flat	2.0–3.7[F] (2.7)	1.9–4.0[F] (2.9)	3.7–5.6[F] (4.7)	28–44[F] (36%)	1.02–1.94[F] (1.3 circ/sec)	0.6–1.1[F] (0.9)	60–110[F] >60 mm/sec	0.7–2.3[F] (1.5)
Adult L. lat			3.5–5.7[F] (4.7)					0.9–2.6[F] (1.7)

Superscripts refer to the following references in the bibliography for this chapter: J = Johnson; M = Meyer RA 1977; H = Hagan; S = Sahn; G= Goldberg; F = Feigenbaum, 3rd ed.; Sol = Solinger.

Abbreviations:

Ao = diameter of the aortic root measured from the leading edge of the anterior wall to the leading edge of the posterior wall of the aortic root.

LA = diameter of the left atrium at the end of ventricular systole, measured from the leading edge of the posterior wall of the aortic anulus to the leading edge of the posterior wall of the left atrium.

LVIDd = left ventricular internal diameter at the end of diastole (R wave of the ECG).

SF = shortening fraction.

mVCF = mean velocity of fiber shortening (circumferences/sec).

LVW = left ventricular wall.

E to F slope = the slope of the part of the tracing of mitral valve motion between the E point and the F point (see Fig. 2–11).

RVID = inner diameter of the right ventricular cavity measured during diastole.

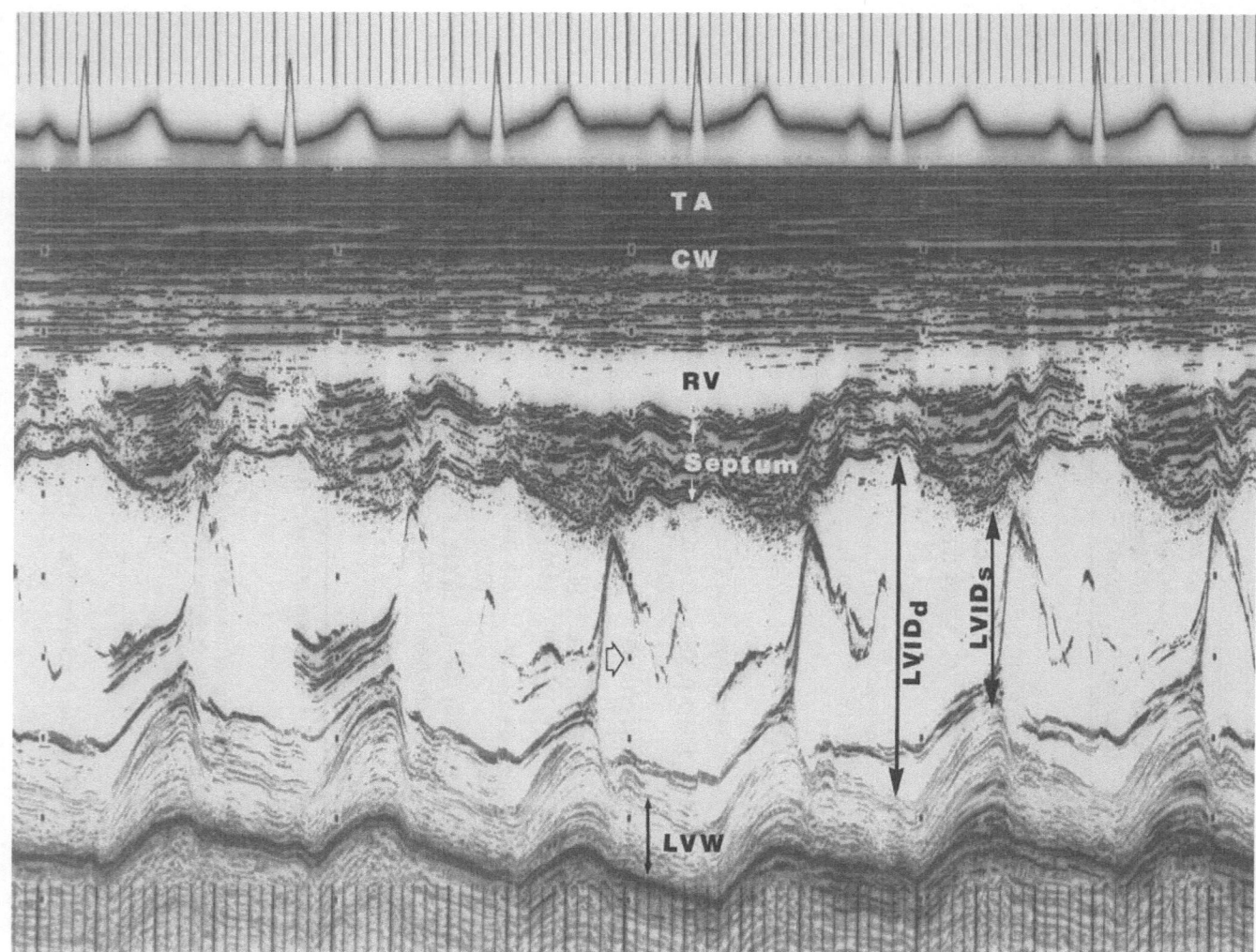

Fig. 2–5. *M-mode (time-motion mode)at the level of the mitral valve and left ventricular cavity.* This image is formed by moving the photographic paper past a screen which displays the B-mode similar to Fig. 2–2. Depth markers (*open arrow*) indicate 1 cm of tissue depth, occurring at 1-second intervals. The transducer artifact (*TA*) and chest wall (*CW*) are the first echoes. Right ventricular free wall is observed, on occasion, just beyond the chest wall, but more often it is obscured. The right ventricular cavity (*RV*) is defined next, then the interventricular septum. The left ventricular cavity is bounded by the septum anteriorly and the LV free wall (*LVW*) posteriorly. The mitral valve can be detected as it moves within the left ventricle. Normally the septum moves posteriorly and the ventricular free wall moves anteriorly to compress the left ventricular cavity during ventricular systole. The mitral apparatus and chordae tendineae are easily distinguished from the LV endocardium, since the endocardium moves most rapidly. The internal diameter of the left ventricle in diastole ($LVID_d$) and in systole ($LVID_S$) are used to calculate shortening fraction and mean velocity of circumferential fiber shortening (mVCF). $LVID_d$ is measured at the time of the R wave of the electrocardiogram, while $LVID_S$ is measured either at the peak of motion of the LV wall or the peak of motion of the septum.

letters *A* through *F* are generally used to designate the positions of the anterior mitral leaflet during various phases of its motion so that each phase can be described and quantitated: *A* represents the peak of atrial kick; *B* the onset of ventricular systole; *C* the mitral closing motion; *D* the onset of rapid opening motion; *E* the peak of the opening; and *F* the end of the initial closing slope. Measurements of the amplitude of the D to E motion have been used to estimate volume of the flow during rapid filling or alternatively the flexibility of the valve in mitral stenosis. The E–F slope has been used as an indicator of mitral stenosis, although it has been shown to correlate poorly with severity of the stenosis. The E–F slope may also be reduced with poor compliance of the left ventricle. It has been suggested, therefore, that this motion of the mitral valve reflects the rate of filling of the left ventricle.

To visualize the *tricuspid valve* (Fig. 2–12) the transducer is angled steeply to the right. In some adults this valve cannot be imaged even though the subject reclines on his or her left side. The tricuspid valve moves like the mitral valve but is placed more anteriorly. Because of poor visualization, only qualitative statements are generally made regarding the M-mode image of the tricuspid valve (e.g., presence or absence, position relative to the mitral valve).

Quantitative M-mode images of the *left ventricle* (LV)

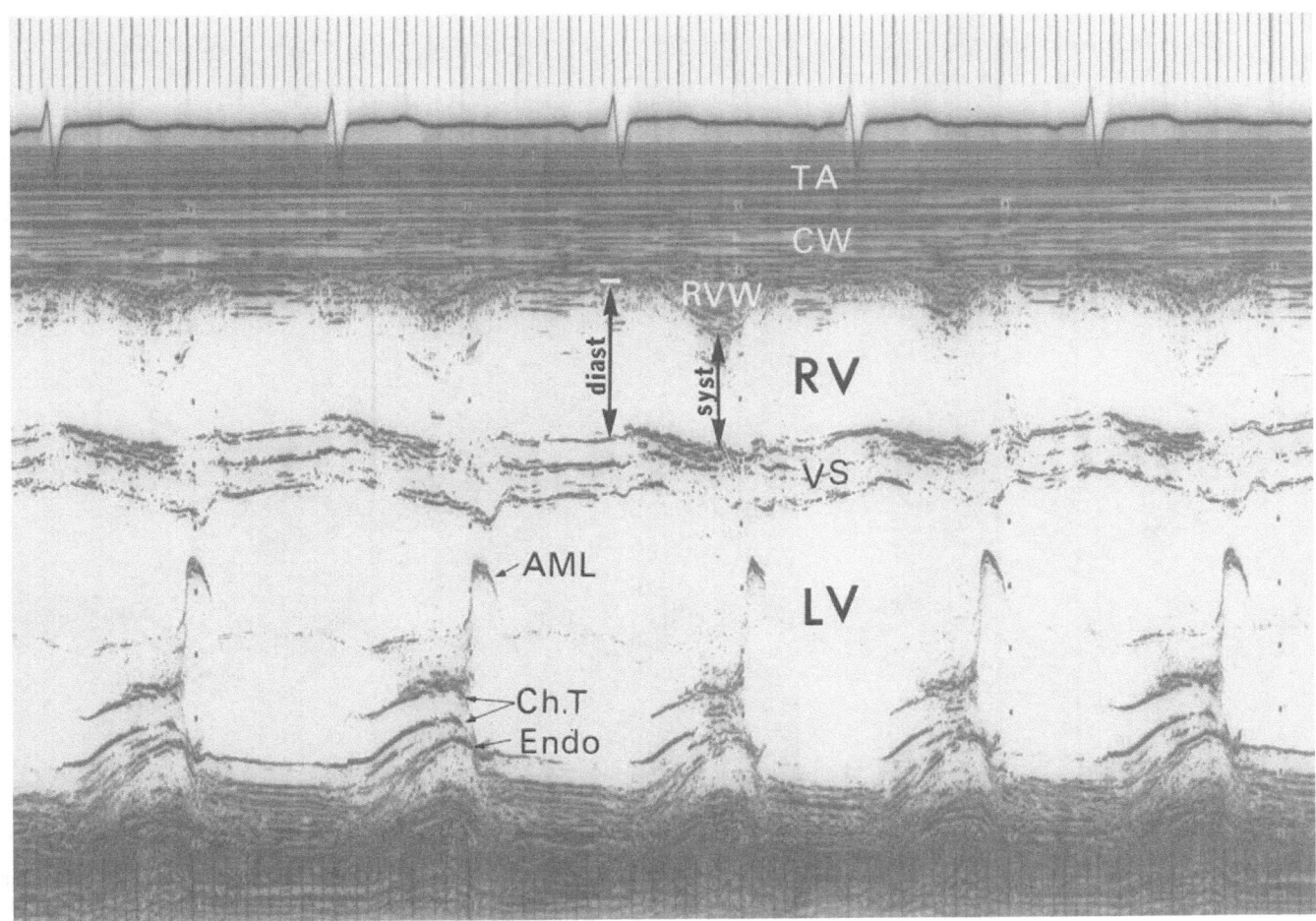

Fig. 2–6. *Measurement of right ventricular diameter by M-mode recording through the right ventricle (RV) and left ventricle (LV) at the level of the tip of the mitral valve (AML). The right ventricular wall (RVW) is well demonstrated so that the RV internal diameter in systole (syst) and diastole (diast) can be measured.* It is important to be consistent in positioning the patient for this measurement (e.g., the RV diameter may increase if the patient lies with the right side up). *TA* = transducer artifact; *CW* = chest wall; *VS* = ventricular septum; *Ch.T* = chordae tendineae; *Endo* = endocardium.

are normally obtained just beyond the tips of the mitral leaflets in adults (Fig. 2–5). In children the standard image of the LV is obtained higher up where the mitral leaflets are easily identified. During systole the septum and LV posterior wall (LVPW) move toward one another. The LV end-diastolic dimension is measured on the R wave of the ECG, and the LV systolic dimension is measured at the peak of upward motion of the LV wall or the peak of downward motion of the ventricular septum (these two measurements are usually nearly identical). The septal thickness and LV free-wall thickness should be measured during diastole, when both sides of the septum are well delineated and the endocardium and epicardium of the

LV free wall are also easily observed. On occasion the septum and LV free wall must be measured on separate tracings. Normal measurements of septal thickness, LV wall thickness, LV diameter, and LV contractions are found in Table 2–1. M-mode echocardiographic dimensions correlate well with angiographic volume determination in healthy young individuals. If dilatation or asynergy is present the correlation between M-mode diameters and angiographic measurements is poor. Thus the operator should determine carefully in each patient whether it is appropriate to use M-mode measurements to estimate LV volume, mass and function. (See section on LV performance, p. 54.)

The *RV internal diameter* (RVID) is measured from

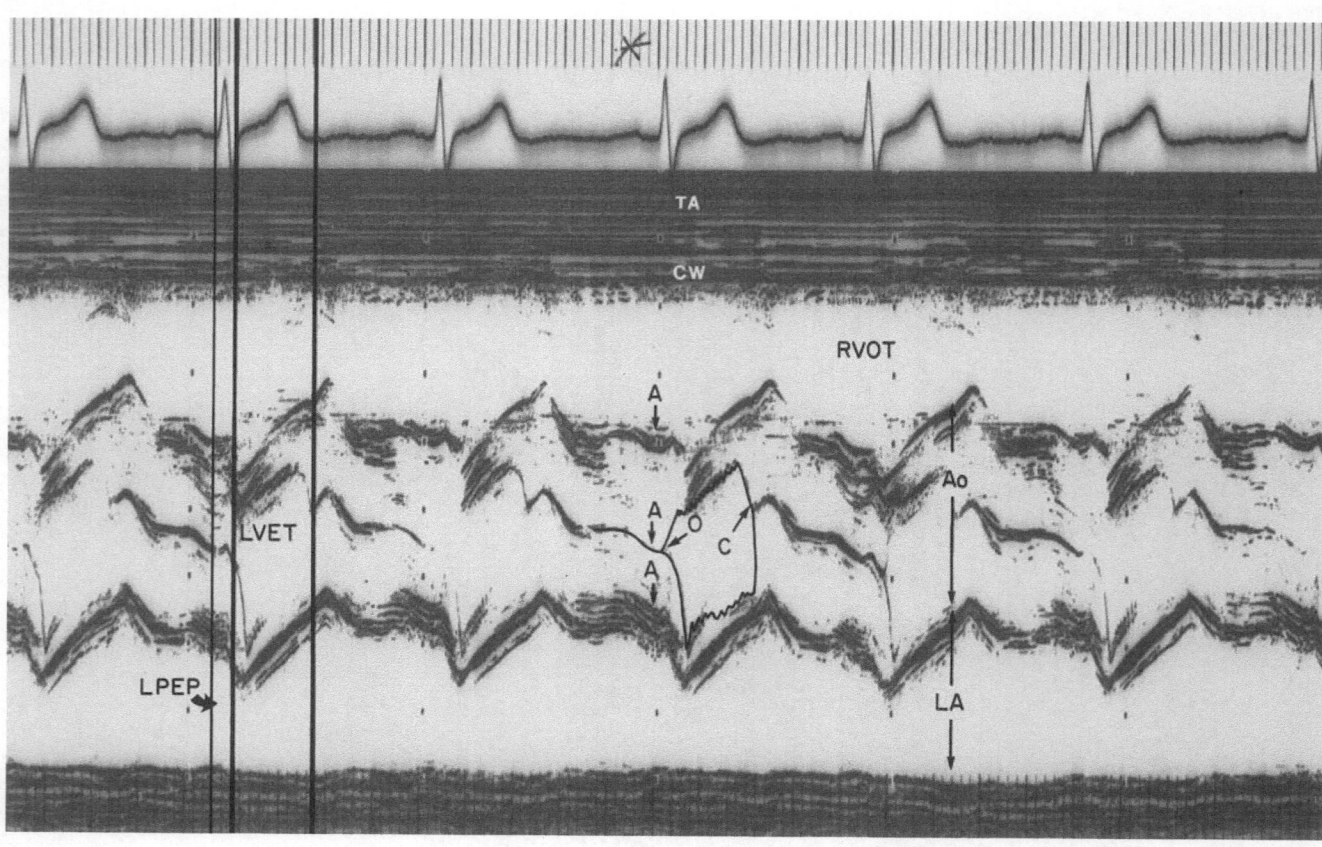

A

Fig. 2–7, A–C. *Aortic valve.* **A** Normal aortic valve in a 16-year-old boy. The anterior and posterior walls of the aorta (*Ao*) move in parallel, while the aortic valve leaflets move toward and away from the transducer during systole. During diastole the leaflets coapt in the middle of the aortic root. Anterior to the aorta is the right ventricular outflow tract (*RVOT*) and posterior to it is the left atrium (*LA*). The atrial "kick" (*A*) is characterized by a posterior dip on the anterior and posterior walls of the aortic root as well as on the coapted leaflets. An idealized parallelogram is traced over one beat and systolic time intervals are indicated. The preejection period for the left ventricle (*LPEP*) is 60 msec and the LV ejection time (*LVET*) is 260 msec. *O* = opening of the valve; *C* = closing of the valve. **B** *Normal aortic valve* showing the third leaflet fluttering in the middle of the aortic root throughout systole (*arrows*). **C** *Fibrotic aortic valve.* The leaflets are thickened. Note multiple echoes during diastole. The leaflets do not meet the anterior or posterior wall of the aortic root during systole. Courtesy of Naftali Neuberger, M.D.

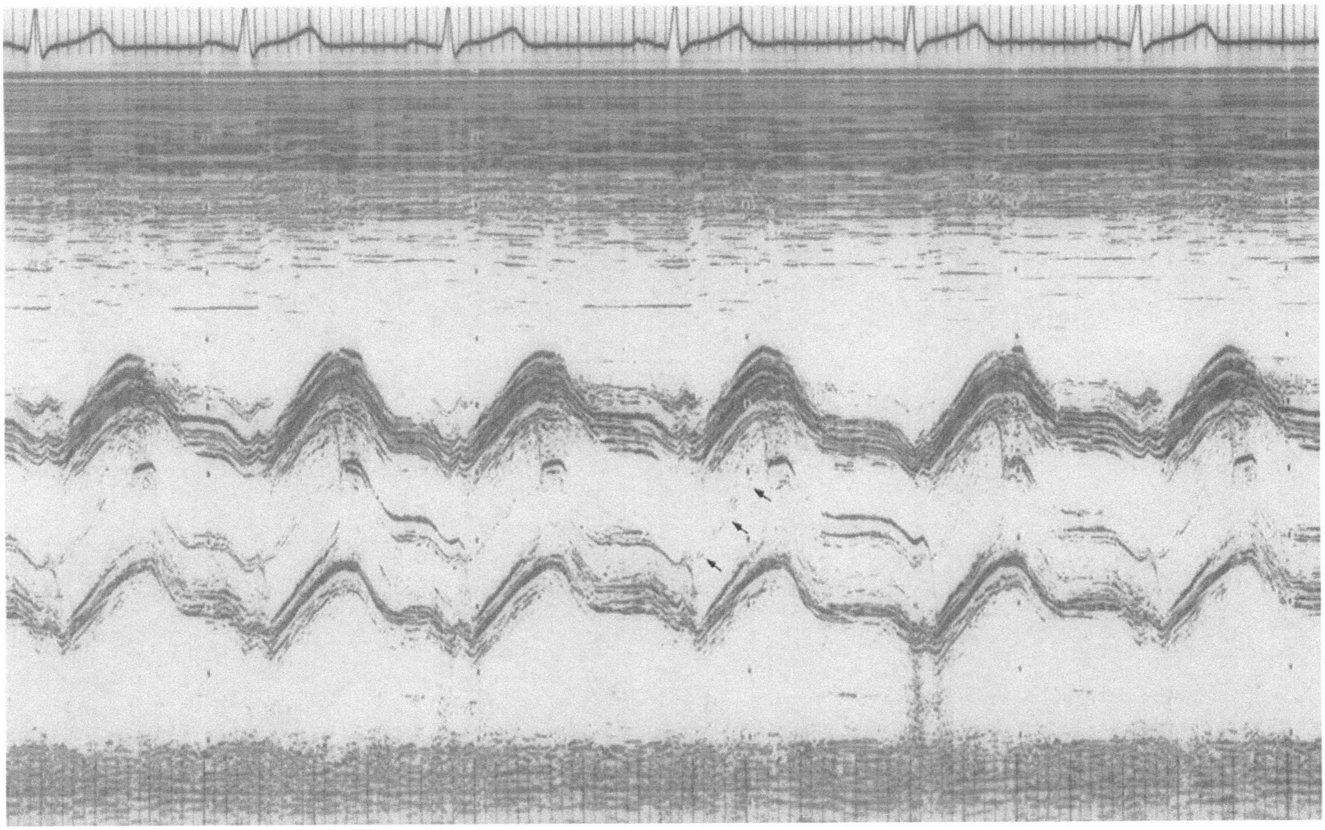

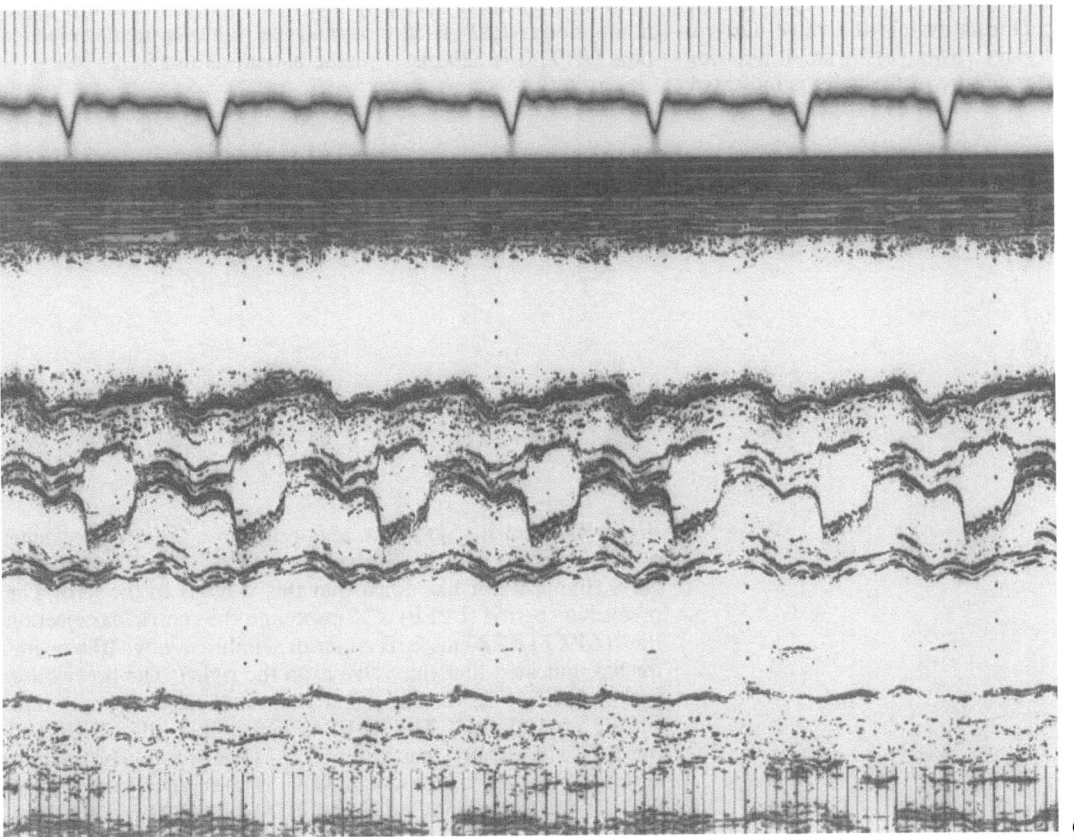

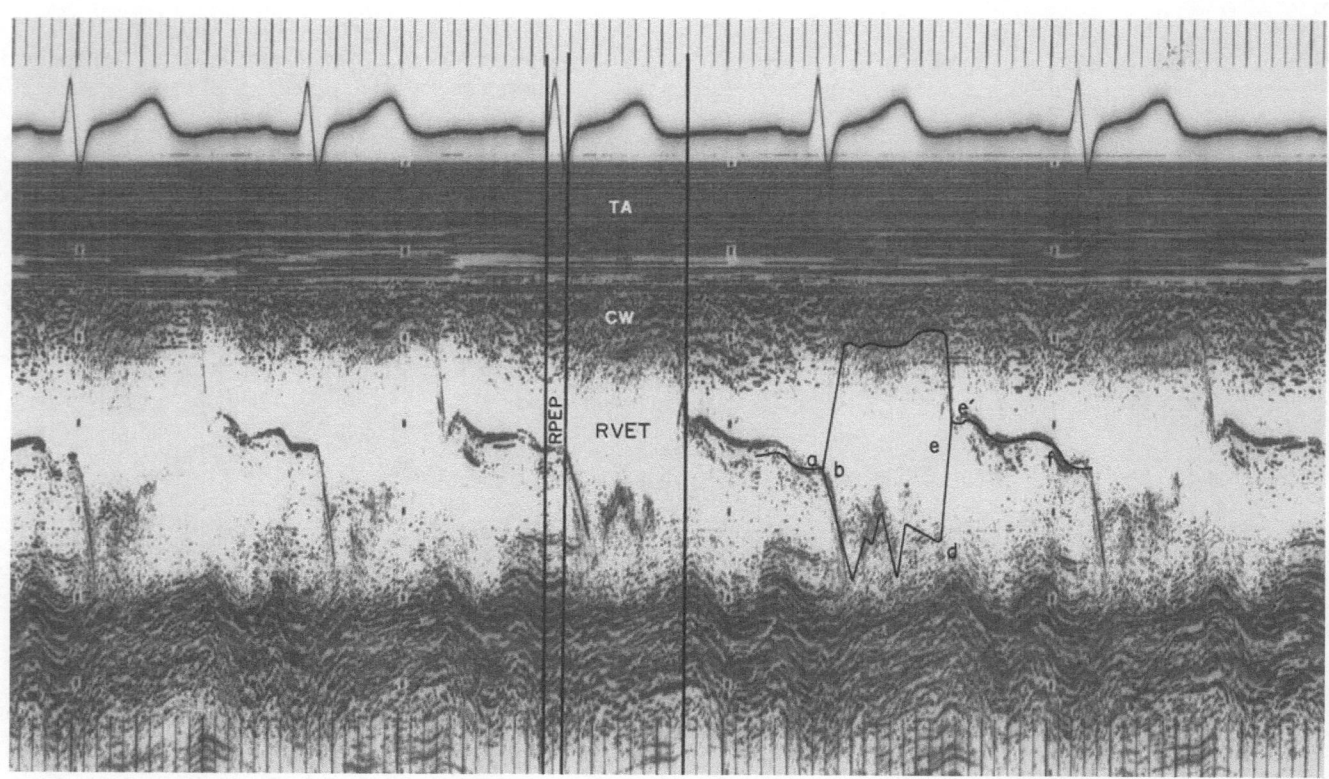

Fig. 2–8. *Normal pulmonary valve.* The small letters are those conventionally applied to pulmonary valve motion. During diastole the coapted leaflets move slowly posteriorly (*f*). The atrial "kick" (*a*) is clearly identified. At onset of ventricular ejection (*b*) the valve opens abruptly. During systole the valve flutters. At the end of systole (*d*) the valve closes (*e*). A small anterior motion present on occasion after closure of the valve is indicated by *e'*. It is rare to record an idealized parallelogram of pulmonary valve motion in adults, because the valve is imaged through the right ventricular outflow tract. Therefore both leaflets move away from the transducer during systole. The right ventricular preejection period (*RPEP*) is 50 msec and the right ventricular ejection time (*RVET*) is 320 msec. (Same patient as in Fig. 2–7A)

Fig. 2–9, A and B. *Systolic time intervals in a 2-day-old cyanotic male.* (The time lines are 10 msec apart.) **A** Posterior semilunar valve (the operator has noted that this valve is to the left). The preejection period (*LPEP*) is 55 msec, and the ventricular ejection time (*LVET*) is 180 msec. **B** Anterior semilunar valve (the operator has indicated that this valve is on the right). The preejection period (*RPEP*) is 70 msec, and the ventricular ejection time (*RVET*) is 150 msec. The RPEP is longer than the LPEP, and the RVET is shorter than the LVET. Thus it is likely that the anterior (right-sided) semilunar valve is the aortic valve. These findings represent strong evidence for D-transposition of the great vessels.

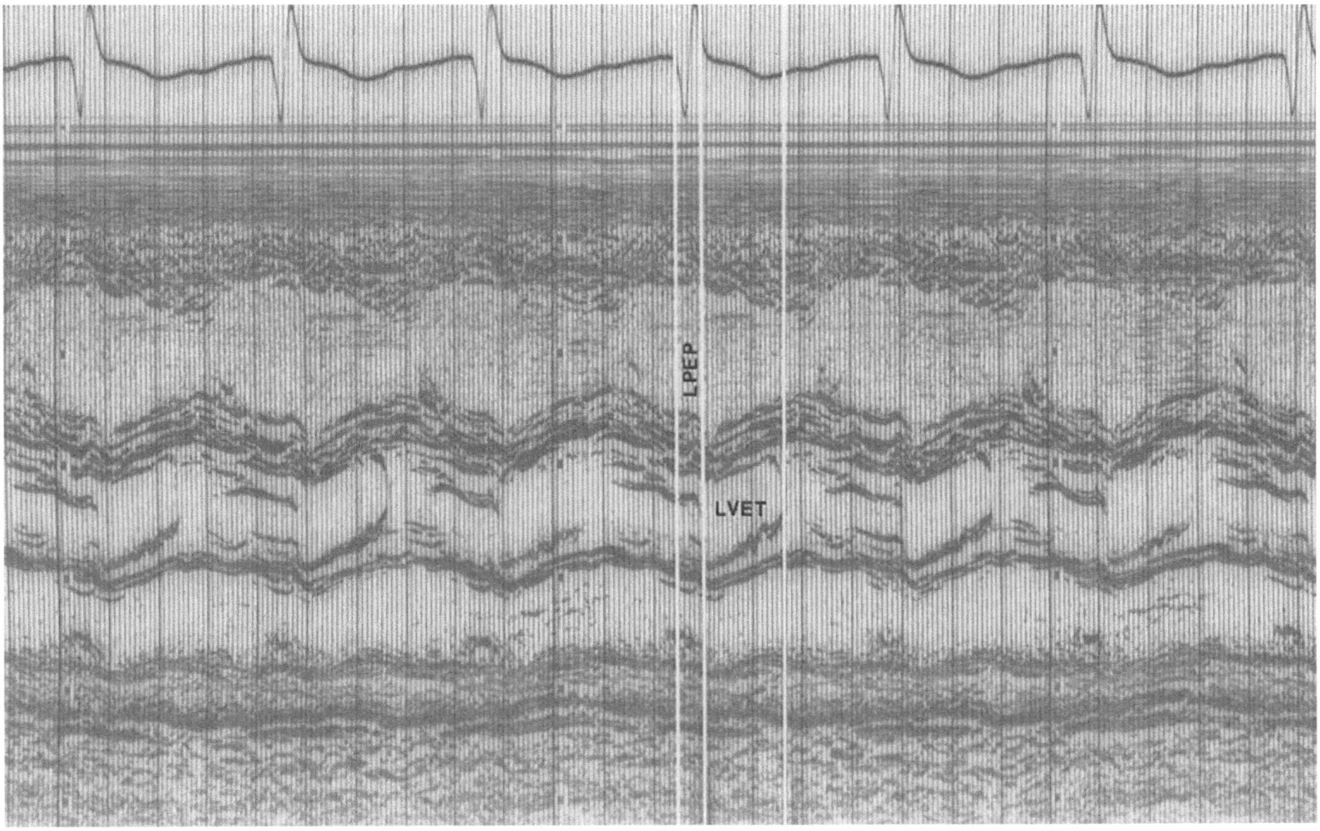

A

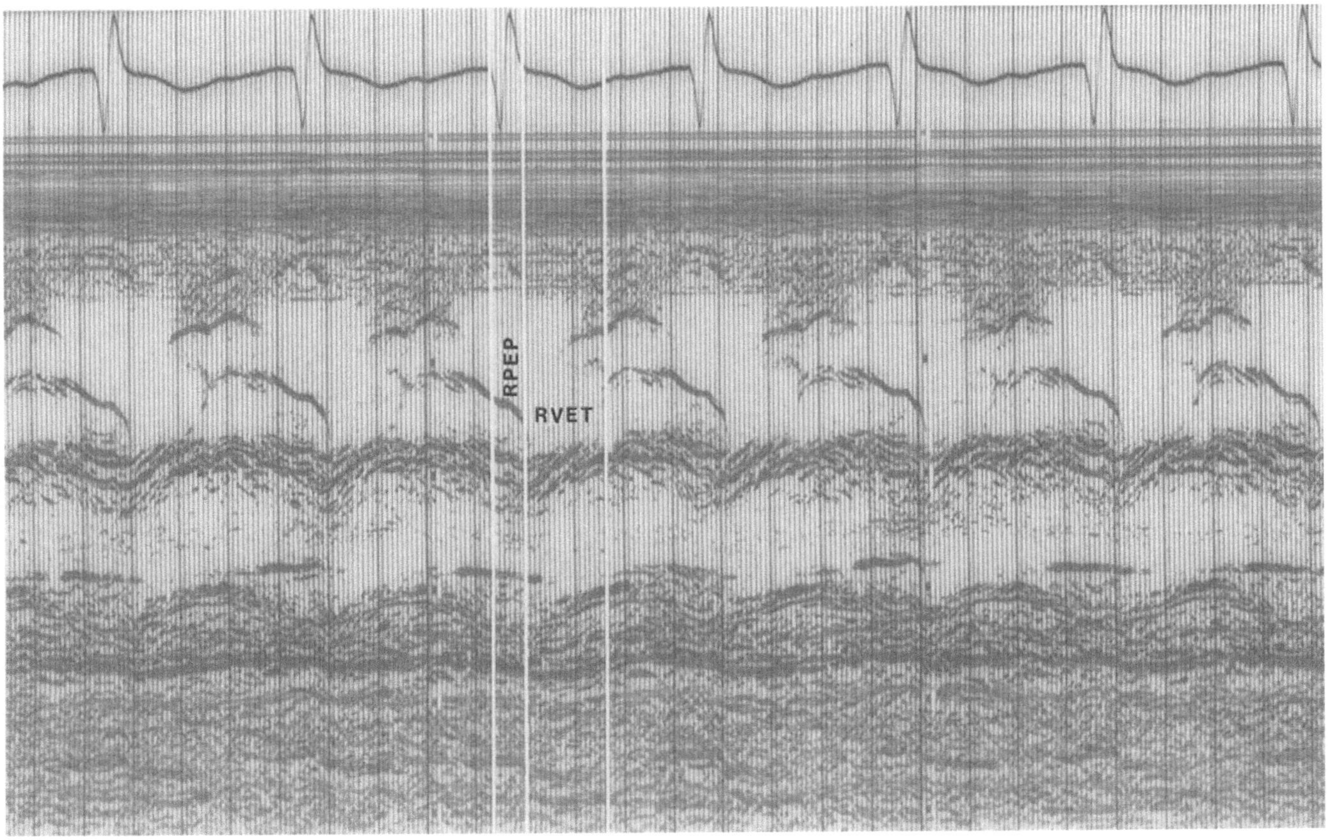

B

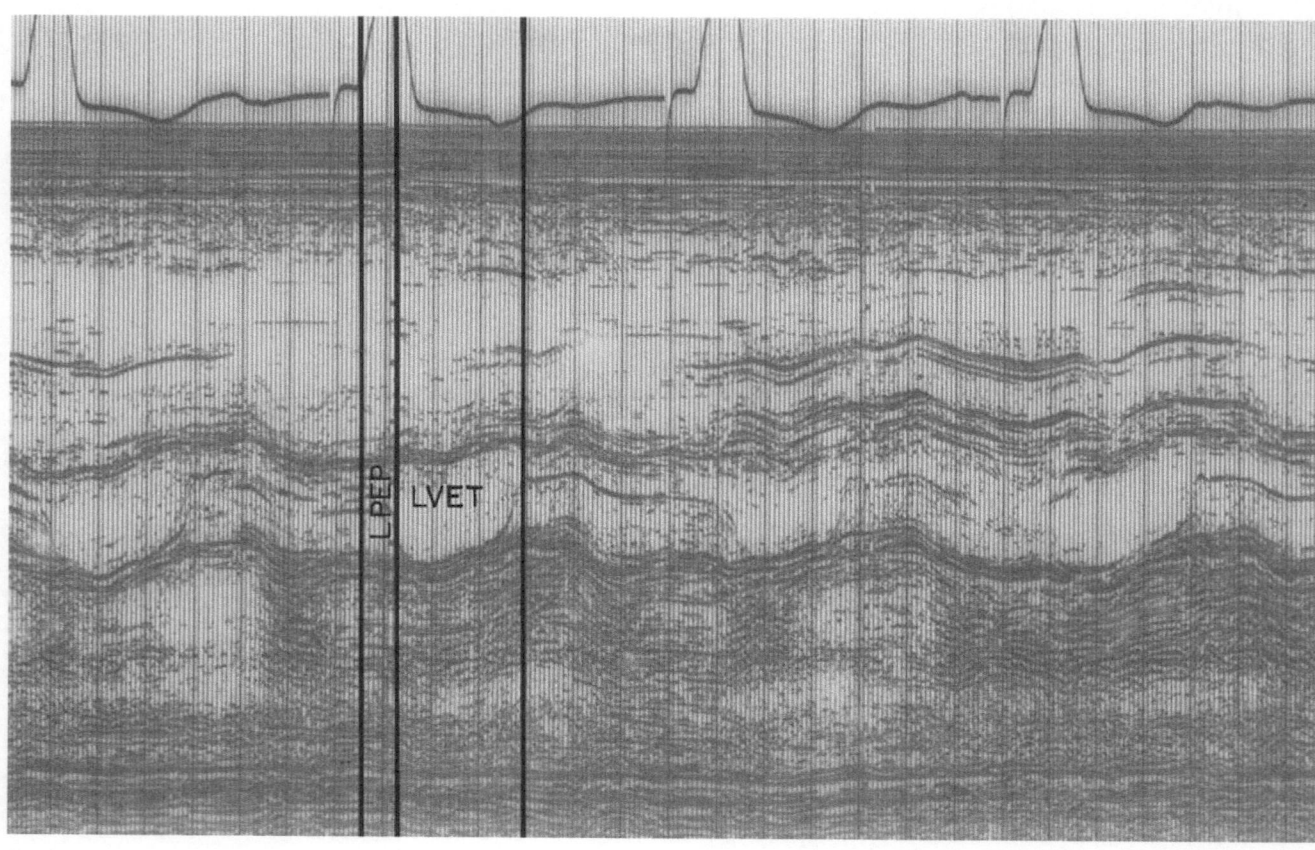

A

B

◀ **Fig. 2–10.** *Systolic time intervals in a 6-year-old child with L-transposition and complete heart block (note pacemaker impulse).* The anterior (left-sided) semilunar valve (*frame A*) has a preejection period (*PEP*) of 175 msec and a ventricular ejection time (*VET*) of 190 msec. The posterior, right-sided valve (*frame B*) has a PEP of 70 msec and a VET of 260 msec. The PEP of the anterior valve is longest, and the VET is shortest. The anterior valve is considered to be the aortic valve. The operator has indicated that the anterior valve is on the left side. The diagnosis, therefore, is L-transposition of the great vessels. Time lines are 10 msec apart.

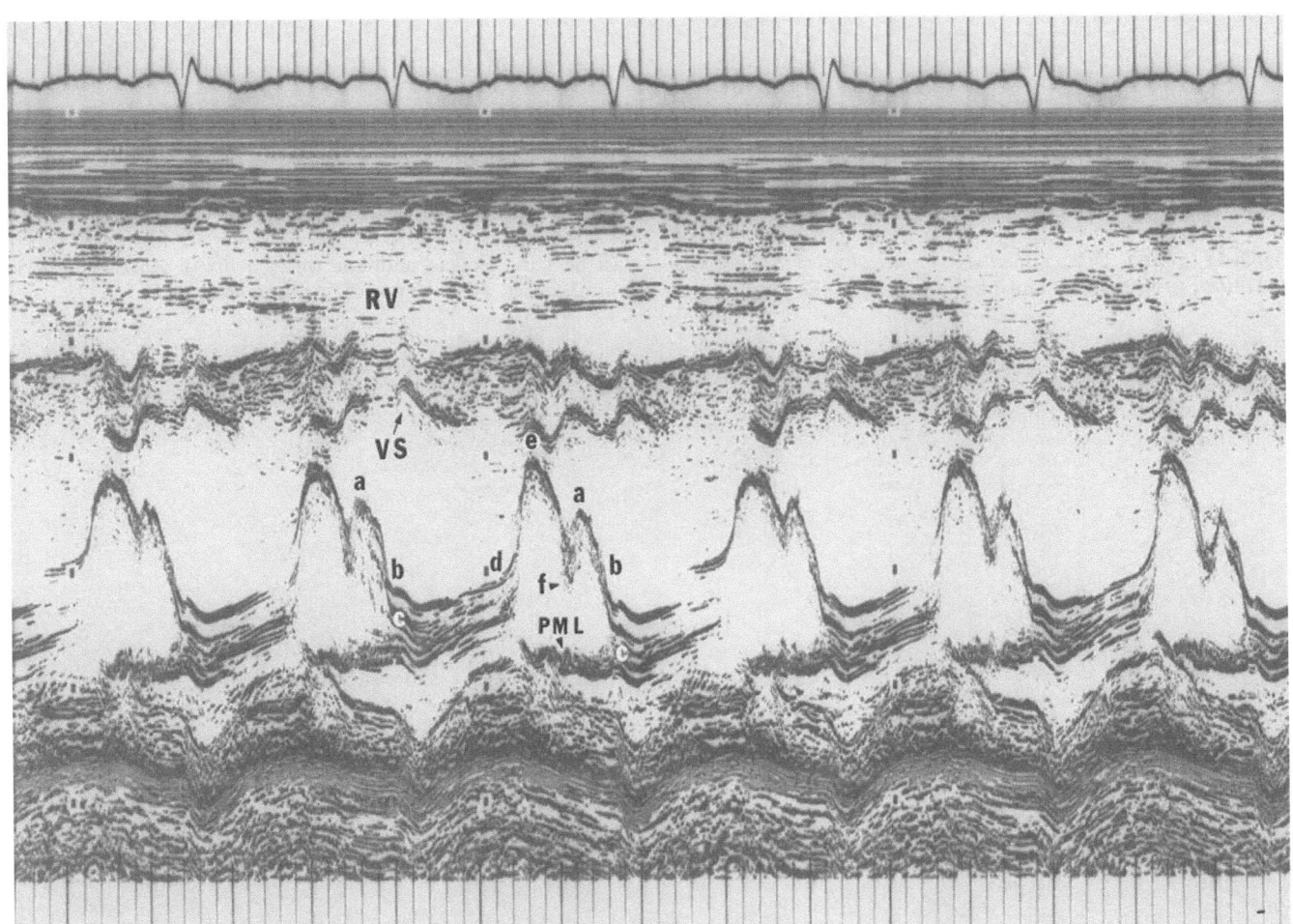

A

Fig. 2–11, A and B. A *Normal mitral valve in a 2-year-old child.* The lower case letters are those conventionally applied to motion of the anterior mitral leaflet. Thus *a* represents atrial "kick"; *b* represents onset of ventricular contraction; *c* represents mitral closure; *c–d* represent ventricular systole; *e* represents the peak of the opening motion during early diastole; *f* is the point at which the mitral valve falls posteriorly at the end of rapid filling. The posterior mitral leaflet (*PML*) moves in an opposite direction. The amplitude of PML motion is much less than that of the anterior mitral leaflet. *VS* = ventricular septum, *RV* = right ventricular cavity. (*Continued on next page.*)

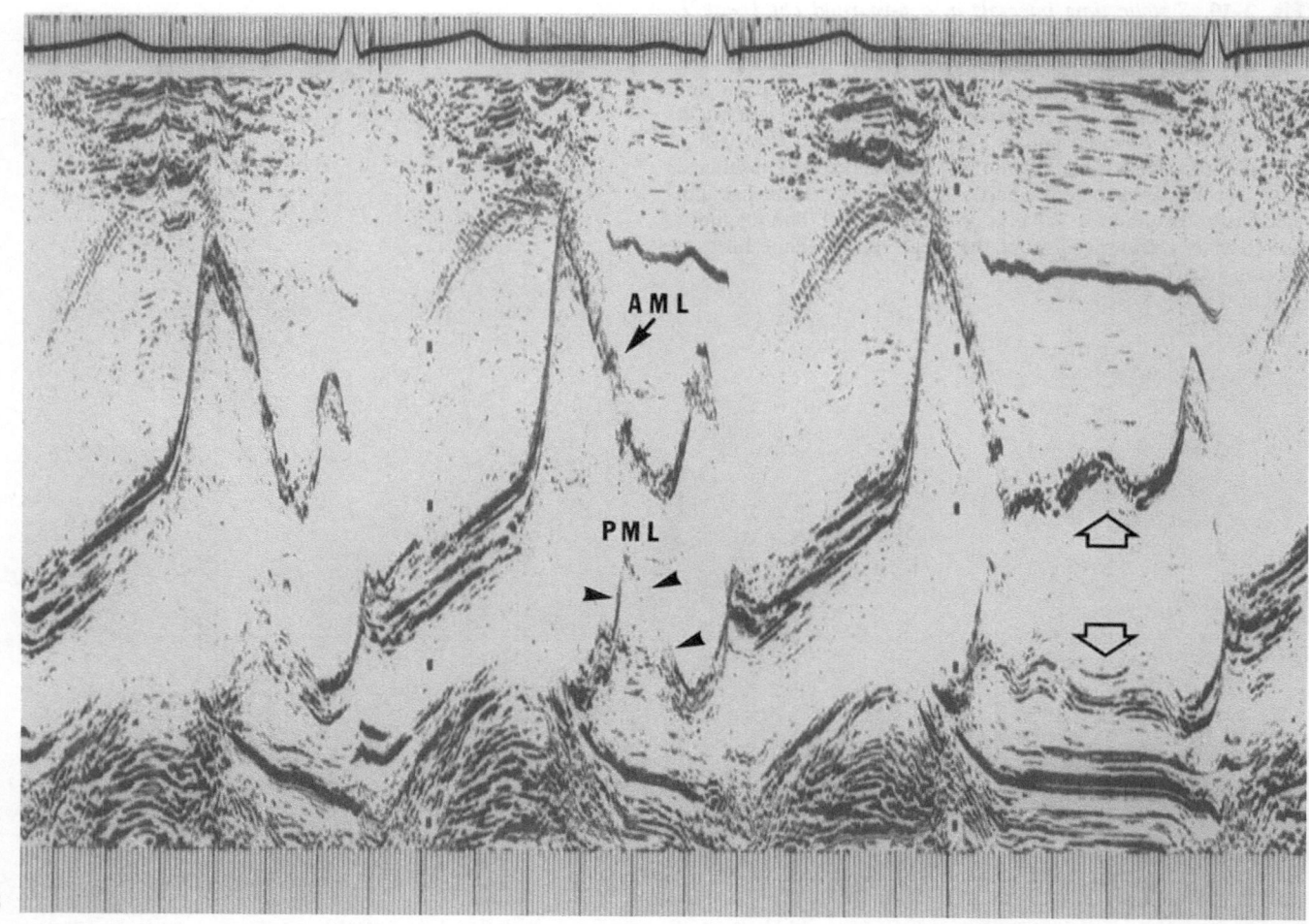

B

Fig. 2–11 (Cont.). B *Magnified view of mitral valve to show posterior mitral valve motion.* During the long diastolic period in the last beat the leaflets undulate (*open arrows*). *AML* = anterior mitral leaflet, *PML* = posterior mitral leaflet.

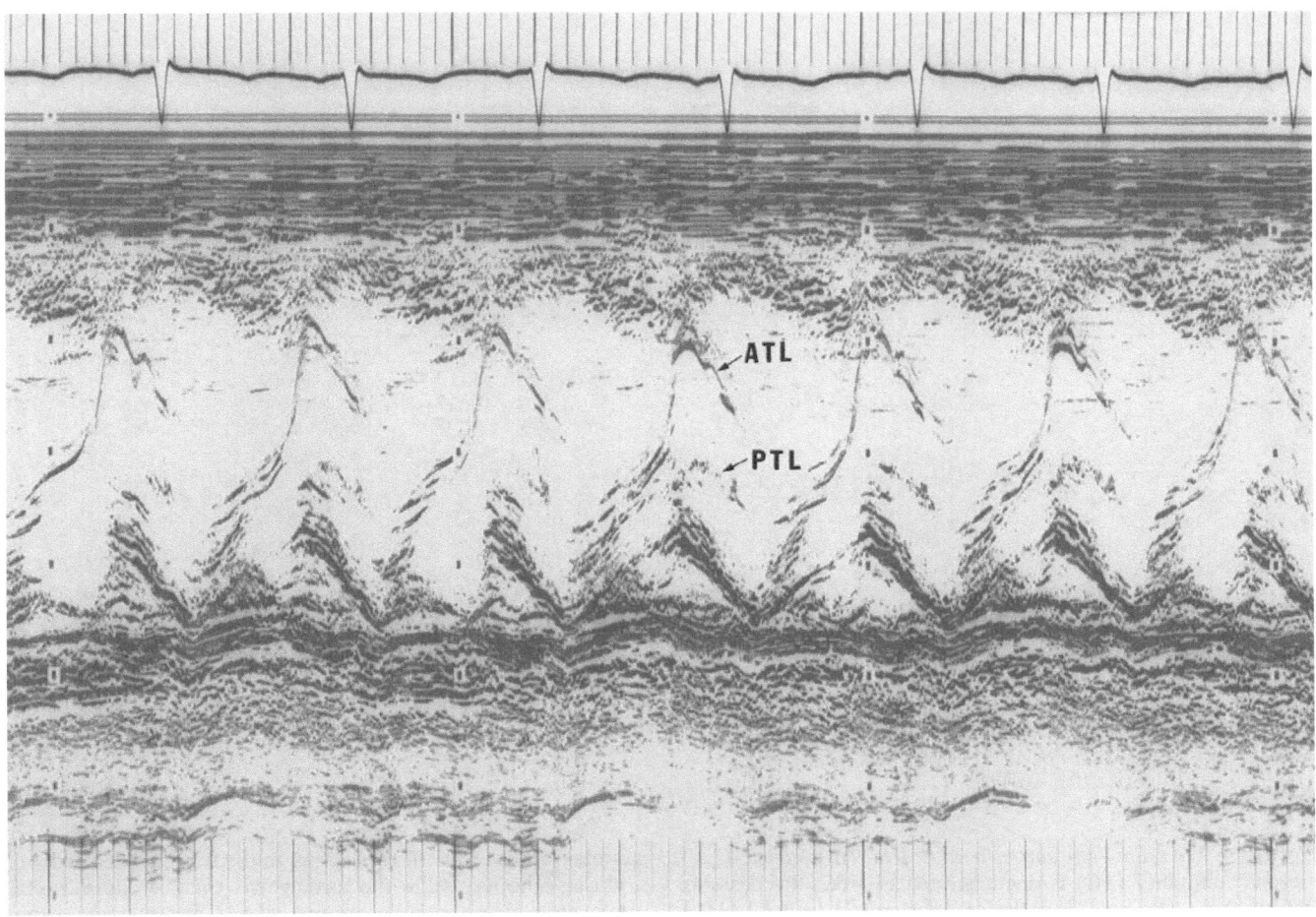

Fig. 2–12. *Normal tricuspid valve. M-mode echocardiogram as observed in an infant or young child.* This image is obtained by directing the transducer from the left third or fourth intercostal space far medially under the sternum. In adults and older children it is difficult or impossible to image this valve even though the patient rotates into the left lateral decubitus position. The pattern of motion of the tricuspid valve is similar to that of the mitral valve. The leaflets imaged are probably the anterior tricuspid leaflet (*ATL*) and the posterior tricuspid leaflet (*PTL*).

the M-mode trace from which quantitative LV images are obtained. The diameter is measured from the inner surface of the anterior wall of the RV to the front of the ventricular septum in mid diastole (Fig 2–6). If the RV free wall cannot be measured then the RV cavity size (RVD) is estimated by measuring from the back of the chest wall to the front of the ventricular septum. It is important to be consistent in positioning the patient for measurements of RV size. The right ventricular cavity appears larger when the subject is lying on the left side because the heart moves more to the left and the RV falls more into the path of the ultrasound beam.

Composite M-Mode Views (Arc Scans)

Evaluation of congenital heart defects by M-mode echocardiography requires careful notation indicating the position and angle of the transducer required to visualize each valve or chamber. The spatial relationships between the structures are determined by recording continuously while the transducer is swept through an arc (arc scan). Typical recordings include arc scans from the aortic valve through the mitral valve to the LV (Fig. 2–13), from the pulmonary valve through the RV outflow tract to the tricuspid valve (Fig. 2–14), and from mitral to tricuspid valves (Fig. 2–15). By using arc scans the presence or absence of aortic to mitral fibrous continuity or overriding of the aorta can be recognized (Fig. 2–16). The location as well as the type of aortic stenosis can also be identified.

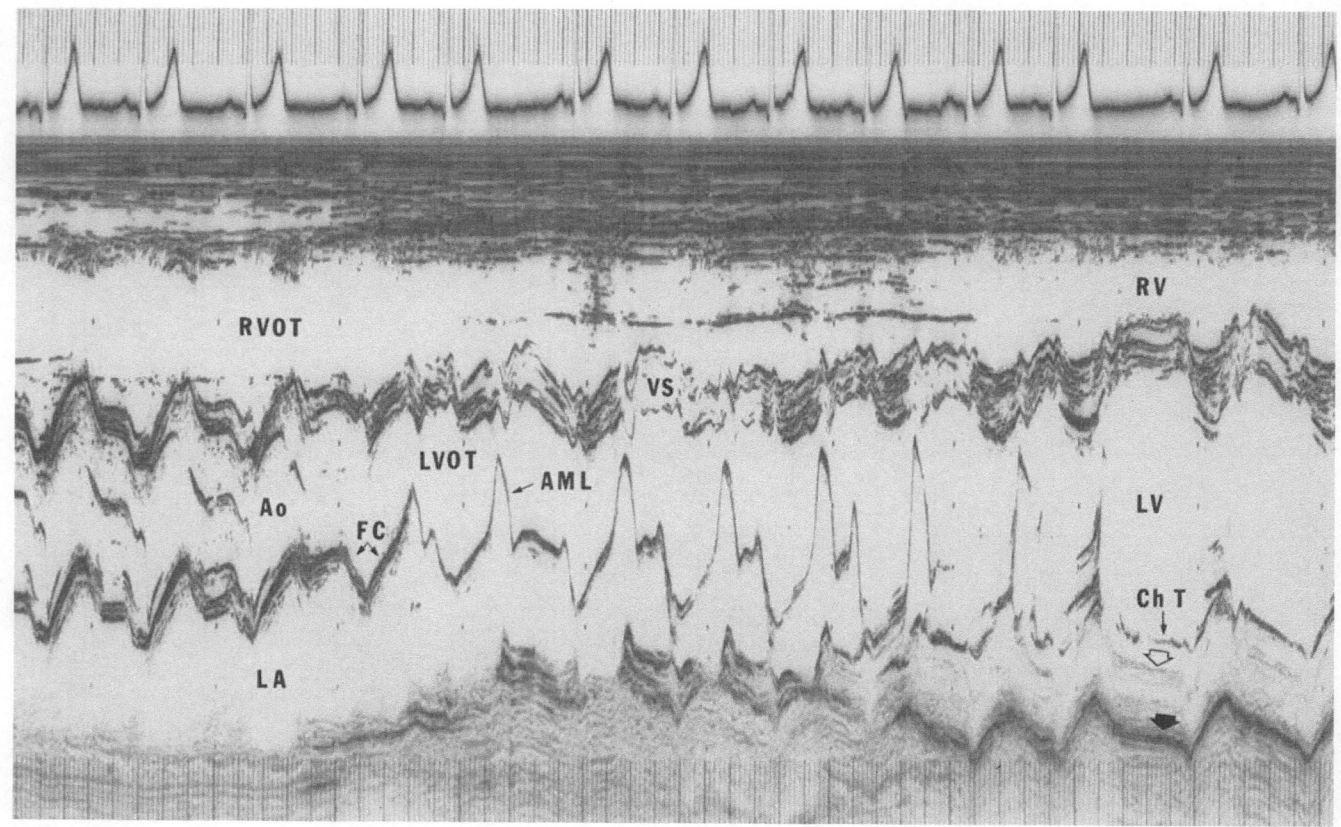

Fig. 2–13. *Arc scan from aortic root (Ao) to left ventricle (LV).* Fibrous continuity (*FC*) is demonstrated between the posterior wall of the aortic root and the anterior mitral leaflet (*AML*). The normal continuity between the anterior wall of the aortic root and the ventricular septum (*VS*) is also noted. The left ventricular outflow tract (*LVOT*) is measured during ventricular systole from the back of the septum to the front of the aorticomitral ring echo just below the aortic valve. *Ch T* = chordae tendineae, *open arrow* = endocardium, *closed arrow* = epicardium plus pericardium, *RV* = right ventricle, *RVOT* = right ventricular outflow tract, *LA* = left atrium.

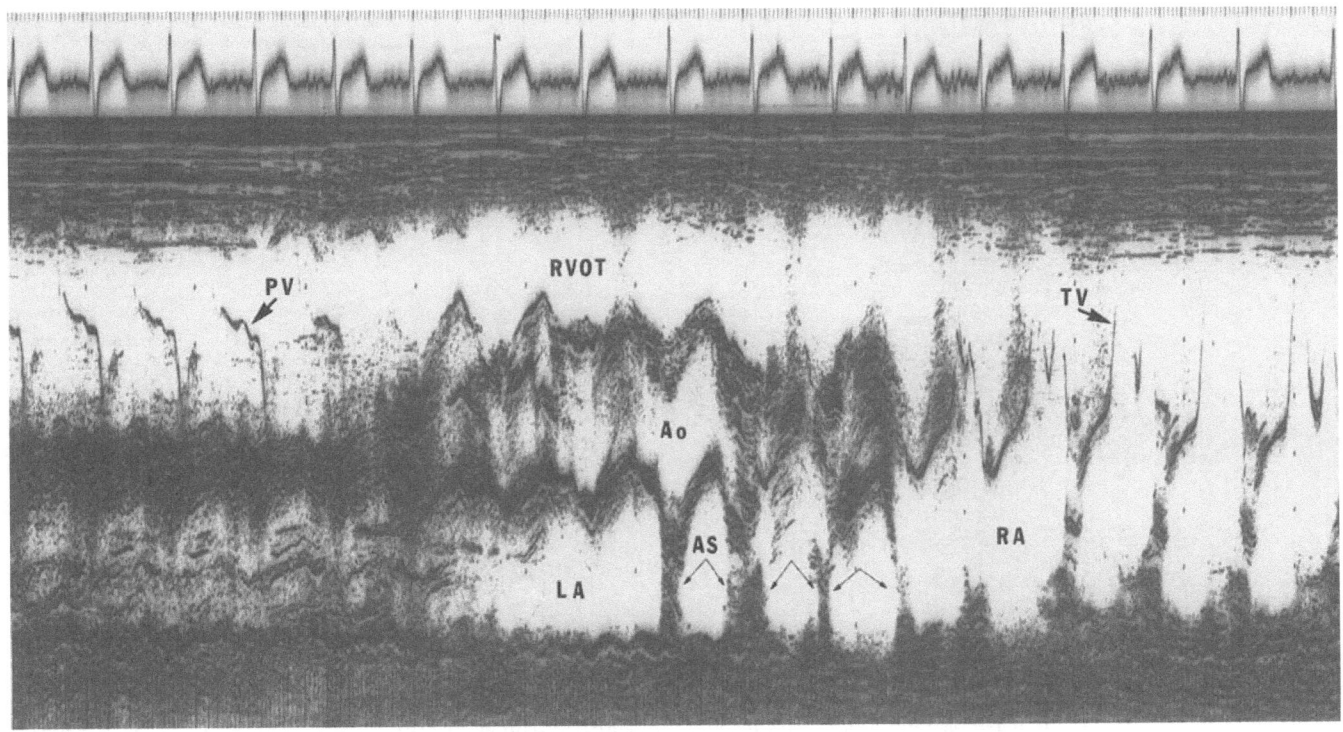

Fig. 2–14. *Arc scan from pulmonary valve (PV) to tricuspid valve (TV).* The operator has noted that the transducer has been swept from a leftward and superior direction in a rightward and inferior course, constituting the normal orientation of the right ventricular outflow tract (*RVOT*) as it wraps around the front of the aortic root (*Ao*). In back of the heart the scan traverses the left atrium (*LA*), the atrial septum (*AS*) and the right atrium (*RA*). (see Fig. 2–4).

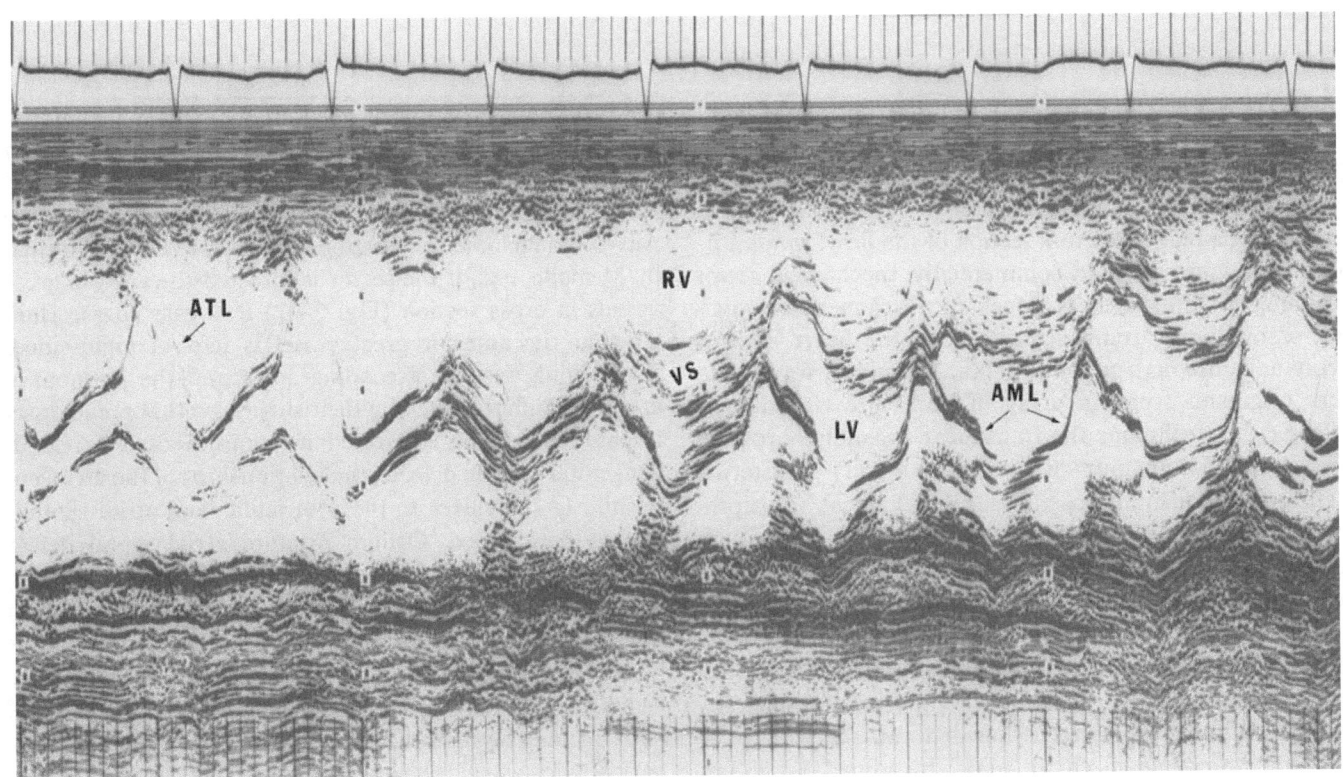

Fig. 2–15. *M-mode arc scan from the tricuspid valve to the mitral valve in a 4-year-old-boy.* The transducer was angled through an arc from a rightward direction to a leftward direction. The tricuspid valve is anterior to the mitral valve. The ventricular septum (*VS*) separates the two valves. *ATL* = anterior tricuspid leaflet; *AML* = anterior mitral leaflet; *RV* = right ventricle; *LV* = left ventricle.

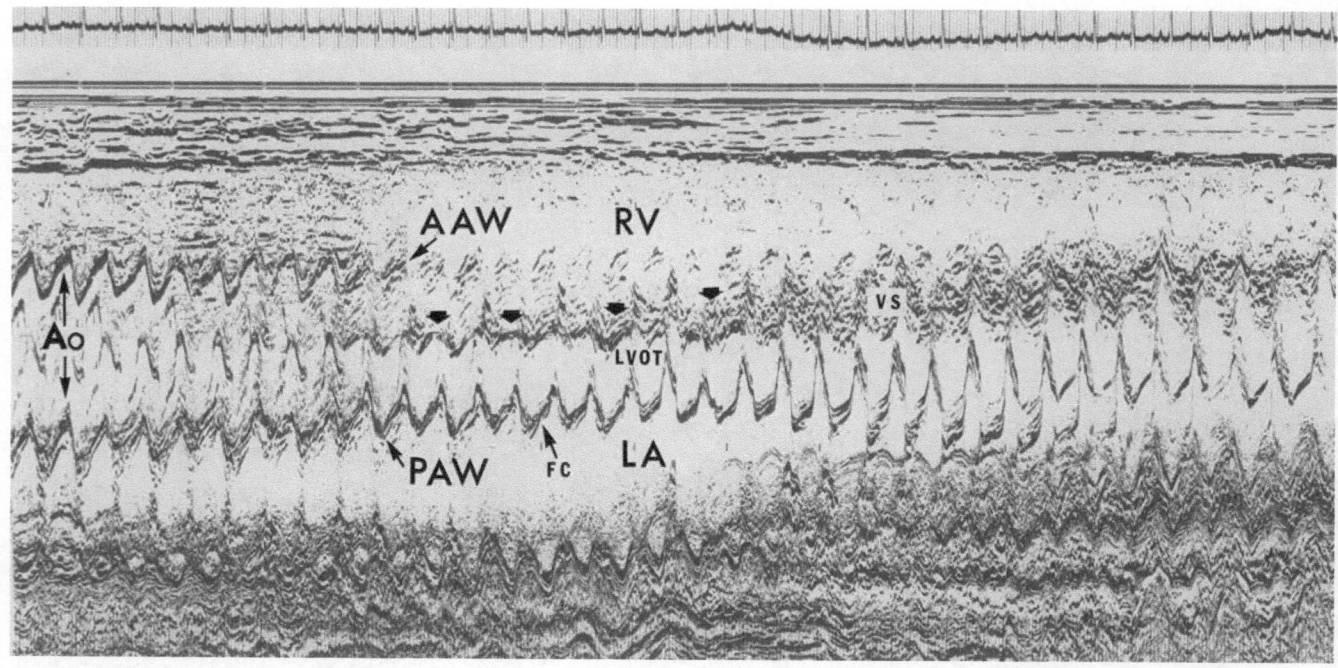

Fig. 2–16. *Arc scan from the aortic root (Ao) across the left ventricular outflow tract (LVOT) in a 1-month-old infant with tetralogy of Fallot.* The aorta overrides the ventricular septum. Overriding of the aorta is also present in instances of truncus arteriosus. If the pulmonary valve is visualized tetralogy of Fallot is likely; however, inability to image the pulmonary valve does not exclude tetralogy of Fallot. It is therefore difficult to arrive at a definite diagnosis of truncus arteriosus by M-mode scans. *AAW* = anterior aortic wall; *PAW* = posterior aortic wall; *closed arrows* and *VS* = ventricular septum; *FC* = mitral-aortic fibrous continuity, *LA* = left atrium.

Real-Time Two-Dimensional Imaging of the Heart

Real-time cardiac images consist of rapid arc scans of the heart, built up in rapid succession (30 frames/sec) so as to produce a real-time cross section of the heart in motion. Two techniques are used commercially: mechanical sector scanning and phased array. Mechanical scanners use rotating or oscillating transducers to scan the heart. Phased array units use high-speed switching to guide a wave front that originates from an array of miniature transducers. Using either technique the transducer assembly is rotated and angled within four "echo windows": (1) parasternal (left fourth to fifth intercostal space), (2) apical, (3) suprasternal notch, and (4) subxiphoid. Figures 2–17 through 2–30 are representative diagrams and cross sections of the normal heart as shown by 2–DE.

Indications for 2-DE are similar to those for M-mode. In many instances, both methods are necessary. The advantages of 2-DE over M-mode are that interrelationships between structures are better delineated and that shapes of structures are recognized in 2-DE. In adults, 2-DE has been superior to M-mode in recognizing intracardiac masses that are not pedunculated, including sessile tumors, sessile vegetations, and apical thrombi (Fig. 2–31). In ischemic heart disease, 2-DE is useful in recognizing asynergy, although it is not as accurate as nuclear techniques in quantitating abnormalities of wall motion or ejection fraction.

In congenital defects the relationships between the valves and chambers are better demonstrated by 2-DE than by M-mode, e.g., if the sector is directed toward the great vessels in cross section (Fig. 2–32) it is easy to ascertain whether the anterior great vessel is left- or right-sided. In the long axis the ascending aorta and the pulmonary artery are differentiated by their shapes, so that great vessel orientation can be confirmed in complex cases. Also in congenital cardiac defects, the relationships of the atrioventricular (A-V) valves to the ventricular and atrial septum can be determined. Ostium primum atrial septal defect can be differentiated from A-V communis, and straddling A-V valve can be recognized. Coarctation of the aorta is not diagnosed by M-mode but can be detected by 2-DE from the suprasternal notch. Total anomalous pulmonary venous return may be suspected on M-mode, but specific patterns may be recognized on 2-DE. The origins of coronary arteries can also be imaged by 2-DE in normal individuals, in instances of anomalous left coronary artery and in coronary artery aneurysm secondary to Kawasaki disease.

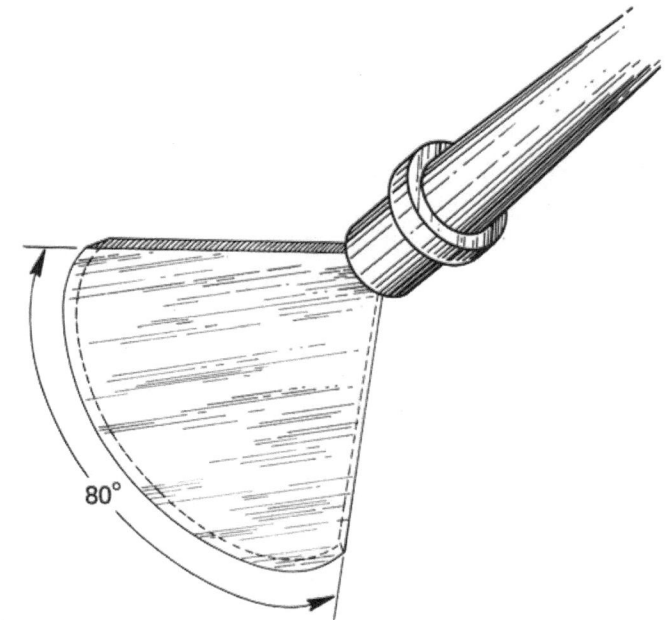

A

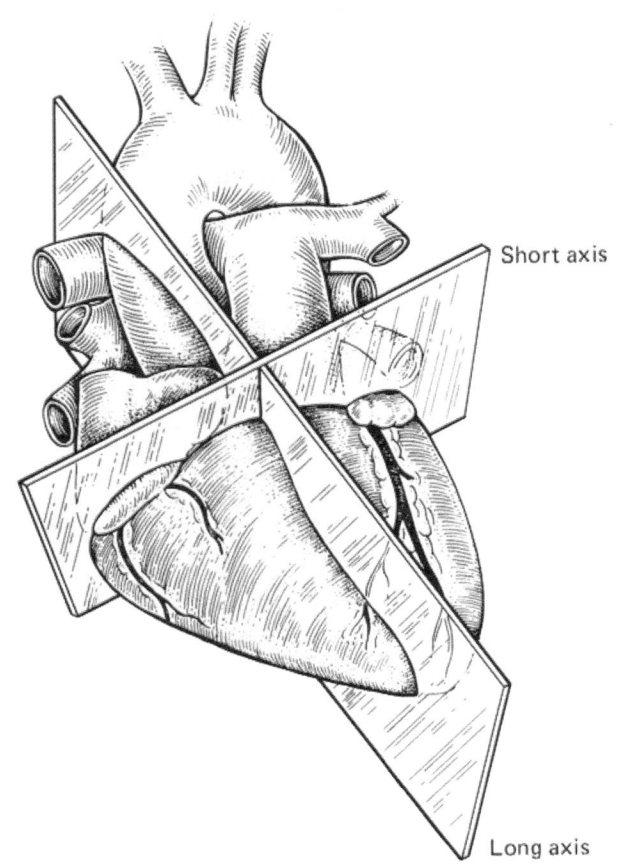

Short axis

Long axis   B

Fig. 2–17. *Diagrams of the heart with tomographic sections frequently used in two-dimensional echocardiography.* **A** is a diagram of a transducer for two dimensional scanning. Either a mechanical sector scanner or an electronic phased array may be used. The device scans repeatedly through an arc to produce repetitive pictures of a section of the heart. The plane of the section is determined by the position of the transducer with respect to the heart. **B** shows two planes commonly used for echocardiographic examination, a long axis view and a short axis view. **C** shows the long axis of the left ventricle (Fig. 2–18). With slight angulation, cuts through the right ventricle are also possible (Figs. 2–21, 2–22). (*Continued on next page.*)

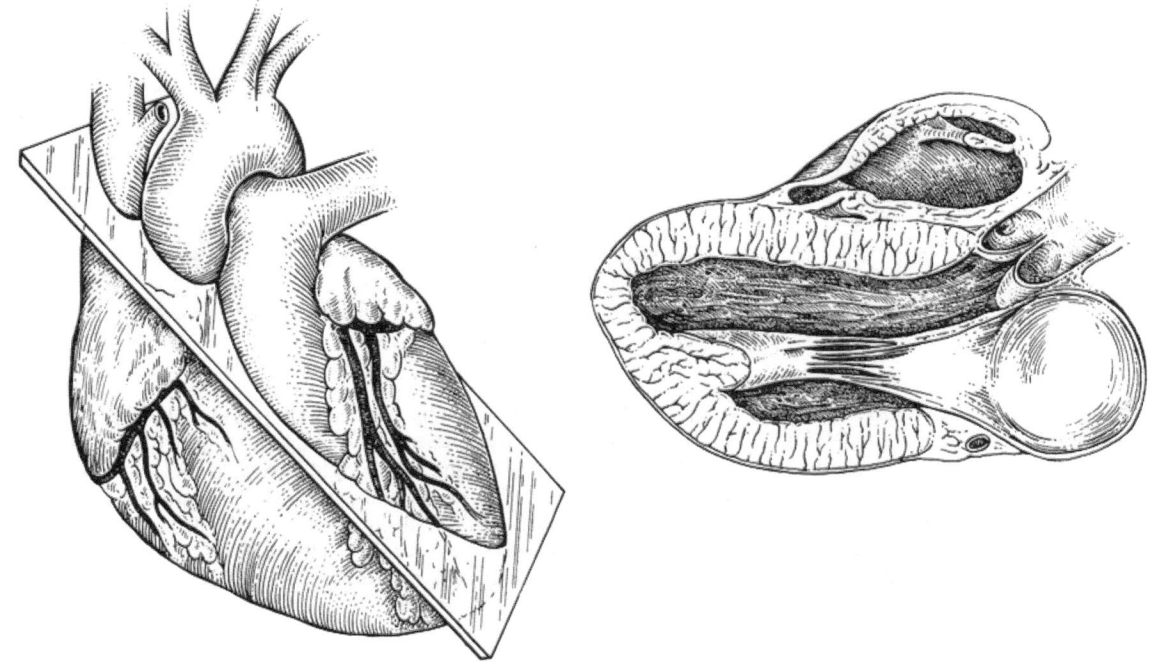

C

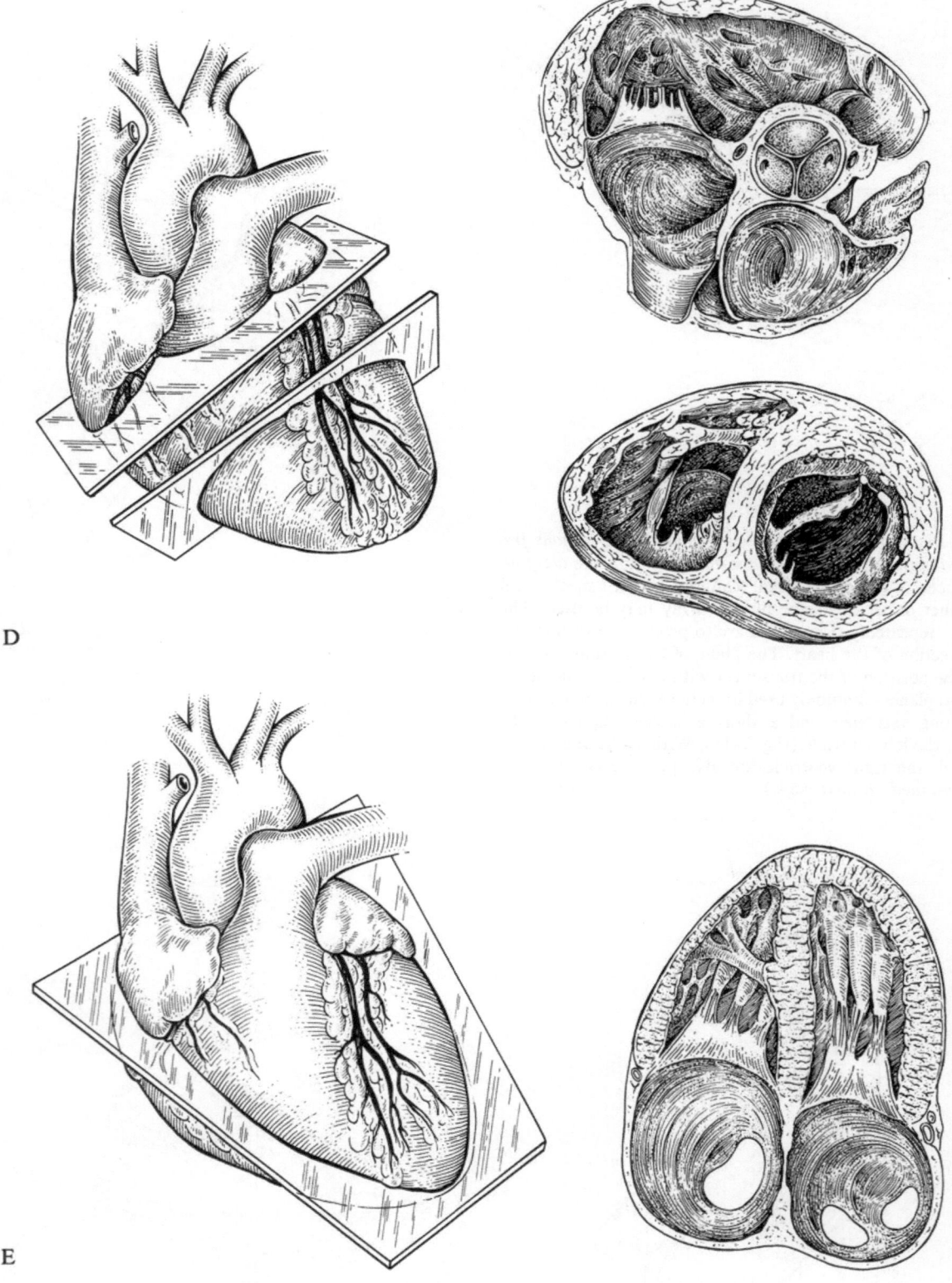

D

E

Fig. 2–17 (*Cont.*). **D** indicates short axis views at the level of the aortic valve and left ventricular cavity (Fig. 2–20). By angling the transducer, cuts across any level of the left ventricle can be obtained (see also Fig. 2–19). **E** indicates a four-chamber view, which can be approximated from the apex (Fig. 2–25) or from the subxiphoid position (Fig. 2–28). By rotating the transducer 90° in the apical position, an apical two-chamber or "RAO-equiv-alent" view is obtained (Fig. 2–26). In the subxiphoid position the transducer can be angled anteriorly from the four-chamber view to image the right ventricle and outflow tract in either a coronal or sagittal plane. Other angulations in the subxiphoid position will bring into view the left ventricular outflow tract and the aortic arch, or alternatively, the right atrium and superior vena cava (see also Figs. 2–36B, 2–39D).

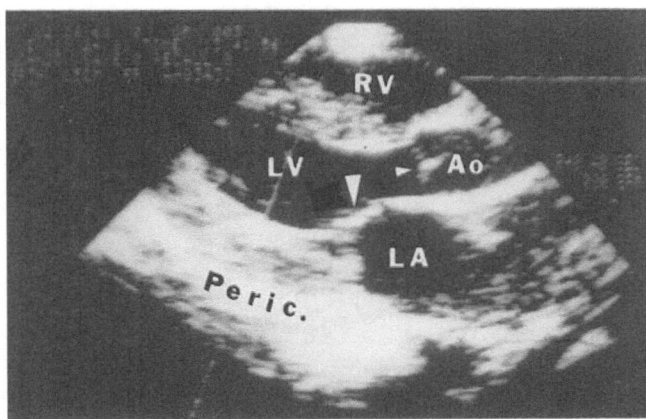

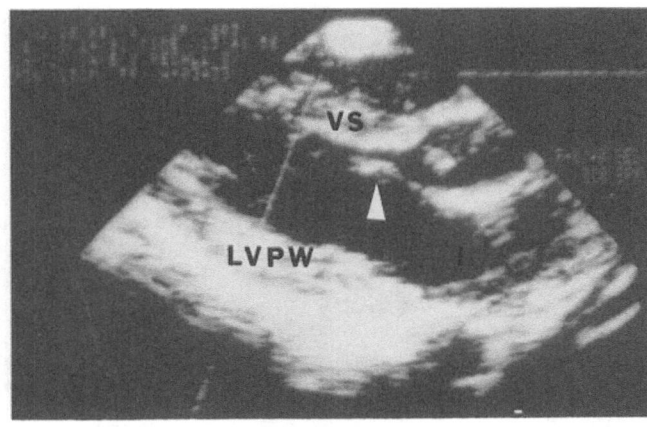

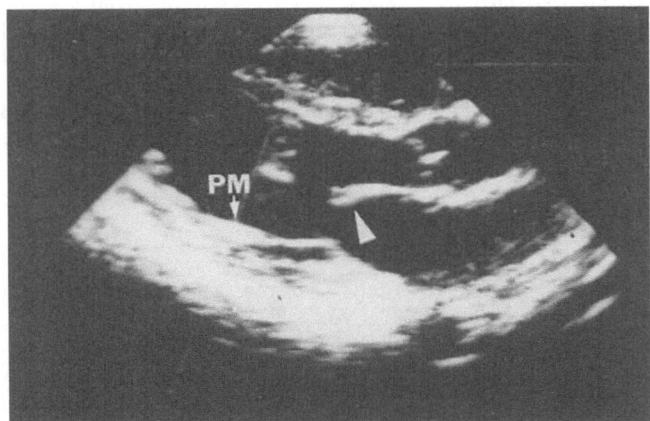

Fig. 2–18, A–C. *Long axis view, left ventricle.* **A** end systole; **B** early diastole; **C** late diastole. In **A** the left ventricle (*LV*), right ventricle (*RV*), aortic root (*Ao*), left atrium (*LA*) and pericardium (*peric*) are identified. *The small arrowhead* points to the aortic valve and the *large arrowhead* identifies the mitral valve. In **B** the mitral valve is widely open during the rapid filling phase (the E point on M-mode). The *large arrowhead* points to the tip of the anterior mitral leaflet. The ventricular septum (*VS*) and the left ventricular posterior wall (*LVPW*) are labeled. In **C** the left ventricle is increased in size. The mitral valve is partially open. The *large arrowhead* indicates the tip of the anterior mitral leaflet. The posterior mitral leaflet is shorter than the anterior leaflet and is attached by way of chordae tendineae to the posterior papillary muscle (*PM*).

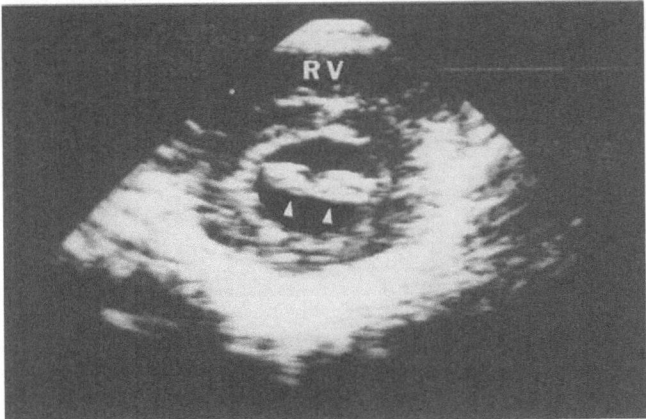

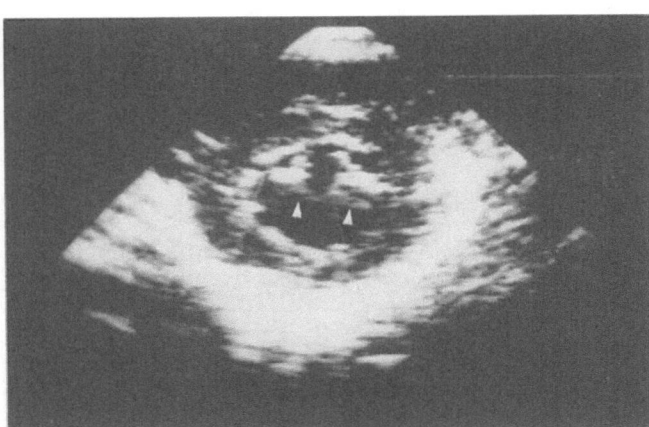

Fig. 2–19, A–C. *Short axis view of the left ventricle at the level of the mitral valve.* **A** late systole; **B** early diastole; **C** late diastole. In this section the left ventricle is outlined as a circular structure. The dense inner ring represents the endocardium, and the relatively lucent ring around it is the myocardium. In **A** the closed mitral valve (*arrowheads*) is visualized as a double horizontal line within the left ventricle. The right ventricle (*RV*) is anteriorly situated. In **B** the mitral valve is widely open (rapid filling phase). The *arrowheads* point to the tip of the anterior mitral leaflet (the posterior mitral leaflet is not identified). In **C** the left ventricle is larger (end diastole), and the mitral valve is partially open. These images were obtained during phases of the cardiac cycle similar to those in Fig. 2–18.

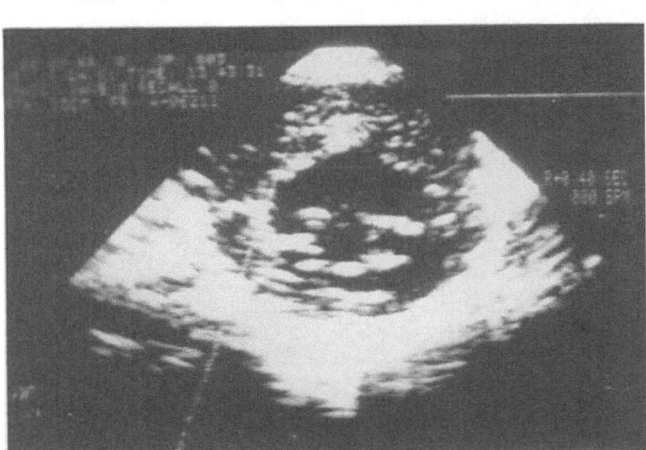

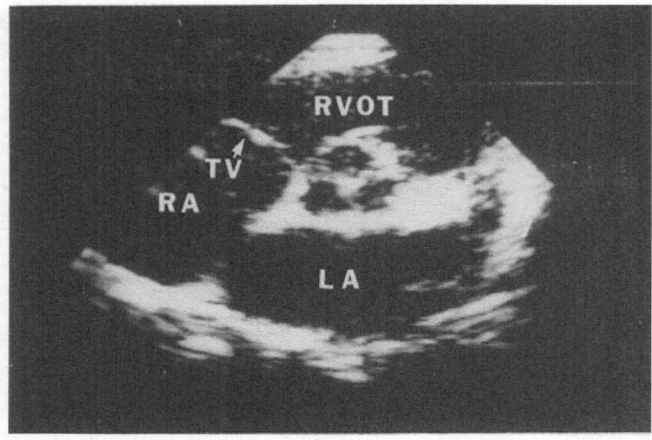
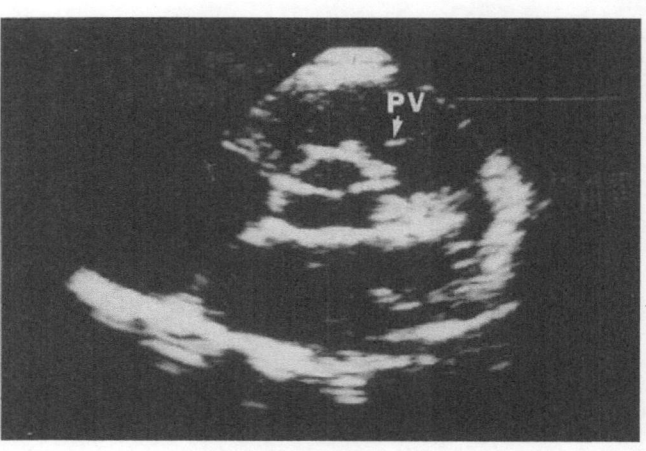

A

B

Fig. 2–20. *Parasternal short axis view at the level of the aortic valve.* The aortic valve is represented by a circular structure. The three commissures are demonstrated in *A* (the "Mercedes Benz sign"). The tricuspid valve (*TV*, frame **A**) is to the right of the aortic valve, while the pulmonary valve (*PV*, frame **B**) is anterior and to the left of the aortic valve. The right ventricular outflow tract (*RVOT*) wraps around the front of the aortic root. The right atrium (*RA*) and left atrium (*LA*) are defined posteriorly and are separated by a few echoes representing atrial septum. (Note: In this patient the left atrium is enlarged.) The atrial septum is poorly identified in this view because it is nearly parallel to the echo beam and echoes are not reflected back. See Figs. 2–4 and 2–17D, which also demonstrate the normal relationship of the aortic root, right ventricular outflow tract and pulmonary valve.

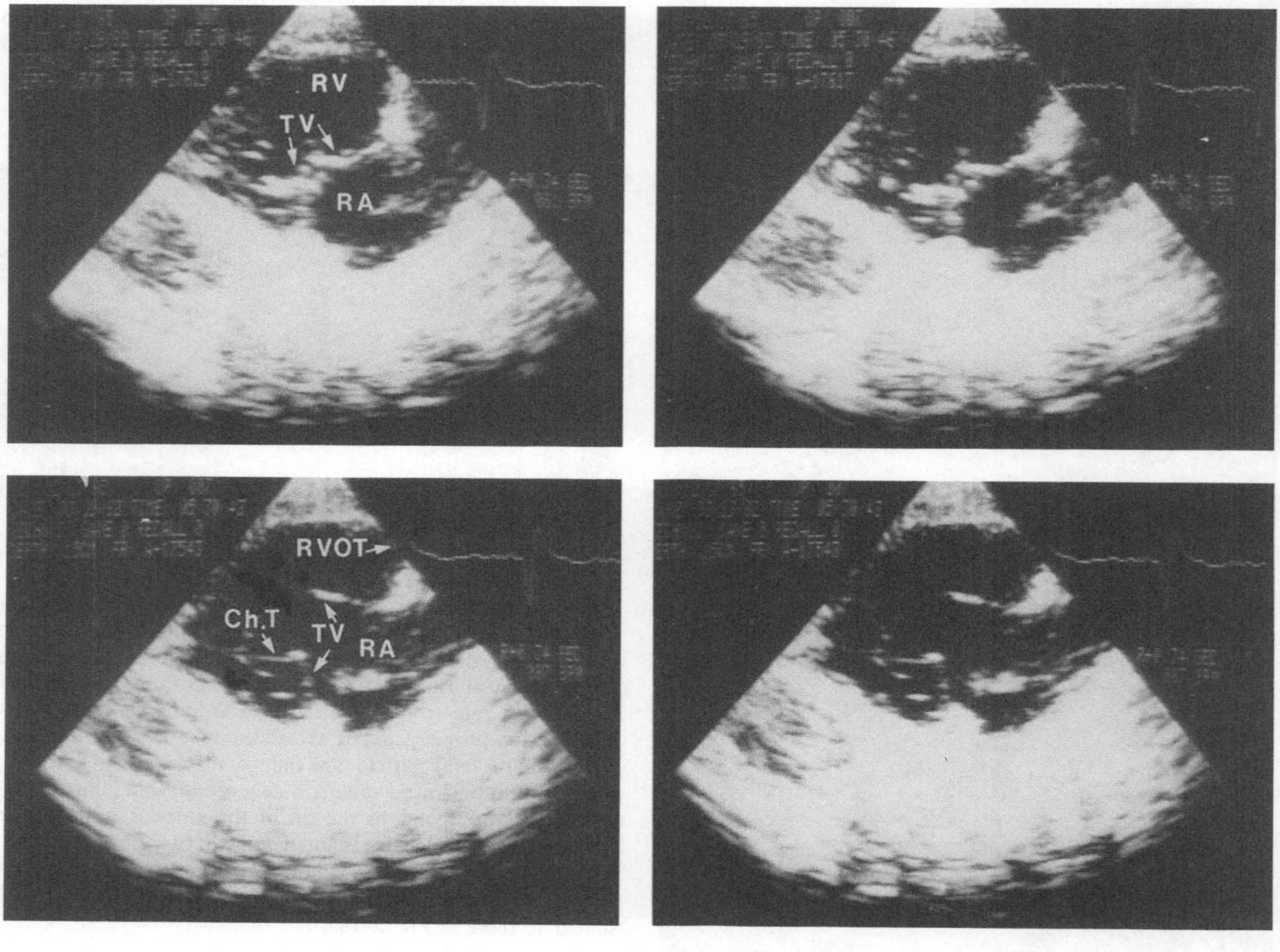

A

B

C

D

Fig. 2–21, A–D. *Parasternal long axis view of RV inflow tract.* **A** and **B** systole; **C** and **D** diastole. This image is obtained by angling the transducer steeply to the right from the long axis view of the left ventricle (see Fig. 2–18). The tricuspid valve (*TV*) is well delineated as is the right ventricular body (*RV*). The right ventricular outflow tract (*RVOT*) extends toward the patient's left (cephalad). *Ch.T* = chordae tendineae. *RA* = right atrium.

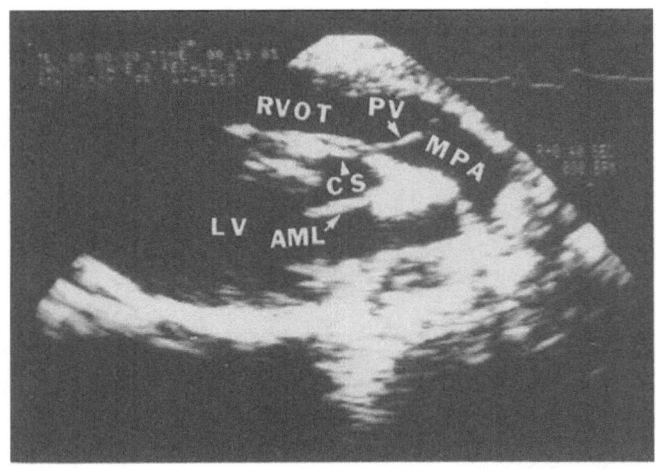

A

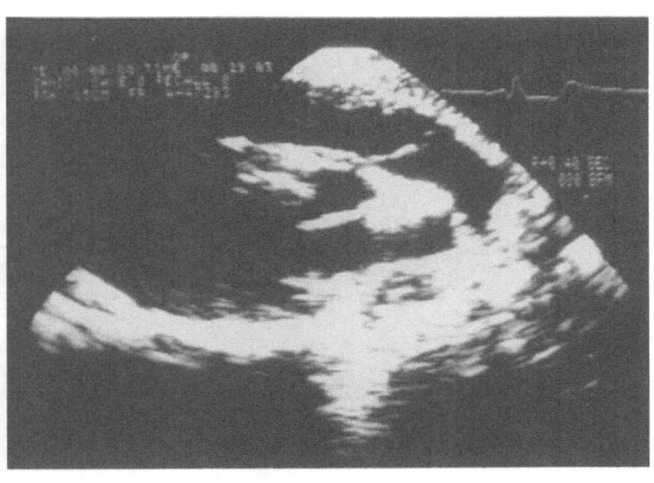

B

Fig. 2–22, A and B. *Parasternal long axis view of the right ventricular outflow tract (RVOT).* **A** with labels; **B** without labels. This image is obtained by rotating the transducer clockwise from the long axis view of the left ventricle illustrated in Fig. 2–18.

The conus septum (*CS*) is identified here with a corner of the left ventricular cavity (*LV*) and the anterior mitral leaflet (*AML*). *PV* = pulmonary valve; *MPA* = main pulmonary artery.

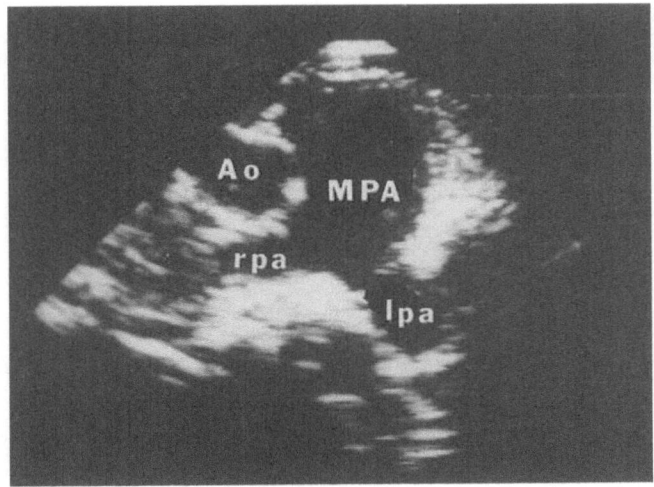

A

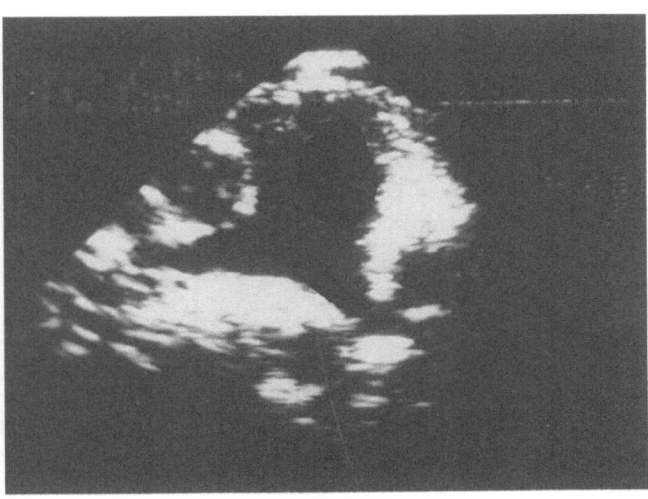

B

Fig. 2–23, A and B. *Parasternal view of the main pulmonary artery (MPA).* **A** with labels; **B** without labels. The origins of the right pulmonary artery (*rpa*) and left pulmonary artery (*lpa*)

are defined. This view is obtained by rotating the transducer clockwise and angling it toward the left from the short axis view of the aortic root (see Fig. 2–20). *Ao* = aorta.

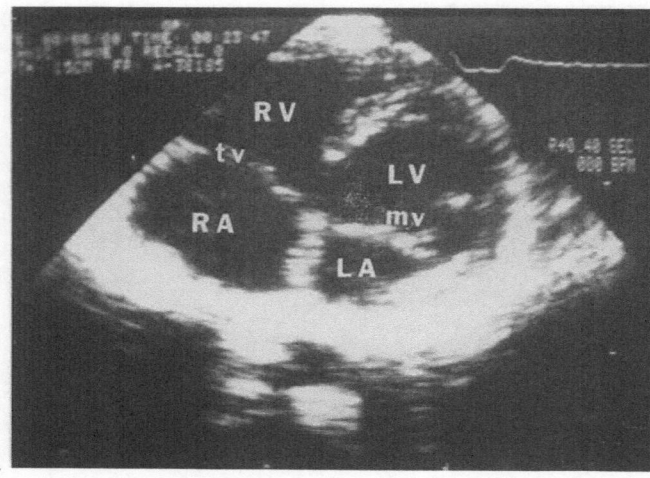
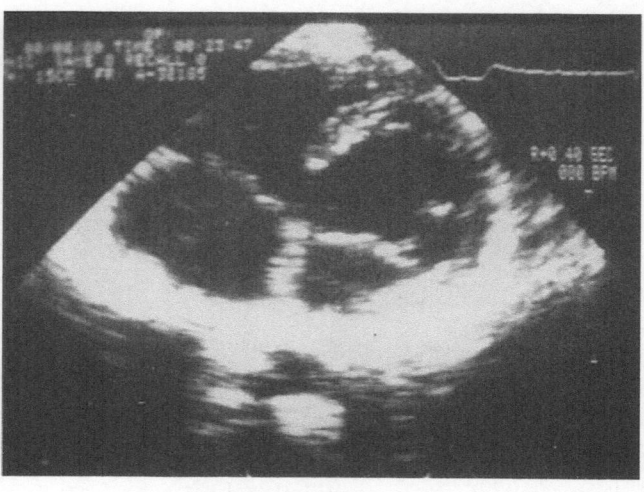

A   B

Fig. 2–24, A and B. *Parasternal oblique four-chamber view.* **A** with labels; **B** without labels. This view is obtained by rotating the transducer about 90° in a clockwise direction from the long axis view of left ventricle without changing the angle. The mitral valve (*mv*) and left ventricular cavity (*LV*) remain in view. Rotation of the transducer brings the tricuspid valve (*tv*) and the right ventricular cavity (*RV*) into view. The tricuspid valve inserts on the ventricular septum slightly distal to the point at which the mitral valve attaches. The atrial septum is clearly identified between the right atrium (*RA*) and left atrium (*LA*). Note dropout in the ventricular septum near the A-V valves—a normal phenomenon that does not necessarily indicate ventricular septal defect.

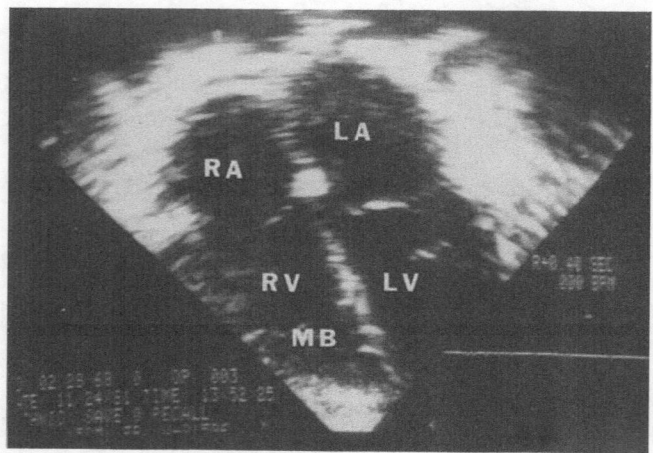
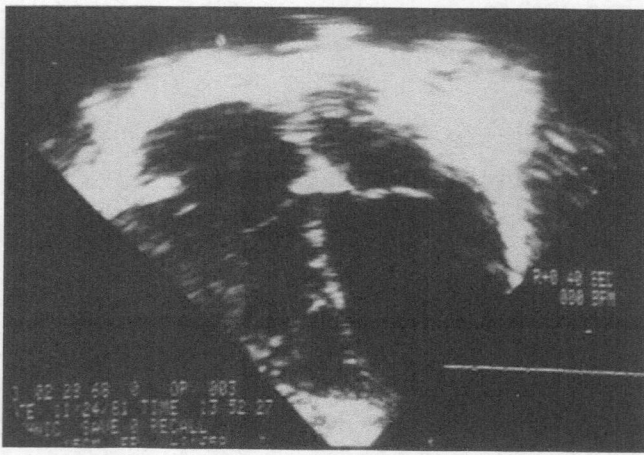

A   B

Fig. 2–25, A and B. *Apex four-chamber view.* **A** with labels; **B** without labels. The image is shown as suggested by the American Society of Echocardiography Committee on Nomenclature and Standards. The apex of the heart is at the bottom of the image. The right ventricle (*RV*) is on the right as if the examinee were facing the examiner. (This image may also be presented with the apex at the top of the screen.) The subject is reclining steeply on the left side with the transducer placed on the apical impulse and directed toward the individual's right shoulder. The transducer is then rotated so that the sector is perpendicular to the ventricular septum, which will then appear as a nearly vertical density in the middle of the screen. The RV is identified by the moderator band (*MB*). The motion of the A-V valves is similar to the motion of the wings of a bird in flight. This view is especially useful for examining the A-V valves in individuals suspected of having Ebstein anomaly or endocardial cushion defects. It is also useful for echo cardiographic contrast studies because all four chambers are in view simultaneously. *RA* = right atrium; *LA* = left atrium; *LV* = left ventricle.

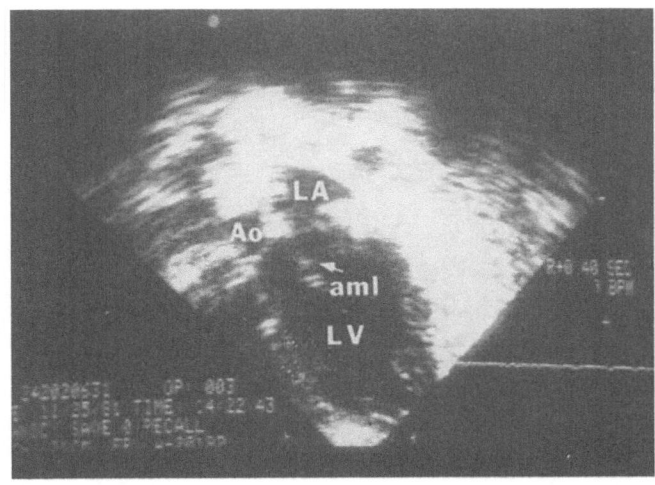

A

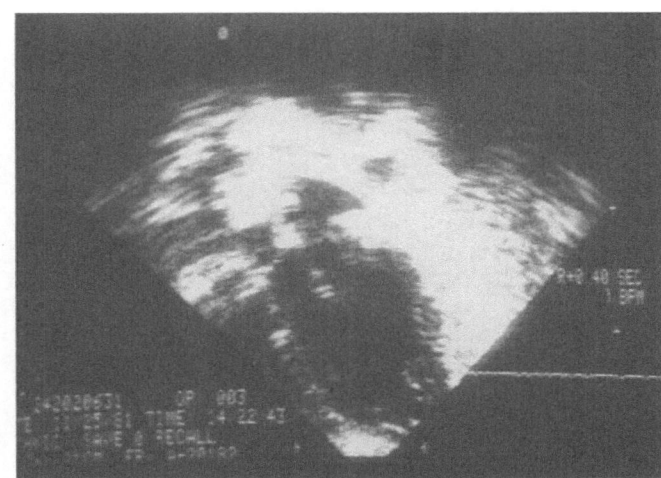

B

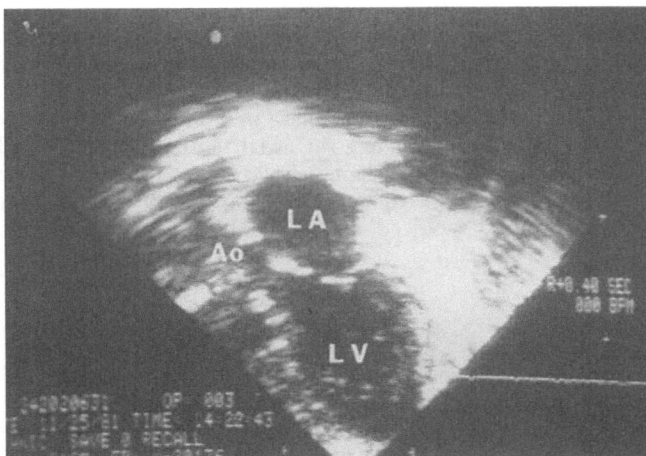

C

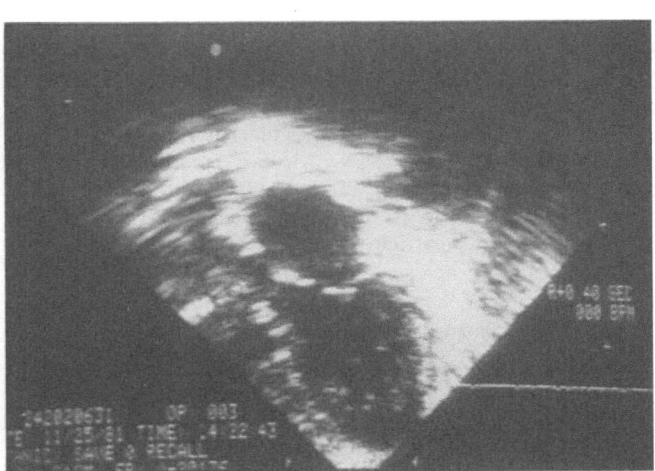

D

Fig. 2–26, A–D. *Apex two-chamber view.* **A** and **B** diastole; **C** and **D** systole. The transducer is rotated 90° from the position used to obtain Fig. 2–25. This image may also be presented with the apex at the top of the screen. In **A** and **B** the mitral valve is open. *aml* = anterior mitral leaflet. In **C** and **D** the mitral valve is closed. The endocardium can be identified, although faintly. With some interpolation a LV volume determination can be obtained from this view using geometrical analysis similar to that used for LV volume by angiography. This view may also be used to assess wall motion as the segments of the septum and the wall correspond to those defined by the RAO view of a left ventriculogram. *Ao* = ascending aorta; *LA* = left atrium. Note: In order for this image to correspond with an RAO view (RAO equivalent view) it should be reversed right to left.

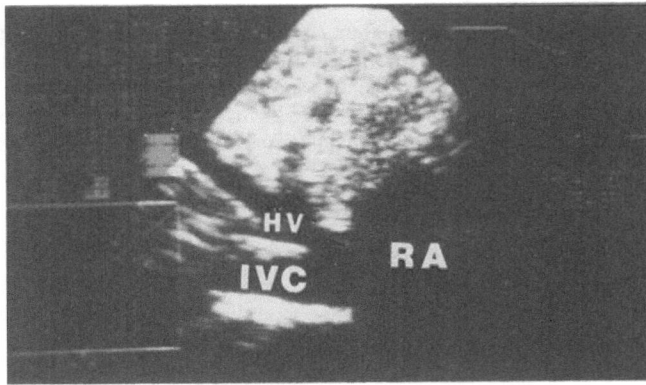

A

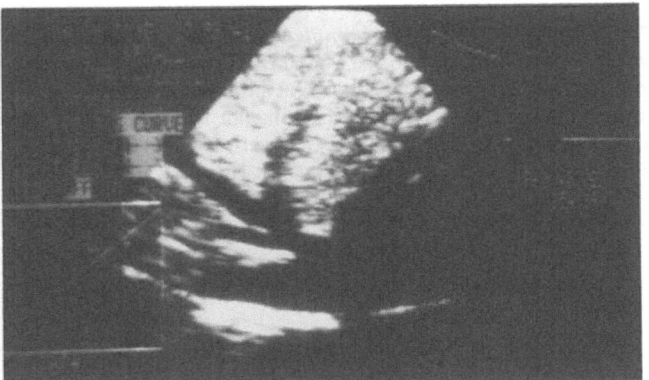

B

Fig. 2–27, A and B. *Subxiphoid view of inferior vena cava.* **A** with labels; **B** without labels. The liver parenchyma is closest to the transducer. The hepatic veins (*HV*) join the inferior vena cava (*IVC*) as it enters the right atrium (*RA*). This image helps to identify the right atrium in the subxiphoid four-chamber view (Fig. 2–28).

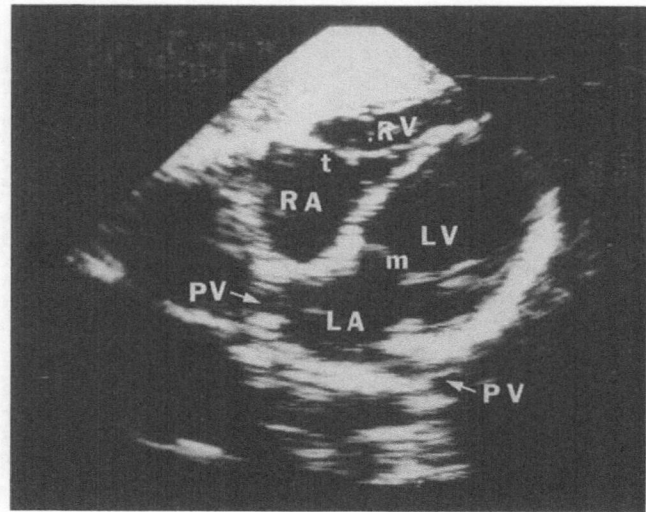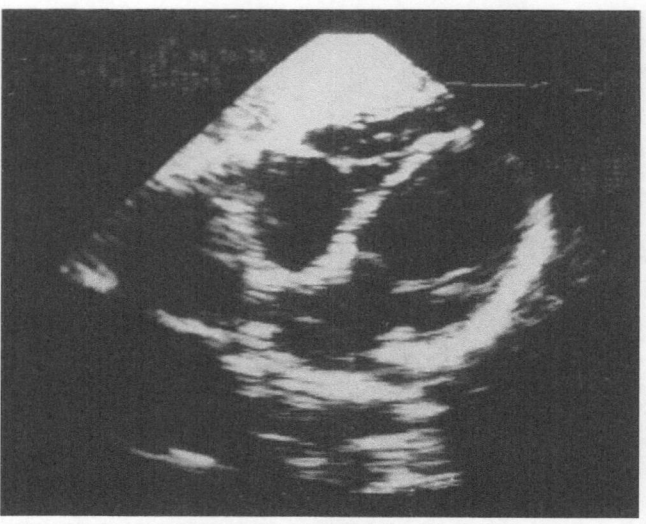

A   B

Fig. 2–28, A and B. *Subxiphoid four-chamber view.* **A** with labels; **B** without labels. The subject is supine. The image is obtained by directing the transducer from the subxiphoid window toward the subject's left shoulder. The transducer is rotated so that the sector is perpendicular to the ventricular septum. This image is presented so that the origin of the sector is at the top of the screen. The chamber closest to the transducer is the right ventricle (RV), while the left ventricle (LV) is farther from the transducer and therefore appears lower on the screen. The transducer is angled posteriorly so that the atria and pulmonary veins are demonstrated. The ventricular septum and the atrial septum are perpendicular to the echo beam and reflect well. This view is therefore especially useful in evaluating the atrial septum in atrial septal defects and endocardial cushion defects, among other congenital anomalies. RA = right atrium; LA = left atrium; PV = pulmonary vein; m = mitral valve; t = tricuspid valve.

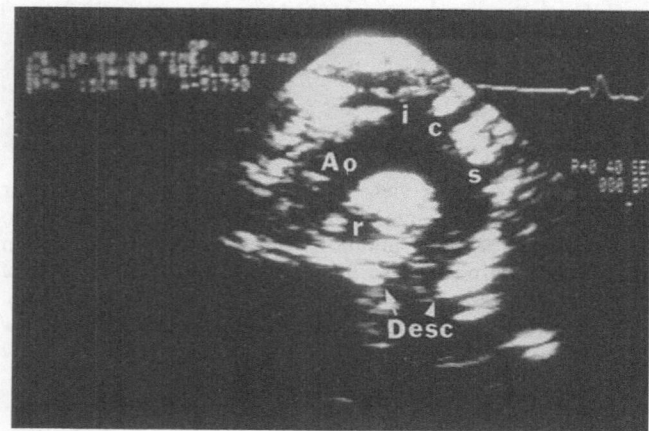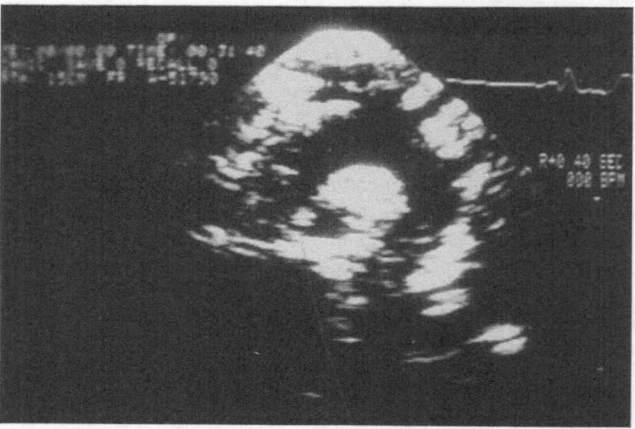

A   B

Fig. 2–29, A and B. *Suprasternal notch view of aortic arch.* **A** with labels; **B** without labels. The aortic arch (Ao) is visualized together with its branches—the right innominate artery (i), left common carotid artery (c), left subclavian artery (s). The right pulmonary artery (r) is beneath the aortic arch. The size of the right pulmonary artery is maximized as the transducer is angled toward the left. Three to four centimeters of descending aorta (*Desc*) are visualized. This view of the aorta identifies coarctation of the aorta, dilatation of the ascending aorta and dissection of the aorta. A right aortic arch is recognized if the transducer is angled toward the right and posteriorly instead of toward the left and posteriorly.

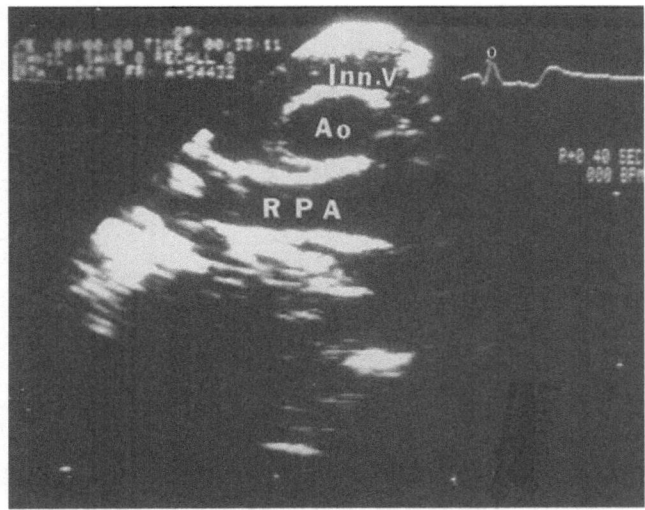

A

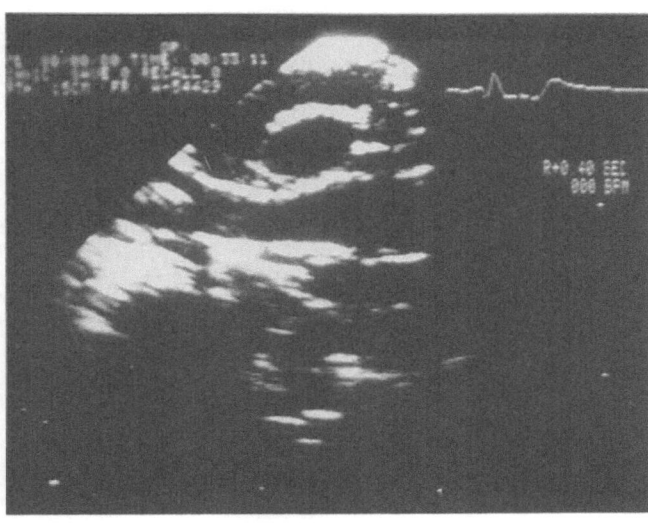

B

Fig. 2–30, A and B. *Suprasternal notch view of the aorta and right pulmonary artery.* **A** with labels; **B** without labels. The transducer is directed caudally from the suprasternal notch with the sector rotated so that it cuts a transverse section. In this examinee the innominate vein (*Inn.V*) is the structure closest to the transducer, while the aortic arch (*Ao*) presents as a circle. The right pulmonary artery (*RPA*) passes from left to right under the arch. This view together with that obtained in Fig. 2–29, aids in estimating the size of the right pulmonary artery in cyanotic patients. Angulation toward the right in this location brings into view the superior vena cava.

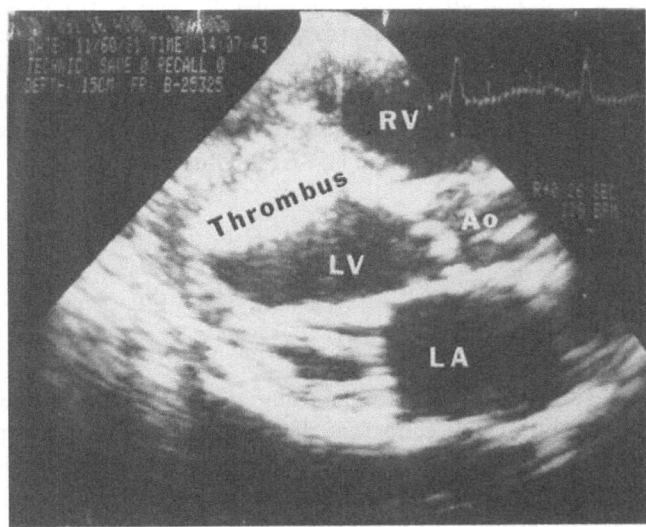

A

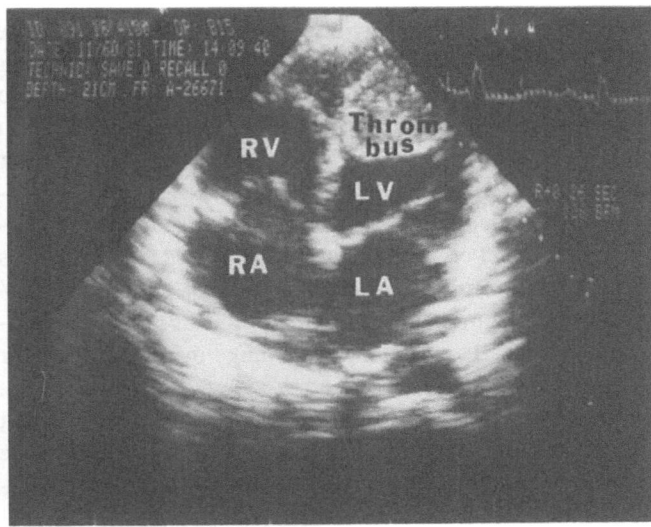

B

Fig. 2–31, A and B. *Apical thrombus.* **A** parasternal long axis view of left ventricle (*LV*); **B** apex four-chamber view (inverted as compared to Fig. 2–25). Akinesis of the anteroapical wall is present, associated with an apical thrombus, which is probably semiliquid. The luminal wall of the thrombus undulates as the heart moves. This thrombus was poorly visualized on M-mode scanning. *RV* = right ventricle; *RA* = right atrium; *Ao* = aorta; *LA* = left atrium. (Courtesy of Maxine Rosoff, M.D.).

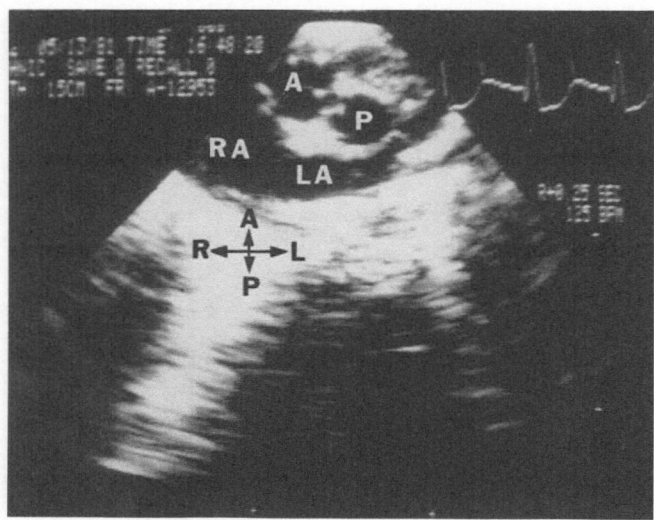

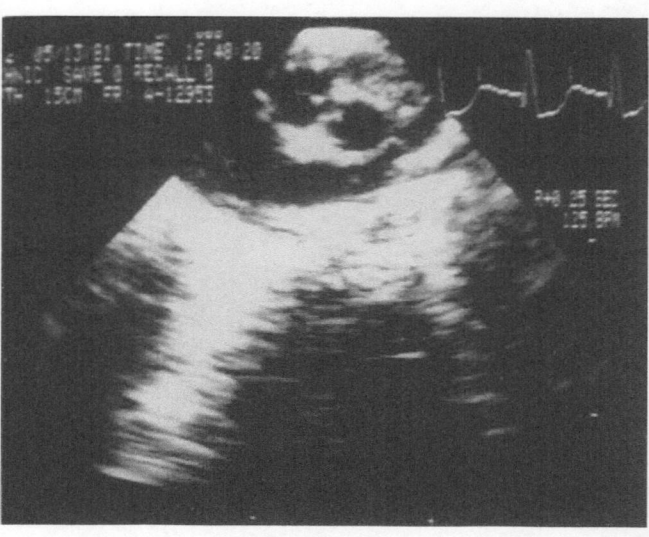

A

B

Fig. 2–32, A and B. *Parasternal short axis view at the level of the great vessels.* **A** with labels; **B** without labels. The anterior semilunar valve is on the right instead of on the left (compare with Figs. 2–4 and 2–20). The great-vessel orientation represented here is consistent with dextrotransposition of the great vessels. A = aortic valve; P = pulmonary valve; RA = right atrium; LA = left atrium.

Left Ventricular Performance

M-mode echocardiography allows measurement of a single left ventricular (LV) diameter (Fig. 2–5), which is similar to the lateral minor diameter used in LV angiograms to calculate LV volume and ejection parameters. Calculation of LV volume from M-mode echo substitutes this minor diameter into formulas derived from those used in angiography. The calculations assume (1) homogeneous LV contraction and (2) constant relationship between the changes in major and minor diameters. Hearts of adults with LV dysfunction cannot be expected to contract in a homogeneous manner. In addition, the change in major diameter relative to the change in minor diameter varies with age and also with the size of the heart. Thus it is not surprising that LV volume, mass, and function derived from M-mode echocardiographic LV diameters has not equaled angiocardiographic volumes in levels of accuracy. Nevertheless, serial changes in individuals and comparisons within well-defined groups have been reported and are clinically useful. Shortening fraction, rather than ejection fraction or cardiac volume derived from M-mode tracings, may be most useful as it relies on the fewest assumptions. The calculation of shortening fraction follows:

$$SF = \frac{LVID_d - LVID_s}{LVID_d} \times 100$$

where

SF = shortening fraction;
$LVID_d$ = Left ventricular internal diameter (diastole);
$LVID_s$ = Left ventricular internal diameter (systole).

Shortening fraction is often expressed as a percentage. Normal values for all ages are presented in Table 2–1. Another value derived from echocardiographic measurements, mean velocity of circumferential fiber shortening (mean VCF), relates to rate of ejection and is calculated from the change in LV dimensions (shortening fraction) divided by the left ventricular ejection time (LVET). Thus,

$$\text{mean VCF} = \frac{LVID_d - LVID_s}{LVID_d \times LVET}$$

Because it is difficult to determine the exact onset of ejection from an LV echogram, left ventricular ejection time (LVET) may be better measured from an aortic valve echogram (Fig. 2–7A). LVET should be obtained while the heart is beating at the same rate and as nearly as possible to the same time (same inotropic state) during which the LV trace is recorded.

Two-dimensional echocardiography has a major potential advantage over M-mode with regard to evaluating LV function. The images are in two dimensions similar to those obtained from angiography and nuclear cardiology. The RAO equivalent view (Fig. 2–26) from the apex and the parasternal LV short axis view (Fig. 2–19) are orthogonal. A number of investigators have subjected such 2-DE images to the same geometrical analysis that has been applied to nuclear scans and to angiograms. The major limitation is that single-frame images fail to show clear endocardial outlines. The outlines therefore have to be drawn in by hand rather than by computer, and many interpolations are necessary. Nevertheless, the results appear promising for estimations of LV ejection fraction and abnormalities of wall motion.

Two-dimensional echocardiography may also prove helpful in studying right ventricular volume and function in individuals with both congenital and acquired heart disease. The apical four-chamber view and the parasternal long axis view of the right ventricular outflow tract are orthogonal. The subxiphoid coronal and sagittal views form another orthogonal pair, which may prove useful in this regard. More work is necessary along this line.

Echocardiography Using Contrast Material

Gramiak et al. described the use of green dye as a contrast medium for echocardiography in 1969. Other liquids such as glucose water and saline can be identified as they mix with the blood in the cardiac chambers. Valdez-Cruz et al. described the use of venous blood that has been withdrawn into a syringe and immediately reinjected into a peripheral vein. After venous injection the "contrast effect" can be followed as the blood flows through the heart. If a right-to-left shunt exists, echo-reflective blood will be noted transiently within a left-sided chamber. If the right-to-left shunt is at the atrial level, echo-reflective blood will be present in the left atrium, left ventricle, and aorta. A left-to-right shunt at the atrial level can be identified on 2-DE as unopacified blood pours into the right atrium, displacing the echo-reflective blood (negative contrast effect) (Fig. 7–7). Contrast echocardiography has been used by some as an adjunct along with 2-DE and M-mode systolic time intervals in differentiating cyanotic heart defects in neonates from severe persistent fetal circulation. Diagnosis of tricuspid atresia may also be facilitated by contrast echocardiography because the characteristic sequence of filling of the chambers can be demonstrated (i.e., RA→LA→LV).

Increased Pulmonary Artery Pressure

Hirschfeld et al. found that elevation of pulmonary artery pressure correlated with lengthening of the right ventricular preejection period (RPEP) and shortening of the right ventricular ejection time (RVET) or an increase in the ratio RPEP/RVET. A RPEP/RVET of 0.30 or greater suggests PA pressure elevation (normal RPEP/RVET = 0.16 – 0.30; mean = 0.24). The same authors report that this relationship between systolic time intervals and pulmonary pressure also exists in D-transposition of the great vessels (where the left ventricle pumps blood to the lungs). Their experience suggests that one might be able to predict pulmonary resistance in cases of left-to-right shunt and follow its progress by means of serial measurements of pulmonary systolic time intervals. If pressure seems high the study may be repeated while the subject breathes a high concentration of oxygen. (See section on ventricular septal defect in Chapter 7.)

Doppler Echocardiography

The Doppler effect on reflected ultrasound has been used for medical diagnosis for about as long as has imaging ultrasound. This effect was first described by Christian Johann Doppler in 1842 to explain the change in the color of light from a star depending upon the motion of the star relative to an observer on earth. For any given transmitted frequency, an observer will sense a higher frequency if the object is moving toward the observer and a lower frequency if the object is moving away from the observer. The spectrum of light from a star moving away from earth is shifted toward the lower frequency (more red), whereas the spectrum from a star moving toward earth is shifted toward a higher frequency (more violet) compared to the spectrum of light emitted by the star. A Doppler shift can also be demonstrated for radio waves (radar) and is used to measure the speed of automobiles. A common experience with the Doppler effect on sound waves is that of listening to a train whistle. As the train approaches, the whistle has a higher pitch and as the train passes and moves away from the observer the pitch of the whistle rapidly falls.

Two ultrasound techniques employing the Doppler effect are in general use today. These are continuous wave Doppler and pulsed Doppler.

Continuous Wave Doppler Ultrasound

Continuous wave Doppler requires two transducers, one transmitting continuously, the other receiving the returning scattered signals. It is thought that red blood cells or minor irregularities in the concentration of red blood cells serve as the reflectors. Continuous wave Doppler was first used to detect presence or absence of blood flow. Together with an inflatable cuff a Doppler instrument was then used to determine blood pressure. Later, the frequency shift was quantitated and plotted against time in order to determine velocity of flow. Throughout this book, velocity toward the transducer is plotted above the zero line and velocity away from the transducer plotted below the line.

The frequency shift relates to the velocity of flow by a formula called the Doppler equation:

$$\Delta f = \frac{2 f_o V \cos \theta}{c} \qquad (1)$$

or

$$V = \frac{c \times \Delta f}{2 f_o \cos \theta} \qquad (2)$$

where V = velocity of flow (m/sec); c = the speed of sound in blood (approximately 1540 m/sec); Δf = frequency shift (Hz); f_o = transmitted frequency (Hz). θ = the angle between the ultrasound beam and the direction of flow. The angle is estimated from the simultaneous 2-dimensional echocardiographic (2-DE) image (Fig. 2–33A)

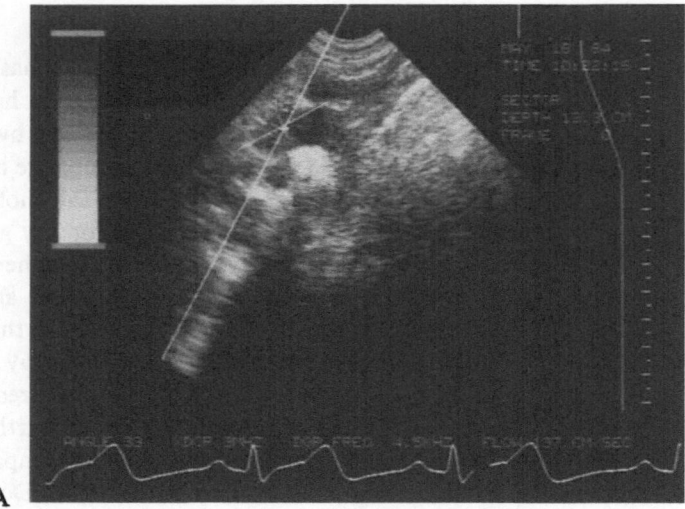
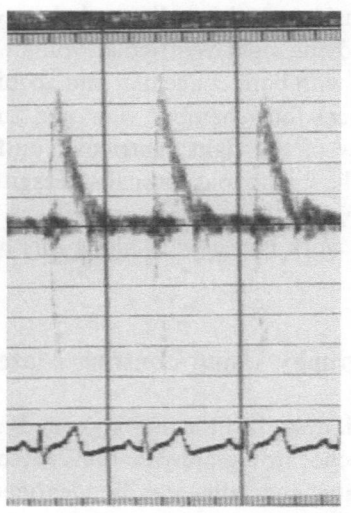

A   B

Fig. 2–33. *Range gating in pulsed Doppler echocardiography.* **A** two-dimensional image of the ascending aorta with the Doppler cursor superimposed. **B** Print-out of the Doppler frequency shift versus time in this location. The horizontal bar in **A** indicates the depth along the cursor which is sensed by the machine after each burst of energy. This spot, called the sample volume, was placed in the ascending aorta. The shorter oblique line was applied by the operator to indicate the angle of incidence. The transmitted frequency is indicated (*XDCR*). The peak Doppler frequency shift (*DOP FREQ*) was obtained by the operator from the print-out in **B**. The computer then calculated the velocity (*FLOW*). In **B** the Doppler frequency shift versus time corresponds to velocity of blood in the aorta. This curve is familiar because it approximately parallels a pressure curve, and a flow curve, in the same location.

even though the angle is defined in three dimensions. The angle in the third dimension (the azimuthal angle) is minimized by angling the transducer to optimize the visual and auditory signal.

Recently analog and digital methods have been used to analyze the spectrum of returning frequencies in order to better estimate maximum and mean velocities and to analyze complex signals returning from areas where disturbance of flow occurs. The most successful of these methods are the Fast Fourier Transform (FFT, digital) and the CHIRP-Z transform (analog).

The advantage of continuous wave Doppler is that it imposes no limitation in the frequency shift and therefore there is no limit on the velocity which can be sensed. Very high velocities are encountered in valvar regurgitation and in valvar stenosis. The disadvantage of continuous Doppler is that it does not differentiate depth, so that Doppler shifts from the entire volume of tissue encountered by the beam are returned to the receiving transducer. If one is looking for only the highest velocity signals, and if only one possible source of high velocity signals is within the beam (e.g., one area of stenosis), then continuous Doppler is preferable.

Pulsed Doppler Ultrasound

The technique of pulsed Doppler ultrasound allows the machine to define a specific distance from the transducer from which the Doppler shift will be sampled. This is called range gating (Fig. 2–33). Range gating is useful in localizing a flow disturbance or high velocity jet, or to determine the direction of flow in a small area within the heart called the "sample volume." Pulsed Doppler devices generate bursts (or pulses) of sound and sample backscattered energy during a discrete interval between the bursts. The timing of the receiving cycle determines the depth of the sample. Only one transducer is necessary, and therefore an imaging transducer can also be used for pulsed Doppler examination. In addition, pulsed Doppler allows an M-mode image to be made simultaneous with the Doppler signal. This aids in verifying the location being sampled. A disadvantage of pulsed Doppler ultrasound is that the pulse repetition frequency (PRF) limits the range that can be sampled as well as the frequency shift (and the velocity) that can be sensed. Once each burst of energy leaves the transducer, the machine must wait until the backscattered signal returns from the sampled depth before it can send out a new burst of energy.

The relationship of range to PRF is described by the following formula:

$$R = \frac{c}{2\,PRF} \tag{3}$$

where c = velocity of sound in blood (1.54×10^5 cm/sec); PRF = the pulse repetition frequency (Hz); and R = the range (cm). The factor of 2 allows the sound to travel to the target and to return from the target. The maximum frequency shift is related to the PRF by this formula:

$$\Delta f = \frac{PRF}{2} \tag{4}$$

because accurate processing requires a sampling frequency at least twice the highest frequency measured. The maximum detectable Doppler shift is sometimes called the Nyquist limit. Thus, as the PRF is reduced in order to interrogate at a greater depth, the maximum detectable frequency is reduced. Table 2–2 shows maximum depth and maximum detectable velocity relative to PRF for transducers commonly used for Doppler examinations. Table 2–3 shows maximum velocities detected by Doppler ultrasound at each orifice in the heart in adults and children. As can

Table 2–2. Maximum Range and Velocity for Pulsed Doppler Systems

Transducer frequency (mHz)	PRF (kHz)	Maximum range (cm)	Maximum velocity at specified depth (m/sec)
5	15	5.1	2.0 at 3cm
	10	7.7	1.2 at 5cm
3.5	10.5	7.3	1.7 at 5 cm
	7	11.0	1.2 at 7cm
2.5	10	7.7	2.4 at 5cm
	5	15.4	1.7 at 7cm

Table 2–3. Maximum Velocities in Normal Children and Adults

	Children	Adults
Mitral	0.78 (0.44–1.28)	0.90 (0.6–1.3)
Superior vena cava	0.51 (0.28–0.80)	
Tricuspid	0.60 (0.5–0.8)	0.50 (0.3–0.7)
Right ventricular outflow	0.76 (0.5–1.05)	0.75 (0.6–0.9)
Pulmonary artery	0.90 (0.7–1.1)	0.75 (0.6–0.9)
Left ventricular outflow tract	1.00 (0.7–1.2)	0.90 (0.7–1.1)
Aorta	0.97 (0.60–1.54)	1.35 (1.0–1.7)

From Hatle L, Angelsen B (1985) *Doppler Ultrasound in Cardiology* Philadelphia, Lea and Febiger, p 93; and Goldberg SJ, Allen HD, Marx GR, Flinn CJ (1985) *Doppler Echocardiography*. Philadelphia, Lea and Febiger, pp 33–54.

be appreciated from this table, the Nyquist limit for even the lowest frequency transducer can be exceeded if velocities are increased because of high flow or because of stenosis. If frequencies above the Nyquist limit are encountered, wrapping occurs, with the peak of the envolope appearing below the baseline. (see Fig. 2–34A). Three methods are used to circumvent the limitations of pulsed doppler. The first is to use a transducer with a lower frequency. The 2-D images will be degraded but will still allow verification of position. Second, for any given transducer, frequency up to twice the Nyquist limit can be accommodated by shifting the zero line to the edge of the page, effectively "cutting and pasting" the peak back on top of the curve (Fig. 2–34B). The third method involves increasing the PRF without regard for range resolution (high PRF). The machine continues to transmit bursts of energy without waiting for the previous signal to return and processes signals when not transmitting. Thus, range resolution is lost; however, maximum detectable velocity is increased (Fig. 2–35).

Doppler Ultrasound with 2-Dimensional Imaging

Both continuous and pulsed Doppler ultrasound are often used in combination with 2-D imaging ultrasound in order to identify the region within the heart which is being sampled (Fig. 2–33). Systems using separate transducers for Doppler and for imaging provide a continuous view of the Doppler signal simultaneous with the 2-D image. Those using a single transducer for both functions allow intermittent updating of the 2-D image during the Doppler examination in order to verify the location of the Doppler sample volume. All the examples of Doppler tracings in this book are produced by a pulsed Doppler device having the same transducer for 2-D imaging and for Doppler interrogation. High PRF is used to accommodate high velocity of flow. The signals are analyzed by FFT.

A new approach called multigate Doppler allows a color overlay representing Doppler shifts across either the M-mode or the 2-D image.

Fig. 2–34. *Wrapping (or "aliasing") occurs when the frequency shift exceeds the Nyquist limit.* A Doppler frequency shift versus time of a sample volume directed into the ascending aorta from the subxyphoid location. The combination of a 5 mHz transmitted frequency and a low-pulse repetition frequency (PRF) results in a limit of frequency shift (Nyquist limit), which fails to accommodate a normal velocity. The envelope is therefore truncated at the edge of the paper, and its peak wraps around to appear at the top of the page above the zero line. One method of avoiding this artifact is by moving the zero line to the edge of the paper as in **B**, thus effectively "cutting and pasting" the tops onto the velocity envelopes. This effectively doubles the frequency shift that can be sensed. (Horizontal calibration lines are 0.5 kHz. Time lines are 0.04 sec apart.)

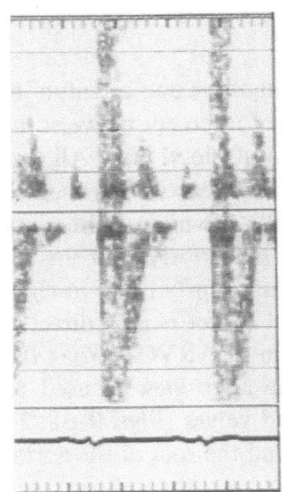
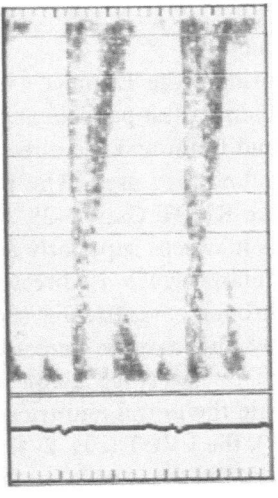

A   B

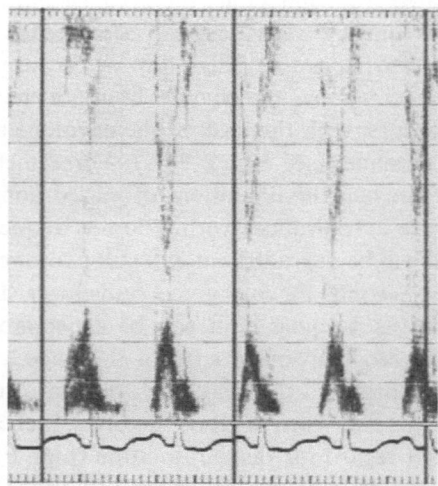

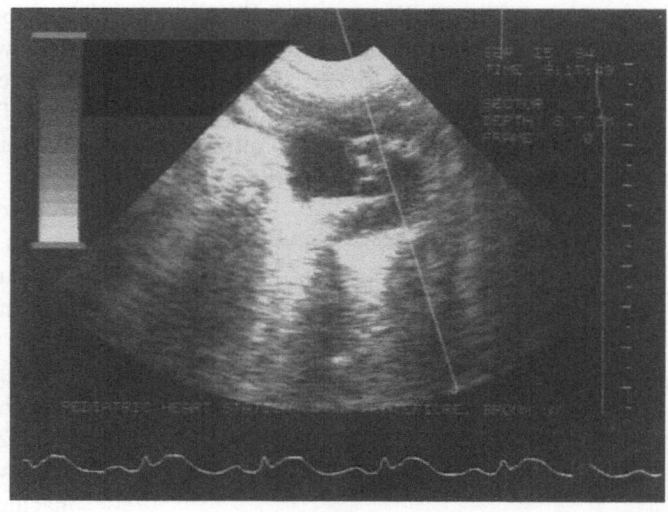

Fig. 2–35. A Doppler tracing from the ascending aorta (subxiphoid view) in a 4-day-old infant with aortic stenosis. Each horizontal calibration line indicates a 2 kHz frequency shift. Each heavy vertical line indicates one second. **B** The two-dimensional echocardiogram verifies the position of the Doppler sample volume just above the aortic valve. After the area of high velocity (the jet) has been localized by range-gated pulsed Doppler, the pulse repetition frequency (PRF) is increased in order to ascertain the maximum Doppler shift (velocity). From the peak velocity the pressure difference across the valve can be calculated. In this patient the Doppler shift is 12 kHz using a 3 mHz transducer. The angle of incidence is approximately 30°. Substituting in Formula (2) the corresponding peak velocity is 3.60 m/sec. Using Formula (5) the corresponding pressure difference is 50 mmHg. This agreed closely with the finding at cardiac catheterization.

Normal Patterns of Velocity vs Time

The patterns of Doppler flow signals from the orifices and chambers of the heart are readily recognizable (Figs. 2–36 to 2–45). Once the location for Doppler sampling is identified by imaging, the signal is optimized by watching the Doppler signal rather than the 2-D image. In addition, the Doppler shift is within the audible range, so that the Doppler signal may be optimized by listening for the clearest audible signal. Laminar flow will yield a narrow spectrum (relatively few frequencies) and will have a clear tonal quality and a pitch that is proportional to the velocity of flow (a higher velocity produces a higher frequency shift and a higher pitched auditory signal) (Fig. 2–35). A sample from an area of flow disturbance will yield a broad spectrum and a harsh sound (Fig. 2–46). The walls of vessels and chambers move more slowly, yielding groaning or crunching sounds, while the motions of valves produce high-pitched clicks and squeaks (Fig. 2–42).

Technique

In performing the Doppler examination one attempts to obtain the smallest possible angle of intercept between the ultrasound beam and the direction of blood flow. All cardiac windows are used. The parasternal view is used to image the RVOT (Fig. 2–39 A–B), the main pulmonary artery as it sweeps superiorly and posteriorly, and the tricuspid inflow which is directed anteriorly. Left-to-right shunt through a ventricular septal defect is also directed anteriorly and may be detected in the RVOT from the parasternal view (Fig. 2–46). The apex view is used to interrogate the mitral and tricuspid valves (Figs. 2–38, 2–41, 2–47), the LVOT (Fig. 2–42) and the root of the aorta.

The subxiphoid position allows interrogation of the inferior vena cava, superior vena cava (Fig. 2–36), and the pulmonary veins. The apex and subxiphoid positions provide the best windows for identifying left-to-right shunts through an ASD (Fig. 2–48). The subxiphoid position also allows the beam to be directed parallel to the RVOT and main pulmonary artery (Figs. 2–39C-D, 2–40). Reversal of flow or continuous flow in the main pulmonary artery due to a patent ductus arteriosus may be recognized either in this view or in the parasternal view. Similarly, the high velocities secondary to valvar or infundibular pulmonic stenosis are often best identified in the subxiphoid view. The subxiphoid view is also used to examine flow in the ascending aorta, the descending aorta and the abdominal aorta (Figs. 2–35, 2–43C and 2–45). Decreased pulsatility and/or continuous flow (diastolic augmentation) in the abdominal aorta are signs of coarctation of the aorta (Fig. 2–49), while reversed flow in the abdominal aorta during diastole indicates a left-to-right shunt through a patent ductus arteriosus or a systemic to pulmonary shunt (Fig. 2–50). The suprasternal notch is used to examine flow in the ascending aorta and in the aortic arch (Figs. 2–43, 2–44). The SVC and right pulmonary artery are also accessible from this location.

Interpretation of Doppler Signals

The returning signals are analyzed qualitatively for laminar flow or disturbed flow. A clean, narrow, smooth curve (envelope) represents a narrow frequency spectrum associated with laminar flow. A wide spectrum, which often completely fills the area under the curve of maximum velocity is characteristic of disturbed flow, usually associated with

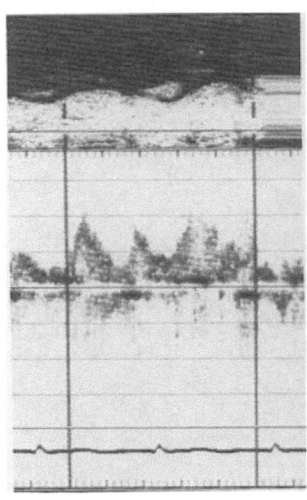
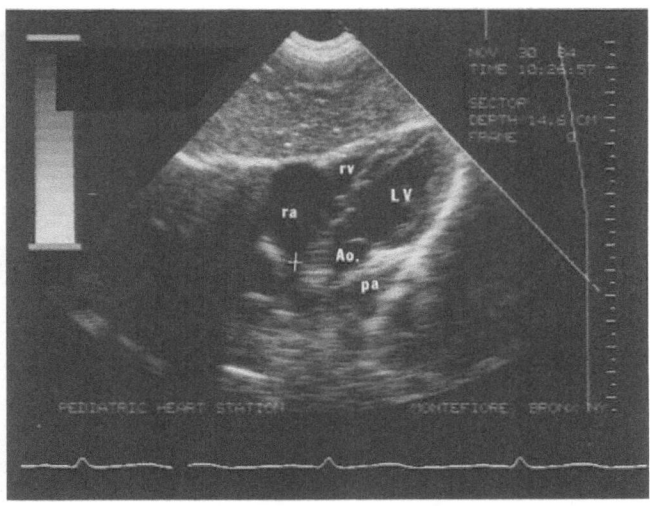

A   B

Fig. 2–36. *Normal Doppler tracing in the superior vena cava.* **A** Tracing of the Doppler frequency shift versus time for a sample volume directed into the superior vena cava from the subxiphoid position. **B** Two-dimensional image to verify the position of the sample volume (*cross*). The flow is toward the transducer and therefore above the baseline. The pattern is reminiscent of the venous pressure waves with two peaks of velocity for each cardiac cycle. Calibration marks indicate 1 kHz. *ra* = right atrium; *rv* = right ventricle; *LV* = left ventricle; *Ao* = ascending aorta; *pa* = main pulmonary artery.

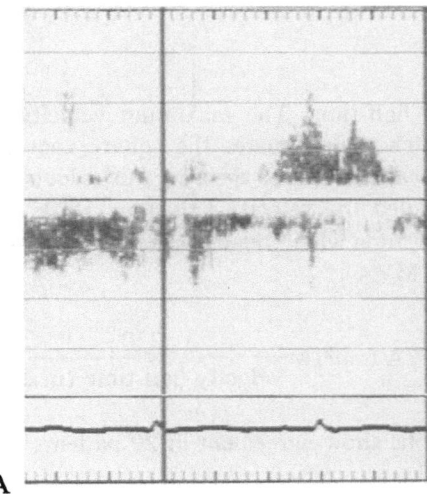
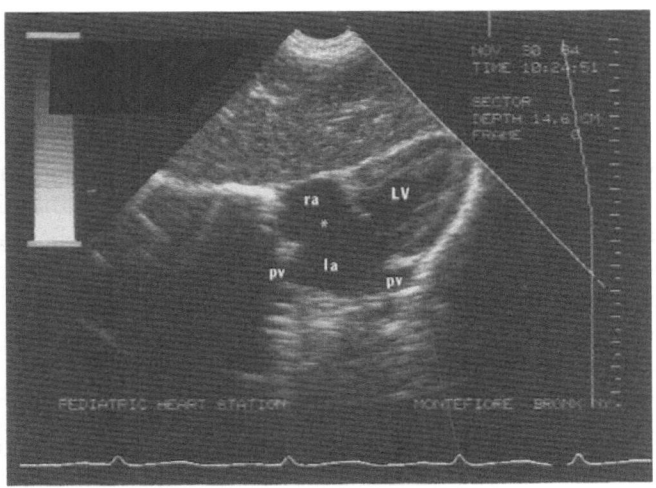

A   B

Fig. 2–37. *Normal Doppler tracing in the right atrium.* **A** Doppler frequency shift versus time from the right atrium near the foramen ovale. **B** Two-dimensional image to verify the position of the sample volume (transverse image from the subxiphoid window). The transducer is angled slightly posteriorly from Fig. 2–36. The sample volume was at the center of the *asterisk.* Flow is bidirec- tional changing direction with respiration. This nondescript pattern is normal for this location because flow in this area is normally perpendicular to the Doppler beam. Compare with Fig. 2–48 which shows the pattern of velocity in a patient with atrial septal defect. *ra* = right atrium; *la* = left atrium; *LV* = left ventricle; *pv* = right and left pulmonary veins.

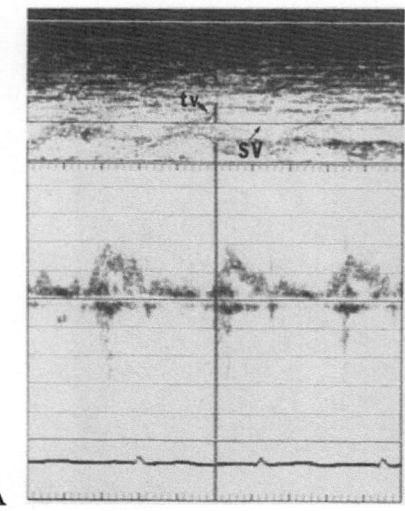
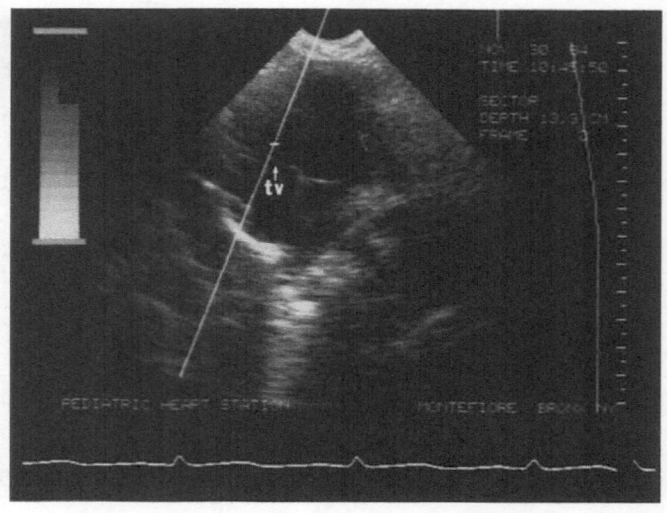

Fig. 2–38. *Normal Doppler tracing in the tricuspid valve.* **A** Pattern of Doppler frequency shift versus time for a sample volume directed from the apex window (4-chamber view) into the right ventricle just below the tricuspid valve. **B** The two-dimensional image to verify the position. The flow is toward the transducer during diastole and has two peaks, the first peak during early filling and the second peak during atrial contraction. The maximum frequency shift is 1.4 kHz, corresponding to a maximum velocity of 0.4 m/sec. The degraded M-mode tracing at the top of the frame shows the tricuspid valve (*tv*) and the Doppler sample volume (*SV*) just inside the right ventricle.

an abnormal or stenotic opening (Fig. 2–40C). In addition the signals are evaluated quantitatively for maximum or peak velocity, which is the highest velocity attained during the cardiac cycle, and for mean velocity, which is the area under the curve of velocity divided by the time to trace the curve. Mean velocity is calculated by use of a planimeter or a computer and digitizing device.

Velocity Related to Pressure Gradient Velocity has been found to correspond reliably with pressure differences across any orifice by the formula:

$$P_1 - P_2 = 4V^2 \qquad (5)$$

Where $P_1 - P_2$ = the pressure difference across the orifice; V = velocity calculated from the Doppler equation. In order to accurately determine pressure differences from Doppler frequency shift care must be taken to find the jet through the stenotic orifice and to record the maximal frequency shift just above the valve. This will produce a clean envelope and a high pitched audible signal (Fig. 2–35). A position slightly off center will produce only spectral dispersion indicating parajet flow disturbance.

The relationships between Doppler velocity and pressure difference has been extensively documented for aortic stenosis and pulmonic stenosis. It has also been found useful in evaluating the difference between RV and LV pressure in patients with VSD. If tricuspid regurgitation is present the pressure in the RV can be estimated from the peak velocity of the regurgitant flow. The pressure difference across the mitral valve in mitral stenosis is also accurately estimated by this method, and severity can be predicted from a calculation of velocity half-time, which corresponds

to pressure half-time. The maximum velocity is divided by 1.4 (which approximates the square root of 2). The time from peak velocity to the time this calculated velocity occurs is called the velocity half-time. Hatle reports the following formula which relates velocity half-time to mitral valve area (MVA):

$$\text{MVA (cm}^2\text{)} = \frac{220}{\text{velocity half-time (msec)}} \qquad (6)$$

Hatle's graphs show agreement in 20 patients with mitral stenosis.

Velocity Related to Volume of Flow Mean velocity along with a measurement of the area of an orifice by 2-D imaging allows an estimation of blood flow through an orifice. The formula for this relationship follows:

$$\bar{V} \text{ (cm/sec)} \times A \text{ (cm}^2\text{)} \times 60 \text{ sec/min} = \dot{Q} \text{ (cm}^3\text{/min)}. \qquad (7)$$

Where $\bar{V}$ = mean velocity (after correction for angle of incidence); A = area of the orifice measured by 2-DE; $\dot{Q}$ = flow across the orifice. The calculation assumes a flat velocity profile such that all the blood within the orifice moves with the same velocity. For instance, assuming no aortic stenosis is present, the mean velocity in the ascending aorta along with the area of the aortic root from a short axis view will allow an estimation of cardiac output. Systemic venous return can be estimated from mean velocity across the tricuspid valve along with a measurement of the area of the tricuspid valve.

In patients with left-to-right shunts pulmonary blood flow can be estimated from the velocity and the area of

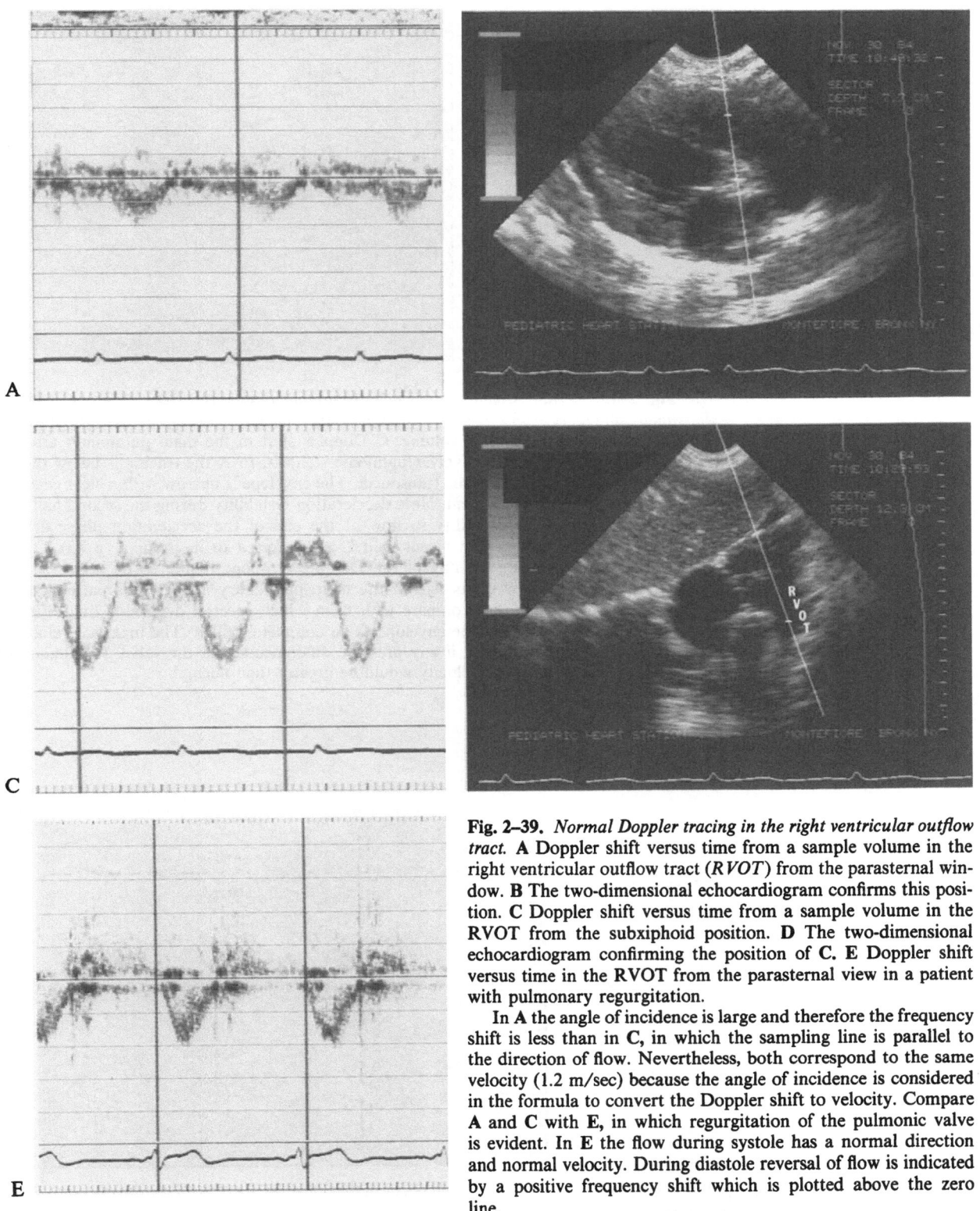

Fig. 2–39. *Normal Doppler tracing in the right ventricular outflow tract.* **A** Doppler shift versus time from a sample volume in the right ventricular outflow tract (*RVOT*) from the parasternal window. **B** The two-dimensional echocardiogram confirms this position. **C** Doppler shift versus time from a sample volume in the RVOT from the subxiphoid position. **D** The two-dimensional echocardiogram confirming the position of **C**. **E** Doppler shift versus time in the RVOT from the parasternal view in a patient with pulmonary regurgitation.

In **A** the angle of incidence is large and therefore the frequency shift is less than in **C**, in which the sampling line is parallel to the direction of flow. Nevertheless, both correspond to the same velocity (1.2 m/sec) because the angle of incidence is considered in the formula to convert the Doppler shift to velocity. Compare **A** and **C** with **E**, in which regurgitation of the pulmonic valve is evident. In **E** the flow during systole has a normal direction and normal velocity. During diastole reversal of flow is indicated by a positive frequency shift which is plotted above the zero line.

the pulmonic valve or from velocity and area of the mitral valve. (Note: estimated flow across the mitral valve has been less reliable than estimated flow for other orifices.) Regurgitant fractions are estimated by comparing the antegrade mean velocity with the retrograde velocity across the orifice. For instance, in a patient with aortic insufficiency, the ratio of the mean reverse velocity during diastole (regurgitant velocity) to the mean forward velocity (ejection velocity) during systole should correspond to regurgitant fraction. Another possibility might be to subtract diastolic mitral flow (forward flow) from systolic aortic flow (forward flow plus regurgitant volume) to calculate regurgitant flow. These last techniques have not had wide use, and further studies are needed.

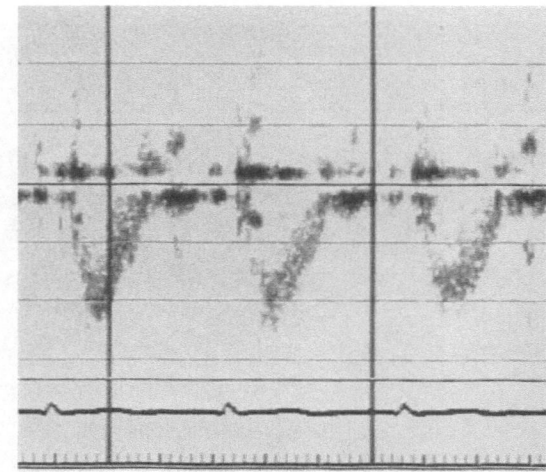
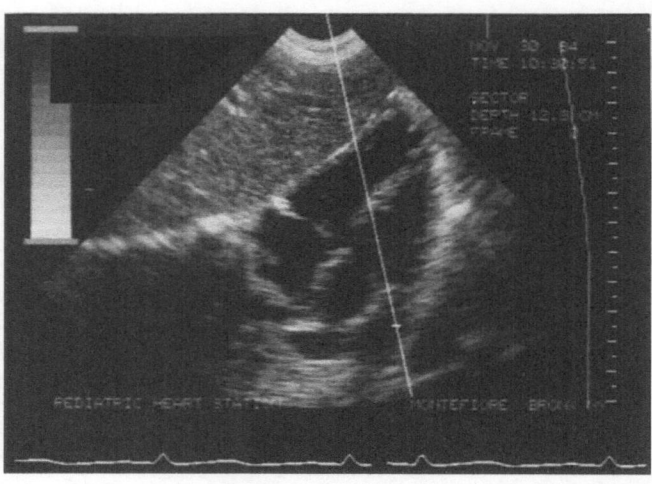

A   B

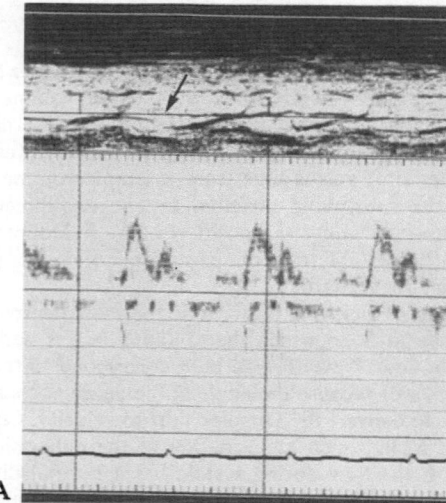

Fig. 2–40. *Normal Doppler tracing in the main pulmonary artery.* **A** Doppler shift in the main pulmonary artery. **B** The two-dimensional image from the subxiphoid window confirming the position of the sample volume. **C** Doppler shift in the main pulmonary artery in a 3-year-old girl with minimal valvar pulmonic stenosis. In **A** the tracing is below the zero line because flow is away from the transducer. The envelope is narrow with a clear center because no flow disturbance is present. Note deceleration instability during the second half of systole. This term refers to instability in flow at the end of the acceleration phase described by Macdonald and Helps in a visual model, and referred to in Berman (p 45). Deceleration instability may cause widening of the Doppler envelope in the aortic arch, the right and left ventricular inflow tracts and in the main pulmonary artery. This pattern of widening does not signify stenosis. Compare with *C* in which spectral dispersion due to mild valvar pulmonic stenosis causes the envelope to be completely filled. The maximal velocity in **C** is normal, indicating minimal if any pressure difference across the valve. If pulmonic stenosis were significant then the velocity would be greater than normal.

C

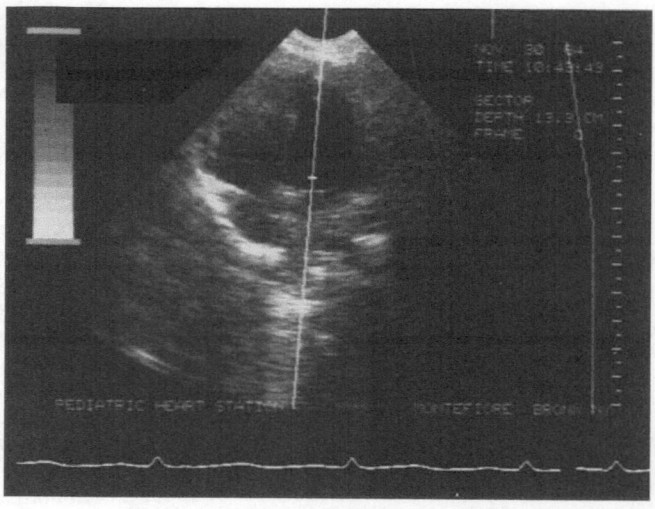

A   B

Fig. 2–41. *Normal Doppler tracing in the mitral valve.* **A** Doppler shift just below the mitral valve with simultaneous M-mode tracing in a child with no cardiac defect. **B** Two-dimensional image confirming the position of the sample volume. The transducer is at the apex of the heart (apex 4-chamber view). In this normal individual the tracing has two peaks similar to that of the tricuspid valve, with a maximum Doppler shift of 2 kHz corresponding to a peak velocity of 1.3 m/sec using a transmitted frequency of 3 mHz. The sample volume line (*arrow*) superimposed on the degraded M-mode tracing indicates that the Doppler tracing comes from a location just below the mitral valve. In the presence of mitral stenosis the flow disturbance and an increased velocity

will occur in this location. Reversed flow during systole just above the mitral valve may indicate mitral insufficiency or may be caused by normal systolic flow in the aortic root, which is immediately adjacent to the left atrium. The sample volume may stray into the left ventricular outflow tract during systole in spite of careful positioning of the transducer. In order to differentiate mitral insufficiency from normal flow in the left ventricular outflow tract it is helpful to rotate the transducer into a 2-chamber view of the left ventricular outflow tract (next figure) and place the sample volume again in the left atrium. Compare this tracing with Fig. 2–47 which depicts mitral insufficiency recognized by scanning across the mitral anulus behind the mitral valve.

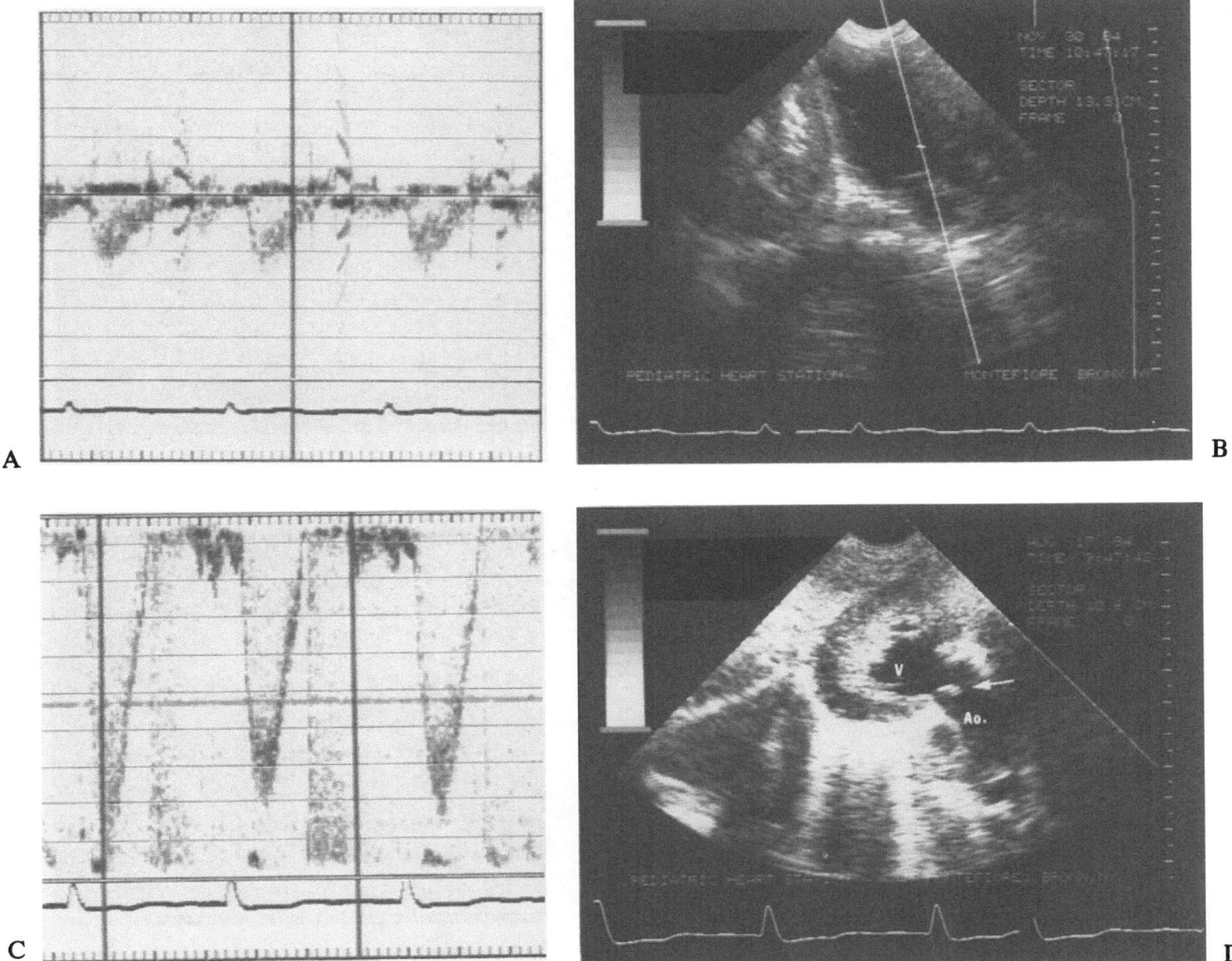

Fig. 2–42. *Normal Doppler tracing in the left ventricular outflow tract.* **A** Doppler shift in the left ventricular outflow tract from the apex two chamber view (**B**). Note that flow here is away from the transducer. It is sometimes difficult to distinguish flow in the left ventricular outflow from flow in the left ventricular inflow. Mitral flow appears as flow toward the transducer during diastole and may be mistakingly interpreted as aortic insufficiency. If the sample volume is directed close to the ventricular septum, the flow from the mitral valve is usually avoided. Compare with **C**, a Doppler tracing below the aortic valve in an infant with single ventricle and aortic insufficiency. During diastole a large positive Doppler shift is identified corresponding to a large pressure difference between the aortic root and the ventricular cavity during diastole. **D** is the 2-D image used to direct the Doppler sample volume. The aortic valve (*arrow*) is thickened. *V* = ventricle; *Ao* = aortic root.

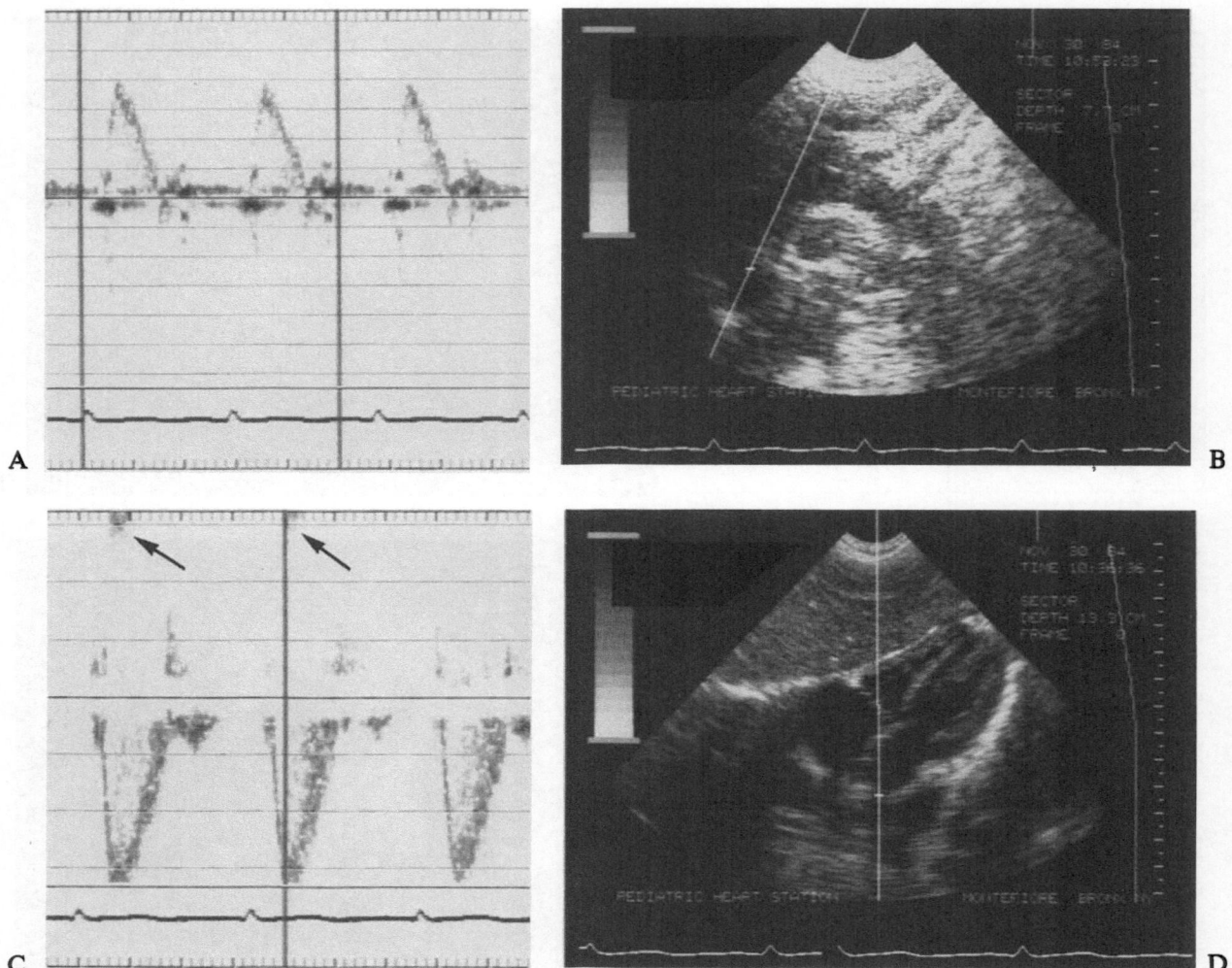

Fig. 2–43. *Normal Doppler tracing in the ascending aorta.* **A** Doppler shift in the ascending aorta from the suprasternal notch view of the aortic arch (**B**). **C** Doppler shift in the ascending aorta from the subxiphoid view (**D**). The information obtained from each view is equivalent. Note wrapping (aliasing) in **C**. The low-pulse, repetition frequency required to reach the ascending aorta from the subxiphoid view without range ambiguity reduces the maximum frequency that can be sensed. Therefore, the envelope is truncated at the bottom of the page and the peak wraps around to appear at the top of the image (*arrows*).

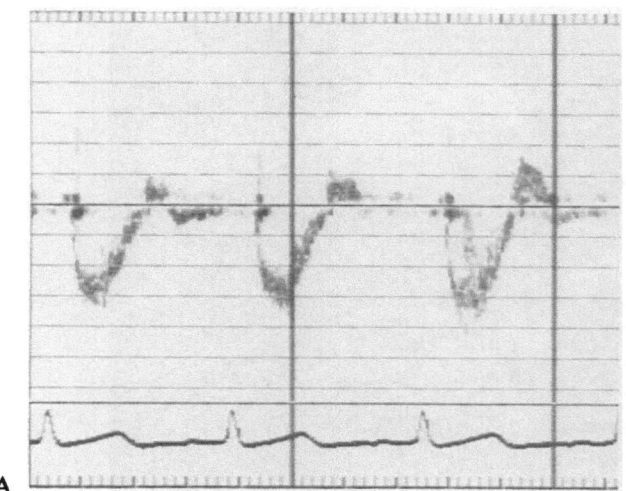
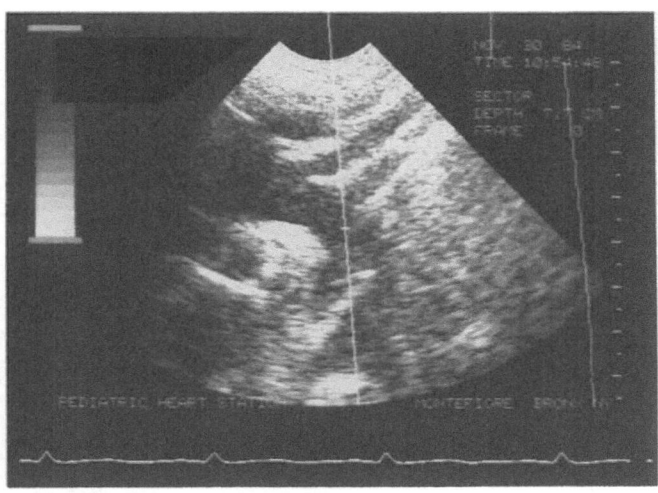

A   B

Fig. 2–44. *Normal Doppler shift in the aortic arch.* **A** Doppler shift in the aortic arch just beyond the left subclavian artery from the suprasternal notch view **(B).** Flow is away from the transducer during systole. A very short period of reversal of flow in early diastole is normal in the ascending aorta and arch and does not indicate aortic insufficiency. Note widening of the envelope during mid-systole. This is a frequent finding in this location and is considered to be caused by deceleration instability (McDonald and Helps), and not by a pathologic disturbance of flow.

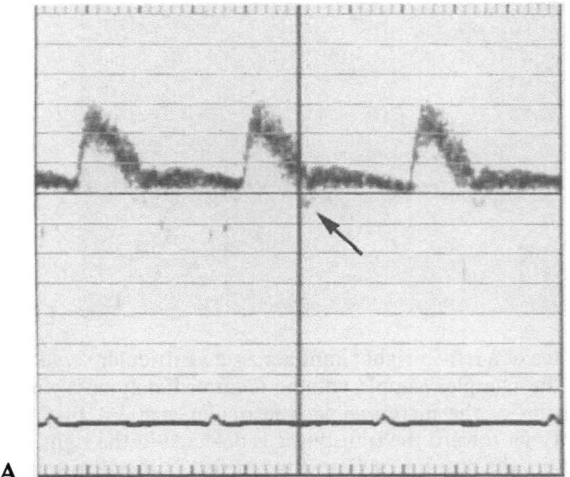
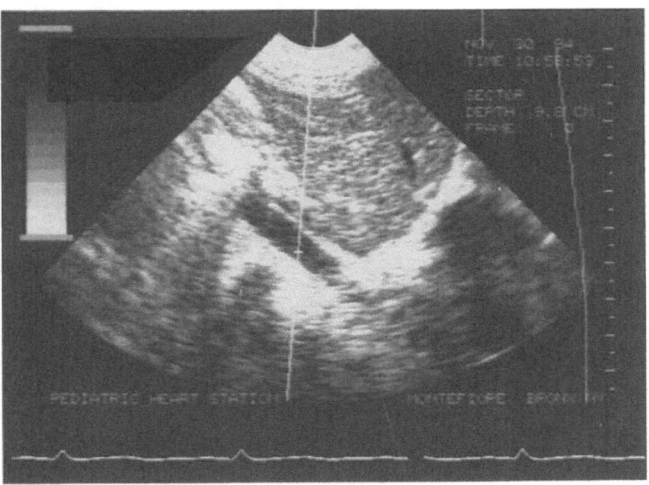

A   B

Fig. 2–45. *Normal Doppler tracing in the abdominal aorta.* **A** Doppler shift in the abdominal aorta. **B** the corresponding 2-D image from the subxiphoid view, pointing cephalad. The angle of incidence is large, and therefore the frequency shift is less than those in the ascending aorta or in the arch where the beam was nearly parallel to the flow. In this location, as in the ascending aorta and in the aortic arch, a momentary reversal of flow is often noted in early diastole (*arrow*).

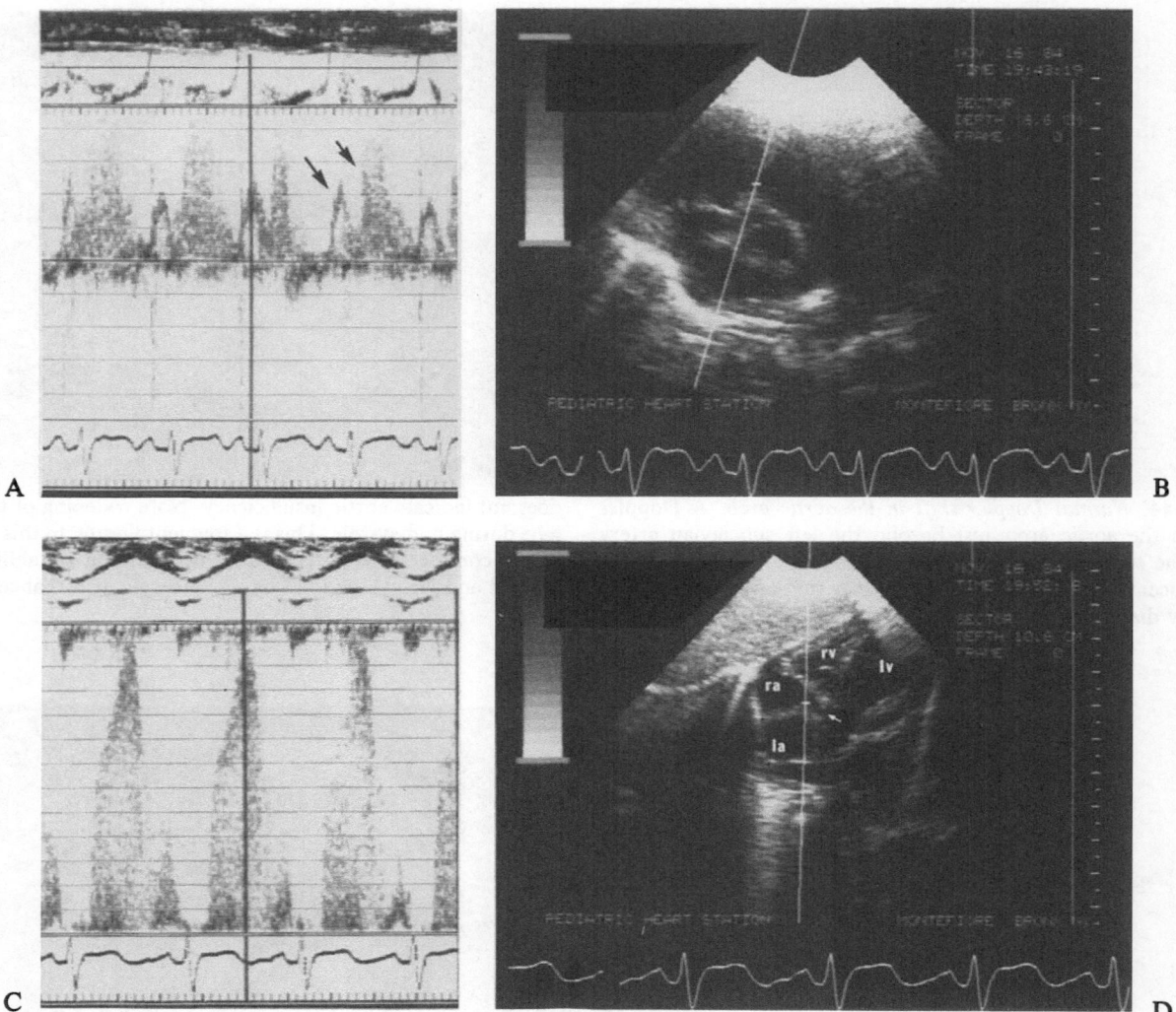

Fig. 2–46. *Doppler tracings and two-dimensional echocardiograms in a two week old girl with ventricular septal defect and left ventricular to right atrial communication.* **A** Doppler shift in the right ventricular outflow tract next to the tricuspid valve. **B** The corresponding two-dimensional image of a short-axis view of the right ventricular outflow tract. **C** The Doppler tracing in the right atrium. **D** The subxiphoid two-dimensional view to verify the position of **C**. In **A** the flow pattern of the tricuspid valve is normal during diastole (*longer arrow*). During systole, flow is again directed toward the transducer (*shorter arrow*) indicating presence of a left-to-right shunt across a ventricular septal defect. In **B** the Doppler sample volume is immediately adjacent to an aneurysm of the membranous ventricular septum. In **C** a high velocity jet toward the transducer is detected in the right atrium. **D** verifies the position of **C** next to a defect in the atrioventricular portion of the membranous ventricular septum (*arrow*). (See the section on left ventricular to right atrial communication for a description of the anatomy of the two parts of the membranous septum.) *lv* = left ventricle; *la* = left atrium; *ra* = right atrium; *rv* = right ventricle.

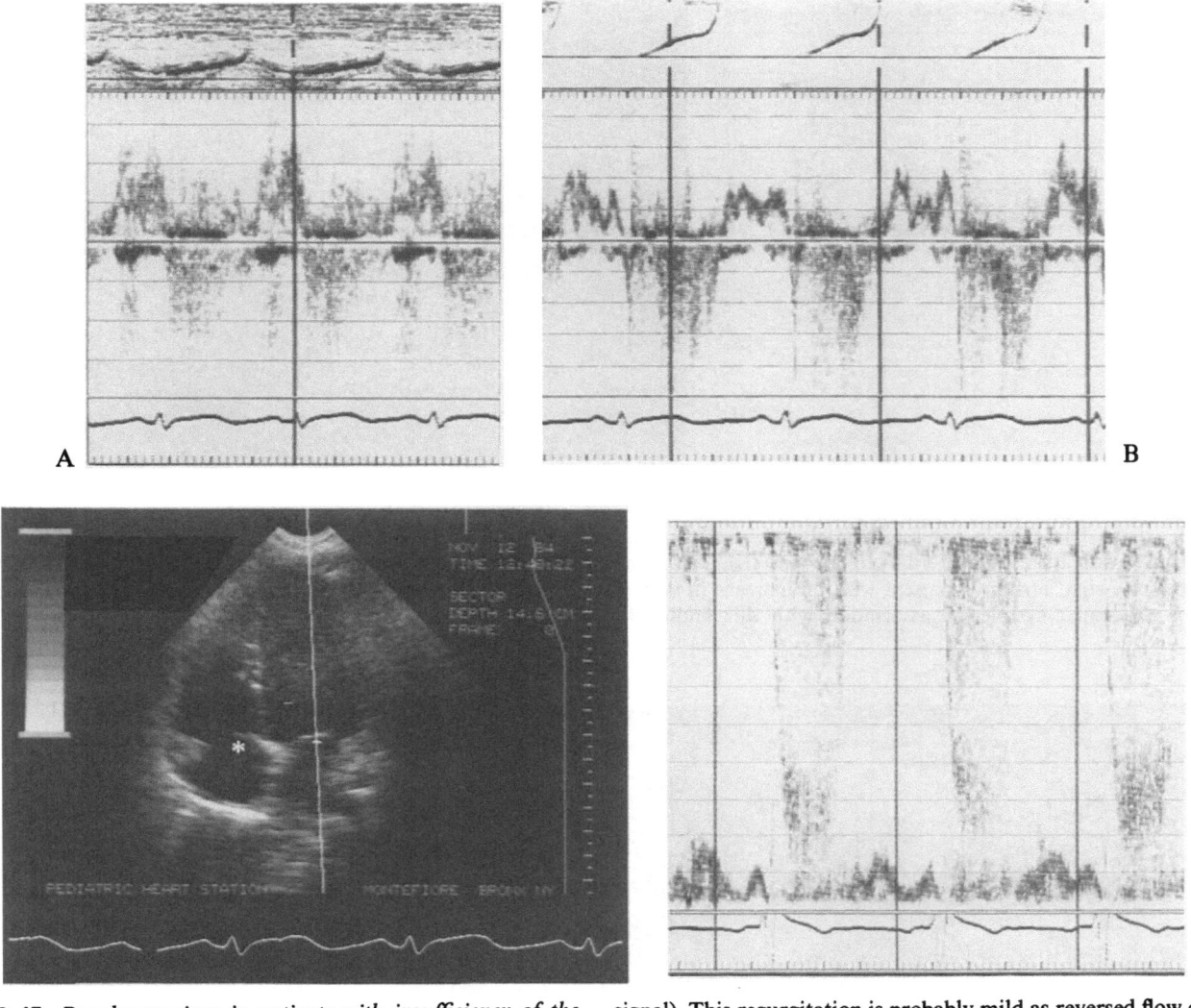

Fig. 2–47. *Doppler tracings in patients with insufficiency of the tricuspid and mitral valves.* **A, B** and **C** are from a 12-year-old girl who had infective endocarditis previously. **A** is from the right atrium just above the tricuspid valve and **B** is from the left atrium just above the mitral valve. The apex 4-chamber-view (**C**) shows the position of the sample volume used to demonstrate mitral insufficiency. The sample is moved to location just above the tricuspid valve (*asterisk*) in order to demonstrate tricuspid insufficiency. In tracings **A** and **B** the regurgitant flow moves away from the transducer during systole. The auditory signal is harsh with high pitched overtones even though the recorded frequency shift is not high. It is likely that only part of the spectrum has been printed here because the energy level of the higher frequency signals was too low to be sensed by the machine. (The continuous wave technique may have picked up the rest of the

signal). This regurgitation is probably mild as reversed flow could not be sensed when the sample volume was moved farther into the left atrium than is depicted in the two-dimensional image. **D** is a tracing from a sample volume above the mitral valve from the apical window in a 6-year-old child who has mitral insufficiency but no congestive heart failure after repair of atrioventricularis communis (A-V communis). A broad spectrum with a high peak frequency shift is recorded immediately above the mitral valve, and can also be sensed far superior near the top of the left atrium. Note: In order to accomodate the high velocity of the regurgitant flow the zero line was shifted to the edges of the paper. Thus, diastolic flow toward the transducer is plotted from the bottom of the page pointing upward, and the regurgitant jet away from the transducer is plotted at the top of the page pointing downward.

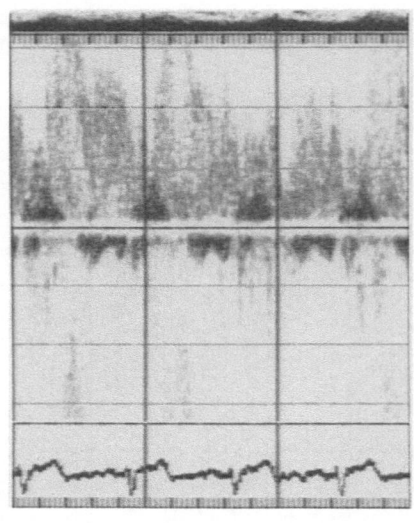 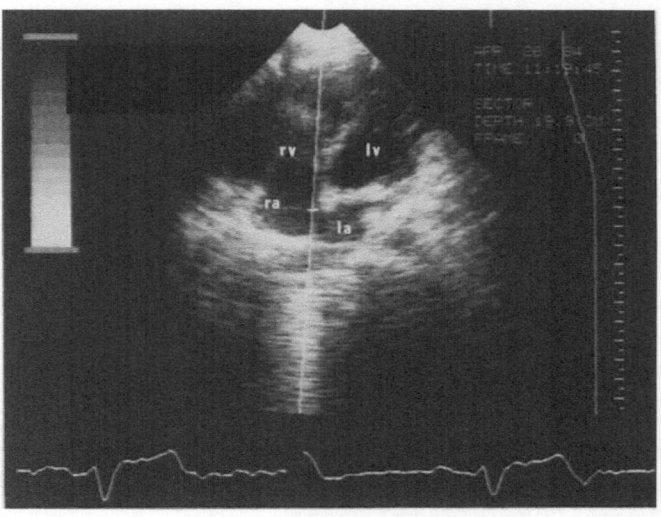

Fig. 2–48. A Doppler tracing in a 14-year-old boy with an atrial septal defect. The sample volume is in the right atrium near the atrial septum from a parasternal oblique view (**B**). Continuous flow into the right atrium is present with an increase in velocity during ventricular systole. In association with this finding the velocity and calculated flow may be increased in the tricuspid valve and in the pulmonic valve. Compare this with the normal Doppler tracing near the atrial septum (Fig. 2–37). *rv* = right ventricle; *lv* = left ventricle; *ra* = right atrium; *la* = left atrium.

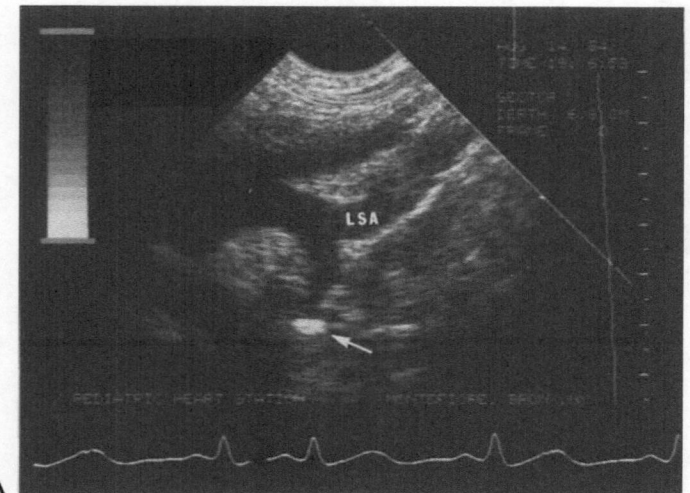 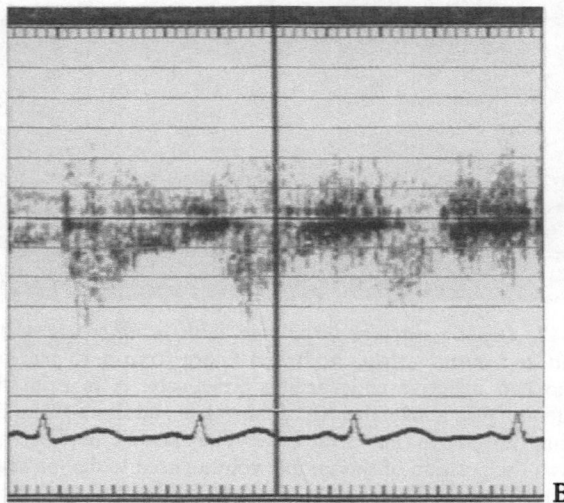

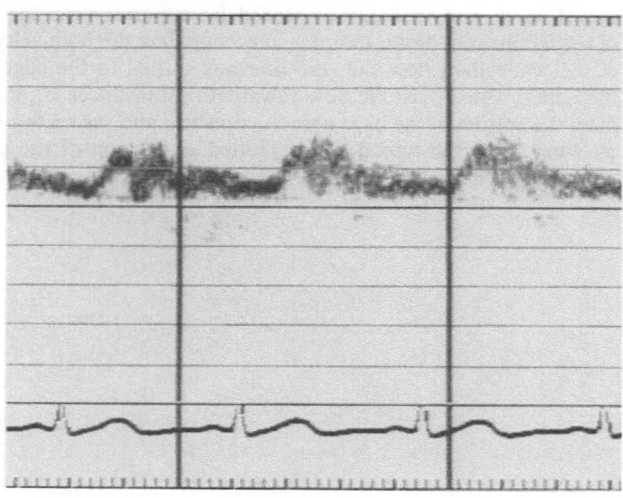

Fig. 2–49. Two-dimensional echocardiogram findings and Doppler tracings in a 5-year-old boy with coarctation of the aorta. **A** The two-dimensional echocardiogram from the suprasternal notch shows a dilated left subclavian artery (*LSA*) and a narrow aortic isthmus. The posterior shelf comprising the coarctation is represented as a highly reflective surface (*arrow*). The Doppler tracing in the isthmus (**B**) shows a marked flow disturbance, and continuous flow. The Doppler tracing from the abdominal aorta (**C**) shows decreased pulsatility during systole and forward flow into the abdominal aorta during diastole (diastolic augmentation) (i.e., the tracing remains above the baseline throughout diastole). This flow may represent the contribution from collateral vessels which bypass the coarctation. Abnormally diminished pulsatility and antegrade flow during diastole (diastolic augmentation) are present in the abdominal aorta in patients with coarctation of the aorta, while reversal of flow during diastole indicates presence of a patent ductus arteriosus, systemic to pulmonary communication or arteriovenous fistula (see also Fig. 2–50).

Fig. 2–50. *Doppler tracing from the abdominal aorta in a 7-day-old premature infant showing reversal of flow during diastole* (arrows). This phenomenon occurs in the abdominal aorta and also in the cerebral arteries in patients with large patent ductus arteriosus or with large systemic to pulmonary shunts placed surgically as palliation for cyanotic congenital heart defects. The reversal of flow is due to emptying of the blood into the pulmonary artery through the patent ductus arteriosus or surgical shunt during diastole. Continuous flow was present in the main pulmonary artery (not shown).

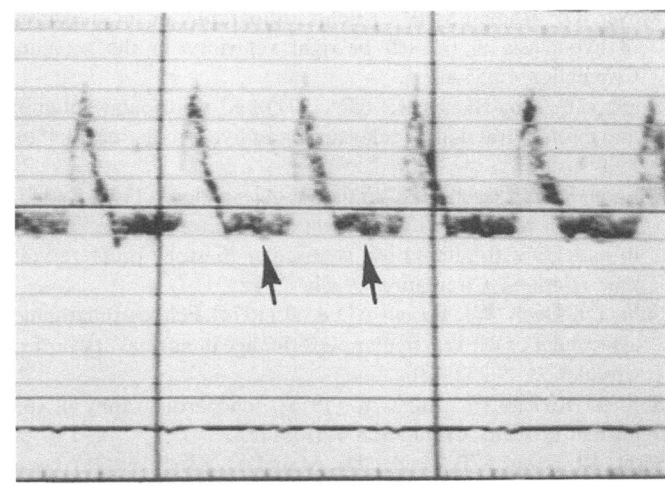

Bibliography

General References

Arvidsson H (1961) Angiocardiographic determination of left ventricular volume. Acta Radiol 56:321–339

Chung KJ, Alexson CG, Manning JA, Gramiak R (1973) Echocardiography in truncus arteriosus: The value of pulmonic valve detection. Circulation 48:281–286

Davis RH, Feigenbaum H, Chang S, Konecke LL, Dillon YC (1974) Echocardiographic manifestations of discrete subaortic stenosis. Am J Cardiol 33:277–280

Dodge HT, Sandler H, Ballew DW, Lord JD (1960) The use of biplane angiocardiography for the measurement of left ventricular volume in man. Am Heart J 60:762–776

Dodge HT, Sandler H, Baxley WA, Hawley RR (1960) Usefulness and limitations of radiographic methods for determining left ventricular volume. Am J Cardiol 18:10–24

Feigenbaum H (1981) Echocardiographic measurements and normal values: Echocardiography, 3rd ed. Lea & Febiger, Philadelphia, pp. 549–563

Fisher EA, Sepehari B, Lendrum B, Luken J, Sevitsky S (1981) Two dimensional echocardiographic visualization of the left coronary artery in anomalous origin of the left coronary artery from the pulmonary artery. Circulation 63:698–704

Folland ED, Parisi AF, Moynihan PF, Jones DR, Feldman CL, Tow DE (1979) Assessment of left ventricular ejection fraction and volumes by real-time, two dimensional echocardiography: A comparison of cine angiographic and radionuclide techniques. Circulation 60:760–766

Fortuin NJ, Hood WP, Craige E (1972) Evaluation of the left ventricular function by echocardiography. Circulation 46:26–35

Fortuin NJ, Hood WP, Sherman ME, Craige E (1971) Determination of left ventricular volumes by ultrasound. Circulation 44:575–584

Gibson DG (1971) Measurement of left ventricular volumes in man by echocardiography—Comparison with biplane angiographs. Br Heart J 33:614

Gillam LD, Hogan RD, Foale RA, Franklin TD, Newell JB, Guyer DE, Weyman AE (1984) A comparison of quantitative echocardiographic methods for delineating infarct-induced abnormal wall motion. Circulation 70:113–122

Goldberg SJ, Allen HD, Sahn DJ (1980) Pediatric and adolescent echocardiography; A handbook, 2nd ed. Yearbook, pp 435

Gramiak R, Shah PM, Kramer DH (1969) Ultrasound cardiography: Contrast studies in anatomy and function. Radiology 92:939–948

Griffith JM, Henry WL (1974) A sector scanner for real-time two-dimensional echocardiography. Circulation 49:1147–1152

Hagen AD, Deely WJ, Sahn D, Friedman WF (1973) Echocardiographic criteria for normal newborn infants. Circulation 48:1221–1226

Henry WL, DeMaria A, Gramiak R, King DL, Kisslo JA, Popp RL, Sahn DJ, Schiller NB, Tajik A, Teichholz LE, Weyman AE (1980) Report of the American Society of Echocardiography Committee on Nomenclature and Standards in Two-Dimensional Echocardiography. Circulation 62:212–217

Hirschfeld S, Meyer R, Schwartz DC, Korfhagen J, Kaplan S (1975) Measurement of left and right ventricular systolic time intervals by echocardiography. Circulation 51:304–309

Kaye HH, Tynan M, Hunter S (1975) Validity of echocardiographic estimates of ventricular size and performance in infants and children. Br Heart J 37:371–375

Kotler NM, Mintz GS, Segal BL, Parry WR (1980) Clinical uses of two-dimensional echocardiography. Am J Cardiol 45:1061–1082

La Corte M, Harada K, Williams RG (1976) Echocardiographic features of left ventricular inflow obstruction. Circulation 54:562–566

Levine RA, Gibson TC, Aretz T, Gillam LD, Guyer DE, King ME, Weyman AE (1984) Echocardiographic measurement of right ventricular volume. Circulation 69:497–505

Linhart JW, Mintz GS, Segal BL et al (1975) Left ventricular volume measurements of echocardiography. Fact or fiction? Am J Cardiol 36:114–118

Meyer RA, Stockert J, Kaplan S (1975) Echocardiographic determination of left ventricular volumes in pediatric patients. Circulation 51:297–303

Meyer RA, Schwartz DC, Covitz W et al (1974) Echocardiographic assessment of cardiac malposition. Am J Cardiol 33:896–903

Meyer RA, Kaplan S (1972) Echocardiography in the diagnosis of hypoplasia of the left or right ventricles in the neonate. Circulation 46:55–64

Pombo JF, Troy BL, Russel RO (1971) Left ventricular volumes and ejection fraction by echocardiography. Circulation 43:480–490

Quinones MA, Gasch WH, Waisser E, Alexander J (1974) Reduction in the rate of diastolic descent of the mitral valve echogram in patients with altered left ventricular diastolic pressure volume relations. Circulation 49:246–254

Sahn DJ, Deely WJ, Hagan AD et al (1974) Echocardiographic assessment of left ventricular performance in normal newborns. Circulation 49:232–236

Solinger R, Elbl F, Minhas K (1973) Echocardiography in the normal neonate. Circulation 47:108–118

Tajik AJ, Seward JB, Hagler DJ, Mair DD, Lie JT (1978) Two-dimensional real-time ultrasonic imaging of the heart and great vessels. Technique, image orientation, structure identification and validation. Mayo Clin Proc 53:271–303

Valdez-Cruz LM, Pieroni DR, Roland JM, Varghese PJ (1976) Echocardiographic detection of intracardiac right-to-left shunts following peripheral vein injections. Circulation 54:558–562

Von Ramm OT, Thurstone F (1976) Cardiac imaging using a phased array ultrasound system. Circulation 53:258–267

Weyman AE, Franklin TD, Hogan RD, Gillam LD, Wiske PS, Newell J, Gibbons EF, Foale RA (1984) Importance of temporal heterogeneity in assessing the contraction abnormalities associated with acute myocardial ischemia. Circulation 70:102–112

Zaky A, Nasser WK, Feigenbaum H (1968) A study of mitral valve action recorded by reflected ultrasound and its application in the diagnosis of mitral stenosis. Circulation 37:789–799

M-Mode Measurements

Baylen BG, Meyer RA, Kaplan S, Ringenburg WE, Korfhagen J (1975) The critically ill premature infant with patent ductus arteriosus and pulmonary disease—an echocardiographic assessment. J Pediatr 86:423–432

Baylen BG, Meyer RA, Korfhagen J, Benzing G, Bubb ME, Kaplan S (1977) Left ventricular performance in the critically ill premature infant with PDA and pulmonary disease. Circulation 55:182–188

Epstein ML, Goldberg SJ, Allen HD, Konecke L, Wood J (1975) Great vessel, cardiac chamber, and wall growth patterns in normal children. Circulation 51:1124–1129

Feigenbaum H (1981) Echocardiography, 3rd edition. Philadelphia, Lea and Febiger, pp 550–551

Goldberg SJ, Allen HD, Sahn DJ (eds) (1975): Pediatric and adolescent echocardiography, a handbook. Chicago, Year Book Medical Publishers, Inc.

Hagen AD, Deely WJ, Sahn D, Friedman WF (1973) Echocardiographic criteria for normal newborn infants. Circulation 48:1221–1226

Johnson GL, Breart GL, Gewitz MH, Brenner JI, Lang P, Dooley KJ, Ellison RC (1983) Echocardiographic characteristics of premature infants with patent ductus arteriosus. Pediatrics 72:864–871

Meyer RA (1977) Pediatric echocardiography. Philadelphia, Lea and Febiger, pp 69, 292

Meyer RA, Kaplan S (1972) Echocardiography in the diagnosis of hypoplasia of the left or right ventricles in the neonate. Circulation 46:55–64

Meyer RA, Stockert J, Kaplan S (1975) Echographic determination of left ventricular volumes in pediatric patients. Circulation 51:297–303

Sahn DJ, Deely WJ, Hagen AD, Friedman WF (1974) Echocardiographic assessment of left ventricular performance in normal newborns. Circulation 49:232–236

Silverman NH, Lewis AB, Heymann MA, Rudolph AM (1974) Echocardiographic assessment of ductus arteriosus shunt in premature infants. Circulation 50:821–825

Solinger R, Elbl F, Minhas K (1973) Echocardiography in the normal neonate. Circulation 47:108–118

Doppler Echocardiography

Abbasi AS, Allen MW, DeCristofaro D, Ungar I (1980) Detection and estimation of the degree of mitral regurgitation by range-gated pulsed Doppler echocardiography. Circulation 61:143–147

Alverson DC, Edridge M, Dillon T, Yobek SM, Berman W (1982) Noninvasive pulsed Doppler determination of cardiac output in neonates and children. J Pediatr 101:46–50

Baker DW (1970) Pulsed untrasonic Doppler blood flow sensing. IEEE Trans Sonics-Ultrasonics SU 17(3):170

Barker FE, Baker DW, Nation AW, Strandness DE, Jr. Reid JM (1974) Ultrasonic duplex echo Doppler scanner. IEEE Trans Biomed Eng BME-21(2):109

Barron JV, Sahn DJ, Valdes-Cruz LM, Lima CO, Goldberg SJ, Grenadier E, Allen HD (1984) Clinical utility of two-dimensional Doppler echocardiographic techniques for estimating pulmonary to systemic blood flow ratios in children with left to right shunting atrial septal defect, ventricular septal defect or patent ductus arteriosus. J Am Col Cardiol 3:169–178

Berger M, Berdoff RL, Gallerstein PE, Goldberg E (1984) Evaluation of aortic stenosis by continuous wave ultrasound. J Am Col Cardiol 3:150–156

Brodersen RW, Hewes CR, Buss DD (1976) A 500 stage CCD transversal filter for spectral analysis. IEEE Trans. (CHIRP-Z transform) Electron Dev. ED 23:143–152

DeKnecht S, Daniels O, Reneman RS (1983) Non-invasive assessment of pulmonary valve stenosis with a multigate pulsed Doppler system. Br Heart J 50:592–593

Diebold B, Peronneau P, Blanchard D, Colonna G, Guermonprez JL, Forman J, Sellier P, Maurice P (1983) Non-invasive quantification of aortic regurgitation by Doppler echocardiography. Br Heart J 49:167–173

Diebold B, Touati R, Blanchard D, Colonna G, Guermonprez JL, Peronneau P, Forman J, Maurice P (1983) Quantitiative assessment of tricuspid regurgitation using pulsed Doppler echocardiography. Br Heart J 50:443–449

Doppler CJ (1842) Uber das farbige Licht der Doppelsterne. Abhandlungen der Koniglishen Bohmischen Gesellschaft der Wissenchoften II:465

Esper RJ (1982) Detection of mild aortic regurgitation by range-gated pulsed Doppler echocardiography. Am J Cardiol 50:1037–1043

Fisher DC, Sahn DJ, Friedman MJ, Larson D, Valdes-Cruz LM, Horowitz S, Goldberg SJ, Allen HD (1983) The mitral valve orifice method for noninvasive two-dimensional echo Doppler determinations of cardiac output. Circulation 67:872–877

Franklin DL, Schlegel W, Rushmer RF (1961) Blood flow measured by Doppler frequency shift of backscattered ultrasound. Science 134:564–565

Gentile R, Stevenson G, Dooley T, Franklin D, Kawabori I,

Pearlman A (1981) Pulsed Doppler echocardiographic determination of time ductal closure in normal newborn infants. J Pediatr 98:443–448

Goldberg SJ, Allen HD, Marx GR, Flinn CJ (1985) Doppler echocardiography. Philadelphia, Lea and Febiger, pp 33–54

Grenadier E, Sahn DJ, Valdes-Cruz LM, Allen HD, Lima CO, Goldberg SJ (1984) Two-dimensional echo Doppler study of congenital disorders of the mitral valve. Am Heart J 107:319–325

Hatle L, Angelsen B (1985) Doppler ultrasound in cardiology. Lea and Febiger, Philadelphia, p 93

Hatle L, Brubakk A, Tromsdal A, Angelsen B (1978) Noninvasive assessment of pressure drop in mitral stenosis by Doppler ultrasound. Br Heart J 40:131–140

Hatle L, Angelsen B, Tromsdal A (1979) Noninvasive assessment of atrioventricular pressure half-time by Doppler ultrasound. Circulation 60:1096–1104

Hatle L (1984) Noninvasive methods of measuring pulmonary artery pressure and flow velocity. Cardiology, an international perspective. Plenum Press, New York, p 783–790

Jenkins GM, Watt DG (1968) Spectral analysis. London, Holden Day

Kitabatake A, Masuyama T, Asao M, Tanouchi J, Morita T, Ito H, Hori M, Inoue M, Abe H (1983) Color visualization of intracardiac flow abnormalities by multigated Doppler technique. In: Spencer M (Ed): Cardiac doppler diagnosis. The Hague, Martinus Nijhoff, pp. 309–318

Kitabatake A, Inoue M, Asao M, Ito H, Masuyama T, Tanouchi J, Morita T, Hori M, Yoshima H, Ohnishi K, Abe H (1984) Noninvasive evaluation of the ratio of pulmonary to systemic flow in atrial septal defect by duplex Doppler echocardiography. Circulation 69:73–79

Kosturakis D, Goldberg SJ, Allen HD, Loeber C (1984) Doppler echocardiographic prediction of pulmonary arterial hypertension in congenital heart disease. Am J Cardiol 53:1110–1115

Lima CO, Sahn DJ, Valdes-Cruz LM, Allen HD, Goldberg SJ, Grenadier E, Barron JV (1983) Prediction of the severity of left ventricular outflow tract obstruction by quantitative two-dimensional echocardiographic Doppler studies. Circulation 68:348–354

Lima CO, Sahn DJ, Valdes-Cruz LM, Goldberg SJ, Barron JV, Allen HD, Grenadier E (1983) Noninvasive prediction of transvalvular pressure gradient in patients with pulmonary stenosis by quantitative two-dimensional echocardiographic Doppler studies. Circulation 67:866–871

McDonald DA, Helps EPW (1959) Streamline flow in veins. London, Wellcome Foundation Film Library. Quoted by: Berman W, Jr. (1983) Pulsed Doppler ultrasound in clinical pediatrics. New York, Futura Publishing Co., p 45

Magnin PA, Stewart JA, Myers S, Von Ramm O, Kisslo JA (1981) Combined Doppler and phased-array echocardiographic estimation of cardiac output. Circulation 63:388–392

Martin CG, Snider AR, Katz SM, Peabody JL, Brady JP (1982) Abnormal cerebral blood flow patterns in preterm infants with a large patent ductus arteriosus. J Pediatr 101:587–593

Meijboom EJ, Valdez-Cruz LM, Horowitz S, Sahn DJ, Larson DF, Young KA, Oliveira Lima C, Goldberg SJ (1983) A two-dimensional Doppler echocardiographic method for calculation of pulmonary and systemic blood flow in a canine model with a variable-size left-to-right extracardiac shunt. Circulation 68:437–445

Meyer RA, Kalavathy A, Korfhagen JC, Kaplan S (1982) Comparison of left to right shunt ratios determined by pulsed Doppler/2D-echo (DOP/2D) and Fick method. Circulation 66 (Suppl II): 232 (abstract)

Miyatake K, Okamoto M, Kinoshita N, Ohta M, Kozuka T, Sakakibara H, Nimura Y (1982) Evaluation of tricuspid regurgitation by pulsed Doppler and two-dimensional echocardiography. Circulation 66:777–784

Oliveira Lima C, Sahn DJ, Valdez-Cruz LM, Allen HD, Goldberg SJ, Grenadier E, Vargas-Barron J (1983) Prediction of the severity of left ventricular outflow tract obstruction by quantative two-dimensional echocardiographic Doppler studies. Circulation 68:348–354

Oliveira Lima C, Sahn DJ, Valdez-Cruz LM, Goldberg SJ, Vargas-Barron J, Allen HD, Grenadier E (1983) Noninvasive prediction of transvalvular pressure gradient in patients with pulmonary stenosis by quantitive two-dimensional echo Doppler studies. Circulation 67:866–871

Patel AK, Rowe GG, Thomsen JH, Dhanani SP, Kosolcharoen P, Lyle LE, Thomsen JH (1982) Pulsed Doppler echocardiography in diagnosis of pulmonary regurgitation: Its value and limitations. Am J Cardiol 49:1801–1805

Quinones MA, Young JB, Waggoner AD, Ostojec MC, Ribeiro LGT, Miller RR (1980) Assessment of pulsed Doppler echocardiography in detection and quantitation of aortic and mitral regurgitation. Br Heart J 44:612–620

Rabiner LR, Gold B (1975) Theory and application of digital signal processing. Englewood Cliffs, N.J., Prentice Hall (Fast Fourier Transform)

Serwer GA, Armstrong BE, Anderson PAW (1980) Noninvasive detection of retrograde descending aortic flow in infants using continuous wave Doppler ultrasonography. J Pediatr 97:394–400

Shub C, Dimopoulos IN, Seward JB, Callahan JA, Tancredi RG, Schattenberg TT, Reeder GS, Hagler DJ, Tajik AJ (1983) Sensitivity of two-dimensional echocardiography in the direct visualization of atrial septal defect utilizing the subcostal approach: Experience with 154 patients. J AM Col Cardiol 2:127–135

Stamm BR, Martin RP (1984) Quantification of pressure gradients across stenotic valves by Doppler ultrasound. J Am Col Cardiol 2:707–718

Stevenson JG, Kawabori I, Guntheroth WG, Dooley TK, Dillard DH (1979) Pulsed Doppler echocardiographic detection of obstruction of systemic venous return after repair of transposition of the great arteries. Circulation 60:1091–1095

Stevenson JH, Kawabori I, Dooley TK, Guntheroth WG (1978) Diagnosis of ventricular septal defect by pulsed Doppler echocardiography. Sensitivity, specificity, and limitations. Circulation 58:322–326

Valdes-Cruz LM, Horowitz S, Mesel E, Sahn DJ, Fisher DC, Larson D (1984) A pulsed Doppler echocardiographic method for calculating pulmonary and systemic blood flow in atrial level shunts: validation studies in animals and initial human experience. Circulation 69:80–86

3 Cardiovascular Nuclear Medicine

Richard M. Steingart and John P. Wexler

Principles of Cardiovascular Nuclear Medicine

The development of radionuclide imaging systems, low energy and easily available isotopes, and small dedicated minicomputers for the acquisition and processing of nuclear medicine data were necessary conditions for the new field of cardiovascular nuclear medicine. This new field combines the imaging of radiology with the quantitative capacities of nuclear medicine to provide a noninvasive means for serial evaluation of the anatomy and physiology of the cardiovascular system. This chapter will describe the field of cardiovascular nuclear medicine, detailing both the methodology and applications.

Acquisition and Analysis of Data

Detection Devices. In theory, data obtained by cardiovascular nuclear medicine may be acquired by any device capable of detecting gamma rays. In practice, three devices are used: the Anger camera, the multicrystal camera and probes. Both the Anger camera and the multicrystal camera are imaging devices capable of producing numerical and visual information, while the probe is a nonimaging device used only for determining quantitative information.

All three devices detect photons in the same way. A photon (or gamma ray) strikes a sodium iodide crystal that is optically coupled to a photomultiplier tube (Fig. 3–1). This excites the crystal and causes a small burst of light to be emitted by the crystal. The intensity of that emitted light is proportional to the energy of the photon striking the crystal. The photomultiplier tube, excited by the light from the crystal, generates a voltage that is proportional to the energy of the gamma ray that struck the crystal. A counter then integrates the rate at which the photomultiplier tube is being excited. This integral corresponds to the number of photons per second striking the detector.

The Anger camera (Fig. 3–2) is composed of a single crystal ¼–½ in. thick and 7–15 in. in diameter. Either 37 or 61 photomultiplier tubes in hexagonal array are interfaced to the back of the crystal. When a photon strikes the face of the Anger camera, light is detected only by those photomultiplier tubes in the proximity of the excited crystal segment. Thus, not only is the photon detected, but its site of origin is localized. The major advantages of the Anger camera are its imaging qualities. Because only a single continuous crystal is used, images may be obtained from the camera with extremely high resolution.

The multicrystal camera (Fig. 3–3) is a rectangular array of multiple 1 cm × 1 cm sodium iodide crystals. The light output of each crystal is detected by a group of photomultiplier tubes in a manner that enables localization of events to a single crystal. The major advantage of the multicrystal camera is its ability to accept significantly higher count

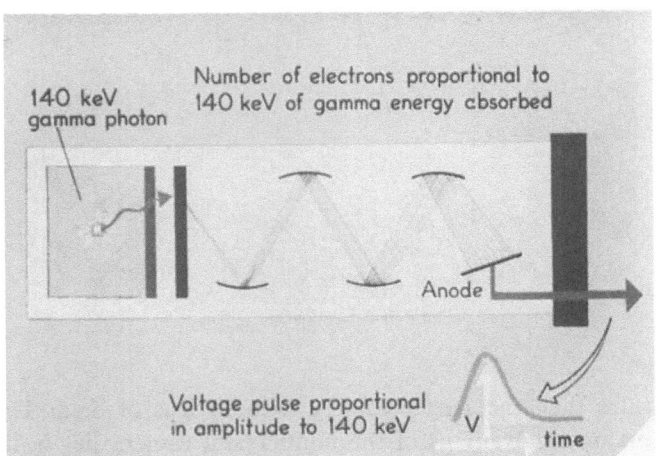

Fig. 3–1. *The conversion of gamma photon emission into an electrical impulse.* A gamma photon (in this schematic, 140 keV in energy) strikes the crystal. Light from the crystal is detected by the photomultiplier tube. The photomultiplier tube produces electrons whose numbers are proportional to the energy of the gamma photon. The voltage of the pulse produced by the anode of the photomultiplier tube is proportional to the energy of the photon that struck the crystal. Reproduced with permission of the Editors, and Nuclear Associates, Inc.

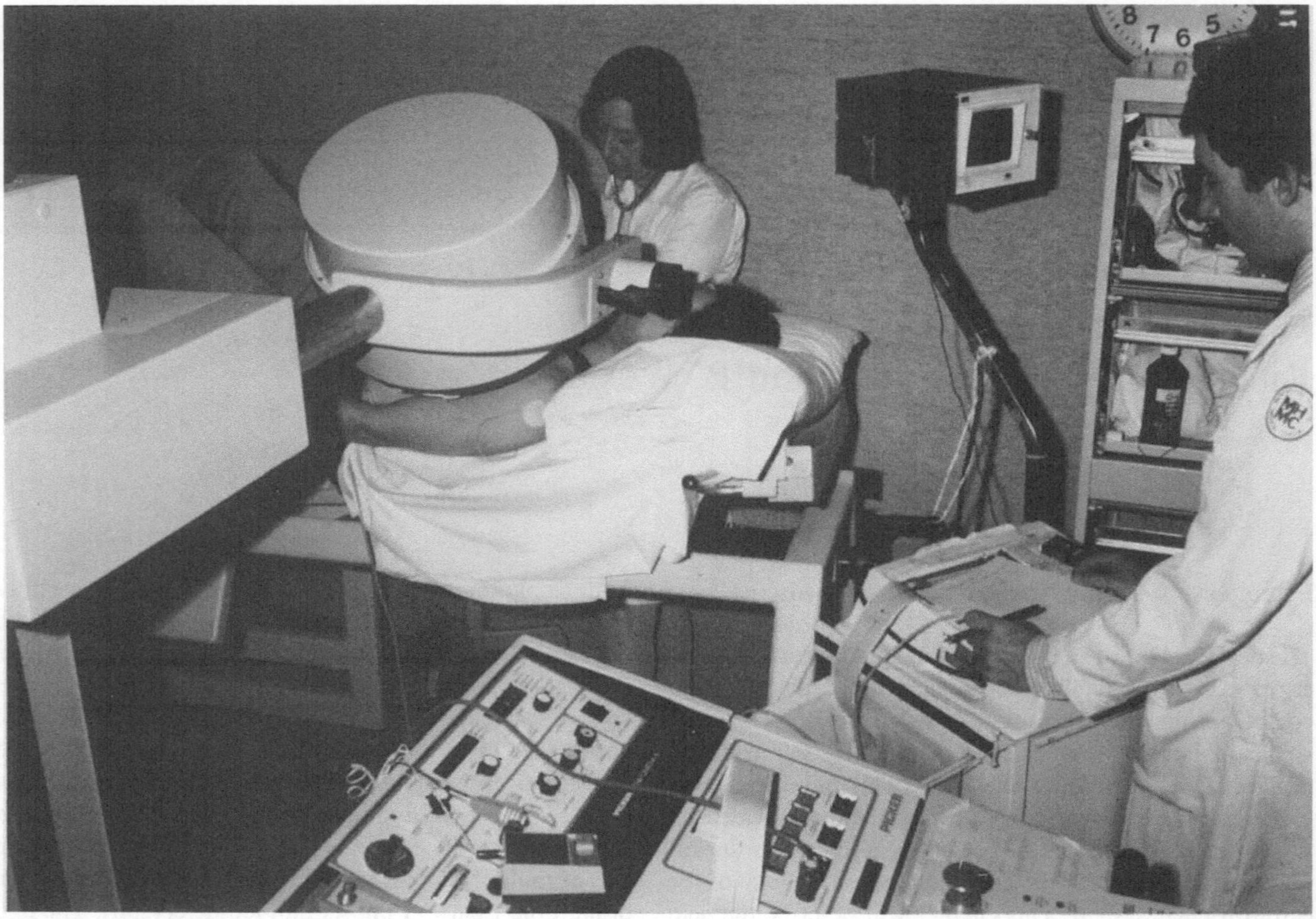

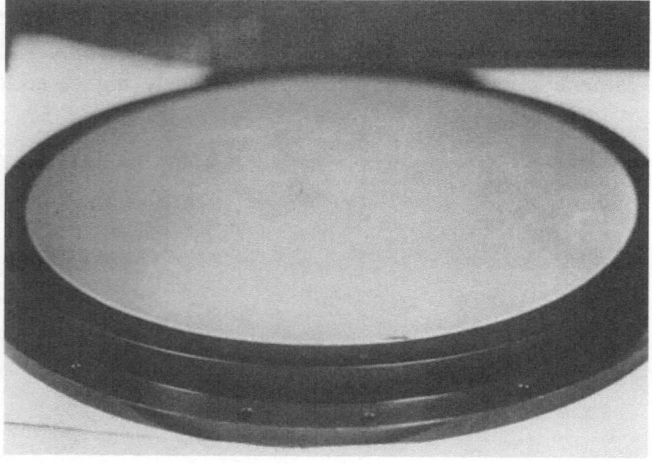

A

B

Fig. 3–2. **A** *Portable Anger camera.* LAO position preparatory to supine gated radionuclide ventriculography. **B** *Anger camera crystal.* The collimator is removed; the crystal is circular, 15 in. in diameter.

rates than the Anger camera without loss of data. The major disadvantage of the multicrystal camera lies in its spatial resolution being less than that obtained with the Anger camera.

The nonimaging scintillation probe (Fig. 3–4) has a single crystal about 2 in. in diameter with a single photomultiplier tube. Because the probe has only a single photomultiplier tube, no spatial information is available; however, probe systems are more sensitive than either the Anger camera or the multicrystal camera and are thus able to be used for cardiovascular nuclear medicine with amounts

of isotope smaller (20%) than the other imaging devices use.

The Anger camera can be utilized for both thallium and technetium imaging. The multicrystal camera is used only for first-pass determinations of left ventricular function, while probe systems can be used either for first-pass or gated determination of left ventricular function.

Photons originating from within the patient are subject to interaction with tissue on their path out of the body. This interaction can change the energy level of the photon and deflect its path. Thus photons may appear to originate

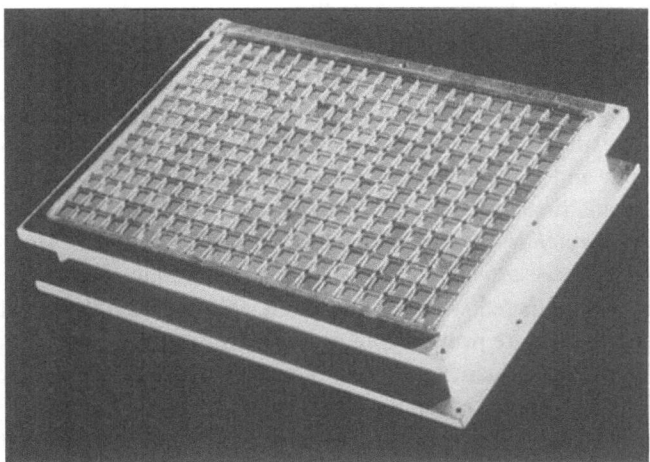

Fig. 3–3. *Scintillation detector of a multicrystal camera.* Note the 294 individual, square crystals that make up the rectangular detector array. Each square is an individual crystal. Courtesy of Baird Atomic, Inc., Valley Stream, New York.

from a source removed from their site of origin. To ensure accurate localization of photon sources, all detection devices described in the foregoing use both collimation and pulse height analysis. A collimator is a lead shield with multiple holes, placed in front of the detection device. These holes and the lead between them effectively allow only photons arising perpendicular to the face of the detecting device to strike the sodium iodide crystal, thus eliminating the detection of photons that are scattered within the body. The smaller the diameter of the holes in the collimator, the greater the spatial resolution of the imaging system. Simultaneously, the smaller the diameter of the collimator hole, the less sensitive is the imaging device. Probe systems are equipped with conical wide-bore collimators to enable high sensitivity at the cost of spatial resolution.

The pulse height analyzer examines the magnitude of the voltage arising from the photomultiplier tubes. The voltage is directly proportional to the frequency of light emanating from the crystal, which in turn is proportional to the energy of the interacting photon. Since photons lose energy as they interact within the body, by accepting photons whose energy levels are within 15%–20% of the normal energy of the emitted photons, the pulse height analyzer reduces the probability that an accepted photon represents scatter.

Radiopharmaceuticals A radiopharmaceutical used for cardiovascular nuclear medicine ideally should satisfy the following criteria: (1) It should produce only gamma rays or x-rays that are energetic enough to penetrate overlying tissue with minimal scatter and attenuation but whose energy is limited so as to be easily detected with available devices; (2) its effective (physical and biological) half-life is long enough to allow reasonable time for measurements but not so long as to create an undue radiation burden to the patient; and (3) either by itself or combined with another radiopharmaceutical it is able to localize predominantly in the structures to be studied with little or no localization in adjacent structures. Such localization may be functional or anatomical. Of the available radiopharmaceuticals, technetium-99m and thallium-201 best meet these criteria for cardiovascular imaging.

Technetium 99m. Technetium 99m is the daughter of molybdenum 99, with a half-life of 6 hours and with the positive attribute of emitting a single 140 keV photon that is highly abundant. These two properties—a short half-life and easy availability—are desirable for cardiovascular nuclear medicine as well as for general nuclear medicine imaging. Technetium 99m is eluted from the molybdenum 99 generator as the monovalent anion TcO_4^- (pertechnetate), which does not satisfy criterion 3 above because it does not selectively localize to structures being studied. Technetium 99m must therefore be combined with a suitable carrier for use in cardiovascular nuclear medicine imaging. Technetium 99m (^{99m}Tc) is used for equilibrium blood pool imaging when bound to red blood cells or human serum albumin. ^{99m}Tc is also utilized for first-pass imaging, either as pertechnetate or bound to substrates such as DPTA (diethyltriamine-pentaacetic acid) or sulfur colloid. For the avid imaging of myocardial infarctions it is administered as technetium Tc 99m pyrophosphate. When bound to pyrophosphate the complex is cleared rapidly through the kidneys, and a small fraction of the dose localizes in the infarcted tissue earlier than in the skeleton. Therefore, such imaging is performed 1–3 hours after injection, allowing time for blood clearance and localization in an infarct before marked skeletal uptake occurs. Although the mechanism of uptake is controversial, adequate blood flow to deliver the agent is a necessary condition.

Thallium 201. Thallium 201 is the daughter of lead 201, which is produced by cyclotron bombardment of thallium 203. Thallium 201 has a half-life of 73 hours and decays to mercury, producing mercury x-rays from 69–80 keV, with less abundant gamma peaks at 137 and 165 keV. These 69–80 keV x-rays are of low energy, and therefore the probability of scatter or attenuation within the body is great.

The hydrated radius of the thallous cation closely approximates that of potassium, and it appears that accumulation of thallium by myocardium is related to potassium active transport into the myocardium. In addition, thallium is known to be a potent competitive inhibitor of myocardial membrane sodium-potassium adenosine triphosphatase (ATPase). Although differences exist between the transport of potassium and thallium, myocardial accumulation of thallium 201 is directly proportional to myocardial blood flow, with a high extraction fraction.

The linear relationship between myocardial blood flow and myocardial accumulation of thallium forms the basis of the ability for thallium to distinguish among normally perfused myocardium, hypoperfused myocardium (resting or exercise induced) and infarcted myocardium. Normally perfused myocardium accumulates thallium uniformly. Accumulation of thallium in hypoperfused or infarcted myocardium is markedly less than in surrounding normal tissue.

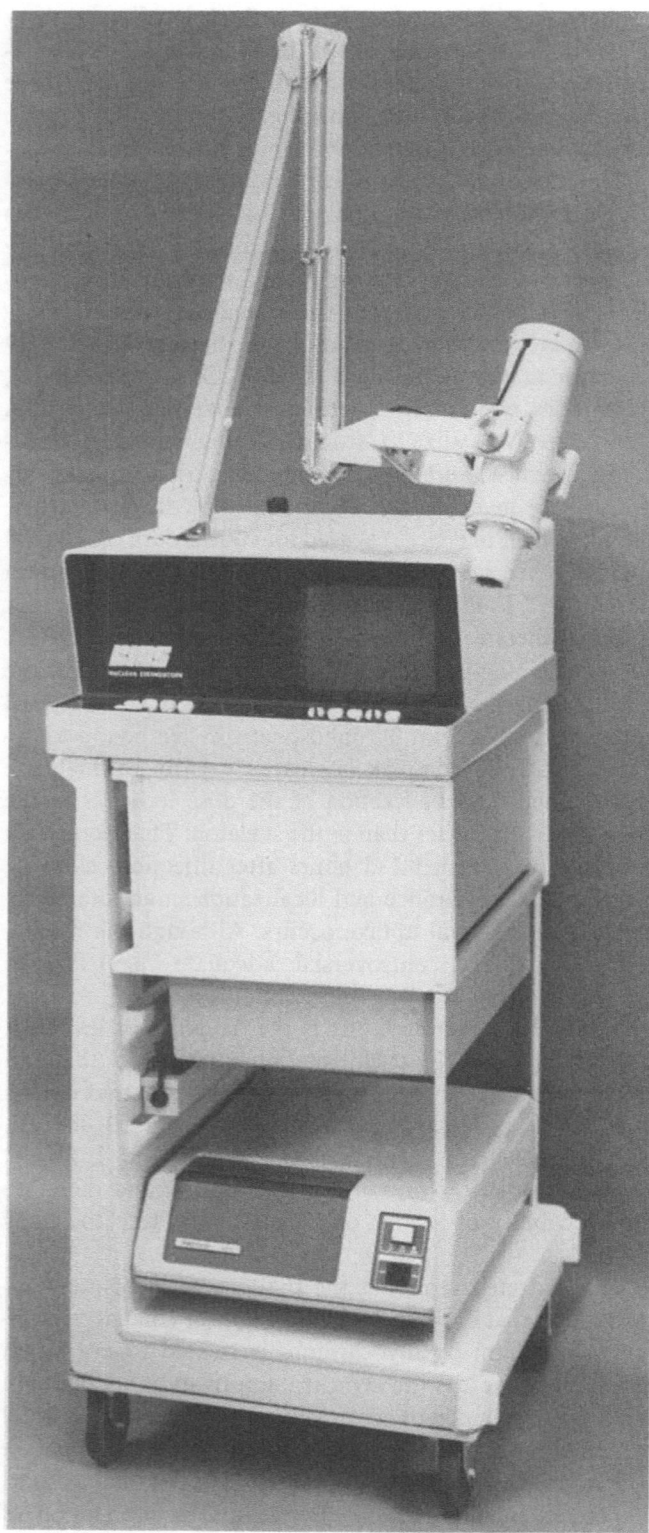

Fig. 3–4. *A nonimaging, gated, scintigraphic probe.* Note that this device is mobile. The single crystal probe detector is suspended from a free-moving arm that allows the probe detector to be positioned in space. The console contains a small video screen for the display of data as well as controls for acquisition and processing of information by the self-contained microcomputer. A video copier is seen on the bottom of the cart, permitting copies of the studies to be made. The system depicted is the Nuclear Stethoscope™ Cardiac Probe, a trademark of Bios Inc., Valhalla, New York.

The disadvantages of thallium are: (1) its low energy, which results in significant distortion due to scatter; (2) the low ratio of target (myocardium) to background (e.g., lung, diaphragm, skeletal muscle); and (3) its high cost.

Usual doses and radiation burden for patients given thallium and technetium are presented in Table 3–1.

Acquisition of Data and Data-Processing Methods.
Radionuclide Angiography—Gated and First-pass Methods. The essential principle of this technique is that the counts detected within the various chambers of the heart at any time are proportional to the volume of that chamber. The various quantitative parameters describing ventricular function are based on this assumption.

The most commonly determined parameter is the left ventricular ejection fraction, which represents the percentage of the left ventricular volume ejected during systole and thus acts as an index of the efficiency of contraction of the ventricle. Left ventricular ejection fraction is defined by the formula $LVEF = (EDV - ESV)/EDV$ where LVEF = left ventricular ejection fraction and EDV and ESV = end-diastolic and end-systolic volumes respectively.

Two distinct methods have evolved for determining ventricular function parameters by the use of cardiovascular nuclear medicine techniques: The first-pass technique and the equilibrium technique. In the first-pass technique a bolus of isotope is injected intravenously. Images of the precordium are obtained at a frame rate (usually 50 msec/frame), which is rapid enough to detect the changes in ventricular volume over a series of systoles. As the isotope traverses the chambers of the heart it is diluted by nonlabeled blood. Isotope does not appear in the left ventricle until after it has cleared the right ventricle. This temporal separation is used to isolate events within the left ventricle from the remainder of the heart (see Fig. 3–5). Corresponding information from several sequential cardiac cycles during the peak concentration of isotope within the ventricle is added and a representative cycle developed. This representative cycle permits calculation of the ejection fraction after appropriate correction for extraventricular counts.

In contrast, the gated technique uses isotope that has achieved equilibrium within the blood pool, accounting for the designation of equilibrium or gated blood pool scanning (GBPS). For determination of ejection fraction by this method, precordial images are obtained in the left anterior oblique projection, which best segregates right from left ventricular activity. Because the counts within the ventricle at any time are small with this method, it is necessary to add corresponding segments of as many as several hundred sequential heart beats to acquire enough counting data for achievement of statistical accuracy. This study is accomplished in the following manner: It is assumed that at equilibrium mechanical events within the heart are reproducible and that these mechanical events can be coupled with the ECG. Acquisition of the precordial image is therefore synchronized to the QRS complex. Each cardiac cycle is divided into segments (usually 16–32), and the data from each segment are held discretely within com-

Table 3–1. Usual Doses and Radiation Burden with Thallium and Technetium

Agent	Usual administered dose (mCi)	Radiation dose (rads)	
		Target organ(s)	Whole body
^{201}Tl	1.5	2.2 (kidney)	0.36
^{99m}Tc Pyrophosphate	15	0.68 (bone)	0.65
^{99m}Tc Red blood cells	20	1.5, 0.66 (heart, marrow)	0.38

puter memory. When the next QRS complex is detected, corresponding segments are added to the relevant existing data within the memory. This part of the study permits a sequence of images to be acquired that have adequate counting data to provide statistically valid visual and numerical information. When gated studies are acquired in the LAO projection, separation of counts from the two ventricles occurs. Such data, however, may be acquired in any projection. Because gated studies may be presented in cine format it is possible by using multiple views to visualize and evaluate regional wall motion.

Advantages and disadvantages exist in each of the methods. First-pass angiography permits visualization of the right and left ventricle with little or no overlapping of adjacent structures. Gated angiography requires positioned segregation of the ventricles, which may be difficult or impossible to achieve by the first-pass technique. A single first-pass study may be performed with as little as 10 mCi of isotope, whereas gated studies are often performed with 20–30 mCi of isotope; however, the gated study permits repetitive determinations with no additional isotope needed for each acquisition. This difference between the two methods is particularly important when interventional studies are performed that require multiple acquisitions.

In patients with reduced cardiac output (e.g., congestive heart failure), dilution of the bolus may impede first-pass scanning, while the gated study is usually free from this constraint. On the other hand, the gated study is dependent on a stable ventricular rhythm; first-pass techniques are less dependent. Finally, whereas the gated study can be performed using a standard Anger camera, the first-pass study is best performed on a multicrystal camera. As indicated in the foregoing, the multicrystal camera is not optimal for imaging, usually being dedicated to first-pass radionuclide angiography. Since this chapter emphasizes radionuclide cardiovascular anatomy, the discussion will center on gated methods, which provide better spatial resolution.

^{201}Tl Scintigraphy. ^{201}Tl scintigraphy is usually performed with stress testing. After ^{201}Tl injection at peak stress, continued maximal exercise is important to ensure myocardial distribution of ^{201}Tl when flow disparity is most marked in patients with obstructive coronary artery disease. Soon after injection, distribution is proportionate to regional blood flow; ^{201}Tl then "redistributes" proportionately to myocardial mass. Therefore, imaging should begin as soon as possible after exercise (5 minutes or less). Storage of

data should include both photographic film and digital computer memory for image enhancement. Counts of 300,000–600,000 per image are obtained, effecting a compromise between completion of multiple views prior to significant redistribution and statistical validity. Studies are then repeated several hours later to assess redistribution.

Computer enhancement of ^{201}Tl images probably increases the accuracy of the technique. Since ^{201}Tl is a physiological flow marker, computer processing of images should be geared to reflect myocardial ^{201}Tl kinetics. However, the myocardial images obtained in vivo reflect background as well as myocardial kinetics. Several conflicting methods for background analysis have been proposed, ranging from no correction to 20% count subtraction or weighted interpolated background correction. It is safe to say that the ideal method has yet to be developed. Currently empiric validation of these methods versus catheterization standards for coronary artery disease should be used.

Technetium Tc 99m Pyrophosphate Imaging of Infarcts. Imaging is started 1–3 hours after injection, with data being acquired on photographic film with images in the anterior, left anterior oblique and left lateral projections. Although computer algorithms are available for rib and blood pool subtraction, most centers rely on interpretation of photographic images (see section, Myocardial Infarction: Technetium 99m Pyrophosphate).

Normal Anatomy

Radionuclide angiocardiography is a noninvasive method of viewing the blood pool, providing structural insight into the central circulation. As outlined in the foregoing, standard techniques include first-pass and equilibrium blood pool scanning. Although offering less optimal spatial resolution, first-pass imaging can clearly delineate individual cardiac chambers and great vessels through temporal separation.

Radionuclide Angiography *First-Pass Scanning.* Figure 3–5 traces the transit of a compact ^{99}Tc bolus (< 0.5 cc) in the anterior projection from a peripheral injection. The bolus is first detected in the right innominate vein and superior vena cava, and next entering the right atrium and right ventricle, which is pyramid shaped. The pulmonary phase follows. The final phase is entry into the left atrium via the pulmonary veins, left ventricle and aorta.

The quality of first-pass studies is critically dependent on the rapid transit of a finite volume of tracer through the circulation. Factors that prolong transit time or disrupt

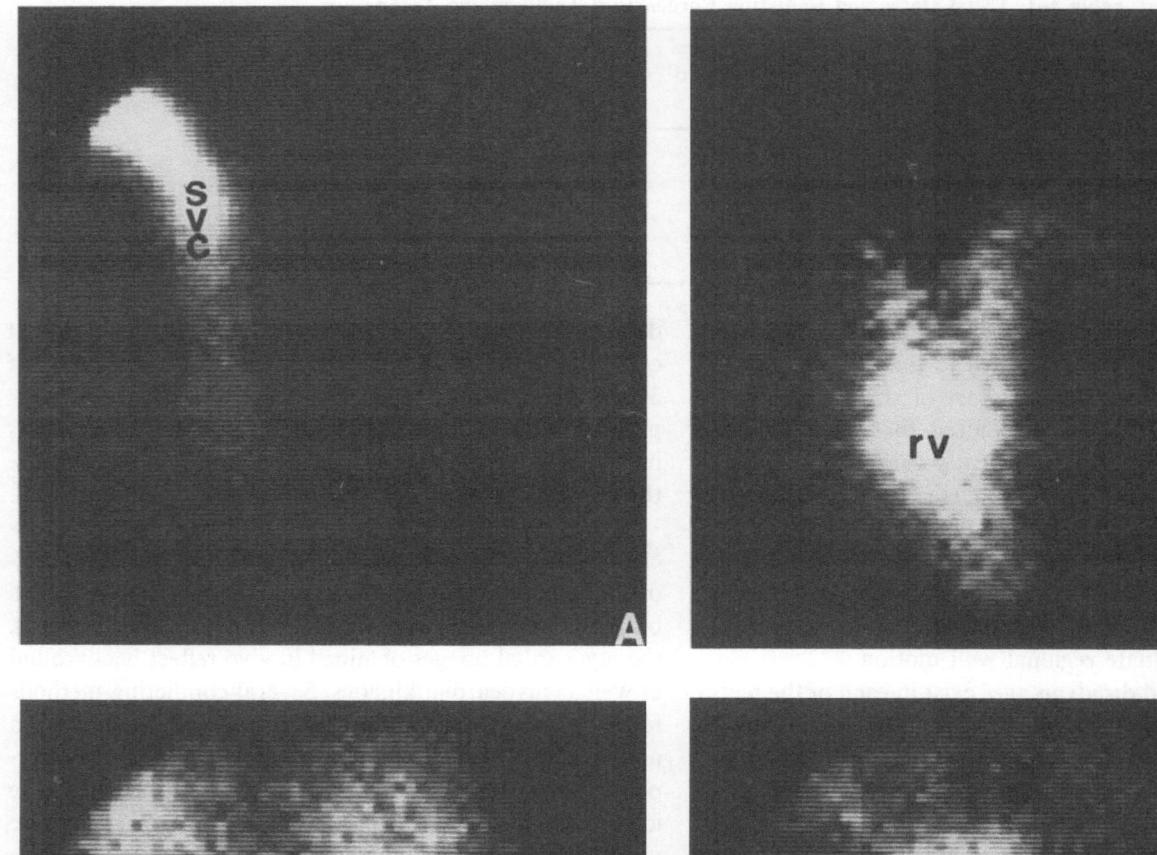

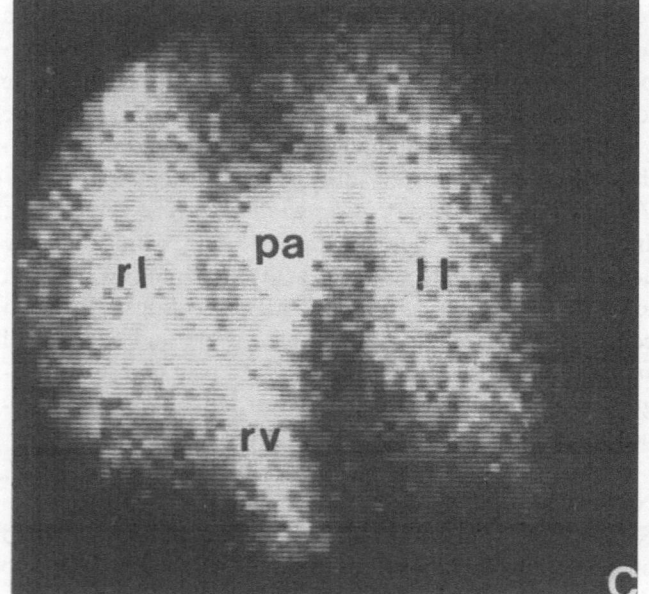

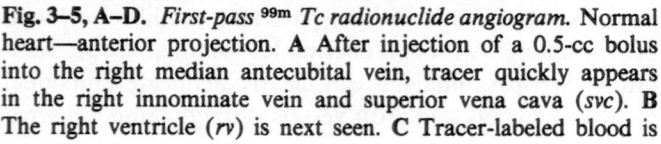

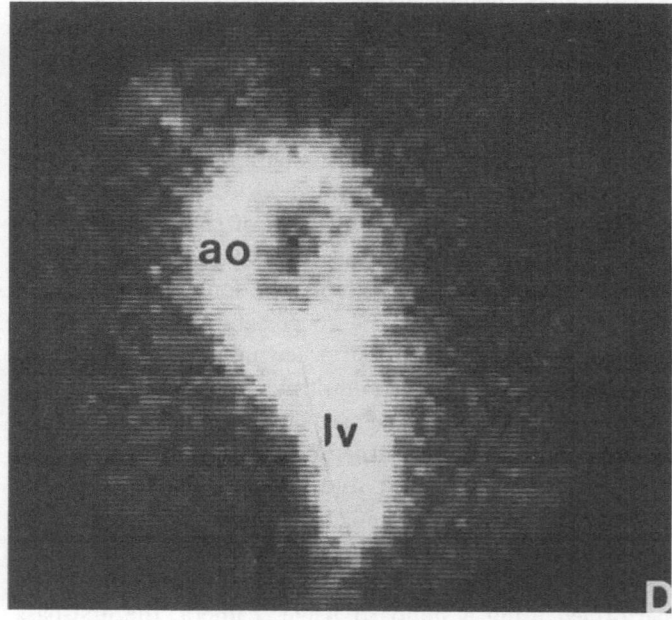

Fig. 3–5, A–D. *First-pass* ^{99m} *Tc radionuclide angiogram.* Normal heart—anterior projection. **A** After injection of a 0.5-cc bolus into the right median antecubital vein, tracer quickly appears in the right innominate vein and superior vena cava (*svc*). **B** The right ventricle (*rv*) is next seen. **C** Tracer-labeled blood is ejected into the pulmonary artery (*pa*) and right and left lungs (*rl* and *ll*). **D** Tracer clears from the right side of the heart and the lungs as the left ventricle (*lv*) and aorta (*ao*) are observed in isolation.

the bolus impair the temporal separation of cardiac structures and reduce the value of this technique.[5] Tricuspid regurgitation is a prime offender as the tracer washes in and out of the right atrium, mixing with a large volume of nonlabeled blood while fragments of the now diluted bolus are transported to the pulmonary arteries and left-sided circulation. Therefore no single chamber is outlined in temporal isolation (Fig. 3–6). Mitral regurgitation will produce similar overlap of image during the levophase, with isotope simultaneously in the left atrium, left ventricle

and aorta for much of the study. Overt low-output states will simulate these effects, as the bolus may trail out into a larger volume of blood while the isotope slowly traverses the central circulation. If visualization of left-sided chambers alone is desired, injection of the isotope directly into the pulmonary artery via the distal port of a Swan-Ganz catheter may enhance results. Figure 3–7 shows such an injection into the right pulmonary artery in the LAO projection.

Raw data from first-pass studies (collected in list mode)

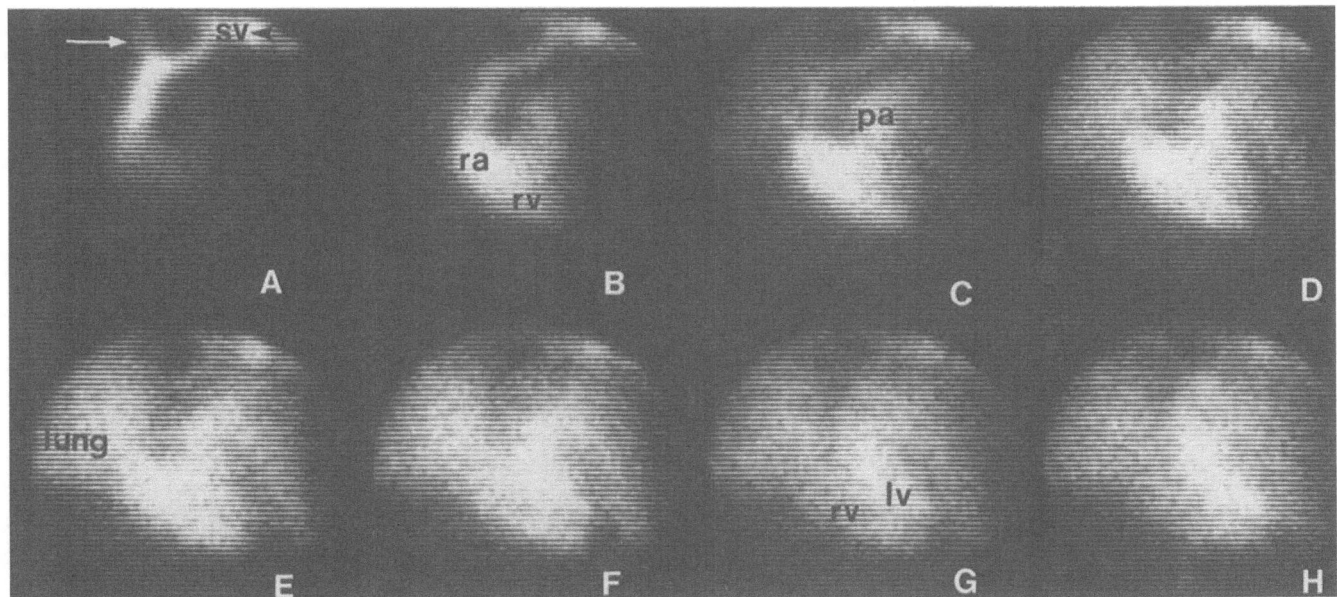

Fig. 3–6, A–H. *Tricuspid regurgitation.* First-pass ⁹⁹ᵐTC radionuclide angiogram from a patient whose tricuspid valve was surgically removed—anterior projection. **A** After injection of a bolus into the left median antecubital vein, tracer is noted in the left subclavian vein (*sv*), left innominate vein and superior vena cava. *White arrow* indicates systolic reflux into contralateral innominate vein, a consistent finding in severe tricuspid regurgitation. **B** Right atrium (*ra*) and right ventricle (*rv*) are identified. **C–E** Tracer in pulmonary artery (*pa*) and lung. **F–H** Tracer enters left heart and aorta, but persistence of tracer is obvious in right atrium, right ventricle and lung.

can be reformatted into gated studies allowing visualization of selected chambers over the course of the cardiac cycle. Such studies provide morphological information similar to that obtained from equilibrium blood pool scanning but

with less count density and therefore less statistical reliability. Nonetheless this method is valuable because it can generate images limited to the right or left side of the heart (Fig. 3–8).

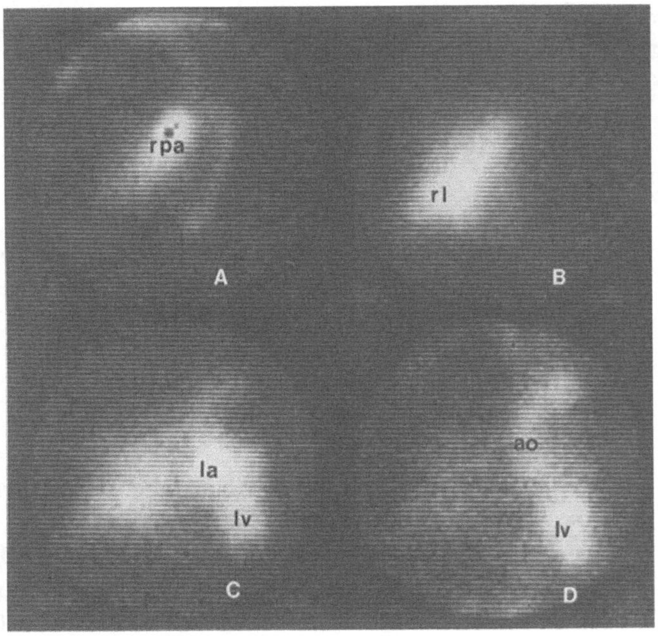

Gated Blood Pool Scanning. With gated blood pool scanning a composite picture of all thoracic blood pool structures is obtained. The resolution depends on the collimator camera-computer system used.[6,7] Figure 3–9 shows anterior, right anterior oblique and left anterior oblique projections commonly used. In general, the anterior projection allows for better left and right ventricular separation than does the RAO view. Separation, however, is enhanced in a left anterior oblique projection with the camera face oriented perpendicular to the plane of the interventricular septum. This view is preferred for quantitative analysis of right and left ventricular function. A caudal tilt in the left anterior oblique projection helps separate left atrium from left ventricle[7] (Fig. 3–10).

Multiple projections are important in gated blood pool scanning to permit identification of regional function, particularly when coronary artery disease is suspected (Fig. 3–11). The normal left ventricle can be likened to a prolate ellipse (the long axis assumed to be twice the short axis). Sequences of normal contraction in biplane projections are depicted in Fig. 3–12. In the anterior projection the anterior and inferior walls approximate one another, while the apex and base move slightly toward one another. Apical motion is often less pronounced than that of the adjacent walls in the normal ventricle. With ventricular dilatation (e.g., aortic regurgitation) this disparity becomes more pronounced, giving the erroneous impression of an isolated,

Fig. 3–7, A–D. *First-pass angiogram—right pulmonary artery injection.* **A** Isotope is injected into the right pulmonary artery (*rpa*) port of a Swan-Ganz catheter—LAO projection. **B** Right lung (*rl*) **C** Left atrium (*la*) and left ventricle (*lv*) are noted in isolation. **D** Tracer enters aorta (*ao*).

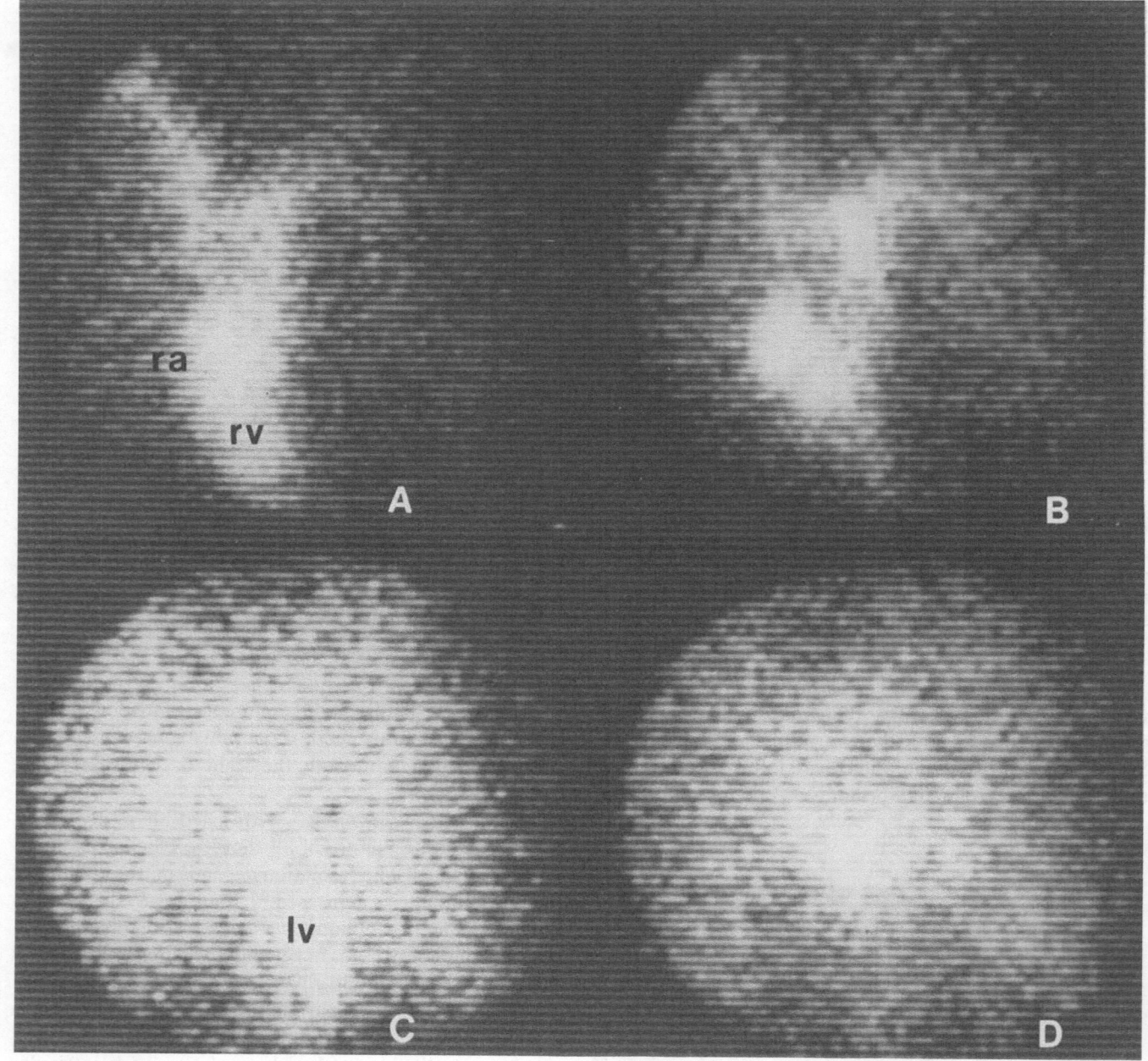

Fig. 3–8, A–D. *Gated radionuclide images, computer generated, from a peripheral first-pass injection.* **A** and **B** End-diastolic and end-systolic frames of the right ventricle (*rv*) and atrium (*ra*). Note the right atrium filling normally in systole. **C** and **D** End-diastolic and end-systolic frames formatted as the bolus traversed the left side of the heart. Resolution is reduced as the bolus has trailed out through the pulmonary circulation, decreasing the left ventricular (*lv*) count rate and creating background activity.

localized, regional abnormality at the apex.[8] Therefore the size of the ventricle must be noted to maximize the accuracy of interpretation of regional wall motion.

A major advantage of gated blood pool scanning over contrast angiographic techniques is the opportunity to image in three dimensions. Motion (or lack thereof) that is non-border-forming (perpendicular to the plane of the image) can be detected in any projection by observing gray scale or color scale changes over the course of the cardiac cycle[9] (Fig. 3–13). This information is particularly impor-

tant during interventional studies when time constraints limit the number of views available for analysis.

Imaging of Myocardial Perfusion with Thallium 201

Thallium 201, a K^+ analogue, is actively transported into muscle via a Na^+-K^+ ATPase. The uptake is so avid that immediately following injection, distribution in the myocardium is limited by flow.[10] Thus, immediately following injection, distribution within the myocardium will reflect blood flow. Figure 3–14 depicts thallium scintigrams in four standard projections, with the ventricular segments

Fig. 3–9, A–F. *Gated blood pool scan (GBPS)—normal heart.* Right anterior oblique (*RAO*) magnified, anterior (*ANT*) full field and left anterior oblique (*LAO*) GBPS. **a, c** and **e** end diastole; **b, d** and **f** end systole. "Zooming" (magnification) is useful for augmenting information contained within the right and left ventricles, while the full field view allows definition of more thoracic blood pool structures. *rv* and *lv* = right and left ventricles; *ao* = aorta; *pa* = pulmonary artery; *upper* and *lower arrows* in *frame c* designate locations of superior vena cava and right atrium.

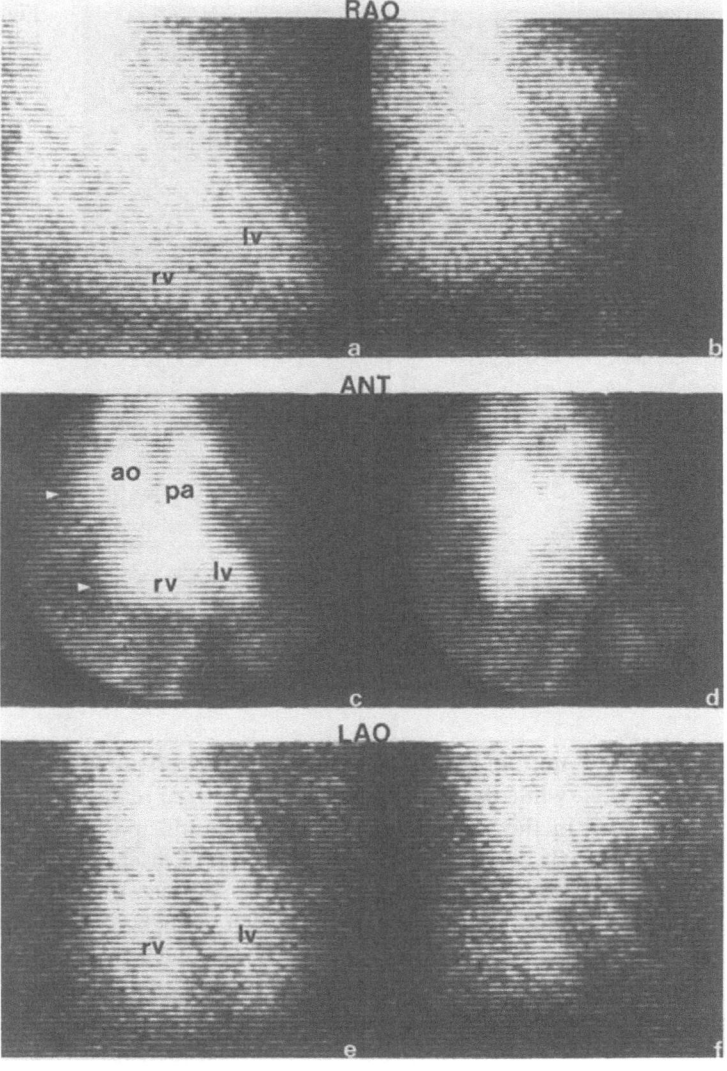

Fig. 3–10. *LAO GBPS with caudal tilt.* End-diastolic (*ED*) and end-systolic (*ES*) frames illustrating the right and left ventricles (*rv* and *lv*). Caudal tilt affords visualization of the "cap" the left atrium (*la*) creates.

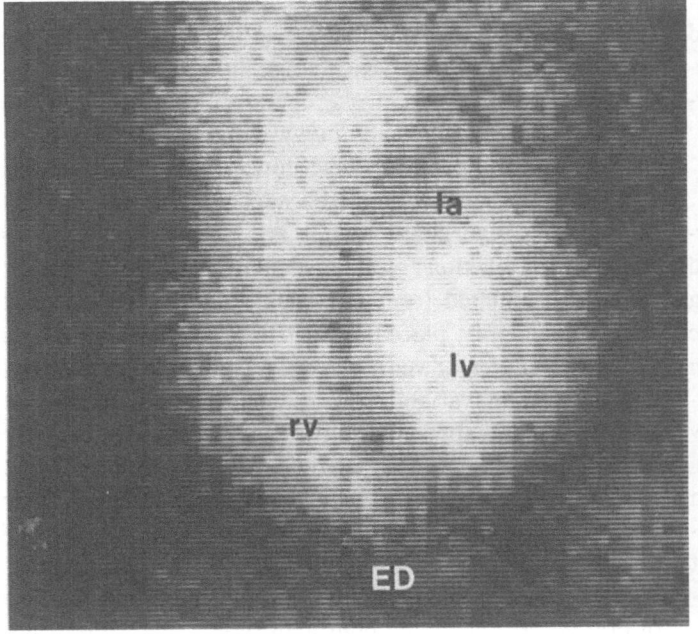
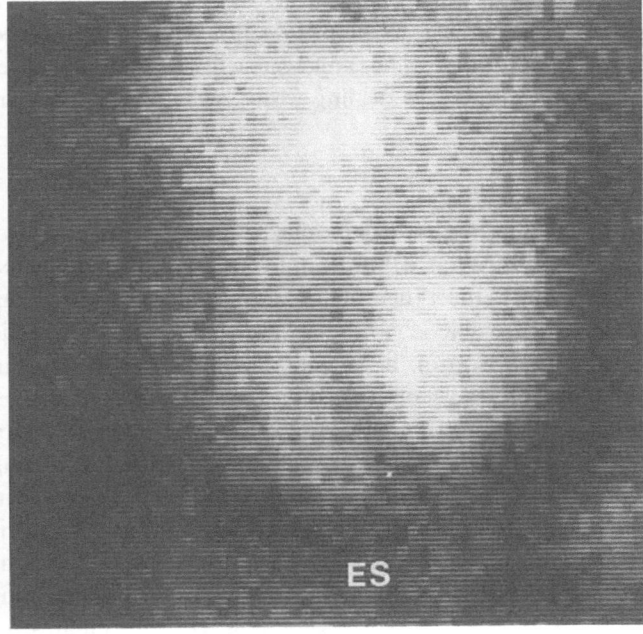

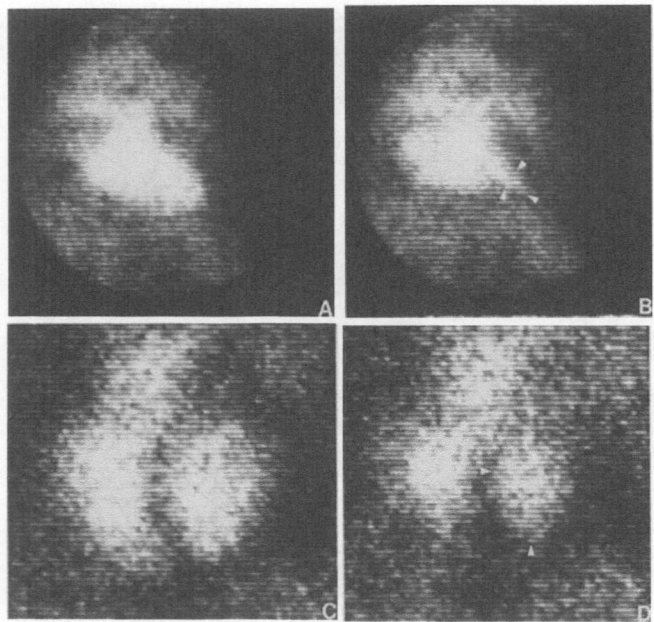

Fig. 3–11, A–D. *Abnormalities of regional wall motion.* Anterior full field (**A** and **B**) and LAO "zoomed" (**C** and **D**) end-diastolic (**A** and **C**) and end-systolic (**B** and **D**) frames from a rest-gated blood pool scan. *Arrows* in LAO systolic frame (**D**) mark subtle wall motion abnormalities in the basal septum and inferoapex. Anterior systolic frame (**B**) reveals extensive akinesia of the inferior wall in this patient with an acute inferior wall myocardial infarct. Multiple projections are useful for detecting and localizing these abnormalities.

indicated. The normal left ventricle appears as a horseshoe-shaped object, while the right ventricle is visualized readily after exercise in the normal individual but should not be delineated clearly at rest except in the presence of disease[11] (Fig. 3–15). The apex of the left ventricle, thinner than the adjacent walls, appears as a small cleft, which may become accentuated when concentric left ventricular hypertrophy is present (Fig. 3–16). Thus the presence of an apical cleft alone does not constitute proof of coronary artery disease (CAD). Further, toward the base of the heart, valve plane merges with myocardium, reducing the normal amount of thallium-containing tissue in the image. Qualitative criteria for pathological defects must therefore consider the size and location of the defect as well as the number of views that confirms its presence. The temporal relationship of imaging and thallium injection also be considered in interpretation of scans. This issue will be discussed subsequently in the section dealing with physiological considerations.

Normal Physiology

Radionuclide Angiocardiography *Resting Function Defined* The heart as a pump must deliver sufficient blood to the tissue to meet their metabolic needs. The determining factors for cardiac performance are preload (end-diastolic volume or pressure), heart rate, afterload (the tension in the wall at the onset of ejection) and contractility. Contractility can be viewed as the force, velocity and capability of shortening of the heart muscle, independent of loading conditions.[12,13] Qualitative radionuclide angiography can provide an indication of the end-diastolic size of the ventricle as a measure of preload. Normally the areas of right and left ventricle are equal. The left anterior oblique projection should be used to assess relative ventricular size.

The rate and extent of wall motion can be used as a rough measure of contractility (Fig. 3–12).

Quantitative Analysis. Recently, gated blood pool scanning has been used to quantitate left ventricular volume.[14-16] By measuring the count rate of ^{99m}Tc per unit blood in a sample drawn during the study and normalizing the background corrected end-diastolic image to the number of beats scanned and the frame duration, Slutsky et al.[16] have developed a regression equation between gated blood pool scan and angiographic left ventricular volume. Such measurements, although not fully accounting for the influence of attenuation on ventricular count rates, have proved useful for comparisons of ventricular volume at rest and during intervention in different patients.

At equilibrium in the normal heart, the output of the two ventricles must be equal. Deviation from unity of the stroke ratio of the two ventricles signifies valve regurgitation or shunting. The stroke count ratio of the left and right ventricle circumvents many of the problems associated with absolute volume determination. But, to date this technique has met with mixed success in detecting and quantitating regurgitant lesions and shunts.[17-19] As contrasted with ejection fraction calculations, the regurgitant index is calculated from non-background-corrected fixed regions of interest placed around the end-diastolic images of the left and right ventricles (Fig. 3–17). Unfortunately, a good deal of variability exists in this ratio in normal individuals, and abnormal ratios correlate only moderately well with catheterization methods. Although promising, these techniques will require further validation before their precise role in clinical practice can be defined.

The ideal measure of contractility is an elusive goal. At the center of the problem is the intimate interrelation of preload, afterload and contractility.[20] The ejection frac-

ANT

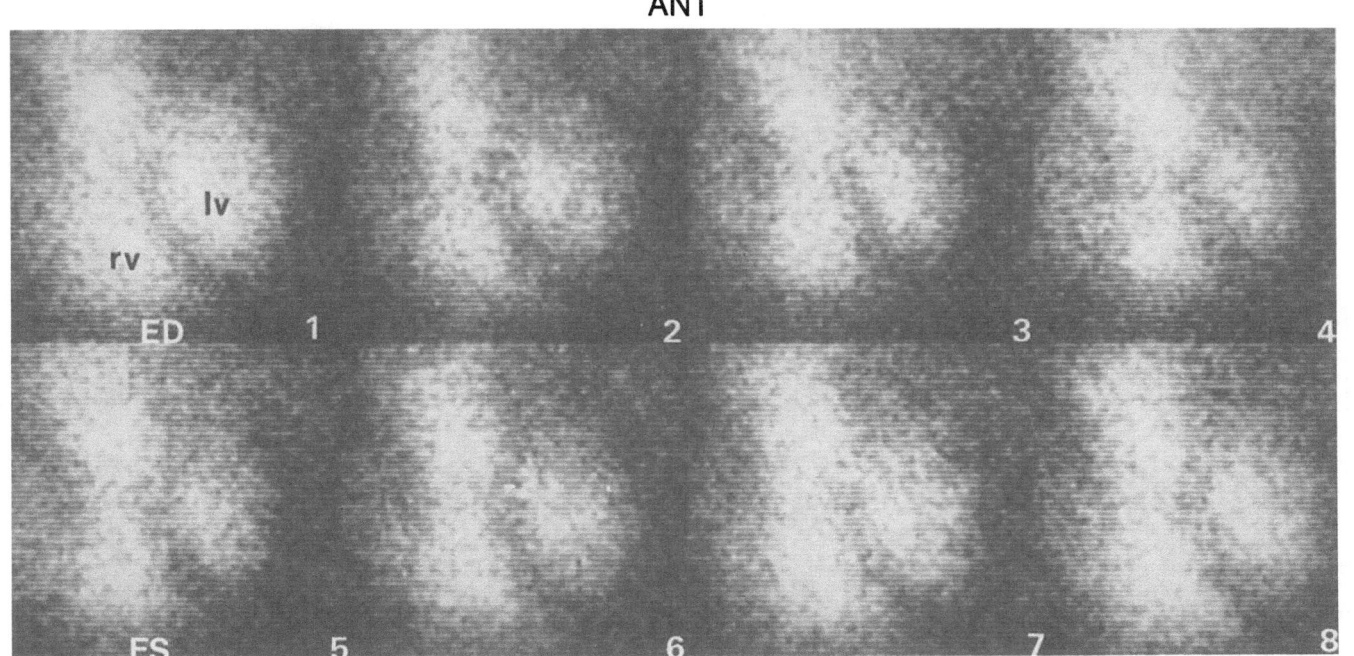

LAO

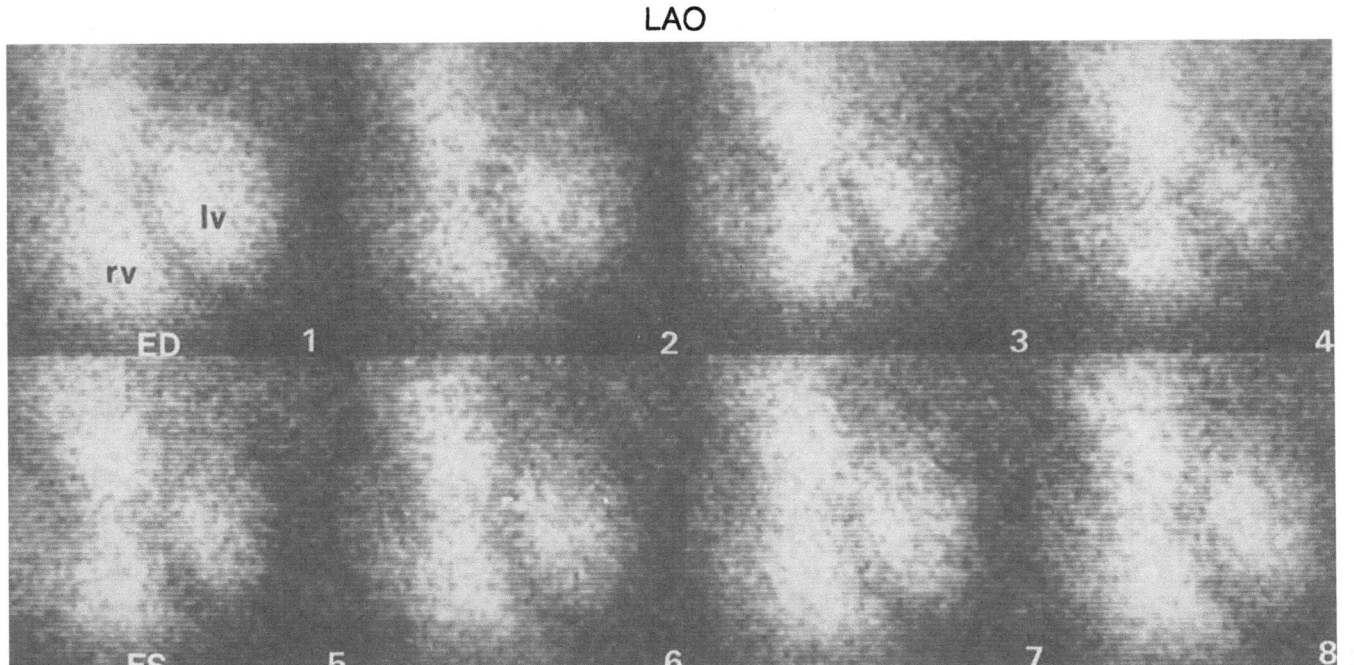

Fig. 3–12, A and B. *Normal contraction sequences.* A "zoomed" anterior and B LAO GBPS. After end diastole (*ED, frame 1*), opposing walls approximate one another, as apex moves toward base (*frames 2–4*) with maximal contraction at *frame 5,* end systole (*ES*). In *frames 6–8,* ventricle fills toward end-diastolic proportions. The spleen (*s*) is well seen in the anterior view.

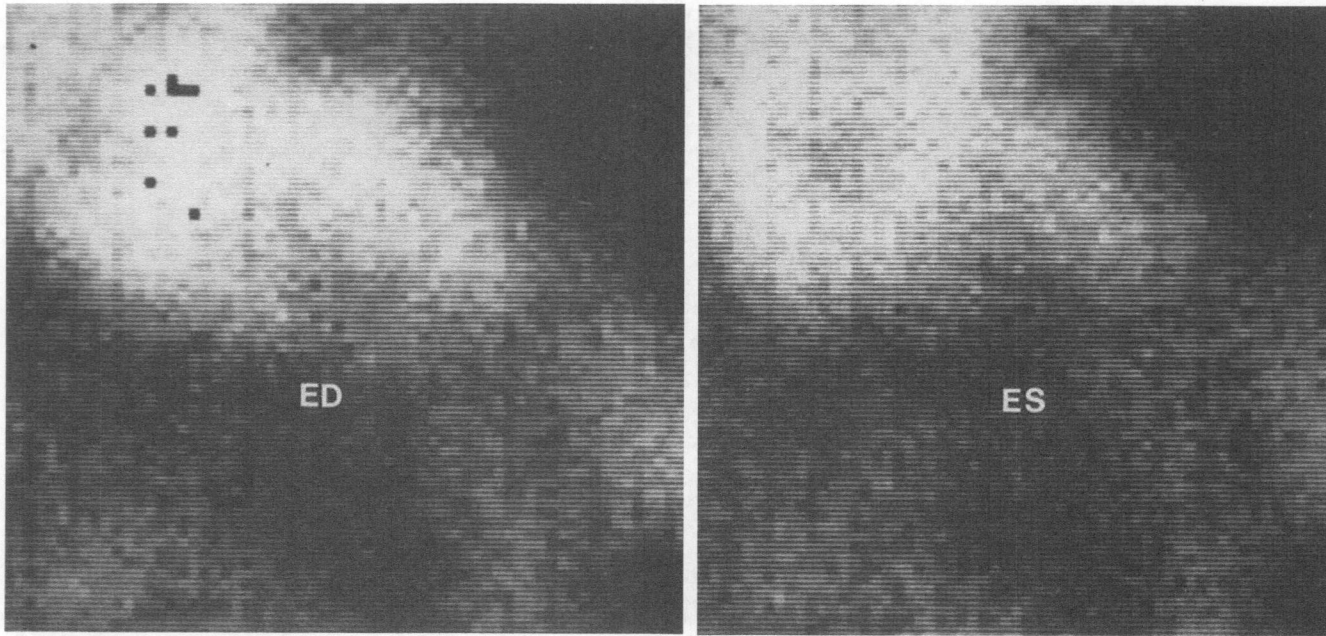

Fig. 3–13. *"Three-dimensional" imaging. End-diastolic (ED) and end-systolic (ES) frames of a GBPS. Although the edge of the left ventricle does not appear to have moved dramatically, a pro*nounced decrease in count intensity over the entire left ventricle is present, indicating ejection of tracer. Such changes in gray scale or color scale provide a three-dimensional view of the heart.

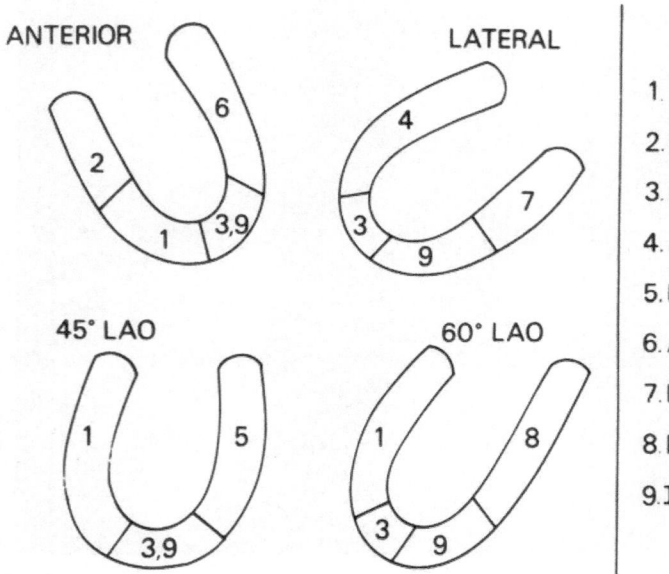

Fig. 3–14. *^{201}Tl scintigraphy.* Representation of the heart in four standard projections used in ^{201}Tl scintigraphy. Leppo J et al (1979) Thallium-201 myocardial scintigraphy in patients with triple-vessel disease and ischemic exercise stress tests. Circulation 59:715. By permission of the American Heart Association, Inc.

1. ANTERIOR SEPTUM
2. POSTERIOR SEPTUM
3. APEX
4. ANTERIOR WALL
5. LATERAL WALL
6. ANTERO–LATERAL WALL
7. POSTERIOR WALL
8. POSTERO–LATERAL WALL
9. INFERIOR WALL

tion, although an imperfect ejection-phase measure of contractility, has proved to be a valuable prognostic tool in patients with valvular and coronary heart disease.[21,22] Radionuclide angiographic ejection fraction (both first-pass and gated) correlates well with contrast angiographic methods[23,24] (Fig. 3–18).

In the authors' laboratory, $EF_{GBPS} = .96\ EF_{cine} + 2.10$.

$N = 36$, $r = 0.92$, $p < .001$. Figure 3–19 depicts the end-diastolic, end-systolic and background regions of interest employed. From time-activity curves generated within these regions, ejection fraction is calculated from the formula EDC-ESC/EDC (corrected for background) = EF, where EDC = end diastolic counts, and ESC = end systolic counts. A normal range for supine resting ejection fraction

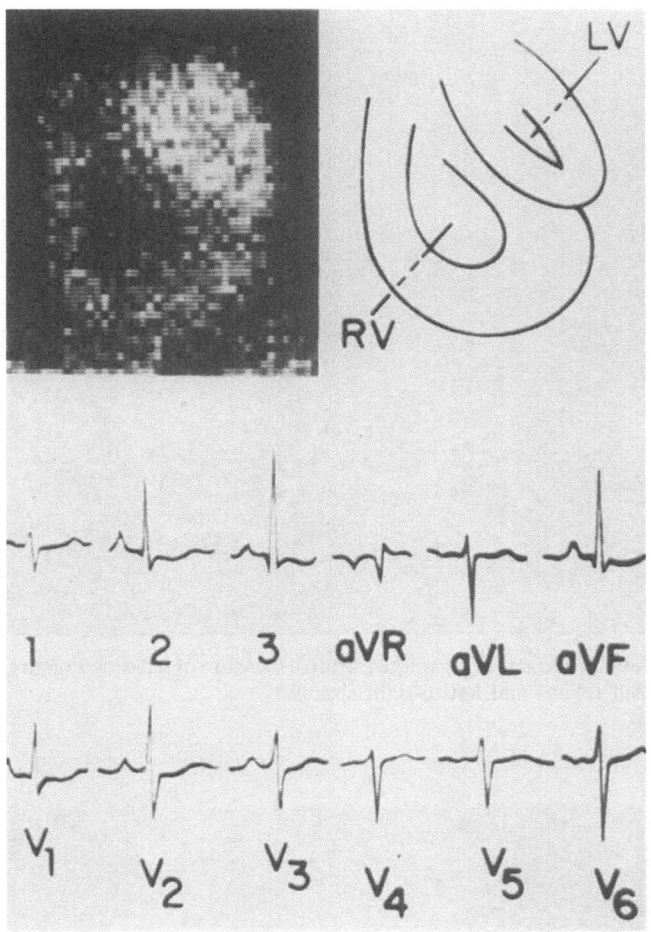

Fig. 3–15. *Resting ^{201}Tl scintigram in right ventricular hypertrophy.* Dilated, thickened right ventricle is apparent. ECG is compatible with RVH. Reprinted with permission from Cohen HA et al (1976) Thallium-201 myocardial imaging in patients with pulmonary hypertension. Circulation 54:792. By permission of the American Heart Association, Inc.

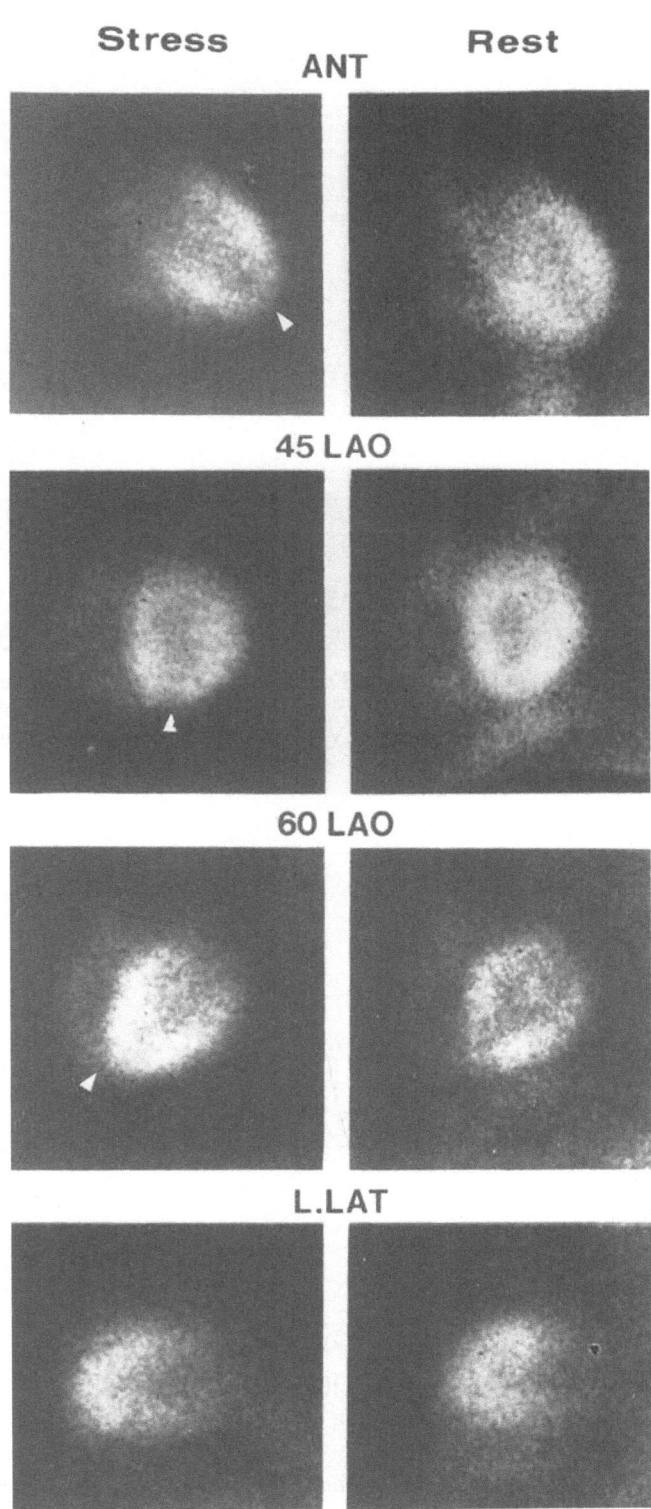

Fig. 3–16. *Normal stress and redistribution ^{201}Tl scintigram.* The patient is a 34-year-old trained athlete with nonanginal chest pain and normal coronary arteries. *Arrows* indicate normal apical cleft, accentuated in this patient by physiological hypertrophy of the adjacent walls. The posterolateral wall, region 7 in the left lateral view, farthest from the camera, is barely visible as the low-energy emissions are attenuated.

in the authors' laboratory is 57%–80%. Despite count-based, computer-generated EF determinations, in a given subject at supine rest, repeated measurements reveal considerable variability in the ejection fraction,[25] which can be attributed to both physiological and technical factors.[26] Of importance, before conclusions are drawn regarding the effects of disease states or interventions on the ejection fraction, the inherent variability of the patient-measurement system should be assessed (Table 3–2).

Experimental work has indicated that ejection phase measures of contractility are independent of preload (at supine rest) but are influenced by the afterload.[27] Thus more accurate measures of the contractile state should incorporate some determination of afterload. One such measure, the end-systole pressure volume index (end-systolic pressure/end-systolic volume), may be superior to the ejection fraction in separating normal from abnormal.[28]

Thus far only global left ventricular function has been considered. The hallmark of coronary artery disease—abnormal wall motion (asynergy)—may or may not affect global measures of left ventricular function.[29] Regional

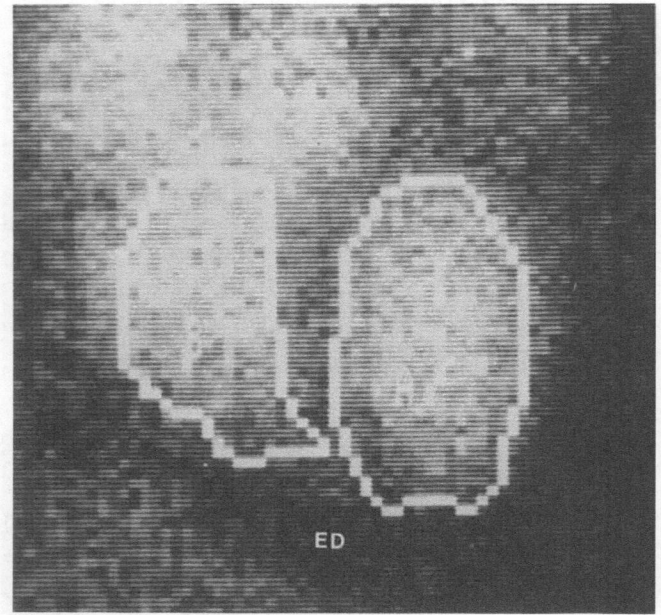

A

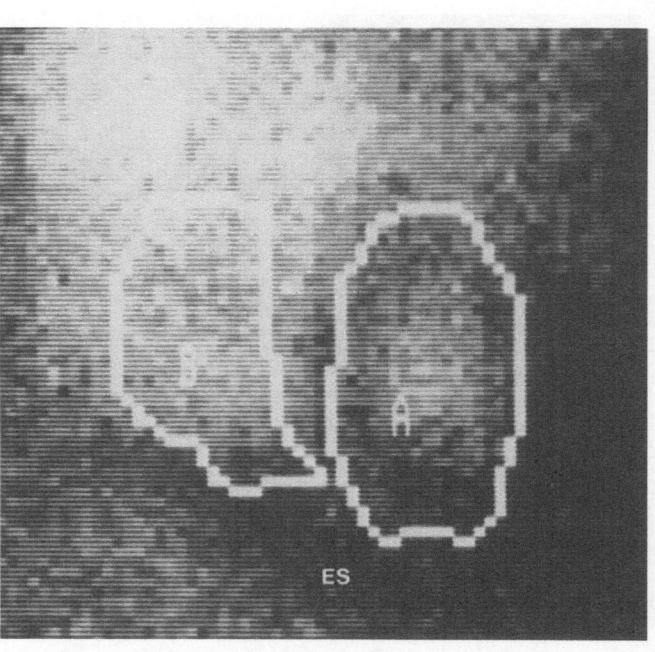

B

Fig. 3–17. *Stroke count ratio. End-diastolic (ED) and end-systolic (ES) frames of an LAO GBPS.* A fixed end diastolic region of interest is used to determine LV and RV stroke counts and their ratio. This ratio is a semiquantitative measure of left-sided regurgitant lesions and left-to-right shunts.

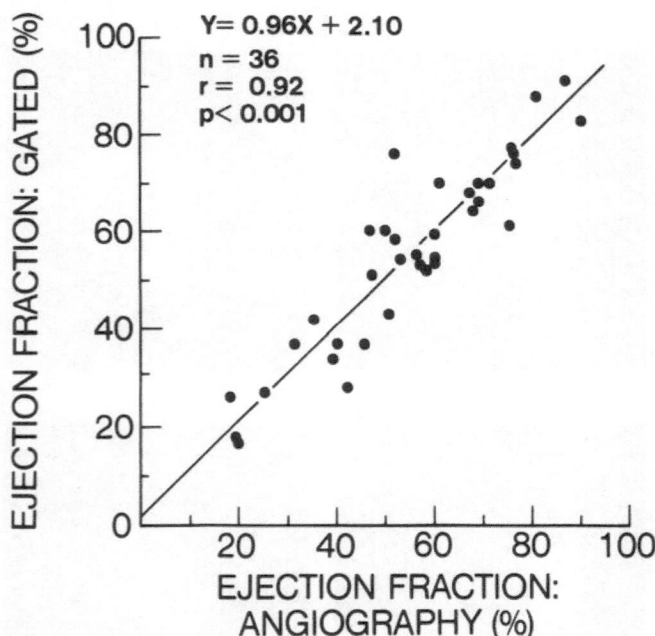

Fig. 3–18. *Correlation of ejection fraction by angiographic and GBPS methods.*

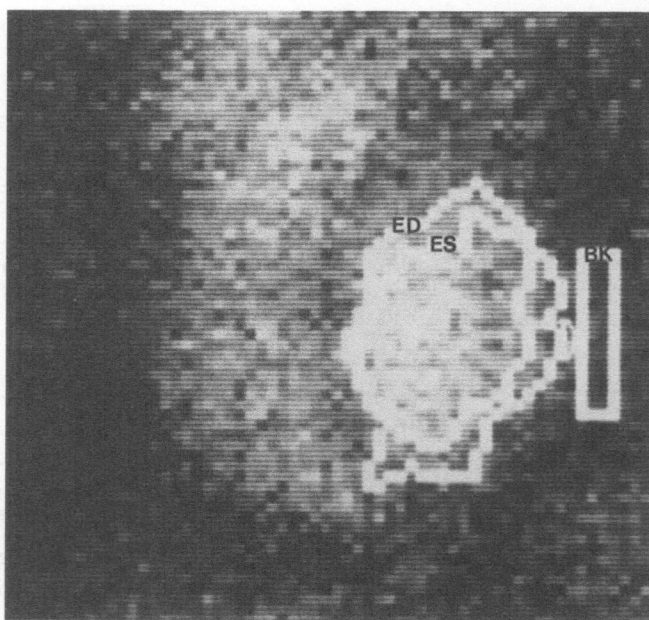

Fig. 3–19. *Ejection fraction.* End-diastolic (*ED*), end-systolic (*ES*) and background (*BK*) regions superimposed on the end-diastolic frame of a GBPS. These "variable" regions are used in the calculation of the ejection fraction.

Table 3–2. Effect of Multiple Ejection Fraction Studies on the Significance of Ejection Fraction Changes

Number of studies		Confidence levels for ejection fraction change*				
Initial (n$_o$)	Final (n$_1$)	60%	80%	90%	95%	99%
1	1	4.2	6.5	8.4	10.1	13.2
1	2	3.9	5.6	7.2	8.7	11.4
1	5	3.3	5.0	6.4	7.8	10.2
1	10	3.1	4.8	6.2	7.4	9.8
2	2	3.0	4.6	5.9	7.1	9.3
3	3	2.4	3.8	4.8	5.8	7.6
5	5	1.9	2.9	3.7	4.5	5.9
10	10	1.3	2.1	2.6	3.2	4.2

* Given a standard deviation of 3.6 EF units for multiple EF determinations at rest in the steady state.

function can be interpreted qualitatively using a rating scale (hypokinesis = decreased but preserved motion; akinesis = absent motion; dyskinesis = paradoxical motion), but objective quantitative computer techniques offer the potential for less interobserver and intraobserver variability. One such quantitative method (Fig. 3–20) divides the ventricle into three zones and utilizes fixed regions of interest and locally weighted backgrounds to calculate regional ejection fraction.[30]

Nongeometrical methods are best suited for study of the right ventricle.[31] Radionuclide techniques have therefore provided new insights into the function of this chamber. First-pass scanning delineates the right ventricle through temporal separation, allowing for definition of contractile function (Fig. 3–5).[32] The key problem in determination of right ventricular ejection fraction by the equilibrium method is definition of valve plane. Functional imaging is most useful in this regard. Since the right atrium and pulmonary artery fill in systole while the ventricle empties, subtraction of the end-diastolic frame from the end-systolic frame (i.e., ESC − EDC) of the right ventricle provides a clearer picture of these structures. Subtraction of the end-systolic image from the end-diastolic frame (e.g., EDC − ESC) produces a stroke volume image. In this manner, functional imaging allows for edge definition of the right ventricle (Fig. 3–21). In this laboratory, RV ejection fraction obtained by GBPS = .86 RVEF$_{cath}$ + 7.8, N = 18, r = 0.95, p < 0.001. The normal values for right ventricular ejection fraction are slightly lower than those for left ventricular ejection fraction.

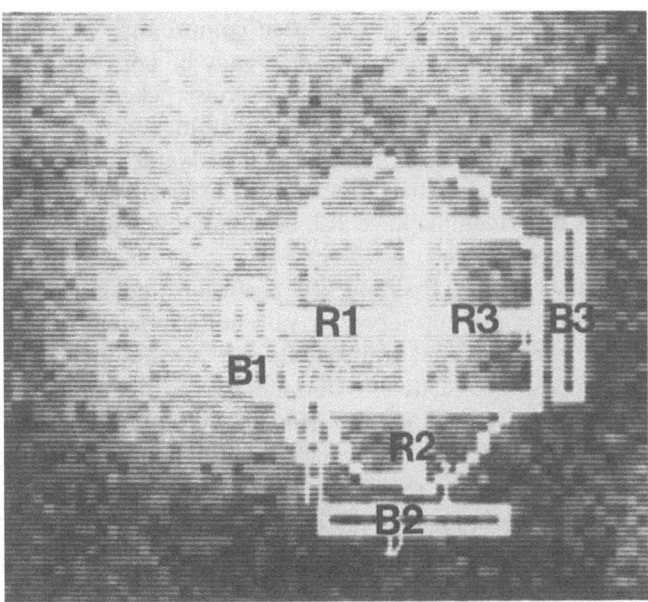

Fig. 3–20. *Regional ejection fraction.* Fixed regions of interest (*R1–R3*) and corresponding backgrounds (*B1–B3*) employed for calculation of regional ejection fraction, a quantitative measure of regional wall motion. *R1* = septal region; *R2* = apical region; *R3* = posterolateral region.

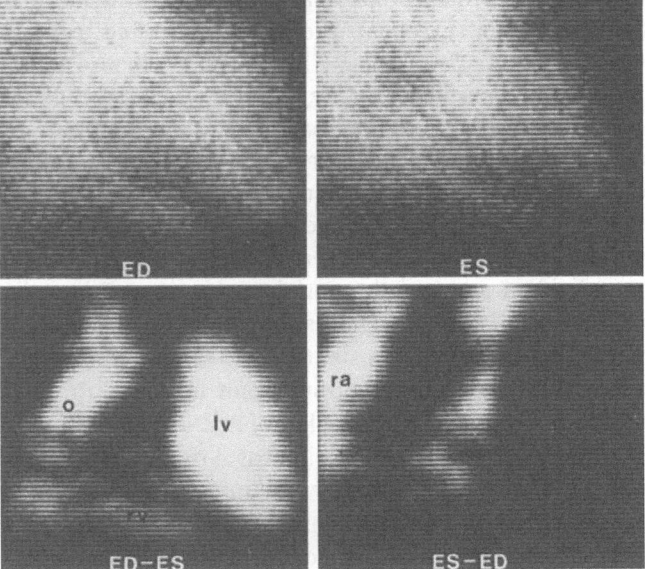

Fig. 3–21. *GBPS functional imaging.* Upper panels are from a shallow LAO view with end-diastolic (*ED*) and end-systolic frames (*ES*). ED–ES (*lower left*) demonstrates stroke volume of the left and right ventricles (*lv* and *rv*) and right ventricular outflow (*o*). ES–ED permits clear visualization of right atrial (*ra*) activity.

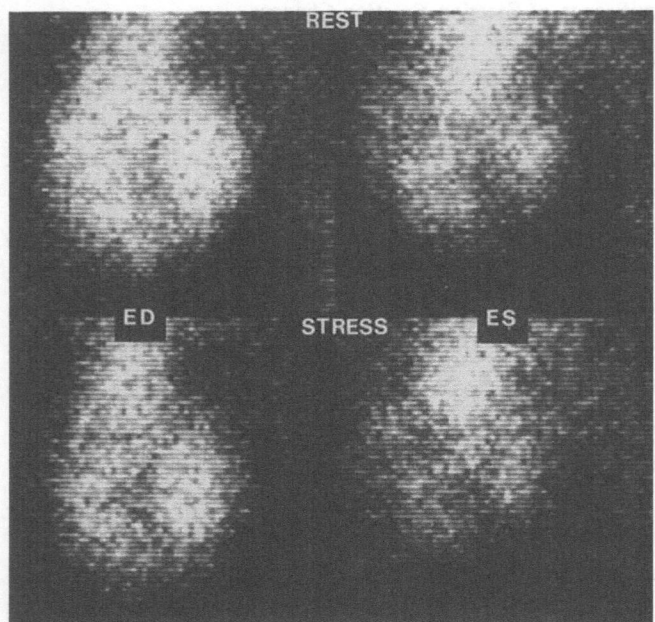

Fig. 3–22. *Normal response to exercise while supine.* Normal supine rest and peak exercise end-diastolic (*ED*) and end-systolic (*ES*) GBPS frames. With stress, ED volume is constant, while ES volume decreases, resulting in an increase in stroke volume and ejection fraction.

Effects of Perturbation. The study of the ventricle at rest touches only a small fraction of cardiac potential. By stressing the ventricle with physiological or pharmacological intervention, cardiac reserve can be tapped and disease states limiting this reserve identified. In the diseased ventricle, therapeutic interventions can also be evaluated at rest and under stress. Of all interventions, dynamic (isotonic) muscular exercise demands maximal cardiac performance and therefore is an excellent means of assessing cardiac reserve.[33] Figure 3–22 depicts the normal response to supine isotonic muscular exercise as assessed by gated blood pool scanning. With supine exercise, cardiac output increases via tachycardia and increased stroke volume. Stroke volume increases through a decrease in end-systolic volume while end-diastolic volume increases slightly or remains constant, ejection fraction therefore rises. At rest, when the individual assumes the upright posture, end-diastolic and end-systolic volumes fall; stroke volume and ejection fraction fall or remain constant (Fig. 3–23). With upright isotonic exercise, cardiac output again increases through tachycardia and increasing stroke volume. However, in this position, end-diastolic volume increases dramatically with exercise, end-systolic volume remains constant or falls slightly, resulting in an increase in the ejection fraction (Fig. 3–24). Segmental wall motion is normally enhanced in both postures during exercise.[26]

Isometric exercise provides a predominant afterload stress on the ventricle[34,35] with little change in heart rate. Since maintenance of a prolonged steady state of sufficient stress is difficult, first-pass techniques are better suited to the study of this intervention. Segmental wall motion and

ejection fraction increase in young subjects but may not increase in normal older individuals.

The influence of drugs can also be evaluated, using radionuclide ventriculography. Nitroglycerin and propranolol, two widely used drugs, have significant influence on left ventricular function and size. Nitroglycerin dilates both resistance and capacitance vessels (predominantly the latter), thus decreasing venous return, which results in a fall in end-diastolic volume and stroke volume. The compensatory response to this drop in stroke volume is tachycardia and increased contractility, resulting in either no change in ejection fraction or an increase (Fig. 3–25). Beta blockers, on the other hand, slow the heart rate and may decrease the ejection fraction in normal individuals.[36] The therapeutic effects of these agents in coronary artery disease will be discussed subsequently.

Quantitative ^{201}**Tl** As already pointed out, distribution of thallium 201 immediately after injection parallels regional blood flow. With time, however, through a process known as redistribution, activity of thallium 201 in the myocardium comes to parallel myocardial mass.[37] Thus if blood flow to a significant mass of viable myocardium is reduced, a transient defect will result (Fig. 3–26). In other words, if these images are then repeated over time, the defect will become less apparent through a loss of thallium from normal tissue and a gain or less rapid loss of thallium from the "ischemic" tissue (Fig. 3–26). On the other hand, infarcted tissue will appear as a persistent defect. The exact mechanism of redistribution of thallium in ischemic tissue remains somewhat controversial.

Since disparity of flow is crucial in thallium 201 imaging, intervention designed to augment differential flow over the heart will enhance the value of the technique. In coronary artery disease, despite stenoses that compromise the coronary artery lumina, segmental flow may be normal at rest through autoregulation.[38] During exercise, when coronary flow may be called upon to increase fivefold, autoregulation of the diseased vessel will be exhausted and a disparity of flow produced.[39] Recently coronary arterial vasodilators such as dipyridamole have also been employed to provoke this disparity.[40]

A limitation of thallium 201 perfusion imaging is the interobserver and intraobserver variability inherent in subjective interpretation. Further, defects are designated by their appearance relative to normal areas, which may lead to false negative readings if ischemia is widespread.[41] Quantitative methods can reduce variability of interpretation while increasing the sensitivity of the method through established criteria for regional activity of thallium. By plotting the relative distribution of thallium 201 activity in a given image, segments falling outside established normal limits can be identified (Fig. 3–27).[42] Further, by plotting activity in segments over time, the patterns of redistribution of thallium 201 may separate normal from abnormal (Fig. 3–26).[43]

SUPINE

UPRIGHT

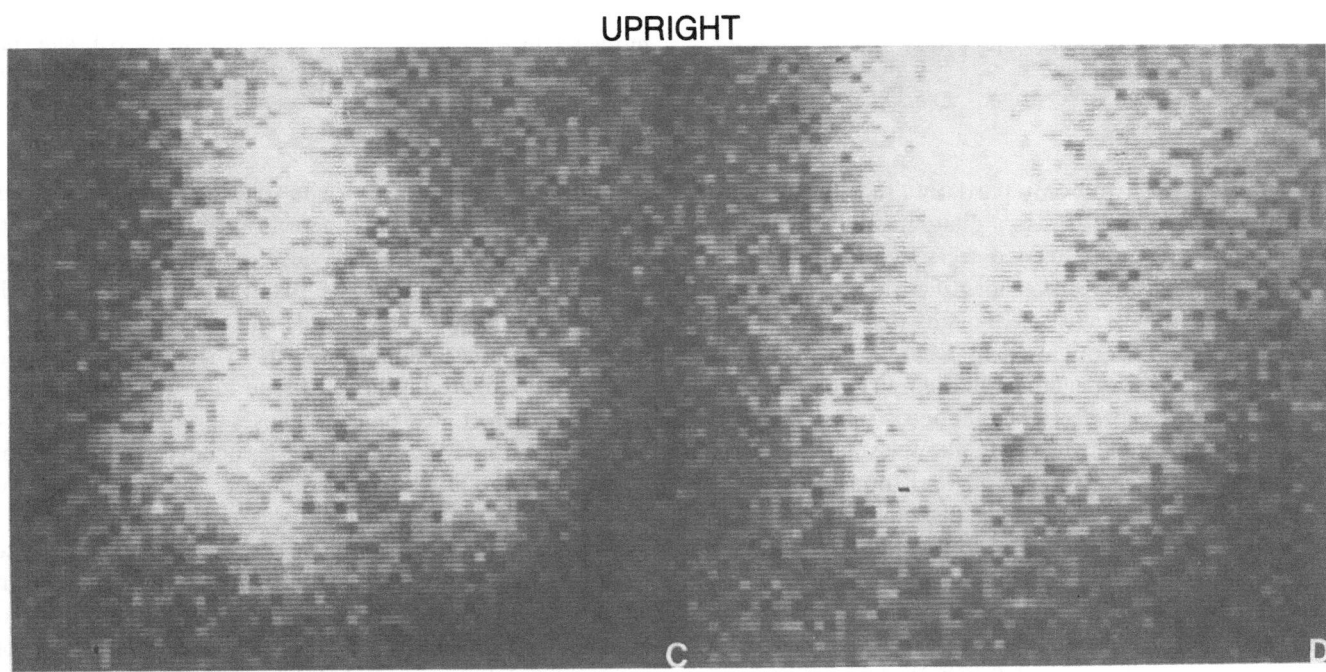

Fig. 3–23, A–D. *Effects of posture on ventricular volume.* LAO projection. **A** and **C** supine and upright resting end-diastolic frames; **B** and **D** end-systolic frames. Volumes decrease on assumption of upright posture.

Ischemic Heart Disease

Ischemia
Ischemic heart disease results from the failure of the coronary circulation to deliver adequate oxygen to the metabolizing tissue. The diagnostic methods employed in cardiovascular nuclear medicine each provide information on a unique aspect of this supply-demand imbalance.

Thallium Scintigraphy *Analysis of Myocardial Thallium Activity.* In patients in whom exercise is not feasible or is contraindicated, myocardial imaging at rest is somewhat useful in detecting coronary artery disease; however, scintigrams recorded after exercise have proved much more sensitive ($r = 0.76$) and specific ($r = 0.89$).[44-46] Figure 3–28A–C demonstrate stress-induced regional perfusion abnormalities. The delayed images (3–4 hours after thallium injection) in fig. 3–28A no longer demonstrate a defect, implying exercise-induced disparity of regional flow but preservation of myocardium, that is, ischemia without infarct. In Fig. 3–28B, a defect in the posterolateral wall is

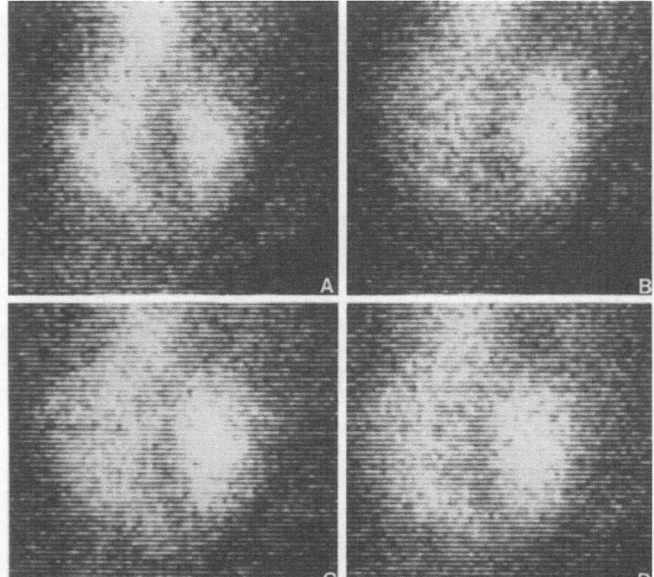

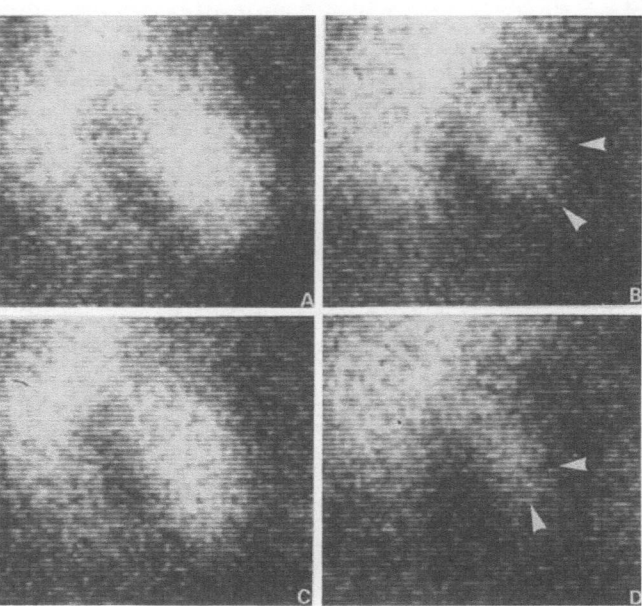

Fig. 3–24, A–D. *Normal end-diastolic volume response to upright exercise.* End-diastolic frame at rest **(A)** and during progressively severe exercise **B–D** in a normal individual. End-diastolic volume increases with upright exercise to levels observed at rest (supine). As with exercise while supine, end-systolic volume decreases.

Fig. 3–25, A–D. *GBPS during angina and response to nitroglycerin.* End-diastolic **(A)** and end-systolic **(B)** LAO frames during a spontaneous anginal episode. *Arrows* indicate regional asynergy in the apical and posterolateral walls. After administration of nitroglycerin the end-diastolic volume is reduced **(C)**, and improvement is noted in the asynergic regions at end systole **(D)**.

present after stress and only partially "redistributes" with rest. Figure 3–28C illustrates a dilated, thin-walled ventricle with fixed rest and stress defects signifying infarction.

Several factors have been identified as causes for false negative thallium scans. Although the level of stress achieved is not as critical as in ECG stress testing, the predictive value of a negative, markedly submaximal thallium test can be expected to be reduced.[47] The "ischemic" zone must be of sufficient size to allow visualization, given the limited resolving capacity of the isotope-camera-computer system.[48] The limitations of the system are compounded by blurring of the image through segmental wall motion, and movement of the whole heart over the cardiac and respiratory cycles. Further a disparity in flow between two regions of myocardium must be on the order of 50% to allow visualization of a defect.[48] Perhaps most importantly, reduction of flow is perceived only relative to areas of normal flow. Therefore, although the sensitivity of thallium scanning for the detection of coronary artery disease increases with the number of vessels involved,[49] it is conceivable that relatively uniform reduction of flow over the heart will result in a normal image. In this regard, quantitative techniques hold promise for the future. Theoretically the behavior of normal and ischemic regions can be characterized by the change in activity over time within these regions[50,51] (Fig. 3–26). It should be emphasized that although quantitative methods are based on sound physiological principles, they are presently undergoing evolutionary changes and their exact roles in clinical scintigraphy require further study.

The most likely causes for false positive thallium scans involve misinterpretation of defects at the base of the heart, which represent plane of the valve, and at the apex, representing normal thinning.[52] Dilatation of the heart with stress in the myopathic ventricle can also give the appearance of an exercise-induced defect. In women, attenuation of counts by overlying breast tissue may give the appearance of a defect. Coronary stenoses graded from 30%–70% by angiography have been associated with thallium defects. The issue of exercise-induced coronary spasm in normal vessels must be evaluated.[53]

Background Analysis. Recently, background activity due to uptake in the lung in poststress images has been shown to correlate reasonably well with elevations of left ventricular end-diastolic pressure during exercise. The finding of an increased lung/heart thallium ratio (Fig. 3–29) may enhance the diagnostic utility of exercise thallium scanning.[54] This may occur because patients with multivessel coronary artery disease tend to have more exercise-induced ventricular dysfunction and therefore higher lung/myocardial ratios.

Rest and Stress Radionuclide Angiography Resting radionuclide ventriculography is quite sensitive for the detection of regional asynergy, a finding characteristic of CAD.[55] Figure 3–30 illustrates an anterior and LAO GBPS from a patient with CAD and resting abnormalities. It is clear, however, that milder degrees of asynergy and some instances of akinesis at rest represent viable but malfunctioning myocardium. Therapeutic intervention aimed at reversing abnormalities of regional wall motion at rest may help to distinguish infarct from ischemia. Figure 3–25 illustrates

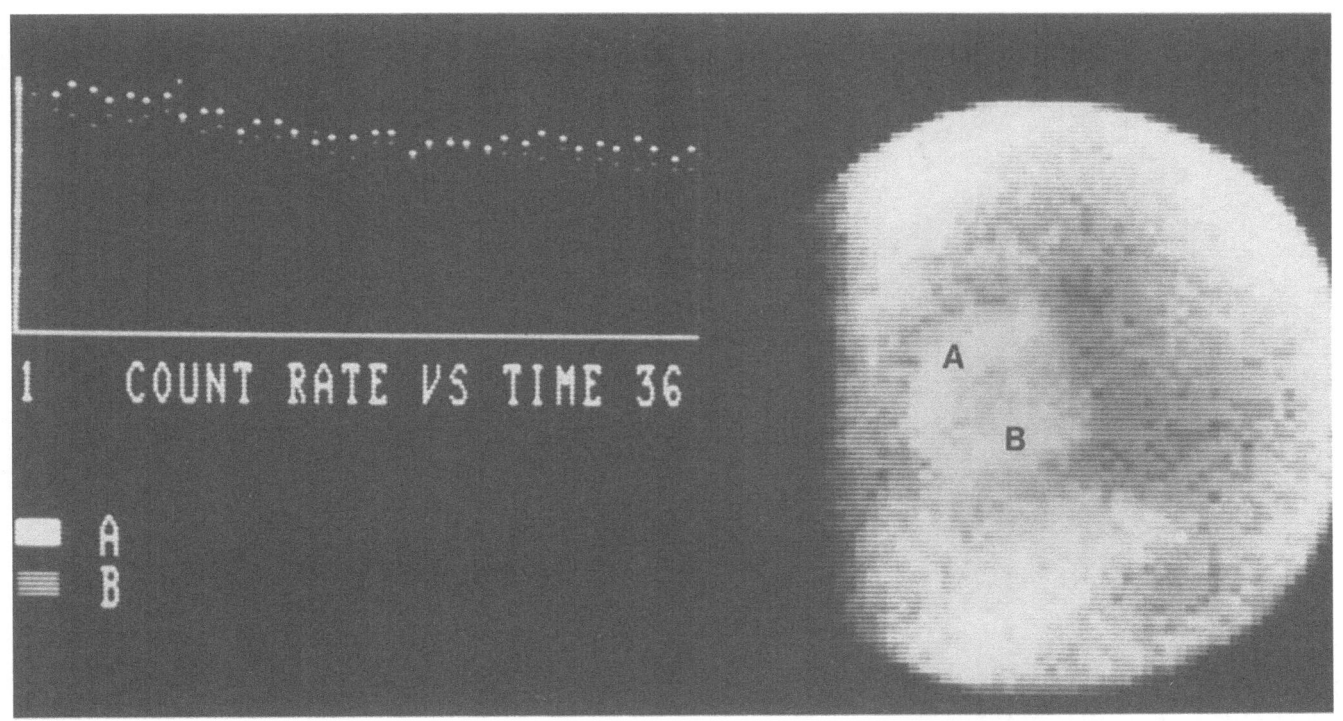

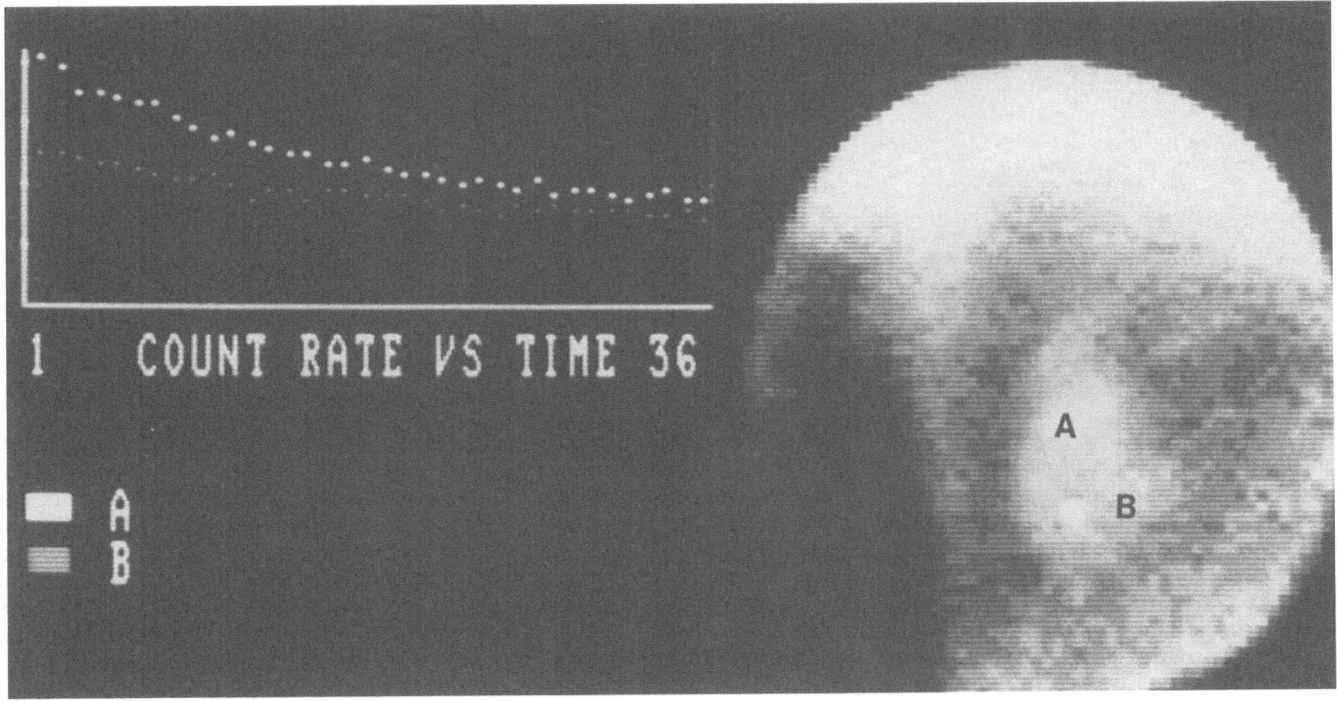

Fig. 3–26, A and **B.** *Quantitative* ^{201}Tl *analysis.* **I** Control experiment. ^{201}Tl was injected intravenously in a dog, exercising maximally on a treadmill. Scintigram at right was obtained during minutes 10–14 after injection of ^{201}Tl. *Regions A and B* demarcate the distributions of the left anterior descending and circumflex coronary arteries respectively. With the camera-animal relationship held constant, scanning was continued for 36 5-minute frames. Graph at left depicts ^{201}Tl activity over time in *regions A and B.* Initial activity is identical in both regions, and the rate of loss is similar. **II** At right is the immediate postexercise scintigram from the same animal after constriction of the circum-flex artery. A qualitative defect is present in *region B.* Quantitative analysis reveals a 35% reduction of counts in *region B,* relative to *A,* in this initial frame. During the 3 hours of scanning, *region B* loses counts more slowly than *region A,* resulting in equalization of activity in both zones. This process of "redistribution" would result in the visual impression of disappearance of the defect in *region B,* i.e., exercise-induced ischemia with redistribution. Were *region B* infarcted, initial counts would be similar to those noted in this example, but the rate of loss over time would parallel that in *region A,* resulting in a persistent defect.

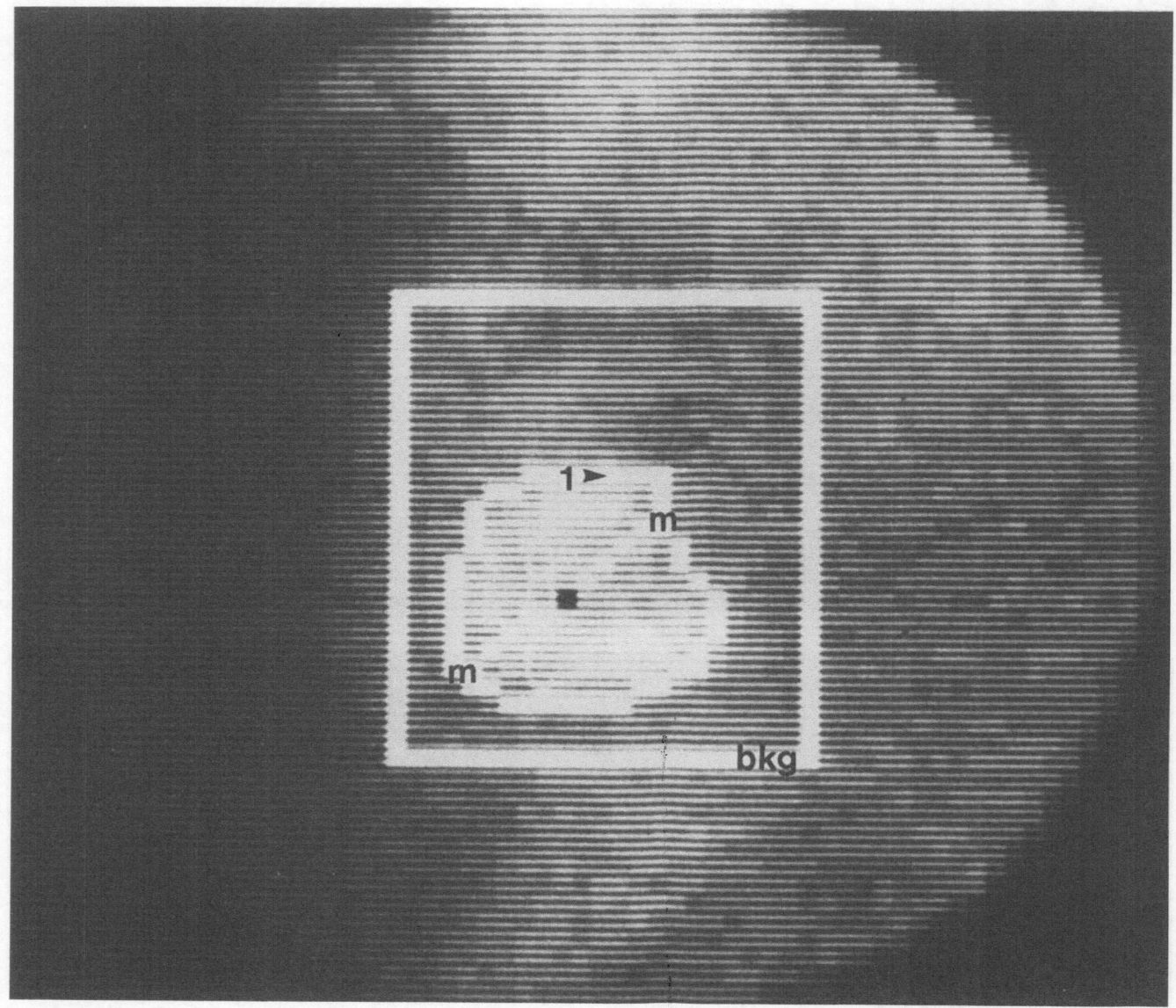

A

Fig. 3–27, A and B. *Circumferential profiles.* **A** Regions of interest employed for generation of circumferential profiles in a dog experiment. Background rectangle (*bkg*) is used for interpolated background correction. Variable region outlines left ventricle. Black pixel represents centroid of left ventricle. Radii are computer drawn from the centroid to each pixel in the ventricular circumference, starting at point 1 and proceeding in a clockwise direction. *m* = the circumferential poles of the major axis. **B** Profile maps, control and postligation. Y axis represents percentage of maximal radius, while x axis depicts sequential radii, starting at point 1 in **A** and proceeding around the ventricle in a clockwise direction. Also noted along the x axis is the percentage of the maximum radial counts that each radius contains. The radii constituting the major axis are labeled. + = 30° increment around the ventricle; *dashed vertical line* = 90° increment. In the control experiment, during minutes 10–14 after ^{201}Tl injection, activity is lowest at the base of the heart (radii 1–13) and at the apex (radii 27–35). After circumflex ligation in the same animal, scanning was again performed during minutes 10–14 after ^{201}Tl injection. Profile maps for control and ligation studies are aligned along the major axis for comparison. Compared with control, an extensive quantitative defect is present in the postligation profile, extending from radius 1 through radii 31–33, i.e., the circumflex distribution.

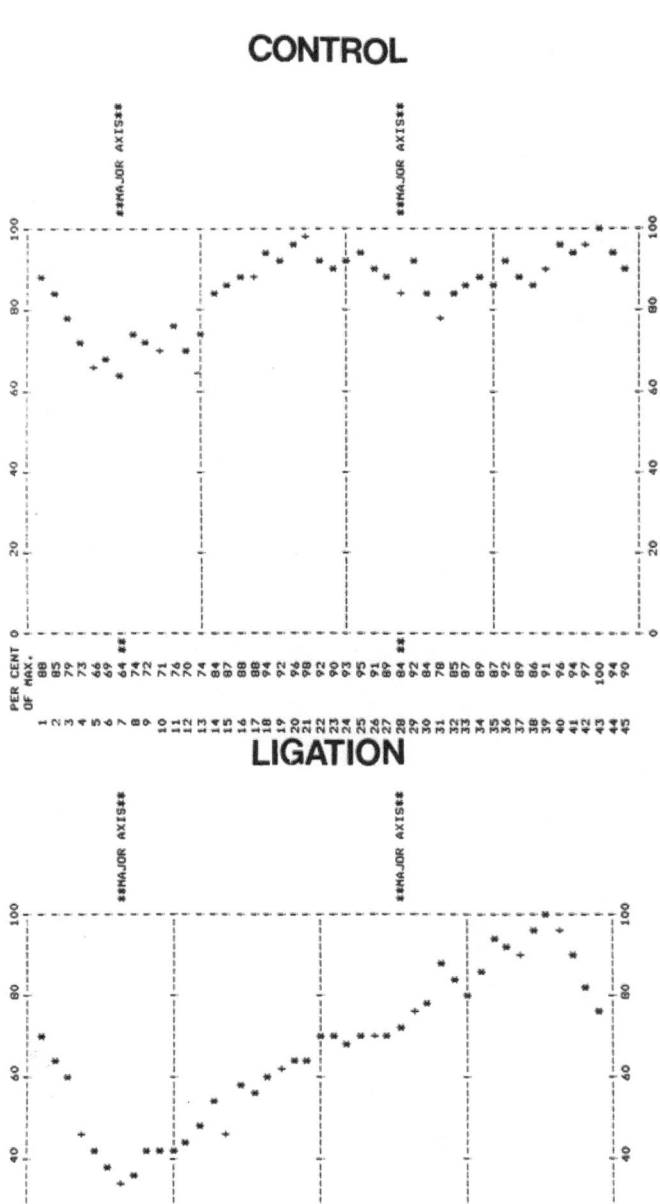

nitroglycerin-induced reversal of abnormalities of regional wall motion through the postulated mechanism of decreased end-diastolic volume and decreased myocardial oxygen demand.

Of great importance to the clinician is the fact that many patients with significant coronary artery disease have normal regional and global left ventricular function at rest. Again, exercise, by increasing myocardial oxygen demand, will result in a supply-demand mismatch if significant coronary artery stenoses are present. The lack of oxygen to the stressed myocardium will result in a decline in regional function and, if sufficiently profound or widespread, will impair global measures of left ventricular function as reflected in the ejection fraction.[56] Figure 3–31 illustrates the abnormal ventricular response to supine exercise in a patient with coronary artery disease who had normal function at rest. With exercise, end-diastolic volume increased and pronounced septal and apical asynergy resulted in a fall in ejection fraction. Exercise-induced abnormalities of regional wall motion are the most specific findings for coronary artery disease, although the rapid time required to acquire data in exercise studies limit resolution. As a result, greater emphasis has been placed on the change in global ejection fraction in response to exercise as a diagnostic criterion. As discussed in the foregoing, however, changes in ejection fraction during intervention must exceed the inherent variability of this parameter at rest if a causal relationship between intervention and ejection fraction change is to be accepted. In their laboratory the authors record three baseline studies and two studies at peak stress. As noted in Table 3–2, a less than 5-unit increase in ejection fraction with stress, accompanied by new or persistent regional wall motion abnormalities are considered indicative of coronary artery disease. With these criteria, the test's sensitivity and specificity both exceed 90%. It is clear, however, that the lack of elevation or a decrease in ejection fraction with exercise is not diagnostic for coronary artery disease. Such a response has been reported in patients with valvular heart disease and cardiomyopathy as well[57] (Fig. 3–32).

Myocardial Infarction

Technetium Tc 99m Pyrophosphate The ideal infarct avid agent should be specific and sensitive in the detection of acute myocardial necrosis such that it can diagnose or exclude acute infarction in patients with chest pain. Unfortunately, positive technetium pyrophosphate scans have been noted in several groups of patients other than those with acute infarcts. Among these are individuals with unstable angina pectoris[58] and a substantial group of individuals without positive cardiac history who, in the process of undergoing undergoing skeletal scans with ^{99m}Tc, show positive myocardial uptake.[59] In the unstable angina population a recent study has shown that so-called false positive pyrophosphate scans may indeed be true positives when serial, highly sensitive and specific CPK-MB (creatine phosphokinase-myocardial band) assays are employed as

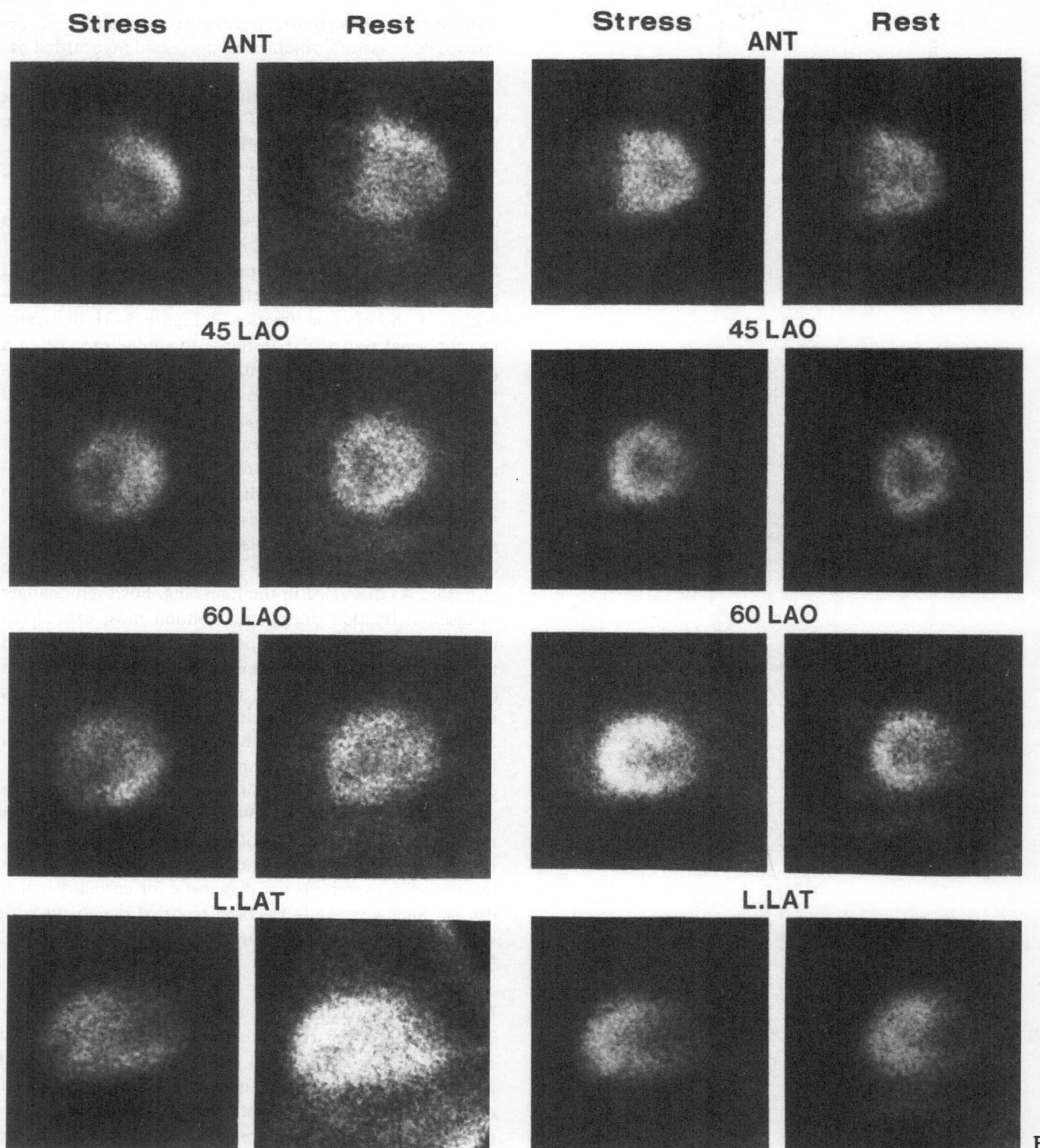

Fig. 3–28, A–C. *Stress and redistribution* ^{201}Tl *images in coronary artery disease.* **A** A defect is noted at stress in the anterior septum, posterior septum and apex. Through redistribution, images obtained some 3 hours later at rest reveal nearly complete "filling in" of the defect, implying exercise-induced ischemia. **B** After stress, a defect is present in the lateral and posterolateral walls in the 45° and 60° LAO images respectively. Only partial filling in of the defect is observed in the delayed images at rest implying infarct and associated ischemia. **C** After stress, a dilated, thin-walled left ventricle is noted with defects in the anterior wall,

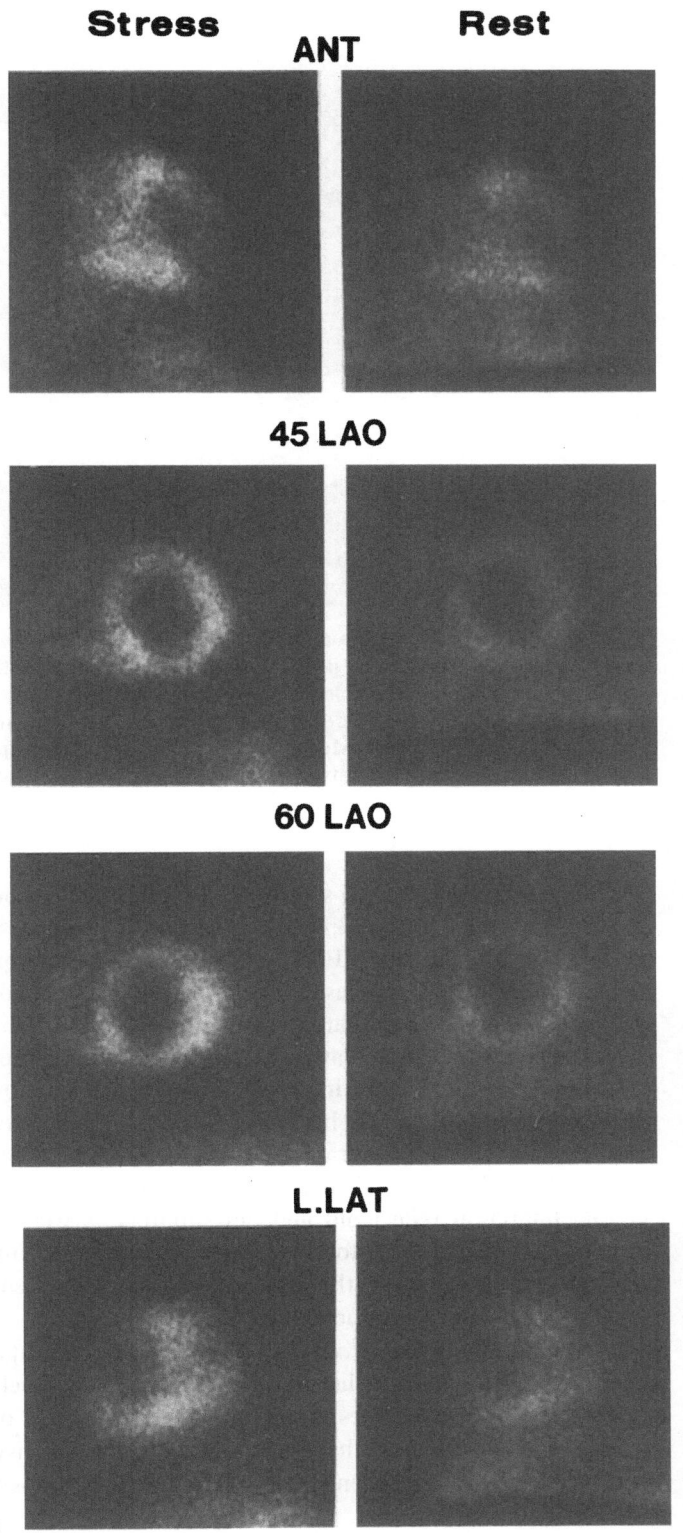

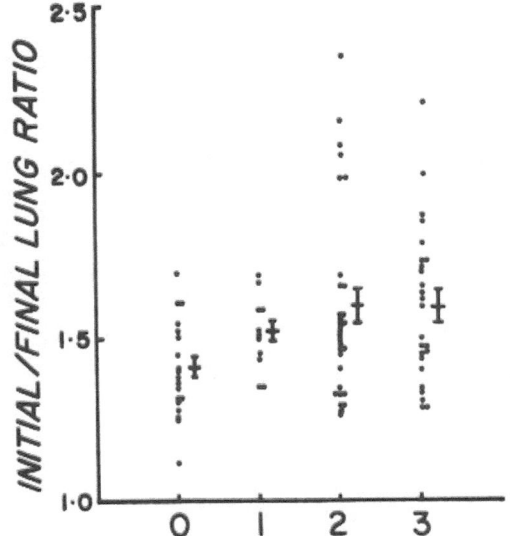

EXTENT OF CORONARY ARTERY DISEASE

Fig. 3–29. *Effect of the extent of coronary artery disease on the initial to final* ²⁰¹*Tl lung uptake ratio.* After stress in patients with CAD; lung to heart ²⁰¹Tl ratios are higher than in normal persons, presumably because of exercise-induced elevations in end-diastolic pressure. With time, lung ²⁰¹Tl "washes out," quickly resulting in higher initial to final ²⁰¹Tl lung ratios. This phenomenon may contribute to the apparent filling in of defects when background subtraction is employed in quantitative analysis of ²⁰¹Tl scintigrams. Reprinted with permission from Bingham JB et al. (1980) Influence of coronary artery disease on pulmonary uptake of thallium-201. Amer J Cardiol 46:821. By permission of the American Journal of Cardiology.

C

anterolateral wall, anterior septum and inferoapical walls. Four hours later, although left ventricular activity is reduced, reduction is uniform, implying that the defects present after exercise represent infarction.

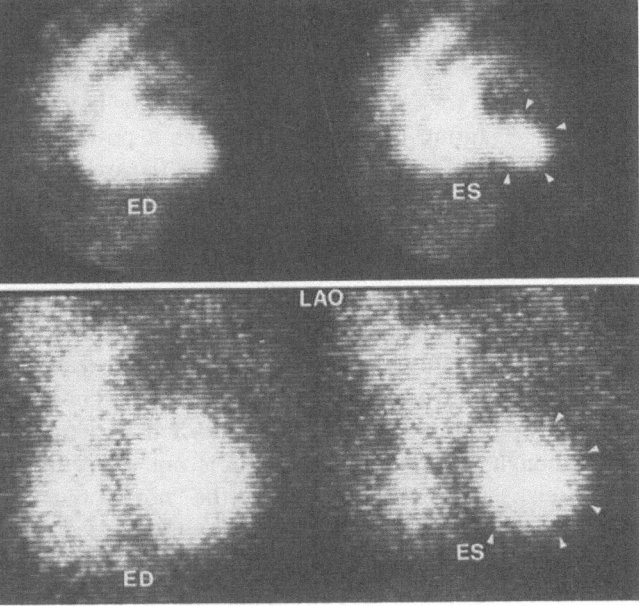

Fig. 3–30. *Ventricular asynergy at rest.* GBPS (resting) anterior and LAO, end-diastolic and end-systolic frames (*ED* and *ES*). *Arrows* demarcate an extensive region of akinesis.

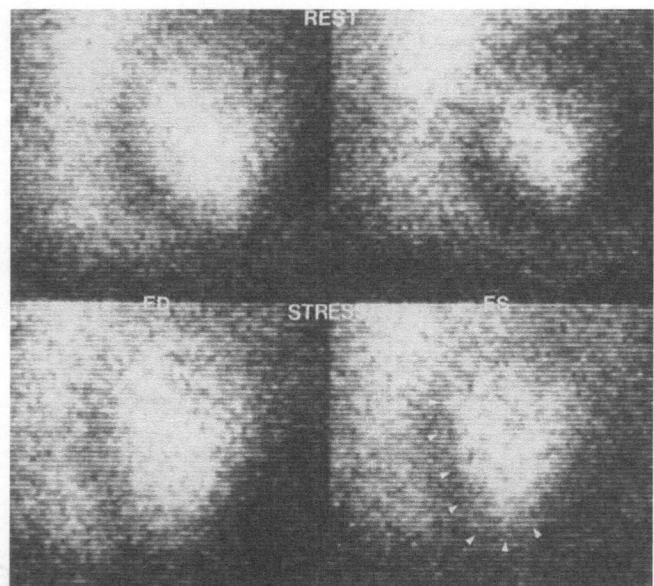

Fig. 3–31. *Exercise GBPS in CAD.* Rest and stress GBPS (supine). End-diastolic and end-systolic (*ED* and *ES*) frames from a patient with coronary artery disease. At rest the ventricle is of normal size and exhibits a normal contraction pattern (EF-64%). With peak exercise (supine) the ventricle dilates, and an extensive region of asynergy is noted in the septum and apex (*EF* = 42%).

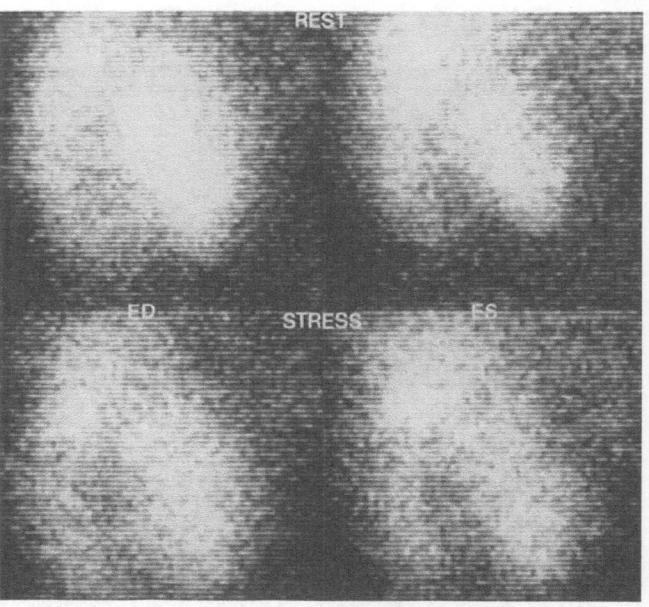

Fig. 3–32. *Abnormal response to exercise in aortic regurgitation.* Format and abbreviations as in Fig. 3–31. In this patient with aortic regurgitation the ventricle is dilated at rest, but the contraction pattern is normal. At peak exercise while the patient is supine the ventricle dilates further. Moderate diffuse hypokinesis is apparent. Patients with cardiomyopathy may have a similar response.

the standard method for comparison.[60] Although its specificity has been questioned, it is clear that technetium 99m scans are highly sensitive in the diagnosis of acute transmural myocardial infarction (MI). Scans will begin to suggest a positive result approximately 6 hours after the onset of symptoms, but maximal sensitivity is attained 2 to 5 days after the event.[61] Interpretation of the scans is qualitative with a 0 to 4+ rating scale commonly used (Table 3-3). A 2+ rating (or greater) signifies a positive test.[61] Various levels of positive results using ^{99m}Tc are illustrated in Fig. 3–33 to 3–35. It should be stressed that scans may be focally or diffusely positive. A 2+ diffuse rating creates difficult problems in interpretation, being a frequent cause of false positive scans. Yet the exclusion of such scans can significantly degrade the sensitivity of the test.[62,63] Causes for 2+ diffuse readings (other than acute transmural MI) include nontransmural MI, persistent blood pool activity, old infarction and, of course, normal variations.[64,65]

Although pyrophosphate uptake is not solely dictated by the size of the infarct, the size of the "hot spot" correlates reasonably well with the size of the infarct as measured by CPK enzyme curve analysis.[66] A large area of 3+ to 4+ uptake or a doughnut pattern indicates extensive infarction and a poor prognosis, as do persistently positive scans.[67,68] On the other hand, false negative scans indicate smaller acute infarcts and a better prognosis.[69]

Thallium 201 Scintigrams at rest (using thallium) are highly sensitive but not specific for the diagnosis of acute MI. The sensitivity is particularly good if scanning is performed within 6 hours of the onset of symptoms.[70] The

lack of specificity is due to scarring from old infarcts and in some instances to severe reductions in flow during rest in the absence of infarcts[71] (Fig. 3–36). Even with infarction the size of the defect decreases with time, perhaps secondary to regression of periinfarction ischemia. Therefore the thallium image obtained late correlates well with other measures of the size of an infarct.[72] Accurate localization of infarcts by thallium 201 has been confirmed by electrocardiography, ventriculography and postmortem studies.[73,74] Since thallium defects in the acute phase of a myocardial infarction reflect old and new infarcts as well as ischemia, they define the total quantity of nonfunctioning myocardium. They may therefore serve as an excellent prognostic indicator for short-term mortality.[75]

Radionuclide Ventriculography The location of segmental abnormalities on radionuclide ventriculography in the setting of acute MI correlates strongly with other means of infarct location. Further, these methods are quite sensitive and specific for the detection of left ventricular aneurysms[76]

Table 3–3. Rating Scale for Technetium Tc 99m Pyrophosphate Infarct Scans

0	= No activity
1+	= Faint activity
2+	= Definite activity but less than that of bone
3+	= Activity equal to bone
4+	= Activity greater than bone

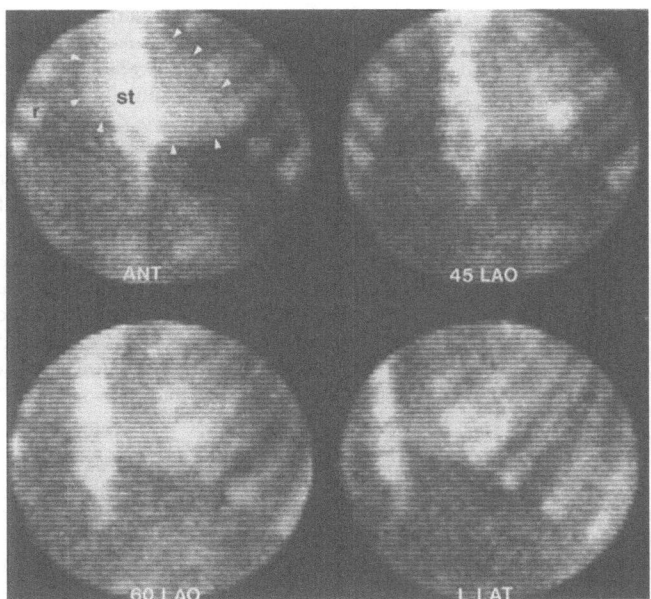

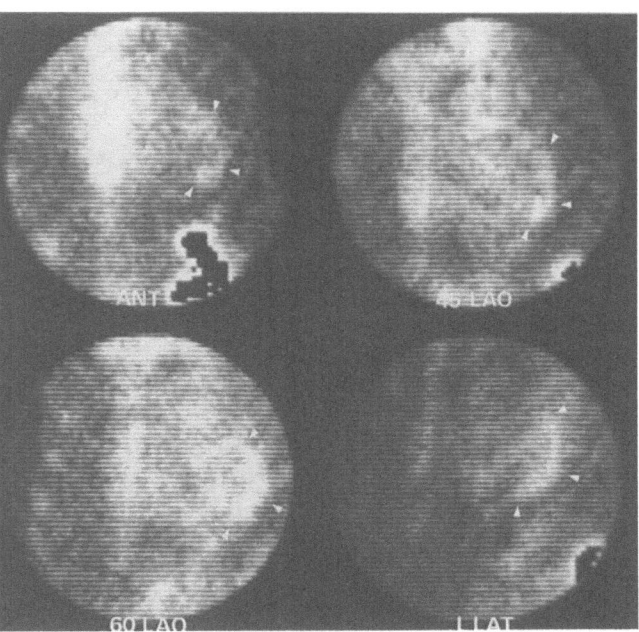

Fig. 3–33. *Pyrophosphate infarct scintigraphy.* A 2+ diffuse ^{99m}Tc pyrophosphate infarct scan in four standard projections. *Arrows* outline what appears to be the entire cardiac silhouette. Imaging of the femoral triangle showed that blood pool activity was not the cause for this finding. (See text for causes for 2+ diffuse readings.)

Fig. 3–35. ^{99m}*Tc infarct scan. Arrows* denote 4+ activity in the anterolateral, posterolateral and lateral walls.

of right ventricular infarction from cardiac tamponade in the setting of inferior wall MI (Fig. 3–38).[78] When first examined, patients with right ventricular infarction may have paradoxical pulse, elevation of jugular venous pressures and equalization of diastolic pressure in all chambers of the heart as manifestations of severe right ventricular failure. In other patients, the dip and plateau pressure pulse in the right ventricle closely mimic that observed in patients with constrictive pericarditis. Findings of right ventricular infarction by gated radionuclide angiography are quite characteristic demonstrating isolated asynergy of the LV inferior wall and basal septum and a dilated, hypokinetic RV. In tamponade or constriction, both the right and left ventricles are small and hypercontractile (Fig. 3–39).[79]

First-pass techniques can detect and quantify acute ventricular septal defects[80] in the setting of myocardial infarction (Fig. 3–40, A and B). A discussion on the quantitation of left-to-right shunts by radionuclide techniques is contained in the section on pediatric applications.

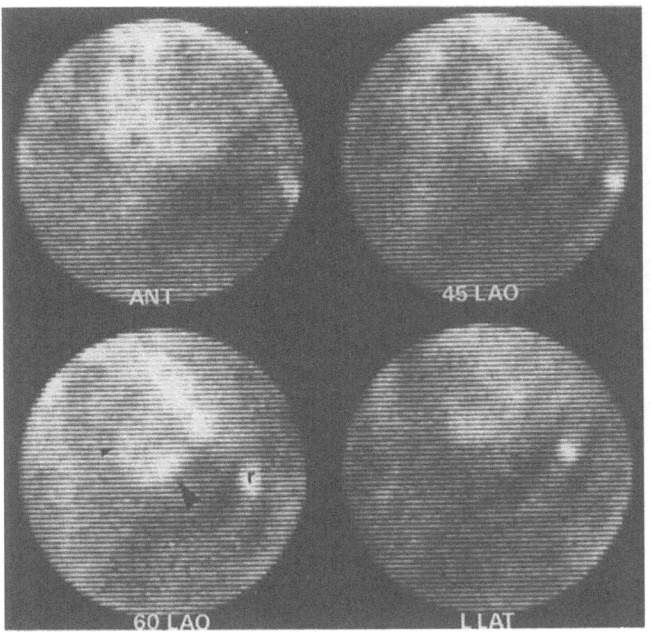

Fig. 3–34. ^{99m}*Tc infarct scan.* Abnormalities are best defined in the 60° LAO projection. *Large arrowhead* indicates 3+ activity in the posterolateral wall; *small arrowhead* indicates 2+ activity in the septum. *r* = increased activity in a rib.

Valvular Heart Disease

A great dilemma in clinical cardiology is the timing of operations in patients with regurgitant valvular lesions.[81] As with coronary artery disease, the extremes of ejection fractions at rest can be used to separate patients with poor and good prognoses. However, the distinction is often imperfect, especially in the middle range of ejection fraction. It would seem reasonable that the response of the left ventricle to stress may help separate those patients with favorable and unfavorable prognoses. However, the measurement of left ventricular performance in the setting of regurgitant valvar lesions is complicated by many factors. The most

(Fig. 3–37). Ejection fraction is depressed in the majority of patients with acute MI, and early improvement in ejection fraction is associated with a relatively good prognosis.[77] In addition, the influence of drugs and mechanical intervention on left ventricular function in acute MI can be assessed (Fig. 3–25). Radionuclide ventriculography has been of particular importance in the differentiation

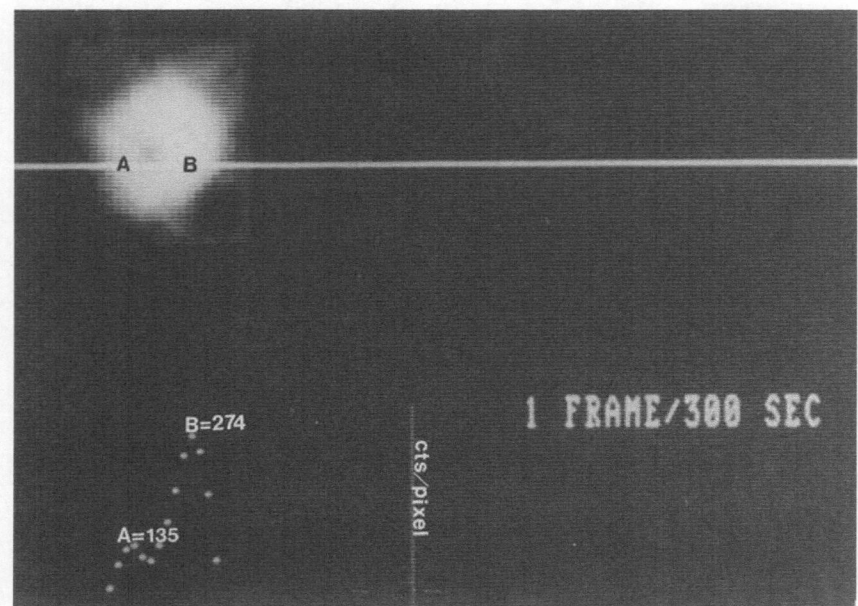

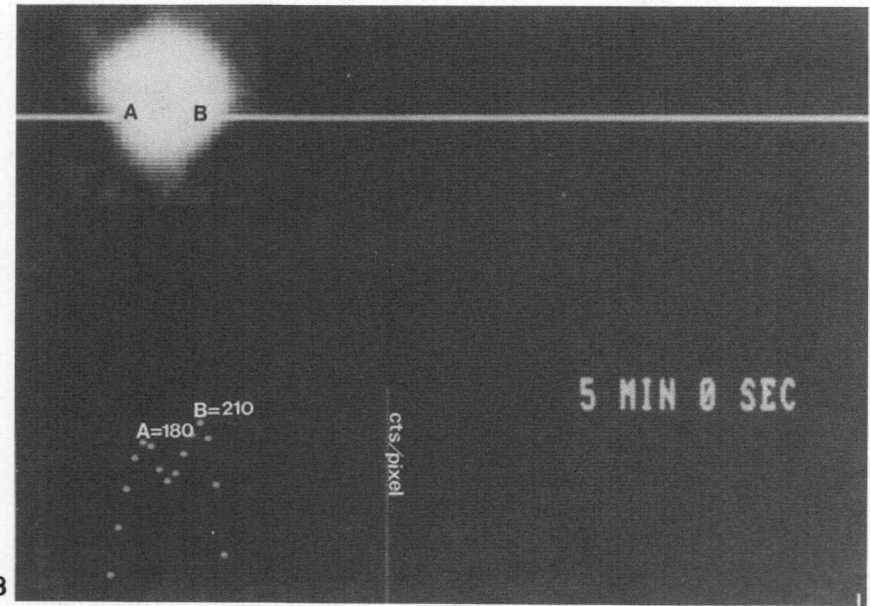

Fig. 3–36, A and B. [201]*Tl scintigram (resting) during an asymptomatic interlude in an elderly man with unstable angina.* **A** In this 45° LAO scintigram obtained early after ^{201}Tl injection, a qualitative defect is seen in the septum (*A*). Horizontal slice (*white line*) through the septum and posterolateral wall (*B*) is used to generate the count profile seen below. Peak counts in region A are 135, while in B they are 274. **B.** Three hours later the defect is no longer observed through an increase in counts in the septum and a decrease in the posterolateral wall. These findings are consistent with reduction of flow at rest in the LAD distribution.

commonly employed measure of left ventricular function is the ejection fraction. It is clear, however, that the ejection fraction reflects not only myocardial contractility but also other factors influencing global ventricular performance. These include heart rate, afterload and preload.[82] In the setting of coronary artery disease, a fall in ejection fraction with supine exercise can be viewed as a mismatch between the contractile state of the left ventricle and the afterload. Preload remains relatively constant. In regurgitant valvular heart disease, preload changes primarily during exercise,

and therefore must be considered in the analysis of left ventricular function during stress. For instance, during exercise in patients with aortic insufficiency left ventricular end-diastolic volume may decrease with tachycardia and a shortened diastolic filling period (Fig. 3–41). This factor may lower the ejection fraction. The simultaneous increase in afterload will also tend to decrease the ejection fraction. Under these circumstances the intrinsic contractility of the heart may or may not be the primary determinant of change in ejection fraction. Similar considerations exist in mitral

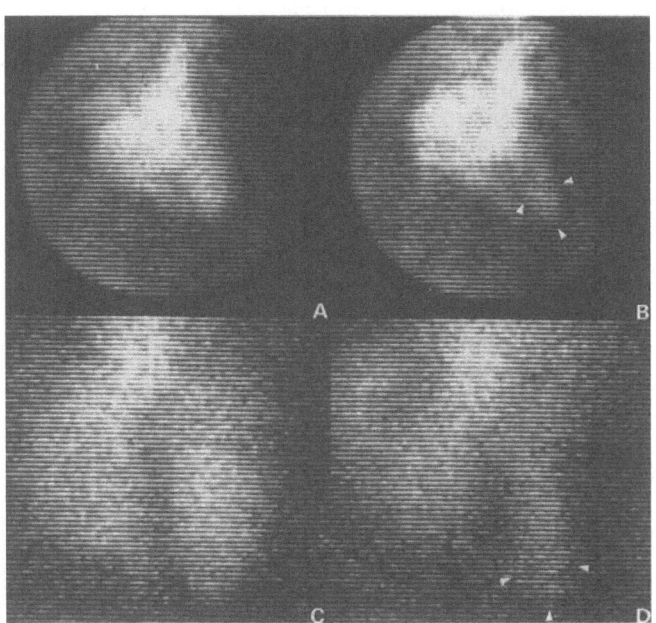

Fig. 3–37, A–D. *Ventricular aneurysm on GBPS* (*resting*). **A** and **C** Anterior and LAO end-diastolic frames and **B** and **D** end-systolic frames with dyskinetic segments indicated (*arrowheads*).

ED   ES

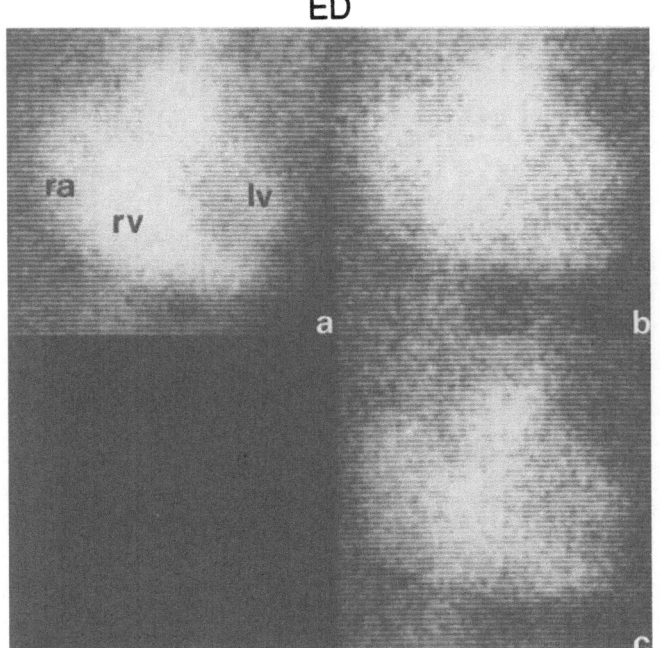

Fig. 3–38. *Right ventricular infarction.* End-diastolic (*ED*) and end-systolic (*ES*) anterior GBPS frames from a patient with an acute inferior wall myocardial infarction and associated right ventricular infarct. Clinical features simulated tamponade. Resting study (**A**) reveals dilated, akinetic right ventricle (*rv*), large right atrium (*ra*) and akinesis of the inferior wall of the left ventricle (*lv*). Therapy with inotropic agents (**B**) and intraaortic balloon pumping (**C**) proved to be of no avail.

regurgitation. Under these circumstances, for a given level of contractility, the ejection fraction would be expected to be higher because of a decrease in afterload that the mitral leak provides.[82] Therefore in the setting of mitral regurgitation, determination of the ejection fraction may lead to overestimation of the contractile function of the left ventricle. Although reports are emerging regarding left ventricular function during exercise in valvular heart disease, the clinical significance of the observations on ejection fraction requires further study.[83]

Radionuclide studies at rest can nevertheless provide valuable diagnostic information in patients with both valvular and pulmonary heart disease. As indicated, the regurgitant index can provide an estimate of the degree of mitral or aortic regurgitation.[17-19] In aortic stenosis the radionuclide blood pool study will offer a measure of left ventricular function in the presence of significant afterload stress. Thickening of the walls can be visualized and relative ventricular size estimated (Figs. 3–42, 3–43). In mitral regurgitation left ventricular size and motion as well as left and

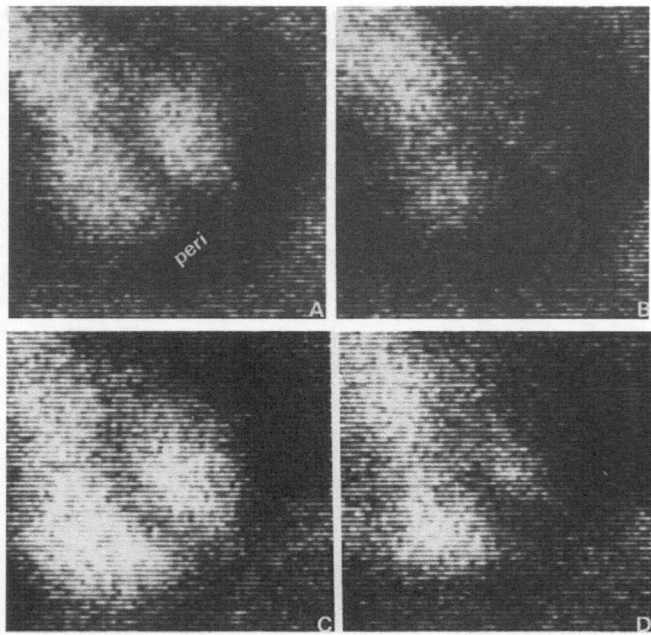

Fig. 3–39, A–D. *Cardiac tamponade.* **A** and **B** LAO GBPS end-diastolic and end-systolic frames. Both ventricles are small and hyperdynamic. Note large clear space around the heart representing pericardial fluid (*peri*), which is free of activity. **C** and **D**: End-diastolic and end-systolic frames after drainage of fluid. The ventricles have dilated to normal size, and the clear space around the heart has partially filled in.

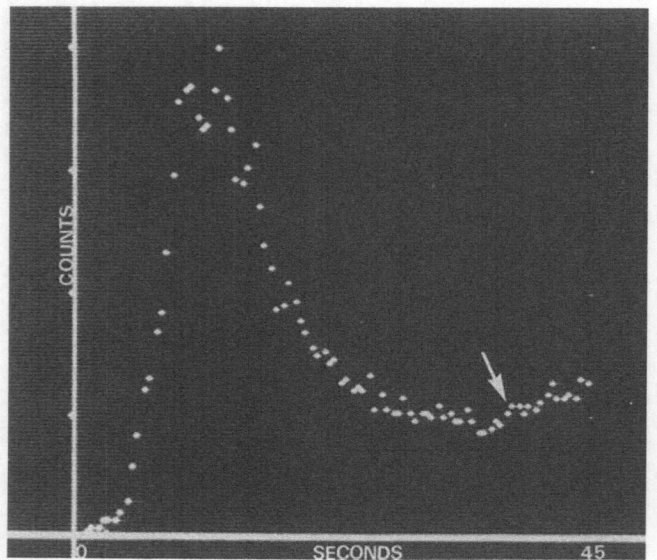

Fig. 3–40, A and B. *Calculations of shunt*—first-pass ⁹⁹ᵐTc time (x axis) vs activity (y axis) curve from a region of interest in the right lung. **A** In a patient without an intracardiac shunt.

Arrow indicates late recirculation of the tracer as it begins its second pass. **B** In a patient with a ventricular septal defect. Early recirculation of tracer is noted.

right atrial size can be estimated. The authors have learned that right ventricular size and function can be a useful clinical guide in mitral stenosis and regurgitation. In general, the systolic function of the right ventricle is inversely related to the afterload. Therefore in states causing pulmonary hypertension the right ventricle is often hypokinetic with a decreased ejection fraction. Figure 3–44 illustrates a dilated hyperkinetic left ventricle and a hypokinetic right ventricle in a patient with mitral regurgitation and pulmonary hypertension.

Left-sided congestive heart failure is often difficult to evaluate in patients with obstructive pulmonary disease.

Gated blood pool scanning or first-pass techniques can be of use in this regard. In the setting of pulmonary disease, the finding of a normal-sized, normally contracting left ventricle in the absence of valvular heart disease militates against a left ventricular component to the patient's symptom complex.[84] An exercise study would be of greater value in excluding a left ventricular contribution to activity-related symptoms.

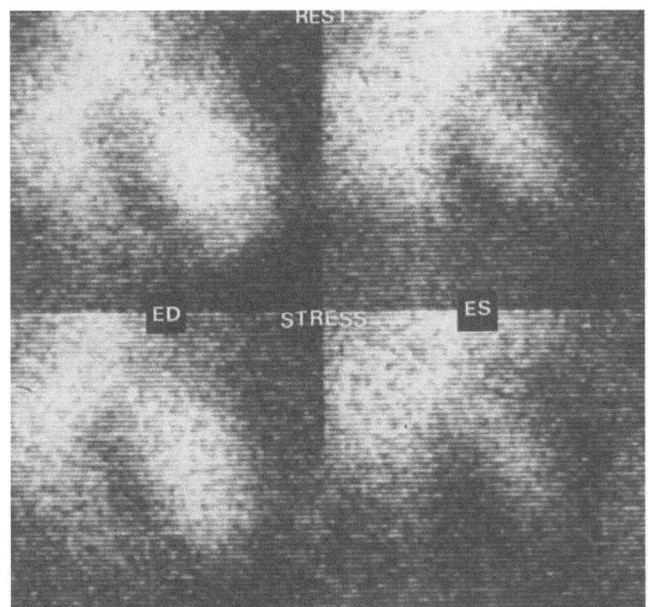

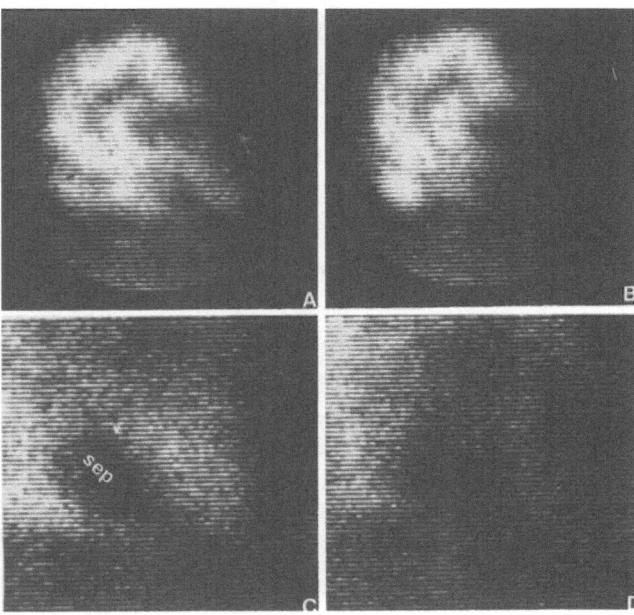

Fig. 3–41. *Normal response to exercise in aortic regurgitation.* Rest and exercise (supine) LAO GBPS in a patient with compensated aortic regurgitation. With exercise, both end-diastolic and end-systolic volumes decrease, resulting in no change or a fall in ejection fraction. In this setting, given the changing load, failure of the ejection fraction to rise may not signify impaired contractility.

Fig. 3–43, A–D. *Idiopathic hypertrophic subaortic stenosis.* Anterior full field (**A** and **B**) and LAO zoomed (**C** and **D**) GBPS (resting) from a patient with idiopathic hypertrophic subaortic stenosis. At end diastole in the LAO view (**C**) disproportionate upper septal (*sep*) thickening is seen. At end systole (**B** and **D**) activity is barely visible in this hypercontractile ventricle.

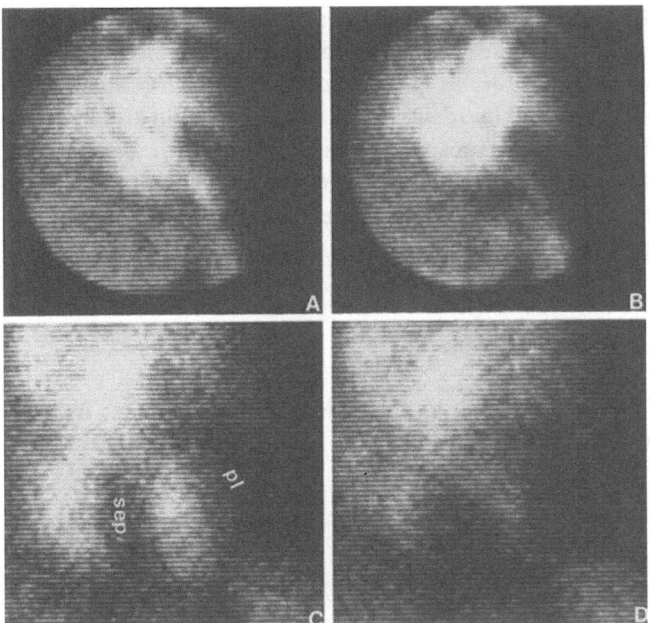

Fig. 3–42, A–D. *Aortic stenosis.* Full field anterior (**A** and **B**) and zoomed LAO (**C** and **D**) GBPS (resting) in a patient with valvular aortic stenosis. At end diastole (**C**), thick septal (*sep*) and posterolateral (*pl*) walls are seen. End-systolic frames (**B** and **D**) reveal a hypercontractile left ventricle.

Pediatric Applications

In children with congenital heart disease, isotope techniques are most useful in the evaluation of left-to-right and right-to-left shunts.[85-87]

In left-to-right intracardiac shunts, pulmonary venous return is shunted to the pulmonary circulation. This shunting may occur singly or in combination at either the great vessel level (e.g., patent ductus arteriosus, aorta-pulmonary window), atrial level (atrial septal defect) or ventricular level (ventricular septal defect). Using first-pass radionuclide angiography, contamination of pulmonary blood flow by pulmonary venous return can be detected and quantified.

Normally after intravenous injection of a bolus of isotope, pulmonary washout is exponential, with rapid clearance of isotope from the lung. In the presence of a left-to-right shunt, recirculation of isotope from the left side of the heart into the pulmonary circulation interrupts this washout, causing either a rise in pulmonary counts or a blunting of the exponential washout. Quantification of the degree of left-to-right shunting can be accomplished by comparing the observed pulmonary washout curve to that which would be expected in the absence of left-to-right shunting (Fig. 3–40A and B).

Unfortunately when a peripheral injection is used the site of left-to-right shunting cannot be detected. The method of peripheral injection is generally used as a screening technique to identify or rule out the presence of left-to-right shunts. However, if selective catheterization is performed it is possible to identify the level of left-to-right

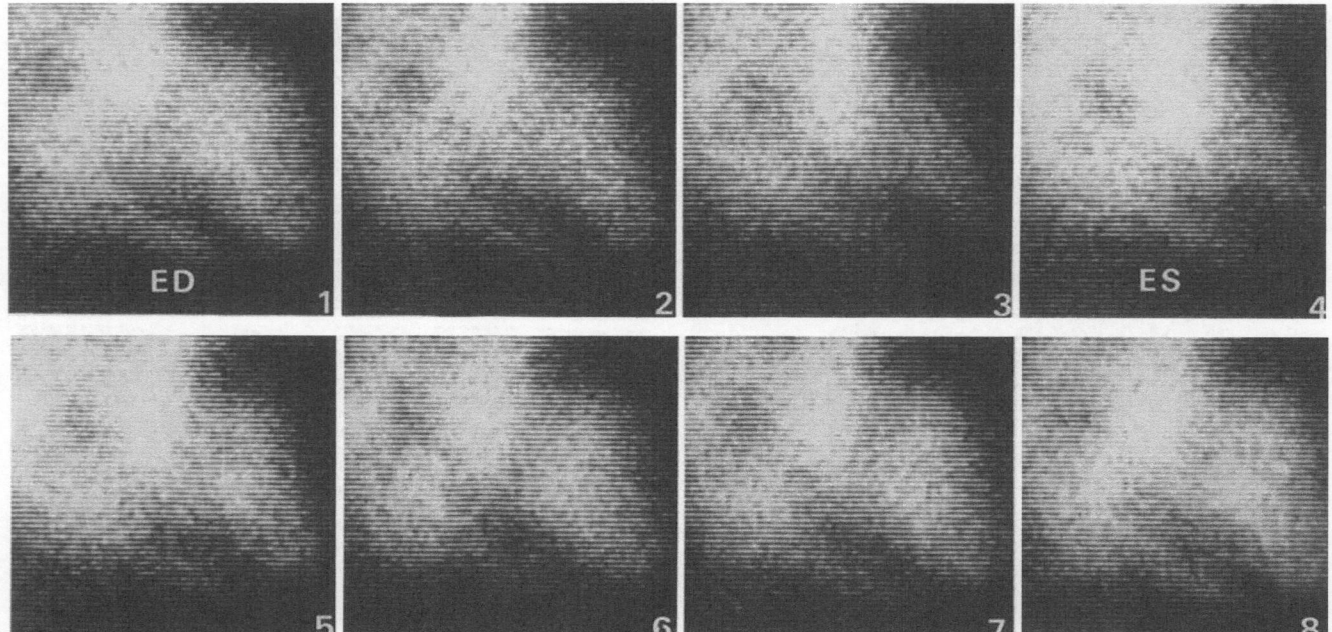

Fig. 3–44. *Mitral regurgitation.* Contraction sequence from an anterior, zoomed GBPS (resting) in a patient with mitral regurgitation. The left ventricle is dilated at end diastole (*ED*). With contraction (2–4), the left ventricle is noted to be hyperkinetic (EF = 80) while the right ventricle is hypokinetic (EF = 30). At catheterization, this patient's pulmonary artery systolic pressure approached systemic levels. Elevated pulmonary artery pressures may lower the right ventricular ejection fraction.

shunting by performing multiple first-pass studies. If this method is used during cardiac catheterization the number of contrast cineangiograms necessary to delineate abnormal anatomy can be reduced.

The detection of right-to-left shunts is also possible using first-pass angiography.[87] Right-to-left shunts are characterized by the shunting of systemic venous return into the systemic arteries. Right-to-left shunts frequently occur at the ventricular level (ventricular septal defect plus pulmonary stenosis) but in complex lesions can occur at either the atrial level (e.g., tricuspid atresia) or at the level of the great vessels (e.g., truncus arteriosus). A right-to-left shunt is detected by identifying the early appearance of a peripherally injected bolus of isotope in the systemic circulation. Quantification of right-to-left shunting is not easily accomplished.

Isotope detection of right-to-left shunts, using selective injection during cardiac catheterization, is particularly useful in evaluating cyanotic congenital heart disease in neonates. In these frequently critically ill babies the length of the procedure as well as radiation exposure can be markedly reduced by identifying the level of right-to-left shunting. Several lesions (e.g., transposition of the great vessels, total anomalous pulmonary venous return, pulmonary atresia) can be identified accurately without contrast angiography by using this technique.

Acknowledgment

The authors wish to thank Matrix Instruments, Incorporated for their help in photographic reproductions.

References

1. Rollo FD (ed) (1977) Nuclear Medicine Physics: Instrumentation and Agents. Mosby, St. Louis
2. Freeman LM, Blaufox MD (eds) (1979) Cardiovascular Nuclear Medicine I. Semin Nucl Med 9:224–319
3. Freeman LM, Blaufox MD (eds) (1980) Cardiovascular Nuclear Medicine II. Semin Nucl Med 10:2–105
4. Freeman LM, Blaufox MD (eds) (1980) Cardiovascular Nuclear Medicine III. Semin Nucl Med 10:115–192
5. Leitl GP, Buchanan JW, Wagner HN (1980) Monitoring cardiac function with nuclear techniques. Am J Cardiol 46:1125–1132

6. Ashburn WL, Schelbert HR, Verba JW (1978) Left ventricular ejection fraction: A review of several radionuclide angiographic approaches using the scintillation camera. Prog Cardiovasc Dis 20:267–284
7. Strauss HW, McKusick KA, Bingham JB (1980) Cardiac nuclear imaging: Principles, instrumentation, and pitfalls. Am J Cardiol 46:1109–1116
8. Lewis RP, Sandler H (1971) Relationship between changes in left ventricular dimensions and the ejection fraction in man. Circulation 44:548–557
9. Borer JS, Bacharach SL, Green MV, Kent KM, Epstein SE,

Johnston GS (1977) Real-time radionuclide cineangiography in the non-invasive evaluation of global and regional left ventricular function at rest and during exercise in patients with coronary artery disease. N Engl J Med 296:839–844

10. Strauss HW, Harrison K, Langan JK, Lebowitz E, Pitt B (1975) Thallium-201 for myocardial imaging: Relation of thallium-201 to regional myocardial perfusion. Circulation 51:641–645

11. Cohen HA, Baird MG, Rouleau JR (1976) Thallium-201 myocardial imaging in patients with pulmonary hypertension. Circulation 54:790–795

12. Braunwald E, Ross J, Sonnenblick EH (1976) Mechanisms of contraction of the normal and failing heart, 2nd ed. Boston, Little, Brown

13. Sonnenblick EH, Strobeck JE (1977) Derived indices of ventricular and myocardial function. N Engl J Med 296:978–982

14. Slutsky R, Karliner J, Ricci D, Schuler G, Pfisterer M, Peterson K, Ashburn W (1979) Response of left ventricular volume to exercise in man assessed by radionuclide equilibrium angiography. Circulation 60:565–571

15. Dehmer GJ, Lewis SE, Hillis LD, Twieg D, Falkoff M, Parker RW, Willerson JT (1980) Nongeometric determination of left ventricular volumes from equilibrium blood pool scans. Am J Cardiol 45:293–300

16. Slutsky R, Karliner J, Ricci D, Kaiser R, Pfisterer M, Gordon D, Peterson K, Ashburn W (1979) Left ventricular volumes by gated equilibrium radionuclide angiography: A new method. Circulation 60:556–564

17. Rigo P, Alderson PO, Robertson RM, Becker LC, Wagner HN (1979) Measurement of aortic and mitral regurgitation by gated cardiac blood pool scans. Circulation 60:306–312

18. Urquhart J, Patterson RE, Packer M, Goldsmith SJ, Horowitz SF, Litwak R, Gorlin R (1981) Quantitation of valve regurgitation by radionuclide angiography before and after valve replacement surgery. Am J Cardiol 47:287–291

19. Lam W, Pavel D, Byrom E, Sheikh A, Best D, Rosen K (1981) Radionuclide regurgitant indices: Value and limitations. Am J Cardiol 47:292–298

20. Ross J (1976) Afterload mismatch and preload reserve: A conceptual framework for the analysis of ventricular function. Prog Cardiovasc Dis 18:255–264

21. Cohn PF, Gorlin R, Cohn LH, Collins JJ (1974) Left ventricular ejection fraction as a prognostic guide in surgical treatment of coronary and valvular heart disease. Am J Cardiol 34:136–141

22. Nelson GR, Cohn PF, Gorlin R (1975) Prognosis in medically-treated coronary artery disease. Circulation 52:408–412

23. Ganz W, Wexler JP, Rabinowitz A, Brenner AI, Steingart RM, Blaufox MD (1980) Methods of improving the precision of left ventricular volume and ejection fraction determination. J Nucl Med 21:48

24. Schelbert HR, Verba JW, Johnson AD, Brock GW, Alazraki NP, Rose FJ, Ashburn WL (1975) Nontraumatic determination of left ventricular ejection fraction by radionuclide angiocardiography. Circulation 51:902–909

25. Ganz W, Wexler JP, Breener AI, Bontemps R, Steingart RM, Blaufox MD (1980) Variability of resting gated ejection fraction. J Nucl Med 21:163

26. Wexler JP, Steingart RM, Blaufox MD (1981) Physiologic intervention in cardiovascular nuclear medicine. Semin Nucl Med 11:68–79

27. Mahler F, Ross J, O'Rourke RA, Covell JW (1975) Effects of changes in preload, afterload and inotropic state on ejection and isovolumic phase measures of contractility in the conscious dog. Am J Cardiol 35:626–634

28. Slutsky R, Karliner J, Gerber K, Battler A, Froelicher V, Gregoratos G, Peterson K, Ashburn W (1980) Peak systolic blood pressure/end-systolic volume ratio: Assessment at rest and during exercise in normal subjects and patients with coronary heart disease. Am J Cardiol 46:813–820

29. Herman MV, Gorlin R (1969) Implications of left ventricular asynergy. Am J Cardiol 23:538–547

30. Maddox DE, Wynne J, Uren R, Parker JA, Idoine J, Siegel LC, Neill JM, Cohn PF, Holman BL (1979) Regional ejection fraction: A quantitative radionuclide index of regional left ventricular performance. Circulation 59:1001–1009

31. Fisher EA, DuBrow I, Hastreiter AR (1975) Right ventricular volume in congenital heart disease. Am J Cardiol 36:67–75

32. Berger HJ, Matthay RA, Loke J, Marshall RC, Gottschalk A, Zaret BL (1978) Assessment of cardiac performance with quantitative radionuclide angiocardiography; right ventricular ejection fraction with reference to findings in chronic obstructive pulmonary disease. Am J Cardiol 41:897–905

33. Smith EE, Guyton AC, Manning RD, White RJ (1975) Integrated mechanisms of cardiovascular response and control during exercise in the normal human. Prog Cardiovasc Dis 18:421–444

34. Lind AR (1970) Cardiovascular responses to static exercise. Circulation 41:173–176

35. Helfant RH, DeVilla MA, Meister SG (1971) Effect of sustained isometric handgrip exercise on left ventricular performance. Circulation 44:982–993

36. Steingart RM, Wexler JP, Blaufox MD (1981) Pharmacologic intervention in cardiovascular nuclear medicine procedures. Semin Nucl Med 21:80–88

37. Pohost GM, Alpert NM, Ingwall JS, Strauss HW (1980) Thallium redistribution: Mechanisms and clinical utility. Semin Nucl Med 10:70–93

38. Gould KL, Lipscomb K, Hamilton GW (1974) Physiological basis for assessing critical coronary stenosis. Am J Cardiol 33:87–94

39. Holmberg S, Serzysko W, Varnauskas E (1971) Coronary circulation during heavy exercise in control subjects and patients with coronary heart disease. Acta Med Scand 190:465–480

40. Gould KL (1978) Noninvasive assessment of coronary stenosis by myocardial imaging during pharmacologic coronary vasodilation I. Physiological basis and experimental validation. Am J Cardiol 41:267–278

41. Leppo J, Yipintsoi T, Blankstein R, Bontemps R, Freeman LM, Zohman L, Scheuer J (1979) Thallium-201 myocardial scintigraphy in patients with triple vessel disease and ischemic exercise stress tests. Circulation 59:714–721

42. Burow RD, Pond M, Schafer AW, Becker L (1979) "Circumferential profiles": A new method for computer analysis of thallium-201 myocardial perfusion images. J Nucl Med 20:771–777

43. Garcia E, Maddahi J, Berman D, Waxman A (1981) Space/time quantitation of thallium-201 myocardial scintigraphy. J Nucl Med 22:309–317

44. Ritchie JL, Zaret BL, Strauss HW, Pitt B, Berman DS, Schelbert HR, Ashburn WL, Berger HJ, Hamilton GW (1978)

Myocardial imaging with thallium-201: A multicenter study in patients with angina pectoris or acute myocardial infarction. Am J Cardiol 42:345–350

45. Ritchie JL, Troubaugh GB, Hamilton GW, Gould KL, Narahara KA, Murray JA, Williams DL (1977) Myocardial imaging with thallium-201 at rest and during exercise. Circulation 56:66–71

46. Bailey IK, Griffith LSC, Rouleau J, Strauss HW, Pitt B (1977) Thallium-201 myocardial perfusion imaging at rest and during exercise. Circulation 55:79–87

47. McLaughlin PR, Martin RP, Doherty P, Daspit S, Goris M, Haskell W, Lewis S, Kriss JP, Harrison DC (1977) Reproducibility of thallium-201 myocardial imaging. Circulation 55:497–503

48. Mueller TM, Marcus ML, Ehrhardt JC, Chaudhuri T, Abboud FM (1976) Limitations of thallium-201 myocardial perfusion scintigrams. Circulation 54:640–646

49. Massie BM, Botvinick EH, Brundage BH (1979) Correlation of thallium-201 scintigrams with coronary anatomy: Factors affecting region by region sensitivity. Am J Cardiol 44:616–622

50. Pohost GM, Zir LM, Moore RH, McKusick KA, Guiney TE, Beller GA (1977) Differentiation of transiently ischemic from infarcted myocardium by serial imaging after a single dose of thallium-201. Circulation 55:294–302

51. Schelbert HR, Schuler G, Ashburn WL, Covell JW (1979) Time-course of "redistribution" of thallium-201 administered during transient ischemia. Eur J Nucl Med 4:351–358

52. Cook DJ, Bailey I, Strauss HW, Rouleau J, Wagner HN, Pitt B (1976) Thallium-201 for myocardial imaging: Appearance of the normal heart. J Nucl Med 17:583–589

53. Boden WE, Bough EW, Korr KS, Benhan I, Gheorghiade N, Caputi A, Shulman RS (1981) Exercise-induced coronary spasm with S-T segment depression and normal coronary arteriography. Am J Cardiol 48:193–197

54. Bingham JB, McKusick KA, Strauss HW, Boucher CA, Pohost GM (1980) Influence of coronary artery disease on pulmonary uptake of thallium-201. Am J Cardiol 46:821–826

55. Okada RD, Kirshenbaum HD, Kushner FG, Strauss HW, Dinsmore RE, Newell JB, Boucher CA, Block PC, Pohost GM (1980) Observer variance in the qualitative evaluation of left ventricular wall motion and the quantitation of left ventricular ejection fraction using rest and exercise multigated blood pool imaging. Circulation 61:128–136

56. Borer JS, Kent KM, Bacharach SL, Green MV, Rosing DR, Seides SF, Epstein SE, Johnston GS (1979) Sensitivity, specificity and predictive accuracy of radionuclide cineangiography during exercise in patients with coronary artery disease. Circulation 60:572–580

57. Borer JS, Bacharach SL, Green MV, Kent KM, Henry WL, Rosing DR, Seides SF, Johnston GS, Epstein SE (1978) Exercise-induced left ventricular dysfunction in symptomatic and asymptomatic patients with aortic regurgitation: Assessment with radionuclide cineangiography. Am J Cardiol 42:351–357

58. Ahmad N, Dubiel JP, Logan KW, Verdon TA, Martin RH (1977) Limited clinical diagnostic specificity of technetium-99m stannous pyrophosphate myocardial imaging in acute myocardial infarction. Am J Cardiol 39:50–54

59. Prasquier R, Taradash MR, Botvinick EH, Shames DM, Parmley WW (1977) The specificity of the diffuse pattern of cardiac uptake in myocardial infarction imaging with technetium-99m stannous pyrophosphate. Circulation 55:61–66

60. Jaffe AS, Klein MS, Patel BR, Siegel BA, Roberts R (1979) Abnormal technetium-99m pyrophosphate images in unstable angina: Ischemia versus infarction? Am J Cardiol 44:1035–1039

61. Parkey RW, Bonte FJ, Meyer SL, Atkins JM, Curry GL, Stokely EM, Willerson JT (1974) A new method for radionuclide imaging of acute myocardial infarction in humans. Circulation 50:540–546

62. Massie BM, Botvinick EH, Werner JA, Chatterjee J, Parmley WW (1979) Myocardial scintigraphy with technetium-99m stannous pyrophosphate: An insensitive test for non-transmural myocardial infarction. Am J Cardiol 43:186–192

63. Willerson JT, Parkey RW, Bonte FJ, Meyer SL, Stokely EM (1975) Acute subendocardial myocardial infarction in patients. Its detection by technetium-99m stannous pyrophosphate myocardial scintigrams. Circulation 51:436–441

64. Berman DS, Amsterdam EA, Hines HH, Denardo GL, Salel AF, Ikeda R, Jansholt A, Mason DT (1977) Problem of diffuse cardiac uptake of technetium-99m pyrophosphate in the diagnosis of acute myocardial infarction: Enhanced scintigraphic accuracy by computerized selective blood pool subtraction. Am J Cardiol 40:768–774

65. Olson HG, Lyons KP, Aronow WS, Kuperus J, Orlando J, Hughes D (1979) Prognostic value of a persistently positive technetium-99m stannous pyrophosphate myocardial scintigram after myocardial infarction. Am J Cardiol 43:889–898

66. Henning H, Schelbert HR, Righetti A, Ashburn WL, O'Rourke RA (1977) Dual myocardial imaging with technetium-99m pyrophosphate and thallium-201 for detecting, localizing and sizing acute myocardial infarction. Am J Cardiol 40:147–155

67. Ahmad M, Logan KW, Martin RH (1979) Doughnut pattern of technetium-99m pyrophosphate myocardial uptake in patients with acute myocardial infarction: A sign of poor long term prognosis. Am. J. Cardiol 44:13–17

68. Olson HG, Lyons KP, Aronow WS, Brown WT, Greenfield RS (1977) Follow-up technetium-99m stannous pyrophosphate myocardial scintigrams after acute myocardial infarction. Circulation 56:181–187

69. Holman BL, Chisholm RJ, Braunwald E (1978) The prognostic implications of acute myocardial infarct scintigraphy with 99m-Tc pyrophosphate. Circulation 57:320–326

70. Wackers FJ, Sokole EB, Samson G, VanDerSchoot JB, Lie KI, Liem KL, Wellens HJJ (1976) Value and limitations of thallium-201 scintigraphy in the acute phase of myocardial infarction. N. Engl J Med 295:1–5

71. Berger BC, Watson DD, Burwell LR, Crosby IK, Wellons HA, Teates CD, Beller GA (1979) Redistribution of thallium at rest in patients with stable and unstable angina and the effect of coronary artery bypass surgery. Circulation 60:1114–1125

72. Smitherman TC, Osborn RC, Narahara KA (1978) Serial myocardial scintigraphy after a single dose of thallium-201 in men after acute myocardial infarction. Am J Cardiol 42:177–182

73. Niess GS, Logic JR, Russell RO, Rackley CE, Rogers WJ (1979) Usefulness and limitations of thallium-201 myocardial scintigraphy in delineating location and size of prior myocardial infarction. Circulation 59:1010–1018

74. Wackers FJ, Lie KI, Sokole EB, Res J, VanDerSchoot JB, Durrer D (1978) Prevalence of right ventricular involvement

in inferior wall infarction assessed with myocardial imaging with thallium-201 and technetium-99M pyrophosphate. Am J Cardiol 42:358–362

75. Silverman KJ, Becker LC, Bulkley BH, Burrow RD, Mellits ED, Kallman CH, Weisfeldt ML (1980) Value of early thallium-201 scintigraphy for predicting mortality in patients with acute myocardial infarction. Circulation 61:996–1003

76. Rigo P, Murray M, Strauss HW, Pitt B (1974) Scintiphotographic evaluation of patients with suspected left ventricular aneurysm. Circulation 50:985–991

77. Rigo P, Murray M, Strauss HW, Taylor D, Kelly D, Wiesfeldt M, Pitt B (1974) Left ventricular function in acute myocardial infarction evaluated by gated scintiphotography. Circulation 50:678–684

78. Lorell B, Leinbach RC, Pohost GM, Gold HK, Dinsmore RE, Hutter AM, Pastore JO, Desanctis RW (1979) Right ventricular infarction. Am J Cardiol 43:465–471

79. Steingart RM (1980) Gated radionuclide ventriculography in the differential diagnosis of right ventricular infarction. J Med Soc NJ 77:597–599

80. Maltz DL, Treves S (1973) Quantitative radionuclide angiocardiography: Determination of Qp:Qs in children. Circulation 47:1049–1056

81. O'Rourke RA, Crawford MH (1980) Timing of valve replacement in patients with chronic aortic regurgitation. Circulation 61:493–495

82. Boucher CA, Okada RD, Pohost GM (1980) Current status of radionuclide imaging in valvular heart disease. Am J Cardiol 46:1153–1163

83. Borer JS, Rosing DR, Kent KM, Bacharach SL, Green MV, McIntosh CJ, Morrow AG, Epstein SE (1979) Left ventricular function at rest and during exercise after aortic valve replacement in patients with aortic regurgitation. Am J Cardiol 44:1297–1305

84. Berger HJ, Matthay RA, Pytlik LM, Gottschalk A, Zaret BL (1979) First-pass radionuclide assessment of right and left ventricular performance in patients with cardiac and pulmonary disease. Semin Nucl Med 9:275–295

85. Anderson PAW, Jones RH, Sabiston DC (1974) Quantitation of left-to-right cardiac shunts with radionuclide angiography. Circulation 49:512–516

86. Parker JA, Treves S (1972) Radionuclide detection, localization and quantitation of intracardiac shunts and shunts between the great arteries. Prog Cardiovasc Dis 13:142–147

87. Treves S, Fogle R, Lang P (1980) Radionuclide angiography in congenital heart disease. Am J Cardiol 46:1247–1255

4 Ischemic Heart Disease

Atherosclerosis of the coronary arteries is the most common cause of clinical ischemic heart disease. The Framingham heart study shows a marked increase in coronary artery disease and myocardial infarction after the age of 40 years.

Coronary atherosclerosis remains asymptomatic for many years in most individuals and permanently so in many. Clinical manifestations occur because of luminal narrowing of a major coronary branch due to (1) progression of the atheromatous process, (2) coronary artery thrombosis, (3) intramural hemorrhage, (4) vasoconstriction (Prinzmetal angina), (5) coronary aneurysms (acquired; congenital); and (6) a combination thereof.

Atherosclerosis is a multifactorial process. Diet high in saturated fat and cholesterol, emotional stress, physical inactivity, hypertension, diabetes, gout, smoking and inherited factors, including hyperlipidemia, play a role in the development of atherosclerosis. The clinical manifestations can be divided into three groups: (1) stable angina pectoris, (2) unstable angina pectoris (preinfarction angina) and (3) acute myocardial infarction.

Other causes of ischemic heart disease and myocardial infarction include aortic stenosis, subaortic stenosis and coronary embolism. Less common causes are anemia and metabolic abnormalities at the cellular or molecular level, which produce chronic hypoxia and damage to the myocardium. Furthermore, the small coronary vessels may be diseased with no involvement of the large coronary arteries.

The major complications of acute myocardial infarction are (1) cardiac arrhythmia, (2) pump failure presenting as cardiogenic shock or congestive heart failure, (3) systemic embolization, (4) ventricular aneurysm, (5) cardiac and interventricular septal rupture, and (6) papillary muscle dysfunction or rupture.

Radiological Examination

The size of the heart in patients with chronic ischemic heart disease, even in cases with advanced coronary artery disease, may be normal on plain films. The presence of cardiomegaly with left ventricular prominence suggests left ventricular dysfunction (asynergy). Left atrial and left ventricular enlargement, particularly with evidence of congestive heart failure, suggests papillary muscle dysfunction. An abnormal bulge of the left heart border may indicate a ventricular (true) aneurysm (Fig. 4–1), whereas a paracardiac mass (Fig. 4–2), particularly in the posterolateral region of the left ventricle, suggests a pseudoaneurysm.

Acute myocardial infarction may result in congestive heart failure with pulmonary vascular redistribution to the upper lobes, perihilar haziness, Kerley B lines, basal interstitial infiltrates and interstitial or alveolar pulmonary edema or both. Development of pulmonary edema after myocardial infarction is usually a poor prognostic sign. The presence of pulmonary edema with a relatively normal heart size suggests papillary muscle rupture (the differential diagnosis includes uremia, mitral stenosis, toxic-gas inhalation, postictal pulmonary edema, drug allergy, pulmonary hemorrhage, heroin intoxication, near-drowning and excess administration of intravenous fluids).

The postmyocardial infarction syndrome (Dressler syndrome) is characterized by an enlarged cardiac silhouette due to pericardial effusion (Fig. 4–3). In addition the development of pleural effusion and pulmonary infiltrates is characteristic. Evidence of congestive heart failure is generally not present. However, in a few patients signs of left ventricular failure, including widening of the superior mediastinum, may be observed. The prime elements of the Dressler syndrome, therefore, are pericarditis, pleuritis and pneumonitis. The syndrome probably represents an autoimmune reaction, initiated by necrotic myocardial tissue, and is reminiscent of the group of postcardiotomy syndromes,

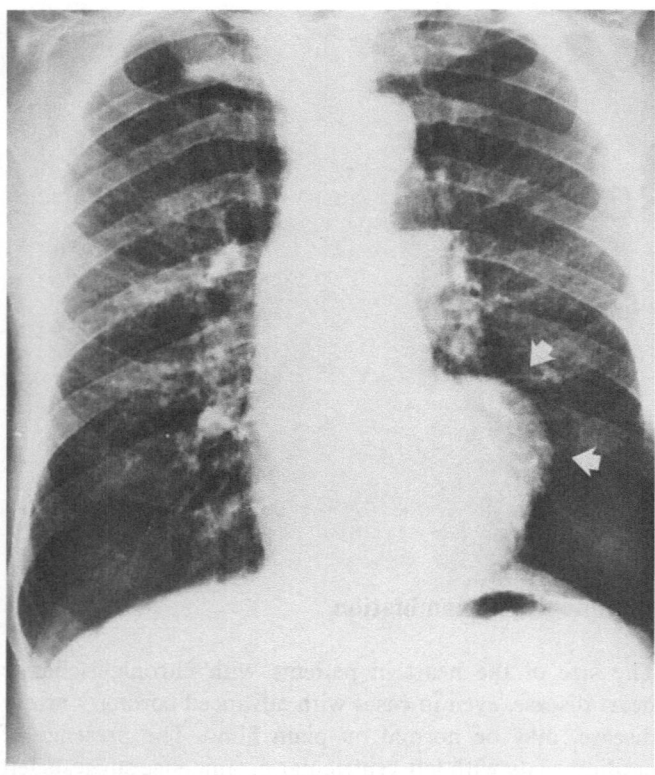

A

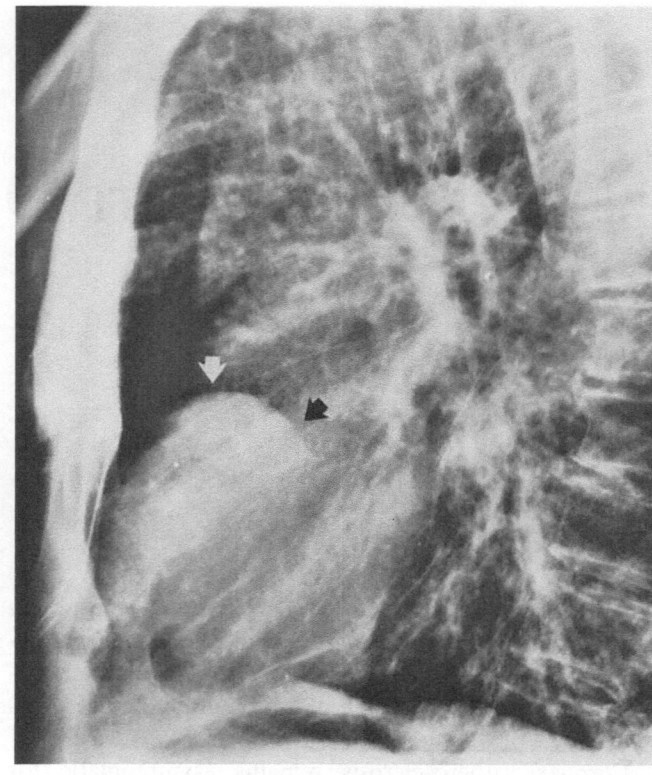

B

Fig. 4–1. *True aneurysm.* PA **(A)** and lateral **(B)** views show a bulge along the anterolateral wall of the left ventricle characteristic of true aneurysms. More often true aneurysms are not identified on plain films or are observed as cardiomegaly (left ventricular enlargement). Dachman A, Spindola-Franco H, Solomon N (1981) Left ventricular pseudoaneurysm: Its recognition and significance JAMA 246:1951–1953

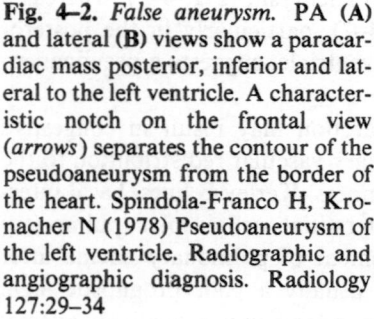

Fig. 4–2. *False aneurysm.* PA **(A)** and lateral **(B)** views show a paracardiac mass posterior, inferior and lateral to the left ventricle. A characteristic notch on the frontal view (*arrows*) separates the contour of the pseudoaneurysm from the border of the heart. Spindola-Franco H, Kronacher N (1978) Pseudoaneurysm of the left ventricle. Radiographic and angiographic diagnosis. Radiology 127:29–34

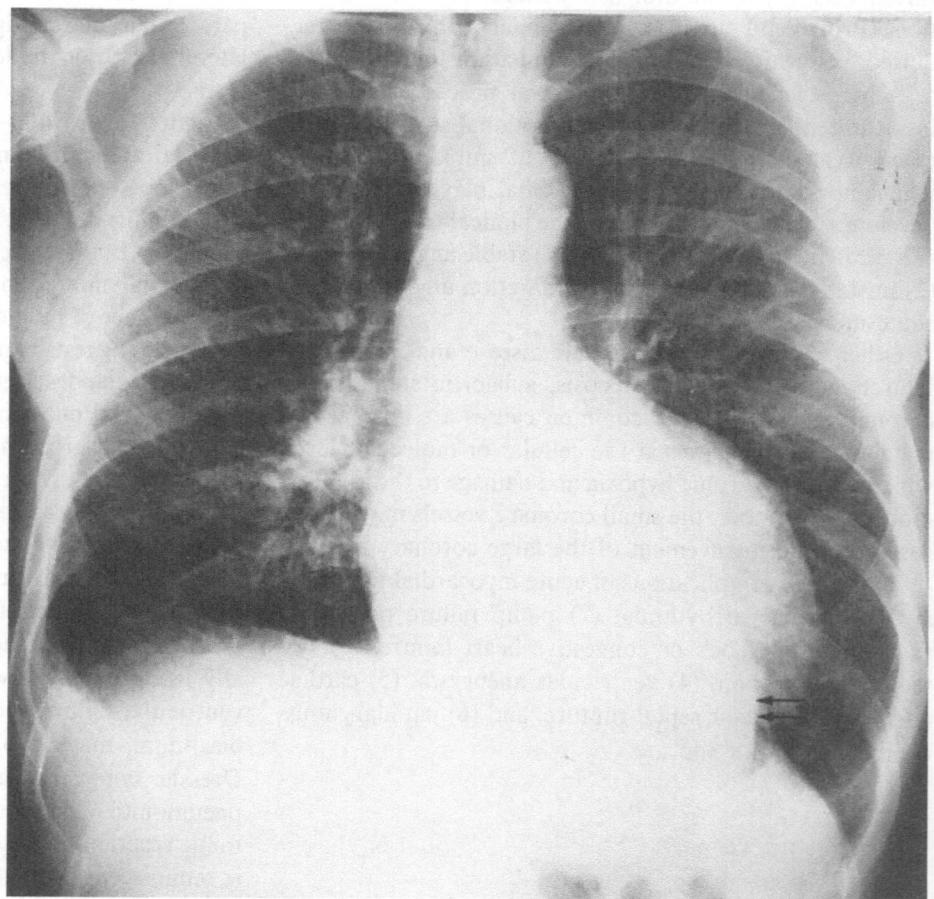

A

the traumatic pericarditis syndrome and the acute pericarditis (idiopathic or viral) syndrome.

Other sequelae (or complications) of myocardial infarction include left ventricular aneurysm, pseudoaneurysm and cardiac rupture. Plain film findings associated with these sequelae are described subsequently in this work. See Figs. 4–41 to 4–45.

Coronary Arteriography

The terms *arteriography* and *angiography* are often used interchangeably, although technically *angiography* refers to veins as well as arteries.

Coronary arteriography deals with the study of the anatomy of the coronary arteries, visualized radiologically by means of contrast medium that has been injected. Coronary arteriography is performed in conjunction with left ventriculography. Here the presence of contrast material within the left ventricle permits determination of the systolic and diastolic volumes of the left ventricle, the ejection fraction, the characteristics of the contractions of the left ventricle, mitral prolapse and some of the other complications of myocardial infarction.

Indications (Table 4–1) The most important indications for coronary arteriography are (1) intractable angina pectoris refractory to medical therapy; (2) preinfarction angina (unstable angina) not amenable to medical therapy; (3)

Table 4–1. Indications for Coronary Arteriography

Ischemic Heart Disease
Symptomatic patients
  Clinical suspicion of angina but not conclusive
  Stable angina
    Inability to tolerate medication
    Reluctance to change life style
    For identification of patients with high-risk lesions
    To assess patency of bypass grafts
  Unstable angina
Myocardial infarction
  Mechanical dysfunction
  Recurrent pain
  Elective for prognosis and therapy
Asymptomatic patients
  Abnormal ECG or stress test
  High-risk occupation

Heart Disease Other Than Ischemic
  Cardiomyopathy, arrhythmia
  Suspected congenital anomaly of the coronary arteries
  Preoperatively in valve surgery
  Preoperatively in congenital heart disease

atypical chest pain; (4) a history of recent multiple myocardial infarctions in a relatively young individual; (5) left ventricular failure due to suspected ventricular aneurysm, postinfarction ventricular septal defect, papillary muscle

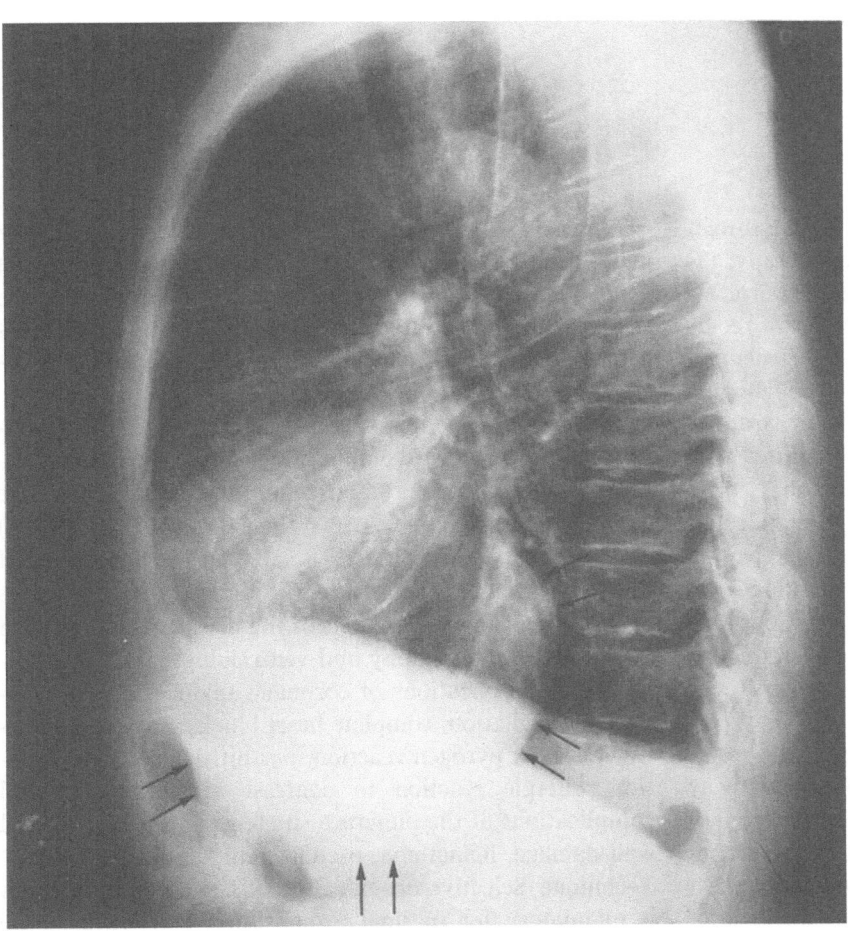

B

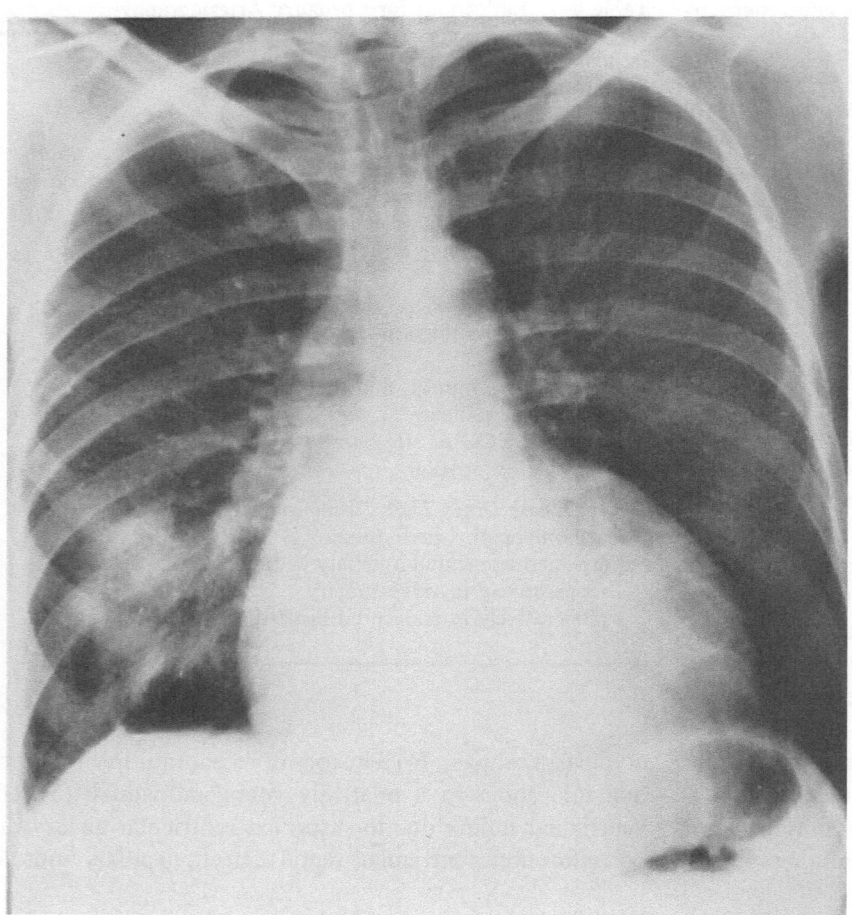

Fig. 4–3. *Dressler syndrome.* Apparent cardiomegaly is caused by pericardial effusion. Pneumonitis and pleural effusion are also present.

dysfunction or cardiomyopathy; (6) recurrent, life-threatening arrhythmia not responding to medical therapy; (7) cardiogenic shock; (8) postoperative assessment of coronary artery bypass surgery, particularly in a patient with recurrent or persistent angina; (9) preoperative assessment of a patient with valvular heart disease, with or without angina and (10) congenital anomalies of the coronary arteries, which include those with physiological abnormalities such as anomalous origin of a coronary artery or coronary arteriovenous fistula and those without physiologic significance but of anatomic importance relative to surgical repair of congenital heart disease (e.g., transposition, tetralogy).

Less common indications for coronary arteriography include mild angina with a distinctly positive exercise test, myocardial infarction in an individual under 40 years (even without residual symptoms) or an abnormal ECG in persons in high risk occupations (e.g., airline pilots).

Contraindications Coronary angiography is a relatively safe procedure in the hands of an experienced coronary angiographic team. The efficacy of this examination is considerable, as observed in the long list of indications. At present no absolute contraindication to coronary arterio-

graphy exists. However, relative contraindications must be kept in mind. These include all intercurrent disorders that could be treated and whose correction would improve the safety of the procedure (e.g., electrolyte disturbance, congestive heart failure, coagulation problems, digitalis toxicity).

Complications The major complications of coronary arteriography are myocardial infarction, stroke, peripheral vascular embolization, thrombosis, and death. The incidence of such complications is less than 1% (0.33%–0.63%) (Adams et al.) and is closely related to the experience of the angiographer, stability of the disease (clinical status of the patient) and the extent of the disease as determined by coronary angiography and ventriculography.

Other complications of coronary angiography are ventricular fibrillation, complete heart block or asystole, vasovagal attack, pyrogen reaction, postnitroglycerin hypotension, allergic reaction to contrast media and arterial complications at the puncture site (e.g., thrombosis, vessel wall damage, hematoma, pseudoaneurysm formation).

Technique Selective opacification of the coronary arteries is mandatory for optimal visualization and for accurate

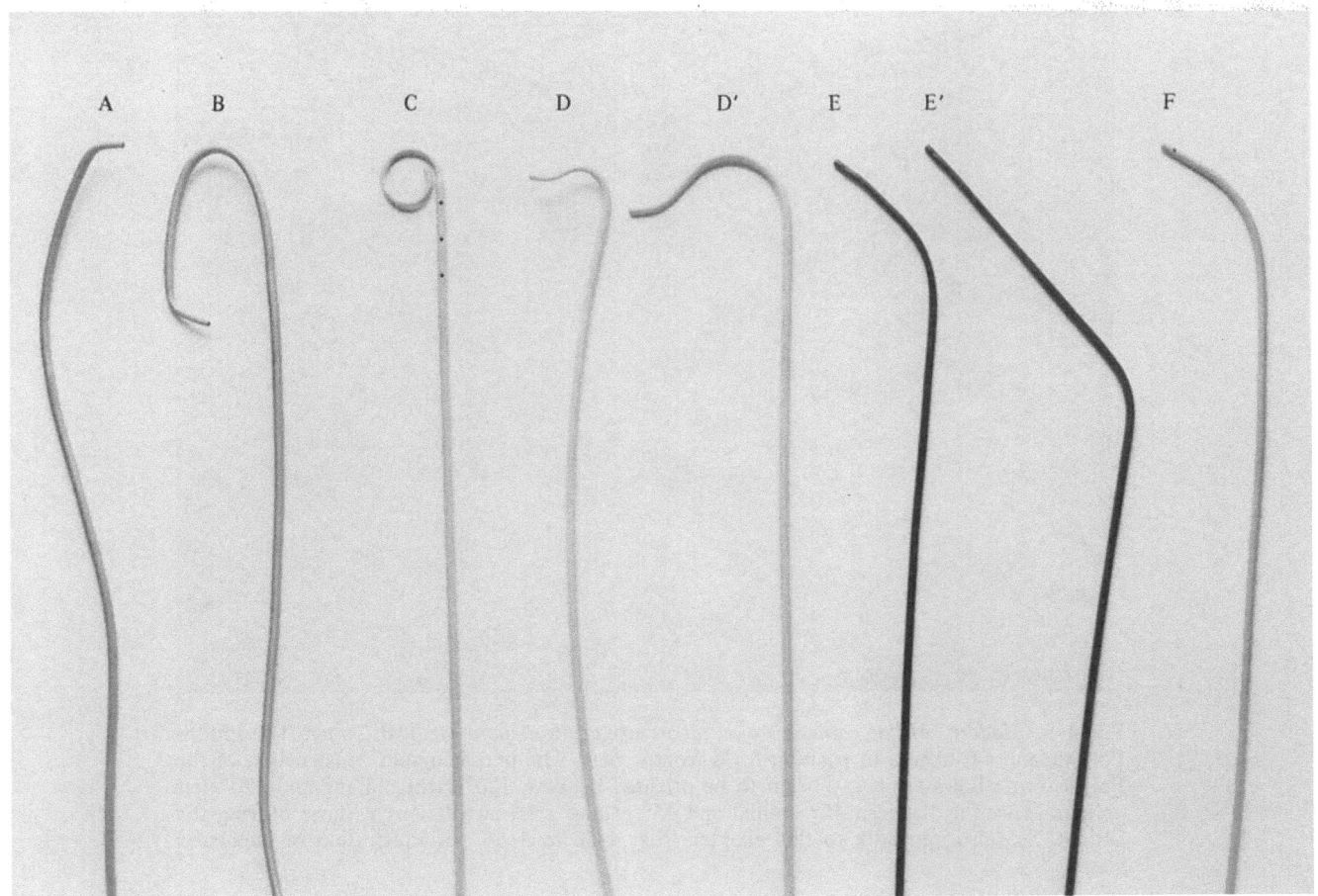

Fig. 4–4. *Catheters used in selective coronary arteriography and left ventriculography. A,* Judkins right coronary; *B,* Judkins left coronary; *C,* pigtail catheter for left ventriculography; *D* and *D'* Amplatz (distal curves of right and left coronary catheters are similar); *E* and *E',* Sones A and B catheter (same catheter is used for right and left coronary arteriography and for left ventriculography); *F,* Schoonmaker used for both coronary arteries.

interpretation. Nonselective studies (sinus of Valsalva injections) are important in those cases in which a diagnosis of coronary ostial stenosis is in question.

At present, two basic approaches exist for selective cannulation of the coronary arteries (selective coronary arteriography)—the retrograde brachial technique and the percutaneous (transfemoral or transaxillary) technique.

The retrograde brachial technique of Sones requires a cutdown and uses a flexible tapered-tipped catheter. Left ventriculography and hemodynamic recordings are obtained with the same catheter. At the Montefiore Medical Center a percutaneous transbrachial approach with an introducer sheath is used, on occasion, thus avoiding a cutdown. The introducer facilitates catheter changes.

Several techniques (e.g., Amplatz, Judkins) use the percutaneous (Seldinger) approach for selective coronary arteriography. The technique of Judkins is the most widely used, requiring preformed separate catheters for the right and left coronary arteries and a pigtail catheter for ventriculography (Fig. 4–4). This technique has the advantage of the ease and speed of the transfemoral approach, permitting consistent selective coronary cannulation with minimal ma-

nipulation. Both cineangiography and rapid serial filming, using large-cut film or 100-mm (or 105-mm) "spot" films can be utilized. Radiological installations (Fig. 4–5) that allow rotation and angulation of the tube and image intensifier are useful to avoid vascular superimposition and to optimally define proximal coronary artery lesions. Physiological monitors for continuous display of the ECG and pressure tracings are required.

Normal Coronary Anatomy

(Also see Appendix to this chapter, Figs 4–58 to 4–64, for angulated views)

Thorough knowledge of the anatomical relationships of the coronary ostia to the root of the aorta and the sinuses of Valsalva is essential for successful coronary artery opacification. The sinuses of Valsalva are named to coincide with the origin of the coronary arteries: right, left, and noncoronary. The right sinus is anterior in location, the left sinus is posterior on the left and the noncoronary sinus is posterior on the right.

Right Coronary Artery (Figs. 4–6, 4–7; also see 4–63, 4–64) The ostium of the right coronary artery (RCA) is lo-

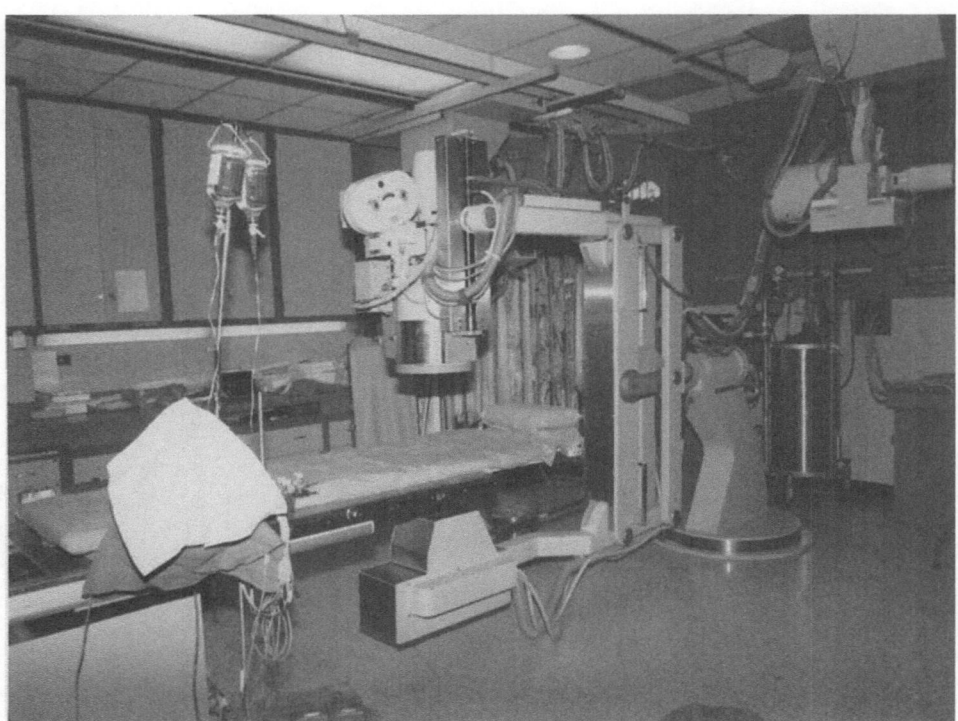

Fig. 4–5. *Modern cardiac catheterization laboratory at Montefiore Medical Center.* The Philips Poly diagnost C-arm is in position for a frontal view. The parallelogram construction of the Poly C-arm allows the x-ray beam to be oriented between 120° right oblique and 120° left oblique as well as between 45° cranial and 45° caudal axial angulations without moving the patient. See also appendix to this chapter (Fig. 4–58 to 4–64) for illustration of angulated views.

RIGHT DOMINANT SYSTEM

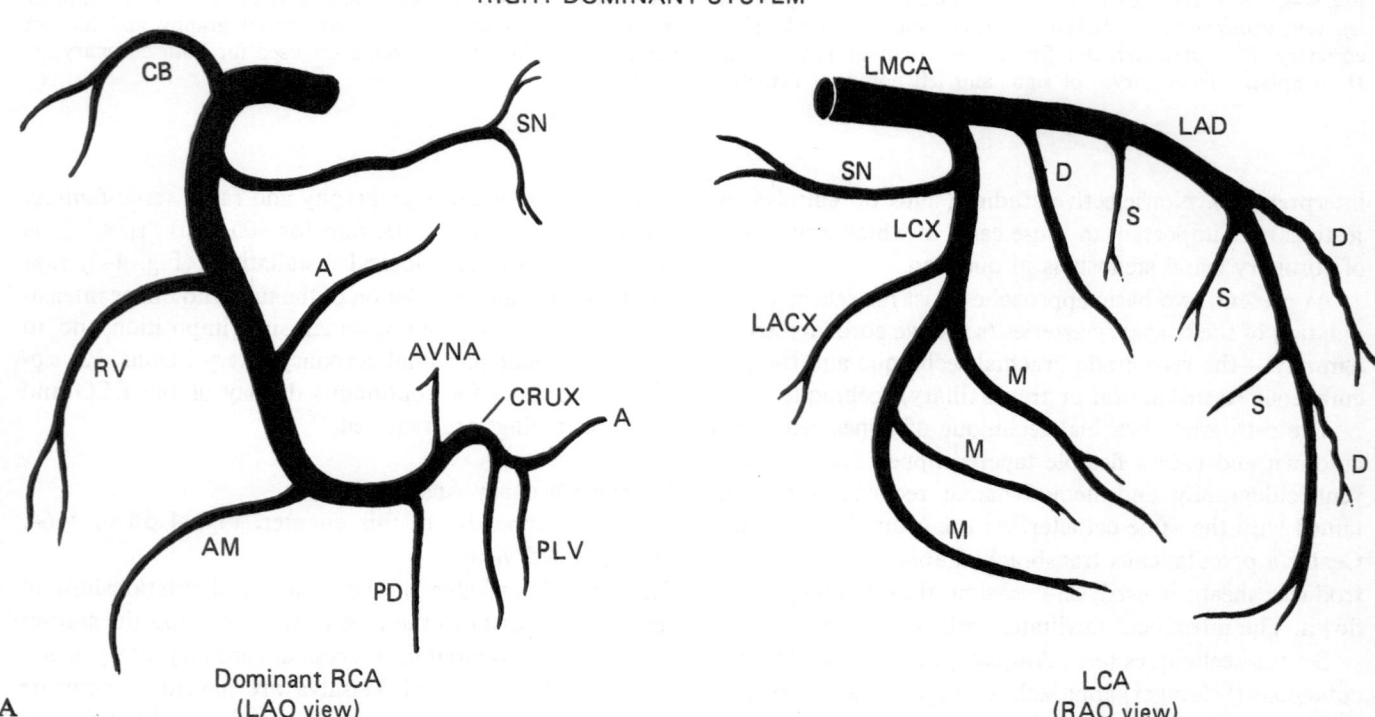

Fig. 4–6. *Normal coronary arteries and coronary artery dominance. Coronary dominance refers to the artery that supplies the diaphragmatic surface of the left ventricle (LV) and the posterior interventricular septum. The RCA is dominant in 80% of cases, the LCA in 9%. In about 11% of cases the circulation is balanced.* **A** *Right coronary artery dominance.* The RCA supplies the poste-

rior interventricular septum by way of the posterior descending artery (*PD*) and the diaphragmatic surface of the left ventricle by way of the crux artery and its posterolateral or posterior left ventricular branches (*PLV*). The crux artery also gives off a small branch to the left atrium. The atrioventricular node artery (*AVNA*) is usually the first branch of the crux artery and serves

LEFT DOMINANT SYSTEM

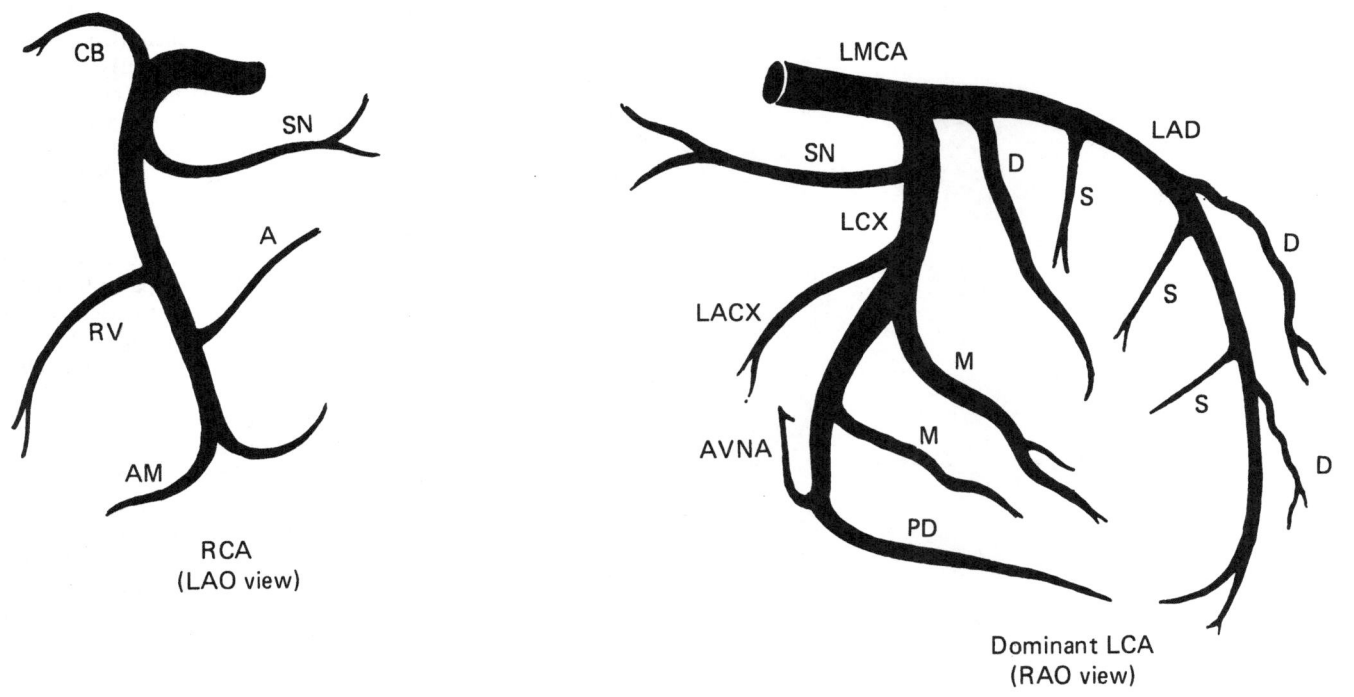

RCA
(LAO view)

Dominant LCA
(RAO view)   **B**

BALANCED CIRCULATION

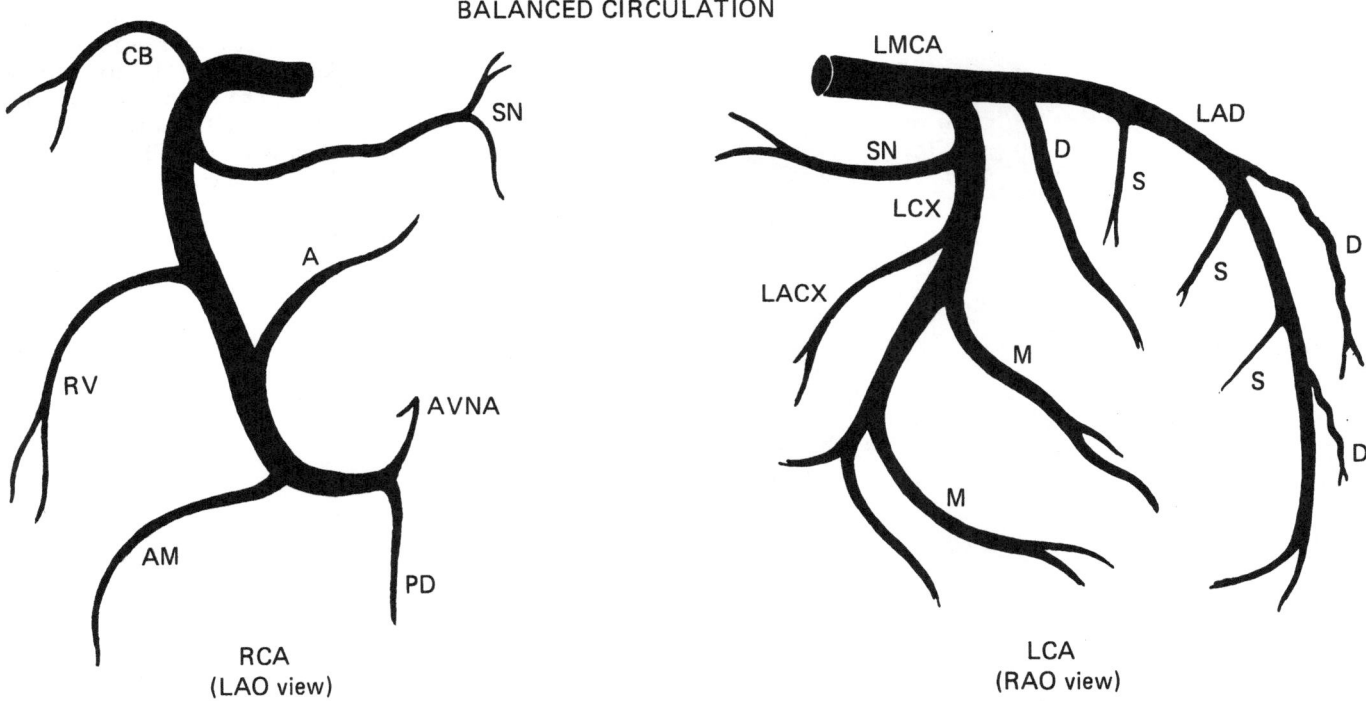

RCA
(LAO view)

LCA
(RAO view)   **C**

as a useful landmark to identify the PD in the LAO view. The PD is the branch just before the AVNA. **B** *Left coronary artery dominance.* The LCA supplies the diaphragmatic wall of the left ventricle by way of marginal branches (*M*) of the left circumflex artery (*LCX*). It also supplies the posterior interventricular septum by way of the *PD,* which is now a branch of the LCX. With LCA dominance a crux artery is absent, and the RCA is small. The AVNA is a branch of the LCX, and the PD is distal to it. **C** *Balanced coronary arterial system.* The diaphragmatic wall of the left ventricle is supplied by marginal branches of the LCX. The posterior interventricular septum is supplied by the RCA by way of the PD. The AVNA may be a branch of the RCA or a branch of the LCX. On occasion, two AVNAs exist, one from the distal RCA and one from the distal LCX.

Note again that no crux artery is present in a balanced system and that the area normally perfused by it is supplied by marginal branches of the LCX. *A* = atrial branch; *AM* = acute marginal branch; *CB* = conus branch or conus artery; *CRUX* = crux artery; *D* = diagonal branch; *LACX* = left atrial circumflex branch; *LAD* = left anterior descending artery; *LCA* = left coronary artery; *LMCA* = left main coronary artery; *RCA* = right coronary artery; *RV* = right ventricular, preventricular or muscular branch; *S* = septal perforator branch (septal artery); *SN* = sinus node artery. (Although the sinus node artery is depicted here as a separate branch from the LCX, it usually occurs as a branch of the LACX.) Spindola-Franco H (1982) Coronary arteriography and left ventriculography. In: Goldberger E (ed) Textbook of clinical cardiology. Mosby, St. Louis, pp 305–325

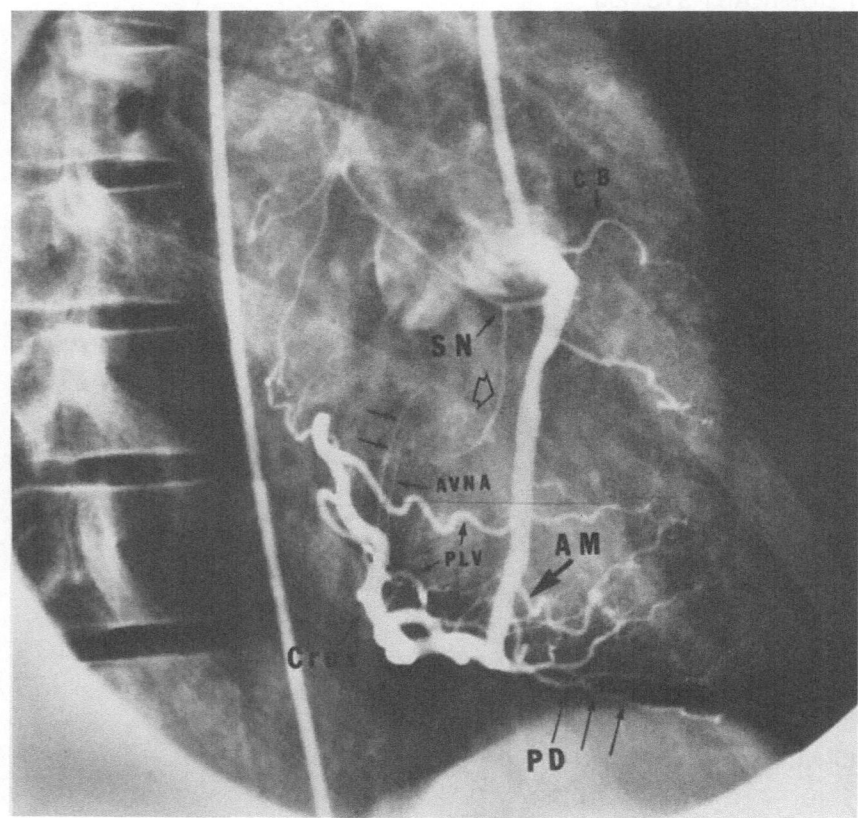

A

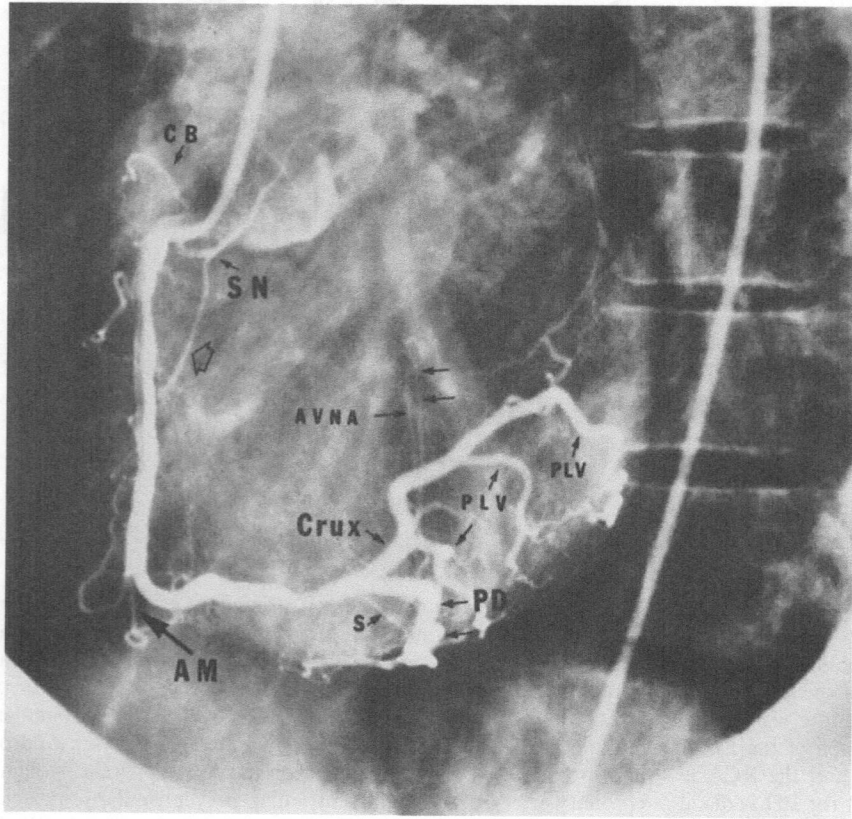

B

Fig. 4–7. *Dominant right coronary artery (RCA).* A RAO view. B LAO view. The first branch is the conus branch (*CB*), which courses anteriorly and superiorly. The second branch is the sinus node artery (*SN*), which courses posteriorly and gives off two small branches, one to the sinus node and one to the posterior wall of the left atrium. In this case the SN also gives off a third branch, which descends around the atrial appendage (*open arrow*). The acute marginal branch (*AM*) is small in this patient. It originates at the acute margin of the right ventricle (compare AM here with Fig. 4–13). The RCA bifurcates distally into two branches, the posterior descending (*PD*) and the crux artery. The PD supplies the posterior interventricular septum (basal septum) via the septal arteries (*S*). The septal arteries from the PD are usually small compared to those from the left anterior descending artery. The crux artery supplies the diaphragmatic wall of the left ventricle by way of posterior left ventricular branches (*PLV*). It also gives off the atrioventricular node artery (*AVNA*), which has a straight vertical course. In this case two parallel AVNAs are noted (see also Fig. 4–9). The PD is recognized by its straight horizontal course along the posterior interventricular sulcus, whereas the crux artery, also known as the "U-turn" artery, loops superiorly. The looping course of the crux artery in the RAO view is very helpful in distinguishing it from the PD during interpretation of cine studies. In the LAO view the PD is identified because it usually precedes the AVNA.

cated in the right sinus of Valsalva at or about the level of the aortic ring; occasionally it may have a higher or lower position. The ostium is in front, either exactly in the center or slightly to the right of the center of the aortic root. Therefore ostial lesions are best studied in the lateral and steep LAO projections.

The RCA, which takes origin from its ostium, passes for a short distance forward between the pulmonary artery and the right atrial appendage and then curves to the right, following the right atrioventricular groove toward the *crux cordis* (the intersection of the atrioventricular and interventricular sulci posteriorly). There the RCA terminates in various ways. If the RCA is dominant (Figs. 4–6, 4–7) it will supply the diaphragmatic and free walls of the right ventricle (right ventricular branches) and almost half of the diaphragmatic surface of the left ventricle via the crux artery through its posterior left ventricular branches. The basal (posterior) interventricular septum is supplied by the posterior descending artery. The RCA also gives branches to the right atrium and to the root of the pulmonary artery and aorta.

The conus branch (CB), the first branch of the RCA, runs anteriorly and superiorly, encircling the outflow tract of the right ventricle at the level of the pulmonic valve. There the CB may anastomose with branches of the left coronary artery (LCA), to form the anastomotic circle of Vieussens. This collateral pathway is of considerable significance in occlusions of either the RCA or the left anterior descending artery (LAD), as a source of blood distal to the occlusion. The CB originates from an ostium separate from that of the RCA in almost 50% of the cases (in some series). It is then known as the third coronary artery (preinfundibular artery of Crainicianu or arteria accessoria of Banchi).

The second branch of the RCA, the sinus node (SN, SA node) artery, originates from the proximal RCA about 60% of the time and from the left circumflex artery 40% of the time. The SA node artery passes superiorly, dorsally and to the right, between the atrial appendage and aorta to encircle the ostium of the superior vena cava. The SA node artery usually bifurcates into a branch to the sinus node (SA node artery proper) and a branch to the posterior wall of the left atrium. Either branch can provide a collateral pathway in an instance of occlusion of the left circumflex or right coronary artery.

The right superior septal artery (RSSA) (Fig. 4–8) is an uncommon (1–3%) but important branch of the RCA. It may arise directly from the proximal RCA, or it may be a branch of the conus artery. The RSSA penetrates the myocardium to run in the parietal branch of the crista supraventricularis, supplying the area of the septum normally perfused by the first septal perforator from the LAD. The RSSA is an important collateral pathway in instances of occlusion of the LAD or posterior descending artery or both.

Right ventricular (muscular or preventricular) branches arise from the RCA, course anteriorly, and supply the right ventricular myocardium. The acute marginal (AM) branch is usually a large preventricular vessel (muscular branch) arising from the RCA at the level of the acute margin of the heart. These muscular or preventricular vessels provide intercoronary and intracoronary collateral flow when coronary occlusion occurs.

At or near the crux of the heart the RCA divides into the posterior descending artery (PD) and crux artery. The PD courses in the posterior interventricular sulcus to anastomose with branches of the anterior descending artery near the apex of the heart. The PD supplies primarily the basal septum (posterior septum) and to a small degree the inferior surface of both ventricles. Important variations of the PD exist in 25% of individuals with RCA dominance; these variations include multiple posterior descending arteries, early origin of the PD and partial supply of the distribution of the PD by the acute marginal or posterior right ventricular branches of the RCA.

The crux artery (on occasion called the U-turn artery) continues past the interventricular sulcus. It supplies posterolateral branches to the diaphragmatic wall of the left ventricle (called posterior left ventricular branches, PLV) and to the atrioventricular node (Fig. 4–9). The bundle of His artery, a branch of the atrioventricular node artery, is frequently visualized on arteriography.

In contrast to a dominant RCA, the nondominant RCA (Fig. 4–10) is small and terminates before the crux of the heart. In such instances the crux artery does not exist. The area ordinarily supplied by the crux artery is perfused by marginal branches of the left circumflex artery (LCX). The PD is also a branch of the LCX.

Left Coronary Artery (Figs. 4–6, 4–11, 4–12, also see 4–58 to 4–62) The left main coronary artery (LMCA) passes forward for a short distance between the base of the pulmonary artery and the left atrial appendage and then divides into two major branches, the left anterior descending (LAD) and the left circumflex artery (LCX). Often the ramus medianus exists as a third branch (Fig. 4–13 C and D, also see Fig. 4–16).

The LAD artery runs in the anterior interventricular sulcus to the apex of the heart, often encircling the apex and terminating in the anterior third of the posterior interventricular sulcus. The LAD supplies branches to the interventricular septum (septal perforators), muscular branches to the anterolateral left ventricular wall (diagonal vessels) and small branches to the anterior surface of the right ventricle. The septal arteries vary in number and size; the first septal perforator usually is the largest and most important vessel. Severe lesions of the LAD before the origin of the first septal artery are more life threatening than lesions located distal to the origin of the first septal vessel. Angiographically, septal arteries usually are observed to arise from the LAD at a 90° angle and to run a straight course, usually ending in a characteristic fork-like configuration. The vessels of the septum represent an important collateral pathway between the RCA and LCA (Fig. 4–13).

The diagonal arteries are branches from the LAD, sup-

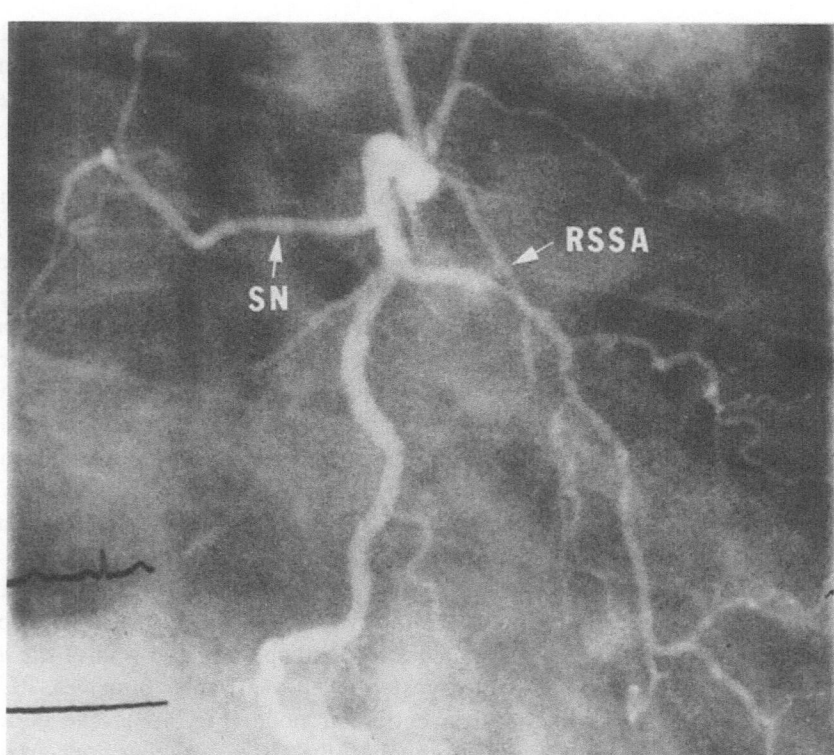

Fig. 4–8. *Right superior septal artery.* **A** RAO view and **B** LAO view of right coronary artery. The right superior septal artery (*RSSA*) arises from the proximal right coronary artery after the conus branch and before the sinus node artery (*SN*). The RSSA perforates the myocardium in the vicinity of the crista supraventricularis to reach the interventricular septum. *SN* = sinus node artery.

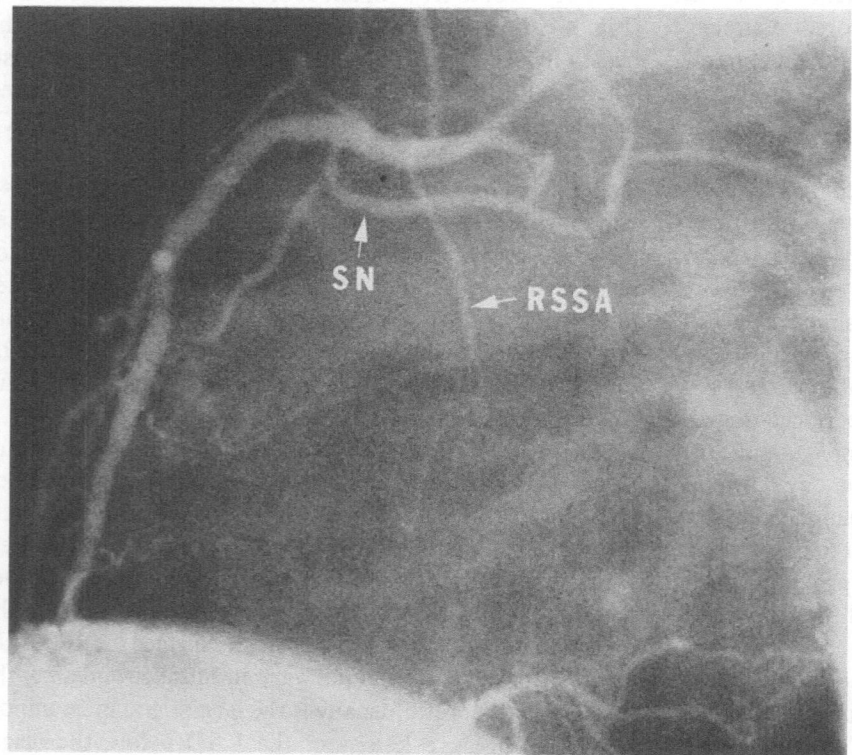

Fig. 4–9. *Atrioventricular node artery (AVNA).* LAO view. A particularly excellent image of the AVNA is illustrated. The bundle of His artery (*His A*) is also clearly noted to branch off from the AVNA at an acute angle. Note that the posterior descending precedes the AVNA. This right coronary artery is dominant because it supplies the posterior interventricular septum via the posterior descending artery and the diaphragmatic wall of the left ventricle via the crux artery and its posterior left ventricular branch (*PLV*). The crux artery and its single PLV are small in this patient. Note also that the sinus node artery (*SN*) bifurcates into a branch to the sinus node (*open arrow*) and a branch to the left atrium (*closed arrow*).

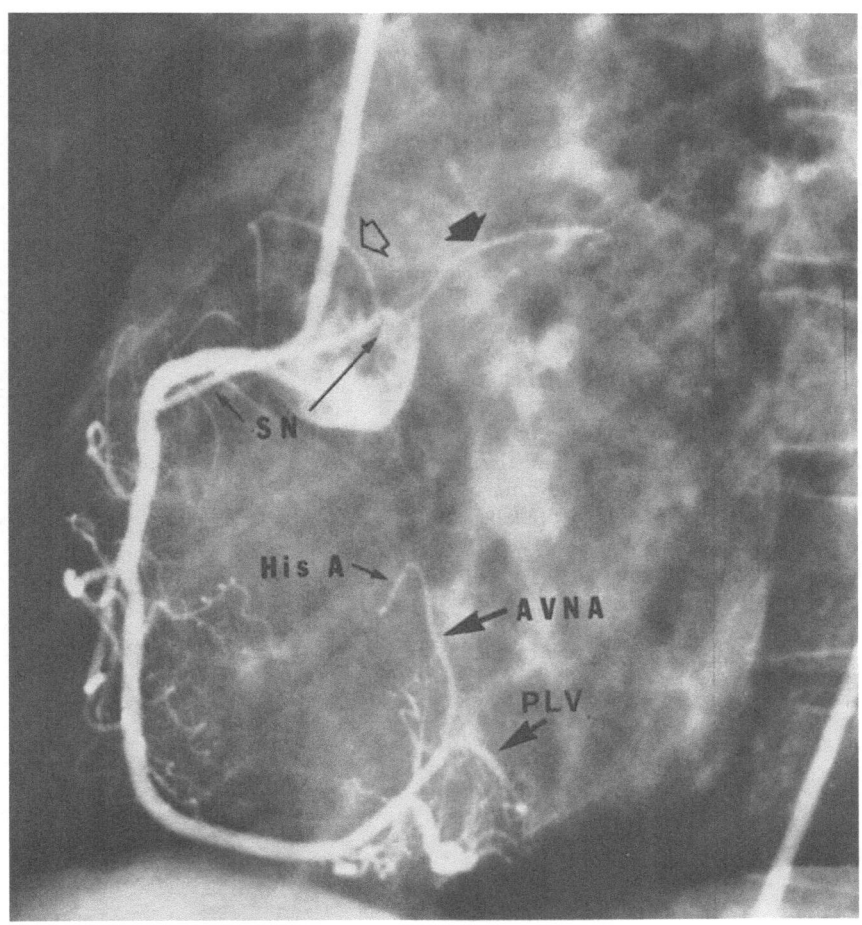

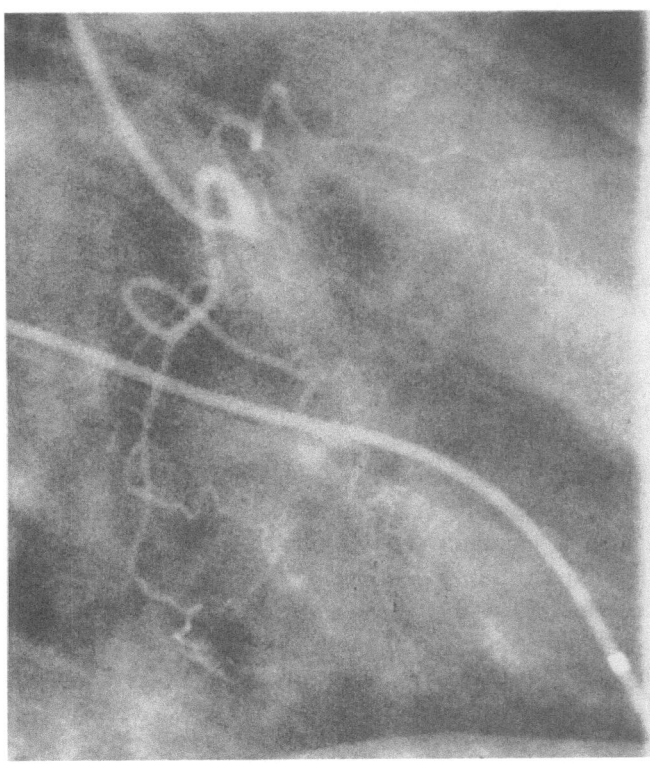

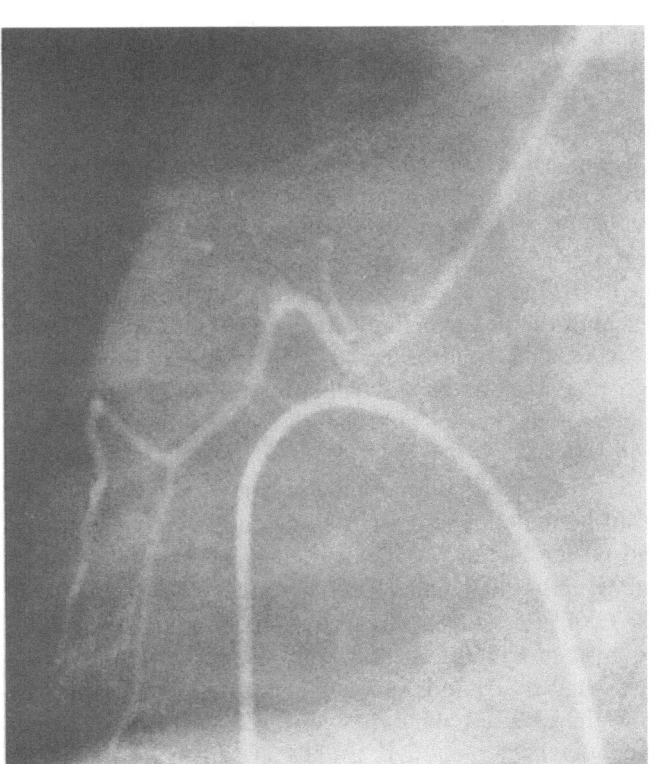

A
B

Fig. 4–10. *Nondominant right coronary artery.* **A** RAO view; **B** LAO view. In contrast to the dominant right coronary artery (Fig. 4–7) the nondominant one is small and terminates before the crux of the heart. Therefore it does not give off a posterior descending or crux artery. The posterior descending artery is a branch of the left circumflex artery. The area supplied by the crux artery is supplied instead by marginal branches of the left circumflex. See also Fig. 4–6.

Fig. 4–11. *Normal nondominant left coronary artery.* **A** RAO view; **B** LAO view; **C** Lateral view. The left main coronary artery (*LMCA*) usually bifurcates into two branches, the left anterior descending artery (*LAD*) and the left circumflex artery (*LCX*). Not infrequently the LMCA divides into three branches, the third branch being designated the ramus medianus (see Fig. 4–13C and D). The LAD courses in the anterior interventricular sulcus and supplies branches to the anterior interventricular septum (septal perforators or septal arteries (*S*), and diagonal branches (*D*) to the anterolateral left ventricular wall. Note the rather straight courses and forked tips of the septal arteries. The LCX runs posteriorly along the atrioventricular groove toward the crux of the heart and gives off marginal branches (*M*) to the posterolateral wall of the left ventricle. The LCX also supplies the left atrium via the left atrial circumflex branch (*LACX*).

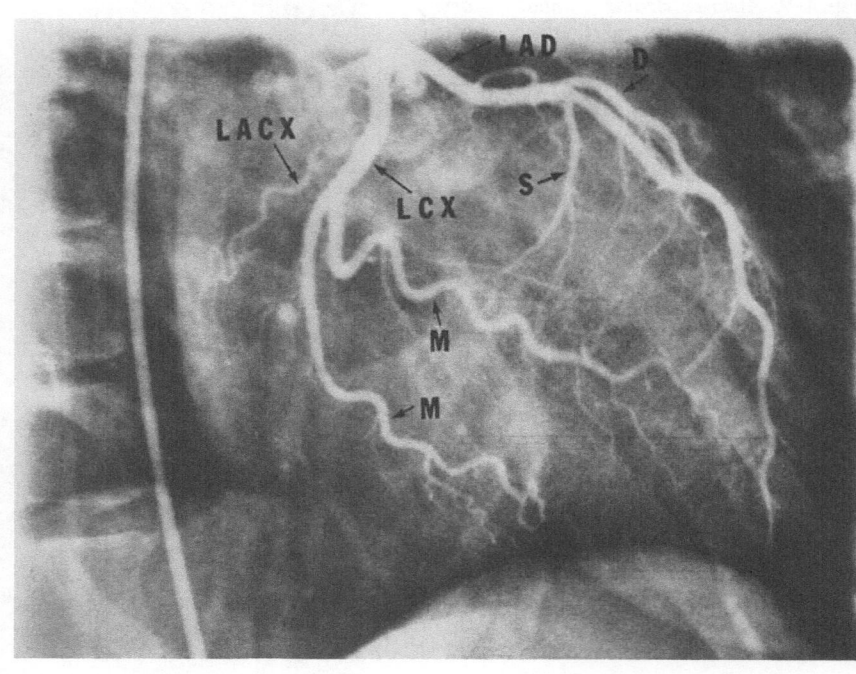

A

plying the left ventricular wall, with an oblique course toward the apex. The caliber of these diagonal arteries and their number are variable, on occasion being even longer and larger than the LAD or LCX. Angiographically the diagonal arteries have a motion opposite from the LAD (crisscross or seesaw motion).

The LCX is a branch from the LMCA, running posteriorly along the atrioventricular groove toward the crux of the heart. In the majority of instances the LCX ends before reaching the posterior interventricular septum. When this vessel reaches the crux area, it usually supplies the distribution of the posterior descending artery and the atrioventricular node. In such instances the LCA is called dominant (Fig. 4–12).

The LCX gives off muscular (marginal) (Fig. 4–11) and atrial branches. The marginal branches supply the lateral and posterolateral surface of the left ventricle, varying in size, length and number. The left atrial circumflex artery (LACX) is usually a large vessel, commonly originating from the proximal LCX to supply the left atrium. In other cases the left atrium is supplied by multiple small branches from the LCX. In about 40% of cases, the SA node artery is a branch of the LCA, usually arising from the LCX, and on occasion from the LMCA.

Kugel's artery (*arteria anastomotica auricularis magna*) is a branch from the proximal LCX, which runs in the atrioventricular plane at the base of the interatrial septum;

it may anastomose with the SA node artery and AVNA. Kugel's artery is usually observed as a collateral pathway in occlusions of either the right or left coronary arteries. In practice a collateral pathway noted frequently on angiography between the SA node artery (from the RCA) and the AVNA (from the crux artery) is also called Kugel's artery (Fig. 4–14).

The ramus medianus (RM)(Fig. 4–13C and D) is a branch of the LMCA, running diagonally across the midportion of the anterior left ventricular wall. On occasion the RM is observed to arise from the proximal LAD (large diagonal branch) or from the proximal LCX (obtuse marginal branch).

Variations in Coronary Artery Anatomy

Anatomical variants of the coronary arteries include high origin of the coronary arteries, single coronary artery (Fig. 4–15), myocardial bridging (Fig. 4–16), ectopic origin of a coronary artery (e.g., separate ostia for the RCA and the conus artery; LCX arising from the RCA—Fig. 4–17), congenitally small vessels, anomalous origin of a coronary artery from the pulmonary artery (see Fig. 4–55) and anomalous lung supply from the coronary circulation ("pulmonary steal" syndrome) (see Fig. 1–13).

Spindola-Franco et al. have described 23 cases of an entity called *dual LAD* (Fig. 4–18). In this variant two branches supplied the usual distribution of the LAD. A

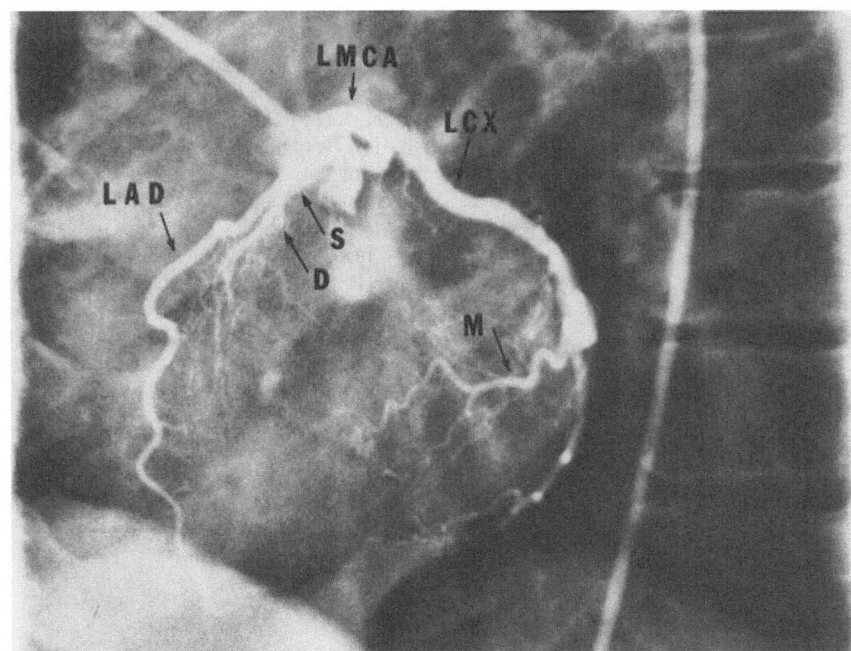

B

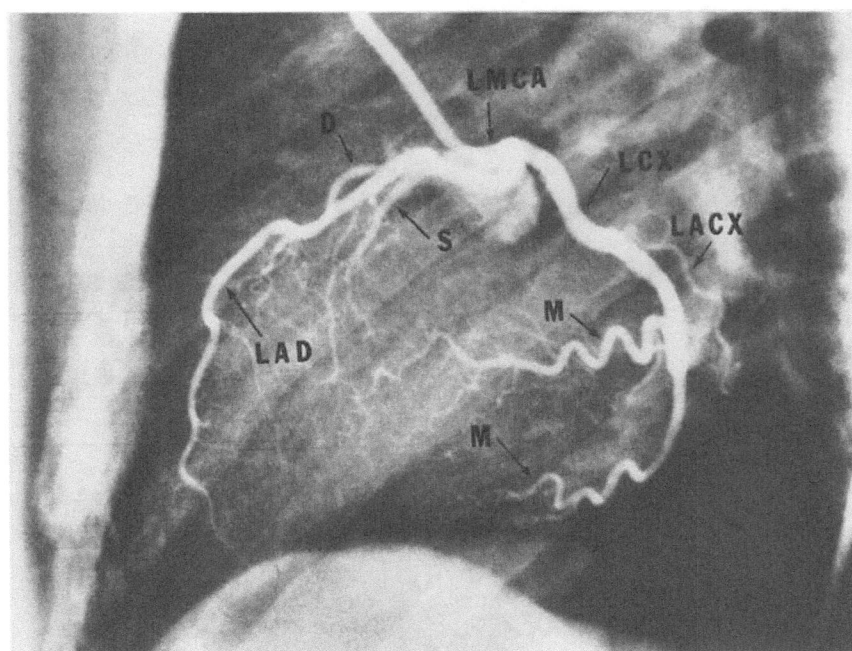

C

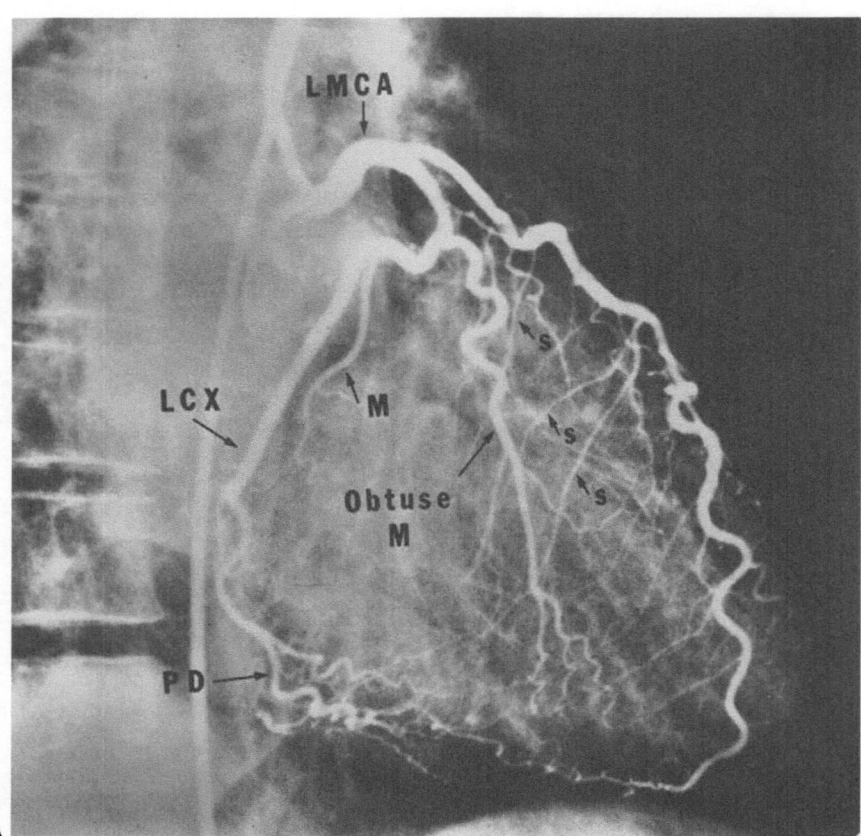

A

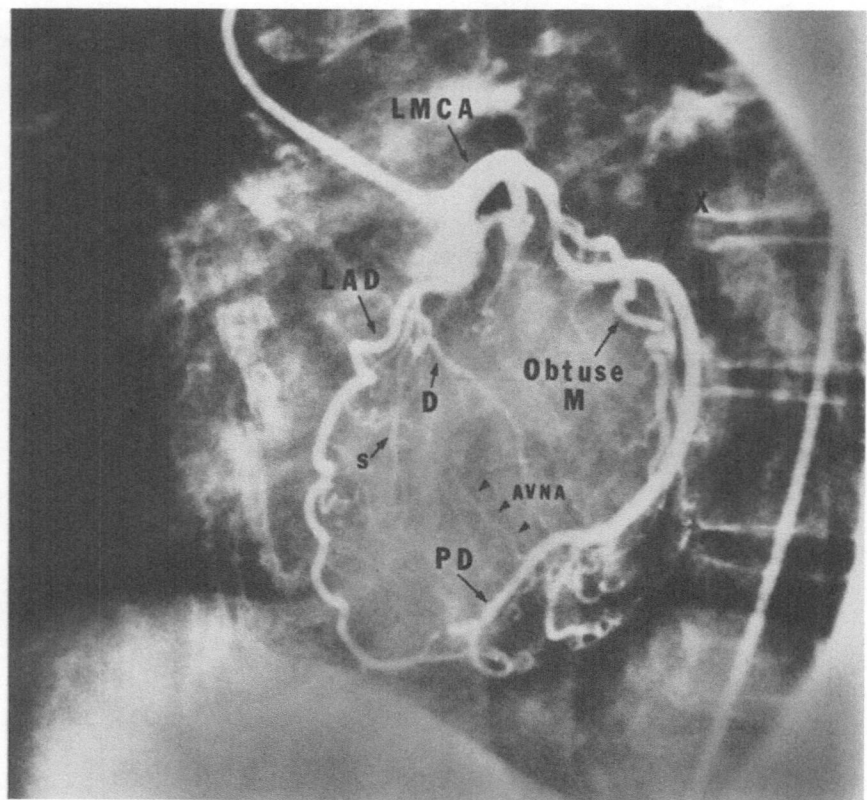

B

Fig. 4–12. *Dominant left coronary artery.* **A** RAO view; **B** LAO view. The posterior left ventricular wall is supplied by the left circumflex artery (*LCX*) via the marginal branches (*M*). The LCX supplies the posterior interventricular septum by way of the posterior descending artery (*PD*). Note that the atrioventricular node artery (*AVNA; arrowheads*) antecedes the PD. The first marginal branch is called an obtuse marginal because it courses in the plane of the ramus medianus (see Fig. 4–13C and D). *D* = diagonal branch; *LAD* = left anterior descending artery; *LMCA* = left main coronary artery; *S* = septal perforator branch. (See also Fig. 6–8.)

Fig. 4–13. *Septal collateral flow.* **A** RAO and **B** LAO views of right coronary artery; **C** lateral and **D** LAO views of left coronary artery. The right coronary artery gives off numerous large septal arteries (*S*) which provide collateral flow to the left anterior descending artery (*LAD*). There is dual supply to the posterior interventricular septum because the acute marginal branch (*AM*) is large and gives off branches to the posterior ventricular septum. The posterior descending artery (*PD*) is small. The LAD is severely stenosed in its proximal portion and opacifies segmentally because of dilution from unopacified blood from septal collaterals seen in frames A and B. The marginal branches (*M*) of the LCX are also severely stenosed. Note that the LMCA trifurcates in this patient. The third branch is called the ramus medianus (*RM*). If the ramus medianus arises from the LCX it changes its name to "obtuse marginal branch" (see Fig. 4–12). If the ramus medianus takes its origin from the LAD it becomes a diagonal branch. *AVNA* = atrioventricular node artery; *CB* = Conus branch or conus artery; *CRUX* = crux artery; *D* = diagonal branch; *LMCA* = left main coronary artery; *LCX* = left circumflex artery; *M* = marginal branch; *PLV* = posterolateral or posterior left ventricular branch; *RV* = right ventricular, preventricular, or muscular branch; *SN* = sinus node artery. Spindola-Franco H. In Goldberger E (ed.) Textbook of clinical cardiology. Mosby, 1982, pp. 305–325.

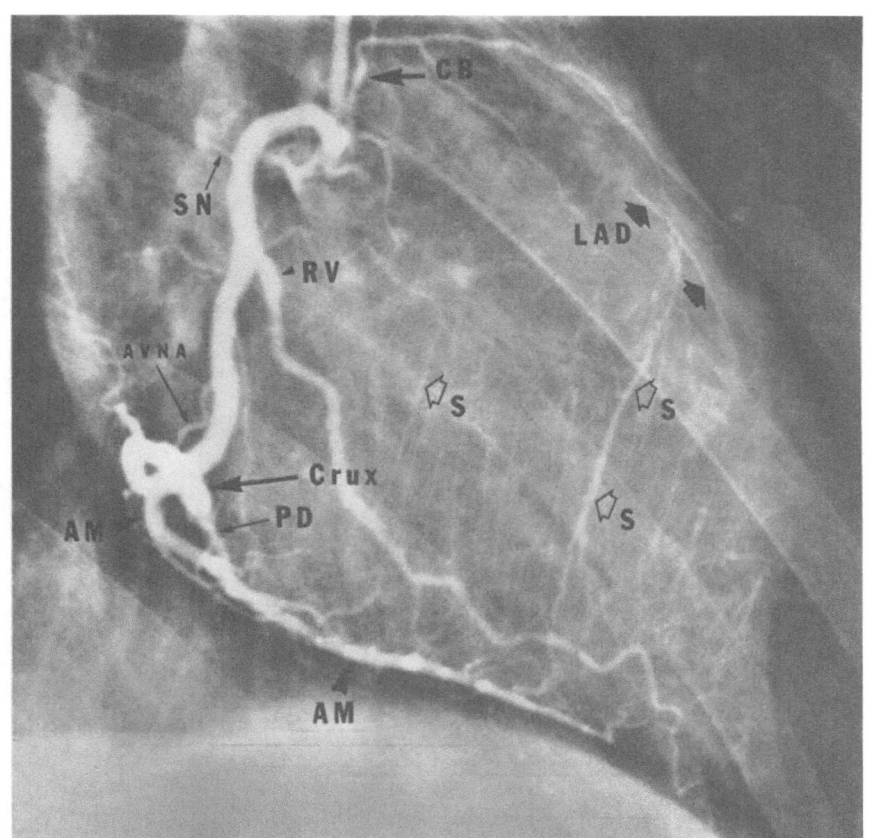

A

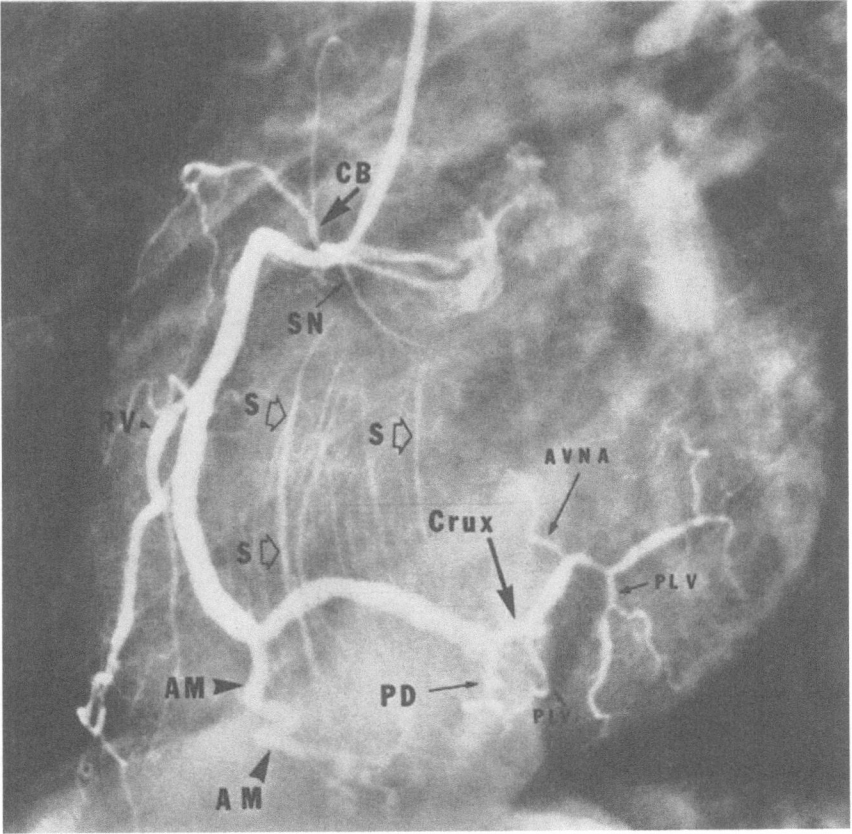

B

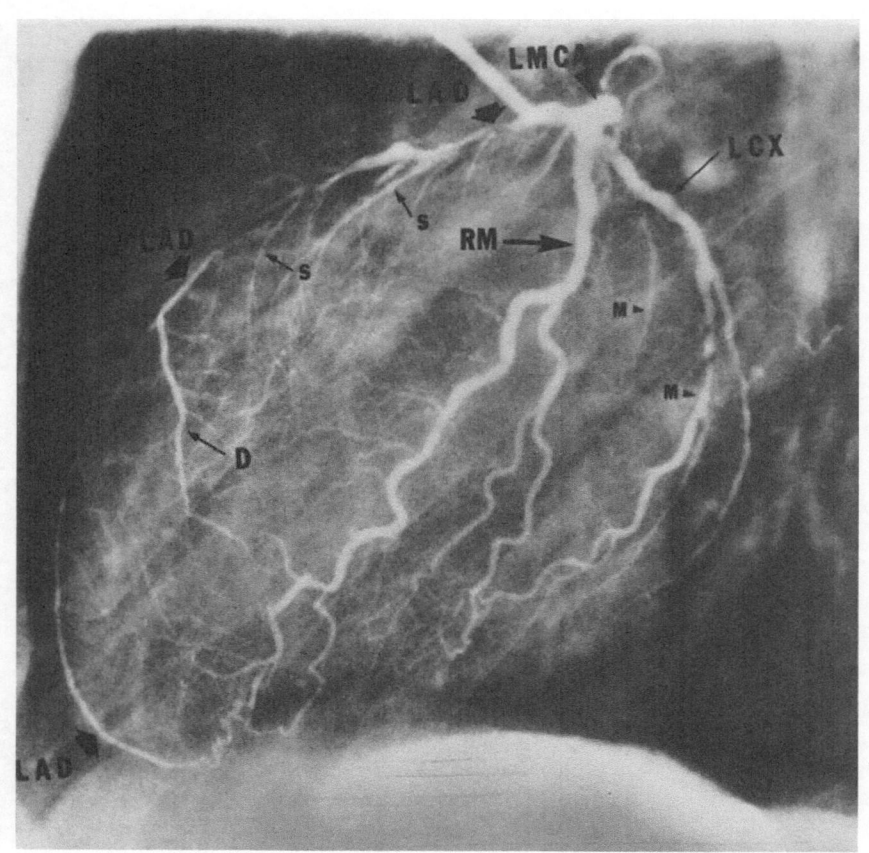

C

Fig. 4–13 (*Cont.*).

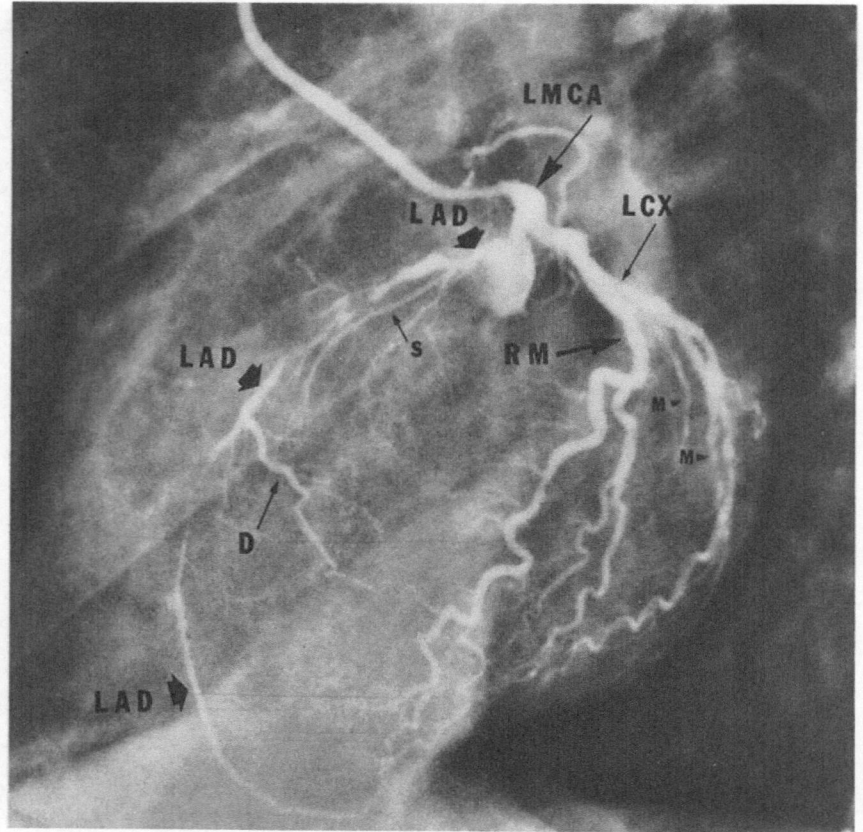

D

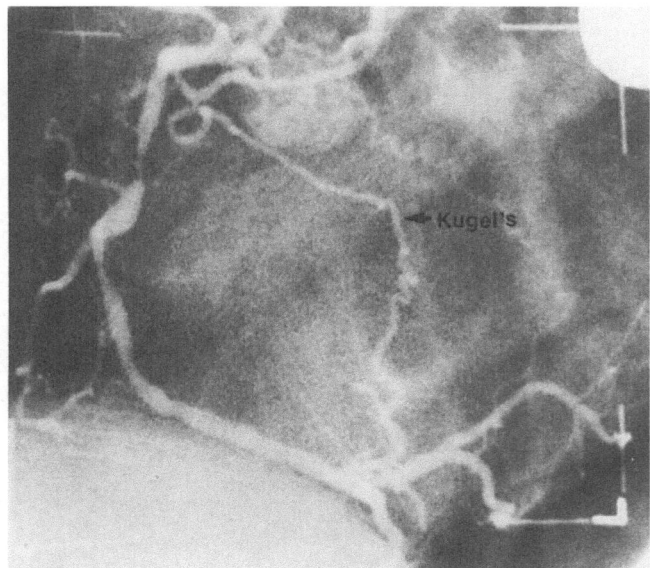

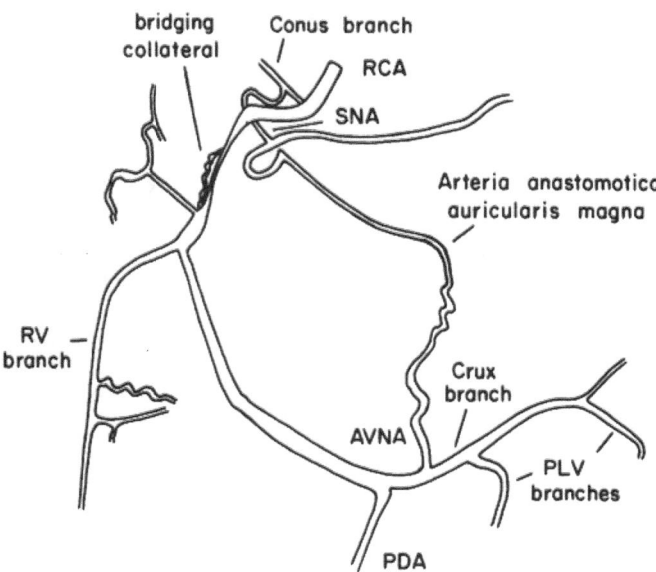

Fig. 4–14. *Kugel's artery* (arteria anastomotica auricularis magna). LAO view of right coronary angiogram. The Kugel's artery is a collateral pathway connecting the sinus node artery (*SNA*) to the A-V node artery (*AVNA*). It serves as a collateral pathway to the distal RCA. Note also that the RCA is occluded distal to the conus artery and reconstitutes by way of multiple bridging collaterals. *RV branch* = right ventricular branch; *PDA* = posterior descending coronary artery; *PLV branches* = posterior left ventricular branches.

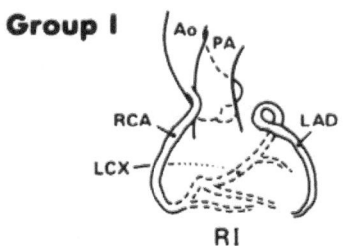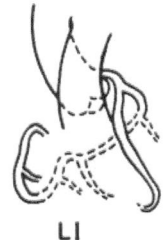

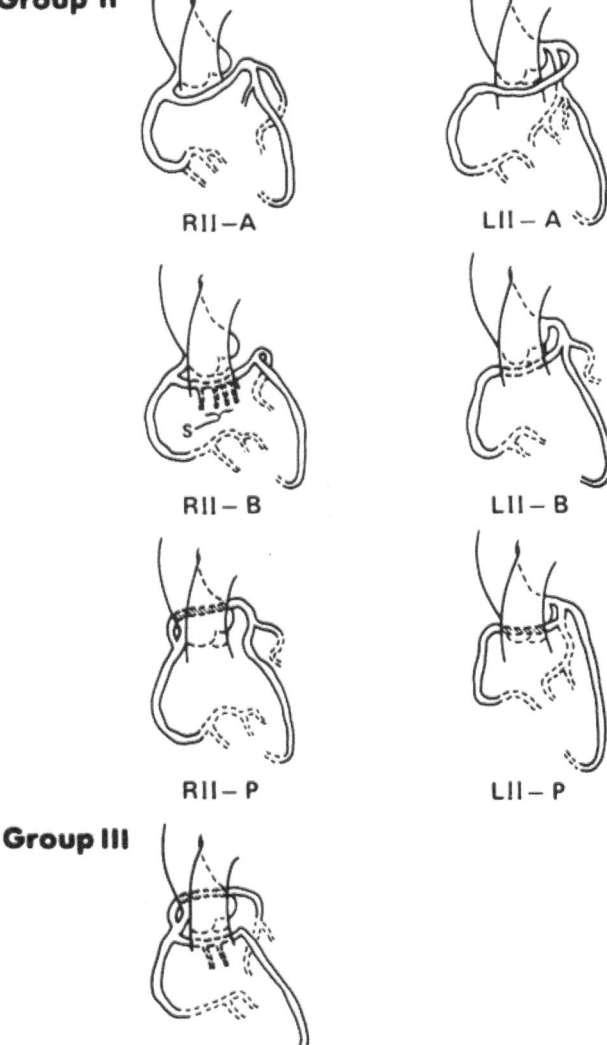

Fig. 4–15. *Single coronary artery.* A single coronary artery may arise from the left or right sinus of Valsalva. In *group I* the right or left single coronary artery continues past the crux of the heart within the atrioventricular groove to supply the area normally perfused by the contralateral coronary artery distribution. In *group II-A* a large branch of the single coronary artery crosses anterior to the pulmonary artery. In *group II-B* the large trunk passes between the aorta and pulmonary artery, while in *group II-P* the large trunk crosses posterior to the aorta. *Group III* includes subtypes with two smaller vessels that supply the contralateral distribution. One branch crosses between the great vessels, and one crosses behind the great vessels. *Group II-P,* in which the trunk passes between the great vessels, may be a cause of sudden death as a result of compression of the artery by the aorta and pulmonary artery. R = right; L = left; Ao = aorta; PA = main pulmonary artery; LAD = left anterior descending coronary artery; LCX = left circumflex coronary artery; RCA = right coronary artery; S = septal arteries; A = anterior, B = between, and P = posterior to the great vessels. Shading of the transverse trunk indicates this artery courses posterior to the aorta. Lipton MJ et al. (1979) Isolated single coronary artery: Diagnosis, angiographic classifications, and clinical significance. Radiology 130:39–47

123

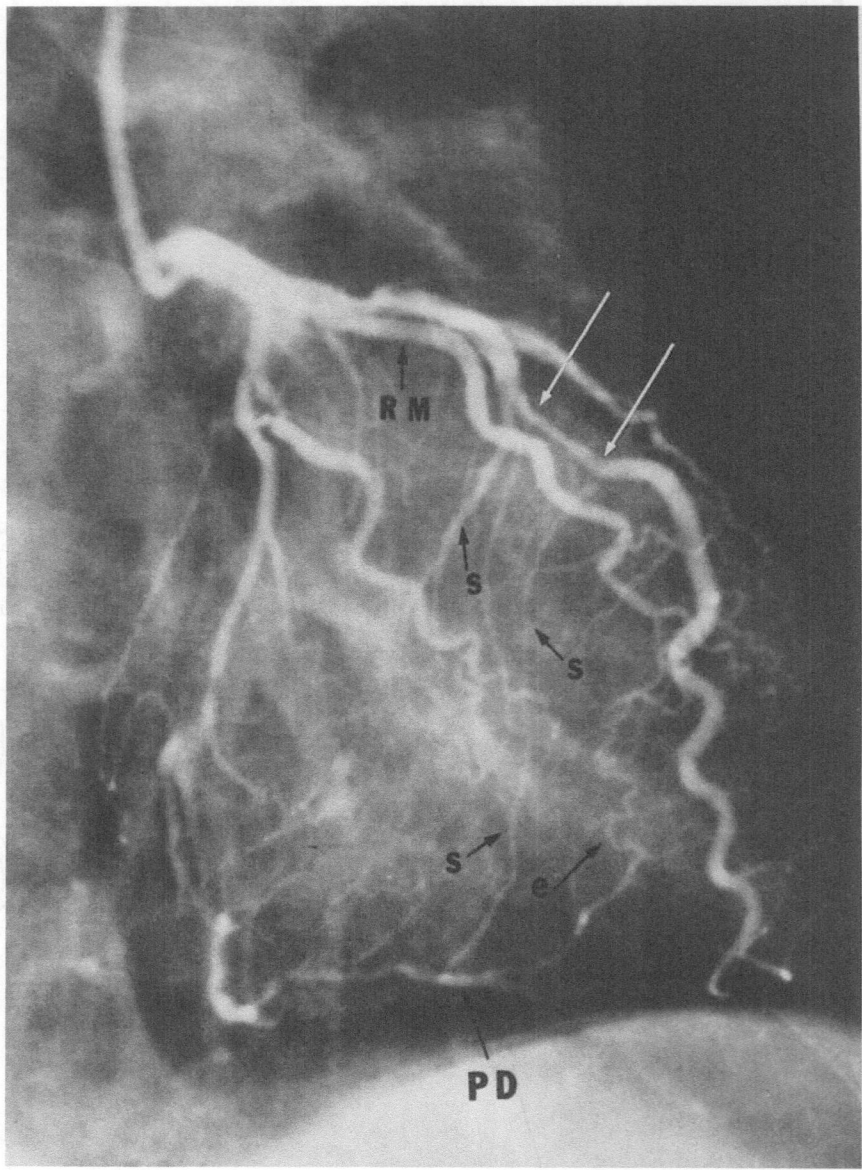

A

Fig. 4–16. *Myocardial bridging or "milking" of a coronary artery.* RAO view of left coronary artery; **A** systole; **B** diastole. Note the long segment of marked narrowing of the left anterior descending artery during systole, which completely disappears during diastole. This segment is embedded in the myocardium with an overlying myocardial bridge (*long arrows*). Observe also reconstitution of the posterior descending artery (*PD*) by septal (*S*) and epicardial (*e*) collaterals. The left atrial circumflex branch provides flow to the crux artery via the atrioventricular node artery. The right coronary angiogram showed occlusion of that vessel. *RM* = ramus medianus.

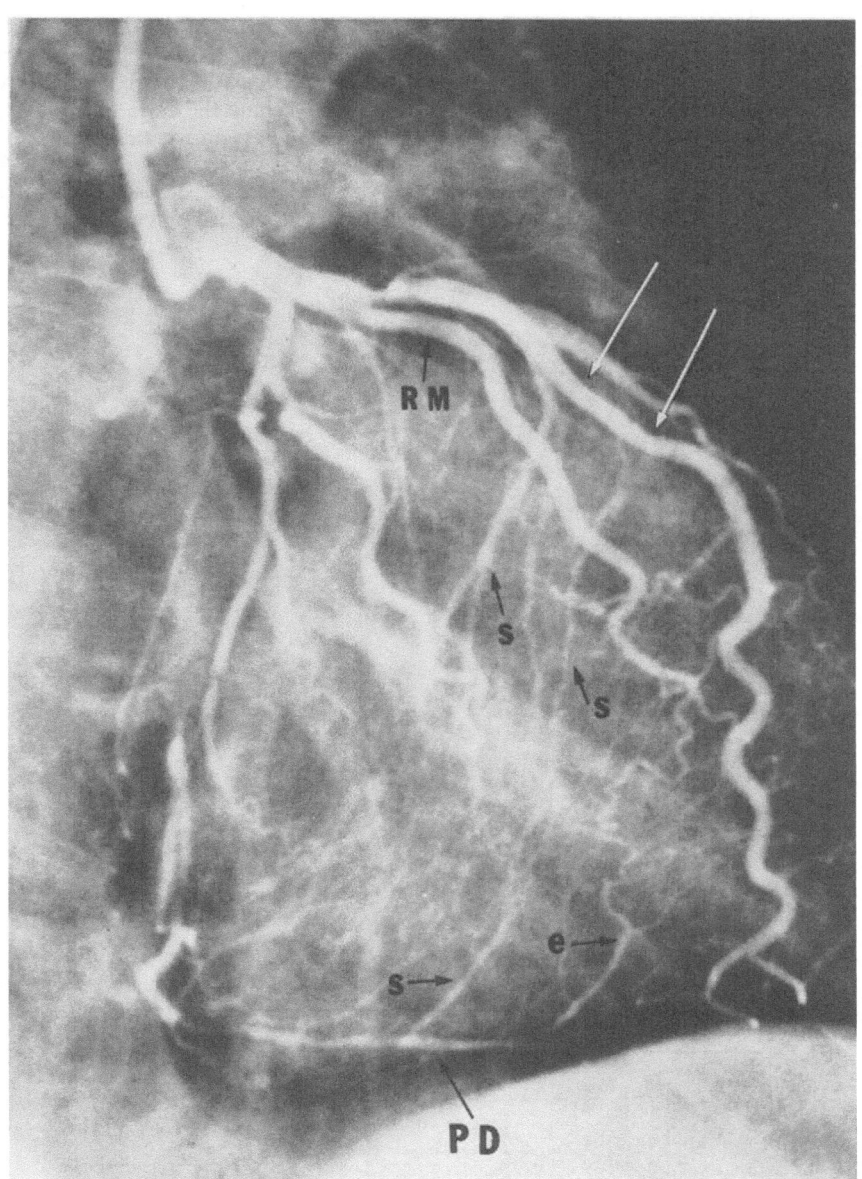

B

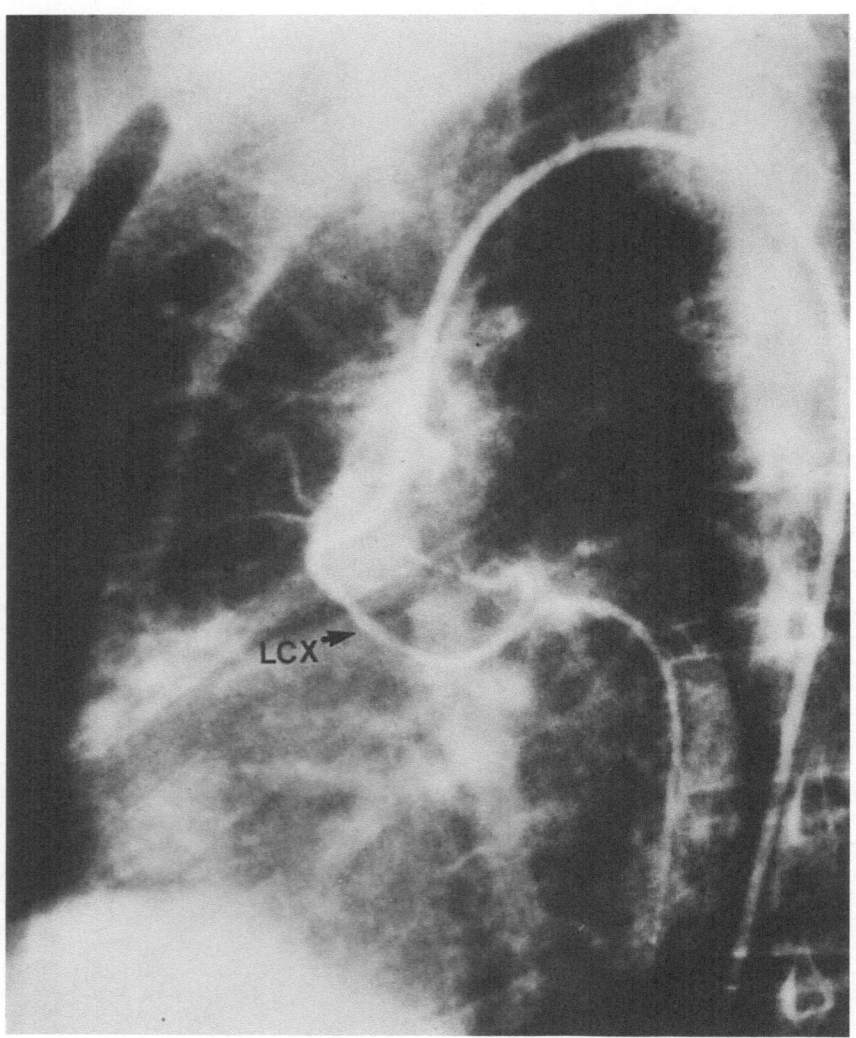

Fig. 4–17. *Left circumflex artery arising from right coronary artery.* LAO view of selective angiogram of the left circumflex artery (*LCX*), a branch of the right coronary artery passing behind the aorta to reach the left atrioventricular groove and supply the posterolateral left ventricular wall. The RCA proper is not visualized because the catheter is selectively in the left circumflex artery.

Fig. 4–18. *Dual left anterior descending artery (LAD) variants.* In types I, II and III the LAD proper (*LAD$_p$*) divides into two branches: the short LAD (*S-LAD*) and the long LAD (*L-LAD*). The S-LAD runs within the interventricular sulcus but terminates well before the apex. The L-LAD runs initially outside the interventricular sulcus but reenters the sulcus to assume the course of the LAD distally. In type I the L-LAD runs along the left ventricular surface. In type II the L-LAD runs along the right ventricular surface. In type III the L-LAD runs within the interventricular septum. In type IV the LAD$_p$ and S-LAD form a single very short vessel situated high in the interventricular sulcus. The first septal perforator and proximal diagonal branches are given off by this vessel. The L-LAD is a branch of the right coronary artery (RCA). The first portion of the L-LAD is formed by a transverse trunk that courses anteriorly to the infundibulum and makes a sharp turn to descend along the anterior interventricular sulcus, while giving off septal and left ventricular diagonal branches. (*Cont.*)

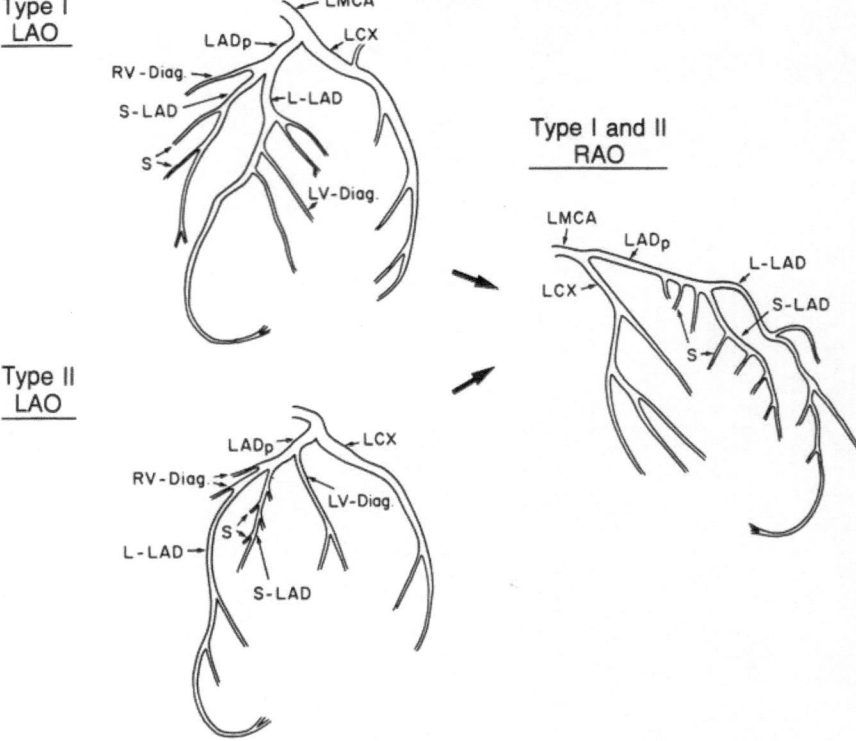

Type III
LAO

Type III
RAO

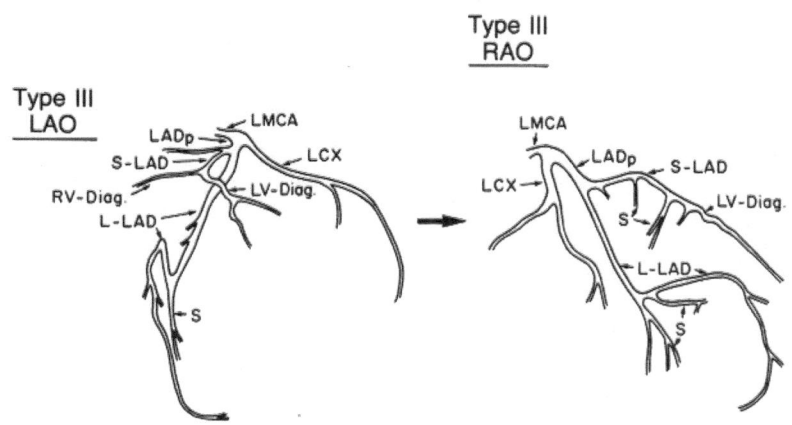

Fig. 4–18 (*Cont.*) *LCA* = left coronary artery; *LMCA* = left main coronary artery; *LCX* = left circumflex artery; *LV-Diag* = diagonal branch to the wall of the left ventricle; *S* = septal artery; *RV-Diag* = diagonal branch to the wall of the right ventricle. *Diag* = diagonal branch; *septal* = septal artery; *RV-branch* = right ventricular branch. Spindola-Franco H et al (1983) Dual left anterior descending coronary artery: Angiographic description of important variants and surgical implications. Am Heart J 105:445–455

Type IV
LCA
RAO

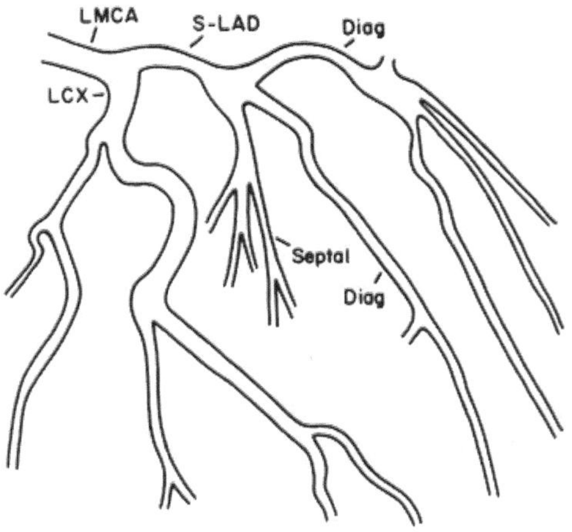

Type IV
LCA
LAO

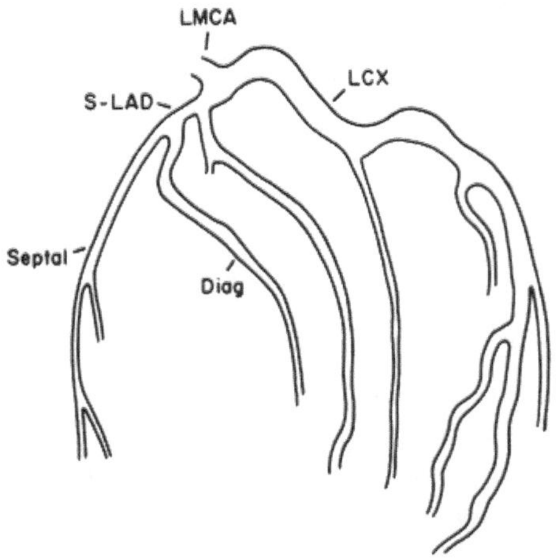

Type IV
RCA
RAO

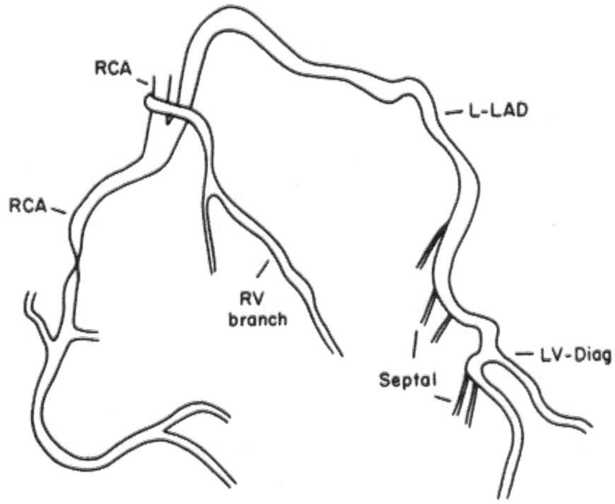

Type IV
RCA
LAO

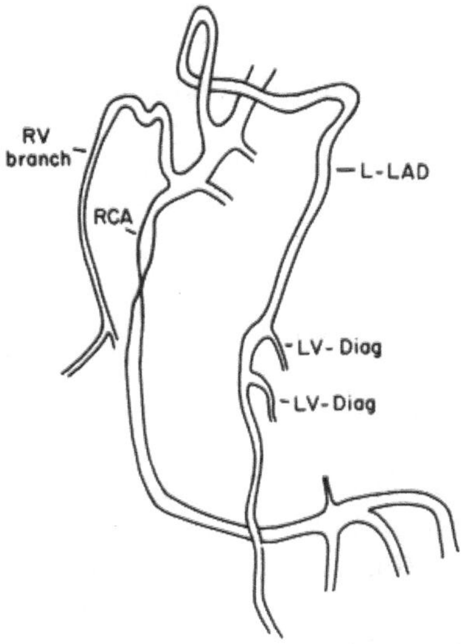

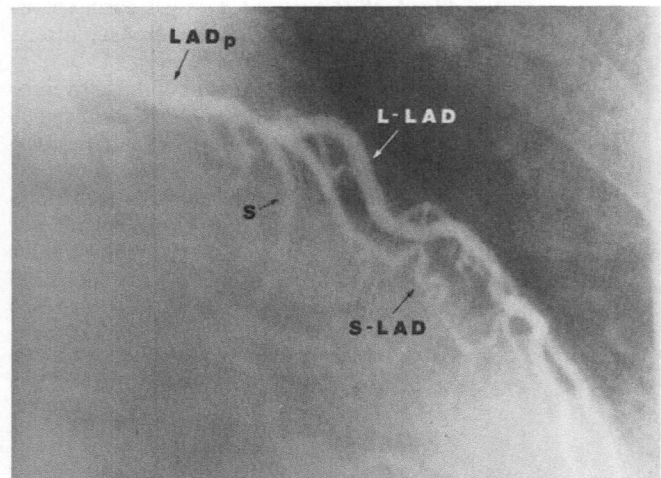

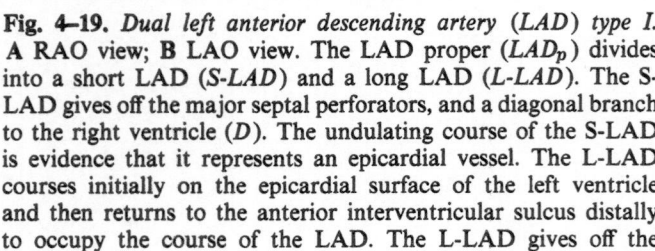

A

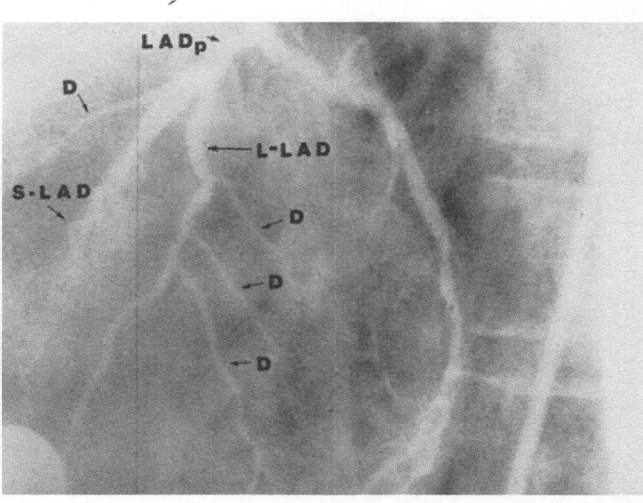

B

Fig. 4-19. *Dual left anterior descending artery (LAD) type I.* A RAO view; B LAO view. The LAD proper (*LADₚ*) divides into a short LAD (*S-LAD*) and a long LAD (*L-LAD*). The S-LAD gives off the major septal perforators, and a diagonal branch to the right ventricle (*D*). The undulating course of the S-LAD is evidence that it represents an epicardial vessel. The L-LAD courses initially on the epicardial surface of the left ventricle and then returns to the anterior interventricular sulcus distally to occupy the course of the LAD. The L-LAD gives off the diagonal branches to the left ventricle. Note the apparent "avascular" area between the S-LAD and L-LAD and the gap between the S-LAD and the L-LAD within the interventricular sulcus. In the RAO view the left circumflex artery is not included in the area filmed. Spindola-Franco H et al (1983) Dual left anterior descending coronary artery: Angiographic description of important variants and surgical implications. Am Heart J 105:445–455

short branch (the short LAD) terminated proximally within the anterior interventricular sulcus (AIVS) on the surface of the heart. A second branch (the long LAD) had a variable course outside the AIVS and returned to the AIVS distally. The long LAD arose from the LAD proper (LADₚ) in 21 cases (Figs. 4–19, 4–20) and from the RCA in 2 cases (Fig. 4–21). The initial course of the long LAD was along the left ventricular surface (17 cases— Fig. 4–19), or along the right ventricular surface (three cases), or within the ventricular septum (three cases—Fig. 4–20).

Recognition of a dual LAD is important so that the correct vessel is grafted at the time of myocardial revascularization. Dual LAD can also help in understanding the discrepancies between lesions of the coronary artery and cardiac abnormalities. As an example, the report by Spindola-Franco et al. includes a case of an acquired ventricular septal defect (VSD) of the apical septum with a normal (short) LAD. The occlusion occurred in a branch (the long LAD) that traveled initially along the left ventricular surface and assumed the course of the LAD distally.

A parallel diagonal branch (Fig. 4–22) may give off branches to the ventricular septum, but nevertheless is not included among the varieties of dual LAD because a paral-

lel diagonal branch does not reenter the interventricular sulcus to assume the distal course of the LAD.

Coronary Occlusion Arteriography

Selective injection of contrast medium into the coronary arteries significantly alters the hemodynamics within the coronary arterial bed. This phenomenon is most dramatic when the catheter occludes the coronary artery in patients with spasm of the coronary artery, with a small coronary vessel, or with luminal narrowing of a proximal coronary artery due to disease. Various unusual coronary vascular patterns may be identified during occlusion arteriography (Spindola-Franco et al.). Opacification of the anterior cardiac veins is not observed during injections in the right coronary artery unless the artery is occluded by the catheter. Contrast material normally fills the coronary sinus and middle cardiac vein after selective injections into either the right or the left coronary arteries. On the other hand, when the arterial lumen is obliterated during selective catheterization of the right coronary artery, an intense myocardial blush is followed by early and highly concentrated filling of the anterior cardiac veins mimicking a coronary arteriovenous fistula (coronary pseudoarteriovenous fistula; Fig. 4–23). In other patients occlusion arteriography in

Fig. 4–20. *Dual left anterior descending artery (LAD) type III.* **A** RAO view and **B** LAO view of left coronary angiogram. The LAD proper (*LAD_p*) gives off two branches. The long LAD (*L-LAD*) and the short LAD (*S-LAD*). The S-LAD runs along the anterior interventricular sulcus and gives off diagonals (*D*). The L-LAD runs initially within the interventricular septum. The L-LAD makes a sharp turn (*open arrow*) to emerge beyond the termination of the S-LAD and takes over its course distally (*closed white arrow*). Note the long gap in the interventricular sulcus between the S-LAD and the L-LAD. Spindola-Franco H et al (1983) Dual left anterior descending coronary artery: Angiographic description of important variants and surgical implications. Am Heart J 105:445–455

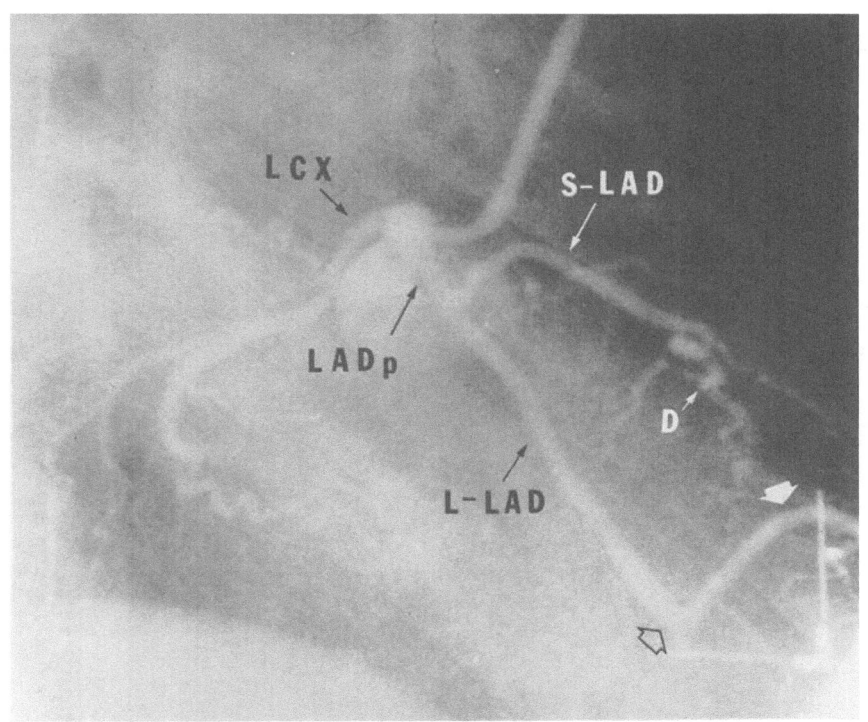

A

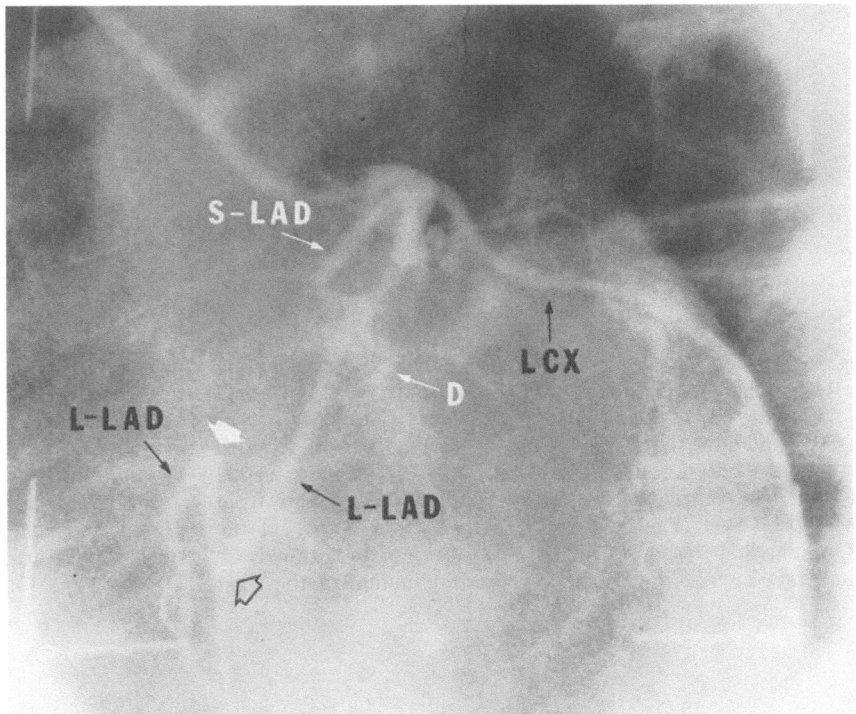

B

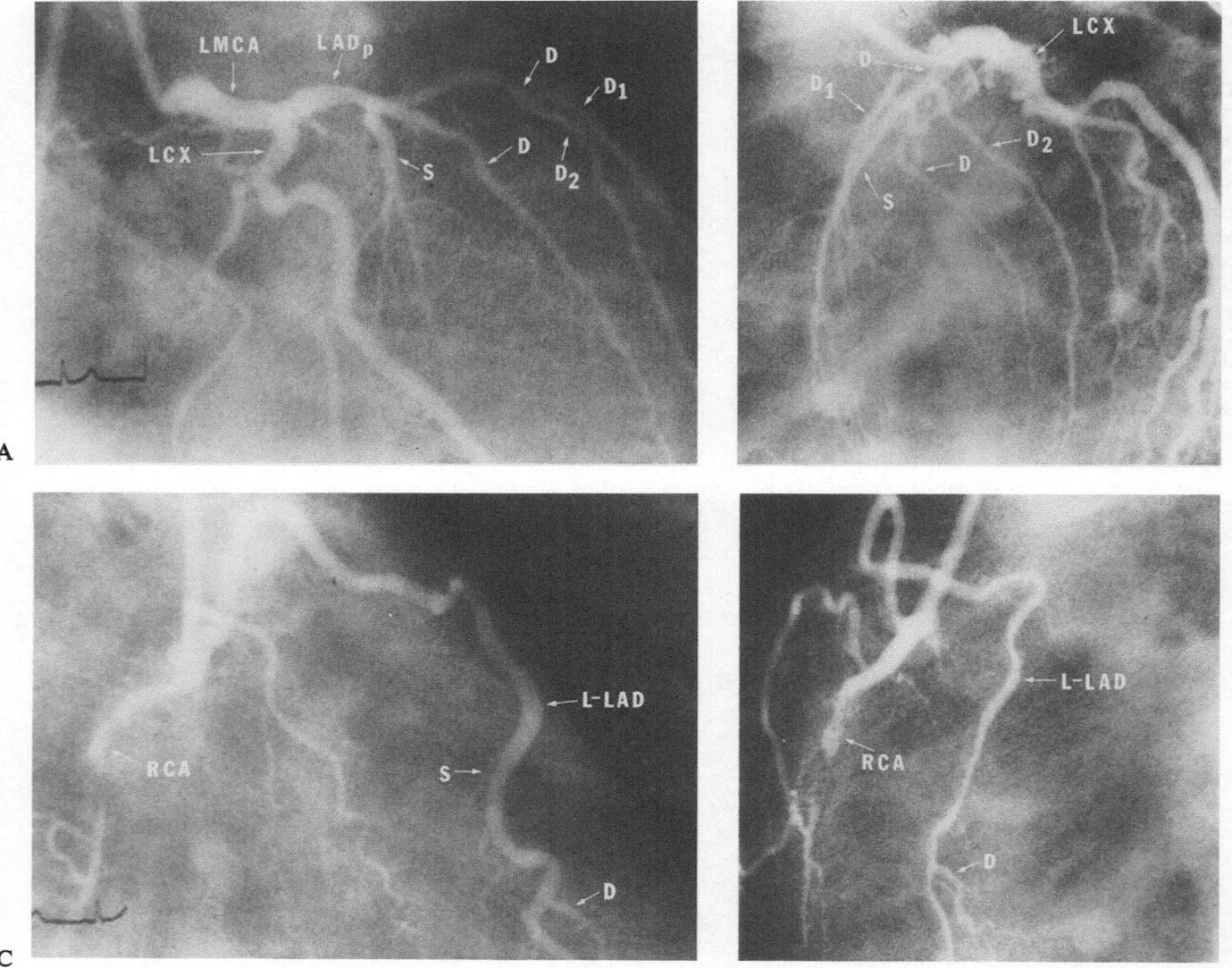

Fig. 4–21. *Dual left anterior descending artery (LAD) type IV.* **A** RAO and **B** LAO views of left coronary artery; **C** RAO and **D** LAO view of right coronary artery (*RCA*). The LAD proper (*LAD$_p$*) and short LAD form a single very short vessel situated high in the anterior interventricular sulcus. The major septal (*S*) and left ventricular diagonal (*D*) branches originate from this short vessel. The long LAD (*L-LAD*) is a branch of the RCA. The first portion of the L-LAD is formed by a transverse trunk that courses anteriorly to the infundibulum of the right ventricle and makes a sharp turn to descend on the anterior interventricular sulcus. The L-LAD gives off septal (*S*) and left ventricular diagonal branches (*D*). *LMCA* = left main coronary artery; *LCX* = left circumflex artery; *D$_1$* and *D$_2$* = superior and inferior branches of the first diagonal. Spindola-Franco H et al (1983) Dual left anterior descending coronary artery: Angiographic description of important variants and surgical implications. Am Heart J 105:445–455

Fig. 4–22. *Parallel diagonal vessel.* LAO view of left coronary angiogram. A large diagonal vessel (*Diag*) runs parallel to the left anterior descending (*LAD*) but does not take over the course of the LAD. Both vessels extend to the apex. This variation should be differentiated from dual LAD type I. There is severe stenosis in the parallel diagonal (*closed arrow*). It will be important to distinguish the two vessels at surgery so that the correct one is grafted. *LCX* = left circumflex artery. Spindola-Franco H et al (1983) Dual left anterior descending coronary artery: Angiographic description of important variants and surgical implications. Am Heart J 105:445–455

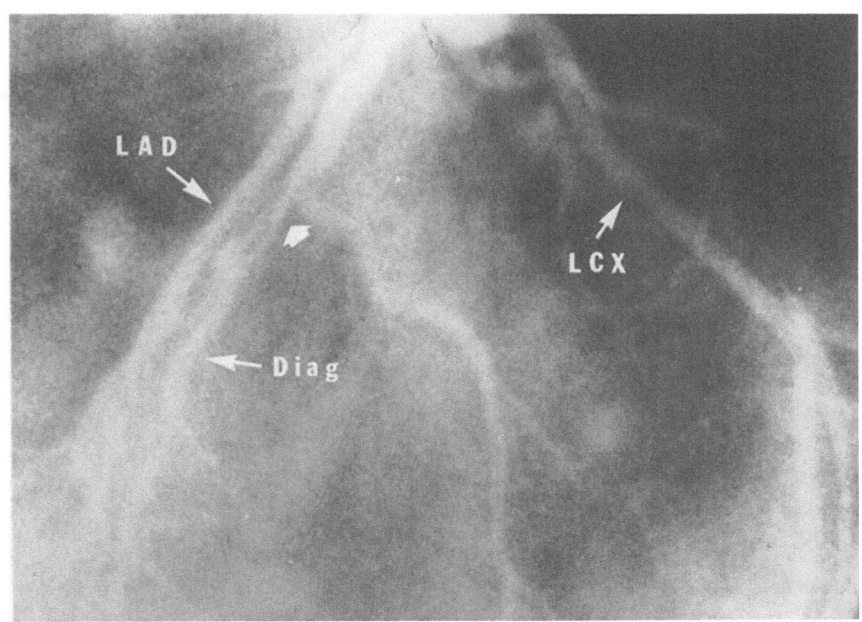

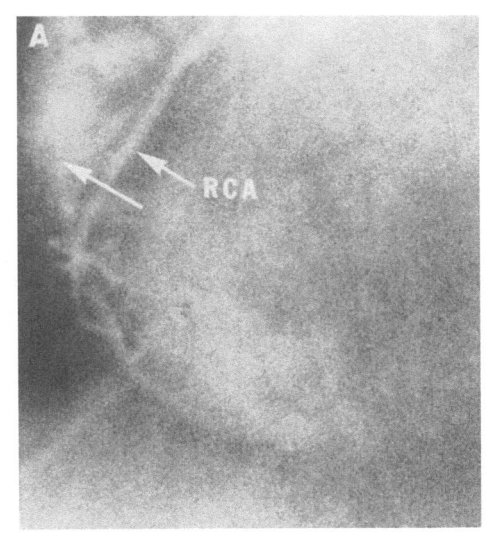

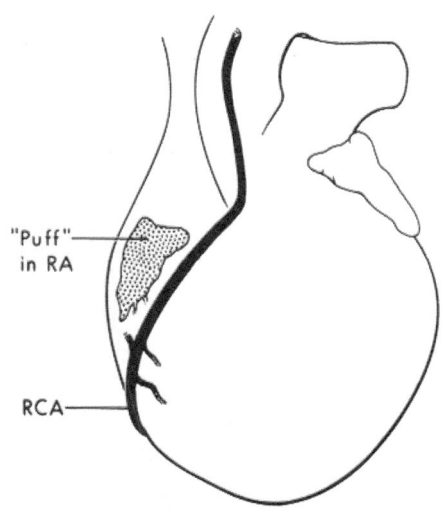

Fig. 4–23. *Occlusion arteriography causing pseudo coronary arteriovenous fistula.* **A** LAO view of right coronary artery (*RCA*) angiogram; **B** diagram of findings in **A**; **C** flush aortogram, same case. Note in **A** and **B** opacification of the right atrium (*RA*) by way of the anterior cardiac veins before the coronary sinus fills, simulating an arteriovenous fistula from RCA to RA. The flush aortogram shows that the RCA is small and that no arteriovenous fistula is present. Spindola-Franco, H et al (1975) Coronary vascular patterns during occlusion arteriography. Radiology 114:59–63

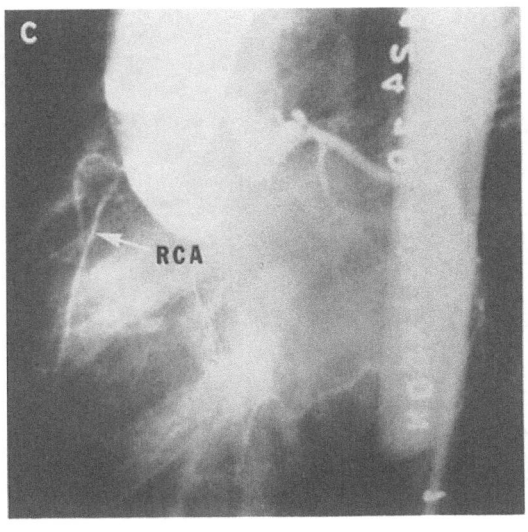

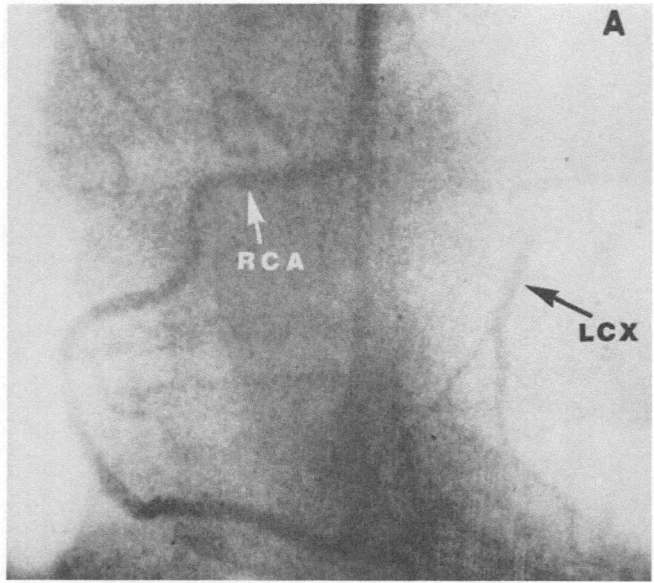

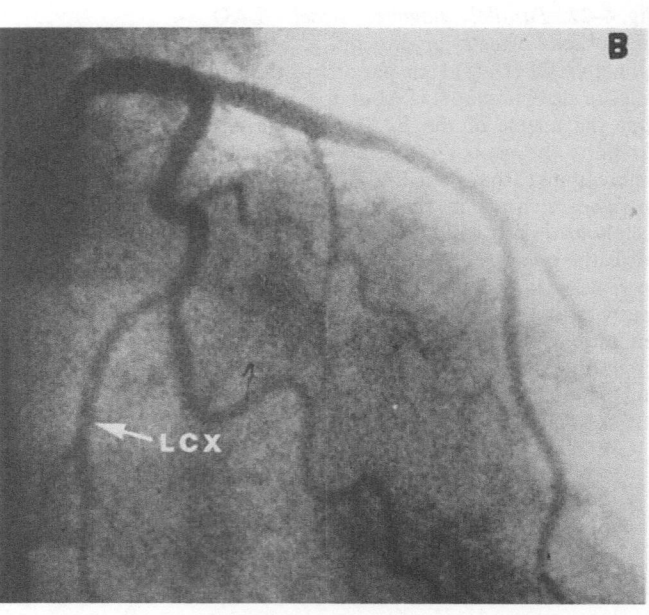

Fig. 4–24. *Occlusion arteriography causing retrograde opacification of the left circumflex artery.* **A** Frontal view of right coronary artery (*RCA*) angiogram; **B** RAO view of left coronary artery angiogram. In **A** the left circumflex artery (*LCX*) opacifies from the RCA, simulating collateral flow and suggesting stenosis or occlusion of the LCX. In **B** the LCX is shown to be normal. Spindola-Franco H et al (1975) Coronary vascular patterns during occlusion arteriography. Radiology 114:59–63

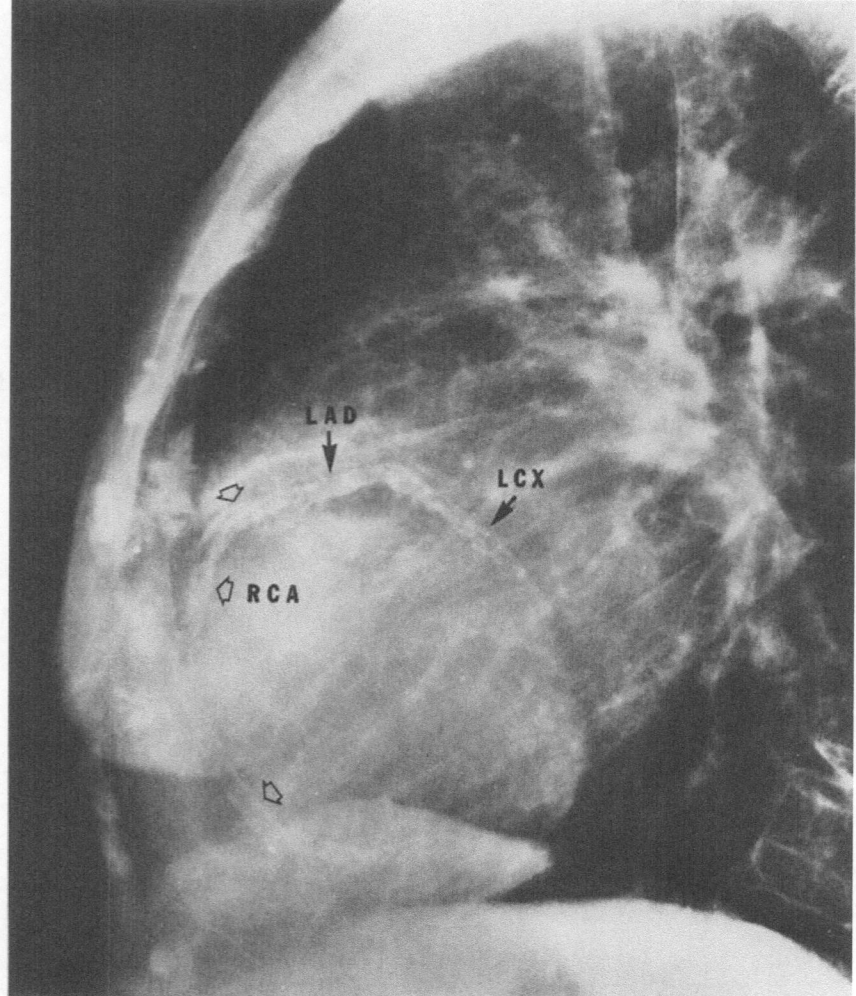

Fig. 4–25. *Coronary artery calcification.* Lateral view of chest roentgenogram demonstrates calcification of the entire left anterior descending artery (*LAD*) and left circumflex artery (*LCX*). The right coronary artery (*RCA*) is also well delineated. The uppermost *open arrow* indicates the origin of the RCA.

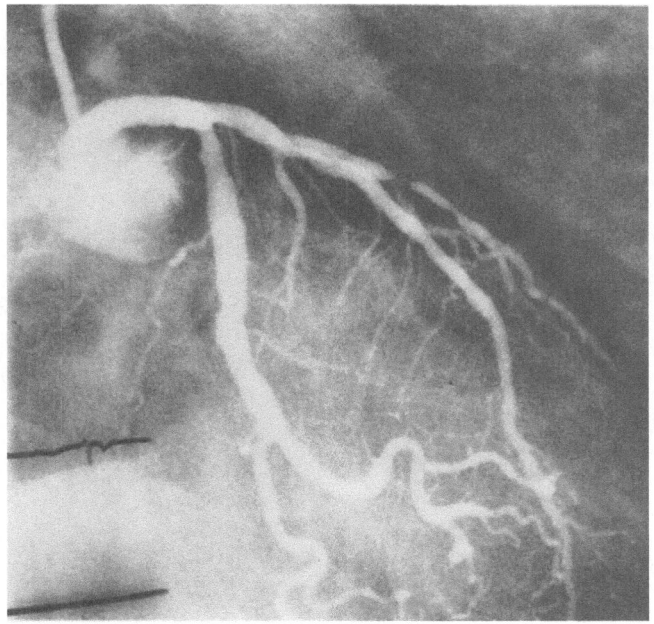

A

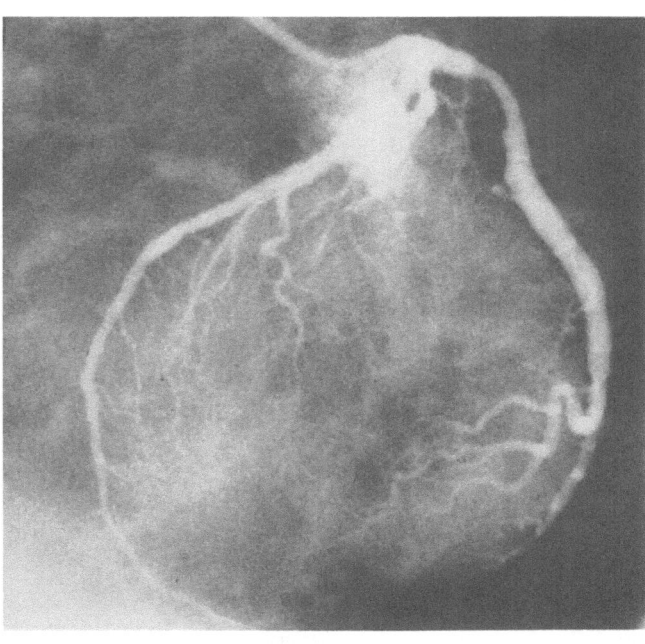

B

Fig. 4–26. *Coronary artery ectasia or arteriomegaly.* **A** RAO view and **B** LAO view of left coronary artery. The left circumflex artery displays diffuse ectasia in its proximal and middle segments.

Diffuse ectasia (arteriomegaly) predisposes to coronary artery thrombosis. Note also diffuse atherosclerotic change in the left anterior descending artery and diagonal vessels.

the right coronary artery results in retrograde opacification of the left coronary arterial system, simulating a stenotic lesion in the left coronary artery (Fig. 4–24).

Roentgen Pathology of Coronary Artery Disease
The coronary arteries should be individually assessed for (1) extent of the disease (e.g., single-, double-, triple-vessel involvement); (2) location (proximal or distal); (3) degree (less or greater than 70% of the arterial lumen); (4) length of the coronary occlusive lesions; (5) anatomy of the vessel distal to the obstruction and (6) status of the myocardium supplied by the affected vessel (left ventricular contraction is assessed by ventriculography). Calcification (Fig. 4–25), focal or diffuse ectasia (arteriomegaly; Fig. 4–26), ulceration (Fig. 4–27) and aneurysm (Figs. 4–28, 4–29) should also be identified and reported.

The *dominance* of either the *RCA* or *LCA* must be indicated (Fig. 4–6). *Coronary dominance* refers to the vessel that supplies the diaphragmatic surface of the left ventricle (LV) and the posterior interventricular septum by way of the crux artery and posterior descending artery (PD) respectively. Right coronary dominance as described in the foregoing occurs in the majority of individuals. Of 2333 coronary angiograms performed at Montefiore Medical Center in 1982 and 1983, 1856 (80%) had a dominant RCA, 207 (9%) had a dominant LCA, and 270 (11%) had a balanced coronary arterial system in which the PD comes from the RCA, but the diaphragmatic wall of the LV is supplied by marginal branches of the LCX.

Fixed coronary artery stenosis is hemodynamically significant when the diameter of the vessel is diminished by more than 75%, when *reciprocating flow* is present or when collateral vessels are apparent. *Reciprocating flow* (Figs. 4–30, 4–31) refers to the phasic alternation of the direction of movement of blood in a coronary artery so that in some phases of the cardiac cycle it is antegrade and in others retrograde (Spindola-Franco et al.). Visualization of reciprocating flow in epicardial vessels is associated with

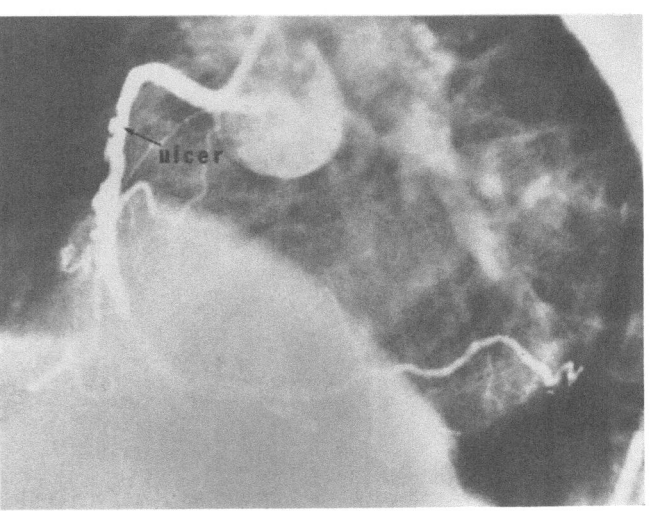

Fig. 4–27. *Atherosclerotic ulcer.* The LAO view of the right coronary artery shows an atherosclerotic ulcer.

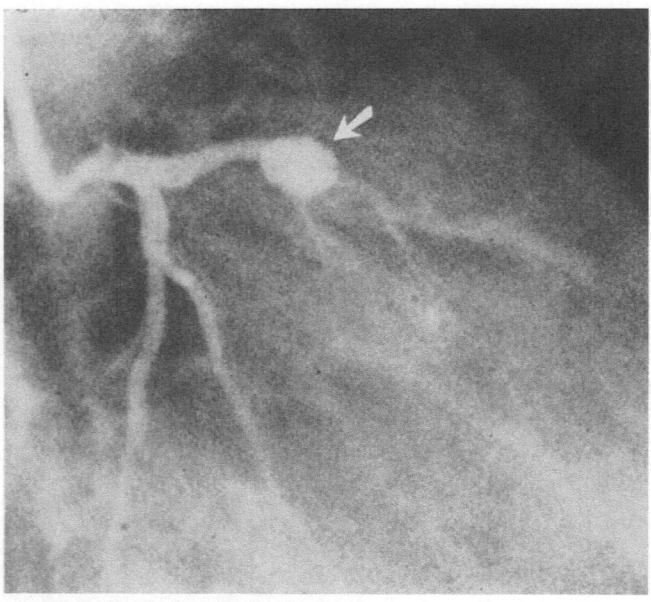

A

B

Fig. 4–28. *Congenital coronary artery aneurysm.* RAO view of left coronary artery. **A** early film; **B** later film. The aneurysm *(arrow)* and the left circumflex artery fill immediately. The left anterior descending artery opacifies after the aneurysm is visualized. On later films (not shown here) the aneurysm remains opaci-

fied after the coronary arteries empty. Congenital aneurysms of the coronary arteries characteristically occur at sites of bifurcations and are characterized by the presence of a narrow neck and smooth walls. A tendency exists for thrombosis to occur in the coronary artery so affected.

greater than 85% coronary stenosis or with occlusion with collateral pathways and a perfusable (viable) capillary bed. Reciprocating flow is not detected in diffusely diseased coronary arteries. Thus, the presence of reciprocating flow should be considered a favorable sign if coronary artery bypass surgery is contemplated.

When hemodynamically significant disease of one or

more coronary arteries is observed, an average annual mortality of 3.3% with single-vessel disease, 6.8% with double-vessel disease, and 11.4% with triple-vessel disease may be anticipated. However, if the one vessel involved is the left main or the left anterior descending artery, the mortality is considerably higher than 3.3%. The presence of asynergy on the ventriculogram doubles the mortality. If an increase in heart volume and a reduction of the ejection fraction are associated, the annual mortality may increase as much as tenfold.

Spasm of the Coronary Arteries (Prinzmetal Variant Angina) Spasm of a coronary artery can be the cause of chest pain and ST-segment elevation in patients with Prinzmetal variant angina (PVA). It is important to differentiate spasm from fixed stenosis because spasm may be managed medically whereas fixed stenosis may require surgery. Symptomatic (spontaneous) spasm of a coronary artery must also be differentiated from catheter-induced spasm, which requires no treatment. Catheter-induced spasm (Fig. 4–32) is asymptomatic and is almost exclusively confined to the RCA. Characteristically, catheter-induced spasm has the appearance of a smooth, concentric, 1- to 2-mm narrowing at the site of the tip of the catheter. This form of spasm disappears after administration of nitroglycerin or after repositioning of the catheter. On the other hand, in patients with PVA, spasm (Fig. 4–33) can occur in any coronary artery, being frequently associated with transient ST changes, angina, hypotension, cardiac dysrhythmias and even cardiac standstill. PVA-induced spasm begins 1–4 mm beyond the tip of the catheter, involving a fairly long segment with an irregular or eccentric appearance, which may simulate fixed obstruction.

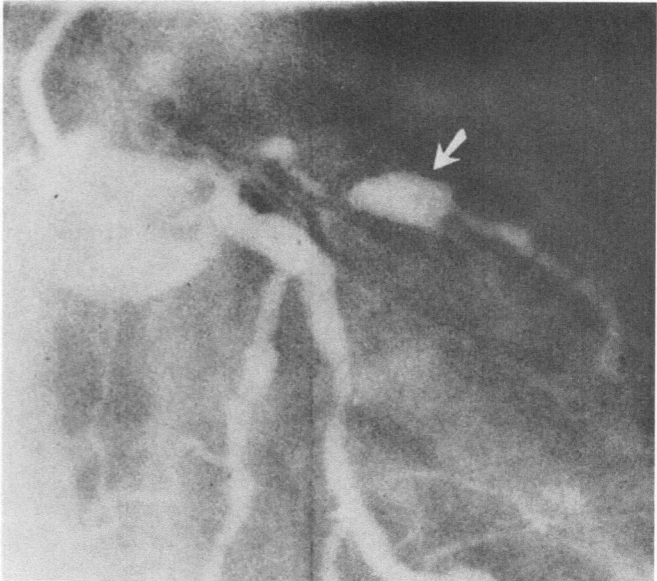

Fig. 4–29. *Acquired coronary artery aneurysm.* RAO view of left coronary artery. This aneurysm *(arrow)* is not related to a bifurcation. The irregular walls and wide mouth are also typical of atherosclerotic aneurysm.

Fig. 4–30. *Patterns of reciprocating flow.* **A** The direction of reciprocating flow related to the events of the heart cycle. Primary epicardial flow is noted in the distal portion of the occluded vessel from collateral flow. During most of the cardiac cycle, blood can be observed to flow toward the lesion (positive direction on the bar graph). During isovolumic contraction the blood may cease to flow or may reverse its direction (negative direction on the bar graph). This flow pattern is identical to the normal pattern of flow in the coronary circulation. The reversal of direction probably reflects both increased intramyocardial resistance to flow and compression of the intramyocardial capillary bed. Reciprocating flow in epicardial vessels is associated with significant localized coronary artery obstruction with a perfusable coronary artery bed. Reciprocal flow is not present in diffusely diseased vessels. Thus its presence should be construed as a favorable sign if coronary bypass surgery is contemplated. **B** Secondary epicardial flow pattern (*S.E.*) represents the reverse of the primary epicardial flow pattern (*P.E.*), apparent after injection into the diseased artery. Antegrade flow occurs in the diseased vessel only during isovolumic contraction. At other times, retrograde motion of the column of opacified blood is present because of collateral flow. In intramyocardial vessels (*I.*) retrograde flow is noted during the ejection period and antegrade flow during the rest of the cardiac cycle. Spindola-Franco H et al (1973) Reciprocating flow in the coronary circulation. Radiology 107:497–504

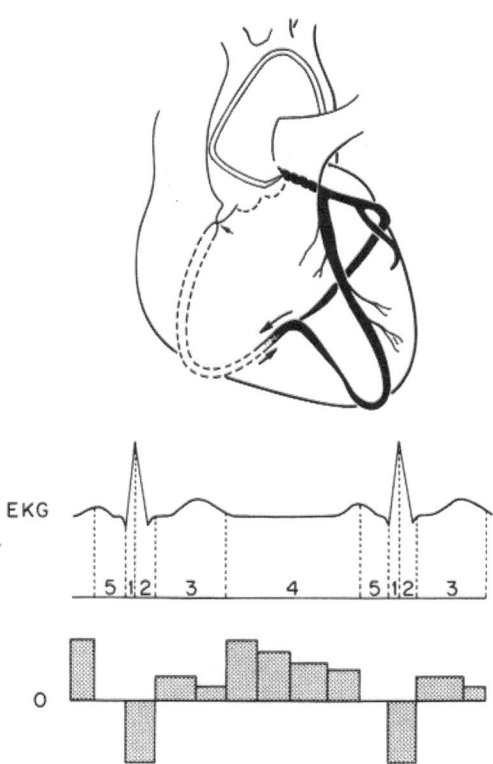

A

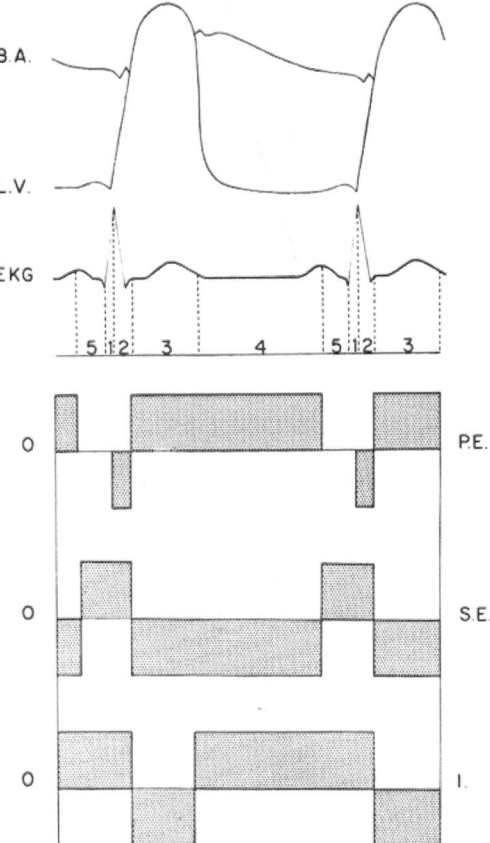

B

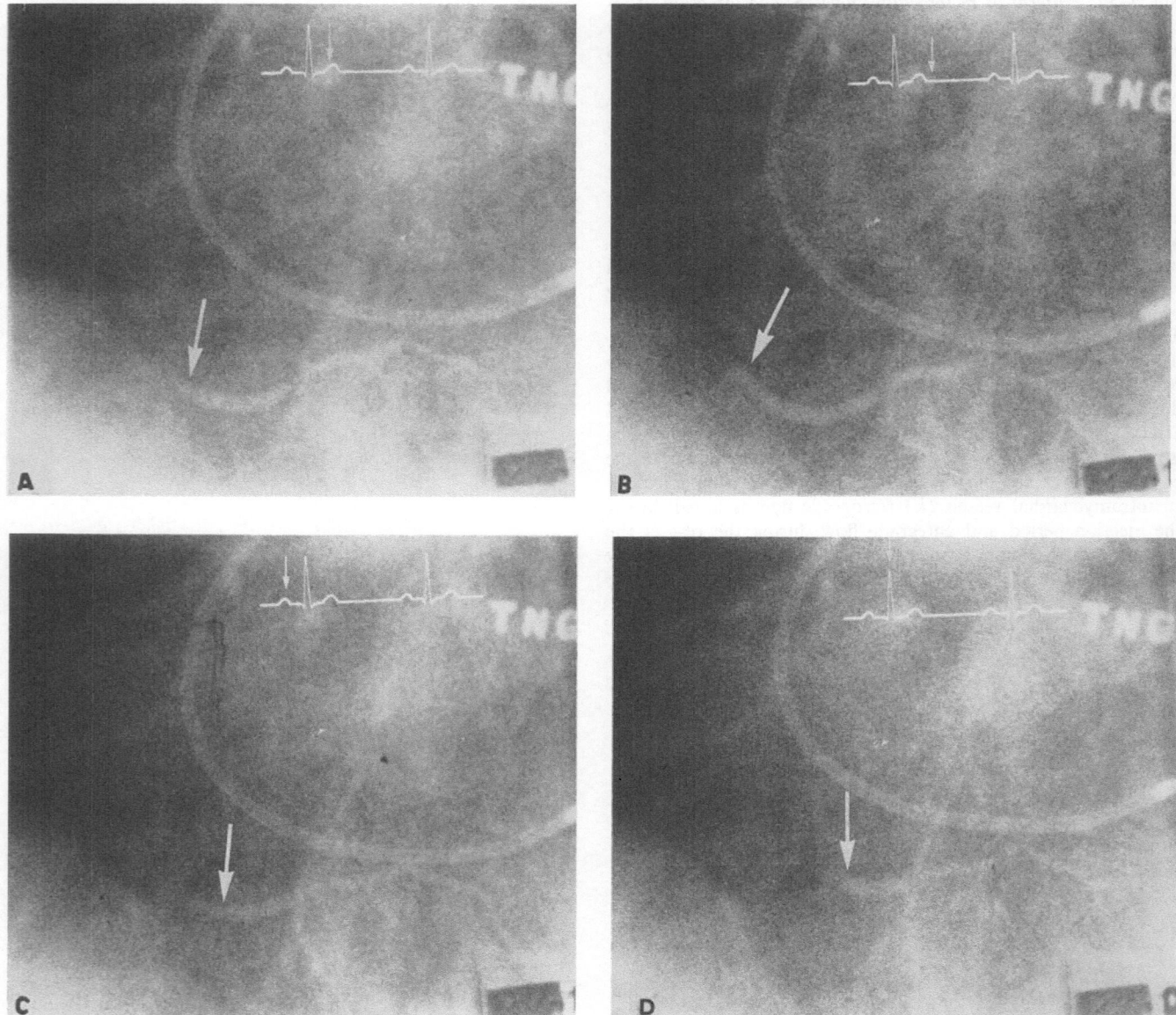

Fig. 4–31. *Reciprocating flow* (*primary epicardial flow pattern*). Cine frames after left coronary artery injection in a patient with occlusion of the proximal right coronary artery. The timing of each frame relative to the cardiac cycle is indicated by *small arrow* above the ECG. The distal right coronary artery is indicated by the *large arrow.* Note the antegrade flow (toward the lesion) during frame **A** (ventricular systole), which is maximal during frame **B** (ventricular diastole). Flow ceases in frame **C** (atrial systole) and reverses during frame **D** (isovolumic contraction). Spindola-Franco H et al (1973) Reciprocating flow in the coronary circulation. Radiology 107:497–504

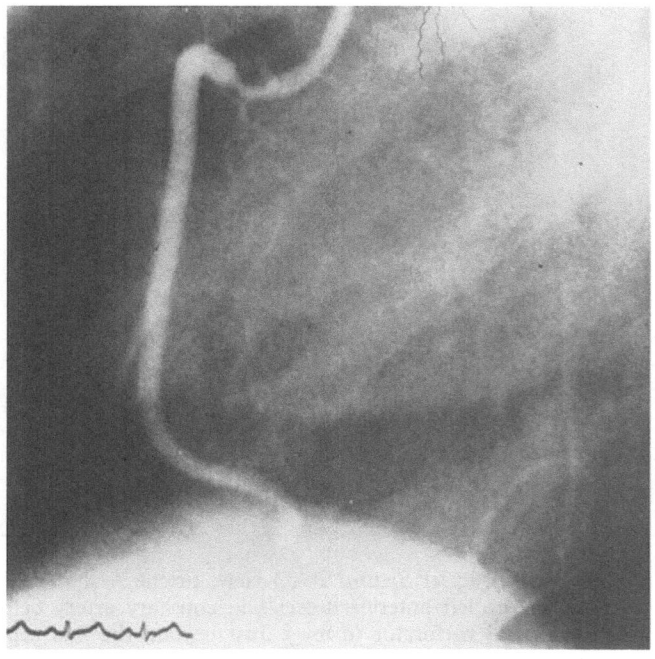

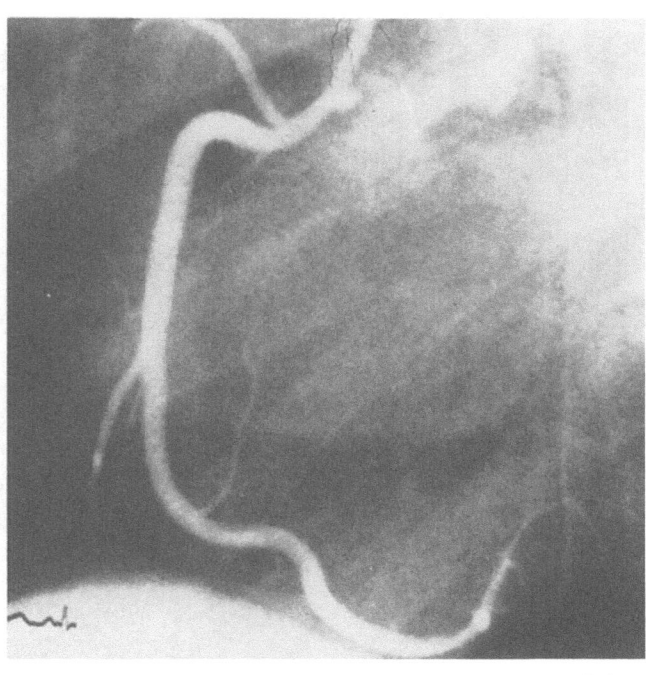

A   B

Fig. 4–32. *Catheter-induced spasm.* LAO view of right coronary artery. Frame **A** Note the spasm identified as a very short segment of narrowing just at the catheter tip. Symptoms and ECG changes were absent. Frame **B** shows resolution after administration of nitroglycerin. Friedman AC et al (1979) Coronary spasm: Prinzmetal's variant angina vs catheter-induced spasm; refractory spasm vs fixed stenosis. Am J Roentgenol 132:897–904

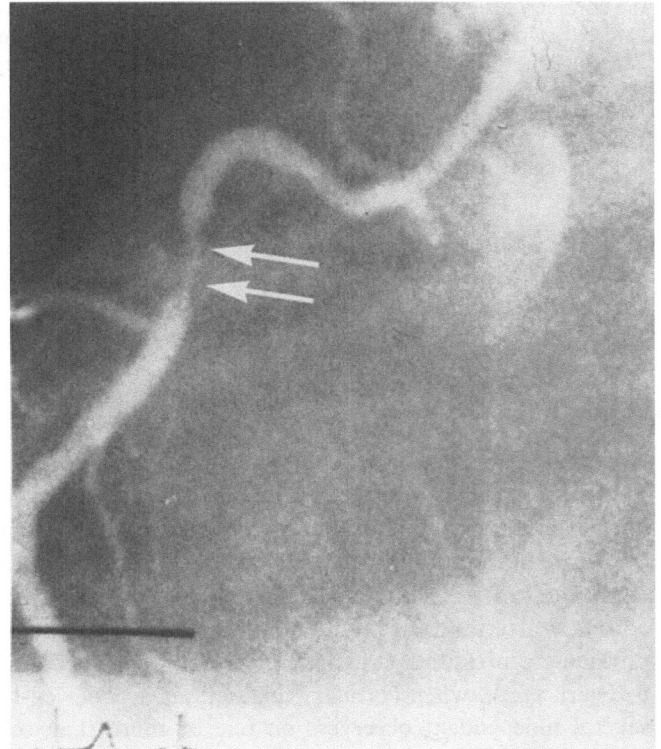

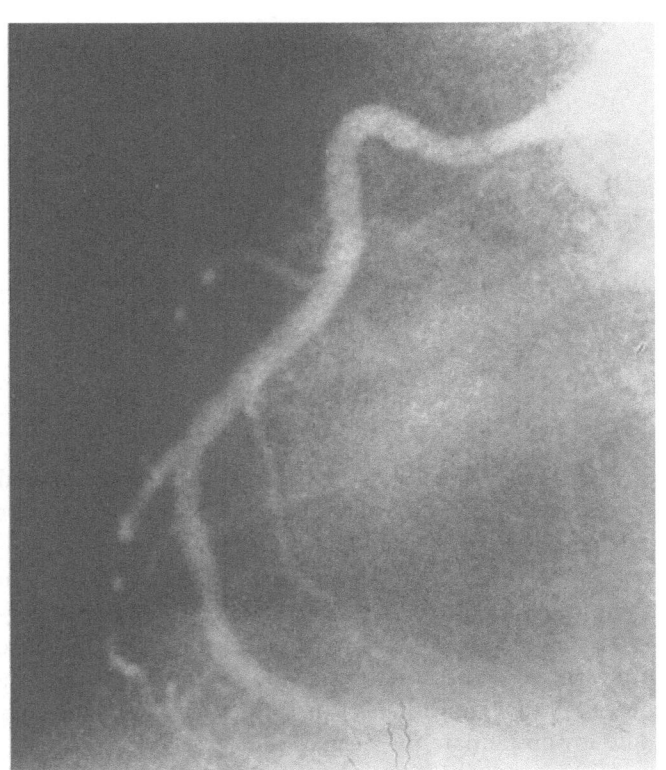

A   B

Fig. 4–33. *Prinzmetal variant angina spasm in the right coronary artery.* Frame **A** LAO view. Observe the long segment of narrowing (*arrows*) with irregular walls 2 cm distal to the catheter tip. Pain in the chest and elevation of the ST segments were associated. After sublingual administration of nitroglycerin the pain and elevation of the ST segment cleared as did the spasm (frame **B**). Friedman AC, et al (1979) Coronary spasm: Prinzmetal's variant angina vs catheter-induced spasm; refractory spasm vs fixed stenosis. Am J Roentgenol 132:897–904

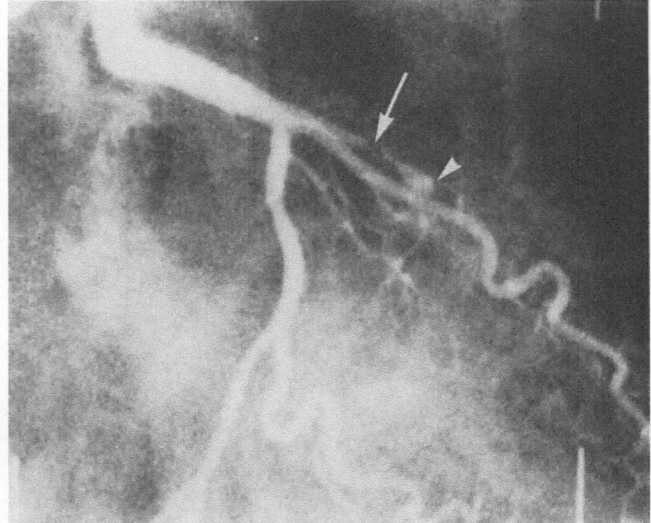

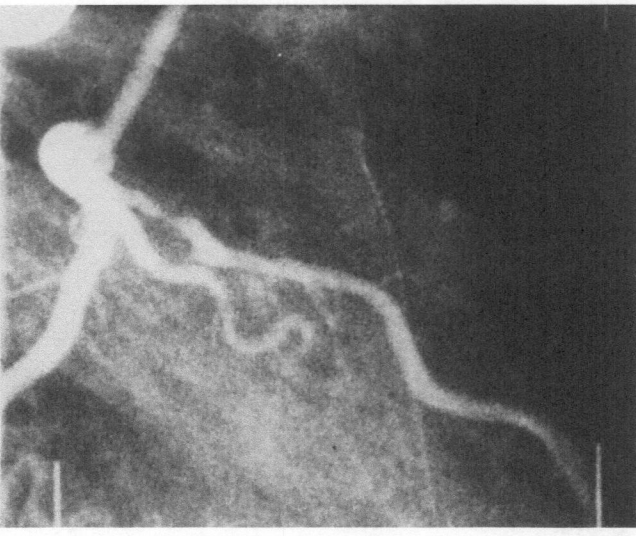

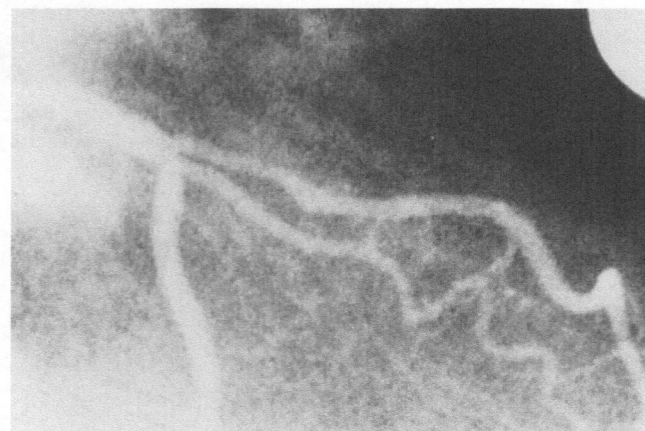

Fig. 4–34. *Refractory Spasm.* RAO view. Frame **A** shows 99% stenosis of the left anterior descending coronary artery before the first septal perforator (*arrow*). Just beyond the first septal perforator the left anterior descending coronary artery is occluded (*arrowhead*). Frame **B** following administration of nitroglycerin shows resolution of the occlusion but persistence of the severe stenosis. In frame **C** during recatheterization because of suspicion of spasm, the left anterior descending artery is normal. **D** and **E** represent diastolic and systolic frames of the left ventriculogram in the RAO view at the time of spasm of the left anterior descending coronary artery. The ventricle is slightly dilated during diastole. During systole the apex and the anterolateral wall are akinetic. Apical dyskinesis was noted on the LAO view (not shown). **F** is a systolic frame from the same patient after resolution of the coronary artery spasm. The contractions of the ventricle have reverted to normal. Friedman AC et al (1979) Coronary spasm: Prinzmetal's variant angina vs catheter-induced spasm; refractory spasm vs fixed stenosis. Am J Roentgenol 132:897–904

In patients with PVA the coronary angiogram should be obtained again after administration of nitroglycerin or calcium channel blockers (e.g., nifedipine, verapamil, diltiazem) to differentiate spasm from fixed obstruction. In some instances spasm in PVA is refractory to pharmacological manipulation (Fig. 4–34). If suspicion of the presence of spasm exists because of the clinical findings, it may be necessary to obtain another coronary arteriogram at a later date to substantiate the diagnosis.

In patients with ischemic symptoms but with normal coronary arteries on angiography, medications such as ergonovine, histamine or methoxamine can be given intravenously to provoke spasm to determine a cause for the symptoms.

Accuracy of Coronary Arteriography

Estimation of the severity of narrowing of vessels on coronary arteriography does not correlate well with the extent of disease in the coronary arteries disclosed in pathological studies unless the pathological studies are carried out on coronary arteries fixed after perfusion with barium gel at physiologic pressures (Plucinski). In addition, according to Björk et al., when coronary angiograms are viewed by several independent observers on one or more than one occasion, considerable intraobserver and interobserver variation is identified in assigning a percentage to the degree of stenosis encountered. Multiple observers interpreting radiological studies together as a group improve their diagnostic accuracy to a significant extent.

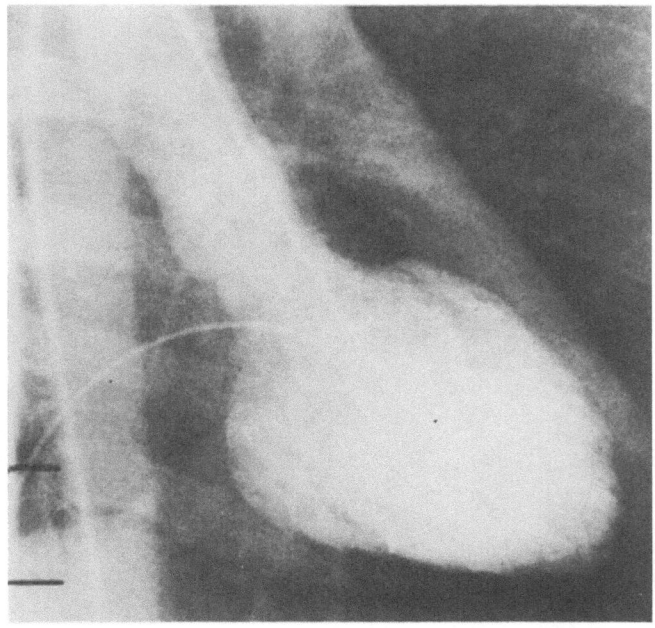

D

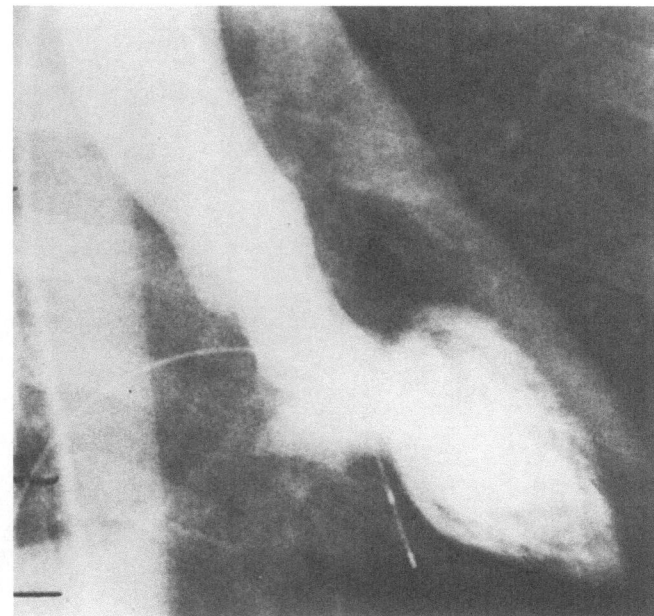

E

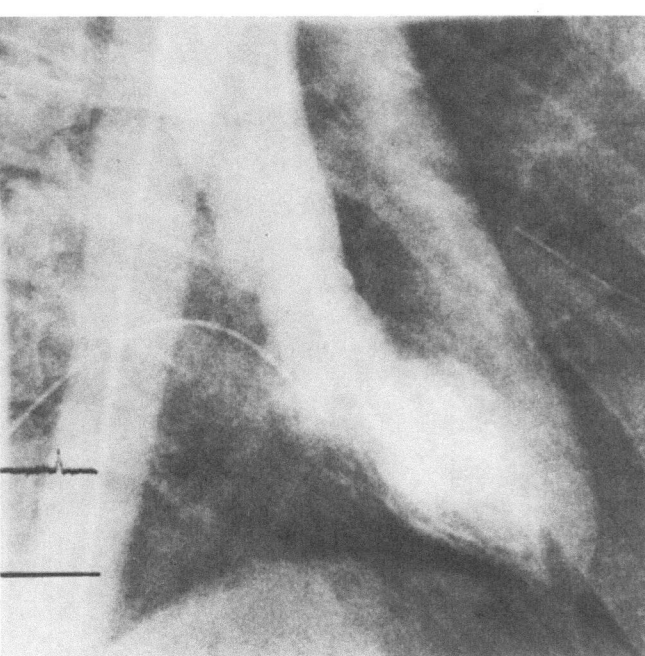

F

Left Ventriculography

Left ventriculography is used to define function (ventricular performance) and structural anatomy (Figs. 4–35, 4–36). Measurements of left ventricular peak systolic and end-diastolic pressures, obtained during ventriculography, represent additional important parameters of ventricular function. Left ventriculography, in addition, is useful in the determination and quantification of the abnormal direction of blood flow, e.g., mitral insufficiency, left-to-right shunts (congenital or acquired), myocardial rupture (false aneurysm).

Left ventriculography usually is performed at rest. However, in special situations, atrial pacing, exercise or adminis-

tration of drugs may unmask abnormal function, not ordinarily appreciated. Angiographic determination of left ventricular volumes involves the analysis of either single-plane (AP or RAO) or biplane (frontal and lateral or RAO and LAO) ventriculograms.

Arvidsson assumed that the shape of the LV could be approximated to an ellipsoid. Thus he measured the long and transverse diameters of the ventricle from the angiogram to calculate the LV volume. This method overestimates the LV volume by approximately 35%. Dodge et al., also assuming the shape of the LV cavity to be ellipsoid, calculated LV volume by measuring the long diameter and the surface area of the ventricular image (area-length technique). Other methods are available for determination of

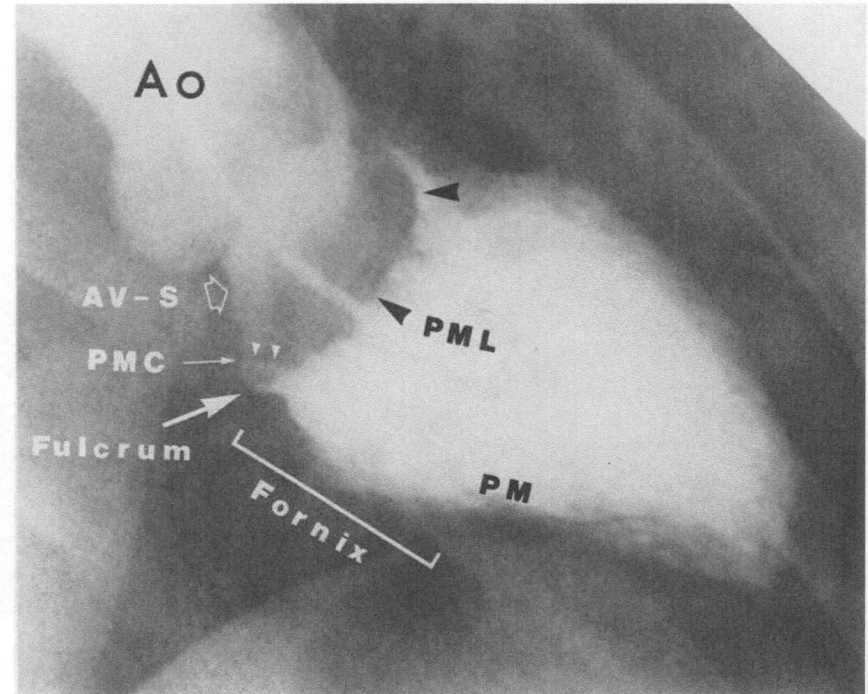

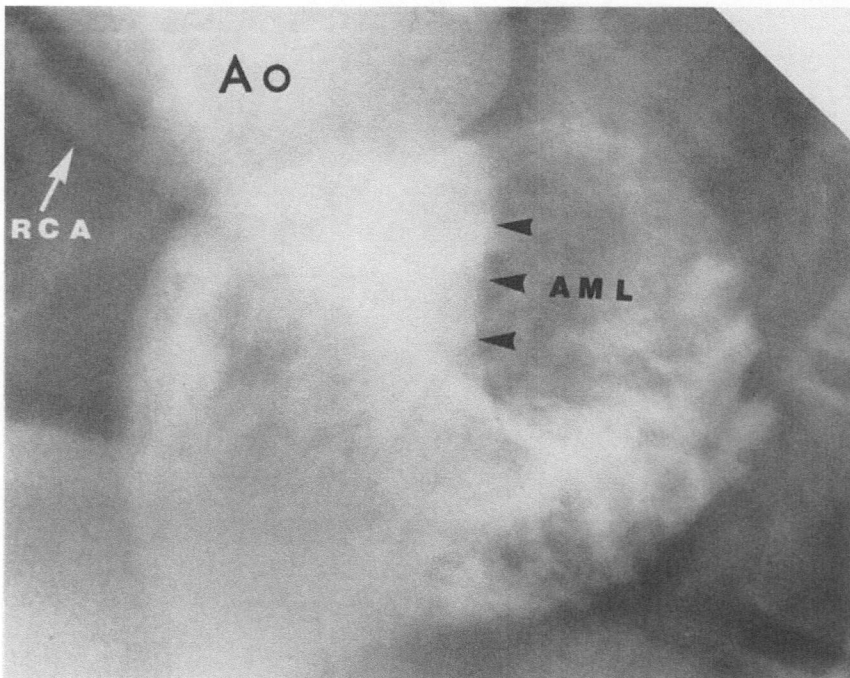

Fig. 4–35. *Normal left ventricle and normal mitral valve apparatus.* **A** RAO view early diastole; **B** RAO view end systole; **C** LAO view diastole; **D** LAO view systole; **E** determination of ejection fraction and analysis of wall motion. The size and contraction are normal. In **A** and **B** the components of the mitral valve are labeled. The *fulcrum* is the point of attachment of the posterior mitral leaflet (*PML*) to the anulus fibrosus. This term is used to describe the lowermost point along the mitral anulus. *Fornix* refers to the portion of the left ventricular wall between the fulcrum and the papillary muscle. It is important to recognize the fulcrum and the fornix when attempting to diagnose abnormalities of mitral motion (e.g., mitral prolapse). The posteromedial commissure (*PMC*) of the mitral valve is identified

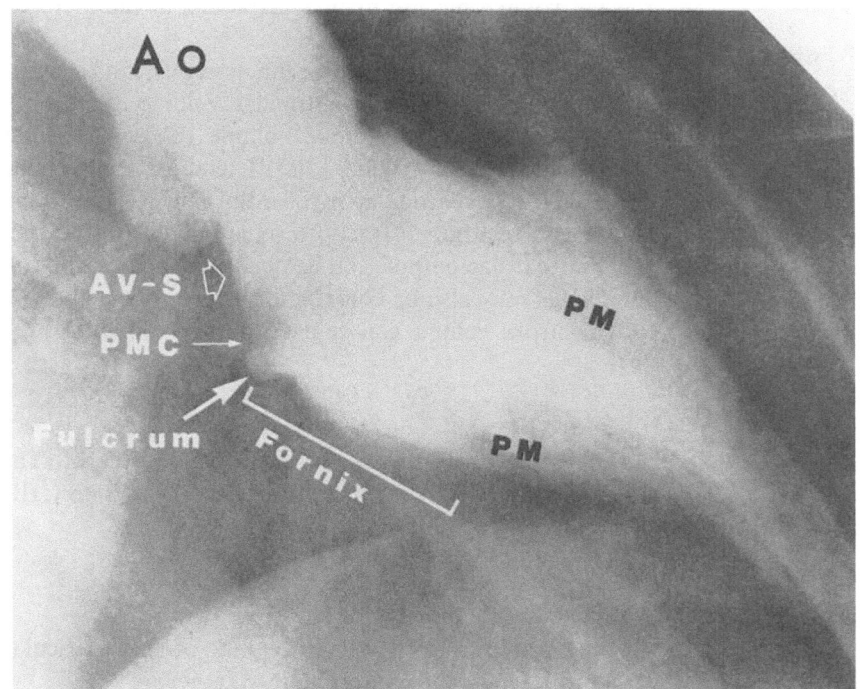

B

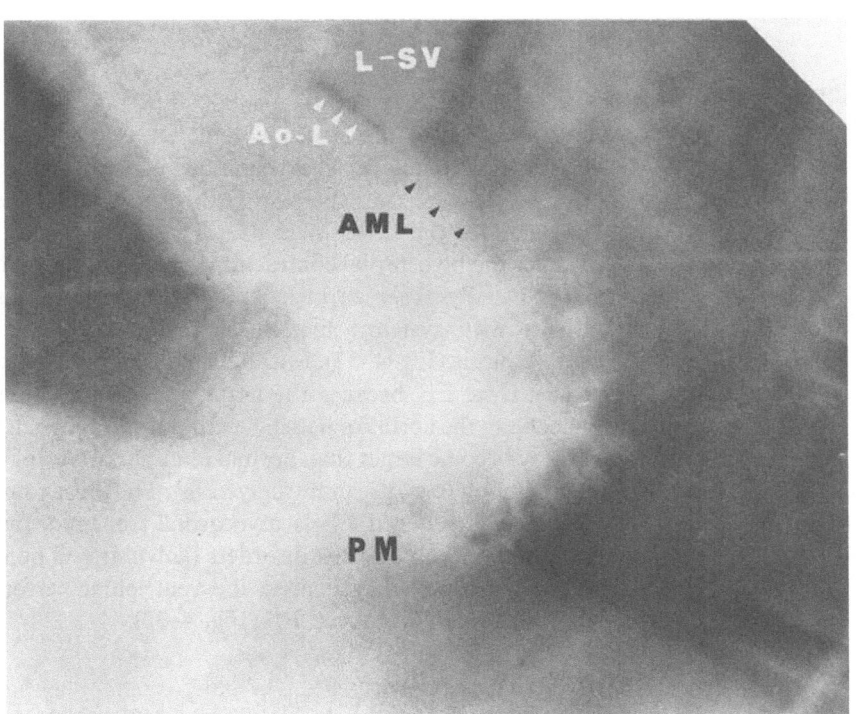

D

as a radiolucent line during systole and diastole. The papillary muscles (*PM*) (anterior and posterior) are best demonstrated during systole. The atrioventricular portion of the membranous septum (*AV-S*) is observed in the subaortic region, being straight or slightly curved. This portion of the membranous septum is affected in patients with endocardial cushion defects and in patients with left ventricular-to-right atrial communication. Compare with left ventricular angiograms in appropriate sections. In **C** and **D** the base of the anterior mitral leaflet (*AML*) and the left aortic leaflet (*Ao-L*) are labeled. Fibrous continuity between the aortic leaflet and the anterior mitral leaflet is demonstrated in **C** diastolic frame). (*Cont.*)

TWO BEAT VENTRICULOGRAM ANALYSIS
BSA = 1.91 (M2) HR = 0(BPM)
CORRECTED RESULTS OBTAINED FROM BEAT 1 ONLY

| | AREA-LENGTH METHOD | | SIMPSON'S RULE | |
	RESULT	RESULT/BSA	RESULT	RESULT/BSA
EDV(CC)	140	73	192	100
ESV(CC)	44	23	64	33
SV(CC)	96	50	128	67
CO(L/MIN)	.00	00	.00	.00
EF	.68		.66	

SYSTOLIC EJECTION RATE	.00	WALL THICKNESS (MM)	.0
REGURGITANT FRACTION	.00	WALL STRESS (DIAST)	0
SPECIFIC COMPLIANCE	.00	WALL STRESS (SYST)	0
COMPLIANCE	.00	LV MASS	0
VCF	.00		

SEGMENTAL WALL MOTION ANALYSIS

		AXIS
	NSC	SHORTENING (%)
ANTEROBASAL	1.14	49.4
ANTEROLATERAL	1.09	50.0
APICAL	1.13	48.8
DIAPHRAGMATIC	.79	20.5
POSTEROBASAL	.57	21.2

EJECTION FRACTION .68

LONG AXIS SHORTENING(%)	28.8
ROTATIONAL ANGLE	1.3
ECCENTRICITY	1.77

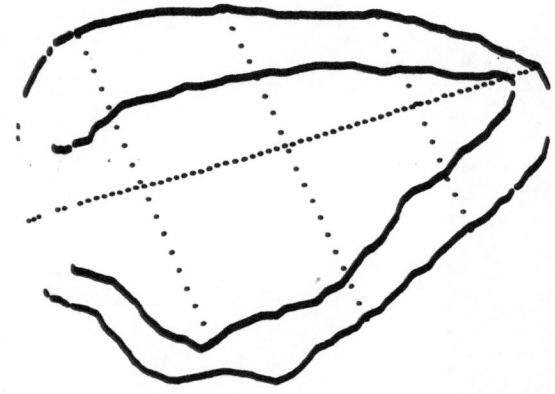

E

Fig. 4–35 (Cont.) In E, a computer printout of left ventricular volumes, ejection fraction and analysis of wall motion from an RAO image of a left ventricular angiogram, the outline of the left ventricular cavity is drawn with a light pen. Some measurements that can be made are listed by the computer. RCA = right coronary artery; Ao = aorta; L-SV = left sinus of Valsalva; NSC = normalized segmental contraction.

the LV volume but are mainly variations in the methods noted in the foregoing.

Several parameters of cardiac function that can be evaluated by measurements of ventricular volume exist. They include the ventricular stroke volume (SV), ventricular work, end-diastolic volume (EDV), end-systolic volume (ESV) and left ventricular myocardial mass. In addition, shunts and regurgitant fractions (angiographic output minus Fick cardiac output) can be quantitated. Pressure-volume loops may also be constructed.

The stroke volume can be determined as follows:

$$SV = EDV - ESV$$

The SV is expressed as milliliters per heart beat. The cardiac output (CO) is the SV times the heart rate (HR) in milliliters per minute:

$$CO = SV \times HR$$

The ejection fraction (EF) is the ratio of left ventricular stroke volume to the end-diastolic volume:

$$EF = \frac{SV}{EDV}$$

The EF expresses the stroke volume as a fraction of the ventricular volume at the beginning of contractions and may be designated as the relative stroke volume. The normal value for the EF is 67 ± 8%. The larger the EF, the stronger the myocardial contraction. An EF larger than normal is usually observed in hypertrophic ventricles, as in patients with systemic hypertension, and aortic and subaortic stenosis (Fig. 4–37). Mitral insufficiency may also result in a large EF, because the left atrium presents less resistance than the aorta. In patients with normal ventricles the EF may become larger than normal after pharmacological manipulation (e.g., use of nitroglycerin). The most common cause of a reduced EF is myocardial ischemia, but a number of other myocardial disorders (valvular and nonvalvular myopathies) may depress the ventricular performance, resulting in a reduced EF (Fig. 4–38).

Left Ventricular Asynergy

In patients with myocardial ischemia the left ventriculogram provides definitive information about the size, shape and function (contractility) of the LV. Determination of the ejection fraction and analysis of segmental wall motion in conjunction with pressure measurements (LV end-diastolic pressure) represent the most useful parameters for the evaluation of recent myocardial infarcts in these patients and are important in predicting the prognosis (longevity) and the potential success of coronary artery bypass surgery.

A normal pattern (synergy) of ventricular contraction is noted in approximately 35% of patients studied for coronary heart disease (Fig. 4–35), whereas the remaining 65%

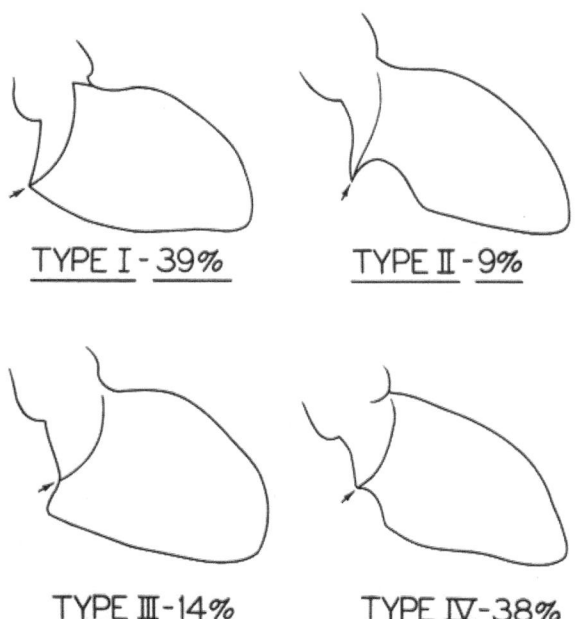

Fig. 4–36. *Four types of normal mitral valve configurations* as observed on RAO view. These variations are distinguished by the position of the mitral fulcrum in protodiastole and by the appearance of the left ventricular fornix during diastole. Types I and II have low fulcra, but type II has a notched fornix. Types III and IV both have high fulcra. The fornix is notched in type IV. Types I and IV are more common than types II and III.

show various manifestations of ventricular *asynergy* (abnormal contraction) at rest. Asynergy usually occurs following myocardial infarction, although it may be present without infarction. The patterns vary from the classical well-delineated bulging aneurysm of the left ventricle to several types and degrees of abnormal wall motion with no change of the overall size of the heart. Asynergy is an important cause of heart failure.

Asynergic segments may be *dyskinetic* (systolic expansion or paradoxical motion), *akinetic* (absence of wall motion) (Fig. 4–39) or *hypokinetic* (decreased wall motion), and the area may be composed of viable (ischemic) myocardium, scar or both. *Asynchrony* may also be observed, which is a disturbed temporal sequence of contraction. On occasion a segment of a normally contracting myocardium that is marginally perfused by a critically stenosed coronary artery may become dyskinetic following administration of nitroglycerin, which diverts or redistributes blood to an area of ischemia (coronary steal syndrome) (Fig. 4–40).

Differentiation of asynergic, ischemic, nonfunctioning myocardium from infarcted muscle may be made by administration of nitroglycerin or norepinephrine or by studying post-extrasystolic potentiation beats. The first two techniques require a second ventriculogram. The potentiated or augmented beat can be compared with a control beat in the same ventriculogram. A positive response to any of these maneuvers (contraction in a previously noted asynergic segment of myocardium) unmasks residual contractile ability and predicts a benefit from myocardial revascularization. Conversely, if normal myocardial contractility is found in subjects at rest with severe coronary artery disease, stress (exercise, atrial pacing, isoproterenol) may precipitate myocardial ischemia and reveal areas of asyn-

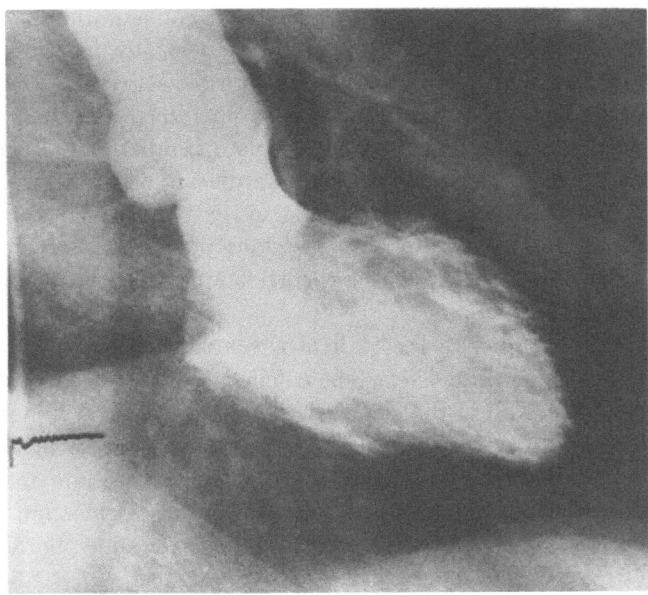

A

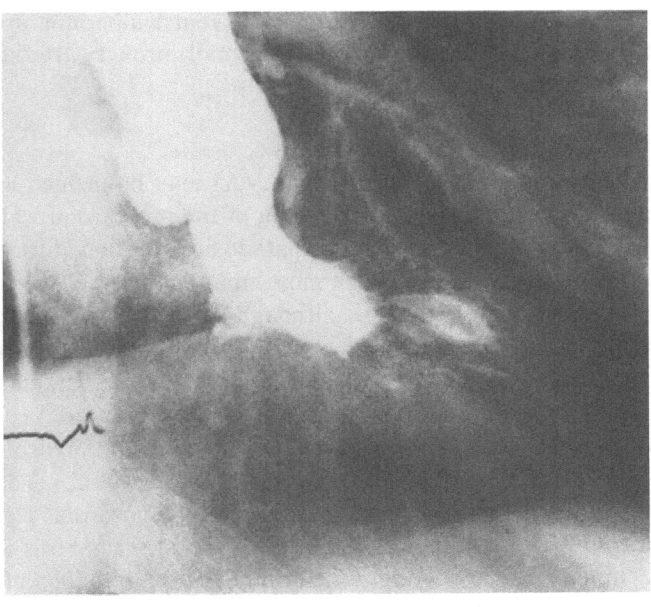

B

Fig. 4–37. *Hyperkinetic left ventricle.* RAO view. **A** diastole; **B** systole. During diastole the left ventricular volume is normal. During systole complete cavitary obliteration with apposition of the papillary muscles is observed. Left ventricular hypertrophy is indicated by thickened left ventricular walls and by prominent papillary muscles and trabeculae. The thickened trabeculae produce the feathery appearance. Compare with Fig. 4–35 which depicts a normal trabecular pattern.

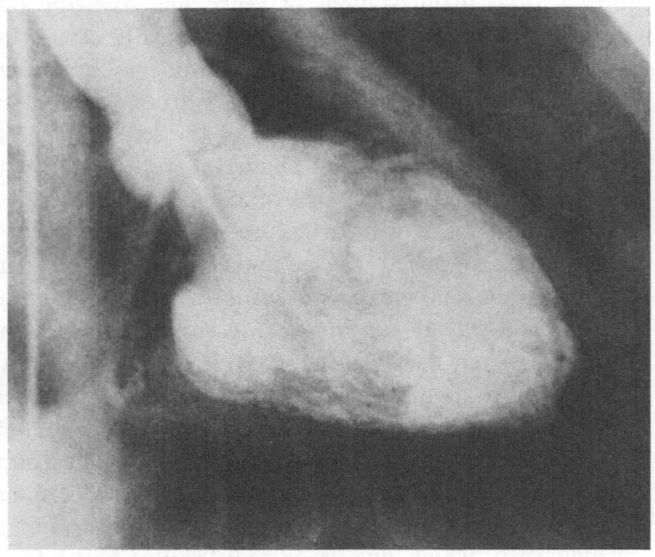

A

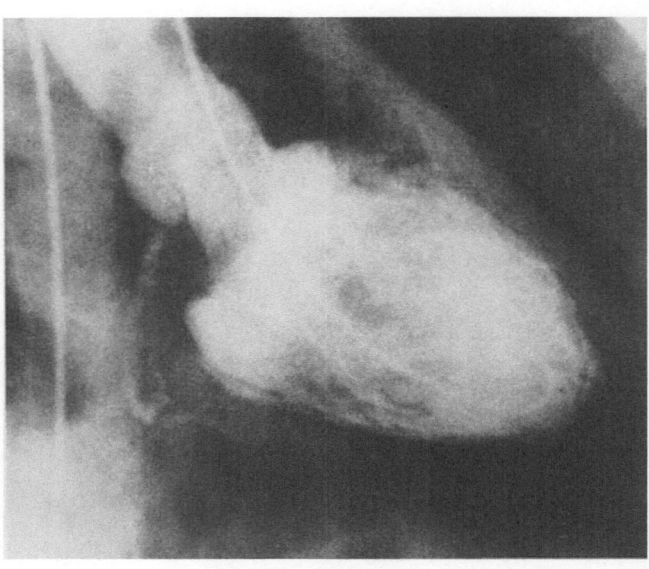

B

Fig. 4–38. *Global hypokinesis.* RAO view. **A** diastole; **B** systole. In a case of cardiomyopathy. The diastolic volume is increased.

During systole the ventricle barely contracts. The ejection fraction is 28%. The coronary arteries are normal (not shown).

ergy. Ventriculographic demonstration of asynergic zones under such conditions suggests deficient focal myocardial perfusion and provides important information concerning the severity or significance of a given coronary artery stenosis.

Abnormal findings on left ventriculography occur not only in coronary artery ischemic heart disease but also in other conditions producing myocardial ischemia (e.g., anemia, metabolic abnormalities at the cellular or molecular level). These disorders produce chronic hypoxemia and injury to the myocardium. In addition, findings similar to myocardial ischemia may be observed in various forms of cardiomyopathies. Abnormal left ventriculograms are also encountered with disease of the small coronary arteries without involvement of large vessels.

Left Ventricular Aneurysm

Aneurysm of the left ventricle (LVA) may be defined as an abnormal bulge or outpouching of the myocardial wall with or without calcification; paradoxical motion during systole may be present. The most common cause of LVA is coronary artery disease although on occasion it may result from congenital defects (e.g., annular subvalvular aneurysm), apical aneurysm of Chagas' disease, trauma (blunt or penetrating), myocardial abscess or bacterial endocarditis. The incidence of aneurysm following myocardial infarction varies from 12%–15% (Abrams et al.). The wall of the aneurysm consists of scarred myocardial elements with fibrosis and calcification. Mural thrombosis is common. The overlying pericardium is usually adherent. The usual location of the ventricular aneurysms is the apex and the anterior wall. A small aneurysm may have little or no hemodynamic effect; however, a large aneurysm (20%–25% of left ventricular area) closely mimics mitral

insufficiency. During systole, blood is transferred into the aneurysmal sac, impairing ventricular ejection. This, in conjunction with a local delay in the development of peak isometric tension, may result in regional dyskinesis with increase in LV work and ineffectual expenditure of energy. The LV compliance is decreased, and a fall in SV and CO occurs.

The chest roentgenogram is usually normal, particularly if the aneurysm is small. When the aneurysm is large, a localized bulge of the left heart border is visible in more than one projection (Fig. 4–1). Frequently a large aneurysm of the apex and lateral wall will blend with a dilated LV, resulting in cardiomegaly of nonspecific configuration. Septal aneurysms are not border forming in any projection and cannot be detected on plain films. Aneurysms of the diaphragmatic wall are usually not identified. Pulmonary vascular redistribution and other plain film findings of cardiac failure are often present. Cardiac fluoroscopy is of little or no value in the evaluation of ventricular aneurysms. Paradoxical or decreased pulsations may be present, or pulsation may be absent, but correlation with ventriculography is very poor.

Calcification of the wall of a ventricular aneurysm is not unusual (Fig. 4–41). The calcification usually involves the inner wall of the aneurysm and appears as curvilinear streaks a few millimeters within the outer margin of the cardiac silhouette. Calcification of the pericardium may have a similar appearance. The pericardial calcification is more peripheral and is noted to involve the outer border of the cardiac shadow.

Angiographic studies (Fig. 4–42) are most accurate in detecting the aneurysmal sac, which may be dyskinetic or akinetic or both. Mural thrombi may be observed as filling defects. Ventriculographic analysis shows an in-

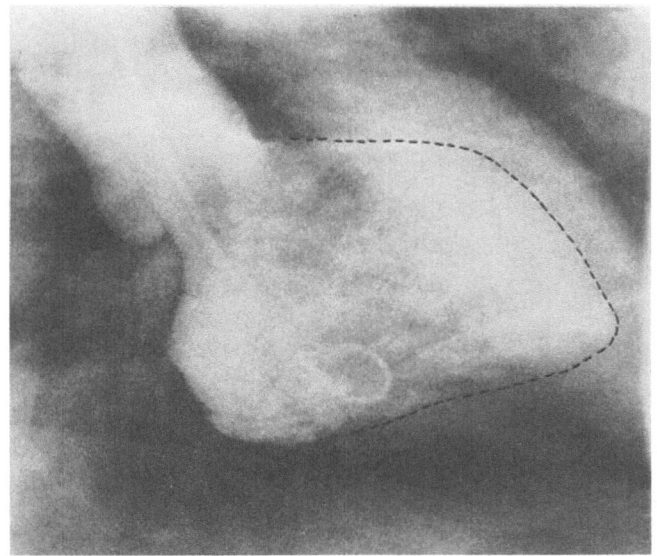

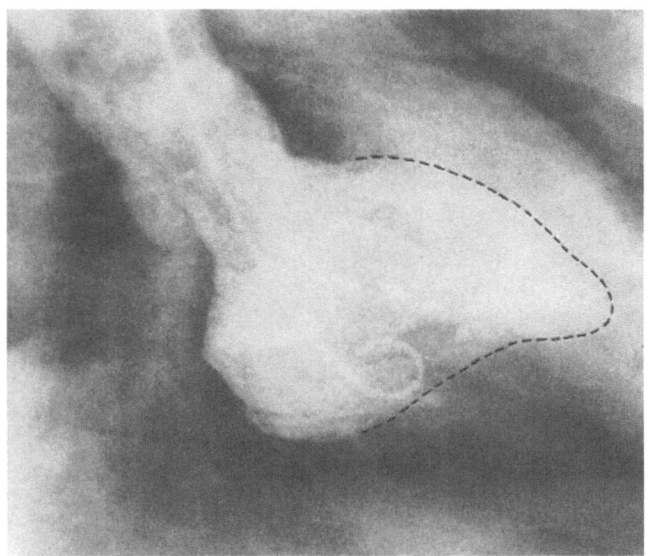

A

B

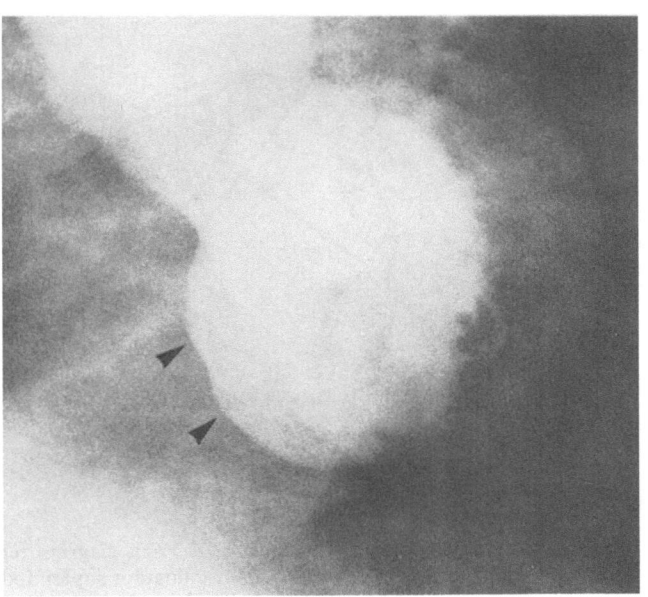

C

Fig. 4–39. *Focal akinesis* in a patient with history of inferior wall myocardial infarction. **A** diastole, RAO view; **B** systole, RAO view; **C** systole, LAO view. During systole the mid and posterior segments of the diaphragmatic wall do not move. In the LAO view the septum bulges during systole (paradoxical motion or dyskinesis) (*arrowheads*).

creased EDV and a reduced EF. Paradoxical motion (dyskinesis) is not a sine qua non feature of LV aneurysms. It may also be present in areas of acute infarction or chronic ischemia of the myocardium.

The differential diagnosis on plain films of an aneurysm that produces a bulge along the left heart border includes false aneurysm (pseudoaneurysm), pericardial cyst, heart tumor (rhabdomyosarcoma), dermoid cyst, thymoma and carcinoma of the pulmonary lingular segment. Angiocardiographic studies may be necessary for differentiation. An aneurysm usually appears on ventriculography as a localized smooth-walled bulge of the contrast medium-filled LV, containing a wide mouth communicating with the LV. Both the aneurysm and the ventricular cavity opacify simultaneously. Conversely, pseudoaneurysm, which is an intrapericardial ventricular rupture contained by adhesive pericardium, has a smaller communication with the LV and opacifies after the ventricular cavity if the injection is made into the LV (Figs. 4–43, 4–44). However, a true aneurysm of the congenital (saccular) type can give the same appearance as a false aneurysm. Differentiation between true and false aneurysms can be made by coronary arteriography (Spindola-Franco and Kronacher). The free wall of a false aneurysm is avascular, whereas the free wall of a true aneurysm contains coronary vessels. The complications of aneurysms and indications for aneurysmectomy are thromboembolism, intractable heart failure and cardiac arrhythmias.

Cardiac Rupture

Rupture of the heart is a common cause (4.7%) of sudden death in the first 2 weeks following myocardial infarction.

Causes of cardiac rupture, other than coronary artery disease, include bacterial endocarditis, myocardial abscess due to septicemia, dissecting aneurysm of the sinus of Valsalva, luetic or tuberculous myocarditis, hydatid disease, malignant disease and trauma.

Cardiac rupture occurs in acute transmural myocardial infarcts. Myocardial perforation depends on the site and extent of the infarct and may occur in any part of the heart. Perforation tends to occur in areas with no collateral circulation or myocardial fibrosis. The typical appearance of the myocardium is that of a dissecting hematoma rather than a tear or "blowout." Cardiac rupture is followed by hemopericardium, cardiac tamponade and sudden death. Rarely is the perforation contained by adhesive pericardium and nonspecific fibrous tissue, thus resulting in a pseudoaneurysm. Unlike a true aneurysm, which seldom ruptures, a pseudoaneurysm frequently does (Dachman et al.). The radiological diagnosis of pseudoaneurysm is of extreme importance since it is amenable to surgical therapy.

Pre-op   Post-op

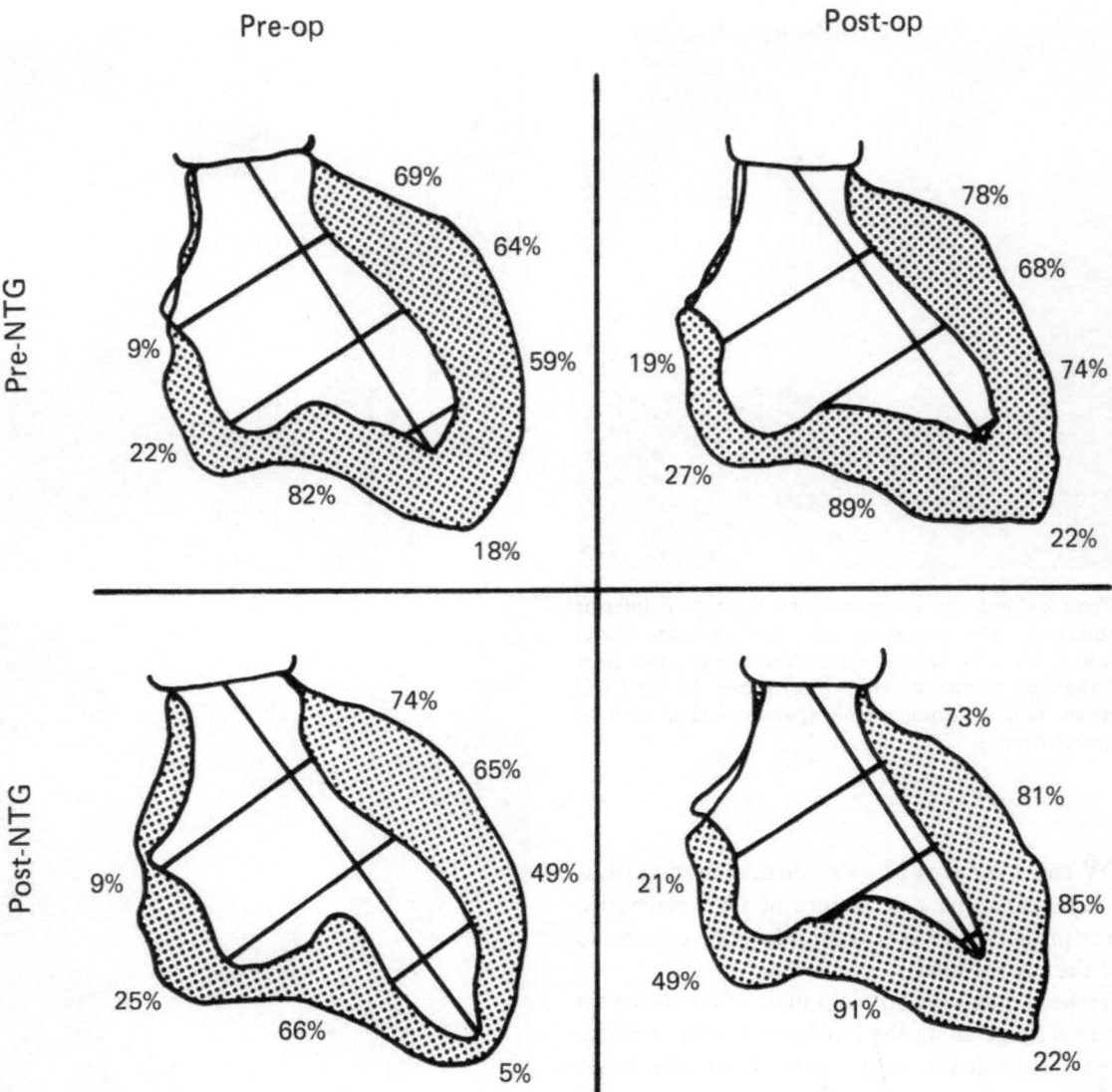

A

Fig. 4–40. *Coronary steal phenomenon.* **A** Each diagram represents a diastolic frame from a left ventriculogram superimposed on a systolic frame, the outer tracing representing diastole, the inner systole. Before surgery, occlusion of the right coronary artery accounted for akinesis of the posterior diaphragmatic wall. The left anterior descending artery (LAD) was severely stenosed as well, with collateral vessels from the LAD to the right coronary artery. Nevertheless, the anterolateral wall was marginally per-fused and moved normally at rest. After administration of nitroglycerin (*NTG*) the anterolateral wall became akinetic and dyskinetic. This effect is probably caused by the redistribution of coronary blood flow away from the distribution of the stenotic vessel during NTG resulting in ischemia of the affected area. After myocardial revascularization the paradoxical response to NTG was no longer observed.

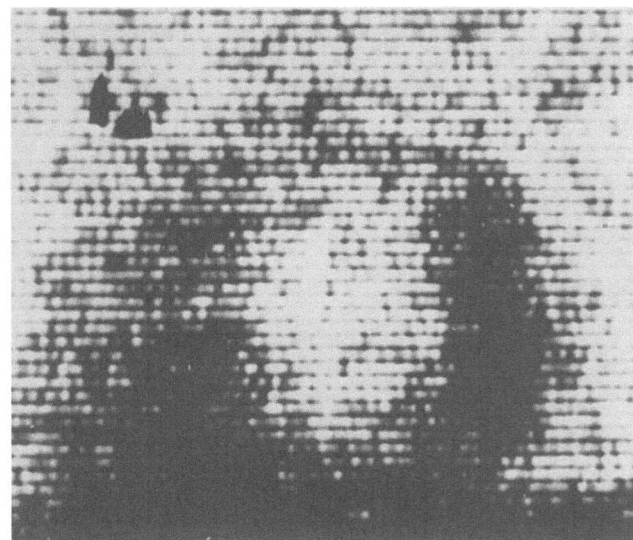

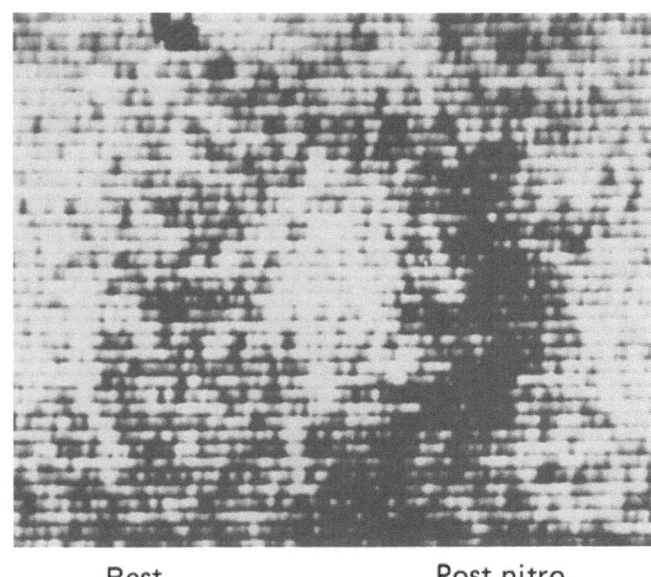

B

Rest   Post nitro

70° LAO

Fig. 4–40 (*Cont*) **B** Radionuclide myocardial perfusion scan, 70° LAO, in same patient. At rest, focal areas of decreased activity are noted in the anteroseptal wall. After administration of NTG the scan shows a distinct worsening of these defects and appearance of new defects in the anteroapical area.

The presence of a paracardiac mass on plain films (Fig. 4–2) should suggest the diagnosis of pseudoaneurysm, especially in a patient who has had a recent myocardial infarct, a history of trauma or a recent ventriculotomy. Demonstration by echocardiography or by ventriculography of a biloculated or multiloculated paraventricular chamber, communicating with the LV by means of a relatively narrow orifice, is suggestive of the presence of a pseudoaneurysm (Fig. 4–44A). However, congenital aneurysms may have a similar appearance. The distinction is made by coronary arteriography (Fig. 4–44B). Demonstration of coronary vessels over the wall of the paraventricular chamber is indicative of the presence of a true aneurysm. In contrast, the free wall of the pseudoaneurysm is avascular on coronary arteriography.

Postinfarction Ventricular Septal Defect

Rupture of the interventricular septum following a transmural myocardial infarction is less common than rupture of the wall of the myocardium (0.5%–1% and 5% respectively). The former is often fatal, accounting for 2% of

the deaths due to myocardial infarction. The rupture usually occurs during the first week after the causative insult. It is usually anteroapical in location (66%) and less commonly posterior. A ventricular aneurysm is associated with the ventricular septal defect (VSD) in 50% of the cases.

Clinically, two modes of presentation exist. In the first, shock and severe heart failure occur soon after the infarct develops. In the second mode, signs of heart failure and sudden development of a holosystolic murmur several days after a myocardial infarct are characteristic. Chest roentgenograms show cardiomegaly with biventricular enlargement. Signs of congestive heart failure, such as pulmonary vascular redistribution, interstitial and alveolar edema are present; however, in spite of the left-to-right shunt, overcirculation may not be evident. Ventriculography (Fig. 4–45) shows a muscular VSD with left-to-right shunting. Biventricular enlargement and myocardial asynergy are present. Mitral insufficiency may be an additional complication.

A VSD following a myocardial infarct carries a grave prognosis. Surgery is nearly always indicated, using a combined surgical approach consisting of repair of the VSD,

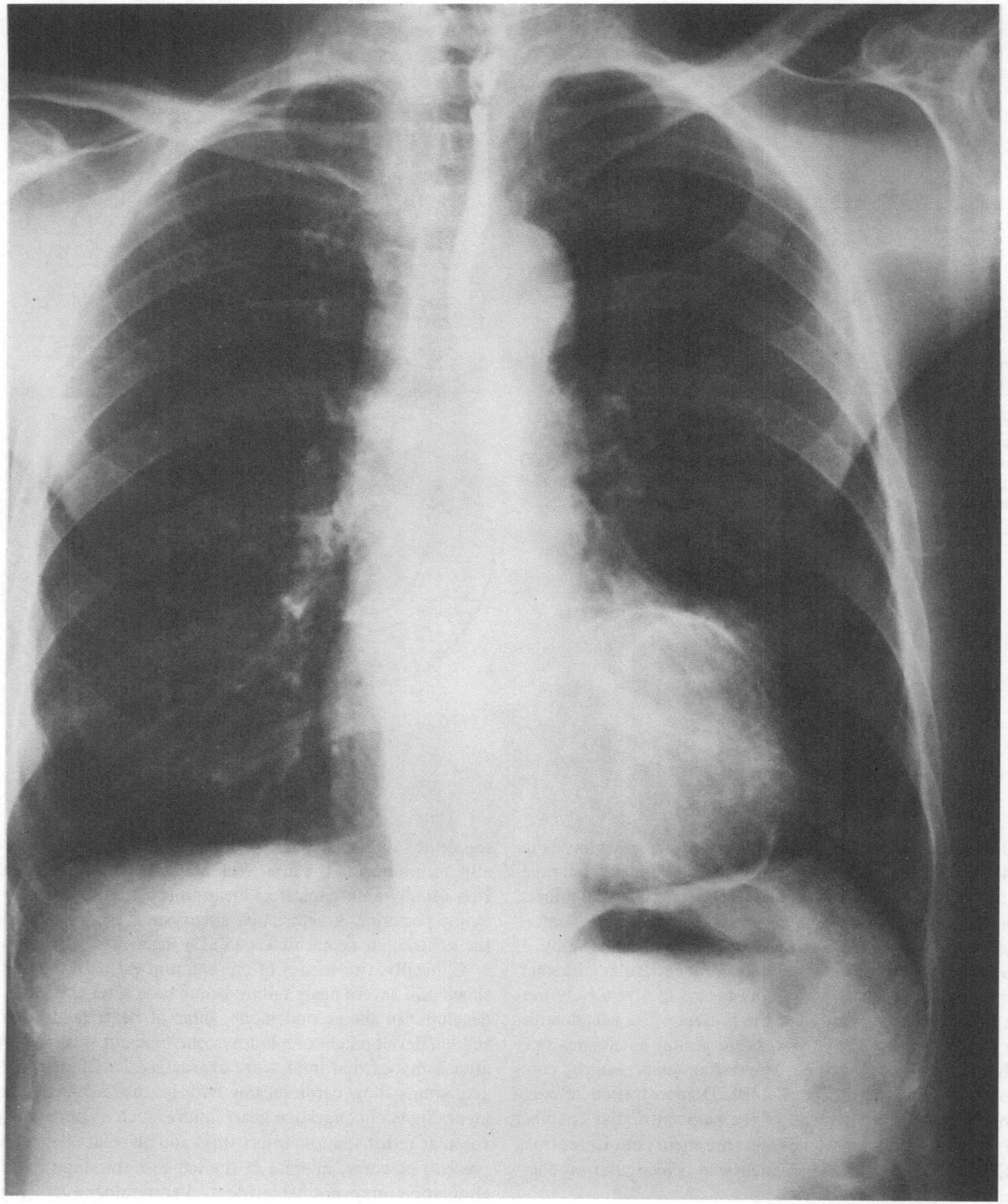

A

Fig. 4-41. *Calcification of a left ventricular aneurysm.* **A** PA view; **B** lateral view; **C** LAO view (page 150). This pattern of calcification is distinguished from pericardial calcification because (1) the calcification is inside the cardiac shadow; (2) it does not follow the outer circumference of the heart but turns inward to follow the outline of the left ventricle; and (3) on the LAO view the calcification follows the curve of the anteroseptal region of the left ventricle.

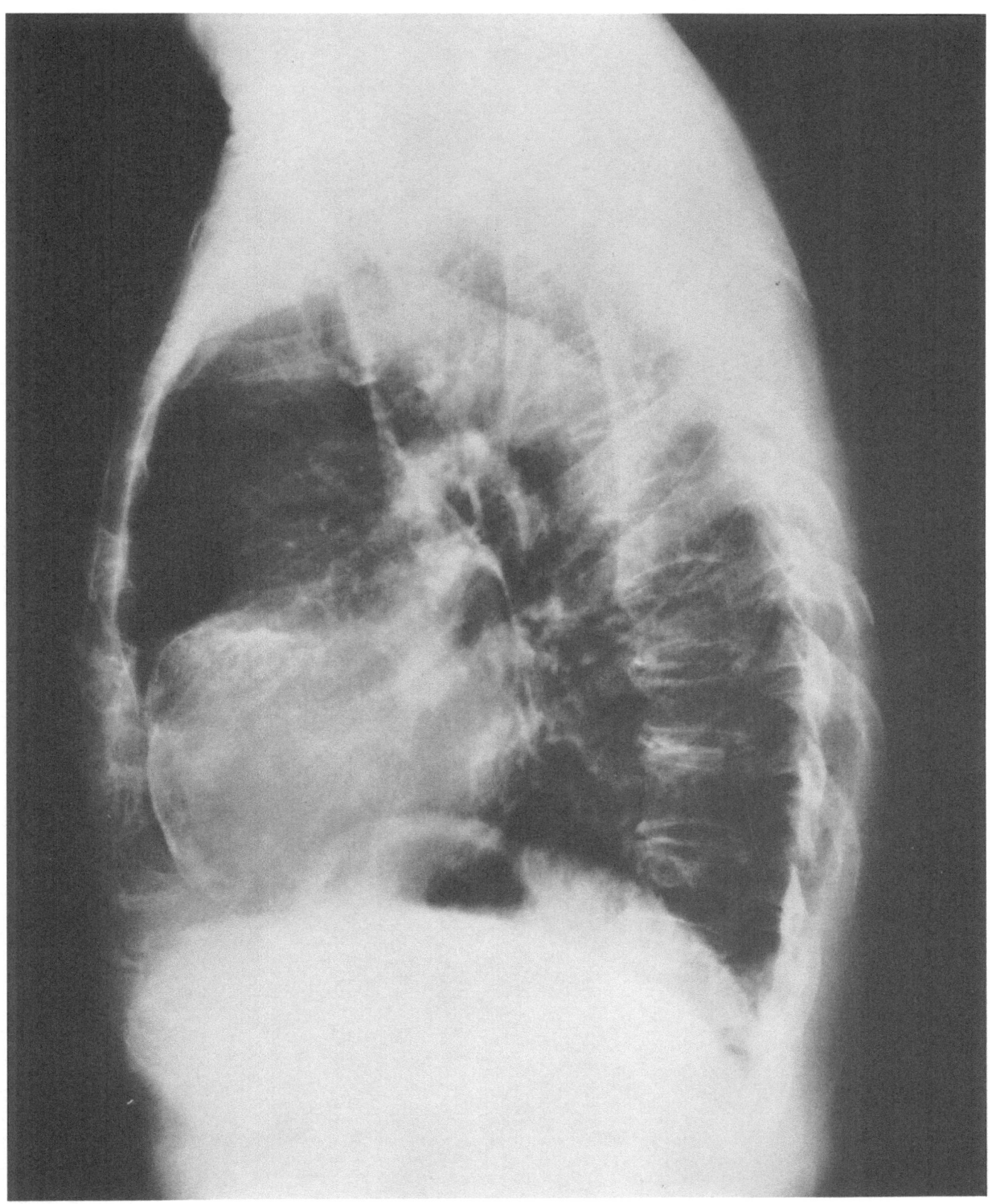

B

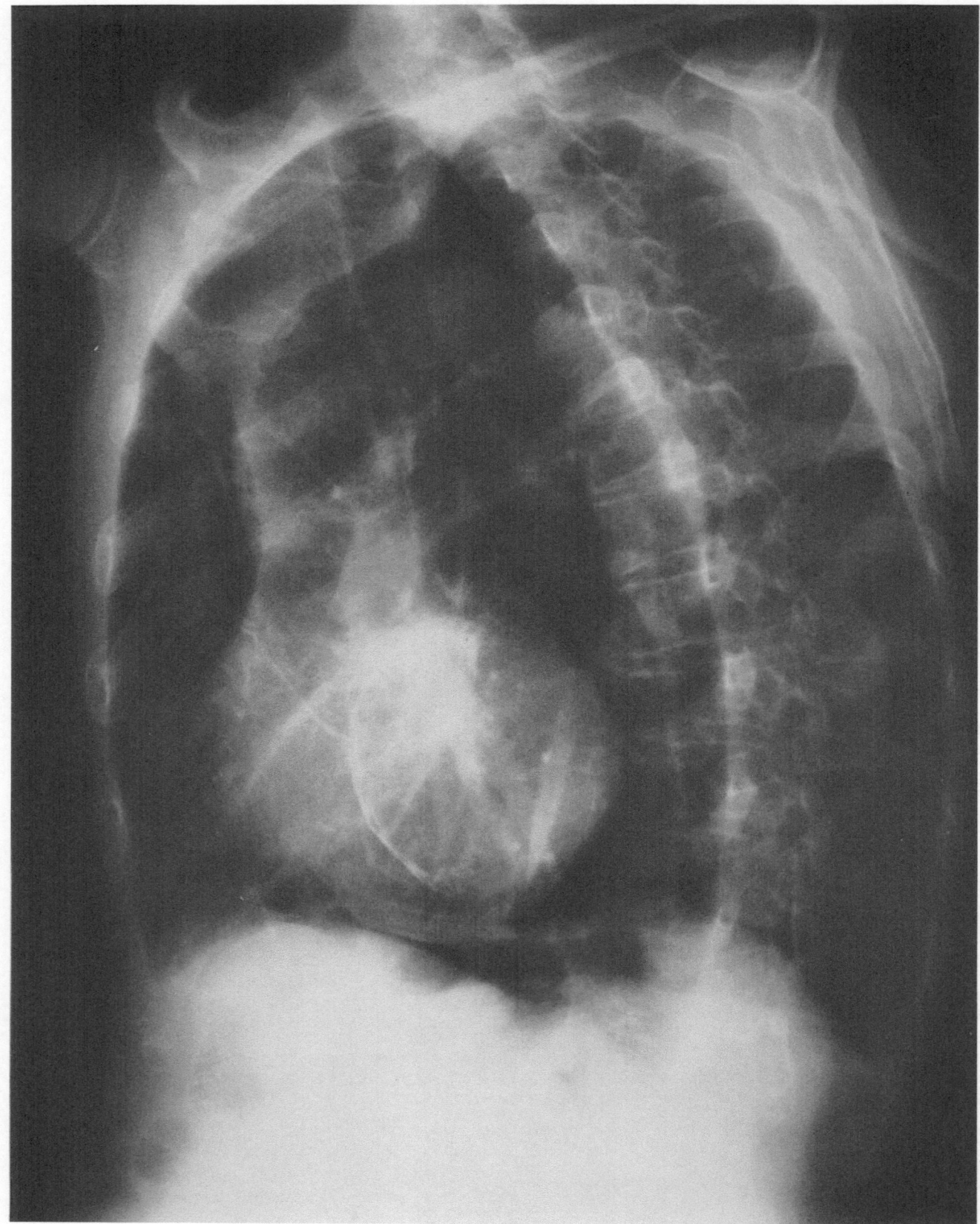

C

Fig. 4-41

Fig. 4–42. *Left ventricular aneurysm.* **A** RAO diastole; **B** RAO systole. The left ventricular volume is large. During systole motion of the anteroapical wall is lacking. Motion studies show paradoxical motion (dyskinesis) of the anteroapical wall. A small apical thrombus is noted.

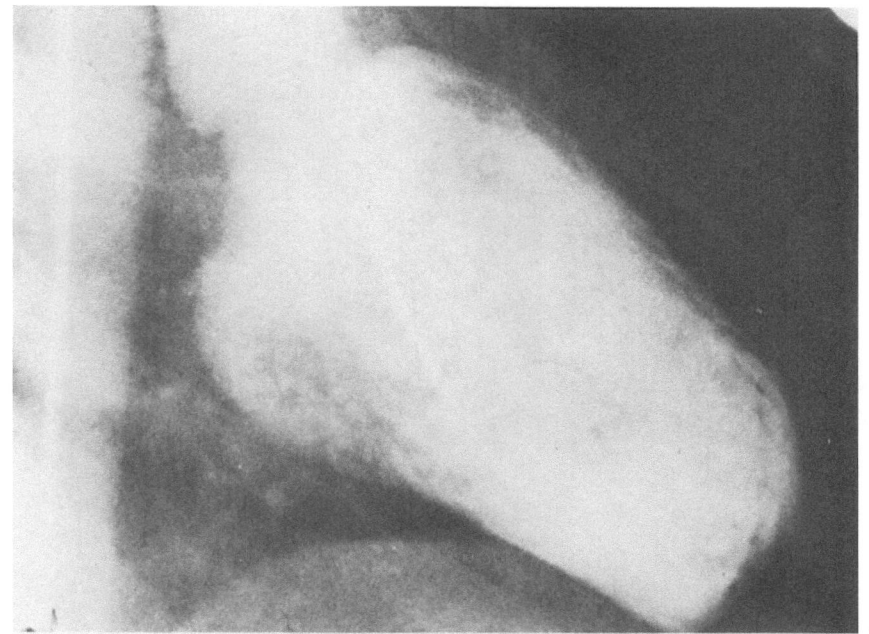

A

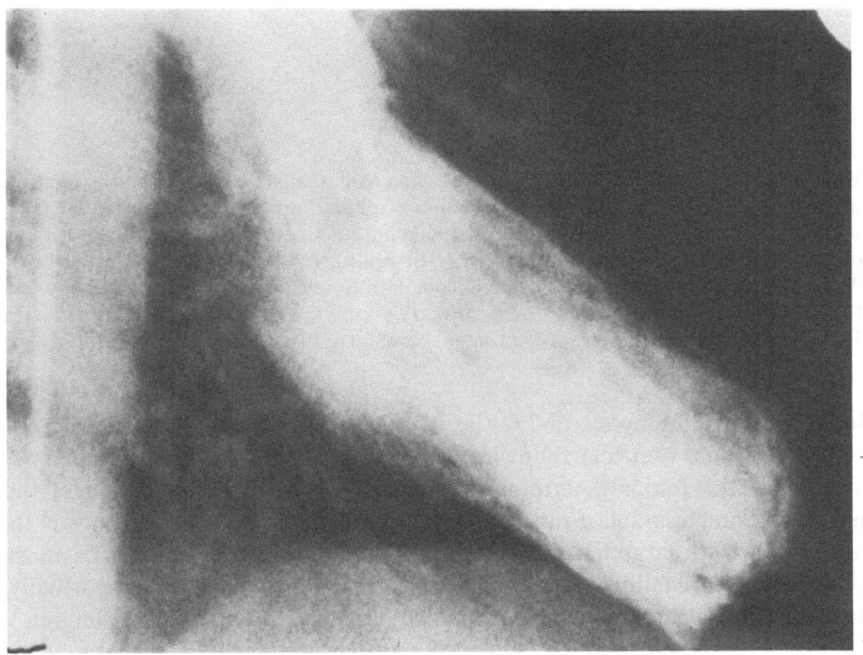

B

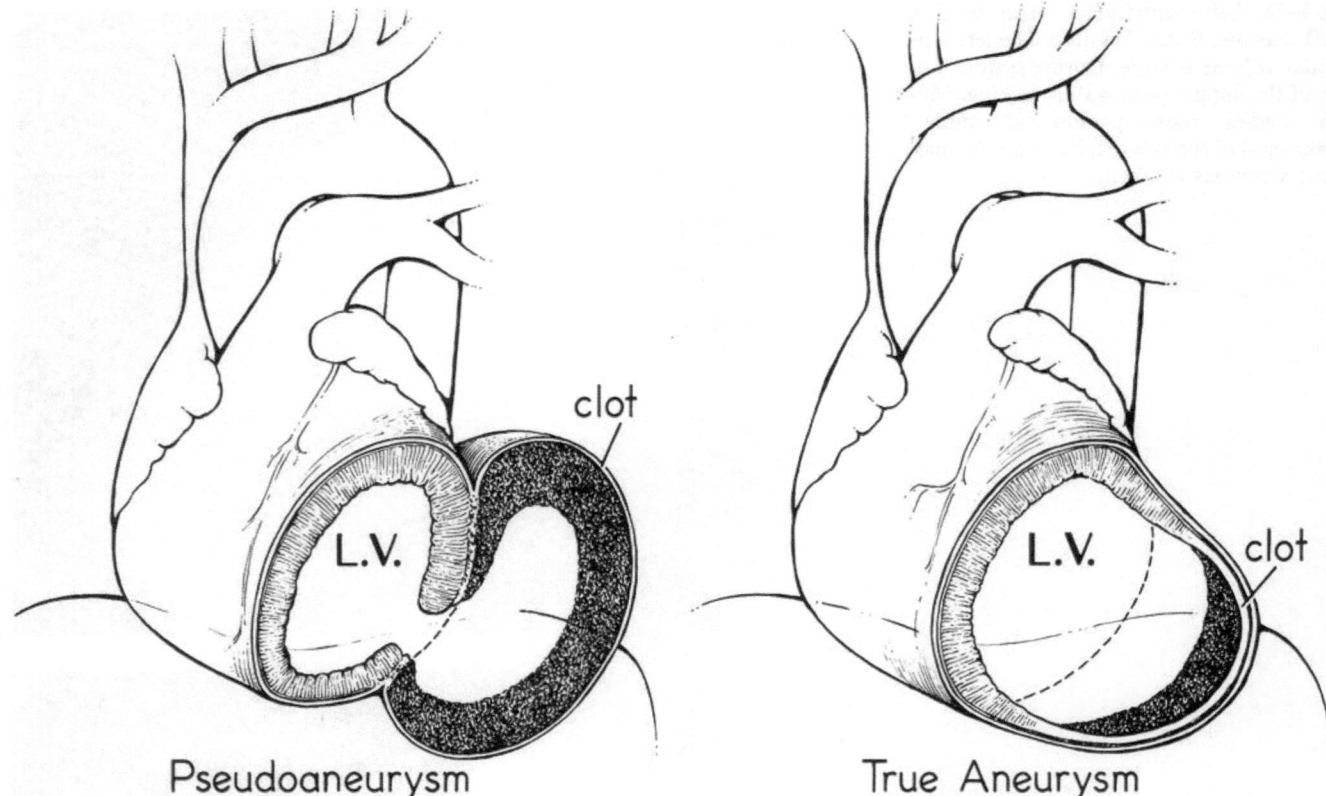

Pseudoaneurysm   True Aneurysm

Fig. 4–43. *Comparison of false aneurysm with true aneurysm of the left ventricle.* **Right** True aneurysm shares a common lumen with the left ventricular (*L.V.*) chamber, having a smooth zone of transition between the two areas rather than a narrow orifice. The wall of the aneurysm is formed from fibrous elements of the infarcted myocardium, and hence coronary vessels are present. **Left** A pseudoaneurysm, representing a contained myocardial rupture, has a relatively narrow communication with the left ventricular (*L.V.*) chamber. The wall is distinct from the myocardium and is composed of adherent pericardium and fibrous tissue without coronary vessels. Clot forms in both because of stasis. Spindola-Franco H, Kronacher N (1978) Pseudoaneurysm of the left ventricle. Radiographic and angiographic diagnosis. Radiology 127:29–34

infarctectomy and myocardial revascularization. The function of the left ventricle following surgery has been described as the major determinant in survival (Killen et al.). Grose and Spindola-Franco studied eight patients with acute VSD with large left-to-right shunts, shock or severe congestive heart failure. All eight patients had right ventricular (RV) dysfunction angiographically and biventricular infarction at surgery. The RV dysfunction was the major cause of death in two cases, and a contributing factor in three. RV papillary muscle rupture was identified in one case.

Papillary Muscle Dysfunction and Rupture
Papillary muscle dysfunction is an electrocardiographic-auscultatory syndrome characterized by a loud late systolic murmur at the apex. The murmur has a diamond-shaped ejection quality. Because of this characteristic murmur, an amyl nitrite test may be necessary to differentiate it from the murmur of aortic stenosis. If the murmur becomes softer after inhalation of the drug, a mitral origin is indicated. The electrocardiogram shows changes in the ST segment, T and U waves. The most common cause of mechanical dysfunction of the papillary muscles is coronary artery disease.

Electrocardiographic evidence indicates that mechanical papillary muscle dysfunction is primarily due to dysfunction of the anterior papillary muscle. However, it is well known that when rupture of a papillary muscle occurs it is most frequently the posteromedial muscle, occurring usually in association with a transmural diaphragmatic infarct. When a papillary muscle fails to contract normally as a result of ischemia (with or without infarction), mitral closure is impaired and insufficiency may result. The plain film manifestations of this abnormality vary according to its severity and chronicity. The chest roentgenogram is usually normal. However, cardiomegaly with LV and left atrial enlargement and pulmonary vascular redistribution may be observed. In the presence of chronic congestive heart failure, enlargement of the right side of the heart is also present. Left ventriculography is important in determining the degree of mitral insufficiency and in evaluating ventricular performance, knowledge of which is essential before corrective surgery and myocardial revascularization are contemplated. Prolapse of the mitral valve may be observed on occasion. True prolapse of the mitral valve usually represents intrinsic myxomatous degeneration of the valve rather than papillary muscle dysfunction. If, however, marked abnormality of wall motion occurs in

Fig. 4–44. *False aneurysm.* **A** Left ventriculogram in the LAO view demonstrates opacification of the pseudoaneurysm (*PA*) via a narrow orifice. *LV* = left ventricle. **B** Left coronary angiogram, LAO view. The coronary arteries do not extend to the wall of the pseudoaneurysm (*PA*). The early capillary phase is observed here as a blush that further outlines the myocardium. The PA remains avascular. Interposed myocardium clearly separates the left ventricular chamber from the paraventricular mass. Spindola-Franco H, Kronacher N (1978) Pseudoaneurysm of the left ventricle. Radiographic and angiographic diagnosis. Radiology 127: 29–34

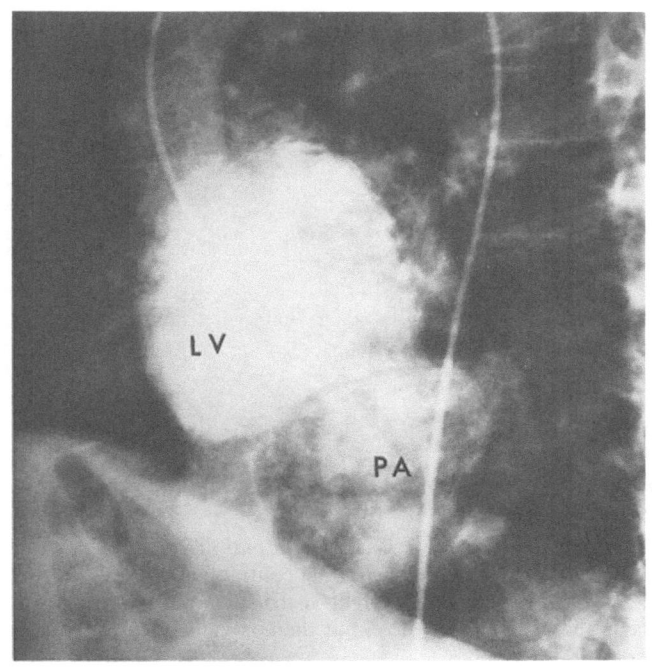

A

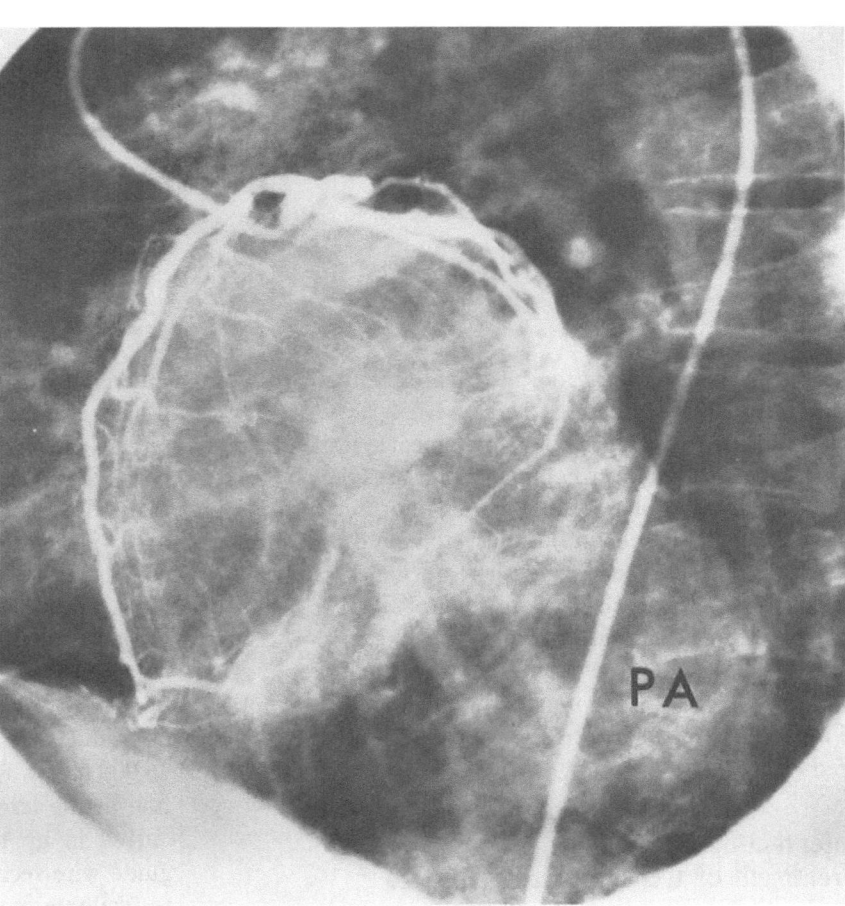

B

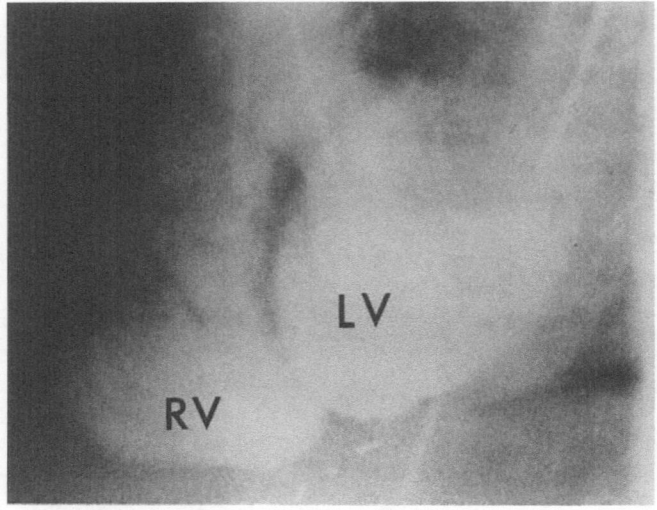

A

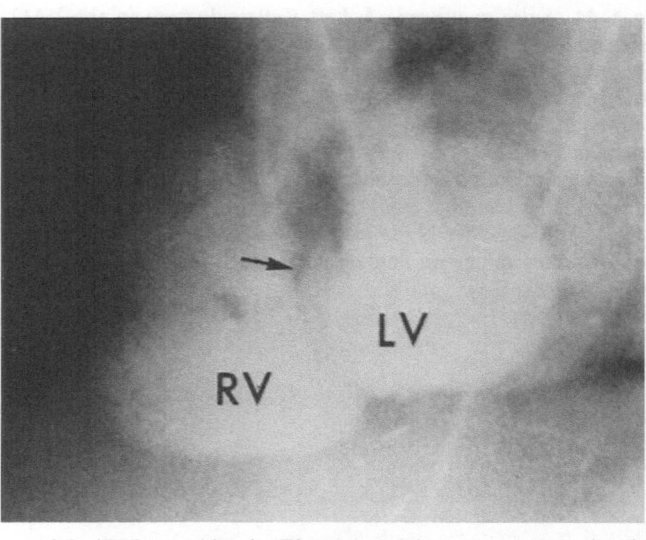

B

Fig. 4–45. *Postinfarction ventricular septal defect.* LAO view. **A** diastole; **B** systole. Note the normal contraction of the left ventricle (*LV*) in this view. The right ventricular outflow region contracts slightly during systole, but the body and apex of the right ventricle (*RV*) are akinetic. The *arrow* points to contrast material shown on cine to be trapped within the ventricular septum. Grose R, Spindola-Franco H (1981) Right ventricular dysfunction in acute ventricular septal defect. Am Heart J 101:67–74

the region of a papillary muscle, then ischemic cardiomyopathy may be regarded as the cause.

The sudden appearance of a loud apical systolic murmur in a patient with myocardial infarction raises the possibility of a ruptured papillary muscle. The murmur is early in onset (with the first sound), holosystolic and possibly crescendo. Pulmonary edema with a normal-sized heart is the usual presentation on plain films. A flail leaflet may be observed on echocardiography (see Fig. 5–66). Severe mitral insufficiency is usually present on angiography. Because of the high (80%) mortality in patients with rupture of a papillary muscle, corrective surgery should be considered.

Interventional Radiology for Treatment of Ischemic Heart Disease

In some patients with acute thrombotic occlusions, intracoronary infusion of streptokinase has proved useful for lysis of thrombus (Fig. 4–46). Furthermore, in patients with acute myocardial infarction, streptokinase appears to limit the size of the infarct, thus reducing mortality.

Streptokinase and urokinase are thrombolytic agents that activate the proenzyme plasminogen, thus promoting the formation of the proteolytic enzyme plasmin. No major difference exists in efficacy between streptokinase and urokinase so streptokinase is preferred because of its lower cost. Urokinase is used in patients with a high antistreptococcal antibody titer. The major risk in use of these drugs is development of hemorrhage. Streptokinase, a nonenzymatic protein excreted by group C beta hemolytic streptococci, has two half-lives: the first occurs at 18 minutes after binding with antistreptokinase antibodies, and the second at 83 minutes. Streptokinase 1000–2000 U/min may be infused selectively for 15–95 minutes in the ischemia-related coronary artery (average duration of infusion is 60 minutes for a total dose of streptokinase of 128,000 ± 36,000 units). Reopening of the occluded vessel or a reduction in the luminal narrowing of subtotal lesions has occurred in up to 80% in some series. In some patients, guide wire recanalization of the lesion may be attempted to facilitate reopening of a vessel. Intracoronary injection of nitroglycerin (NTG) or sublingual administration of nifedipine usually precedes thrombolytic therapy. A bolus of 10,000 units of heparin is given intraarterially at the start of the study. Left ventriculography and coronary arteriography are performed at the beginning and at the end of the procedure. Selective opacification of the ischemia-related artery is performed 30 seconds and 3 minutes after the injection of NTG, and then every 15 minutes during

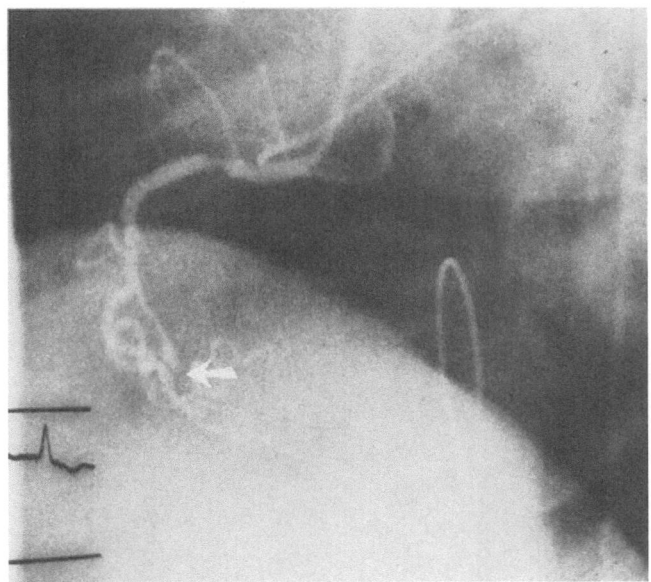

A

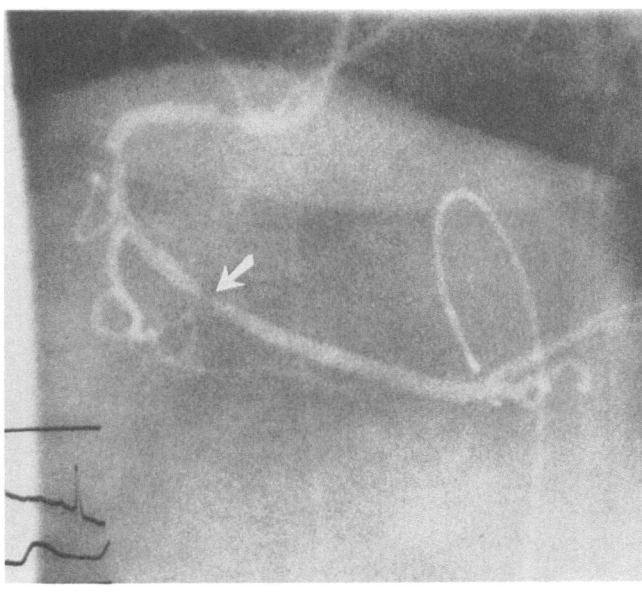

B

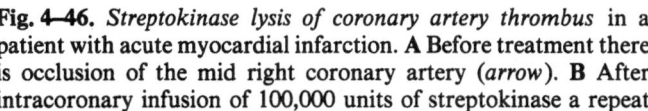

Fig. 4–46. *Streptokinase lysis of coronary artery thrombus* in a patient with acute myocardial infarction. **A** Before treatment there is occlusion of the mid right coronary artery (*arrow*). **B** After intracoronary infusion of 100,000 units of streptokinase a repeat right coronary angiogram shows reopening of the vessel distal to the obstruction. A residual 99% stenosis (*arrow*) is noted. This patient could benefit from angioplasty during this same procedure or during subsequent intervention.

the streptokinase infusion until reopening of the vessel has occurred.

Acylated streptokinase-plasminogen complex has been reported to cause fewer systemic effects on coagulation variables than does streptokinase or urokinase. Tissue plasminogen activator (t-PA), a human enzyme produced by recombinant DNA technique, has also been found to be a clot specific agent. It is administered by intravenous infusion. Advantages of t-PA are lack of antigenicity, selectivity of action on clot, absence of induction of a systemic lytic state, and a short biologic half-life. According to the TIMI (thrombolysis in acute myocardial infarction) study group t-PA is twice as effective in lysing clot from thrombosed arteries as is streptokinase.

Percutaneous Transluminal Coronary Angioplasty

Percutaneous transluminal coronary angioplasty (PTCA) is a nonoperative catheterization method designed for relief of coronary artery obstruction. It is derived from a technique described by Dotter and Judkins in 1964. A balloon-tipped catheter is passed through the stenosis. The balloon is then transiently inflated to 4–7 atmospheres of pressure and the catheter removed after deflation (Fig. 4–47). Gruntzig et al. report a primary success rate (first dilatations) of 85% and an overall success rate of 93% if second dilatations are included.

Initially PTCA was performed in single-vessel disease, but improvement in instrumentation (e.g., steerable guide wires, low profile balloons) and general expertise have broadened its indications to multivessel disease. PTCA in the left main coronary artery has been accomplished with success; however, the risk of in-hospital mortality associated with PTCA is excessive in patients with lesions of the LMCA. Therefore, PTCA is generally not offered to such individuals whether the LMCA lesion is isolated or whether it is in combination with other stenoses (Dorros). Angioplasty for obstruction of coronary artery bypass graft has also been performed successfully (Fig. 4–48). Results indicate that if a coronary artery bypass graft is going to restenose this will occur within 6 months. If occlusion does not occur within this period the vessel will remain patent. Relief of the luminal narrowing and disappearance of the pressure gradient across the lesion are the criteria for successful angioplasty. The indications for angioplasty at present are angina of recent onset refractory to medical therapy, with adequate ventricular function, reversible abnormalities of wall motion and the presence of proximal, discrete, compressible and noncalcified lesions. The incidence of myocardial infarction and death following PTCA is low (less than 3% and 1% respectively). Because of the occasional requirement for emergency bypass graft after PTCA (5% of cases) angioplasty should not be performed without emergency surgical "standby."

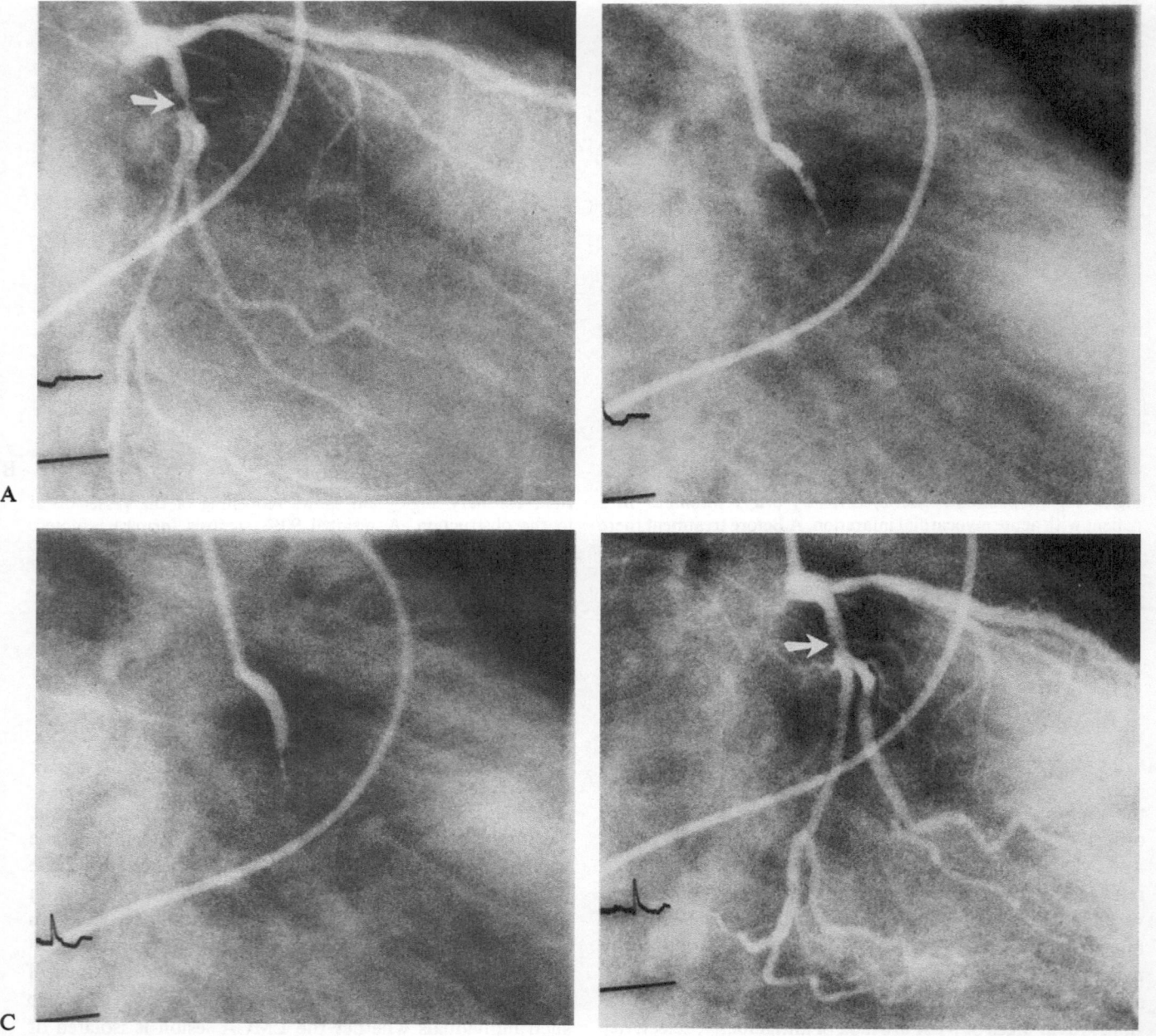

Fig. 4–47. *Percutaneous transluminal coronary angioplasty.* **A** Left coronary angiogram RAO view shows 99% stenosis (*arrow*) of the proximal left circumflex artery. **B** The guiding and the dilating catheters are in place, and the balloon is distended. Note the lucent notch produced by the stenosis. **C** With further distention the lucent defect has disappeared. **D** Postdilatation angiogram demonstrates minimal residual stenosis (*arrow*).

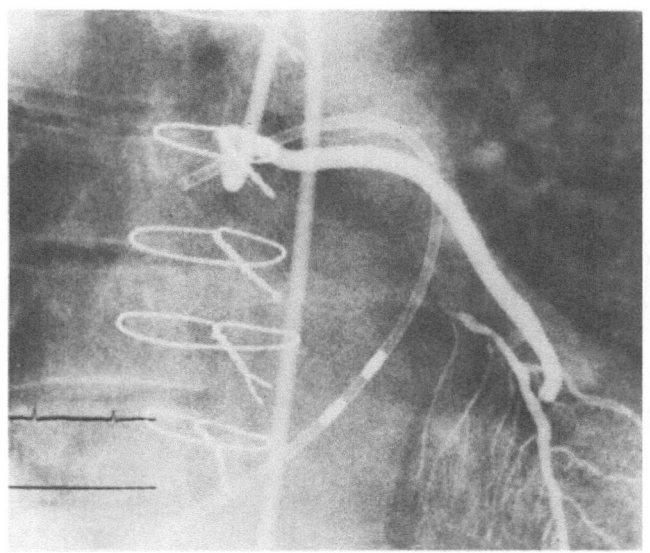

A

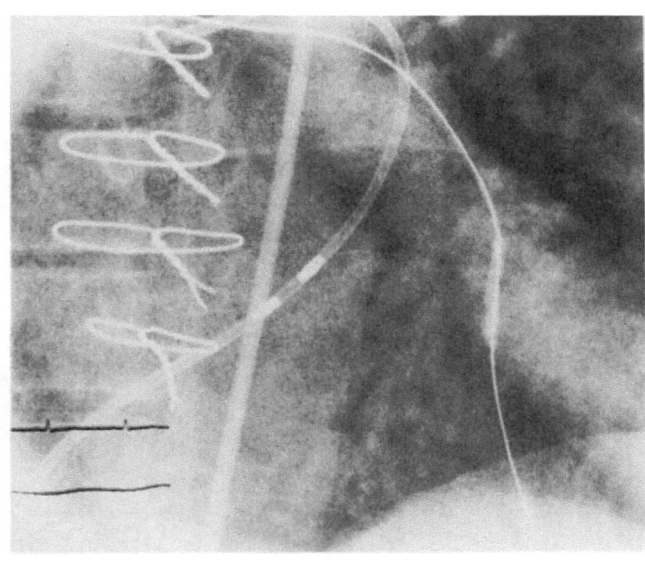

B

Fig. 4–48. *Percutaneous transluminal angioplasty of a stenosis at the distal anastomosis of a coronary artery bypass graft (CABG) to the left anterior descending.* In **A** a 95% stensois is evident. In **B** the balloon catheter is inflated at the site of the stenosis. In **C** opacification of the CABG after dilatation shows minimal residual narrowing.

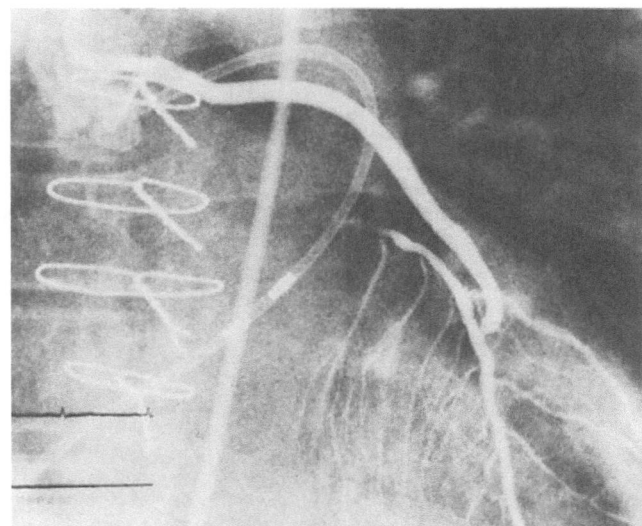

C

Surgical Treatment of Ischemic Heart Disease

For refractory angina pectoris and in some patients with acute myocardial infarction, myocardial revascularization is performed by way of saphenous vein bypass graft (Fig. 4–49) or by anastomosis of the mammary arteries to the coronary arteries. In patients with obstruction of one coronary artery and minimal or reversible LV dysfunction, mortality is less than 2%. Involvement of multiple vessels, stenosis of a long segment and disease of small vessels decrease the success rate as does LV dysfunction or presence of a LV aneurysm. After surgery anginal symptoms are generally relieved. However, controversy exists whether life expectancy is improved. Stenosis or occlusion (thrombosis) occurs within 2 years in up to 15%–20% of patients with saphenous vein bypass grafts (Figs. 4–48, 4–50, 4–51). Surgery for complications of myocardial infarction include repair of false aneurysm (contained cardiac rupture), excision of true ventricular aneurysm, repair of acquired interventricular septal defect and replacement of the mitral valve in patients with rupture of the papillary muscle.

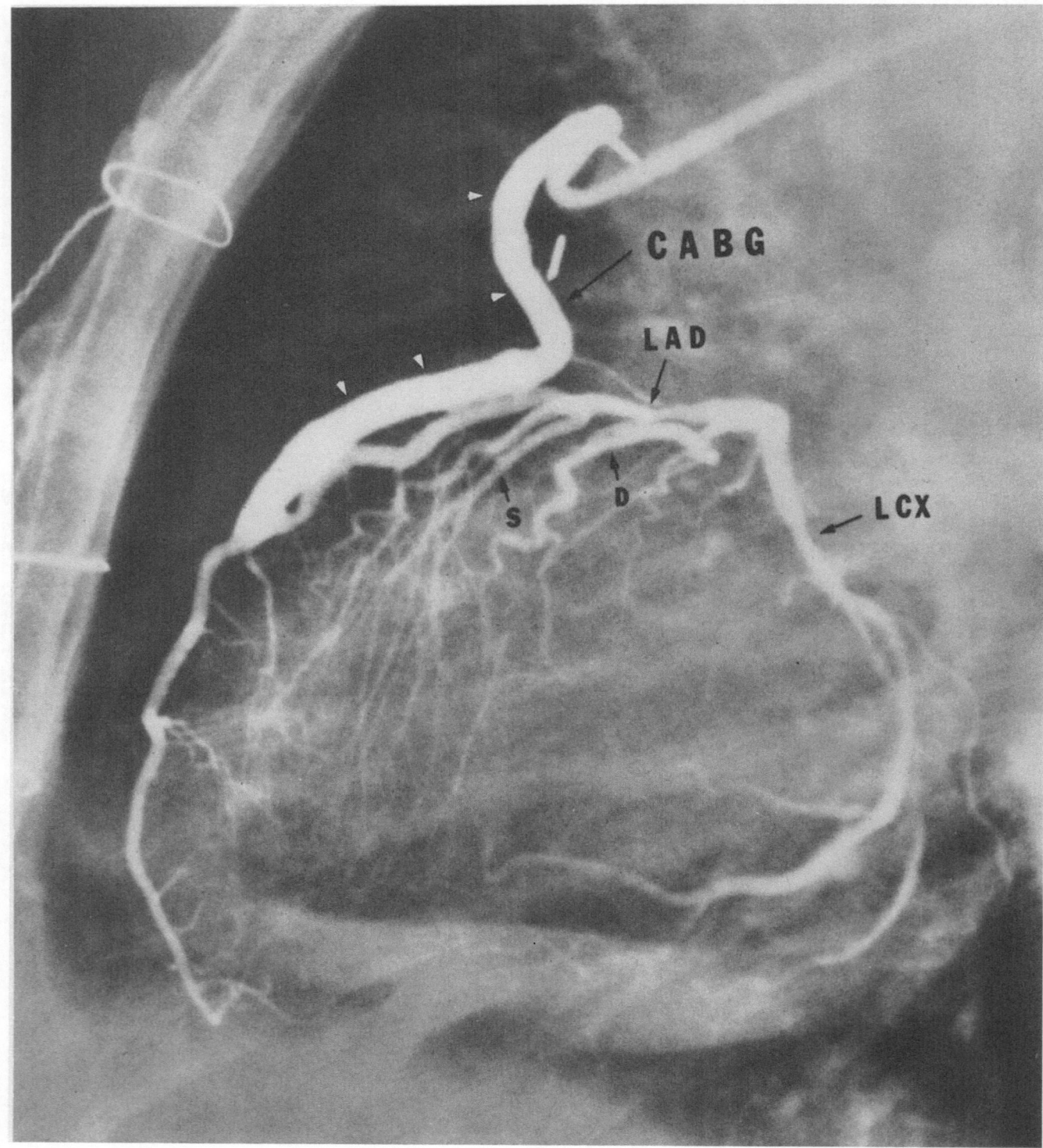

Fig. 4–49. *Patent coronary artery bypass graft (CABG).* Observe the excellent runoff in the graft with bidirectional flow (antegrade and retrograde) into the left anterior descending artery (*LAD*) and left circumflex artery (*LCX*) and branches. Stenosis is present in the proximal LAD. Not shown is complete occlusion of the distal left main coronary artery after selective injection. *S* = septal artery; *D* = diagonal branch. Spindola-Franco H (1982) Coronary arteriography and left ventriculography. In: Goldberger E. (ed.) Textbook of clinical cardiology. Mosby, St. Louis, p 305.

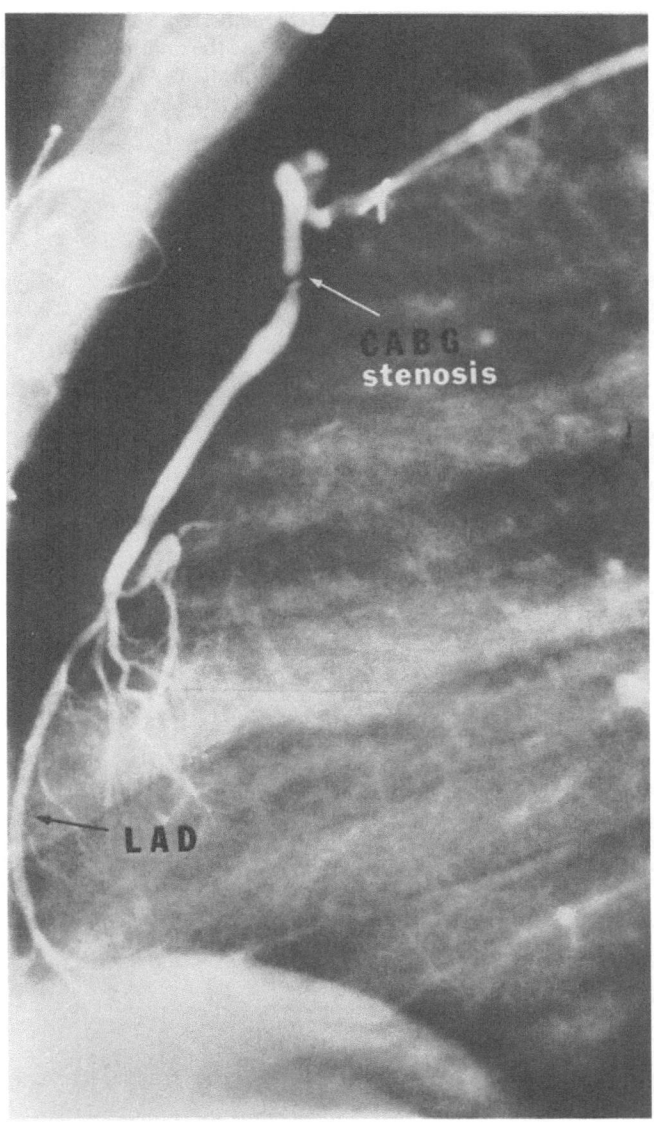

Fig. 4–50. *Stenosis of a coronary artery bypass graft (CABG). Severe stenosis (arrow) has developed in the graft leading to the left anterior descending artery (LAD).*

Ischemic Heart Disease in the Young

In children and young adults, ischemic heart disease can be caused by congenital anomalies of the coronary arteries or by the effects of systemic inflammatory and metabolic disorders. Emboli may occlude the coronary arteries. Occasionally coronary artery insufficiency may result from trauma.

Of the congenital anomalies affecting the coronary arteries, anomalous origin of the LCA from the pulmonary artery is most significant. It is discussed subsequently.

A single coronary artery has been implicated in a few cases of sudden death if a major branch crosses between the aorta and the pulmonary artery.

Kawasaki disease (which seems to be identical to polyarteritis nodosa) is the most common inflammatory disease affecting the coronary arteries. Lupus erythematosus and other collagen vascular diseases also produce vasculitis that occasionally affects the coronary arteries. Degos syndrome is a rare disease that produces atrophic papular lesions of the skin, gastrointestinal ulcerations and, on occasion, coronary arteriolar stenosis. In some metabolic disorders abnormal deposits may obliterate the coronary arteries. Among these are the mucopolysaccharidoses (e.g., Hurler disease), homocystinuria, Fabry disease and pseudoxanthoma elasticum. Progeria produces accelerated atherosclerotic changes. Ehlers-Danlos syndrome may cause aneurysms of multiple arteries, including the coronaries.

Anomalous Origin of the Left Coronary Artery from the Pulmonary Trunk (Bland-White-Garland Syndrome)

Origin of the LCA from the pulmonary artery instead of the aorta is a rare congenital disorder. Origin of both coronary arteries, or even of a single coronary artery, from the pulmonary trunk is exceedingly rare. Anomalous origin of the RCA from the pulmonary trunk is considered a relatively benign defect and is usually an incidental finding at autopsy. Most patients with anomalous origin of the LCA die during the first year of life from myocardial ischemia and congestive heart failure, unless collateral circulation to the LV develops through intercoronary anastomoses. Survival then depends on the flow of oxygenated blood into the LCA from the RCA. Thus a left-to-right shunt from the RCA to the pulmonary artery is present. This shunt is usually of a small volume and has only a minor hemodynamic effect on the LV. Cardiomegaly in these patients is the result of inadequate arterial perfusion of the LV myocardium.

The terms *adult type* and *infantile type* have been used to distinguish between patients who live for many years with virtually no symptoms and those who die during infancy with profound symptoms. A third group of patients is encountered with congestive heart failure who survive early infancy and by 3 or 4 years of age are asymptomatic or nearly so. On plain chest roentgenograms the heart varies from normal or nearly so to massively enlarged (LV) (Fig. 4–52). The left atrium may be enlarged, especially with mitral insufficiency. The degree of pulmonary venous hypertension is usually severe. Dystrophic calcification of the LV may be observed fluoroscopically but is not readily apparent on plain films. The electrocardiogram may show an infarction pattern, left axis deviation and left ventricular hypertrophy. Echocardiography (Fig. 4–53) in symptomatic individuals reveals a dilated hypocontractile LV with normal or decreased thickness of the ventricular wall. If heart failure is present the left atrium is enlarged and mitral valve motion is decreased because of high LV diastolic pressure. These signs indicate myocardial dysfunction and are not specific for anomalous origin of the LCA. Visualization of the anomalous origin of the LCA by 2-D echocardiography has been reported.

Scanning with thallium usually demonstrates LV dysfunction (myocardial ischemia) in infants. In older children, myocardial performance may be normal. Ventriculog-

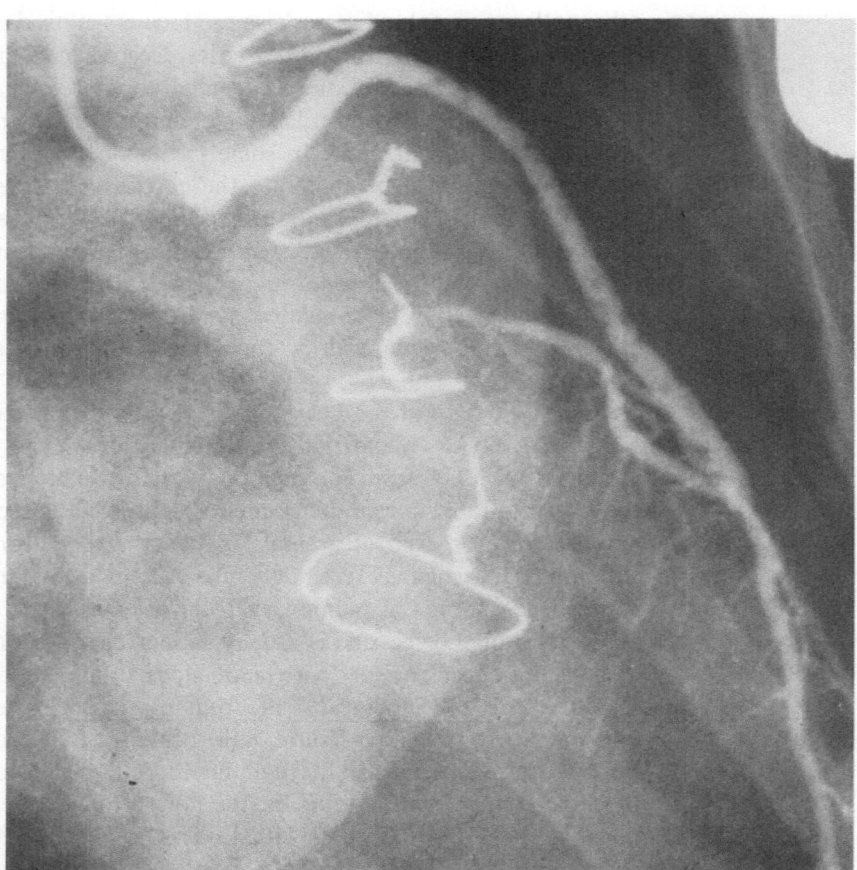

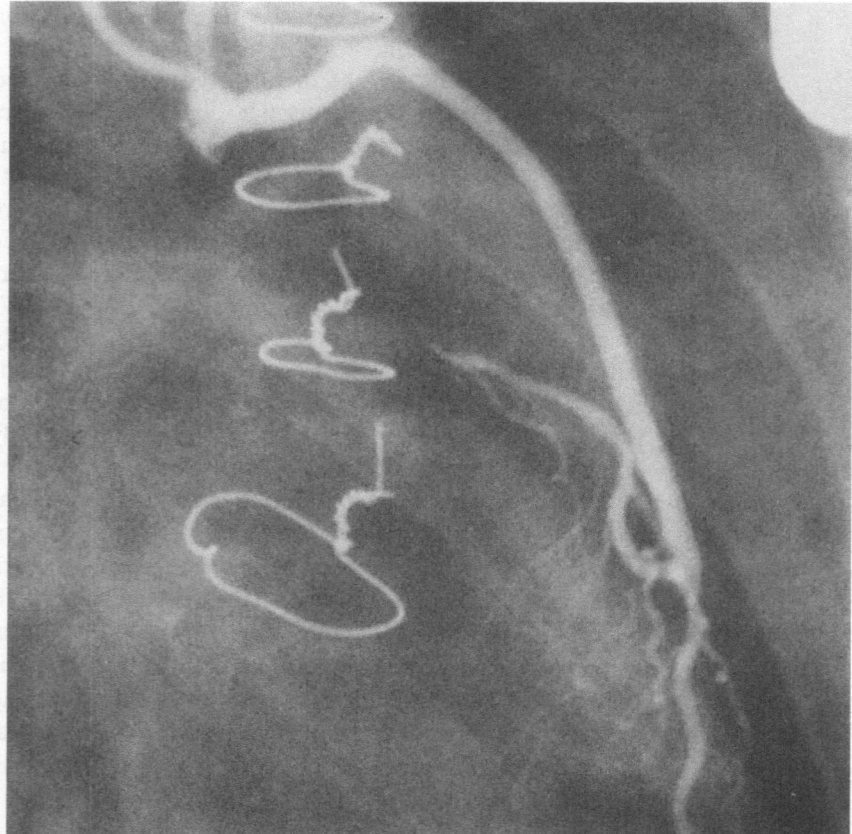

Fig. 4–51. *Thrombosis of coronary artery bypass graft.* **A** Note the multiple filling defects throughout the graft. **B** After heparin therapy the filling defects have disappeared.

Fig. 4–52. *Ischemic cardiomyopathy* in an infant with anomalous origin of the left coronary artery from the pulmonary artery. Frontal roentgenogram. The heart is markedly enlarged because of left ventricular dilatation. Pulmonary venous hypertension is manifested by pulmonary vascular redistribution and perivascular and hilar haze.

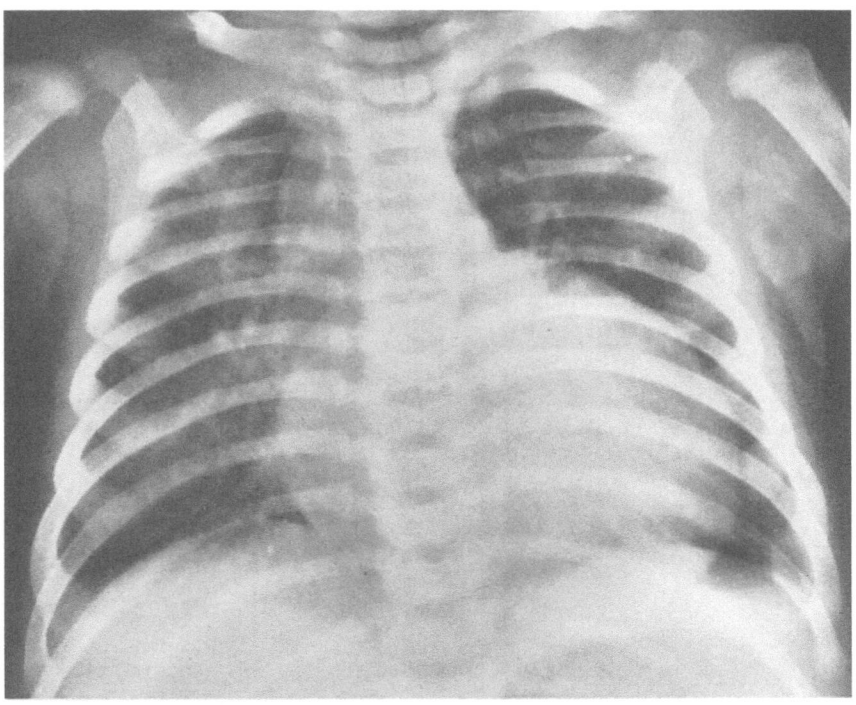

raphy (Fig. 4–54) in sick infants reveals marked LV dilatation with diffuse hypokinesis, akinesis and dyskinesis. Mitral insufficiency (probably secondary to papillary muscle dysfunction or infarction) may also be present. Aortography (Fig. 4–55) or selective coronary arteriography (Fig. 4–55C) shows a large RCA that communicates with the LCA through intercoronary anastomoses. A small left-to-right shunt usually is present, with opacification of the pulmonary artery. Inasmuch as an anomalous LCA arising from the pulmonary trunk carries a high mortality (80%–85%) in symptomatic infants, prompt surgical treatment is indicated. Several surgical methods are available: ligation of the LCA, anastomosis of the left subclavian artery (LSA) to the LCA, direct reimplantation of the LCA into the aorta, and saphenous vein graft (e.g., interposition, bypass). Recently, excellent results have been obtained with two new techniques: (1) retroaortic coronary artery bypass graft, using a free segment of the LSA and (2) transpulmonary arterial coronary artery bypass graft, also using a free segment of LSA.

Kawasaki Disease

Kawasaki disease (mucocutaneous lymph node syndrome) represents an acute inflammatory disease affecting children. A specific causative agent has not been identified. This disease appears to be a variant of or identical with infantile periarteritis nodosa. Cardiac manifestations include myocarditis, pericarditis, endocarditis and angiitis. Aneurysms of coronary arteries and other systemic vessels are observed (Fig. 4–56). Death occurs in approximately 0.6% of patients affected and is caused by myocarditis involving the atrioventricular conduction system or coronary thromboarteritis. Rupture of a coronary aneurysm may occur. Two-dimensional echocardiography (Fig. 4–57) may identify aneurysms at the origins of the coronary arteries. In some centers, coronary arteriography is performed routinely on all infants with this disease since these are at the highest risk for coronary artery involvement. Regression of coronary artery aneurysms has been demonstrated by serial echocardiography and angiography; however, residual thickening of the wall of the affected coronary artery detected by echocardiography may represent fibrosis. Coronary stenosis may be a late sequela. Coronary artery bypass graft may be indicated in some cases. Aspirin has been recommended to prevent coronary thrombosis.

The differential diagnosis of coronary artery aneurysms includes: syphilis, pyogenic infection, atherosclerosis, periarteritis nodosa, scleroderma and Ehlers-Danlos syndrome. Aneurysms may also be of congenital origin. Systemic arterial aneurysms are similar to those associated with Takayasu disease, atherosclerosis, trauma, syphilis and Marfan syndrome.

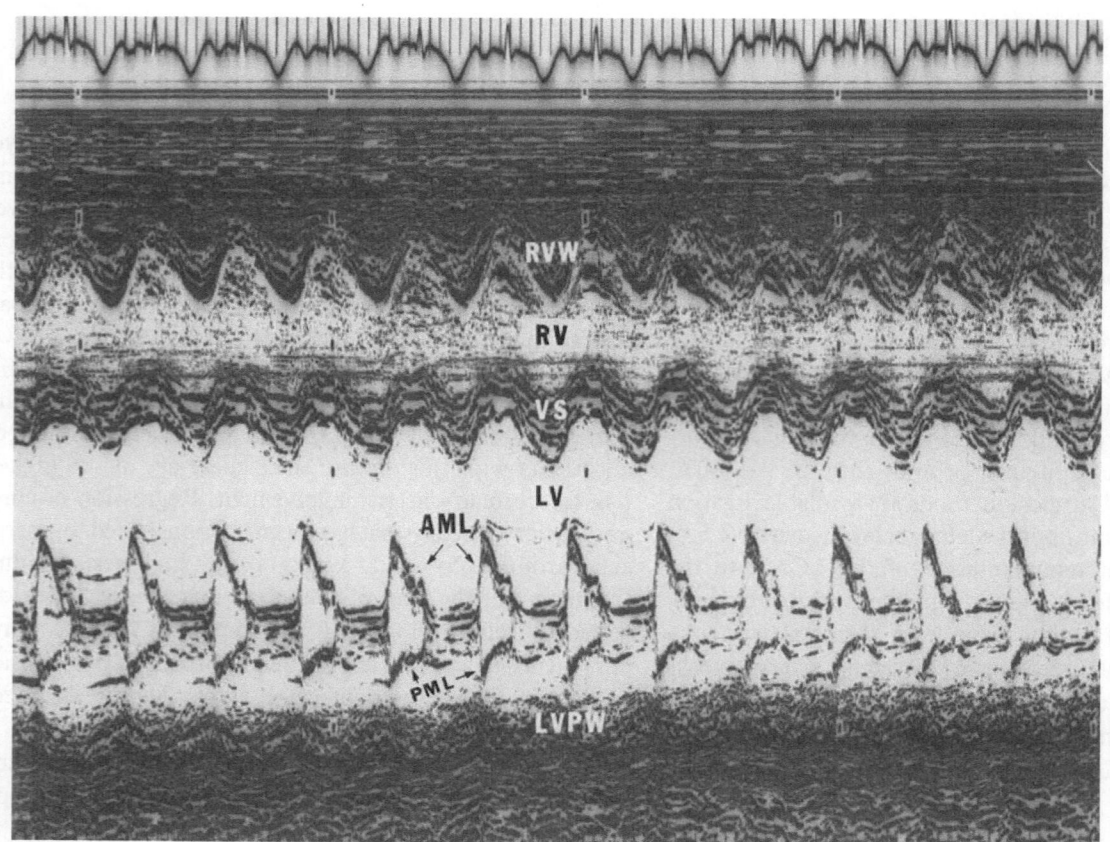

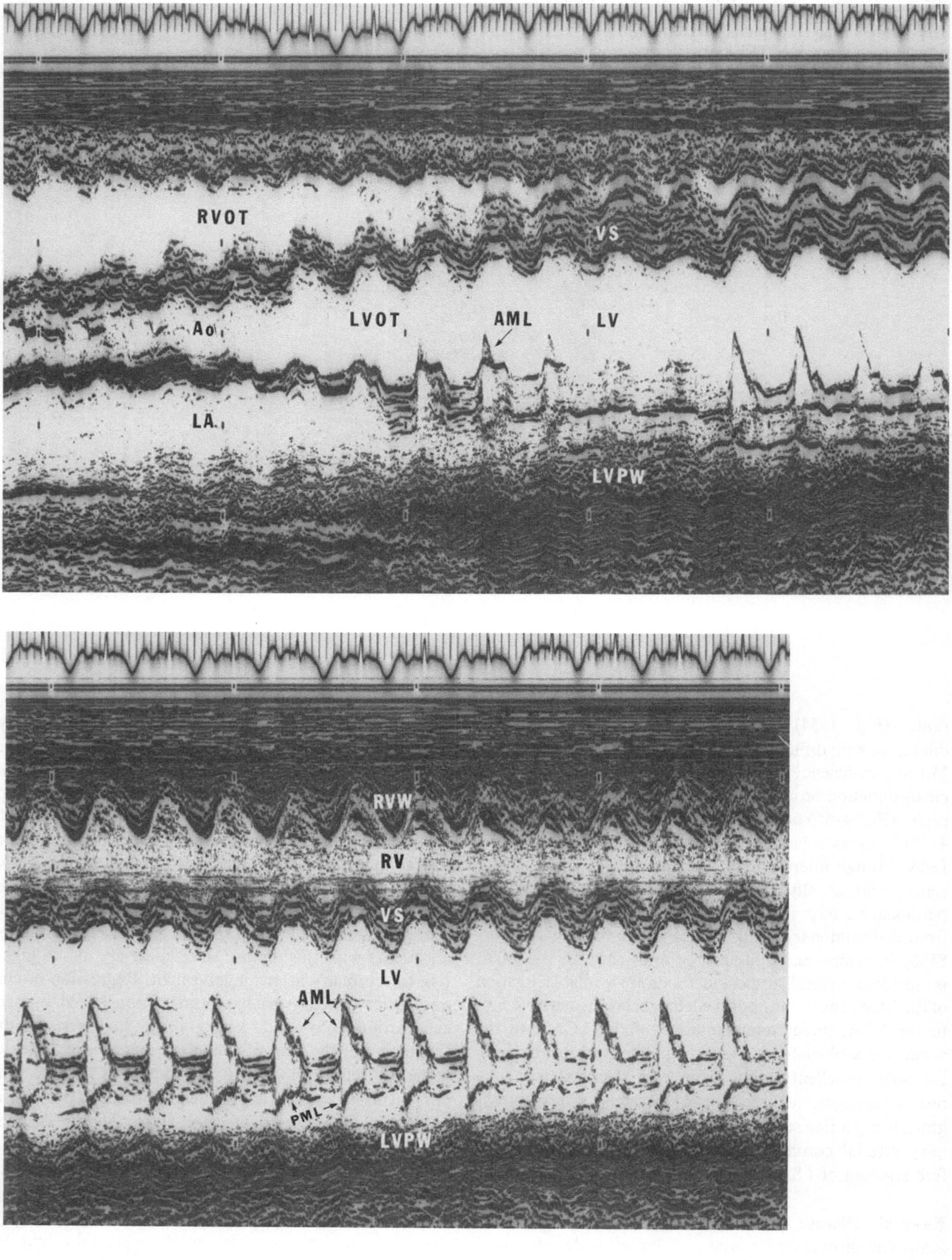

◀ **Fig. 4–53.** *Anomalous origin of the left coronary artery from the pulmonary artery.* **A** Arc scan from aorta (*Ao*) to left ventricular cavity (*LV*); **B** M-mode echogram at the level of the mitral valve. The left atrium (*LA*) is dilated. The left ventricle is large, and the posterior wall (*LVPW*) barely moves. In contrast, the amplitude of motion of the right ventricular wall (*RVW*) and ventricular septum (*VS*) is greater than normal—especially well illustrated in **B.** The grossly impaired motion of the left ventricular wall suggests a segmental dysfunction consistent with ischemic heart disease rather than generalized cardiomyopathy. *RVOT* = right ventricular outflow tract; *LVOT* = left ventricular outflow tract; *AML* = anterior mitral leaflet; *PML* = posterior mitral leaflet.

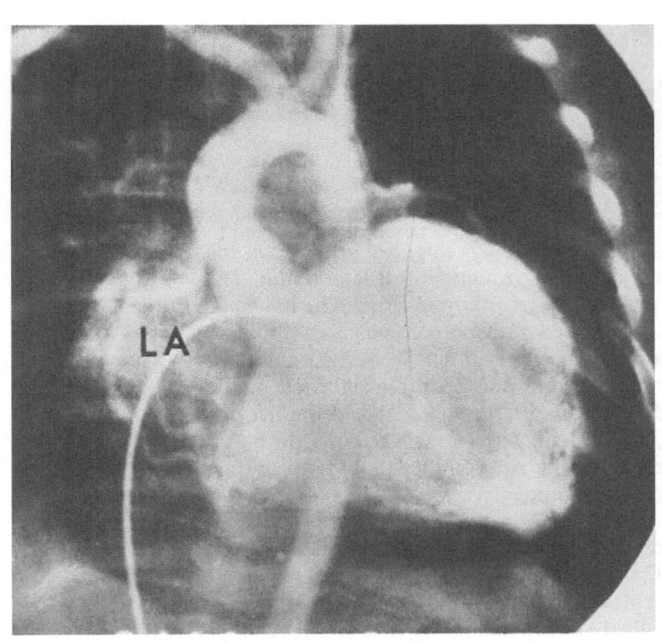

A

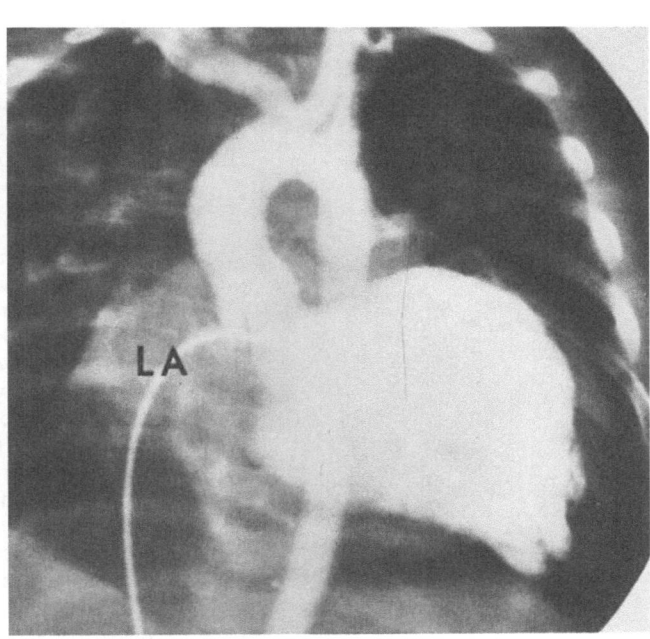

B

Fig. 4–54. *Anomalous origin of the left coronary artery.* Left ventriculogram. **A** diastole; **B** systole. The left ventricle is markedly dilated. During systole only the diaphragmatic wall contracts. The anterolateral wall and apex are akinetic. Dyskinesis of the apex and anterolateral wall were observed on cine film. Mild mitral insufficiency was present. The left atrium (*LA*) is enlarged. (Same patient as in Figs. 4–52, 4–53, and 4–55 A and B.)

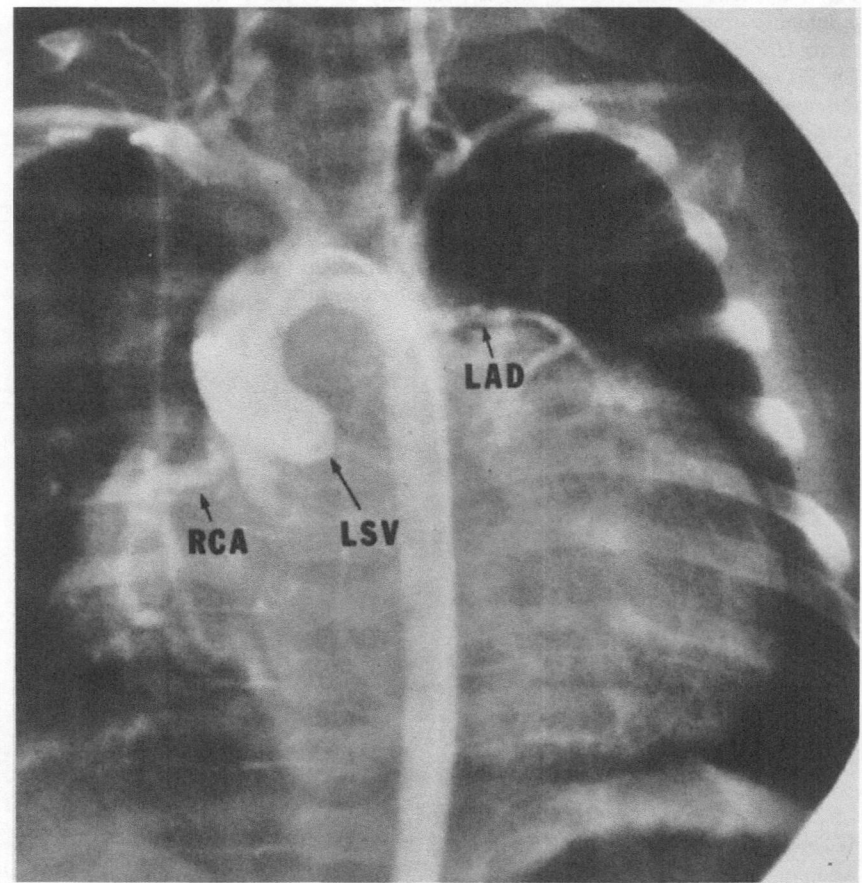

A

Fig. 4–55. *Anomalous origin of the left coronary artery from the pulmonary artery.* Aortogram. **A** frontal film; **B** lateral film. The right coronary artery (*RCA*) arises from the aorta. The left sinus of Valsalva (*LSV*) is well filled with no coronary vessel arising from it. The left coronary artery system fills from the right coronary artery by way of collateral flow with opacification of the left anterior descending coronary artery (*LAD*) and the left circumflex artery (*LCX*). The collateral vessels (*colls.*) are better demonstrated on the lateral film. Also on the lateral film contrast medium is identified in the pulmonary artery. *LMCA* = left main coronary artery.

C Frontal view of a selective RCA angiogram in a 33-year-old woman. The RCA is large. The LCA opacifies by way of extensive septal and epicardial collateral vessels. The pulmonary artery (*MPA*) is also filled densely, indicating that the LCA originates from the main pulmonary artery. *PD* = posterior descending artery; *PLV* = posterior left ventricular branch.

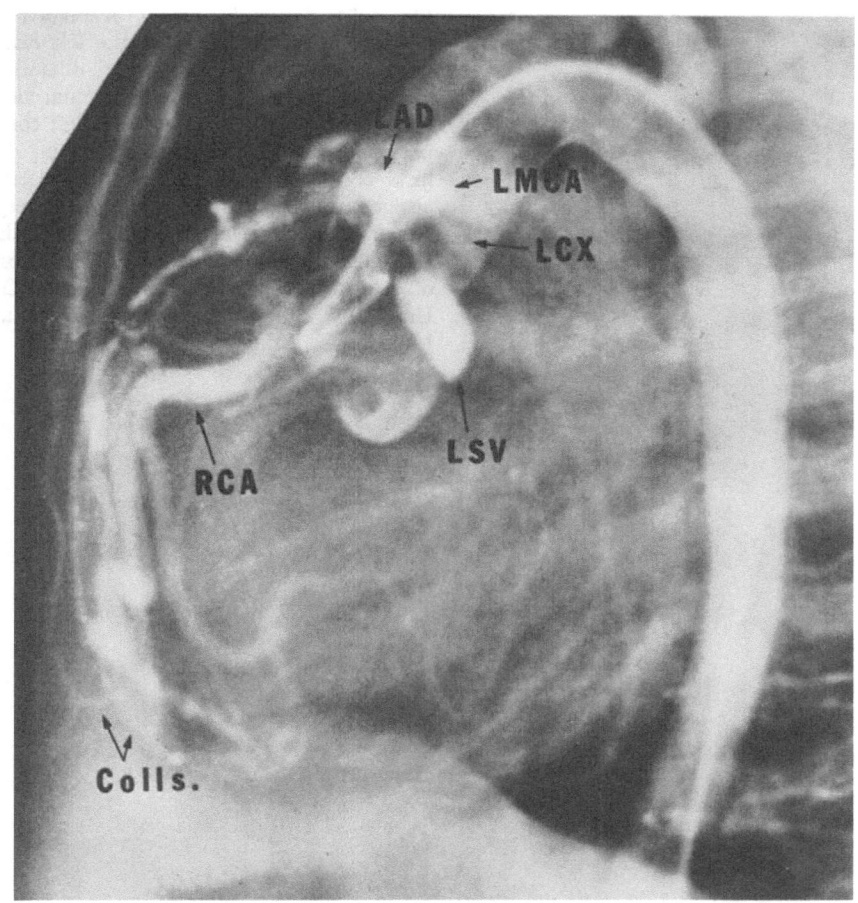

B

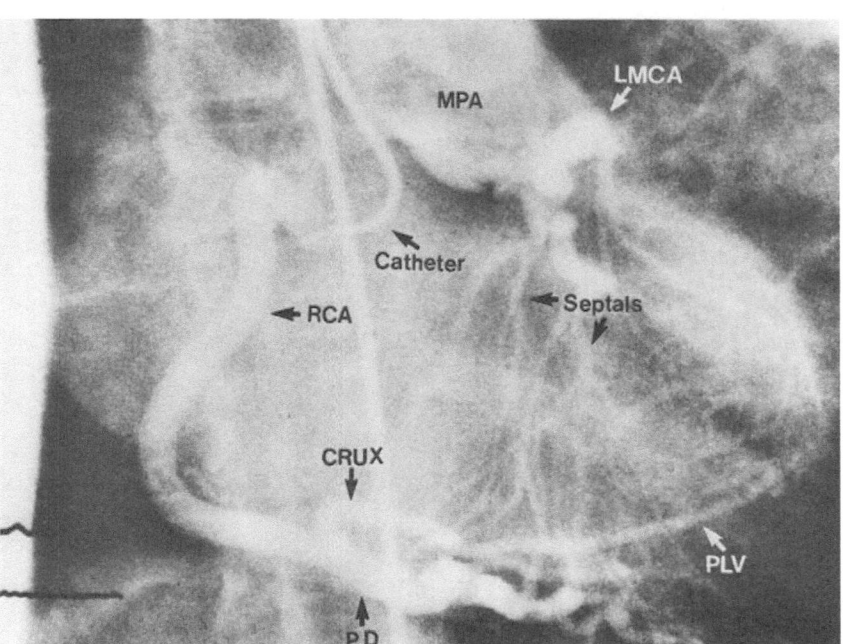

C

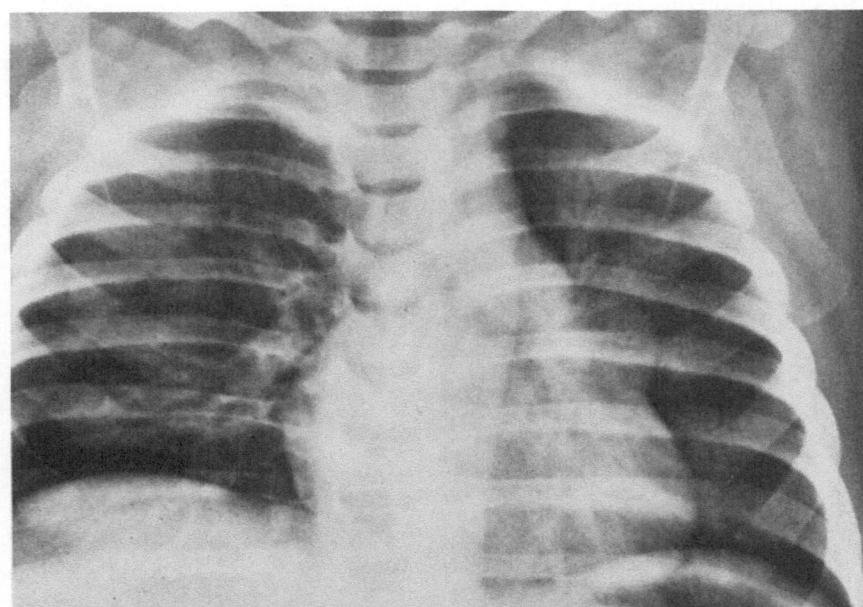

A

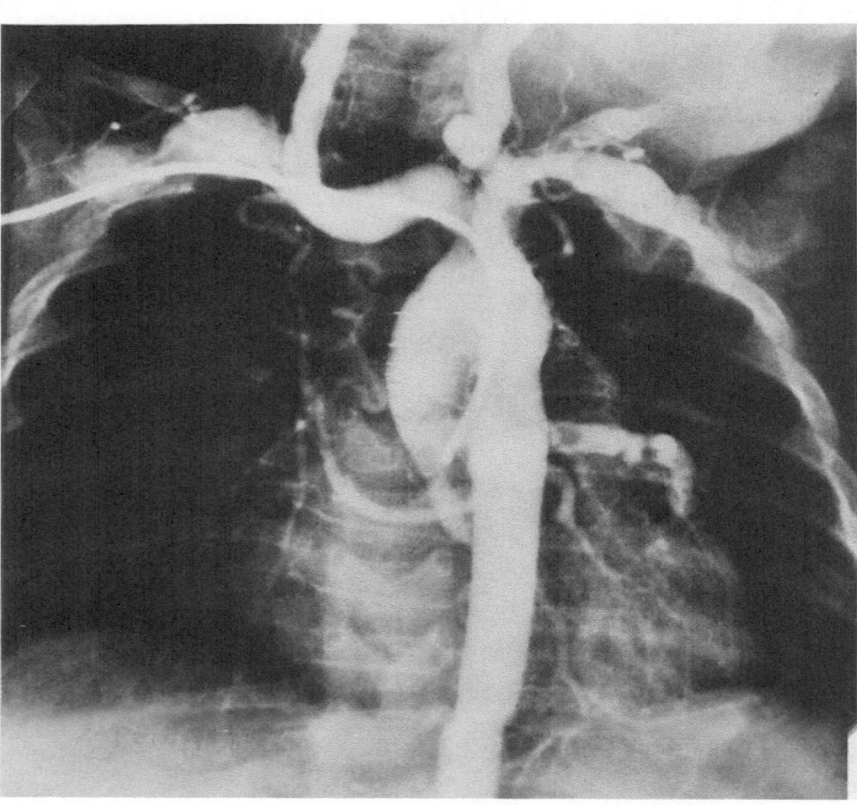

B

Fig. 4–56. *Kawasaki disease.* **A** Plain film of the chest. A bulge along the left heart border is caused by aneurysmal dilatation of the left coronary artery. **B** Frontal view of aortogram. Note ectasia of the left coronary artery and its branches with filling defects consistent with thrombosis. Observe also ectasia of the left subclavian artery. Aneurysms were also observed in the branches of the abdominal aorta. Courtesy of Wilfrido R. Castaneda-Zuniga, M.D., University of Minnesota Heart Hospital, Minneapolis, Minnesota

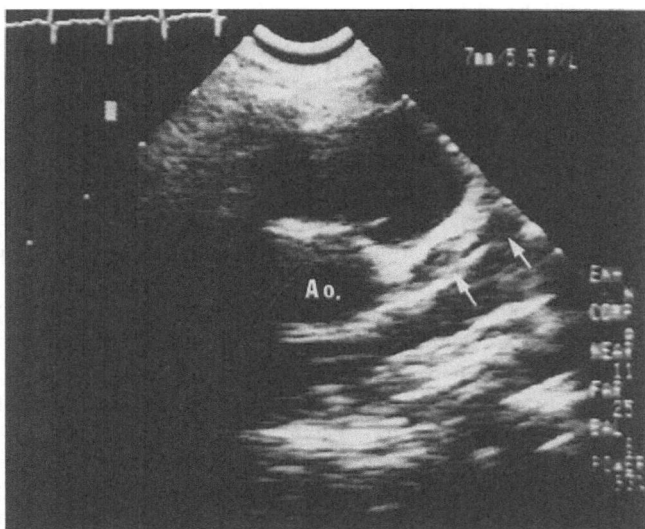

Fig. 4-57. *Aneurysm of the left coronary artery in a 12-month-old boy who had Kawasaki disease 6 weeks prior to the study.* On two-dimensional echocardiography the left coronary artery is dilated with highly reflective walls. The inner surface of the left coronary artery is irregular, with two small aneurysms (*arrows*). *Ao.* = aorta.

Bibliography

Ischemic Heart Disease

Abrams DL, Edelist A, Luria MH, Miller AJ (1963) Ventricular aneurysm: A reappraisal based on a study of sixty-five consecutive autopsied cases. Circulation 27:164–169

Adams DF, Fraser DB, Abrams HL (1973) The complications of coronary arteriography. Circulation 48:609–618

Arvidsson H (1961) Angiocardiographic determination of left ventricular volume. Acta Radiol 56:321–338

Baltaxe, HA, Amplatz K, Levin DC (1973) Coronary angiography. Thomas, Springfield

Baron MG (1971) Post-infarction aneurysm of the left ventricle. Circulation 43:765–769

Bell WR, Meek AG (1979) Guidelines for the use of thrombolytic agents. N Engl J Med 301:1266–1270

Bjork L, Spindola-Franco H, Van Houten XF, Cohn PF, Adams DF (1975) Comparison of observer performance with 16 mm cinefluorography and 70 mm camera fluorography in coronary arteriography. Am J Cardiol 36:474–478

Braunwald E, Morrow AG, Cornell WP, Aygen MM, Hilbish TF (1960) Idiopathic hypertrophic subaortic stenosis: Clinical, hemodynamic and angiographic manifestations. Am J Med 29:924–945

Bream PR, Souza AS Jr, Elliot LP, et al. (1979) Right superior septal perforator artery: its angiographic description and clinical significance. Am J Roentgenol 133:67–73

Carlsson E, Keene RJ, Lee, P, Goerke RJ (1971) Angiocardiographic stroke volume correlation of the two cardiac ventricles in man. Invest Radiol 6:44–51

Chaitman BR, Rogers WJ, Davis K, et al (1980) Operative risk factors in patients with left main coronary artery disease. N Engl J Med 303:953–957

Codini MA, Bardfeld PA, Spindola-Franco H (1976) Paradoxical effect of nitroglycerin on left ventricular wall motion in coronary artery disease. Am J Cardiol 37:127

Collen D, Verstraete M (1983) Systemic thrombolytic therapy of acute myocardial infarction. Circulation 68:462–465

Dachman A, Spindola-Franco H, Solomon N (1981) Left ventricular pseudoaneurysm: Its recognition and significance. JAMA 246:1951–1953

Dodge HT, Sandler H, Ballew DW, Lord JD, Jr (1960) The use of biplane angiocardiography for the measurement of the left ventricular volume in man. Am Heart J 60:762–776

Dressler W (1959) The postmyocardial infarction syndrome. A report on 44 cases. Arch Intern Med 103:28–42

Eliot RS, Bratt GT (1968) The paradox of myocardial ischemia and necrosis in young women with normal coronary arteriograms. Relationship to anomalous hemoglobin-oxygen dissociation (abstr). Am J Cardiol 21:98

Friedman AC, Spindola-Franco H, Nivatpumin T (1979) Coronary spasm: Prinzmetal's variant angina (PVA) versus catheter-induced spasm, refractory spasm versus fixed stenosis. Am J Roentgenol 132:897–904

Friedman HS (1973) Cardiac rupture following myocardiol infarction: A review. Cardiol Dig 8:10–16

Gash AK, Spann JF (1980) Differential diagnosis and treatment of Dressler's syndrome. Pract Cardiol 6:27–32

Gensini GG, Buonanno C, Palacio A (1967) Anatomy of the coronary circulation in living man. Coronary arteriography. Chest 52:125–140

Grose R, Spindola-Franco H (1981) Right ventricular dysfunction in acute ventricular septal defect. Am Heart J 101:67–74

Harrison DC, Isaeff DM, Debusk RF (1972) Papillary muscle syndromes. Disease-a-Month (Jan Issue)

Herman MV, Heinle RA, Klein MD, Gorlin R (1967) Localized

disorders in myocardial contraction. N Engl J Med 277:222–232

James TN (1961) Anatomy of the coronary arteries. Hoeber, New York

James TN (1974) Diseases of the large and small coronary arteries. Arch Intern Med 134:163–176

Judkins MP (1968) Percutaneous transfemoral selective coronary arteriography. Radiol Clin North Am 6:467–492

Kannel WB (1981) Risk factors in established coronary heart disease: Prospects for secondary prevention. Baylor Cardiol Ser 4:7–25

Kannel WB, Sorlie P, McNamara PM (1979) Prognosis after initial myocardial infarction: The Framingham Study. Am J Cardiol 44:53–59

Kasper W, Erbel R, Meinertz T, Drexler M, Rückel A, Pop T, Prellwitz W, Meyer J (1984) Intracoronary thrombolysis with an acylated streptokinase-plasminogen activator (BRL 26921) in patients with acute myocardial infarction. JACC 4:357–363

Keene RJ, Raphael MJ (1970) Mechanical complications of myocardial infarction. Radiologic Aspects. Calif Med 113:11–15

Killen DA, McConahay DR, Crockett JE, Reed WA, McCallister BD, Bell HH (1974) Emergency infarctectomy and closure of ruptured interventricular septum. Arch Surg 109:623–626

Kittredge RD, Gamboa B, Kemp HG (1976) Radiographic visualization of left ventricular aneurysms on lateral chest film. Am J Roentgenol 126:1140–1146

Klein MD, Herman MV, Gorlin R (1967) A hemodynamic study of left ventricular aneurysm. Circulation 35:614–630

Kugel MA (1927) Anatomical studies on the coronary arteries and their branches. I. Arteria anastomotica auricularis magna. Am Heart J 3:260–270

Lipton MJ, Barry WH, Obrez I, Silverman JF, Wexler L (1979) Isolated single coronary artery: Diagnosis, angiographic classification, and clinical significance. Radiology 130:39–47

Loop FD, Cosgrove DM, Lytle BW, Thurer RL, Simpfendorfer C, Taylor PC, Proudfit WL (1979) An 11-year evolution of coronary arterial surgery (1967–1978. Ann Surg 190:444–455

Miller GAH, Kirklin JW, Swan HJC (1965) Myocardial function and left ventricular volumes in acquired valvular insufficiency. Circulation 31:374–384

Miller SW, Spindola-Franco H (1974) Systolic prolapse of the mitral valve. Contemp Surg 5:100–104

Nejat M, Greif E (1976) The aging heart. A clinical review. Med Clin North Am 60:1059–1078

Paulin S (1964) Coronary angiography. A technical, anatomic and clinical study. Acta Radiol suppl 233, pp 11–25

Phillips JH, Burch GE, De Pasquale NP (1963) The syndrome of papillary muscle dysfunction. Its clinical recognition. Ann Intern Med 59:508–520

Plucinski DA, Fishman SJ, Opravil M, Ganote CE, Moran JM, Bulawa WF, Lesch M, Meyers SN (1984) Circulation 70 (Supp II):326

Rentrop P, Blanke H, Karsch KR, Kaiser H, Kostering H, Leitz K (1981) Selective intracoronary thrombolysis in acute myocardial infarction and unstable angina pectoris. Circulation 63:307–317

Seldinger SI (1953) Catheter replacement of the needle in percutaneous arteriography. A new technique. Acta Radiol 39:368–376

Sones FM Jr, Shirery EK (1962) Cine coronary arteriography. Mod Concepts Cardiovasc Dis 31:735–738

Sorlie P (1977) Cardiovascular diseases and death following myocardial infarction and angina pectoris: Framingham study, 20-year follow-up. In: Kannel WB, Gordon T (eds): The Framingham study. DHEW and NIH, Washington

Spencer FC, Glassman E (1973) Preinfarction angina: Current therapeutic considerations. Am J Cardiol 32:382–384

Spindola-Franco H (1978) Plain film diagnosis of congestive heart failure. J Med Soc NJ 75:783–784

Spindola-Franco H, Adams DF, Herman MV, Abrams HL (1973) Reciprocating flow in the coronary circulation. Radiology 107:497–504

Spindola-Franco H, Eldh PA, Adams DF, Abrams HL (1975) Coronary vascular patterns during occlusion arteriography. Radiology 114:59–63

Spindola-Franco H, Grose R (1980) Unusual variants of the left anterior descending artery. Circulation 62:178

Spindola-Franco H, Grose R, Solomon N (1983) Dual left anterior descending coronary artery: Angiographic description of important variants and surgical implications. Am Heart J 105:445–455

Spindola-Franco H, Hooshmand I, Platt RR, Adams DF (1974) Venous visualization during left ventriculography. Radiology 113:587–589

Spindola-Franco H, Kronacher N (1978) Pseudoaneurysm of left ventricle. Radiographic and angiocardiographic diagnosis. Radiology 127:29–34

Spindola-Franco H, Weisel A, Delman AJ (1978) Pulmonary steal syndrome: An unusual case of coronary bronchial pulmonary artery communication. Radiology 126:25–27

The TIMI study group (1985) Special report. The thrombolysis in myocardial infarction (TIMI) trial. Phase I findings. New Engl J Med 312:932–936

Van de Werf F, Ludbrook PA, Bergmann SR, Tiefenbrunn AJ, Fox KAA, De Geest H, Verstraete M, Collen D, Sobel BE (1984) Coronary thrombolysis with tissue-type plasminogen activator in patients with evolving myocardial infarction. N Engl J Med 310:609–613

Percutaneous Transluminal Coronary Angioplasty

Cohen LS (1979) Percutaneous transluminal coronary angioplasty. N Engl J Med 301:1344–1345

Dorros G, Cowley MJ, Janke L, et al (1984) In-hospital mortality rate in the National Heart, Lung, and Blood Institute Transluminal Coronary Angioplasty Registry. Am J Cardiol 53:17c–21c.

Dotter CT, Judkins MP (1964) Transluminal treatment of arteriosclerotic obstruction: Description of a new technique and a preliminary report of its application. Circulation 30:654–670

Gruntzig AR, Senning A, Siegenthaler WE (1979) Nonoperative dilatation of coronary artery stenosis. Percutaneous transluminal coronary angioplasty. N Engl J Med 301:61–68

Kent K, Banka V, Bentivoglio P et al (1980) Percutaneous transluminal coronary angioplasty (PTCA): Update from NHLBI registry (abstr). Circulation 62:160

Ischemic Heart Disease in the Young

Brosius FC, Roberts WC (1981) Coronary artery disease in the Hurler syndrome. Am J Cardiol 47:649–653

Cheitlin MD, McAllister HA, deCastro CM (1975 Myocardial infarction without atherosclerosis. JAMA 231:951–959

Imahori S, Bannerman RM, Graf CJ, Brennan JC (1969) Ehlers-Danlos syndrome with multiple arterial lesions. Am J Med 47:967–977

Morettin LB (1976) Coronary arteriography. Uncommon observations. Radiol Clin North Am 14:189–208

Tsakraklides VG, Blieden LC, Edwards JE (1974) Coronary atherosclerosis and myocardial infarction in association with lupus erythematosus. Am Heart J 87:637–641

Vlodaver Z, Neufeld HN, Edwards JE (1975) Coronary arterial variations in the normal heart and in congenital heart disease. Academic Press, New York

Anomalous Left Coronary Artery

Arciniegas E, Farooki ZQ, Hakimi M, Green EW (1980) Management of anomalous left coronary artery from pulmonary artery. Circulation 62:180–189

Bland EF, White PD, Garland J (1933) Congenital anomalies of coronary arteries: Report of unusual case associated with cardiac hypertrophy. Am Heart J 8:787–801

Bookstein JJ (1964) Aberrant left coronary artery. Am J Roentgenol 91:515–528

Burch GE, DePasquale NP (1962) The electrocardiogram in certain anomalies of the coronary arteries. Am Heart J 64:38–43

Choh JH, Levinsky L, Srinivasan V, Idbeis B, Subramanian S (1980) Anomalous origin of the left coronary artery from the pulmonary trunk: Its clinical spectrum and current surgical management. Thorac Cardiovasc Surg 28:239–242

Finley JP, Howman-Giles R, Gilday DL, Olley PM, Rowe RD (1978) Thallium-201 myocardial imaging in anomalous left coronary artery arising from the pulmonary artery. Am J Cardiol 42:675–680

Gasior RM, Winters WL, Glick H, Sandiford F, Chapman DW, Morris GC, Jr. (1971) Anomalous origin of left coronary artery from pulmonary artery. Treatment by aorto-left coronary saphenous vein bypass. Am J Cardiol 27:215–220

Hawthorne JW, Scannell JG, Dinsmore RE (1966) Anomalous origin of the left coronary artery. N Engl J Med 275:660–663

Menke JA, Shaher RM, Wolff GS (1972) Ejection fraction in anomalous origin of the left coronary artery from the pulmonary artery. Am Heart J 84:325–329

Wesselhoeft H, Fawcett JS, Johnson AL (1968) Anomalous origin of the left coronary artery from the pulmonary trunk. Circulation 38:403–425

Kawasaki Disease

Fujiwara H, Chen C, Fujiwara T, Nishioka K, Kawai C, Hamashima Y (1980) Clinicopathologic study of abnormal Q waves in Kawasaki's disease (mucocutaneous lymph node syndrome). An infantile cardiac disease with myocarditis and myocardial disease. Am J Cardiol 45:797–805

Fujiwara H, Hamashima Y (1978) Pathology of the heart in Kawasaki's disease (mucocutaneous lymph node syndrome). Pediatrics 61:100–107

Fukushige J, Nihill MR, McNamera DG (1980) Spectrum of cardiovascular lesions in mucocutaneous lymph node syndrome: Analysis of eight cases. Am J Cardiol 45:98–107

Hiraishi A, Yashiro I, Kusano H (1979) Noninvasive visualization of coronary arterial aneurysm in infants and young children with mucocutaneous lymph node syndrome with two dimensional echocardiography. Am J Cardiol 43:1225–1233

Hiraishi A, Yashiro K, Oguchi K, Kusano S, Ishll K, Nakazawa K (1981) Clinical course of cardiovascular involvement in the mucocutaneous lymph node syndrome. Am J Cardiol 47:323–330

Chapter 4 Appendix

Angulated Views of Coronary Artery Angiograms

(Figs. 4–58 to 4–64)

In this appendix pictures of the C-arm positioned for standard and angulated views are presented along with corresponding pictures of the coronary catheters and coronary arteriograms. The purpose is to demonstrate the position of the catheter tip and the appearance of the coronary arteries in standard and angulated projections.

The cardiac catheterization laboratory at Montefiore Medical Center contains a Phillips Poly Diagnost C-arm. The parallelogram construction of the Poly C-arm allows the x-ray beam to be oriented between 120° right oblique and 120° left oblique as well as between 45° and 45° caudal axial angulations without moving or supporting the patient.

The following projections are usually obtained by the authors during coronary arteriography. Not all views are obtained on all patients. Replay of the video tape allows the operator to choose appropriate views to demonstrate the lesions.

The left coronary artery is routinely examined in multiple views including the standard RAO view (Fig. 4–58) and LAO view (Fig. 4–61 A and B) and the RAO with cranial tilt (Fig. 4–59), RAO with caudal tilt (Fig. 4–60), and LAO with cranial tilt (Fig. 4–61 C and D). The frontal and lateral views are then performed if needed. Other views described are only performed if indicated (Fig. 4–62).

The right coronary artery is usually studied in the RAO and LAO view, and angulated views are not often needed. In our laboratory we prefer the angulated RAO views (Figs. 4–63 and 4–64) rather than angulated LAO views, although both may be useful in the individual case.

The standard views are performed biplane, thus reducing the number of injections of contrast. Angulated views are done in single plane because the lateral tube in our laboratory does not have axial capability. Table 4–2 is a list of abbreviations used to label the illustrations.

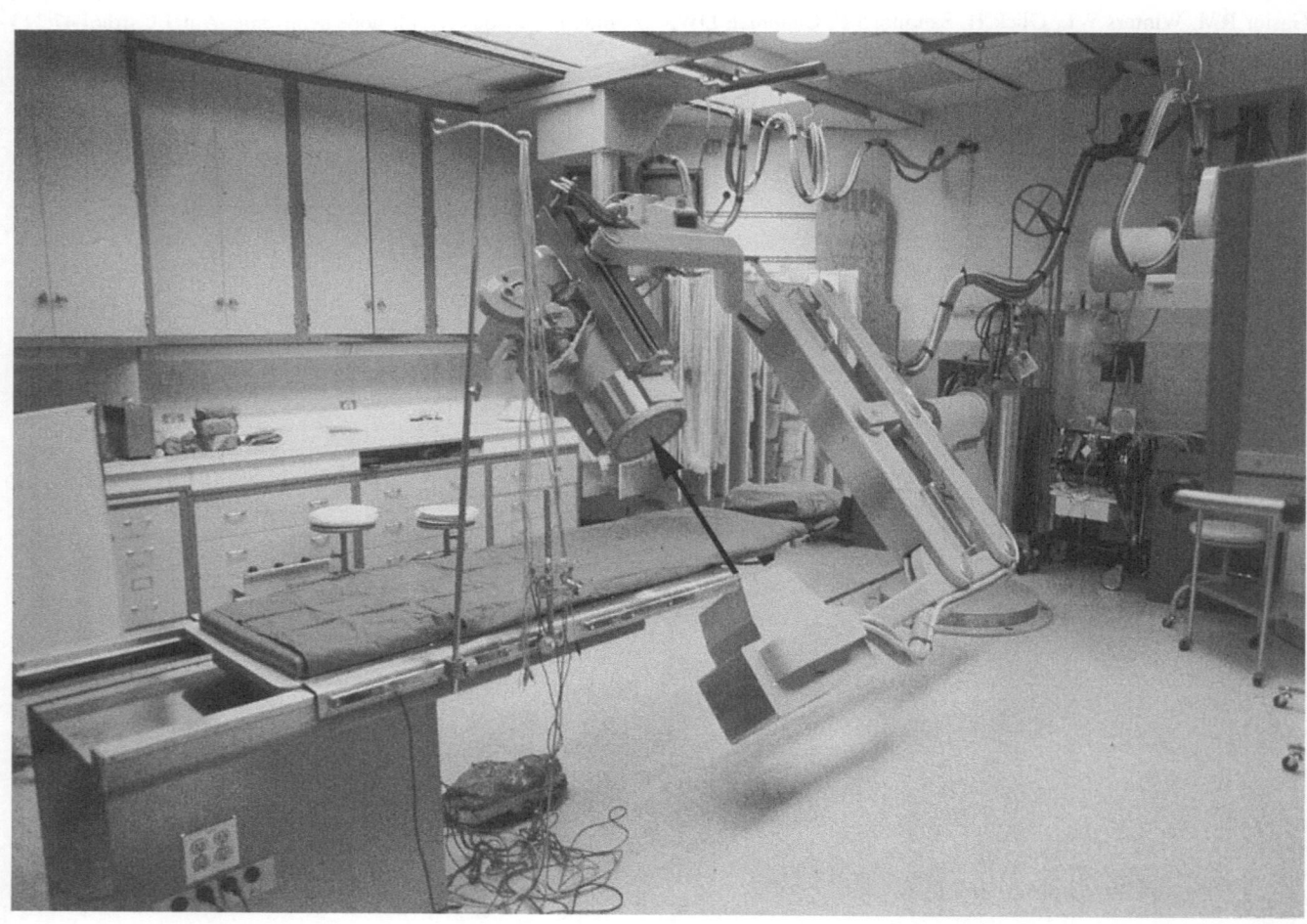

A

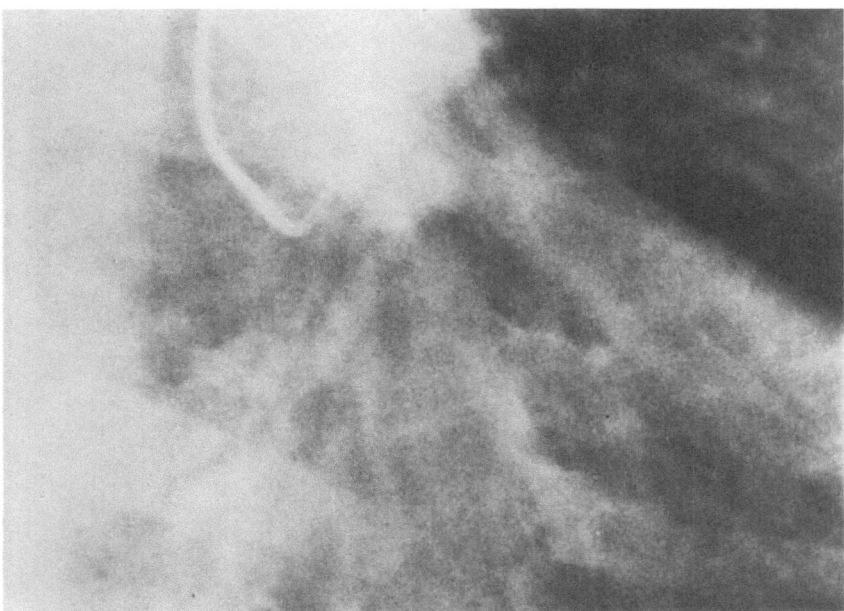

B

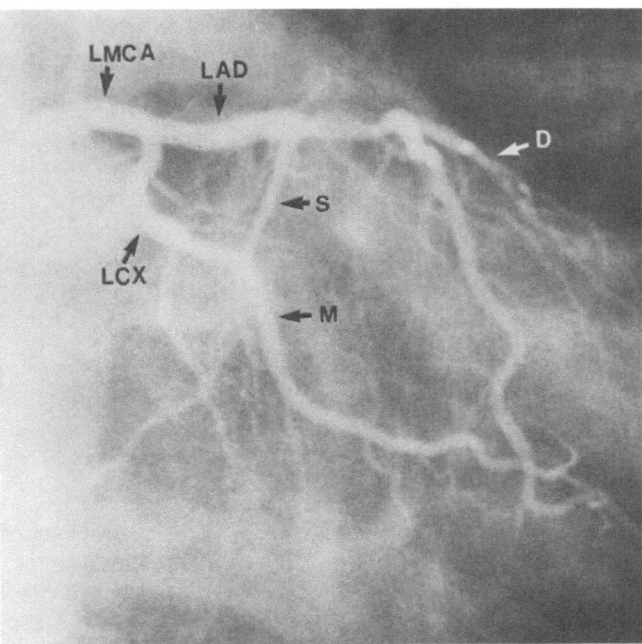

C

Fig. 4–58. *RAO view of the left coronary artery.* In **A** the x-ray tube is below the table on the left. The image intensifier is above the table and on the right. The direction of the X-ray beam is indicated by the arrow. **B** presents the typical appearance of the catheter tip in the left coronary artery. **C** shows the typical appearance of the left coronary artery in the RAO view.

Table 4–2. Abbreviations Found in Illustrations in this Appendix

D = diagonal(s)
LAD = left anterior descending artery
LCX = left circumflex artery
$LMCA$ = left main coronary artery
M = marginal branch(es)
PD = posterior descending artery
PLV = posterior left ventricular branch(es)
RM = *ramus medianus*
RV = right ventricular branch
S = septal(s)

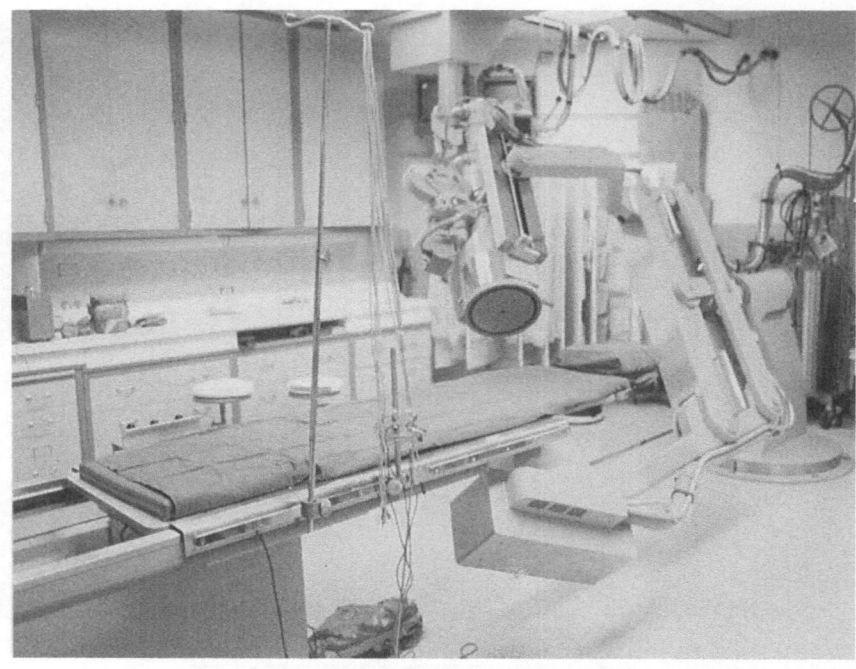

A

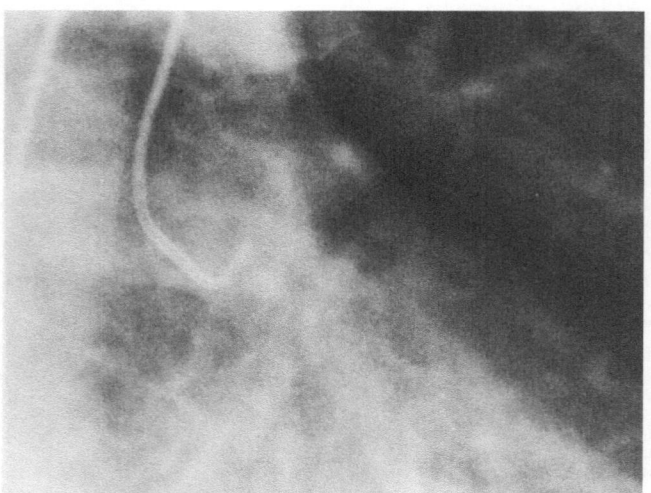

B

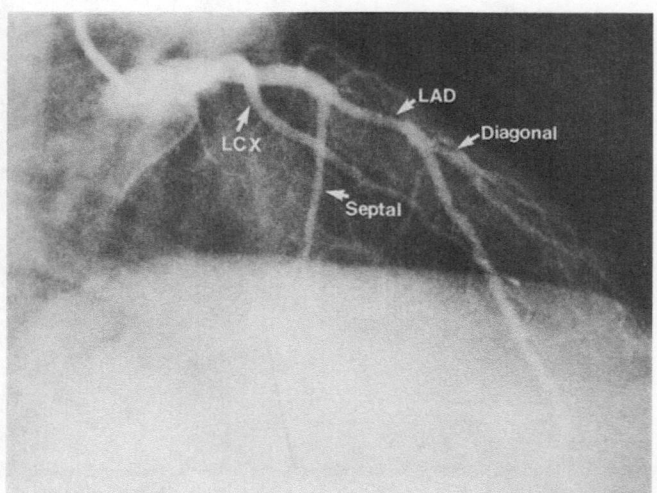

C

D

Fig. 4–59. *RAO view of the left coronary artery with cranial tilt, also known as headward RAO or RAO with caudocranial angulation.* In **A** the C-arm is positioned for the RAO with 20–25° cranial tilt. In **B** the catheter tip in the LCA points superiorly. In **C** the LAD and LCX tend to be close to one another, may be superimposed, or the LCX may cross the LAD to appear above the LAD in contrast to the appearance in the RAO with caudal tilt Fig. 4–60. The RAO with cranial tilt is useful in delineating the entire course of the LAD and the origins of the diagonal and septal arteries. Further headward angulation (greater than 25°) exaggerates the superior position of the LCX and inferior position of the LAD allowing better delineation of the origins of the diagonal and septal branches; however, increased angulation impairs resolution especially in heavy patients. **D** is from a different patient and illustrates the effect of a 30° cranial angulation, giving the LAD the appearance of a denuded spine of a fish with the septal arteries pointing inferiorly and the diagonal branches superiorly. The origin of the septal (*S*) and diagonal

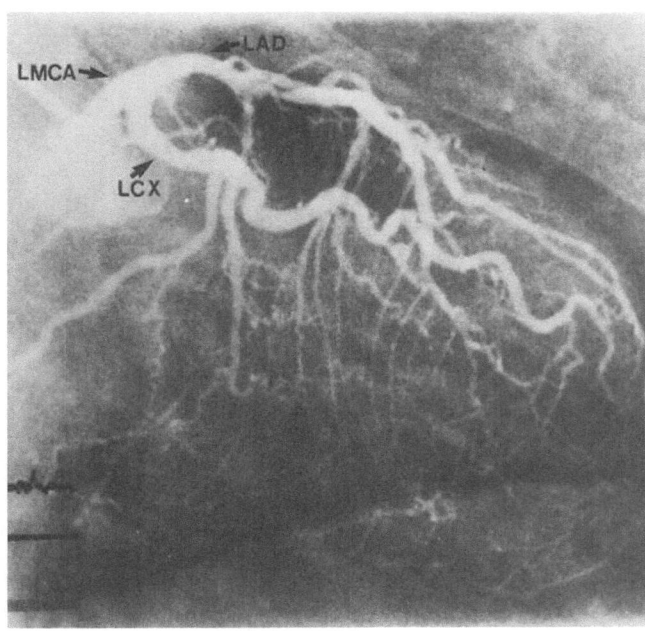

E

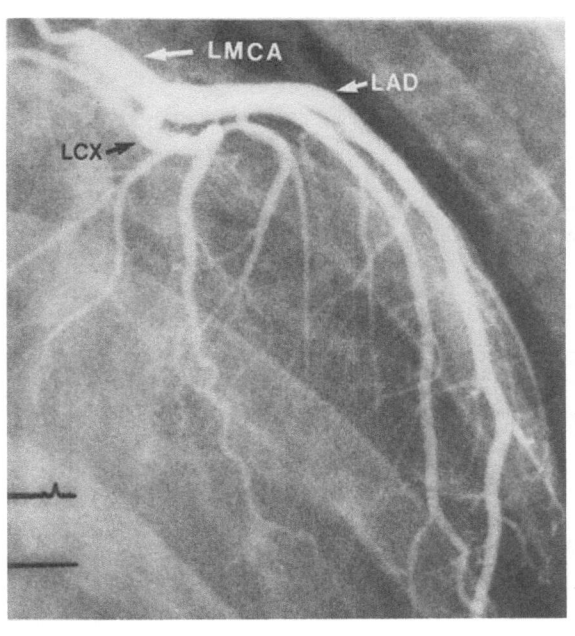

F

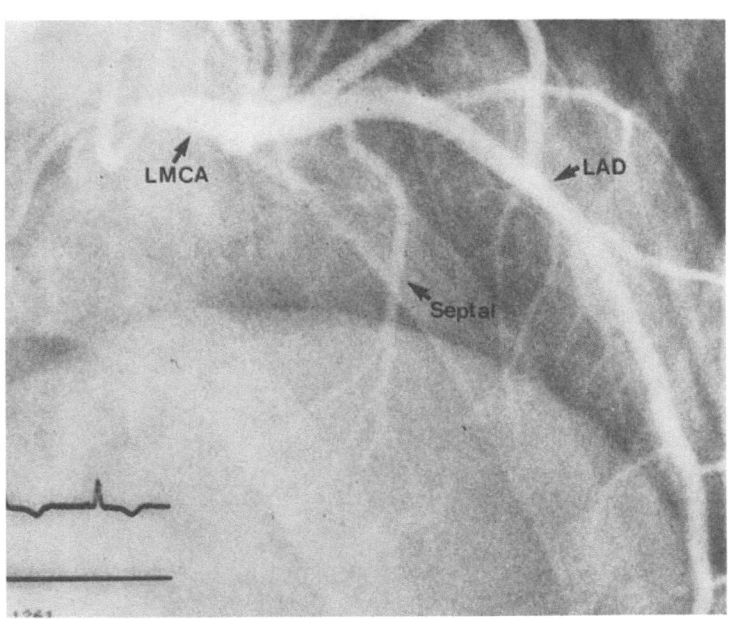

G

(*D*) branches are clearly delineated. **E** is the standard RAO view in the same patient for comparison. In patients with dilated cardiomyopathy the same effect can be achieved without increasing the headward angulation. **F, G** and **H** are from a different patient with dilated cardiomyopathy. In **F,** the standard RAO view, the LAD, the diagonals, and a third vessel are superimposed. It is not possible to determine in this view whether the third vessel is a ramus medianus, an obtuse marginal branch, or a large proximal diagonal vessel. In **G,** the RAO view with cranial tilt, the LCX and the third vessel are superior to the LAD. The entire LAD and the origins of the septals and diagonals can now be assessed individually. **H** is a RAO view with caudal tilt in the same patient showing the opposite effect, with the LCX being inferior and widely separated from the LAD. In this view the third vessel is recognized as a ramus medianus (*RM*) because it takes origin from the distal left main coronary artery (trifurcation). This view allows separation of the origins of the LAD, LCX and the ramus medianus if present. In addition the entirety of the left main coronary artery is visible.

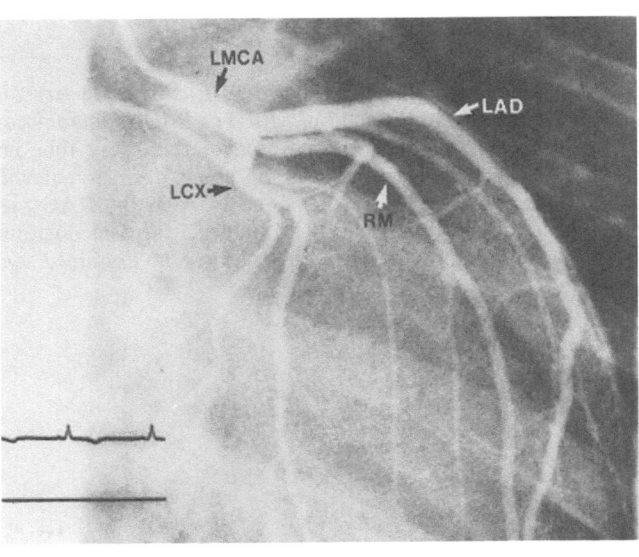

H

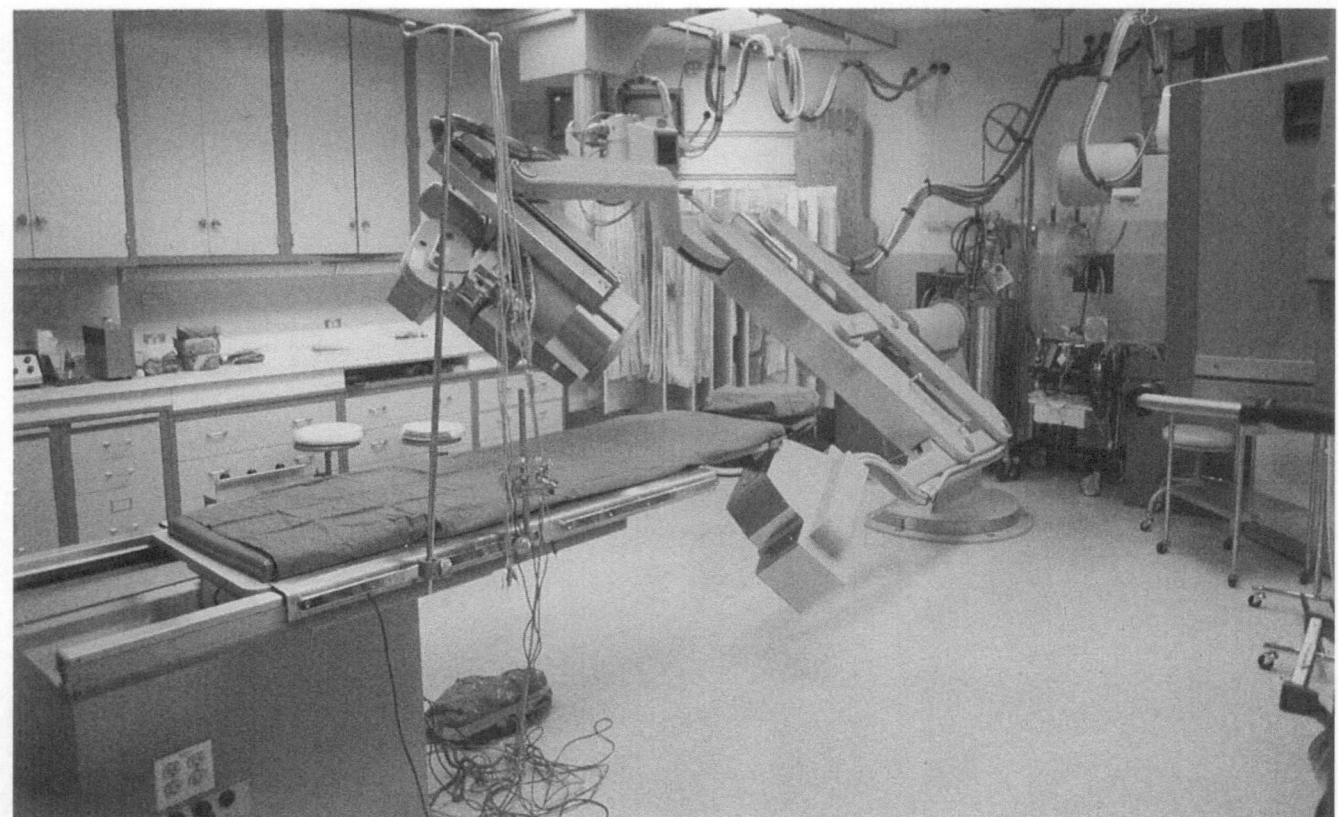

A

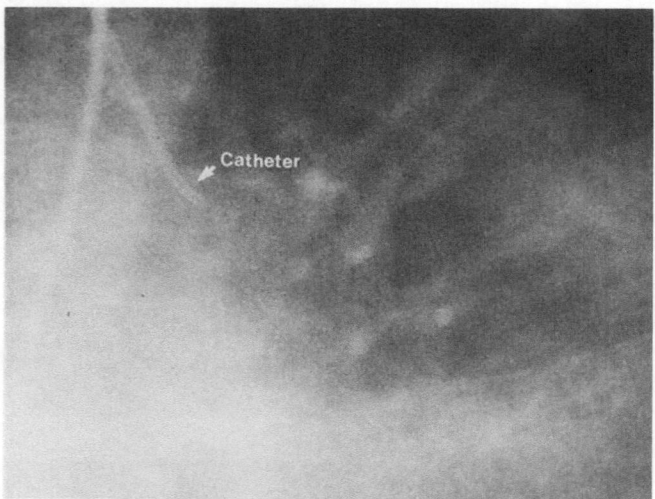

B

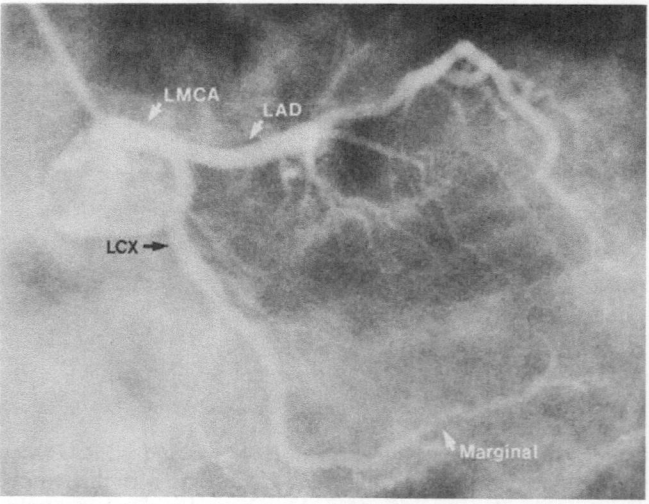

C

Fig. 4–60. *Compound RAO view of the left coronary artery with caudal tilt (also known as footward RAO or RAO with craniocaudal angulation).* **A** shows the position of the X-ray tube and image intensifier. In **B** the catheter tip points down to enter the LCA. **C** shows the appearance of the LCA in the RAO view with caudal tilt. The LAD and LCX are widely separated without overlap of the origins so that each origin can be examined sepa-rately. In addition this view allows differentiation of a ramus medianus, a branch of the distal LMCA, from an obtuse marginal, a branch of the LCX (Fig. 4–59). The middle portion of the LAD forms an angle pointing superiorly reminiscent of the top of a tent, while the LCX and its marginal branch form a similar angle pointing inferiorly (same patient as Figs. 4–58 B and C, and 4–59 B and C).

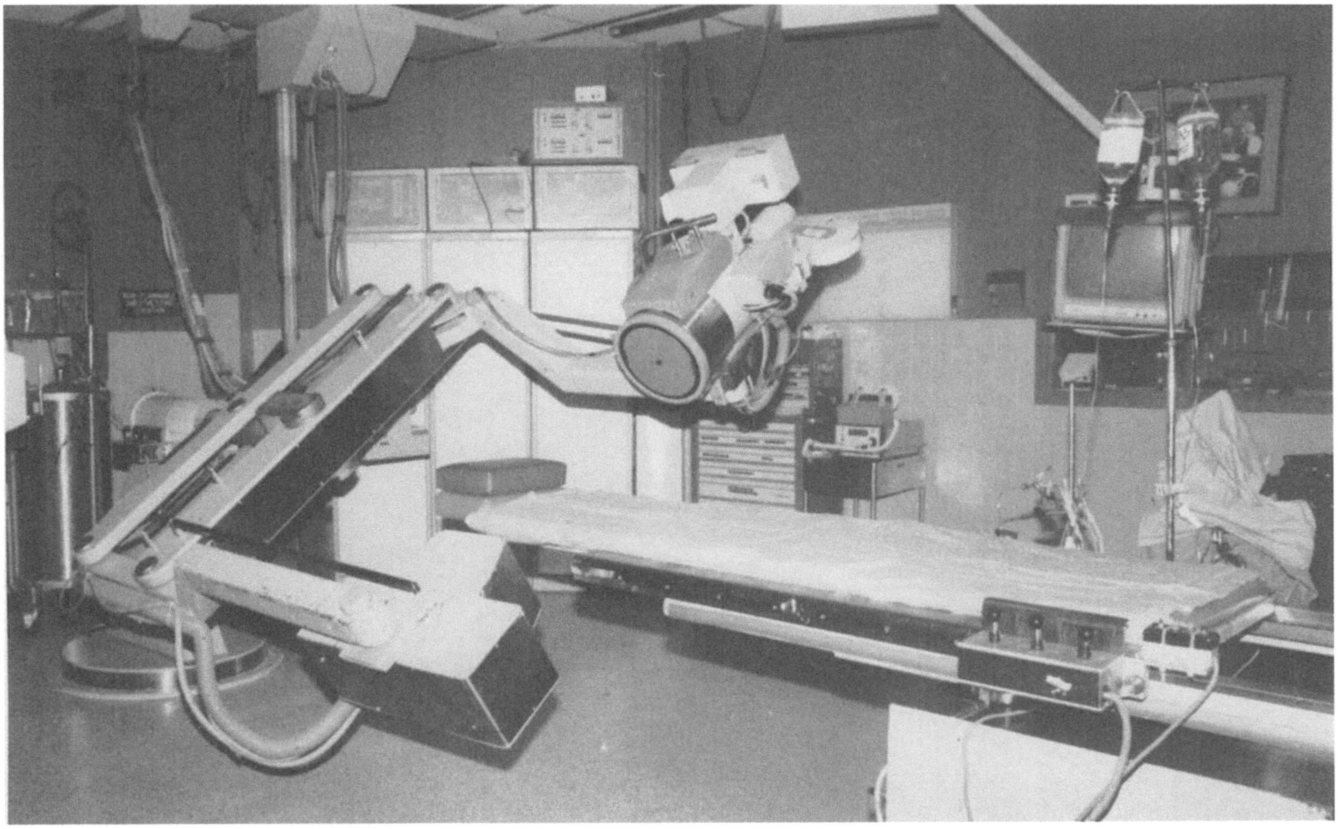

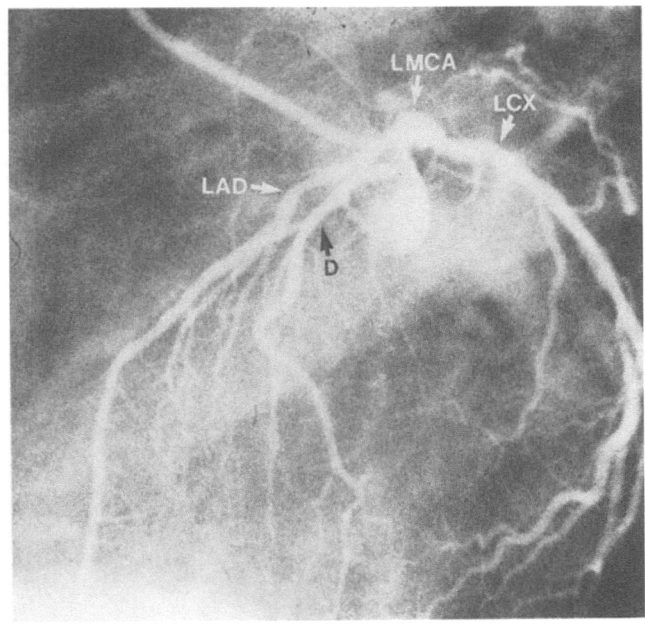

A

Fig. 4–61. *Standard LAO view and LAO view of the left coronary artery with cranial tilt.* The LAO view with cranial tilt is also known as headward LAO, LAO with caudocranial angulation, hepatoclavicular view and four-chamber view. **A** shows the position of the C-arm for a standard LAO view. In **B** the left coronary angiogram in the LAO view shows the left main coronary artery (*LMCA*) on end. The proximal portions of the LAD and the large diagonal branch (*D*) are foreshortened. No stenosis is apparent in this view. (*Cont.*)

B

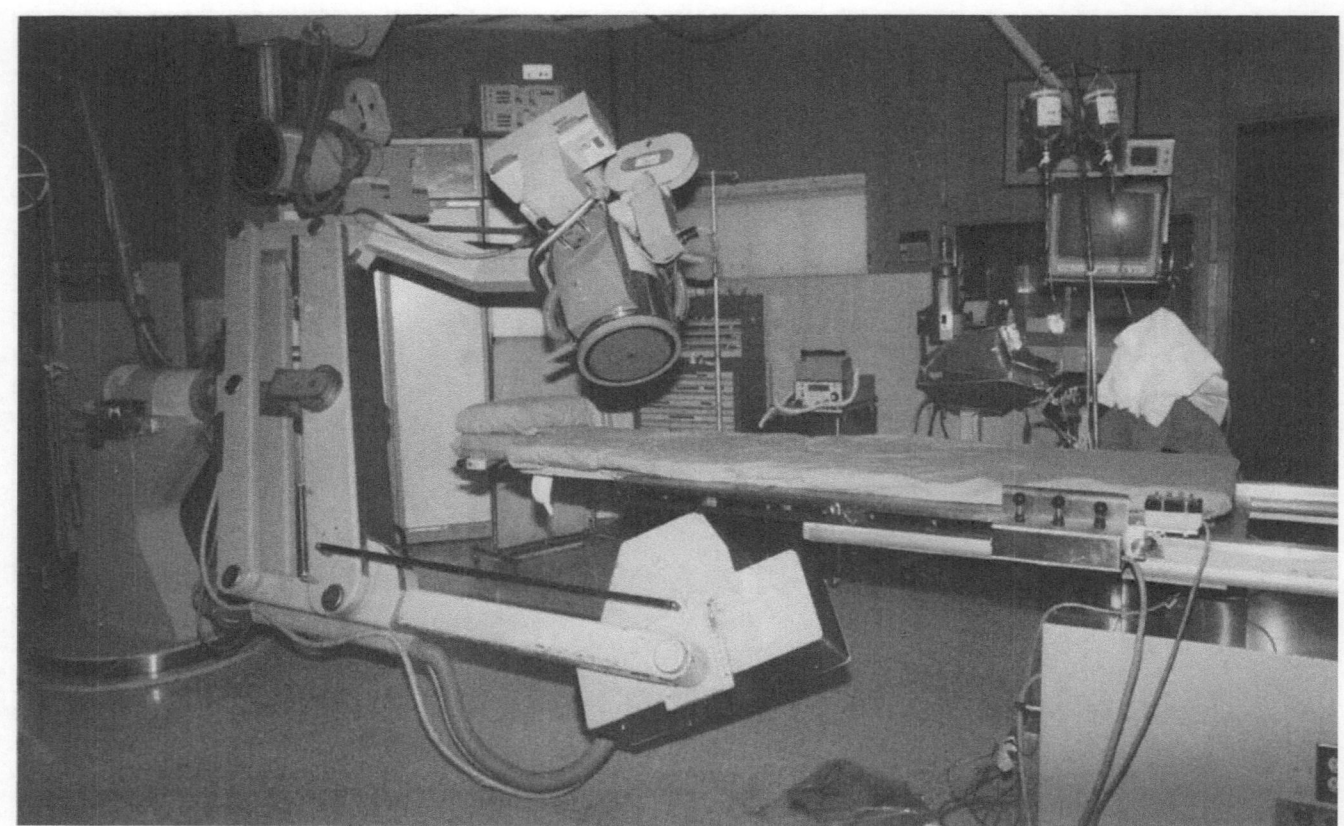

C

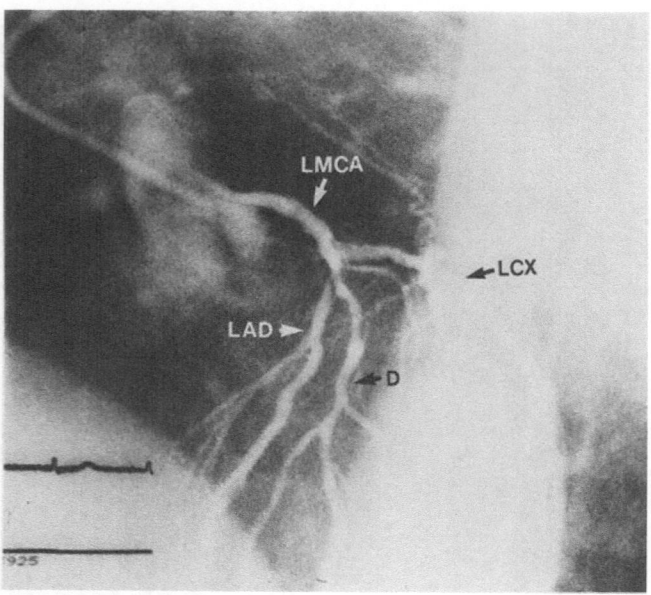

D

Fig. 4–61 (*Cont.*) In **C** the C-arm is positioned for an LAO view with cranial tilt. In **D** the corresponding angiogram of the left coronary artery in the same patient. The LMCA is visualized in its entirety and the proximal portion of the LAD and large diagonal branch are delineated. A significant stenosis of the LAD is now evident just distal to the origin of the large diagonal branch.

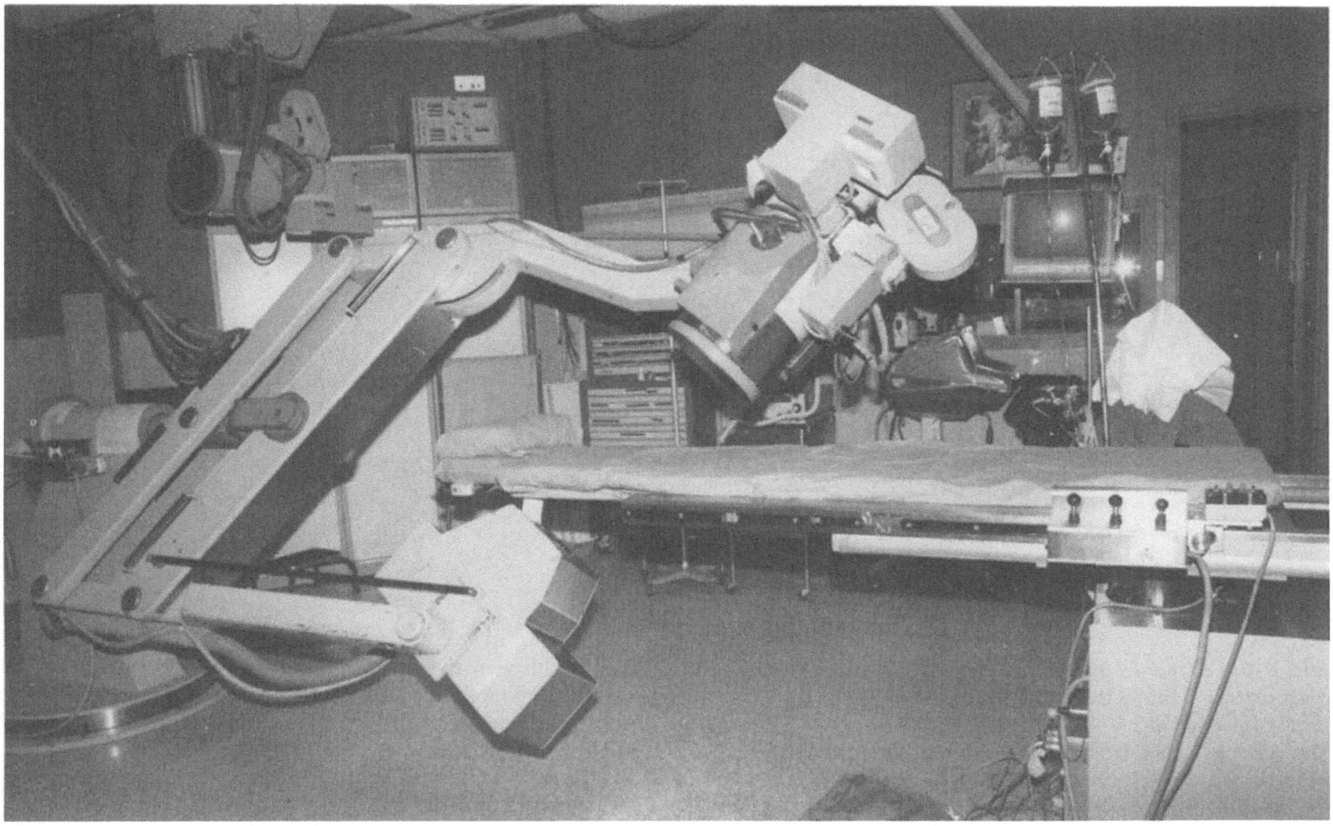

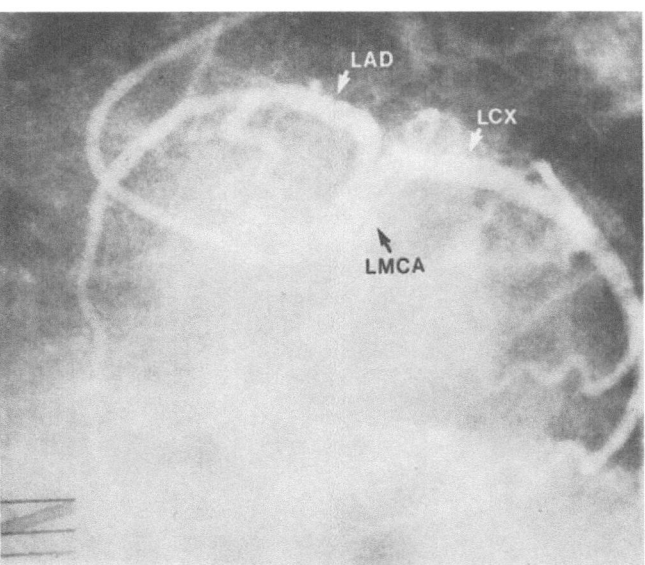

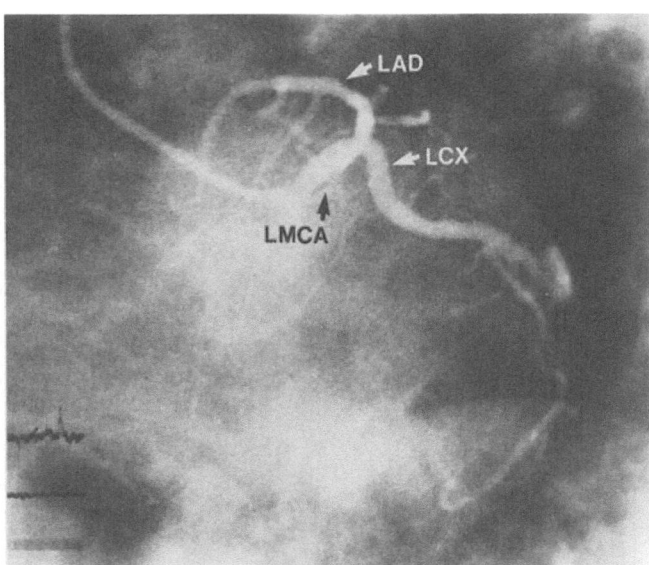

Fig. 4–62. *LAO view with caudal tilt.* This view is also known as footward LAO or LAO with craniocaudal angulation. In **A** the C-arm is positioned for the LAO view with caudal tilt. In **B,** the LAO view of the left coronary artery with caudal tilt, the left main coronary artery points superiorly and the LAD and LCX diverge, so that the origins and proximal portions are separate. The appearance of the LAD and LCX in this view is reminiscent of a bat flying, the left main coronary artery (*LMCA*) being the head and the LAD and LCX being the wings. **C** is an illustration of the same view in a different patient with a short LAD. The right wing of the bat is shorter. The appearance of the LMCA and branches in this view is strikingly different from that observed in the LAO with cranial tilt (Fig. 4–61 C and D).

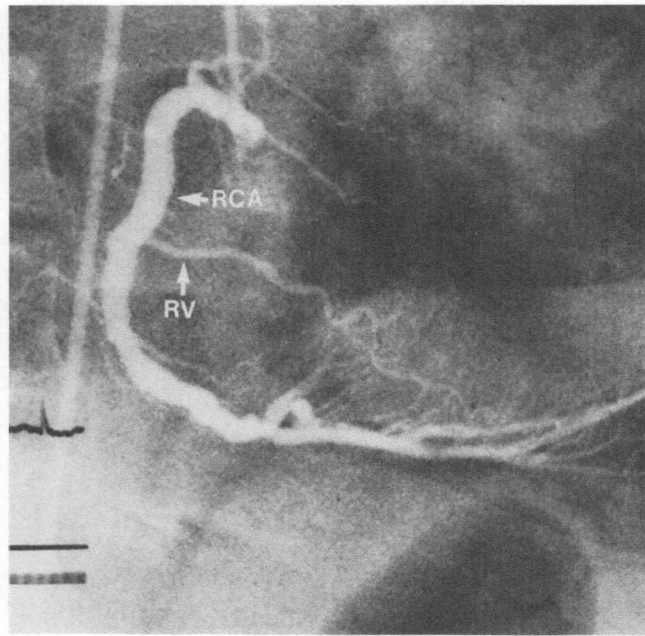
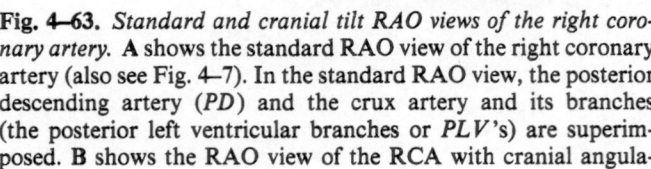

A

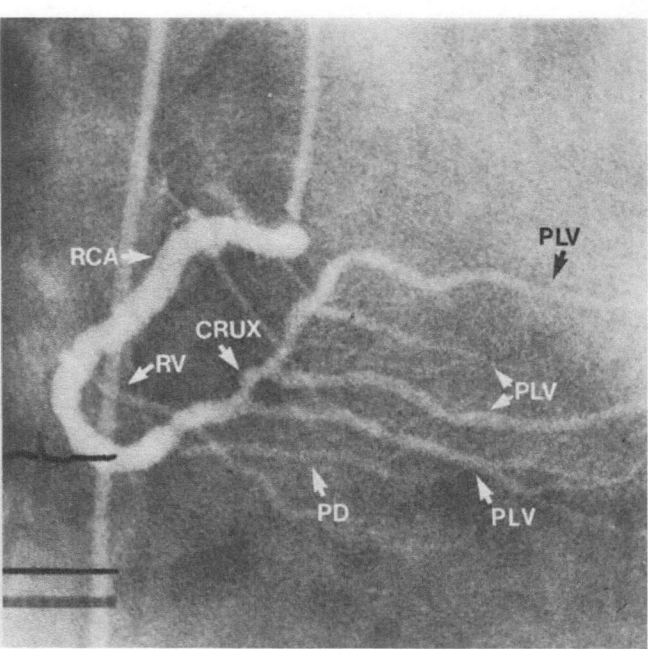

B

Fig. 4–63. *Standard and cranial tilt RAO views of the right coronary artery.* **A** shows the standard RAO view of the right coronary artery (also see Fig. 4–7). In the standard RAO view, the posterior descending artery (*PD*) and the crux artery and its branches (the posterior left ventricular branches or *PLV*'s) are superimposed. **B** shows the RAO view of the RCA with cranial angula-

tion. In this view the crux artery becomes nearly vertical pointing superiorly. The PD and PLV's are separated so that they appear as parallel horizontal lines similar to the steps of a ladder. The PD is at the bottom, with the PLV's above it. The origins are all clearly visualized. *RV* = right ventricular branch arising from the midportion of the right coronary artery.

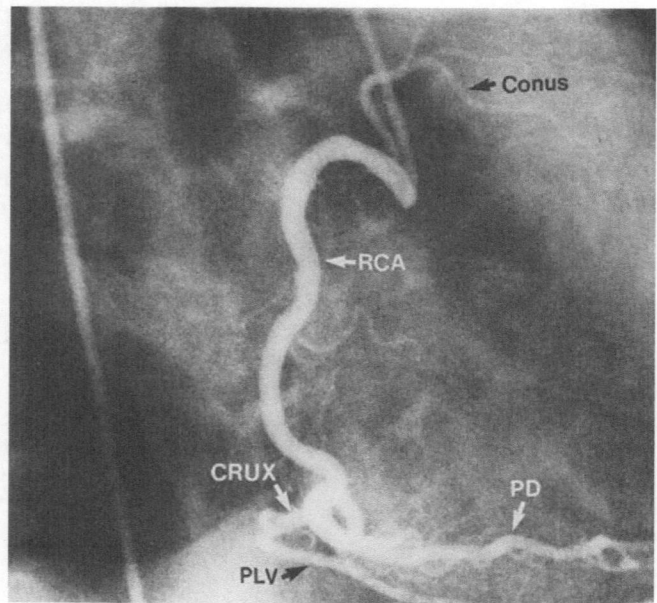

A

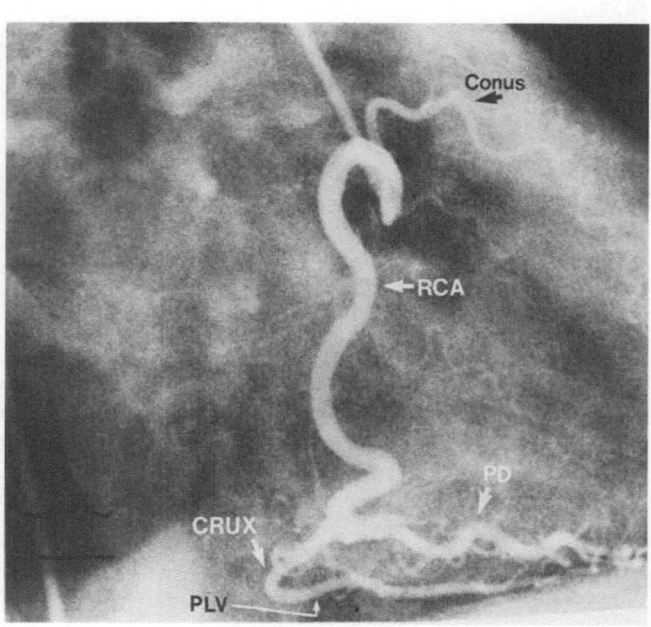

B

Fig. 4–64. *Standard RAO view of the right coronary artery (RCA)* **(A)** *and RAO view with caudal tilt* **(B)**. As in Fig. 4–63, the angulated view (**B**) causes the crux artery to become vertical. The posterior descending artery (*PD*) is now at the top with

the posterior left ventricular branches (*PLV*) projecting below similar to the steps of a ladder. This patient has only one PLV. The distal portion of the RCA, and the origins of the PD and PLV are separated in this view.

5 Valvular Heart Disease

The clinical and hemodynamic manifestations of an abnormality of the semilunar or of the atrioventricular valves are secondary to obstruction or insufficiency of one or more valves.

Valvular heart disease may be congenital or acquired. In some conditions, such as bicuspid aortic valve, a congenital valvular defect is not detected in childhood but presents in adult life once degenerative changes or infection have been superimposed.

Acquired valvular heart disease may be due to chronic or acute inflammatory processes or to degenerative changes. The end result of these disorders is fibrosis, retraction of the leaflets and eventual calcification. Valvular heart disease may also be caused by other congenital defects. For instance, aortic insufficiency may result from a jet of blood from a subaortic membrane. Hypertrophic cardiomyopathy often results in mitral insufficiency because of traction on the chordae tendineae.

The manifestations of valvular heart disease may be simulated by disorders involving surrounding tissues. Aortic stenosis may be mimicked by supravalvular aortic stenosis or subvalvular aortic stenosis. Features of mitral stenosis may be present in instances of left atrial tumor. Poor left ventricular compliance, secondary to restrictive cardiomyopathy, may also prevent filling of the left ventricle so that many features will be reminiscent of mitral stenosis.

Acquired valvular disease usually affects the aortic and mitral valves primarily. The pulmonary and tricuspid valves are usually not primarily affected but may be involved secondarily. In severe mitral valve disease, for instance, severe pulmonary hypertension may result in right ventricular failure and tricuspid insufficiency. In recent years, however, primary involvement of the right-sided valves has been reported in infective endocarditis in drug addicts.

Disorders affecting each valve are discussed separately in this chapter. Congenital bicuspid aortic valve is included here because its manifestations are mostly due to superimposed acquired abnormalities. Other congenital valvular defects are described in Chapter 7.

Aortic Stenosis

Aortic stenosis (AS) may be valvular, subvalvular or supravalvular. The most common causes of valvular AS are rheumatic heart disease and congenital bicuspid aortic valve. Rarely, a congenital bicuspid aortic valve is stenotic from birth, but most cases are not initially stenotic. Fibrosis and calcification occur along "lines of stress" in some instances, so that progressive stenosis ensues. This entity is described separately.

The findings and clinical course of chronic rheumatic AS are indistinguishable from those of aortic valve disease caused by atherosclerosis, rheumatoid arthritis and other collagen vascular diseases. Although isolated aortic valve stenosis may be of rheumatic origin, rheumatic disease is more likely if the mitral valve is also involved. Acute rheumatic valvulitis results in thickening of the valve cusps and a verrucous endocarditis along the edges of the aortic and mitral valves. Initially, aortic insufficiency may occur, usually of mild degree. During healing, fibrosis of the leaflets occurs. Progression of fibrosis shortens the cusps and makes them rigid. Fusion of the commissures decreases the size of the aortic orifice. Calcification occurs within the leaflets initially. Later, calcific masses are deposited on both sides of the aortic leaflets. Infective endocarditis may supervene. The usual chronic course is that of gradual progression of aortic stenosis. Significant aortic insufficiency may be associated.

Acquired bicuspid valve occurs in a fibrotic aortic valve when one commissure, usually the commissure between the right and left cusps, becomes fused by fibrosis. Calcification may develop thereafter. In contrast to the situation in congenital bicuspid valve, an acquired bicuspid aortic valve has well formed sinuses of Valsalva. The pseudo-

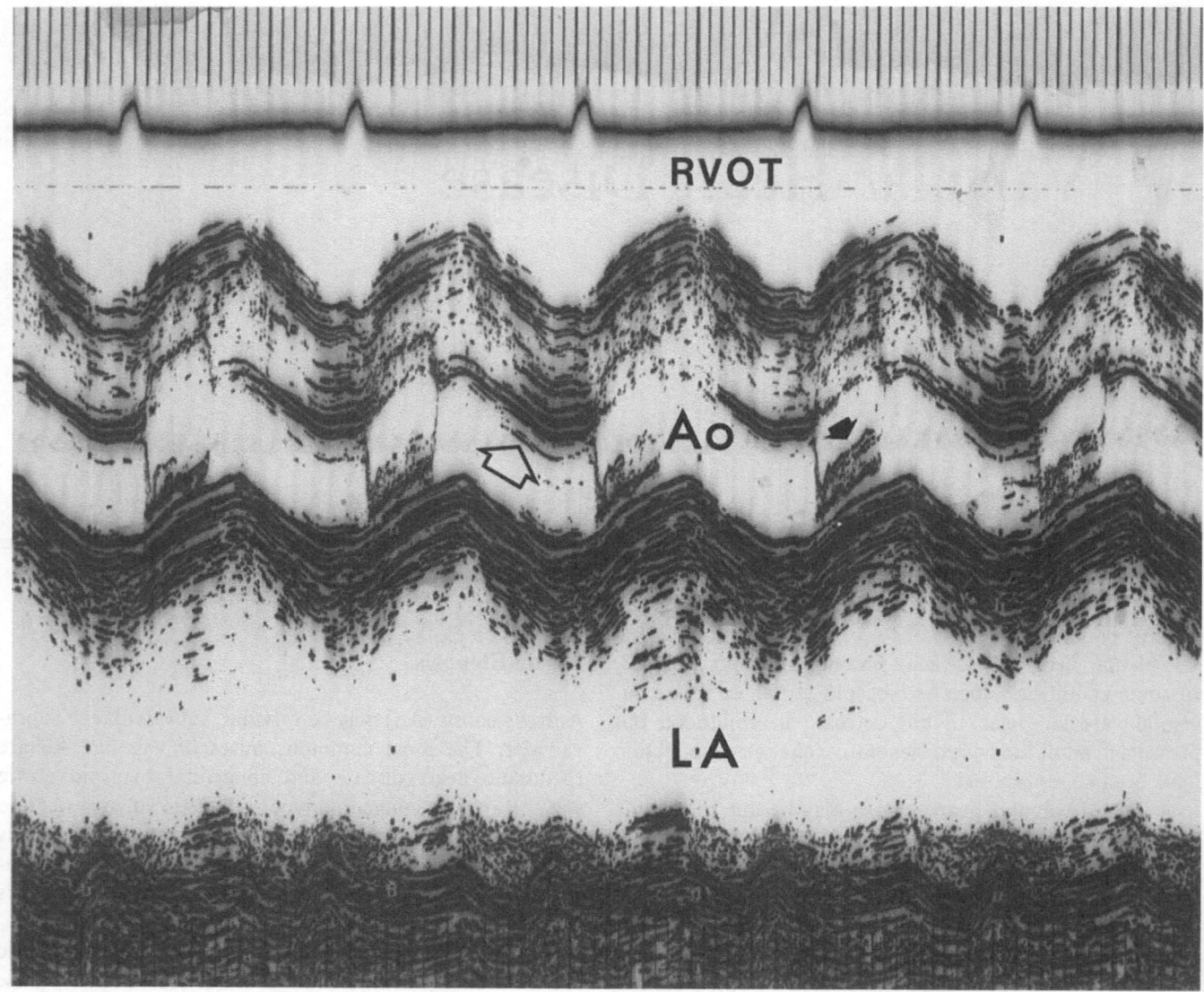

Fig. 5–1. *M-mode echocardiogram in an adult with aortic stenosis.* The valve is in the middle of the aortic root (*Ao*) during diastole. Multiple echoes produced by the leaflets during diastole (*open arrow*) and during systole (*closed arrow*) indicate thickening of the leaflets. During systole the parallelogram of valve motion is visualized more readily than usual because of the limitation of movement of the leaflets. The posterior leaflet opens almost to the aortic wall; the anterior leaflet opens only partially. The valve is likely to be fibrotic but flexible. *RVOT* = right ventricular outflow tract; *LA* = left atrium.

raphe, which represents the fused commissure, extends to the free edge of the leaflet. The fused leaflet is made up of two cusps and therefore comprises more than half the aortic circumference. Valves that are not heavily calcified will have well formed deeply convex sinuses of Valsalva. These findings indicate acquired commissural fusion rather than congenital bicuspid valve.

Clinical Features

The typical murmur of valvular AS from any cause is a harsh systolic ejection murmur at the left mid and right upper sternal borders that may be transmitted to the neck (see Fig. 5–12). An ejection click will be heard if the valve is flexible, but not in calcific AS. With moderate AS a left ventricular heave is palpated while a thrill is felt over the precordium, in the suprasternal notch and over the carotids. With severe AS, pulses may be weak and the pulse pressure narrow. Displacement of the cardiac apex (cardiac enlargement) is a sign of cardiac decompensation. Symptoms of dyspnea on exertion or chest pain occur late in the course. Syncope in an individual with severe AS usually indicates a grave prognosis. Sudden death may occur in some instances of severe AS.

The standard 12-lead electrocardiogram is insensitive to left ventricular hypertrophy and therefore is a poor indicator of progression of disease. T-wave changes on the

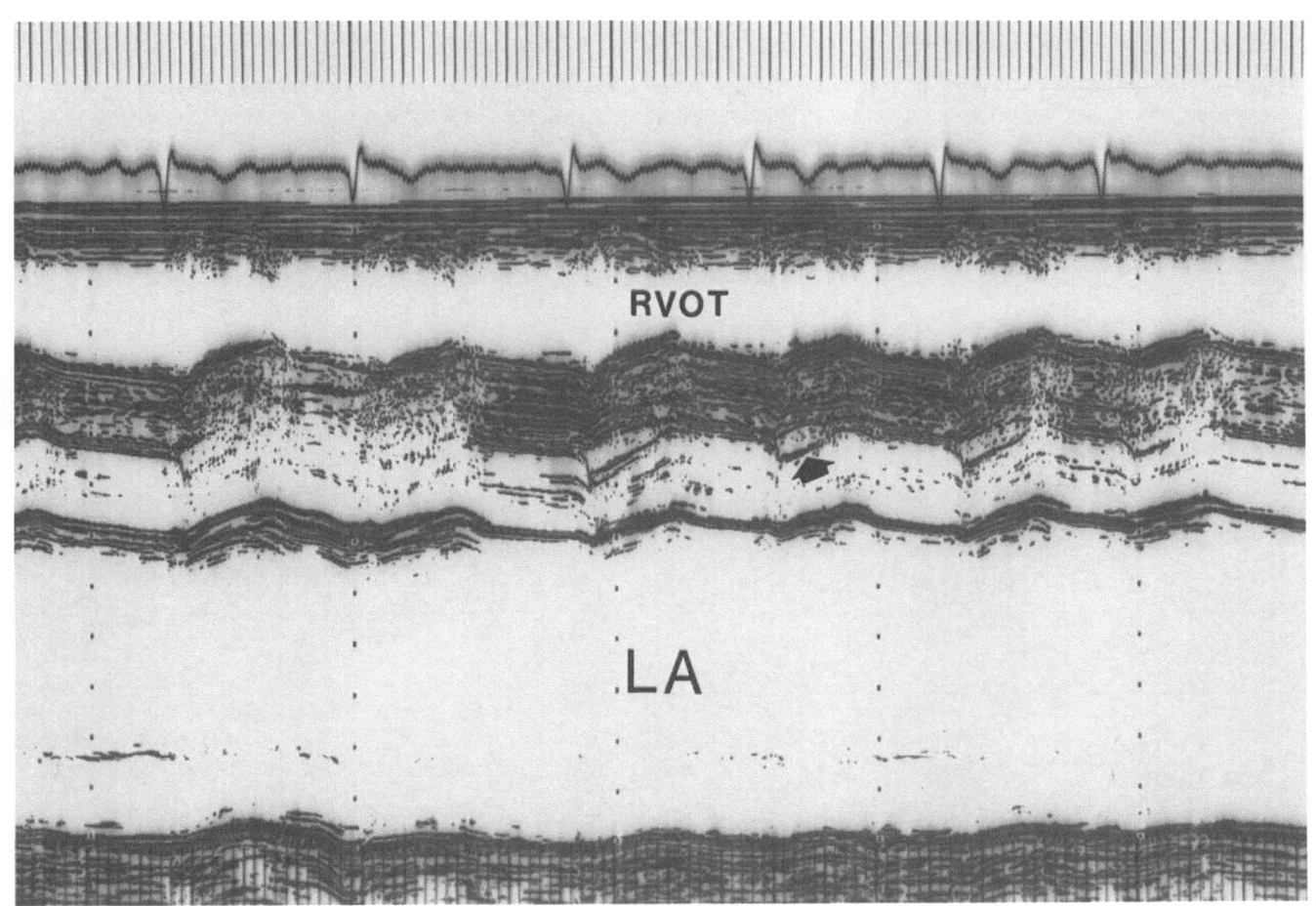

RVOT

.LA

A

Fig. 5–2. *Echocardiograms in three adults with fibrocalcific aortic stenosis.* **A** and **B** M-mode tracings; **C** and **D** long axis, **E** and **F** short axis views of a 2-D echocardiogram. In **A** the parallelogram of the opening of the aortic valve (*arrow*) is narrow because of marked limitation of valve motion. This patient also has mitral valve disease, which accounts for the large left atrium and for the atrial fibrillation noted on the ECG. In **B** the calcified valve appears as a dense cloud of echoes, and the parallelogram of valve motion (*arrow*) is obscured. In **C** and **D**, the long axis view with and without labels, the aortic valve is densely calcified and is immobile during systole. The mitral valve apparatus is also thickened and fibrotic. The left atrium is markedly enlarged.

resting electrocardiogram ("strain pattern") or ST-segment changes on an exercise electrocardiogram indicate that the stenosis is severe.

Echocardiography
On M-mode echocardiography the aortic valve appears thickened with multiple echoes and decreased excursion (Figs. 5–1 and 5–2A; see also Fig. 2–7C). Calcific AS has the appearance of a dense cloud of high-intensity echoes returning from the area of the aortic valve (Fig. 5–2B). The parallelogram of the valve motion may be obscured or obliterated. The thickness of the septum and the left ventricular (LV) free wall is a measure of LV hypertrophy, which correlates with the degree of severity of AS (Fig. 5–3). The ratio of thickness of the LV wall to LV diastolic dimension has been shown to correlate in young people with the severity of stenosis. Decreased LV contractions or LV dilatation indicates myocardial decompensation. Mitral flutter on M-mode echocardiography or evidence by Doppler of reversed flow in the LVOT during diastole in an individual with AS indicates that aortic insufficiency is associated. Thickening of the mitral valve or mitral stenosis is evidence of a rheumatic cause. On 2-D echocardiography the long axis reveals doming or thickening, or both and reduced mobility (Figs. 5–2C and D, 5–4A–D) of the valve. The short axis (Fig. 5–4E and F) may show a cross section of the narrowed orifice, allowing planimetric measurement of its area. Some authors have reported a significant correlation between the area of the valve measured by 2-D echocardiography and area of the valve calculated from hemodynamic data. 2-D echocardiography can also identify associated supravalvular AS, subaortic membrane,

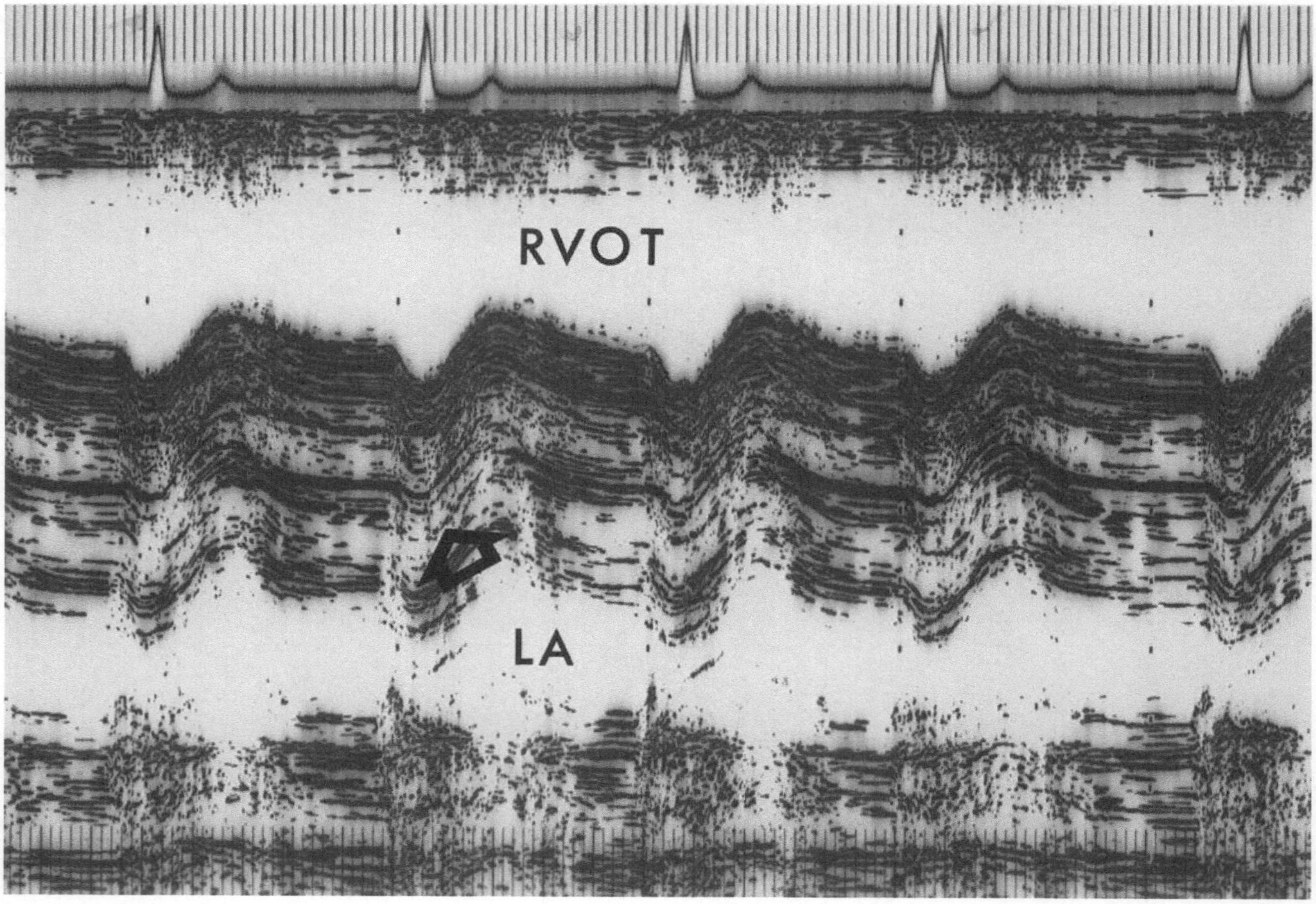

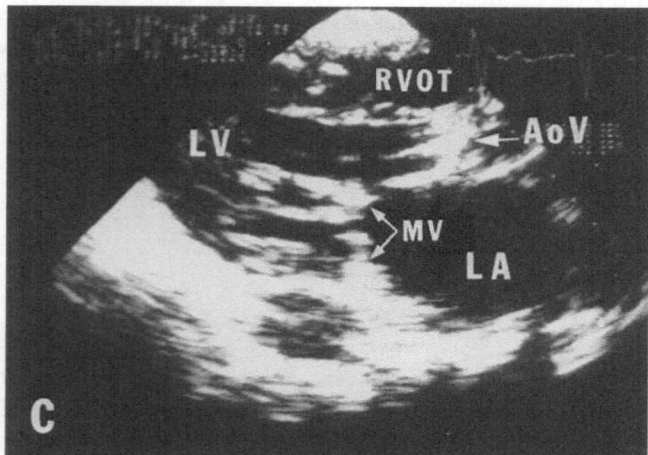

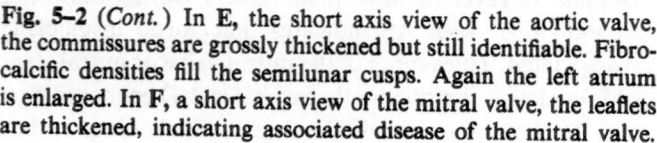

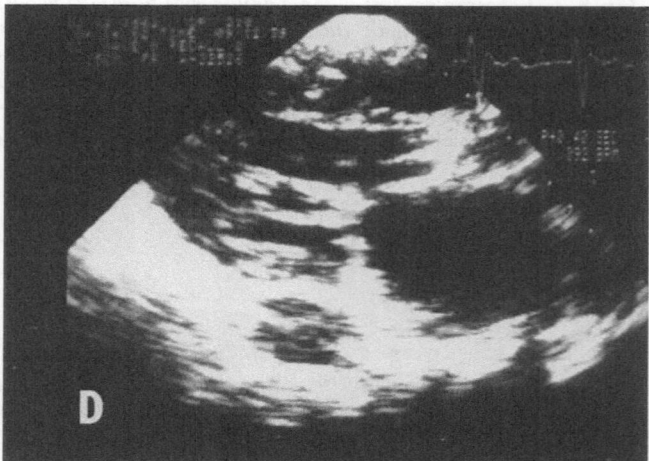

Fig. 5–2 (*Cont.*) In **E**, the short axis view of the aortic valve, the commissures are grossly thickened but still identifiable. Fibro-calcific densities fill the semilunar cusps. Again the left atrium is enlarged. In **F**, a short axis view of the mitral valve, the leaflets are thickened, indicating associated disease of the mitral valve. In the presence of involvement of two valves, a rheumatic etiology should be considered. *RVOT* = right ventricular outflow tract; *LA* = left atrium; *LV* = left ventricle; *AoV* = aortic valve; *MV* = mitral valve; *RV* = right ventricle.

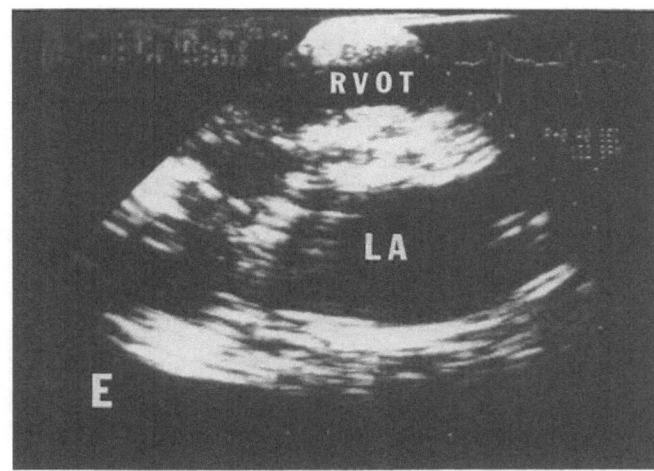

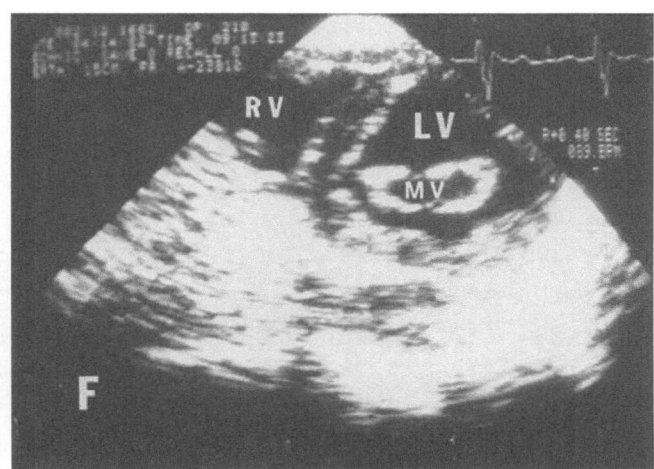

a fibrous tunnel and hypertrophic obstructive cardiomyopathy. Doppler echocardiography, using continuous wave (CW) technique and spectral analysis, has been found accurate in estimating the pressure difference across the valve in children and young adults. In older adults estimation is less reliable because of difficulty in detecting the high frequency components of the Doppler signal.

Radiological (Plain Film) Features
The plain films may be normal, or LV hypertrophy may be reflected as rounding of the cardiac apex (Fig. 5–5). With LV dilatation the left heart border elongates, moving the apex downward and to the left so that it projects below the left hemidiaphragm on the frontal view (Fig. 5–6). Left ventricular dilatation is a sign of cardiac decompensation in pure aortic AS or a sign of volume loading if aortic insufficiency is associated. Thus, failure to determine the presence or absence of associated aortic insufficiency may lead to misinterpretation of the severity of AS on plain films. The aortic arch is usually normal. Dilatation of the ascending aorta (poststenotic dilatation) may or may not be present. If present, it is best demonstrated on the PA view as a convexity of the superior segment of the right heart border (Fig. 5–6A). Poststenotic dilatation of the ascending aorta is also recognized on the LAO projection (Fig. 5–6C) and on occasion in the lateral view. Calcification of the aortic valve is common in adults with AS and is best detected in the lateral, LAO or RAO view (Fig. 5–6). It is poorly visualized or not discernible on the PA view. Mild degrees of calcification are readily demonstrated on cine fluorography. Calcification of acquired AS may appear as three deeply convex lines representing the lines of insertion of the three well-formed sinuses (Figs. 5–6, 5–7). The pseudoraphe (Fig. 5–9) in acquired bicuspid aortic valve appears as a tall slender line on the lateral or LAO view and should be distinguished from congenital bicuspid aortic valve in which the true raphe appears bulbous (Fig. 5–10). Patterns of calcification specific for the

diagnosis of bicuspid aortic valve have been described by Spindola-Franco et al. (see Bicuspid Aortic Valve). Signs of left atrial (LA) dilatation and pulmonary venous hypertension (CHF pattern) in patients with AS are signs of cardiac decompensation, which usually indicate a poor prognosis, particularly without treatment.

Hemodynamics
In valvular AS a systolic pressure gradient exists between the LV and the aorta. In subaortic stenosis the gradient is between the sinus of the LV and its outflow tract, while in supravalvar stenosis the gradient is between the proximal and distal segments of the aorta just beyond the aortic valve. Cardiac output may be well maintained despite severe obstruction. As long as a normal cardiac output is maintained, the peak systolic gradient and LV peak pressure correlate with the severity of the obstruction. A peak valve gradient less than 30 mm Hg indicates mild stenosis; a gradient between 40 and 90 mm Hg, moderate stenosis; and a gradient above 90–100 mm Hg with normal cardiac output, severe stenosis. As cardiac decompensation supervenes the heart is not able to maintain a normal output. As cardiac output decreases the pressure gradient at the valve decreases so that the gradient is no longer a reliable indicator of severity of the stenosis.

In such instances calculation of the area of the valve is helpful, using Gorlin's hydraulic formula:

$$A = \frac{F}{C \times 44.5 \sqrt{\text{mean gradient}}}$$

where A = Valve area (cm²)

   C = Empiric orifice correction factor obtained by comparing the calculated valve area with the valve area measured at surgery (C = 1 for the aortic valve).

Mean gradient is obtained from the planimetered area between the superimposed aortic and left

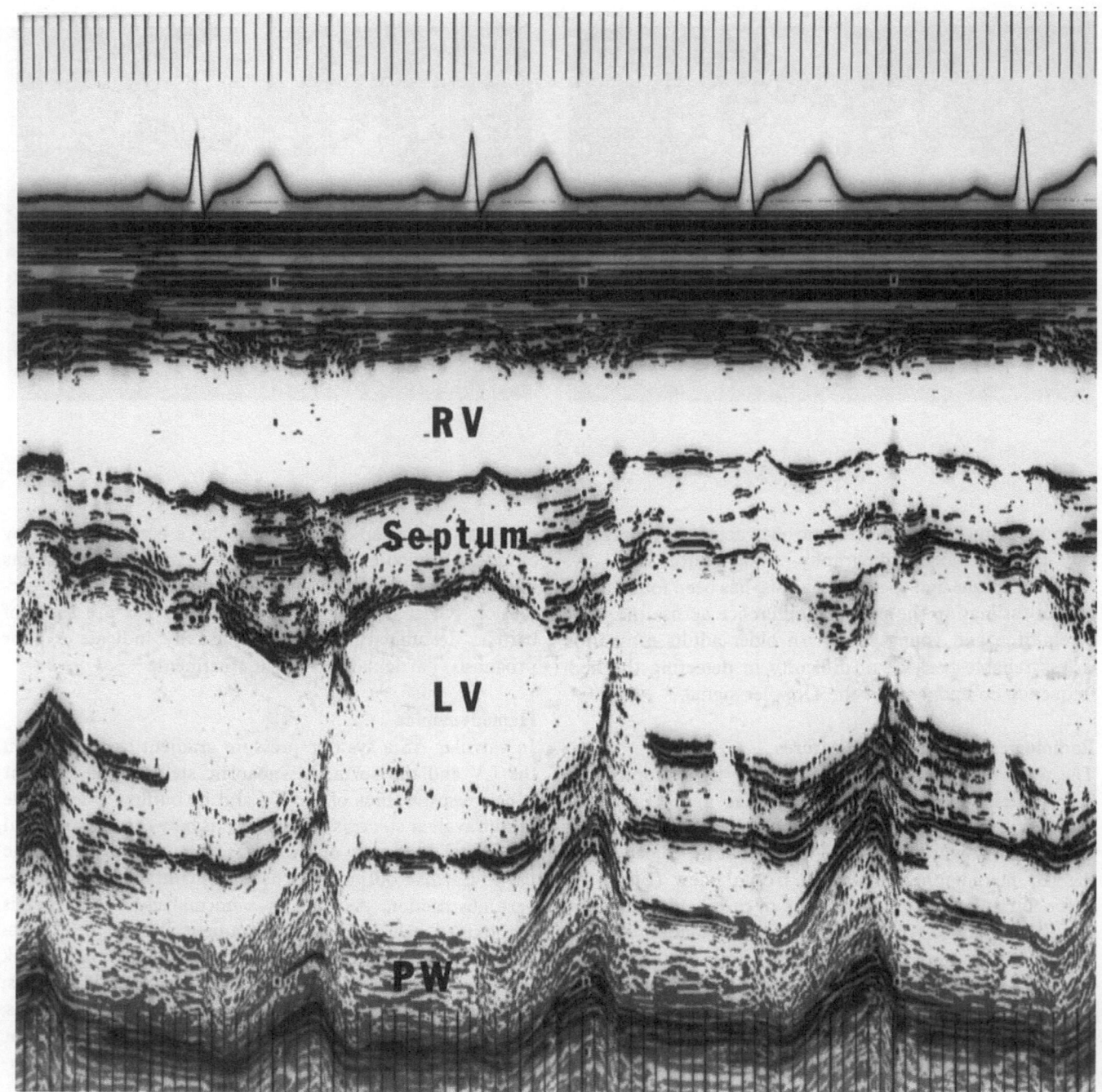

Fig. 5–3. *Left ventricular hypertrophy. M-mode echocardiogram in a young adult with residual moderate aortic stenosis 5 years after valvulotomy.* The septum and left ventricular free wall are thickened, each measuring 1.6 cm (normal approximately 1.0 cm). Left ventricular contractions are normal: Shortening fraction = 40%; mean velocity of circumferential fiber shortening (mVCF) = 1.3 circumferences/sec. *RV* = right ventricle; *LV* = left ventricle; *PW* = posterior wall of left ventricle.

ventricular pressure tracings during systole (mm Hg × sec) divided by the ventricular ejection time (sec)

F = flow rate across the aortic valve obtained from this formula:

$$F = \frac{\text{cardiac output (ml/min)}}{\text{systolic ejection period (sec/min)}}$$

Where the systolic ejection period is the number of seconds per minute during which ventricular ejection occurs (ventricular ejection time × heart rate).

In adults a normal valve area is about 3–4 cm² or 2 cm²/m². A valve area of about 0.6–0.7 cm²/m² is considered a severe narrowing. A valve area of about 0.4 cm²/m² is "critical," generally requiring surgical treatment. The presence or absence of aortic insufficiency must be determined before a valve area is calculated. With aortic insuffi-

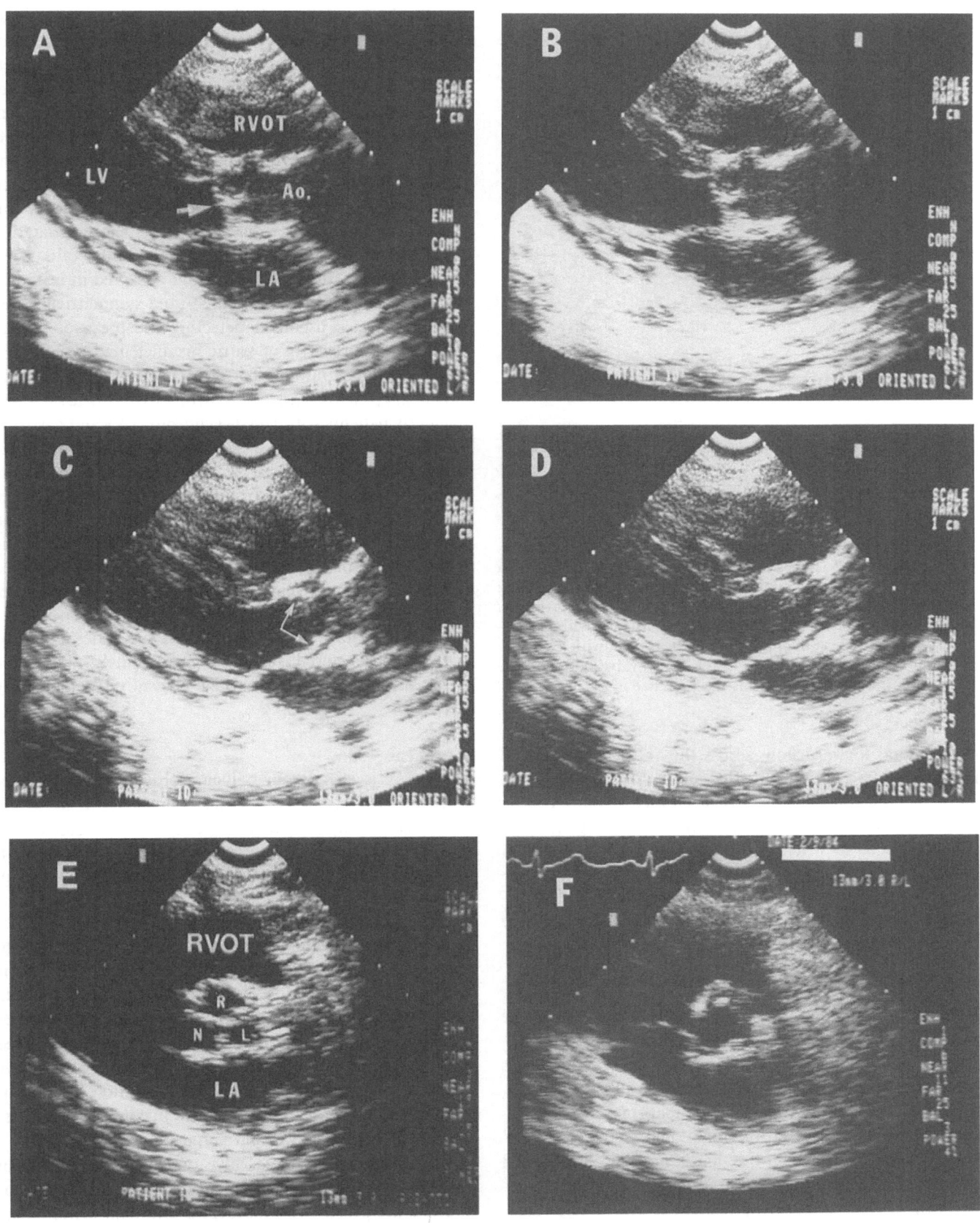

Fig. 5–4. *Two-dimensional echocardiogram in an 11-year-old boy with congenital aortic stenosis.* **A–D** long axis views; and **E** and **F** short axis views. **A** (with labels) **B** (without labels) represent diastole; **C** and **D** represent systole. On the long axis during diastole (**A** and **B**) the aortic valve (*arrow*) is thickened. During systole (**C** and **D**) doming of the valve is noted (*arrows*). On the short axis (**E** and **F**) the aortic valve is thickened, and three commissures are identified during diastole (**E**). During systole (**F**) the orifice of the aortic root has an irregular border and is reduced. *Ao.* = aortic root; *LA* = left atrium; *LV* = left ventricle; *N* = noncoronary cusp; *R* = right coronary cusp; *L* = left coronary cusp; *RVOT* = right ventricular outflow tract.

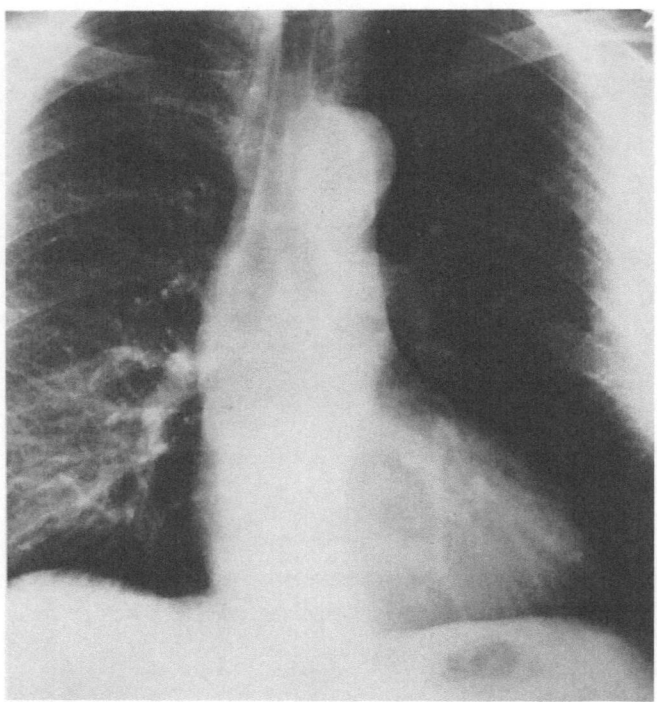

Fig. 5–5 *Posteroanterior roentgenogram of the chest in a 62-year-old man with aortic stenosis.* The heart is mildly enlarged with rounding of the cardiac apex and prominence of the ascending aorta. Rounding of the apex suggests left ventricular hypertrophy. The prominence of the ascending aorta is consistent with poststenotic dilatation. These findings may also be present with hypertension, but extensive calcification of the aortic valve noted on the lateral film (not shown) confirms the presence of aortic stenosis.

ciency, total forward flow across the valve is the sum of forward cardiac output plus the volume of the blood that leaks back into the ventricle (regurgitant volume.) The regurgitant volume must be calculated from the angiographic determinations of volume together with measurements of cardiac output obtained on cardiac catheterization (see section, Aortic Insufficiency). Elevation of the LV end-diastolic pressure or the pulmonary capillary wedge pressure indicates impaired LV performance.

Contrast Studies

Left ventriculography is important in identification of the site of the stenotic lesion (i.e., subvalvar, valvar, supravalvar). A compound axial view (LAO with cranial tilt) is particularly useful in identification of a subaortic membrane (Fig. 7–196C). Mitral involvement (presence and degree) is also assessed, and the functional status of the LV is evaluated. The ejection fraction is normal or increased with AS. If the ejection fraction is depressed (global hypokinesis), valvular cardiomyopathy is the most likely cause. Segmental abnormalities of wall motion, characteristic for ischemic cardiomyopathy, can also occur with valvular cardiomyopathy.

On aortography the degree of thickening, deformity and limitation in motion of the aortic leaflets can be determined readily; however, the appearance of the valve does not necessarily correlate with the severity of the stenosis as indicated by the hemodynamic data. If calcification is not extensive the type of aortic valve (bicuspid or trileaflet) can be determined. The aortogram in acquired AS outlines the three well-formed sinuses of Valsalva. The leaflets are thickened and limited in motion. Doming of the leaflets may be demonstrated in systole with reconstitution of the sinuses of Valsalva in diastole (Fig. 5–8). A jet of unopacified blood entering the aorta during systole is further evidence of moderate or severe AS. Poststenotic dilatation of the ascending aorta (usually asymmetrical) is often present. In contrast, the aortic dilatation observed in instances of cystic medial necrosis is bulbous and symmetrical. Aortography is also useful in detecting the presence of and estimating the severity of aortic insufficiency.

The authors routinely perform coronary arteriography in patients past 40 years of age with valvular heart disease. In elderly patients with Heyde syndrome (AS and gastrointestinal bleeding), selective celiac and superior and inferior mesenteric artery angiography is performed to demonstrate angiodysplasias of the gastrointestinal tract, principally in the right colon. The angiographic hallmark of the lesion is an early draining vein, i.e., a vein that fills during the arterial phase of the study and is more heavily opacified than the rest of the veins draining the bowel. While arteriovenous shunting may be the only positive feature, the malformation itself may be recognized as a series of dilated and tortuous arterial vessels. Approximately 20%–25% of patients with proved vascular ectasia on colonoscopy have AS.

Treatment

Valvotomy is effective in reducing obstruction in the absence of calcification. Care must be taken to incise the commissures only partially, so that all leaflets remain well supported. Nevertheless, severe aortic insufficiency with myocardial decompensation can ensue. Over the long term, fibrosis progresses and the stenosis tends to recur, even if the initial operation is successful.

Replacement of the valve is necessary to relieve the obstruction if a valve is significantly calcified. The risk is low unless myocardial decompensation is present prior to surgery. The necessity for surgery is assessed by clinical judgment. Obviously a valve area of 0.4 cm²/m², associated with symptoms, deserves treatment. Syncope, progressive cardiomegaly, progressive decrease in ejection fraction or abnormalities of wall motion, alone or in combination, presage a poor prognosis without surgery.

Complications of aortic valve replacement, other than intraoperative mortality and perioperative myocardial infarction, are prosthetic endocarditis and dehiscence. Also, for mechanical valve prostheses the special difficulties encountered are structural failure, thrombosis, hemolysis, obstruction and insufficiency. Hemorrhage also occurs, because of the necessity for anticoagulant therapy. Anticoagulants are not necessary with a bioprosthesis; however, the bioprostheses are somewhat less durable than

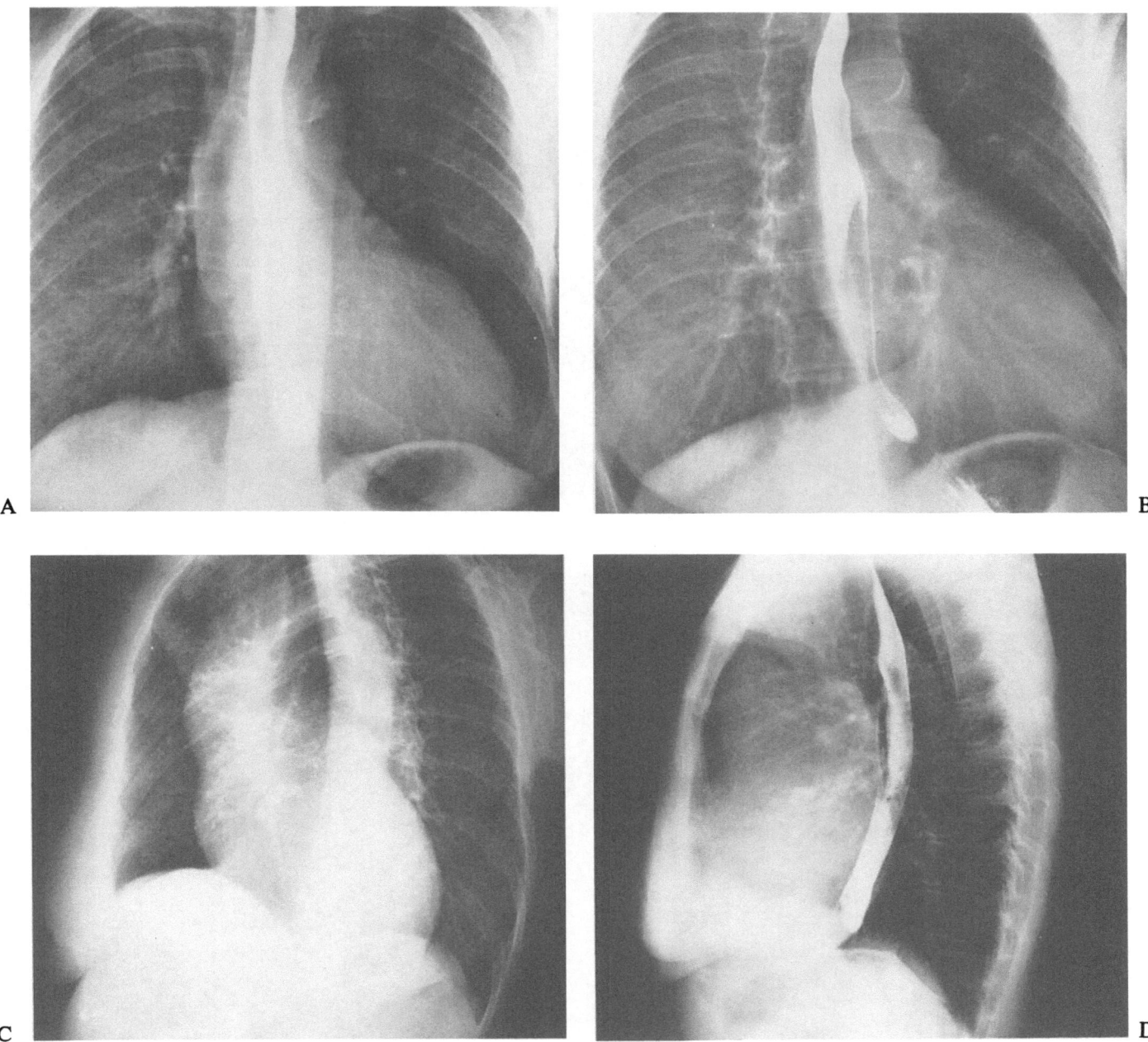

Fig. 5–6. *Roentgenograms of the chest in a woman with calcific aortic stenosis without aortic insufficiency on aortography.* **A** PA film; **B** RAO view; **C** LAO view; **D** lateral film. In the posteroanterior projection (**A**) the left heart border is elongated, with the apex projecting below the left hemidiaphragm. The ascending aorta is prominent. The heavy calcification proven to be present in the aortic valve is not visualized on the frontal plain film. In the RAO projection (**B**) the calcium forms a circular pattern representing the aortic valve while the commissures form a "Mercedes Benz sign" in this view. In the LAO view (**C**) the left ventricle and the ascending aorta are both prominent. The calcified valve is poorly visualized because of underpenetration. In the lateral view (**D**) the dilated ascending aorta narrows the retrosternal clear space. The calcified valve is well appreciated in this view. These roentgenograms demonstrate the position of the aortic valve in the various projections. Enlargement of the left ventricle in a patient without aortic insufficiency indicates early decompensation. If significant aortic insufficiency had been present the ventricular enlargement would have been due to volume loading rather than decompensation.

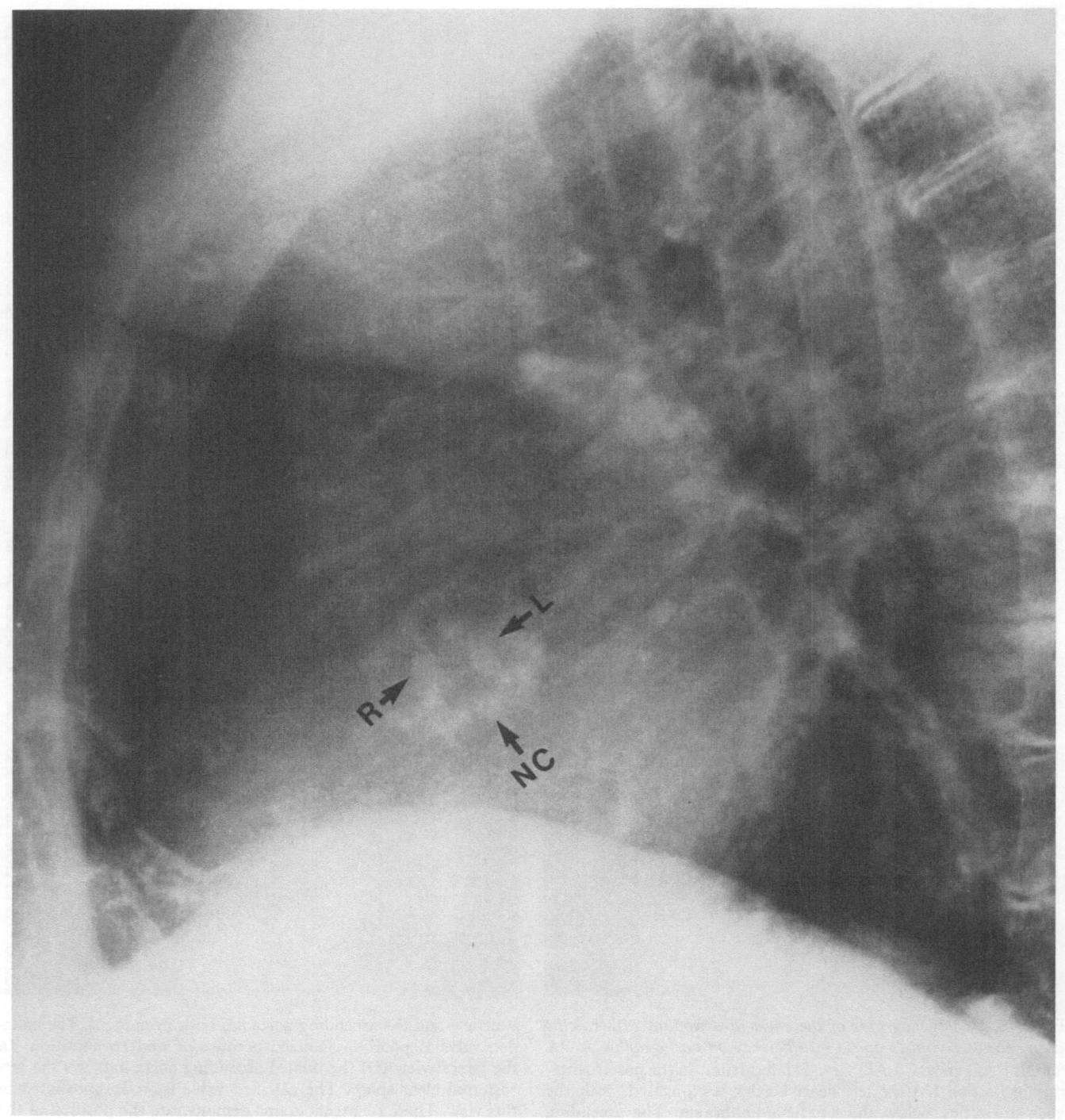

Fig. 5–7. *Lateral roentgenogram of the chest in an 82-year-old woman with calcific aortic stenosis.* The attachments of the three leaflets to the root of the aorta are represented. Compare this image with the pattern of calcification associated with bicuspid aortic valve (Figs. 5–10, 5–16, 5–17) and acquired bicuspid aortic valve (Fig. 5–9). *NC* = noncoronary cusp; *R* = right coronary (or anterior) cusp; *L* = left coronary cusp.

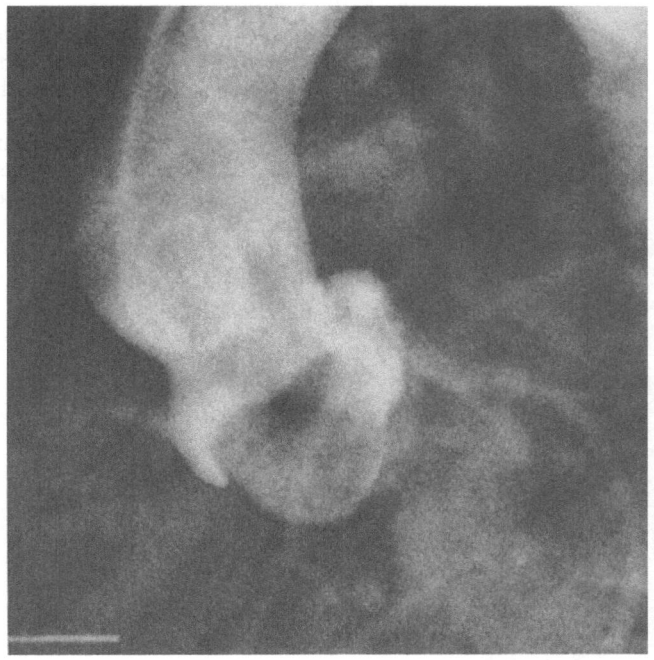

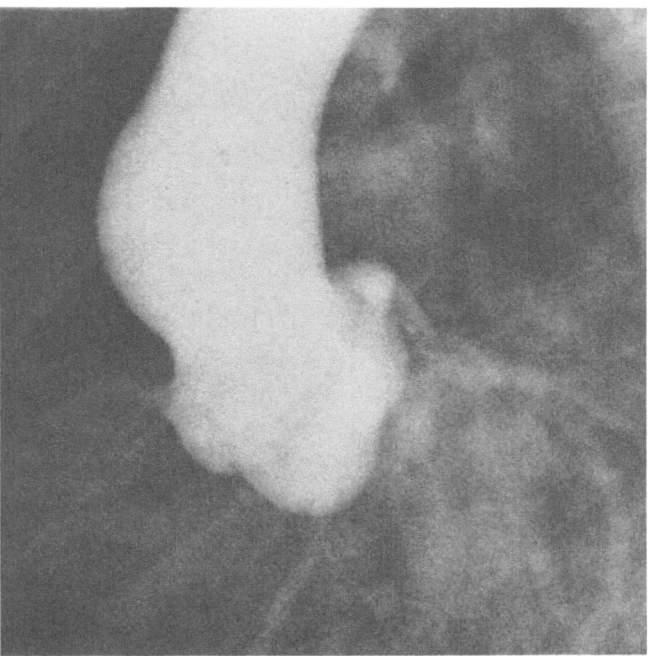

A

B

Fig. 5–8. *Aortogram in an adult male with a stenotic trileaflet aortic valve.* During systole (**A**) doming occurs and a jet of unopacified blood impinges on the anterior lateral wall of the ascending aorta, resulting in asymmetrical dilatation. During diastole (**B**) the three semilunar sinuses are reconstituted.

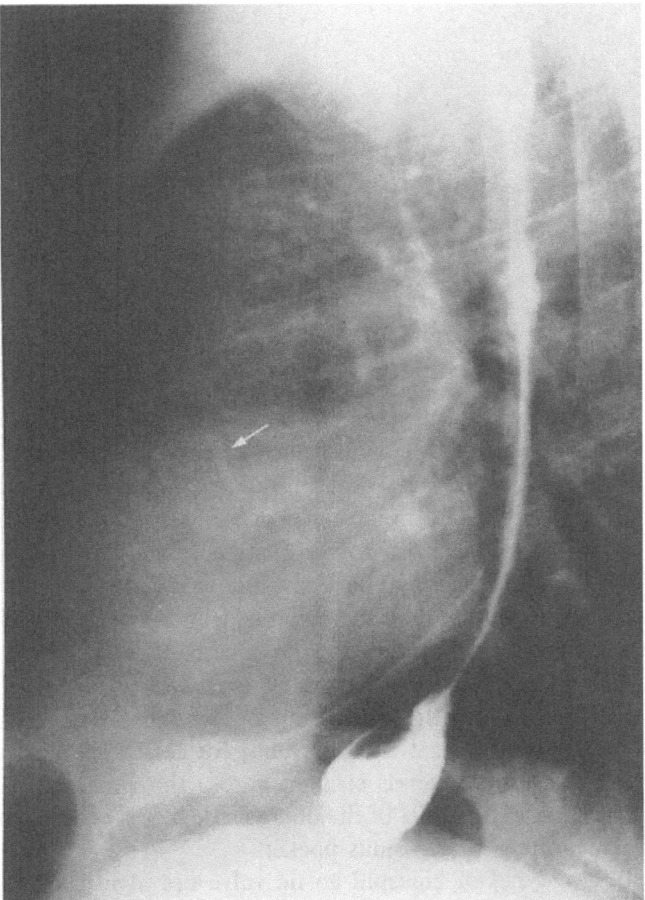

A

5–9. *Acquired bicuspid aortic valve.* **A** Lateral roentgenogram of the chest shows the characteristic linear pattern of the false raphe (or pseudoraphe). **B** Aortogram in diastole demonstrated three well-formed sinuses of Valsalva. Spindola-Franco H et al (1982) Recognition of bicuspid aortic valve by plain film calcification. Am J Roentgenol 139:867–872. Copyright 1982. Reproduced by permission.

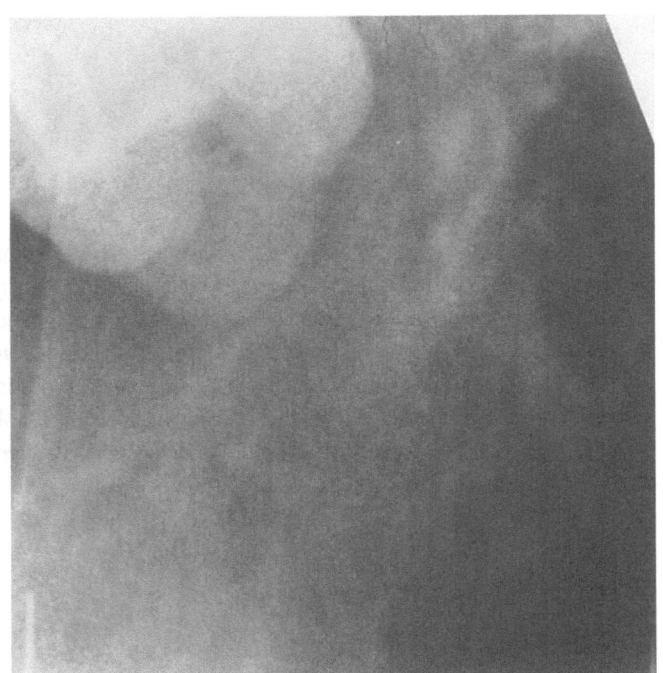

B

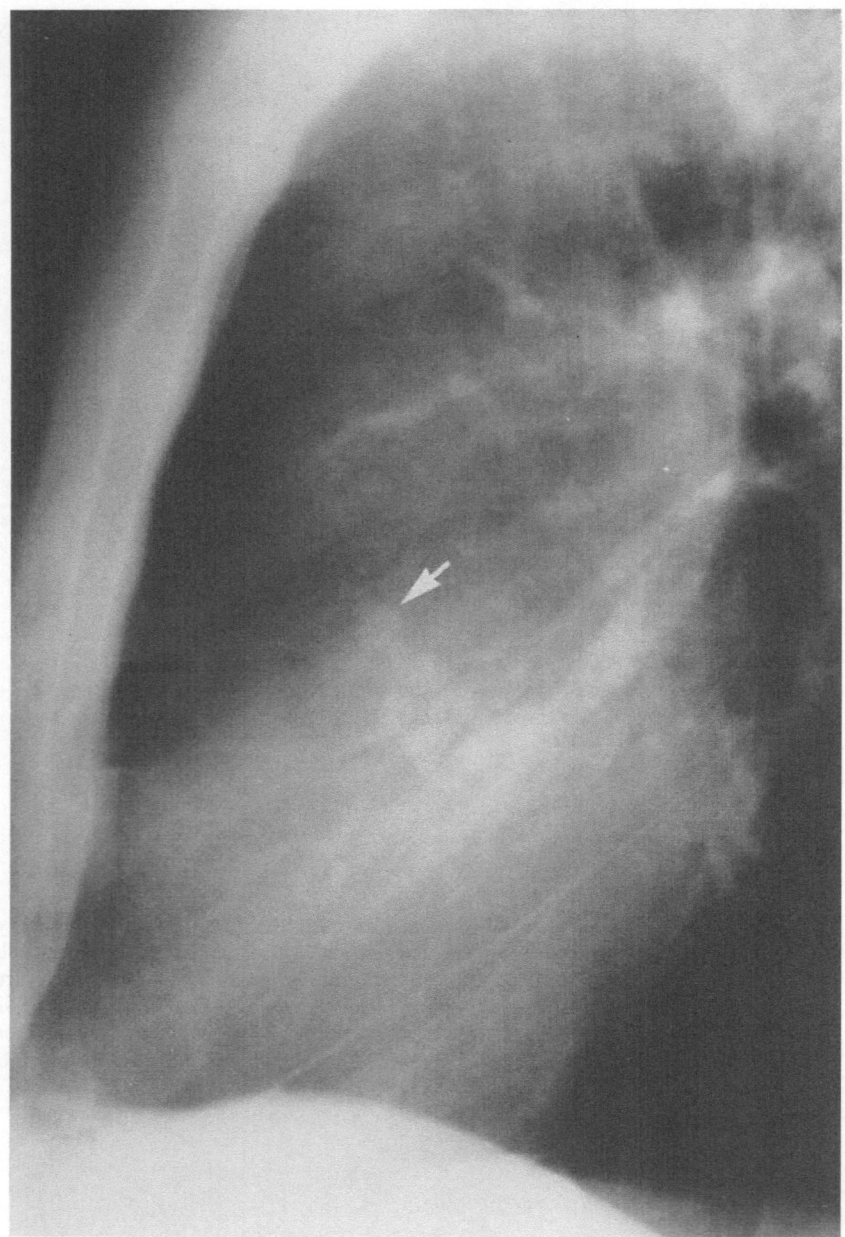

Fig. 5–10. *Lateral roentgenogram of the chest in a patient with a calcified congenital bicuspid aortic valve (type I, see Fig. 5–15).* The bulbous or clublike appearance of the raphe is illustrated (*arrow*). Spindola-Franco H et al (1982) Recognition of bicuspid aortic valve by plain film calcification. Am J Roentgenol. 139:867–872. Copyright 1982. Reproduced by permission.

mechanical valves because of their tendency toward perforation and development of calcification.

Bioprostheses are indicated for individuals who cannot be given anticoagulant agents, for women of childbearing age who plan additional pregnancies and for patients whose anticipated life expectancy from other causes is less than 7 years. Mechanical prostheses are indicated for patients with atrial fibrillation, for patients who require valves of smaller size and for those individuals who wish to reduce their chance of reoperation to a minimum.

Bicuspid Aortic Valve

Bicuspid aortic valve is the most common congenital cardiac defect, occurring in approximately 2% of the general population. A bicuspid aortic valve consists of two major cusps instead of three. One cusp, designated the conjoint leaflet, is divided by a shallow ridge or "raphe" along its aortic aspect. The raphe never extends to the free edge of the leaflet. The other cusp lacks a raphe and is called the nonfused leaflet. The two cusps generally are about equal in size, although the conjoint leaflet may be slightly larger than one normal cusp but smaller than two normal cusps. The circumferential distance between the two commissures around the aortic ring is equal or nearly equal. The sinus of Valsalva of the conjoint leaflet is shallow, and the leaflet extends straight across the aortic anulus. The sinus of Valsalva of the nonfused leaflet is deeply convex, forming a deep sinus pocket.

Two types of bicuspid aortic valve are identified (Fig. 5–11). When right and left cusps are present the commis-

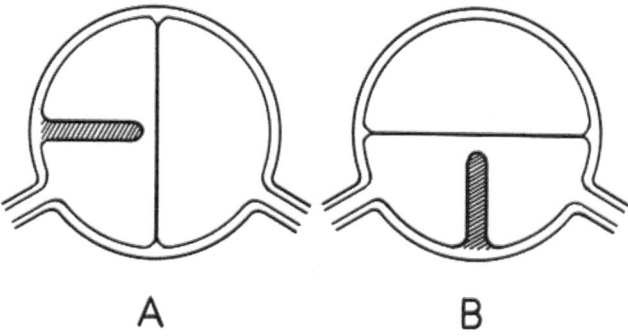

Fig. 5–11. *The two types of congenital bicuspid aortic valves.* In A a right and a left cusp are present, and the commissures are anterior and posterior. The line of coaptation runs from front to back. The raphe is in the right cusp (or conjoint leaflet). One coronary artery arises from each cusp. In **B** the cusps are anterior and posterior, and the commissures are right sided and left sided. The leaflets coapt in a line running from side to side. The raphe is in the anterior cusp (or conjoint leaflet). Both coronary arteries arise in front of the anterior or conjoint leaflet. Spindola-Franco H, et al.: Recognition of bicuspid aortic valve by plain film calcification. Am J Roentgenol 139:867–872. Copyright 1982. By permission.

sures are anterior and posterior and a coronary artery arises from each cusp. The raphe is in the right cusp. When anterior and posterior cusps are present the raphe is located in the anterior cusp. The commissures are right and left sided, and both coronary arteries arise from the aortic root in front of the anterior cusp. Johnson et al. described the frequent occurrence of a short left main coronary artery

and dominance of the left coronary artery in association with bicuspid aortic valve. Congenital bicuspid aortic valve may be differentiated from the acquired form (see subsequent discussion).

Bicuspid aortic valve is usually not stenotic from birth; however, in rare cases, when a bicuspid valve is also dysplastic, it produces a critical degree of AS in infancy. On occasion a congenital bicuspid valve presents in childhood with significant stenosis that generally progresses in severity during childhood and adolescence. A few children may have associated aortic insufficiency secondary to congenital bicuspid valve. In such instances the valves tend to be less fibrotic. Calcification along "lines of stress" may occur at an early age, but by the age of 50–60 years, most valves are heavily calcified. Early calcification appears in the raphe and along the base of the leaflets. Later in life the sinuses of Valsalva become filled with calcific masses, and valve motion becomes severely limited. One pathological study reports that stenosis occurred in 6% of bicuspid valves between the age of 20 and 39 years, in 18%–21% between age 40 and 69 years and in 40% between 70 and 89 years. In 27% of individuals the valves appeared to function normally, even in the oldest age group. Infective endocarditis occurs frequently in bicuspid aortic valves in individuals below age 50–59 years but infrequently in patients with severely calcified valves.

A nonstenotic bicuspid valve produces a characteristic systolic ejection click at the apex (Fig. 5–12). Stenosis is indicated by a systolic murmur in the aortic area that

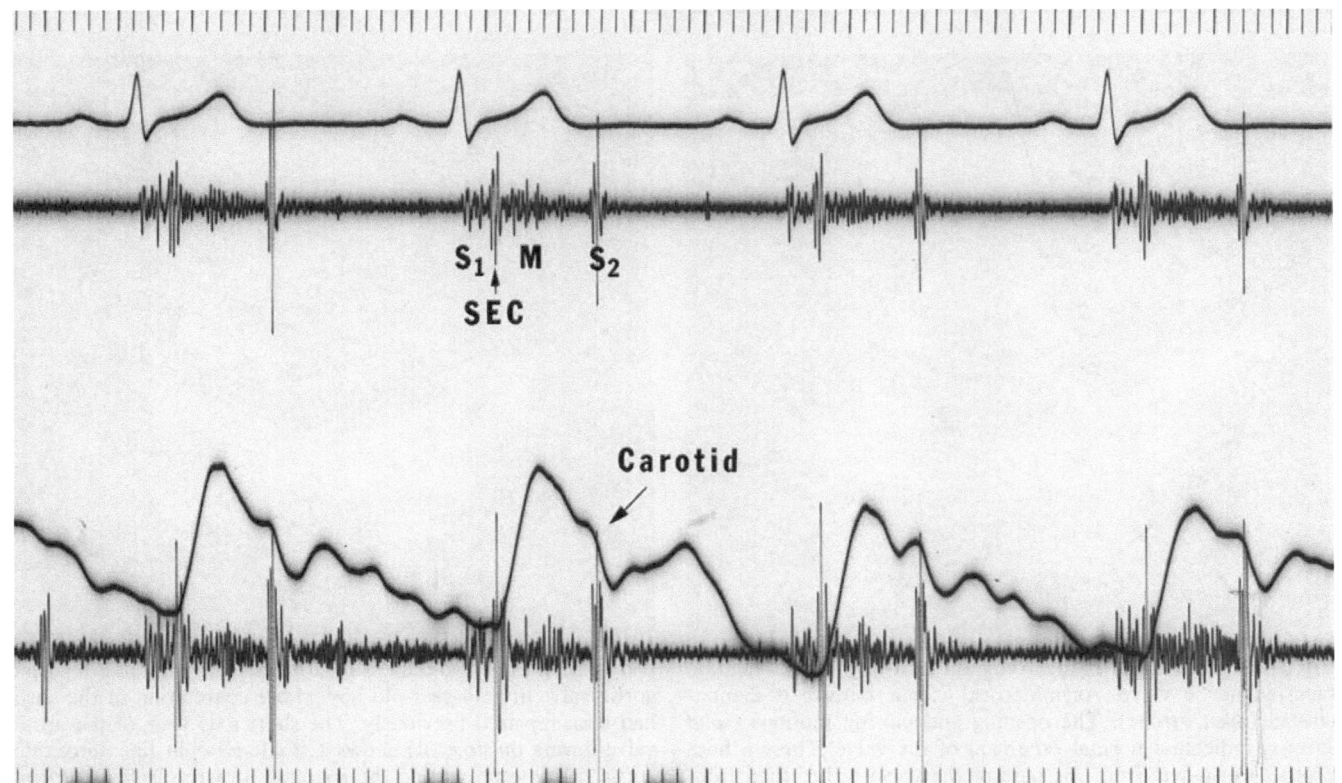

Fig. 5–12. *Phonocardiogram in a young man with aortic stenosis.* A typical systolic ejection click (*SEC*) and a systolic ejection murmur (*M*) are demonstrated. The carotid trace is normal. S_1 = first heart sound; S_2 = second heart sound.

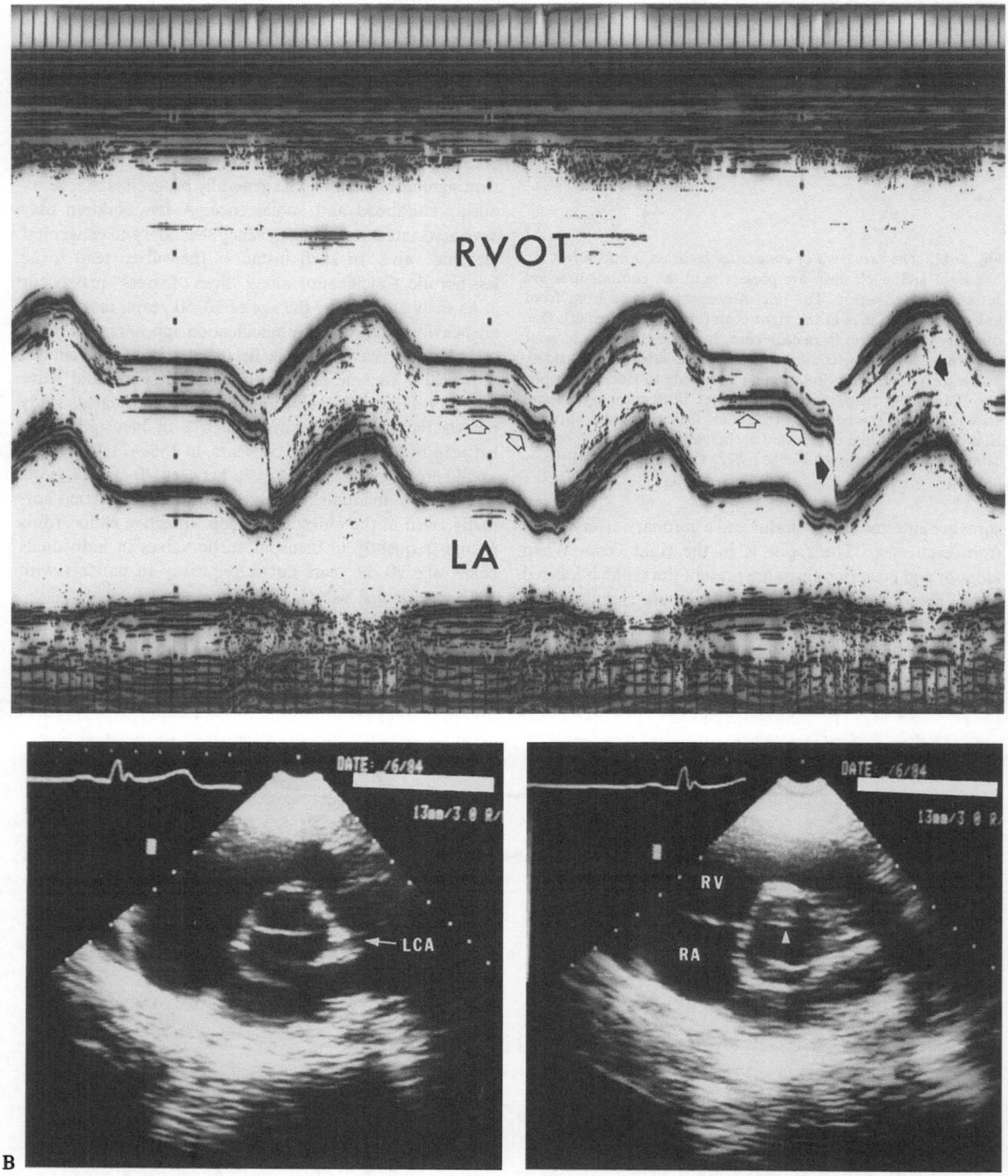

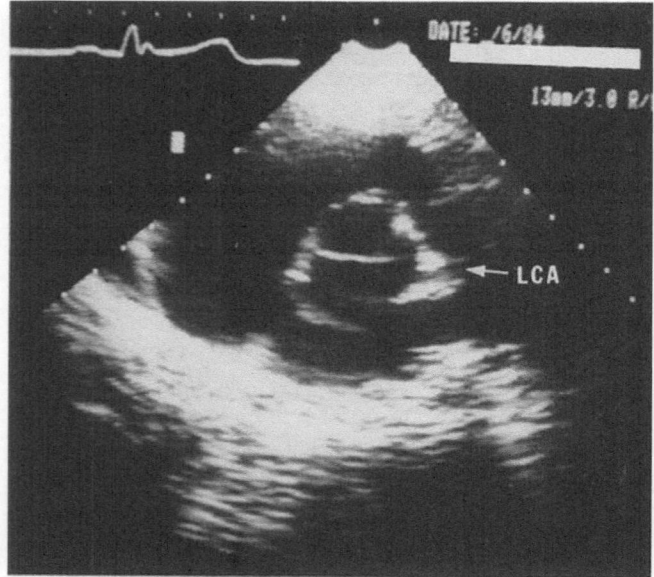

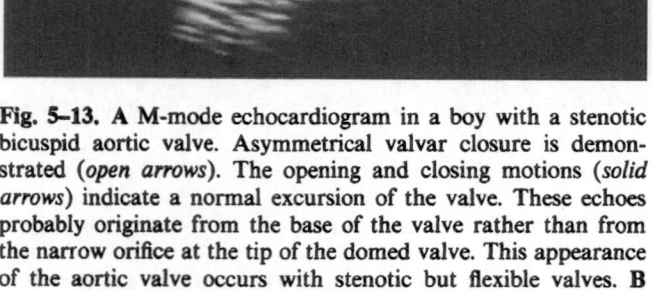

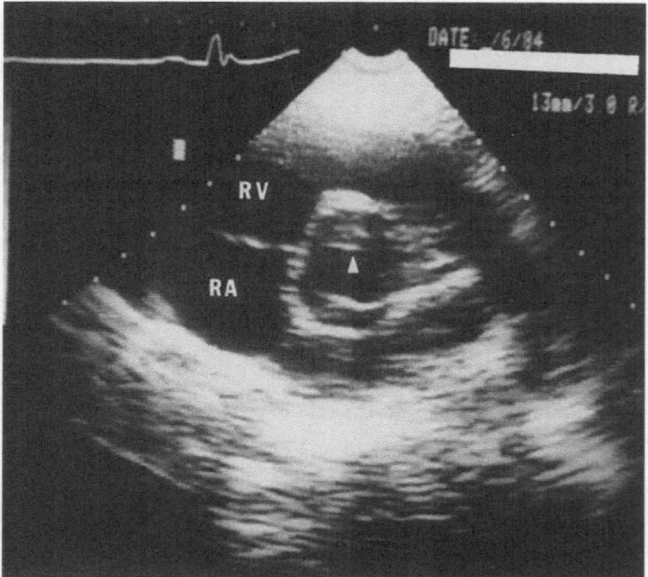

Fig. 5–13. A M-mode echocardiogram in a boy with a stenotic bicuspid aortic valve. Asymmetrical valvar closure is demonstrated (*open arrows*). The opening and closing motions (*solid arrows*) indicate a normal excursion of the valve. These echoes probably originate from the base of the valve rather than from the narrow orifice at the tip of the domed valve. This appearance of the aortic valve occurs with stenotic but flexible valves. **B** and **C** are from a two-dimensional echocardiogram of a bicuspid aortic valve in a 14-year-old boy whose coarctation of the aorta had been repaired previously. The short axis view of the aortic valve during diastole (**B**) shows a single straight line across the aortic orifice representing the coaptation of the leaflets. During systole (**C**) the two leaflets diverge anteriorly (*arrowhead*) and posteriorly.

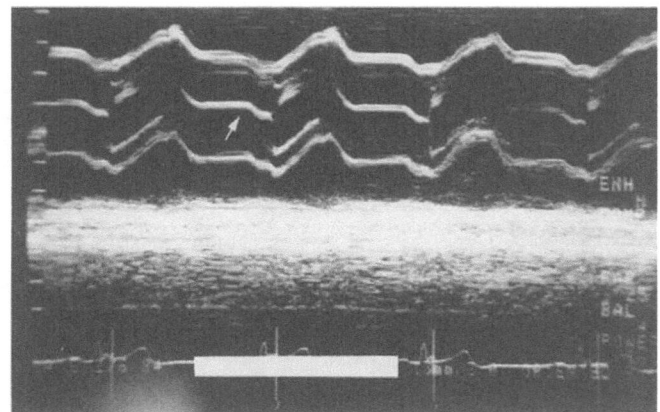

D

Fig. 5–13 (*Cont.*) **D** is the M-mode echocardiogram of the aortic valve in this patient. Note that the line of coaptation (*arrow*) is in the center of the aortic root during diastole. Therefore, this bicuspid aortic valve would not have been recognized by M-mode echocardiography alone. Compare with Fig. 5–4E, a case of aortic stenosis with a trileaflet aortic valve in which an apposition of the free edges of the leaflets form the characteristic "Mercedes Benz" sign during diastole. *RV* = right ventricle; *RA* = right atrium; *LCA* = left coronary artery.

radiates to the carotid arteries. Moderate to severe stenosis is suggested by a thrill in the suprasternal notch and along the carotid arteries. On M-mode echocardiography the finding most characteristic of bicuspid aortic valve is asymmetrical closure of the valve (Fig. 5–13A). On 2-D echocardiography the short axis view of the aortic valve shows the nonfused leaflet and the conjoint leaflet forming a single line of coaptation across the aortic anulus during diastole (Fig. 5–13B). During systole the opening motion of the two leaflets is demonstrated (Fig. 5–13C), in contrast to the "Mercedez-Benz" sign occurring with a normal aortic valve (Fig. 2–20). On aortography (Fig. 5–14) a bicuspid valve is diagnosed when each leaflet of the aortic valve encompasses the entire width of the aortic root in the left anterior oblique or lateral view. The conjoint leaflet forms a slightly curved line across the root of the aorta, while the nonfused leaflet is deeply convex and forms the lower margin of the aortic root. During systole a jet of contrast medium may be apparent, the aortic root being often asymmetrically dilated by the jet against its wall. On occasion, mild aortic insufficiency is present. Severe aortic insufficiency is uncommon with bicuspid aortic valve unless infective endocarditis is superimposed. When heavy calcification is present the sinuses of Valsalva are obliterated and the diagnosis of bicuspid aortic valve can no longer be verified by aortography. In such instances the patterns of calcification observed on plain films (Fig. 5–15) are more likely to be diagnostic than is aortography, the diagnosis being based on the characteristic bulbous appearance of the calcified raphe (Fig. 5–10). The calcified lines of insertion of the shallow conjoint leaflet and of the deeply convex nonfused leaflet also facilitate recognition (Figs. 5–16 and 5–17). In the authors' study of 120 patients with severe calcification of the aortic valve a bicuspid aortic valve was diagnosed in 26 (65%) of 40 patients in whom a bicuspid valve

was observed at surgery. Aortography, on the other hand, was diagnostic in only 25% of cases.

A stenotic bicuspid aortic valve is usually not amenable to commissurotomy because the stenosis is caused by fibrosis and calcification rather than by commissural fusion. A surgical incision to widen the commissure or divide the conjoint leaflet leaves the free edges unsupported, so that aortic insufficiency ensues. When surgical intervention is required in these cases, replacement of the valve is usually necessary.

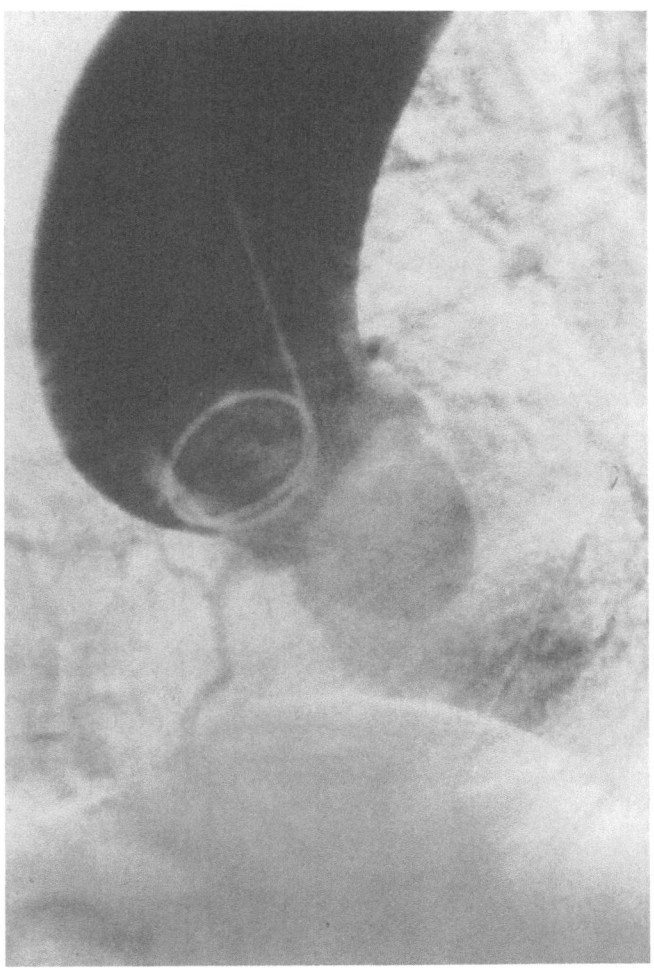

Fig. 5–14. *Aortogram* (*lateral view*) in a congenital bicuspid aortic valve. The single nonfused leaflet encompasses the entire width of the aortic root, forming its deeply convex lower margin. The conjoint leaflet forms a slightly curved line across the root of the aorta. Spindola-Franco H et al (1982) Recognition of bicuspid aortic valve by plain film calcification. Am J Roentgenol 139:867–872. Copyright 1982. Reproduced by permission.

Type I   = 3/40

Type II   = 9/40

Type III   = 10/40

Type IV   = 2/40

Type V   = 2/40

Fig. 5–15. *Patterns of calcification of bicuspid aortic valve and their incidence. Type I,* calcified raphe; *Type II,* calcification of raphe and shallow line of insertion of the conjoint leaflet; *Type III,* calcified raphe and calcification of the lines of insertion of both leaflets (this pattern looks like an upside down mushroom); *Type IV,* calcification of the same structures as in *Type III,* but the calcified aortic ring is rotated, forming a circle on lateral plain chest films; *Type V,* calcification of the shallow conjoint leaflet and deeply convex nonfused leaflet (boat-shape configuration); the raphe is not calcified. Spindola-Franco H et al (1982) Recognition of bicuspid aortic valve by plain film calcification. Am J Roentgenol 139:867–872. Copyright 1982. Reproduced by permission.

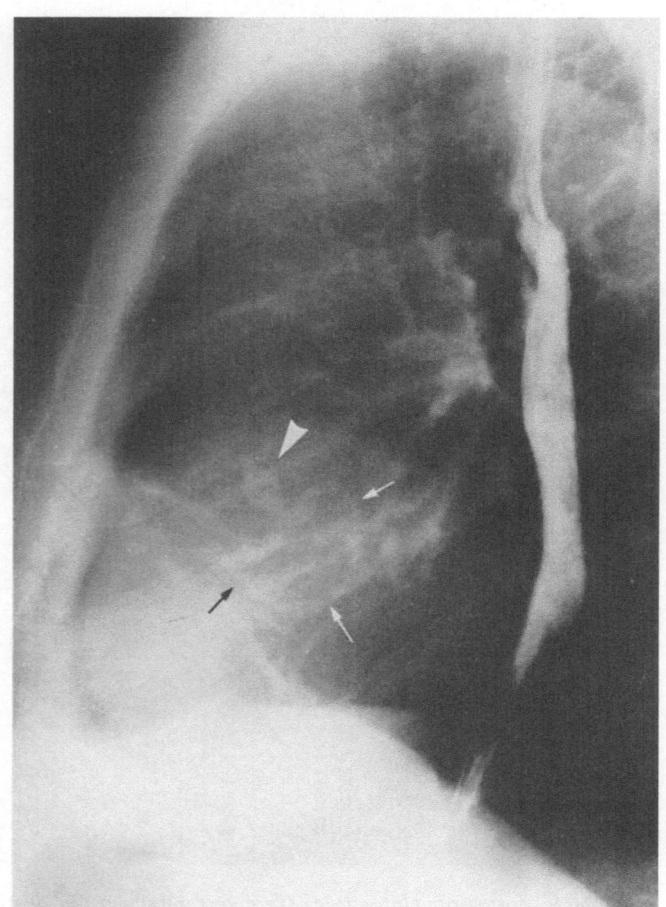

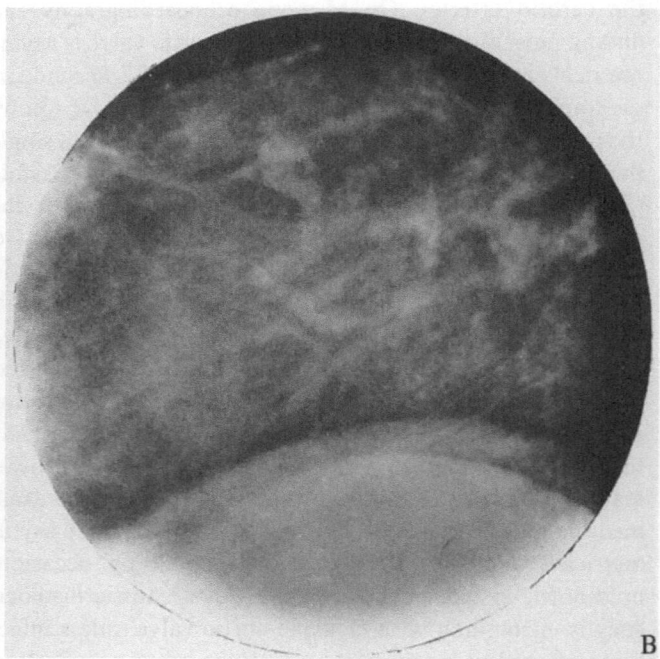

Fig. 5–16. *Roentgenogram of the chest and spot film in a patient with a calcified congenital bicuspid aortic valve (type III).* **A** Lateral view; **B** 100-mm LAO spot film. The bulbous raphe (*arrow head*), the attachment of the conjoint leaflet (unlabeled) and the attachment of the nonfused leaflet (*arrows*) form a characteristic "upside-down mushroom" appearance. Spindola-Franco H et al (1982) Recognition of bicuspid aortic valve by plain film calcification. Am J Roentgenol 139:867–872. Copyright 1982. By permission.

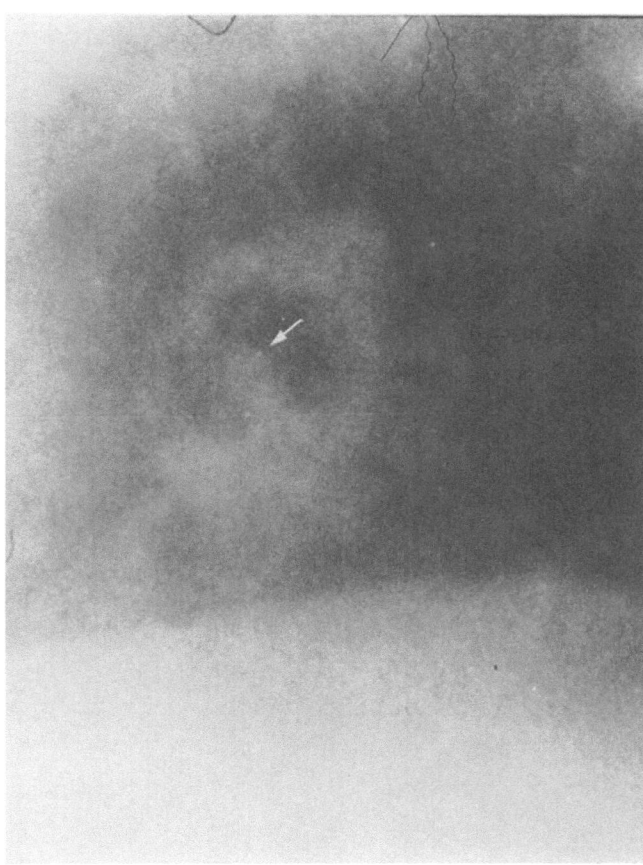

Fig. 5–17. *Left anterior oblique view of a 35-mm cine fluorogram in a patient with a calcified congenital bicuspid valve (type IV). The calcified aortic ring is well demonstrated because of its orientation with respect to the film. The bulbous raphe (arrow) points toward the center.* Spindola-Franco H et al (1982) Recognition of bicuspid aortic valve by plain film calcification. Am J Roentgenol 139:867–872. Copyright 1982. By permission.

Aortic Insufficiency

Although aortic insufficiency (AI) is due chiefly to rheumatic fever, other causes must be considered. These include congenital bicuspid aortic valve, bacterial endocarditis, ventricular septal defect with prolapsing aortic cusp, fenestration of aortic cusps, aortico-left ventricular tunnel, congenital subaortic aneurysm of the left ventricle, ankylosing spondylitis, syphilis, Reiter disease, psoriasis, giant cell aortitis, Takayasu arteritis, Cogan syndrome and systemic lupus erythematosus. AI may be due to systemic hypertension and aortic atherosclerosis, or dissecting hematoma (aneurysm) of the aorta. AI has also been associated with cystic medial necrosis in Marfan syndrome, the mucopolysaccharidoses (e.g., Hurler, Hunter, Scheie, and Morquio syndromes), Ehlers-Danlos syndrome, osteogenesis imperfecta, homocystinuria and Larsen syndrome. AI may also be due to trauma.

Clinical Features
Mild AI is characterized by a diastolic decrescendo murmur beginning after the aortic component of the second sound. Hemodynamically significant AI is indicated by a left ventricular heave and hyperdynamic carotid and peripheral pulses. With severe AI the apical impulse is displaced laterally, indicating left ventricular dilatation. Individuals with mild to moderate AI may remain asymptomatic for many years. Acute deterioration may be secondary to superimposed bacterial endocarditis or acute rheumatic fever. Gradual spontaneous progression is indicated initially by progressive enlargement of the heart or the appearance of pulmonary venous hypertension on plain roentgenograms of the chest. Deterioration of the ejection fraction derived from echocardiography and nuclear studies may also predict myocardial decompensation. Once symptoms have appeared, deterioration is fairly rapid.

Echocardiography
The echocardiographic finding characteristic of aortic regurgitation is flutter of the anterior leaflet of the mitral valve during diastole (Fig. 5–18), representing vibration of the valve secondary to the regurgitant jet. In moderate to severe AI the amplitude of the mitral valve is decreased (Fig. 5–18). Early closure of the valve may be observed in patients with elevated end-diastolic pressure (Fig. 5–19). The LV diastolic diameter and the shortening fraction are increased. LA dilatation may be present. Aortic abnormalities [e.g., bicuspid valve (Fig. 5–13), fibrocalcific deposits (Fig 5–2C), vegetation (also see Fig. 5–61), flail aortic cusp (Fig. 5–19C)] may be identified. Associated dilatation of the aortic root, dilatation of the sinus of Valsalva and aortic dissection may be suggested or even diagnosed by echocardiography. Associated thickening or calcification of the mitral valve may occur because of rheumatic fever. Doppler echocardiography from the apex shows reversal of flow in the left ventricular outflow tract during diastole. With moderate to severe AI a marked reversal of flow is also demonstrated in the aorta (see section on Doppler, Chap. 2).

Radiological (Plain Film) Features
The LV is normal in mild AI. LV enlargement and hypertrophy occur with moderate to severe degrees of AI. LV dilatation is observed on the frontal plain roentgenogram as enlargement of the left lower cardiac contour reflected in the apex projecting below the left hemidiaphragm (Fig. 5–20). On the LAO and lateral projections enlargement of the lower posterior cardiac contour is present. The ascending aorta may be dilated, resulting in prominence of the aortic segment in the frontal-plane and LAO view. The aortic arch and descending aorta may also be prominent. In young patients with LV enlargement and dilatation of the aorta (aortic configuration) valvular disease should be suspected. In the older age group a similar appearance may be due to arteriosclerotic and hypertensive changes.

In complicated AI (LV failure or associated mitral valve disease or both), enlargement of the LA and evidence of

Fig. 5–18. *Mitral valve flutter and left ventricular enlargement in patients with aortic insufficiency.* **A** M-mode echocardiogram in a patient with moderate aortic insufficiency. **B** Magnified image. **C** Left ventricle beyond the mitral valve. Diastolic flutter of the anterior mitral leaflet (*AML*) is demonstrated in **A**. The excursion of the anterior mitral leaflet is reduced by the jet of aortic regurgitation. In **B** the flutter of the anterior mitral leaflet is best delineated. The posterior mitral leaflet (*PML*) does not flutter. In **C** from a different patient the left ventricle (*LV*) is dilated with normal contractions. The septum and left ventricular free wall are thickened. Note flutter of the ventricular septum. *RV* = right ventricle.

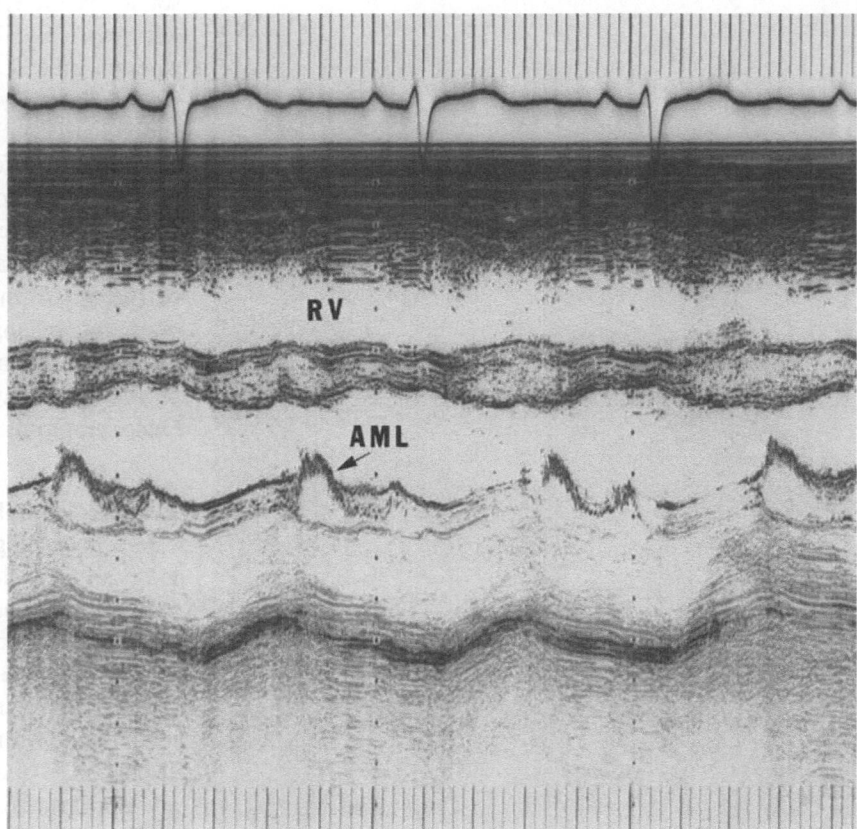

A

B

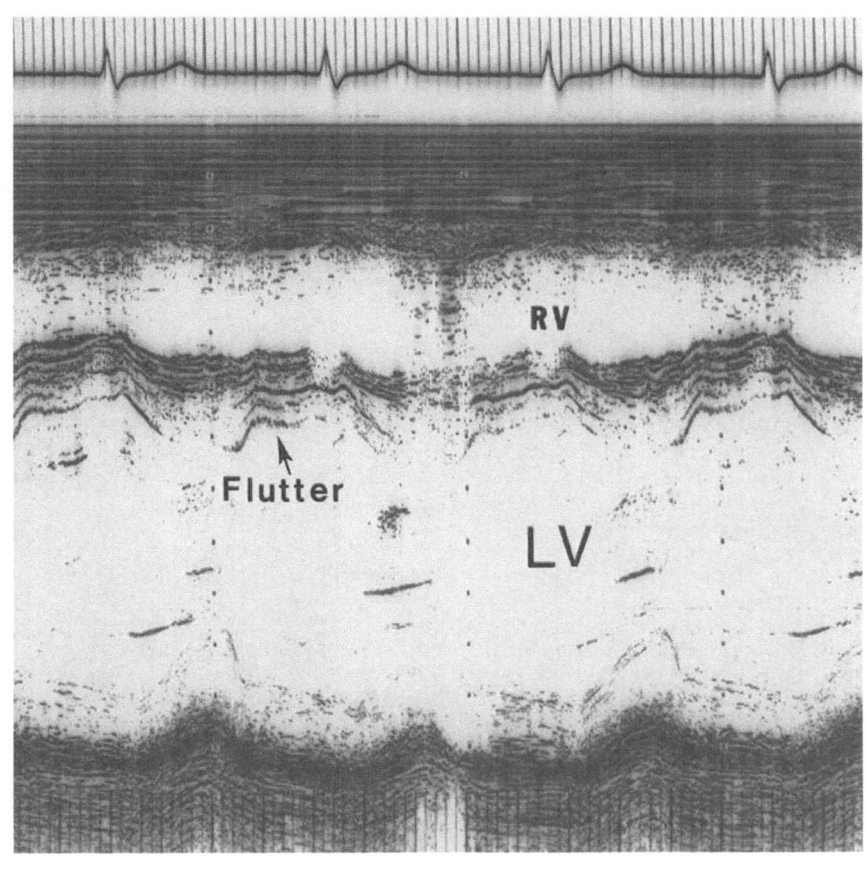

C

pulmonary venous hypertension may be noted. The pulmonary artery and the right-sided chambers of the heart may also become dilated.

Hemodynamics
The magnitude of the insufficiency depends upon the size of the regurgitant opening and the difference between the aortic and LV diastolic pressures. LV stroke volume is increased. The large stroke volume ejected into the aorta (forward cardiac output) causes elevation of the systolic pressure. The regurgitant flow (regurgitant volume) produces lowered aortic diastolic pressure and thus a wide pulse pressure. Severe aortic regurgitation results in decompensation of the LV with elevation of the LV end-diastolic and mean capillary wedge (mean left atrial) pressures. LV dysfunction in the presence of AI is manifested by a decrease in the ejection fraction and an increase in the end-systolic volume. The regurgitant volume (RV) can be calculated as follows:

$$RV = \text{total LV minute output} - \text{forward cardiac output}$$
$$\text{by Fick}$$

$$\text{Total LV minute output} = \text{angiographic stroke volume}$$
$$\times \text{heart rate}$$

Regurgitant fraction (RF) is calculated from this formula:

$$RF = \frac{\text{Regurgitant Volume}}{\text{LV Minute Output}}$$

Contrast Studies
Qualitative assessment of the severity of AI may be obtained from the aortogram. Biplane cine technique is preferable to aortography with serial cut films for estimation of the severity of AI (Fig. 5–21). This assessment is accomplished by observing the rapidity of opacification of the LV with each diastole. The severity is graded mild, moderate, and severe. Mild insufficiency results in incomplete or faint opacification of the LV, which clears in one heart beat. Moderate insufficiency results in opacification of the entire LV, which clears in two or three heart beats. Severe insufficiency is characterized by dense opacification of the LV, which clears slowly after more than three heartbeats, frequently resulting in reopacification of the LV as opacified blood oscillates between the LV and the aorta. The qualitative assessment requires considerable experience because many other factors, such as ventricular performance (hypokinesis or hyperkinesis), ventricular size, and associated aortic stenosis, as well as mitral disease and pharmacologic agents, change the relationship between angiographic dynamics and regurgitant volume. Therefore, any qualitative assessment of aortic insufficiency should be correlated with a quantitative assessment of regurgitant volume (described under the heading Hemodynamics, in this section).

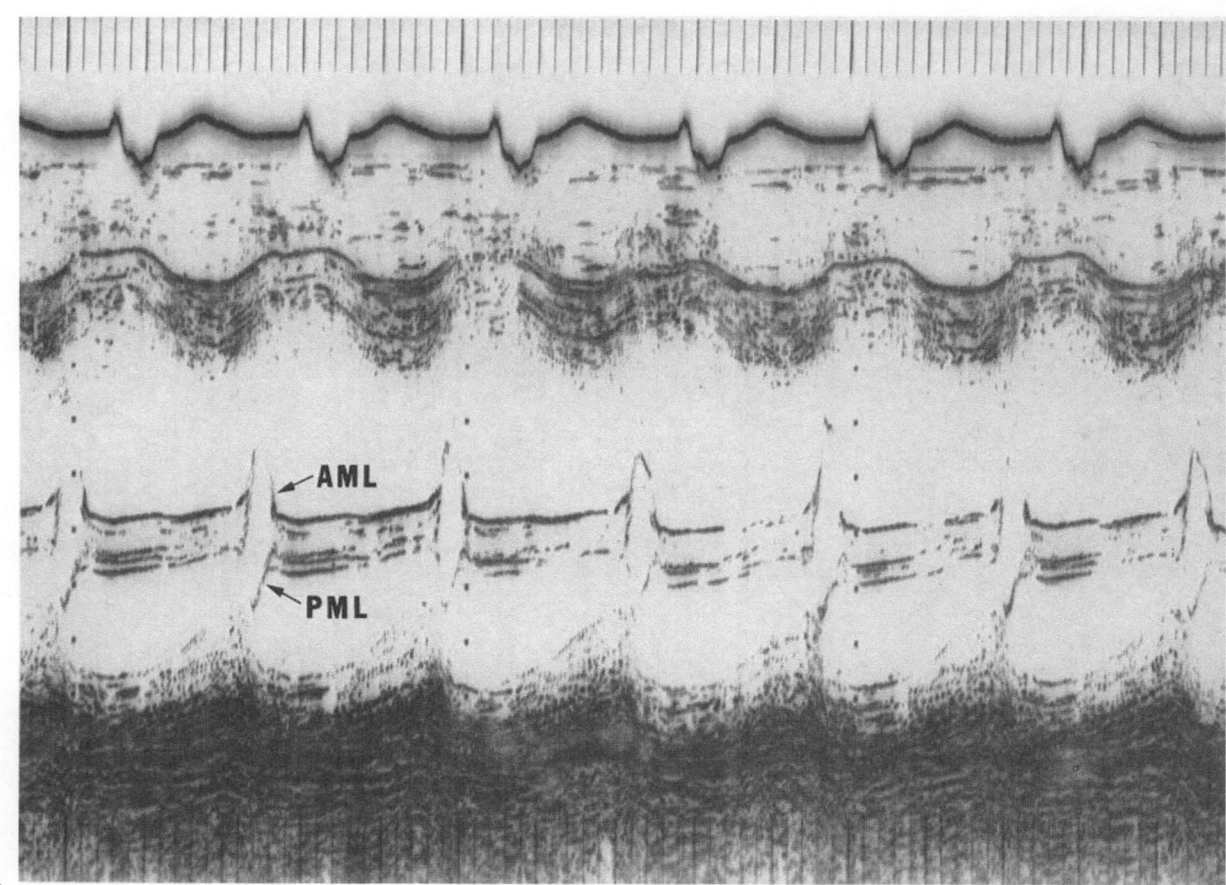

Fig. 5–19. *Acute aortic insufficiency.* Early closure of the mitral valve in an 18-year-old patient in cardiogenic shock, secondary to disruption of a porcine aortic valve prosthesis. **A** M-mode echocardiogram at the level of the mitral valve; **B** M-mode echocardiogram at the level of the aortic valve; **C** arc scan from the aortic valve to the left ventricular outflow tract. In **A** the mitral valve closes prematurely because of high left ventricular diastolic pressure. The left ventricle is dilated. In **B** the aortic leaflet flutters within the aortic root during diastole (*Diast.*). The left atrium (*LA*) is grossly dilated. In **C** the arc scan shows the porcine aortic leaflet (*Ao.L.*) prolapsing into the left ventricular outflow tract (*LVOT*) during diastole. *AML* = anterior mitral leaflet; *PML* = posterior mitral leaflet; *RVOT* = right ventricular outflow tract; *Syst.* = systole; *Ao* = aortic root.

The anatomical abnormality of the aortic valve responsible for the AI may also be elicited from the aortogram (e.g., bicuspid aortic valve, cystic medial necrosis, infective endocarditis, syphilitic aortitis). Other forms of AI and disorders that simulate AI (e.g., ventricular septal defect with prolapsing aortic cusp, aortico-left ventricular tunnel), are discussed in Chapter 7.

Treatment

Ideally one would prefer to intervene prior to the onset of irreversible myocardial decompensation. Once symp-

toms are evident, myocardial decompensation is present, and permanent myocardial damage is likely. Progressive enlargement of the heart on chest roentgenograms may precede symptoms. A large or increasing end-systolic ventricular diameter on echocardiography, a large or increasing end-systolic volume on a gated blood pool scan or a reduction in nuclear ejection fraction during exercise, as compared to the ejection fraction at rest, have also been used as objective criteria for surgical intervention prior to onset of symptoms. Surgical management almost always involves replacement of the aortic valve.

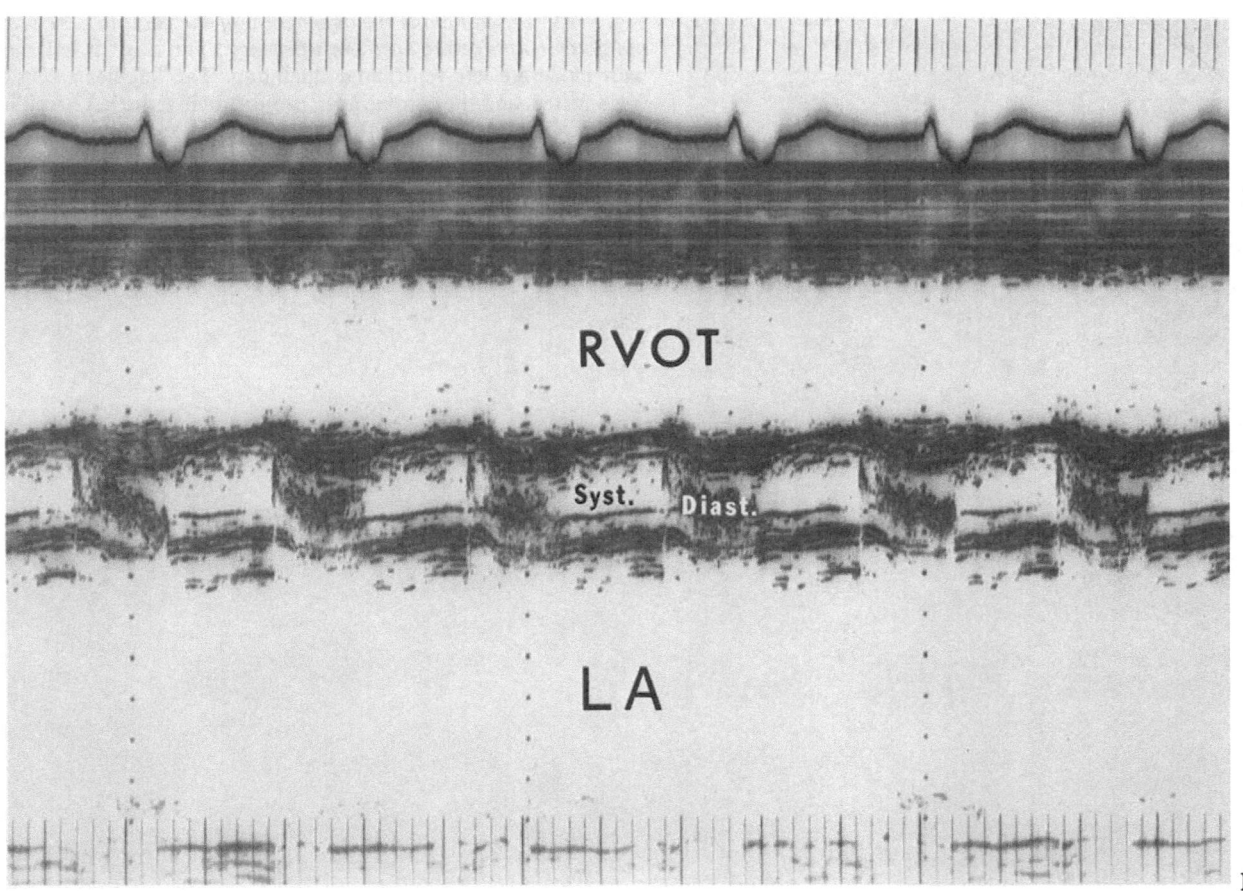

B

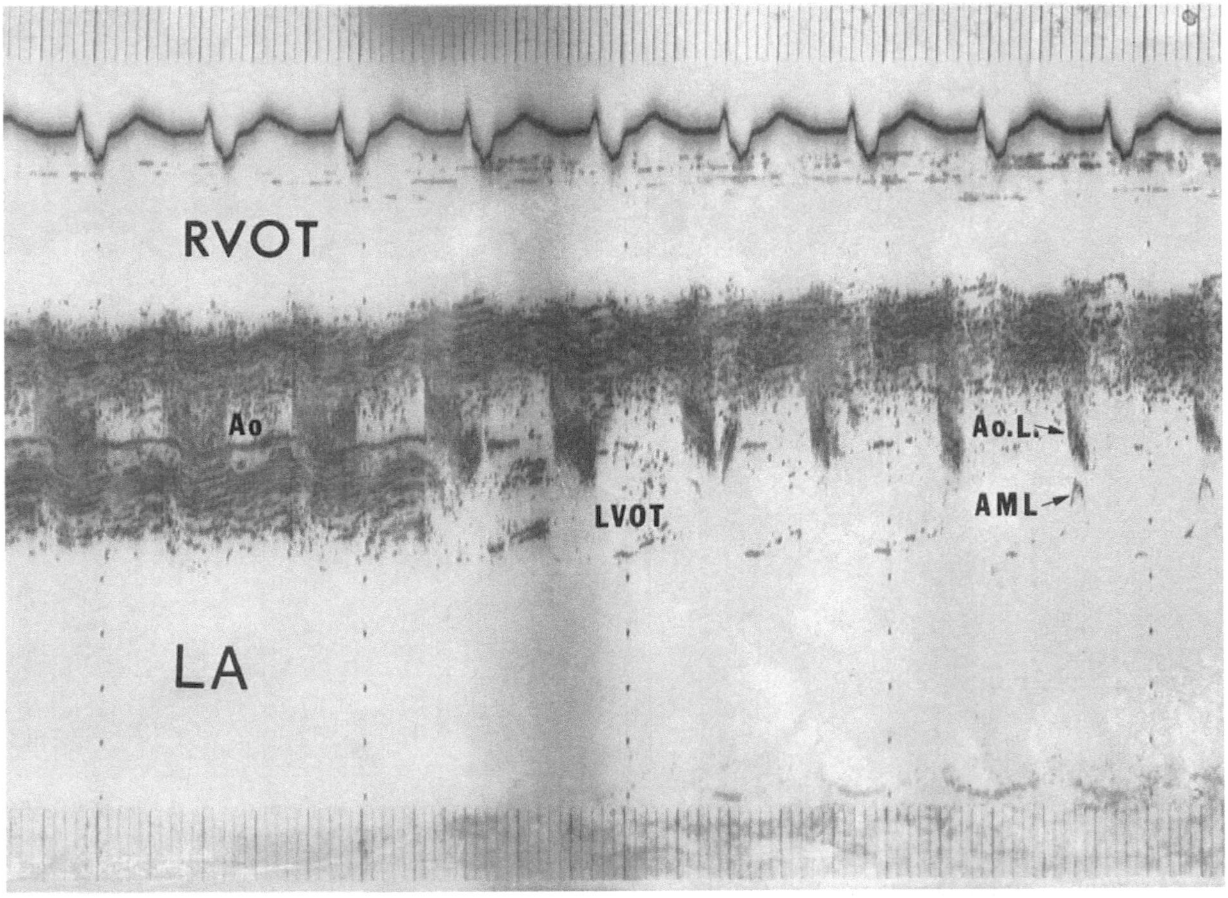

C

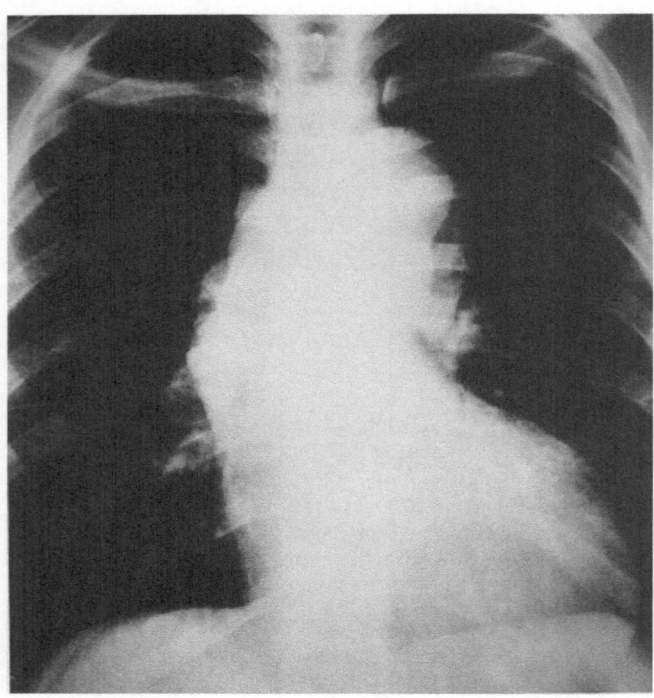

Fig. 5–20. *Frontal plane roentgenogram of the chest in a 31-year-old patient with severe aortic insufficiency.* The heart is enlarged with moderate left ventricular dilatation. The left heart border is elongated, and the cardiac apex projects below the left hemidiaphragm. The ascending aorta and the aortic arch are markedly dilated. Mild pulmonary venous hypertension is indicated by equalization of the caliber of the upper and lower pulmonary vessels. Microscopical examination of surgical specimens of the aortic wall showed giant cell aortitis. See Fig. 5–26 for the aortogram.

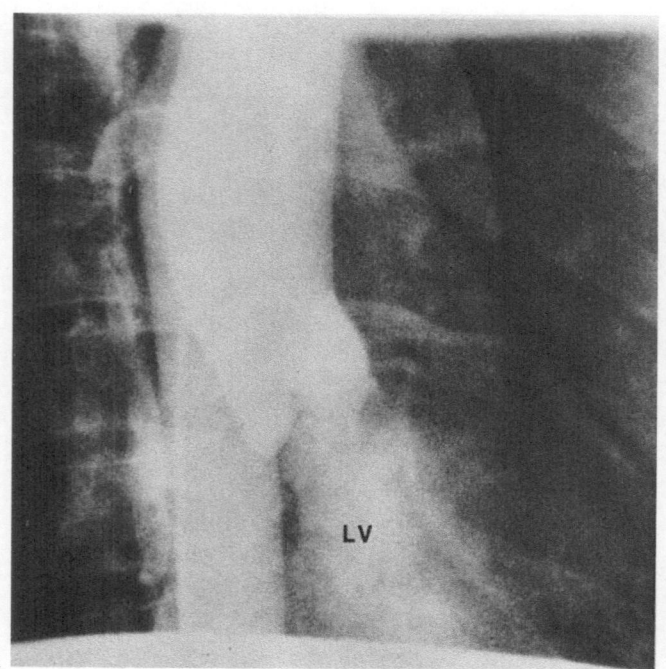

A

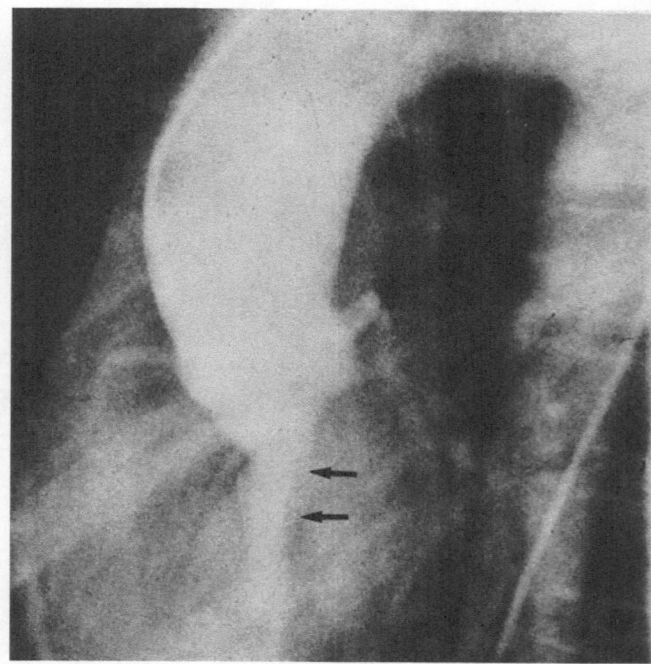

B

Fig. 5–21. *35-mm cine aortogram in a patient with severe aortic insufficiency.* **A** RAO view; **B** LAO view. In **A** the left ventricle fills densely with contrast material after injection into the aortic root. In **B** the regurgitant jet strikes the anterior leaflet of the mitral valve (*arrows*), accounting for flutter of the anterior leaflet on echocardiography and for the Austin Flint murmur, which simulates mitral stenosis in patients with aortic insufficiency. *LV* = left ventricle.

Marfan Syndrome

Marfan syndrome is a generalized disorder of connective tissue involving the skeletal, ocular and cardiovascular systems. The skeletal manifestations include excessively long extremities, arachnodactyly and laxity of joints. Kyphoscoliosis and pectus deformities are common. Subcutaneous fat is sparse. Excessive anterior-posterior dimension of the eye results in myopia and, on occasion, retinal detachment. Later, defects in the suspensory ligaments result in dislocation of the lens. Cardiac manifestations include dilatation, aneurysm and dissection of the aorta due to cystic medial necrosis. Aortic insufficiency may result from aortic dilatation or from myxomatous degeneration of the aortic valve. Myxomatous degeneration of the mitral valve and laxity of the chordae tendineae cause mitral valve prolapse. Accelerated calcification of the mitral anulus has also been reported. Histological studies demonstrate cystic medial necrosis, characterized by mucoid degeneration of elastic fibers and formation of cysts in the media with disruption, fragmentation and rarefaction of the elastica (cystic medial necrosis). Redundancy of smooth muscle masses and dilatation of the vasa vasorum also occur. These findings are usually confined to the aortic root and ascending aorta, resulting in effacement of the sinuses of Valsalva and bulbous (symmetrical) dilatation of the ascending aorta. Dissection and rupture of the aorta are frequent lethal complications. Histological changes in the aortic and mitral valve include disruption and loss of the normal valvular architecture, increase in mucopolysaccharide ground substance and cystic degeneration (myxoid or mucoid in nature). As a result, ballooning or redundancy of the cusps occurs with thinning and fenestration. Histological sections have also shown significant changes in the arteries to the sinus node and atrioventricular node. Associated abnormalities such as coarctation of the aorta, ventricular septal defect, patent foramen ovale, and varicosities of the cardiac and peripheral veins may be present. Bacterial endocarditis may be superimposed. The incidence of hypertension, proteinuria and chronic pyelonephritis is high in patients with Marfan syndrome.

Marfan syndrome is inherited as a dominant trait with variable expression (i.e., the forme fruste of Marfan syndrome); however, in approximately 15% new mutations appear to have developed. Similar pathological changes occur in other disorders such as Ehlers-Danlos syndrome, osteogenesis imperfecta, homocystinuria, Larsen syndrome and the genetic mucopolysaccharidoses (Hurler, Hunter, Morquio, and Scheie syndromes). These changes do not occur in Sanfilippo syndrome. Of interest is the occurrence of cystic medial necrosis of the aorta in rats affected by lathyrism.

Clinical Features

Clinical findings relative to the cardiovascular system include a hyperdynamic precordium and a murmur of aortic insufficiency. Some patients exhibit the characteristic mid systolic click and late systolic murmur of mitral valve prolapse; however, many present with holosystolic murmurs of mitral insufficiency. Progression of the aortic insufficiency is accelerated, and congestive heart failure ensues during young adult life. Acute aortic dissection is especially likely with trauma, with hypertension and during pregnancy. In patients with Marfan syndrome the dissection may be painless (silent dissection). The electrocardiogram may show nonspecific ST-T–wave changes, or it may reflect the excessive volume load placed upon the heart by chronic aortic or mitral insufficiency.

Echocardiography

The echocardiogram may be normal but often indicates dilatation of the root of the aorta. On 2-D echocardiography the sinuses of Valsalva and the proximal segment of the ascending aorta are dilated (Fig. 5–22). Signs of aortic insufficiency (e.g., flutter of the anterior leaflet of the mitral valve, early closure of the mitral valve) are often present. The LV may be dilated. Mitral valve prolapse may be evident as well (see also Fig. 5–50).

Radiological (Plain Film) Features

Abnormalities of the thoracic cage (pectus excavatum) and spine (kyphoscoliosis) may be observed. The LV is usually enlarged with marked prominence of the ascending aorta (Fig. 5–23). Marked dilatation of the sinuses of Valsalva (Fig. 5–24) may cause displacement of the pulmonary artery anteriorly and laterally, producing a bulge in the pulmonary artery segment, reminiscent of dilatation of the pulmonary artery on the PA projection (Fig. 5–25). The dilated sinuses of Valsalva may also produce a double density on the posterolateral roentgenogram, mimicking LA enlargement (Fig. 5–23A). Effacement or obliteration of the normal angle formed by the ascending aorta and base of the heart is often noted on the PA projection (Fig. 5–23). Analysis of the oblique and lateral projections will usually clarify the nature of the abnormality (Fig. 5–23B). Although severe aortic insufficiency due to rheumatic fever may be reminiscent of the foregoing, the rheumatic heart demonstrates true LA and pulmonary artery enlargement secondary to mitral involvement. Pseudo LA enlargement can best be differentiated from true LA enlargement on the LAO and lateral projections. Bulbous dilatation of the root of the aorta will be noted anteriorly, whereas true LA enlargement will be observed posteriorly. Effacement of the angle formed at the waist of the heart by the ascending aorta and the base of the heart is more commonly observed in patients with aortic insufficiency secondary to cystic medial necrosis than in patients with rheumatic aortic valvular disease.

Hemodynamics

Abnormalities in hemodynamics correspond to the severity of the aortic insufficiency. (See section on hemodynamics in aortic insufficiency above.)

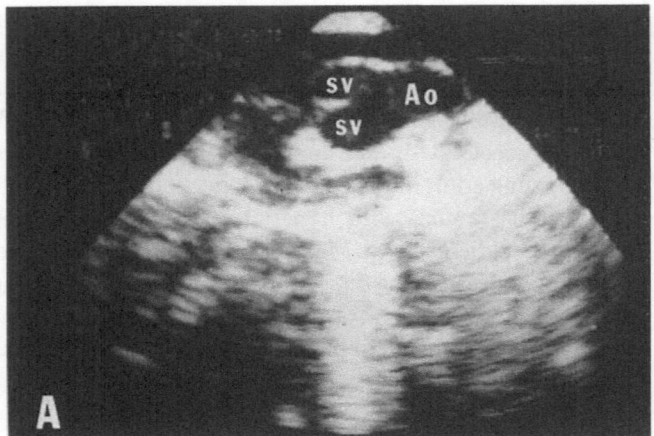
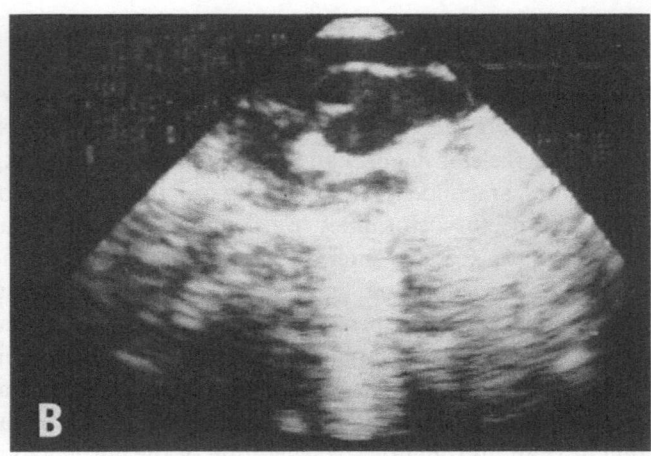

Fig. 5-22. *Two-dimensional echocardiogram of the aortic root in an 11-year-old girl with Marfan syndrome.* **A** with labels; **B** without labels. The sinuses of Valsalva (*SV*) are symmetrically dilated so that the root of the aorta (*Ao*) appears bulbous. **C** M-mode echocardiogram at the level of the aortic valve. The diameter of the root of the aorta (*Ao.*) is 3 cm (normal is 1.7–2.3 cm). The *arrows* indicate the leaflets of the aortic valve. (This is the same patient as in Fig. 5–50). *RVOT* = right ventricular outflow tract; *LA* = left atrium.

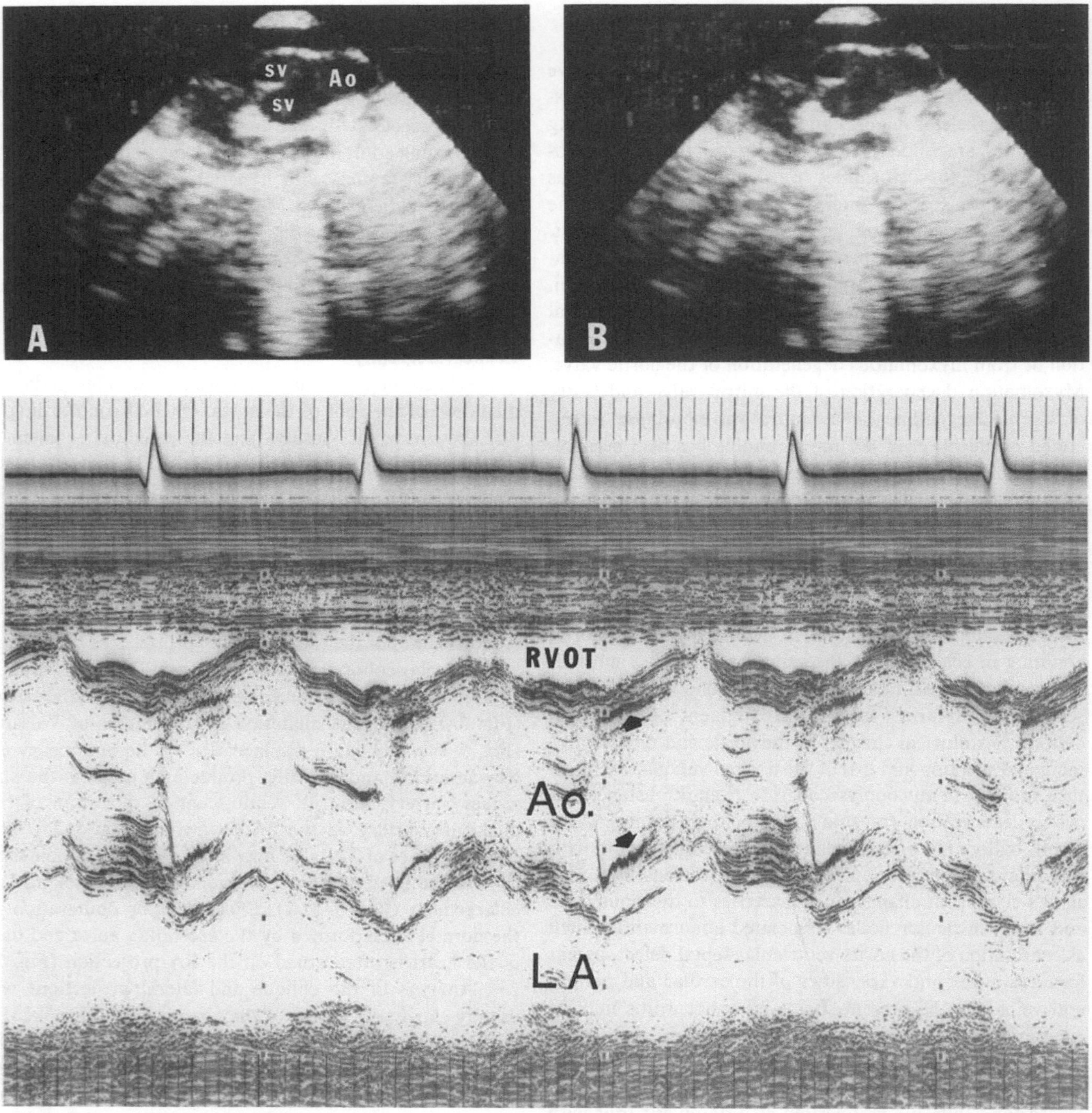

Contrast Studies

The findings on aortography are characteristic of cystic medial necrosis, which occurs in Marfan syndrome and also with other related disorders of connective tissue (Fig. 5–24). The root of the aorta is symmetrically dilated, and the semilunar sinuses are effaced. The appearance of the aortic root is characterized as pear-shaped or onion shaped. The dilatation of the aorta usually does not involve the aortic arch or the origin of the brachiocephalic vessels; however, the descending aorta may be affected. In some instances the proximal portions of the coronary arteries may also be dilated. The branches of the abdominal aorta at their sites of origin may also be affected (e.g., celiac, superior mesenteric, renal arteries). In contrast, in patients with aortic arteritis syndromes, the ascending aorta is uniformly dilated over its entire length, maintaining its tubular appearance (Fig. 5–26) rather than the bulbous shape occurring in Marfan syndrome.

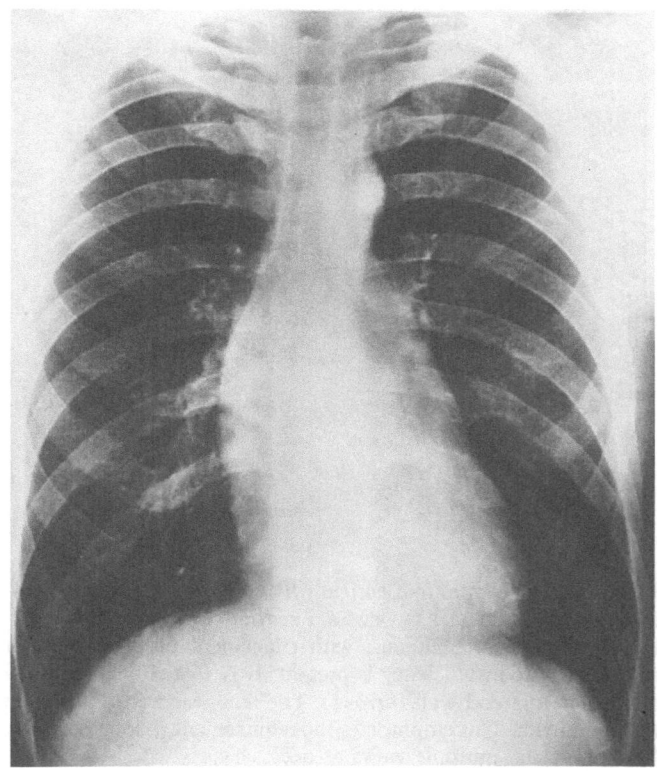

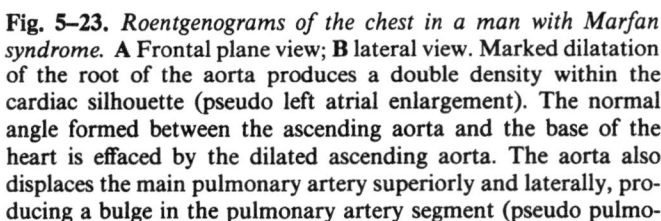

A

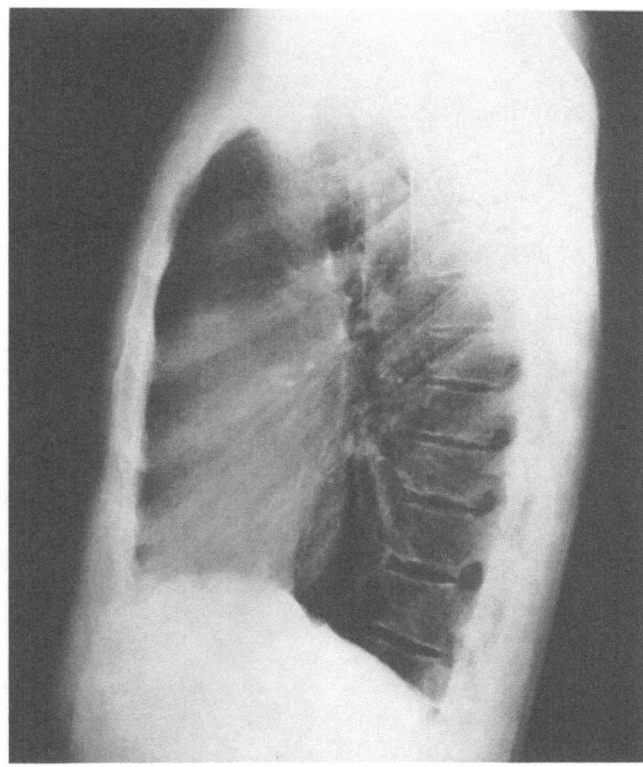

B

Fig. 5–23. *Roentgenograms of the chest in a man with Marfan syndrome.* **A** Frontal plane view; **B** lateral view. Marked dilatation of the root of the aorta produces a double density within the cardiac silhouette (pseudo left atrial enlargement). The normal angle formed between the ascending aorta and the base of the heart is effaced by the dilated ascending aorta. The aorta also displaces the main pulmonary artery superiorly and laterally, producing a bulge in the pulmonary artery segment (pseudo pulmo-

nary artery dilatation) (see also Fig. 5–25). In the lateral film the dilated aortic root obliterates the retrosternal clear space. Thus the lateral film shows that the double density noted on the frontal view is due to the dilatation of the aortic root rather than enlargement of the left atrium. Note that the dilatation of the root of the aorta does not extend into the aortic arch. Mild left ventricular enlargement is present. (Same patient as in Figs. 5–24 and 5–25.)

Intimal flaps (Figs. 5–24B), signifying dissection of the aorta (asymptomatic, or silent dissection), may be difficult to demonstrate, although recognition of these flaps is crucial. Unlike dissection due to hypertension and atherosclerosis, which usually involves the right coronary artery, dissection due to cystic medial necrosis may involve either coronary artery, although involvement of the right coronary artery is more likely. Left ventriculography generally shows a dilated, hyperkinetic ventricle. Late in the course or with acute cardiac decompensation, the LV may contract poorly. Associated prolapse of the mitral valve and mitral insufficiency are also demonstrated. In the authors' experience the combination of dilatation of the aortic root and prolapse of the mitral valve is uncommon. Isolated prolapse of the mitral valve or isolated dilatation of the aortic root is more frequently encountered.

Treatment

Acute aortic dissection or severe progressive aortic insufficiency warrants surgical treatment. Aortic valve replacement with replacement of the dilated ascending aorta, using a composite graft, is recommended. McDonald et al. have

recommended prophylactic replacement of the aortic valve and ascending aorta when the diameter of the aortic root reaches 5.5 cm. On occasion mitral valve regurgitation becomes so severe that the mitral valve requires replacement as well. Postoperative complications frequently encountered in individuals with Marfan syndrome are dehiscence of the prosthetic valve and recurrence of aortic aneurysm.

Mitral Stenosis

Disease of the mitral valve (MV) usually results from rheumatic heart disease. MV disease is rarely congenital in origin. Females are affected by rheumatic mitral stenosis more frequently than are males. Mitral stenosis (MS) is more common than mitral insufficiency (MI). However, MS and MI often occur in the same patient. MS is caused by scarring, thickening, fusion and shortening of the chordae tendineae, resulting in a diaphragm-like funnel-shaped valve with diminished valve excursion. Calcification is frequently present in varying amounts.

On occasion, extensive calcification of the mitral anulus

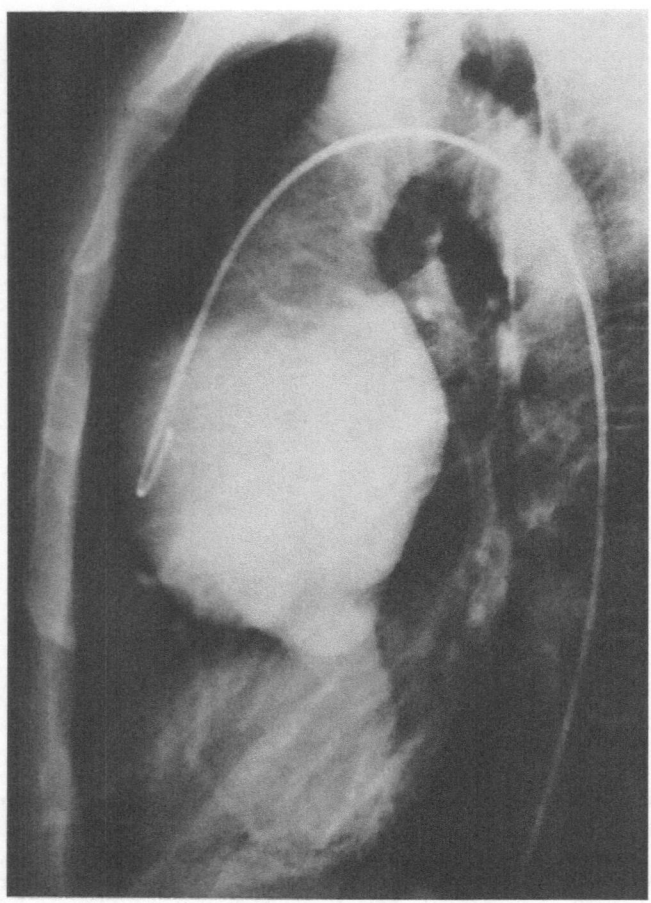

A

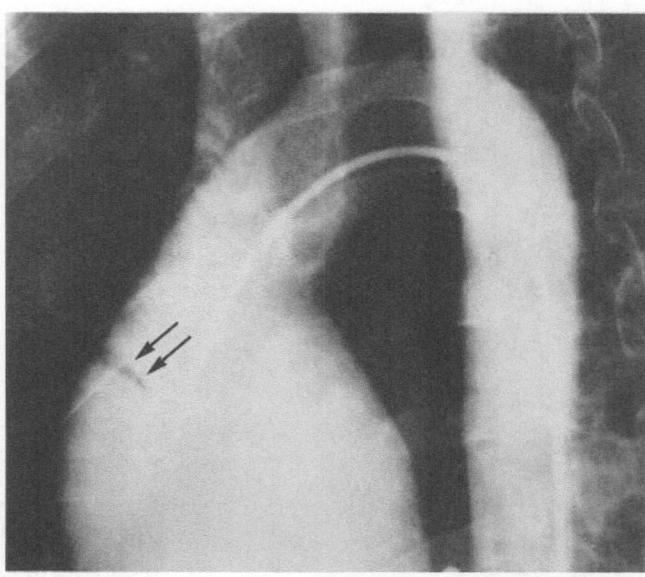

B

Fig. 5–24. *Aortogram in a patient with Marfan syndrome.* A Lateral view; B shallow LAO view. A The root of the aorta is symmetrically dilated and bulbous, with effacement of the semilunar sinuses. Aortic insufficiency is present. B A tear is demonstrated in the anterolateral wall (*arrows*). The tear was not detected on the lateral film. This emphasizes the requirement to look carefully for tears, using multiple views as necessary.

interferes with valvar opening and obstructs the mitral orifice, causing signs and symptoms of MS. The differential diagnosis of MS also includes LA tumor, hypertrophic cardiomyopathy and endomyocardial fibrosis of the LV.

The reduction in the size of the MV orifice increases the resistance to the flow of blood across the MV, causing elevation of the LA pressure. The increased LA pressure is transmitted to the pulmonary veins, pulmonary capillary bed and pulmonary arteries, resulting in elevation of pulmonary artery pressure and resistance. The resulting increased work load on the right ventricle (RV) causes hypertrophy and eventually dilatation of this chamber. The reduced compliance of the hypertrophied RV augments the work load on the right atrium (RA), causing it to enlarge as well. The tricuspid ring may enlarge, causing tricuspid insufficiency. Systemic venous hypertension develops, together with ascites, dependent edema and cardiac cirrhosis. Bacterial endocarditis may be superimposed at any stage of the disease.

Clinical Features
The clinical features of MS relate to the hemodynamic alterations. Dyspnea develops due to the elevated pulmonary venous pressure, while fatigue is secondary to the reduced cardiac output. Individuals with mild degrees of

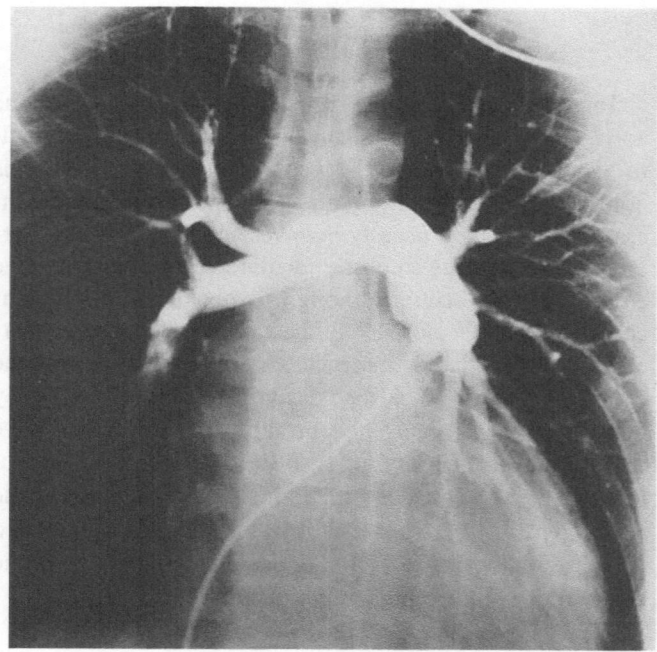

Fig. 5–25. *Pulmonary angiogram in a patient with Marfan syndrome.* The dilated root of the aorta displaces the main pulmonary artery superiorly and laterally, simulating pulmonary artery dilatation or pulmonary hypertension on the frontal roentgenogram of the chest.

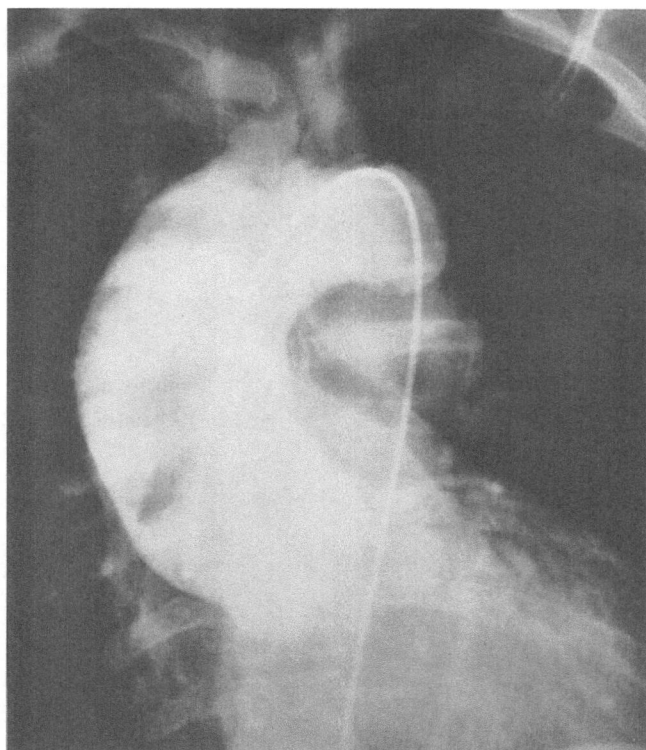

A

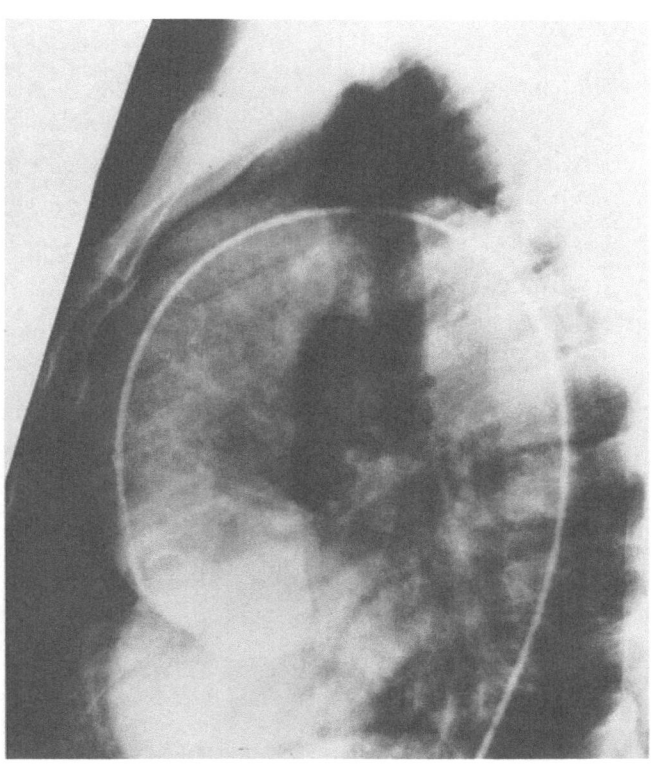

B

Fig. 5–26. *Aortogram in a 32-year-old man with giant cell arteritis and aortic insufficiency.* **A** AP view; **B** lateral view. The ascending and descending aorta are dilated. The arch is also dilated, but to a lesser extent. The root of the aorta and the semilunar sinuses are also dilated. The left ventricle opacifies densely because of severe aortic insufficiency. The coronary arteries are usually dilated in patients with severe aortic insufficiency. This angiogram is from the patient in Fig. 5–20. Compare the appearance of the aorta with that observed on plain roentgenogram of the chest.

MS may be asymptomatic. Dyspnea on exercise is characteristic of moderate stenosis, while dyspnea at rest, orthopnea and signs of pulmonary edema occur with the severe forms of MS. Hemoptysis, due to rupture of bronchial veins may be observed. Pulmonary infections are frequently superimposed. Systemic thromboembolism may occur in less severe forms of MS, becoming more frequent with increasing severity of the MS. Individuals with low cardiac output and atrial fibrillation are especially susceptible to this complication. On occasion a large thrombus forms within the LA cavity, causing acute obstruction of the mitral orifice.

On physical examination, in mild forms of MS a mid diastolic flow rumble, audible at the apex and preceded by an opening snap, is often detected. With progressively severe stenosis the opening snap becomes louder and earlier, tending to disappear as the valve becomes calcified and rigid. In addition, signs of pulmonary hypertension (loud pulmonary second sound) and RV enlargement (RV heave) appear. The diastolic murmur may become louder, and a diastolic thrill may be felt. With severe MS and a subsequent fall in cardiac output, the diastolic murmur may disappear so that only findings relating to the right side of the heart remain. The electrocardiogram shows evidence of LA enlargement or atrial fibrillation. With severe disease of the mitral valve, RV hypertrophy is observed.

Echocardiography

M-mode echocardiography (Fig. 5–27) shows thickening of the MV in MS. The posterior mitral leaflet moves anteriorly at the onset of diastole as if tethered to the anterior leaflet, and both leaflets move gradually posteriorly as the ventricle fills (E-F slope). The slow rate of descent of the MV with MS (decreased E-F slope) is said to reflect slow filling of the LV; nevertheless, the E-F slope does not correlate with the severity of MS. The excursion of the opening motion of the anterior leaflet does, however, correlate with pliability of the valve (a rigid valve will move very little as it opens). On 2-D echocardiography (Fig. 5–28) the

Fig. 5–27. *Mitral stenosis.* M-mode echocardiograms with mild ▶ (**A**) moderate (**B**) and severe (**C** and **D**) stenosis. In **A** the leaflets are thickened, the E-F slope is decreased, and the opening motion is limited; however, the posterior leaflet of the mitral valve (*PML*) moves posteriorly away from the anterior leaflet (*AML*) during diastole. In **B** multiple echoes are present during diastole and the E-F slope is nearly horizontal; however, the opening motion (*D-E* excursion) is normal, indicating a flexible valve. In **C** and **D** the leaflets are markedly thickened and their excursion is decreased. Both leaflets move in parallel, the posterior leaflet moving anteriorly during diastole. The leaflets are not only markedly fibrotic, but they are also probably calcified. *RV* = right ventricle; *IVS* = interventricular septum; *Syst.* = systole

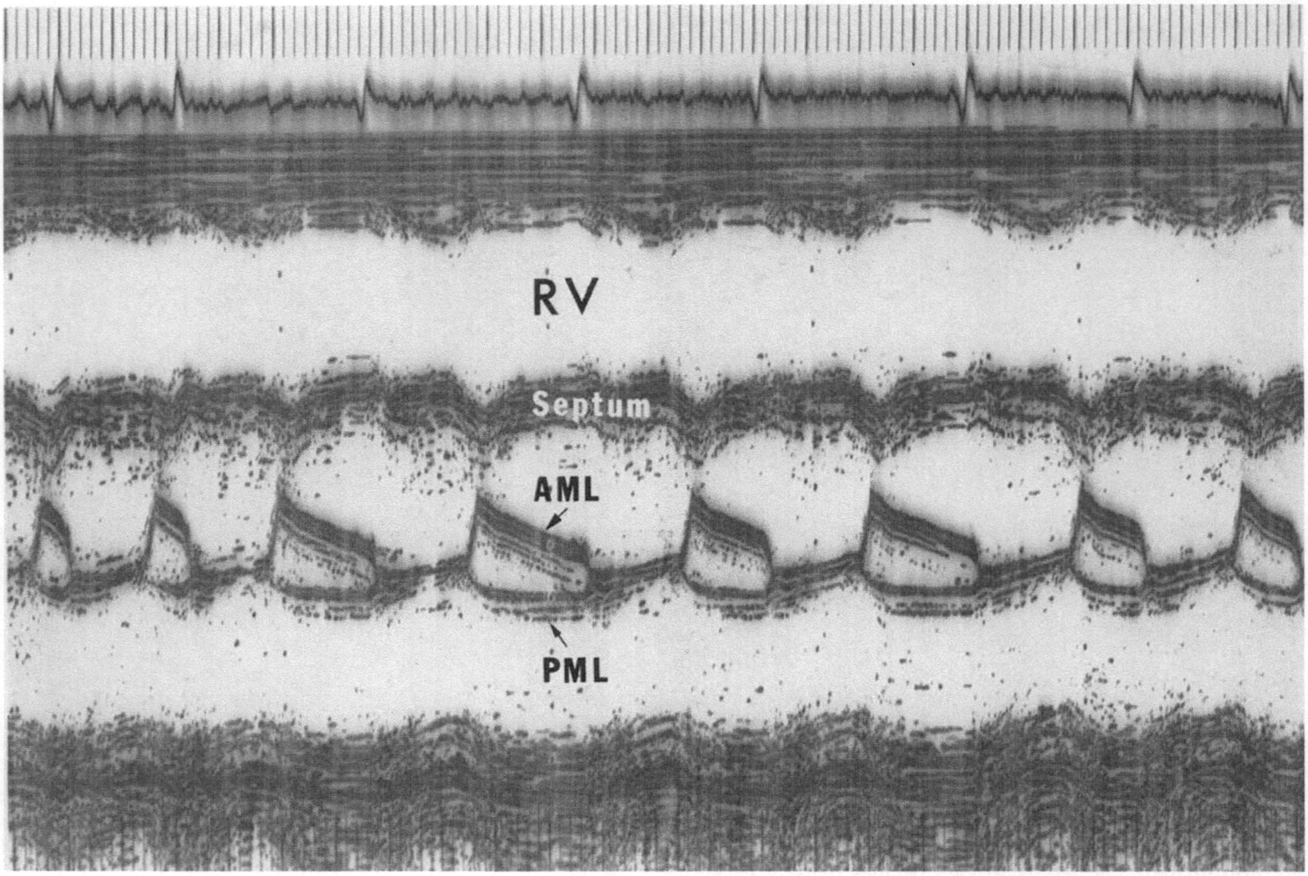

A

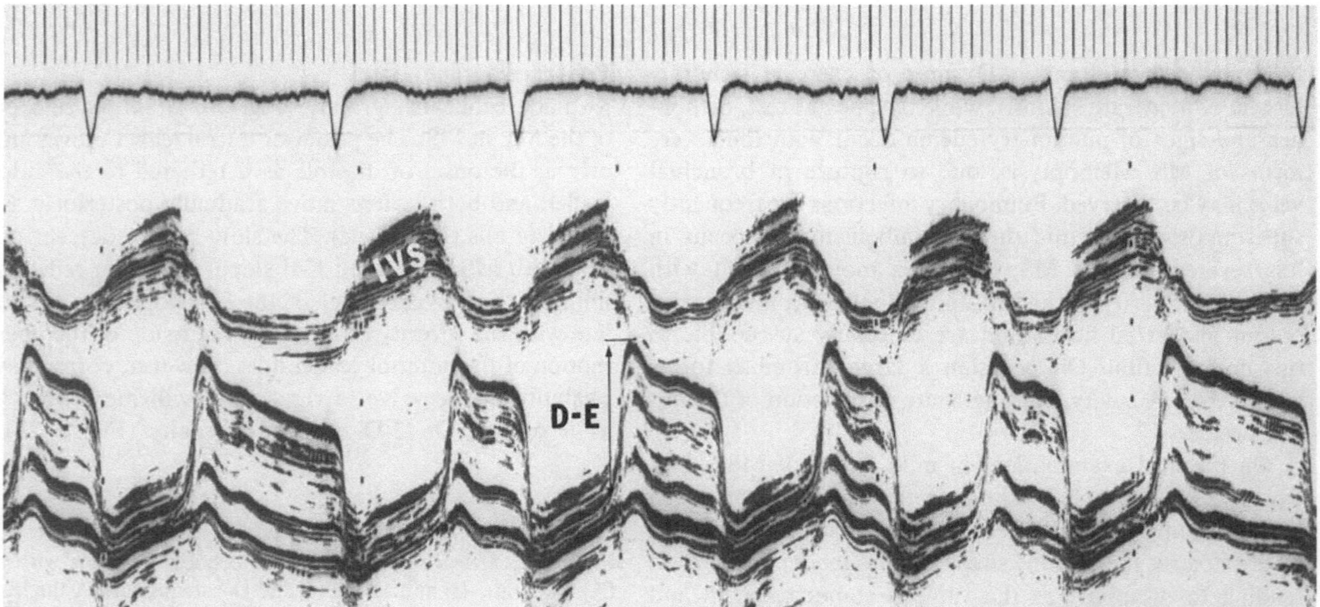

B

Fig. 5–27. *Legend is on preceding page.*

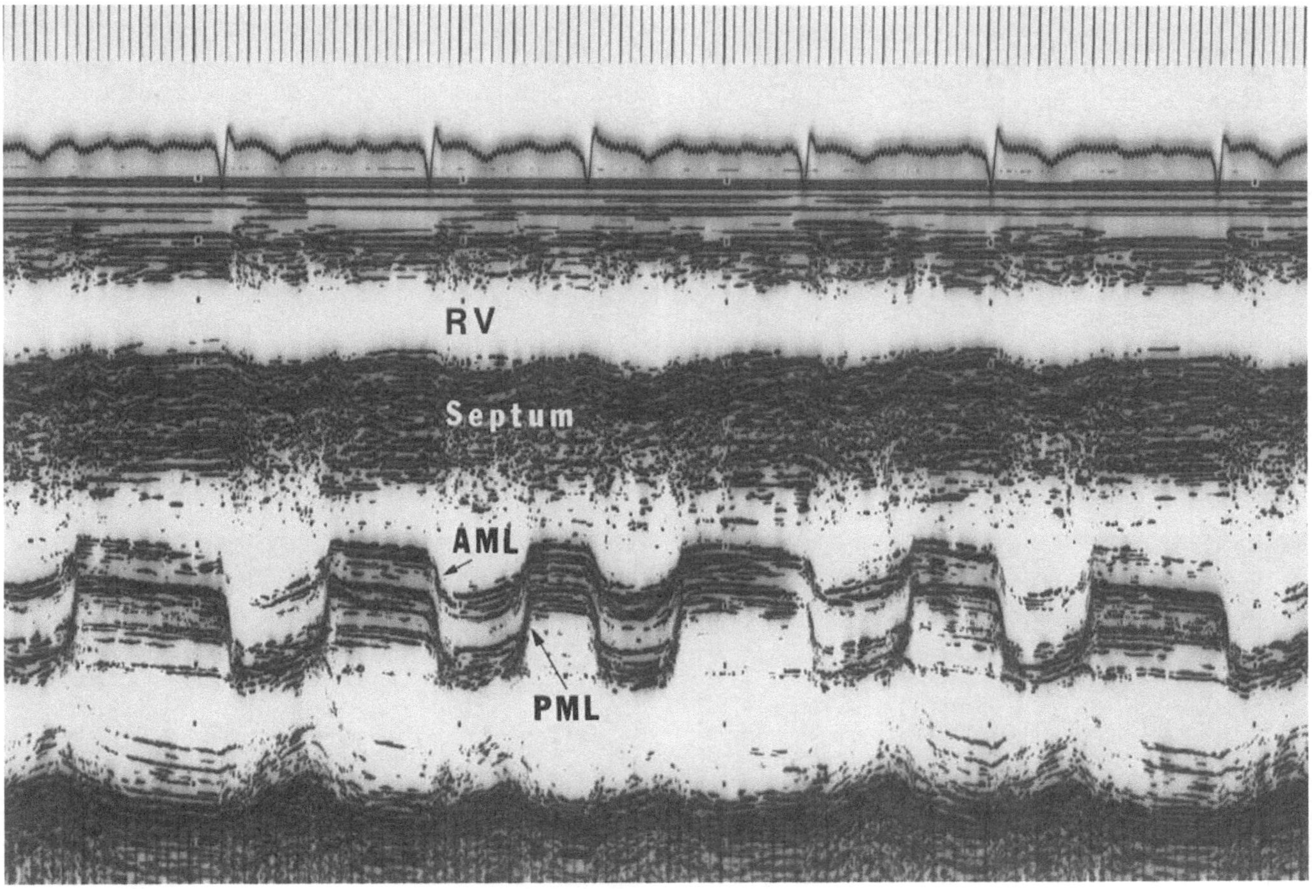

C

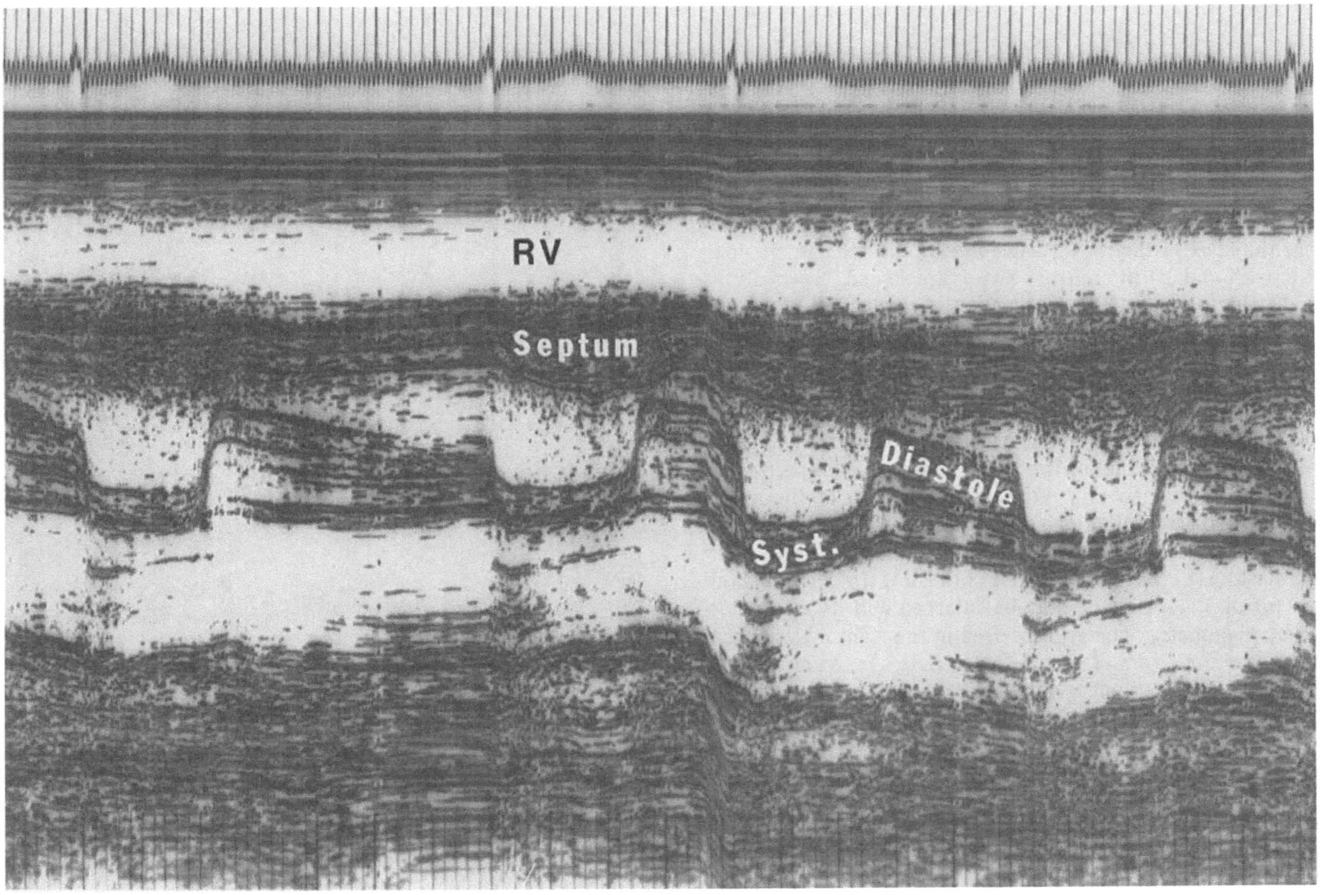

D

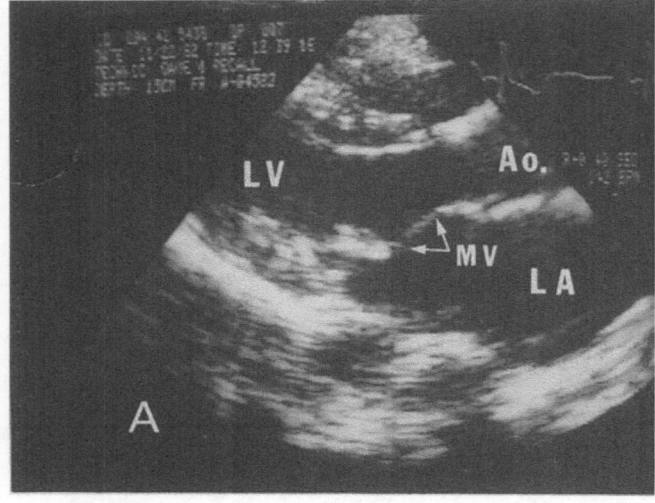

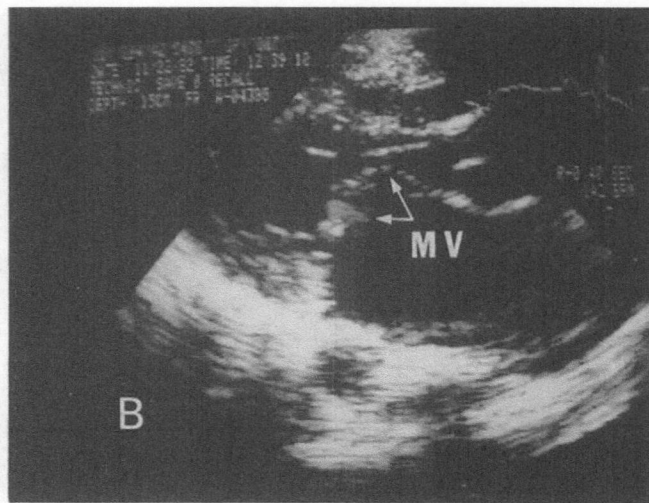

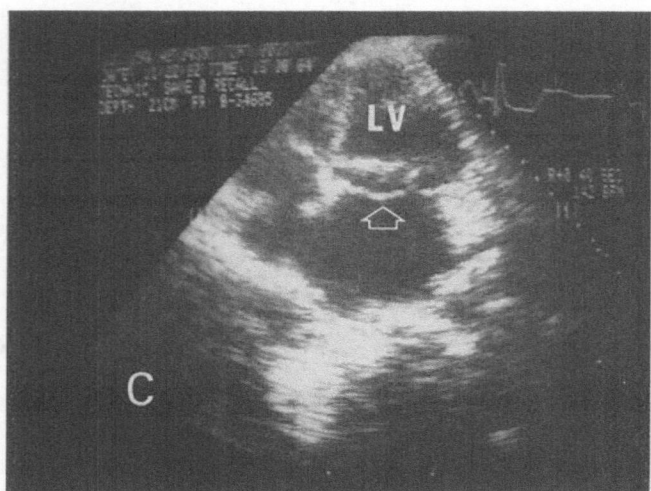

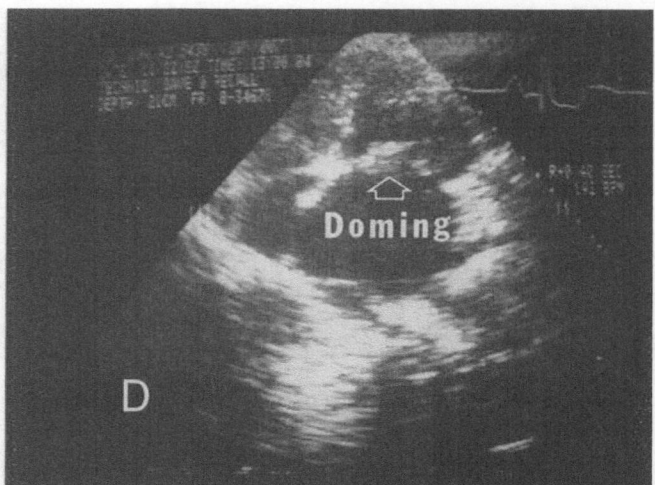

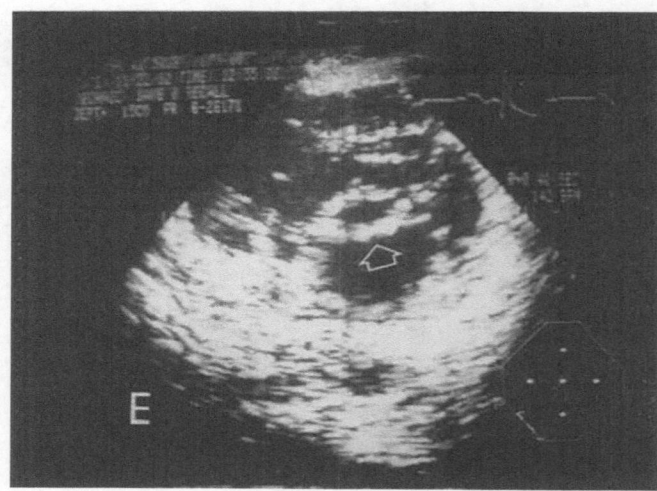

Fig. 5–28. *Mitral stenosis. Two-dimensional echocardiogram in a 35-year-old woman with symptoms of fatigue and dyspnea on exertion.* A Long axis, systole; B long axis, diastole; C four-chamber view, systole; D four-chamber view, diastole; E short axis view at the level of the mitral valve during diastole. In the long axis view (A and B) the mitral valve is thickened, especially its edges. During diastole (B) the excursion of the leaflets is normal. The free edge, however, is tethered so that the anterior leaflet forms an angle or "elbow." The *arrow* points to the anterior mitral leaflet. The mitral orifice is small. In the four-chamber view during systole (C) the mitral valve (*arrow*) forms a slightly curved line across the orifice. The dense echoes on the ventricular side of the anterior leaflet of the mitral valve probably represent side lobes from calcification adjacent to the base of the mitral valve. During diastole (D) the leaflets dome into the left ventricle. The motion of the leaflets is limited. On the short axis view during diastole (E) the narrow orifice of the mitral valve is demonstrated (*arrow*). This image may be enlarged and its area determined by planimetry. The grid inserted in the right lower corner indicates 1 cm × 1 cm. *LV* = left ventricle; *Ao.* = aorta; *MV* = mitral valve; *LA* = left atrium.

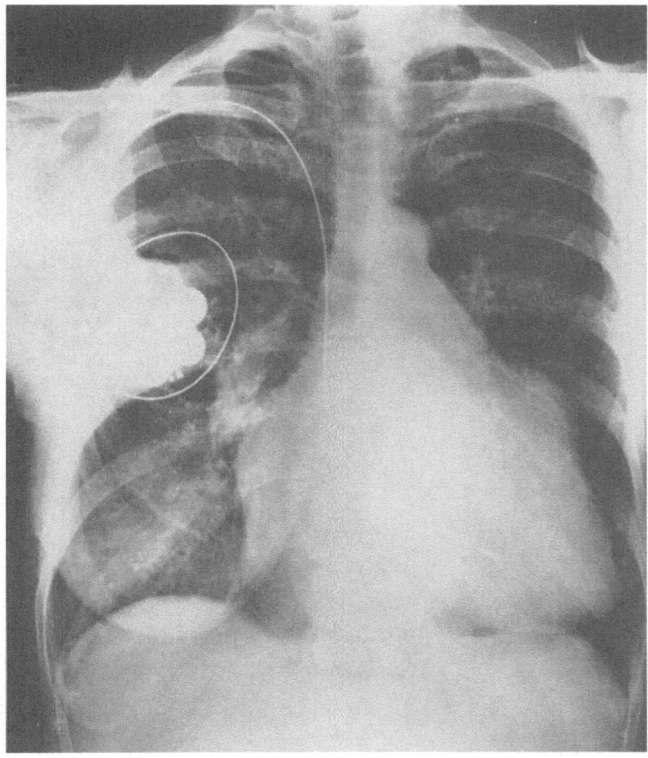

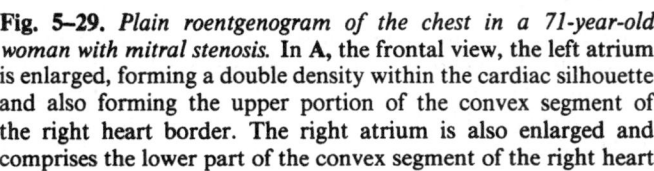

A

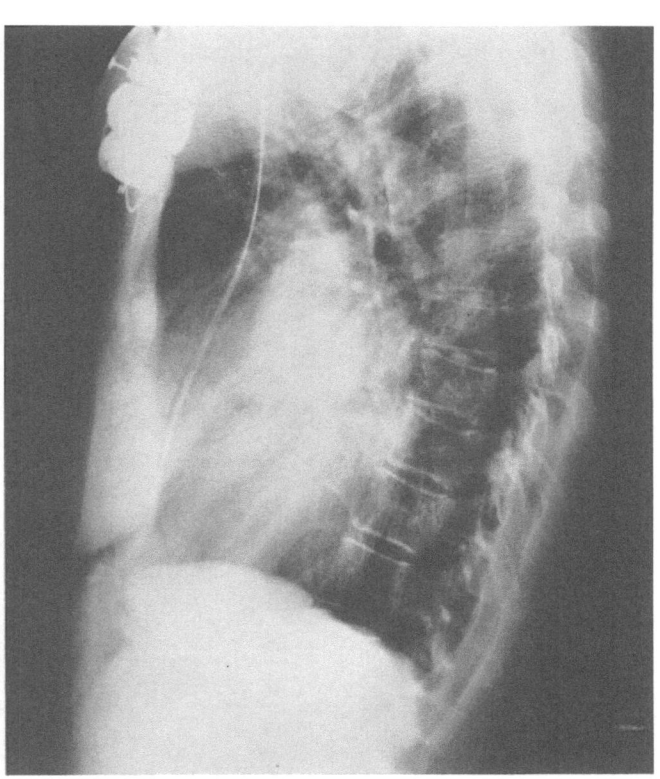

B

Fig. 5–29. *Plain roentgenogram of the chest in a 71-year-old woman with mitral stenosis.* In **A,** the frontal view, the left atrium is enlarged, forming a double density within the cardiac silhouette and also forming the upper portion of the convex segment of the right heart border. The right atrium is also enlarged and comprises the lower part of the convex segment of the right heart border. The opacity of the right atrium is less dense than that of the left atrium. The "third mogul" along the left heart border is formed by the dilated left atrial appendage. **B** On the lateral view the normal retrosternal clear space is obliterated by the enlarged right ventricle and right atrium.

MV is thick and its motion limited; the anterior leaflet domes during diastole. Careful scanning in the short axis may demonstrate the orifice of the MV at the tips of the leaflets. Measurements of the area of this orifice correlate with calculations of valve area based on hemodynamic data and surgical findings. Echocardiography additionally will demonstrate evidence of LA dilatation and RV enlargement if present.

An elevation of the velocity just below the mitral valve by Doppler echocardiography reflects the pressure difference across the valve. A prolonged pressure half-time derived from the Doppler tracing correlates with a small valve area (Hatle).

Radiological (Plain Film) Features

The pulmonary vasculature and the configuration of the cardiovascular silhouette in MS are often characteristic ("mitral heart"), reflecting the pathophysiological changes (Fig. 5–29). The following signs are usually noted on plain films with rheumatic MS: (1) LA enlargement (Figs. 5–30, 5–31), (most common finding); (2) pulmonary venous hypertension; (3) small aortic knob; (4) enlargement of the main pulmonary artery; (5) RV enlargement; (6) RA enlargement; (7) cardiac calcifications (Fig. 5–32) (e.g., MV, LA wall, LA thrombus, wall of LA appendage, pulmonary artery); (8) pulmonary hemosiderosis with pulmonary calcification (Fig. 5–33) and ossification (late findings in pulmonary venous hypertension) and (9) normal sized or small LV. The combination of a normal LV, enlargement of the LA, a prominent pulmonary artery and an inconspicuous aortic arch constitutes the characteristic mitral heart configuration (Fig. 5–29). (See also Chapter 1 for description of pulmonary venous hypertension and cardiac chamber enlargement.)

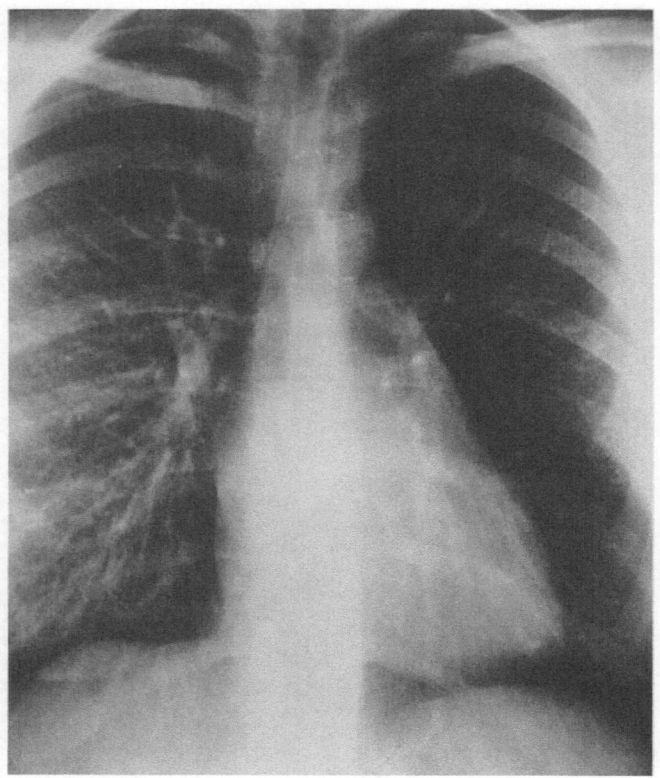

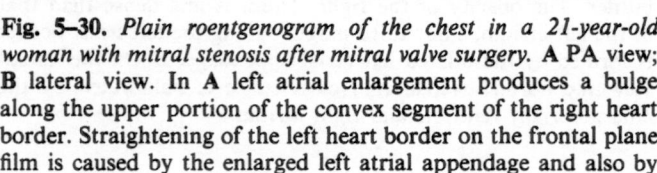

A

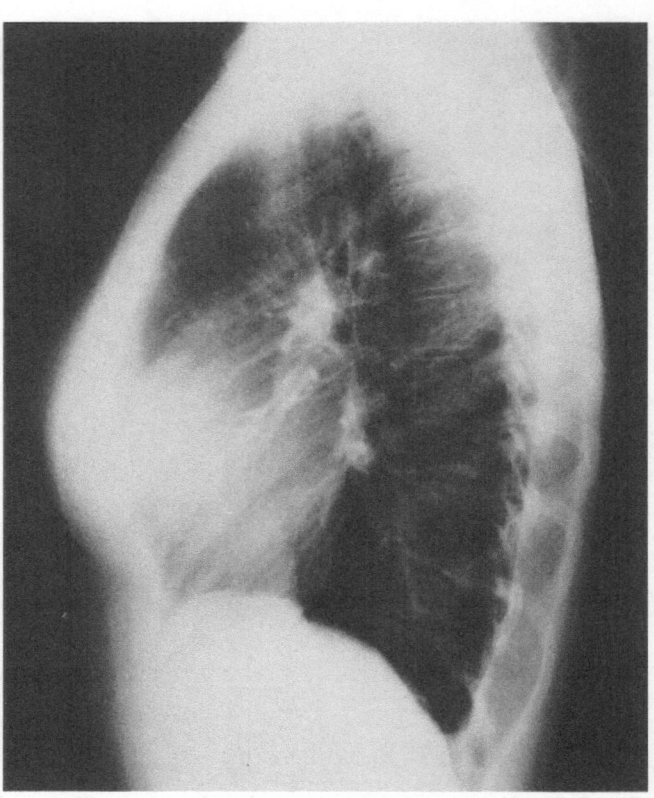

B

Fig. 5–30. *Plain roentgenogram of the chest in a 21-year-old woman with mitral stenosis after mitral valve surgery.* **A** PA view; **B** lateral view. In **A** left atrial enlargement produces a bulge along the upper portion of the convex segment of the right heart border. Straightening of the left heart border on the frontal plane film is caused by the enlarged left atrial appendage and also by mild dilatation of the right ventricle (the outflow tract). On the lateral film (**B**), enlargement of the right ventricular outflow tract partially obliterates the retrosternal clear space. Contrast these subtle findings with classical mitral stenosis illustrated in Fig. 5–29 and with the examples of more exaggerated manifestations of mitral stenosis (Fig. 5–31).

In a large number of patients with MS, MI is associated. Many individuals also have aortic valve disease. The LV does not dilate with pure MS but frequently dilates because of either MI or aortic valve disease. Once this occurs it may be impossible to differentiate between MS and MI on the basis of the plain films alone. Dilatation of the aorta with LV enlargement indicates aortic valve involvement but does not exclude MI. The LA is enlarged in both MS and MI; thus such enlargement is not very helpful in distinguishing between the two entities. Although it has been claimed that a giant LA is characteristic of massive insufficiency and only rarely occurs with pure stenosis, the authors have observed relatively frequently a giant LA in association with pure MS (Fig. 5–34). Aneurysmal dilatation of pulmonary veins (pulmonary varix) is an uncommon finding, being associated with predominant MI (see Fig. 5–47). Calcification of the LA wall represents virtually irrefutable evidence of MS, although rarely it may occur after prosthetic replacement of the MV (Fig. 5–32).

Hemodynamics

In moderate to severe MS, the RV, pulmonary artery and pulmonary artery wedge pressure are elevated. The pulmonary artery wedge pressure, measured simultaneously with the LV pressure, defines the gradient across the valve. The mean valve gradient and the cardiac output are used to calculate the valve area.

The Gorlin Formula for mitral valve area follows:

where A = Valve area (cm²)

$$A = \frac{F}{C \times 44.5\sqrt{\text{mean gradient}}}$$

C = Empiric orifice correction factor obtained by comparing the calculated valve area with the

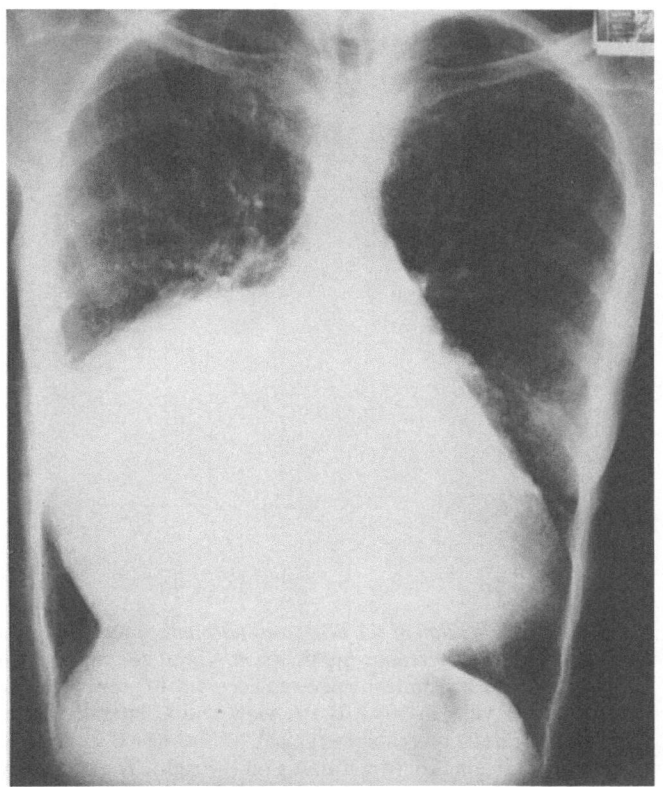

A

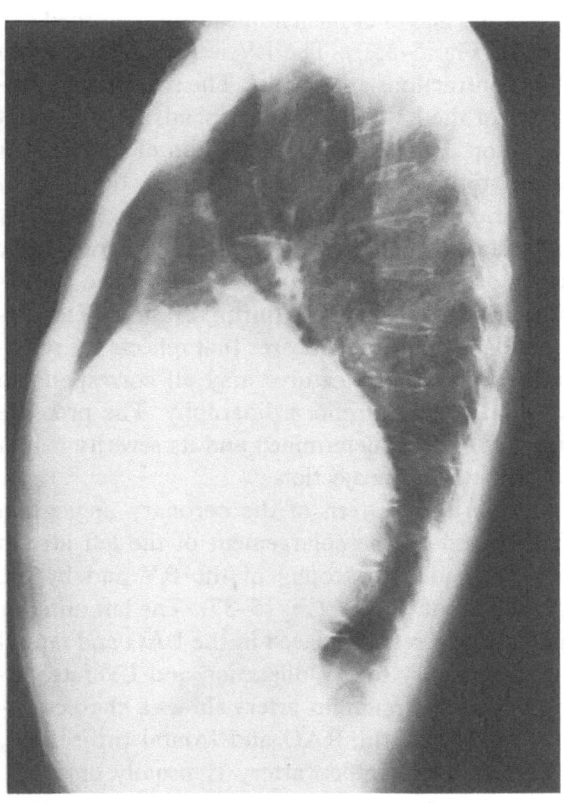

B

Fig. 5–31. *Roentgenograms of the chest in a patient with mitral stenosis and giant left atrium.* **A** *PA view;* **B** *lateral view. On the PA view the left atrium forms the entire right heart border.*

The apex is less dense than usual. In the lateral view the huge left atrium forms the anterior and posterior heart border.

area measured at surgery. (C = 0.85 for the mitral valve). Mean gradient is obtained from the planimetered area between the superimposed left ventricular and left atrial pressure tracings (mm Hg × sec) divided by the diastolic filling period per beat .(sec) measured from the same tracing. (Note: If diastolic filling period per beat is measured from the superimposed aortic and left atrial or pulmonary venous wedge tracings, then C = 0.7).

F = flow rate across the mitral valve (ml/sec) obtained from this formula:

$$F = \frac{\text{cardiac output (ml/min)}}{\text{diastolic filling period (sec/min)}}$$

where diastolic filling period (DFP) is the number of seconds per minute during which filling of the heart occurs. (DFP = diastolic filling period per beat × heart rate).

A MV area of 1.6–2.0 cm² (normal 4–6 cm²) correlates with the presence of mild symptoms. A valve area of 1.0 cm² may be associated with moderate symptoms, and a valve area of 0.5 cm² generally reflects severe symptoms.

Angiocardiography

Selective retrograde opacification of the LV in the RAO (30°) and LAO (70°) projections, using biplane cine technique, is the method of choice for demonstration of diastolic doming of the mitral leaflets (Fig. 5–35A). Varying degrees of obliteration of the radiolucent diastolic filling wave (unopacified blood entering the LV early in diastole) are noted. The MV leaflets are thickened and limited in motion; the papillary muscles and chordae tendineae are thickened and foreshortened (Fig. 5–35B). The LV is usually normal in size, and its contractions are normal. The severity of retrodisplacement of the LV (Fig. 5–36) depends on the extent of RV dilatation. Evaluation of the motion of the anterior leaflet of the mitral valve in the LAO projection is very useful in determination of commissural stenosis. Normally during protodiastole the leaflet opens with a characteristic undulating motion of its free edge. With MS the leaflets pivot open and do not undulate during diastole. The diastolic excursion is limited to a degree that reflects the severity of the stenosis. These features may all correspond to the findings on M-mode echocardiography. The presence of associated MI is best determined and its severity is best estimated in the RAO projection.

The characteristic pattern of the coronary angiogram with MS is caused by the enlargement of the left atrium with dilatation and hypertrophy of the RV and by the retrodisplacement of the LV (Fig. 5–37). The left anterior descending artery is retrodisplaced in the LAO and lateral projections (secondary to RV dilatation and LV retrodisplacement). The left circumflex artery shows a characteristic anterior bowing in the RAO and frontal projections, and the left atrial circumflex artery is usually enlarged. These changes are secondary to LA dilatation. The right coronary artery proper (right circumflex) has a wide sweep (LAO projection) and a longer than normal course, and its branches tend to be large because of RV enlargement. Neovascularity or direct intracavitary drainage (or both) of the atrial branches may be observed, most frequently in the LA appendage (Fig. 5–38). Neovascularity and direct intracavitary drainage in patients with MS have been described in association with thrombus in the LA appendage. In the authors' experience neovascularity and direct intracavitary drainage occur rather frequently in patients with MS, even in the absence of atrial thrombus. The vessels may have formed in response to a thrombus that has since dissolved or embolized, or they may be due to a local phenomenon relating to an abnormality of the wall of the atrium. Neovascularity also occurs in patients with intracavitary tumors, especially left atrial myxoma (Fig. 8–7). The vessels feed the tumor, producing a "blush" inside the heart. Vessels supplying a neoplasm differ from those occurring with mitral stenosis in that they generally originate from sites other than the left atrial appendage.

Treatment

Medical management involves prophylaxis against recurrence of rheumatic fever as well as bacterial endocarditis. Diuretics may relieve symptoms of pulmonary venous hypertension. Digitalis is used to slow the ventricular rate once atrial fibrillation becomes persistent. Anticoagulants are given to patients who are at high risk of embolization.

Surgical treatment consists of mitral commissurotomy or MV replacement, with clots being removed from the LA. On occasion, the LA appendage is removed to reduce the risk of recurrence of thrombosis and embolization.

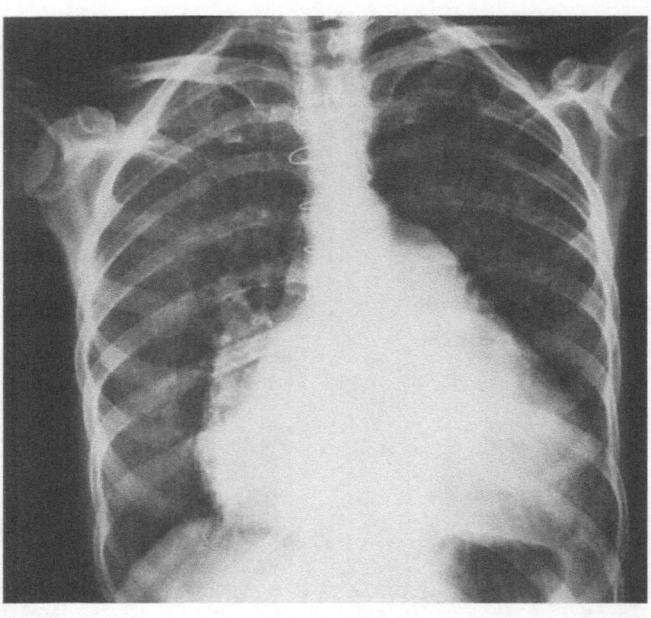

A

Fig. 5–32. *Calcification of the heart and pulmonary vessels caused by chronic pulmonary venous hypertension.* Chest roentgenogram in a woman who had mitral valve replacement for severe mitral stenosis. **A** PA view in 1973; **B** PA view and **C** lateral view in 1981. In **A** the heart presents the typical "mitral heart" configuration. The left atrium is border forming on the right. The convexity of the left heart border is caused by dilatation of the right ventricular outflow tract. The aorta is inconspicuous. By 1981 the entire wall of the left atrium is calcified (**B** and **C**). Calcification of the pulmonary arteries and veins along with pulmonary vascular redistribution indicates chronic pulmonary arterial and venous (precapillary and postcapillary) hypertension. On the lateral film (**C**), calcification of the right ventricular outflow tract is also demonstrated. Calcium in the fornix of the left ventricle (*arrow*) in **B** results from mural thrombosis and scarring after replacement of the mitral valve.

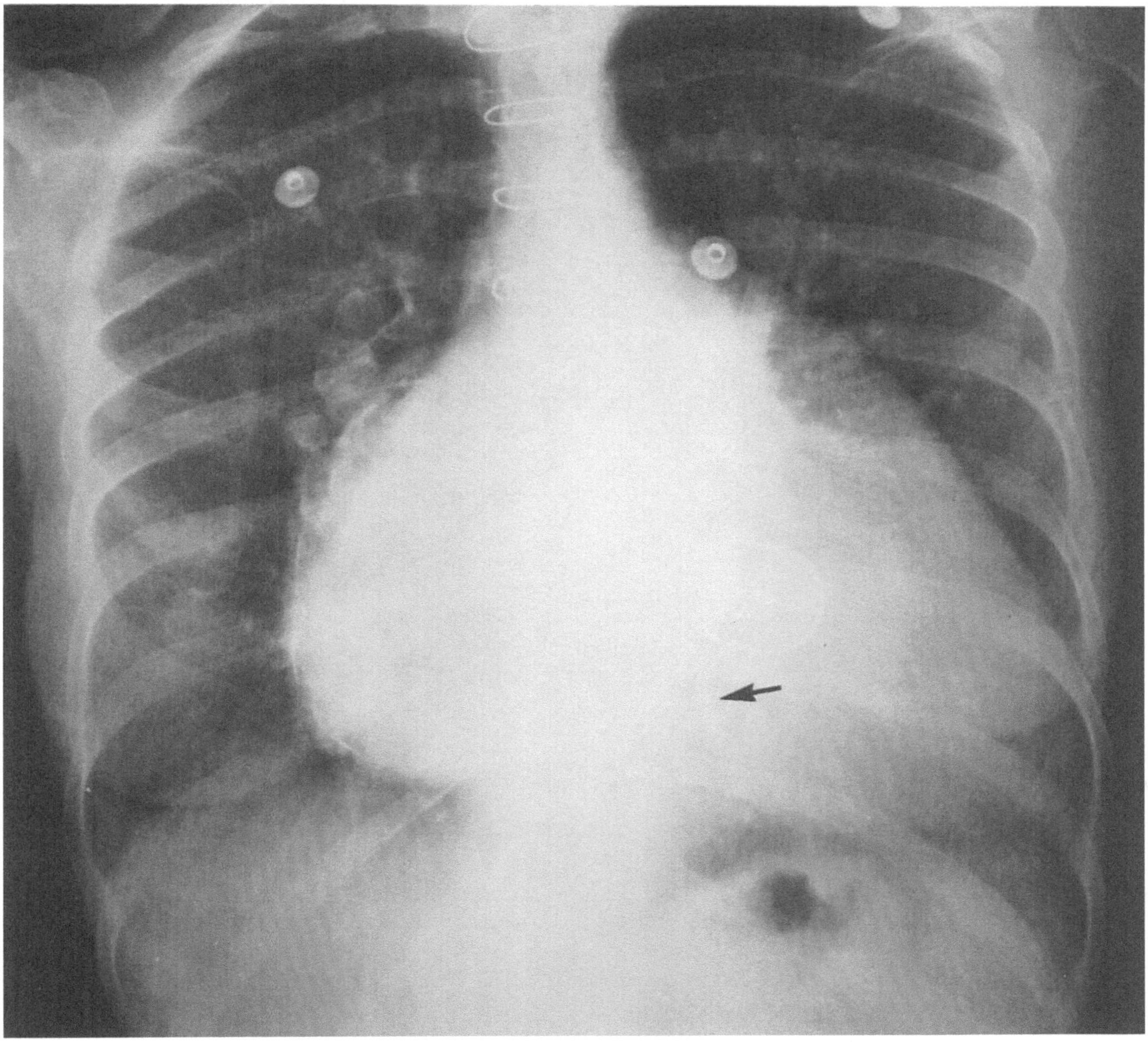

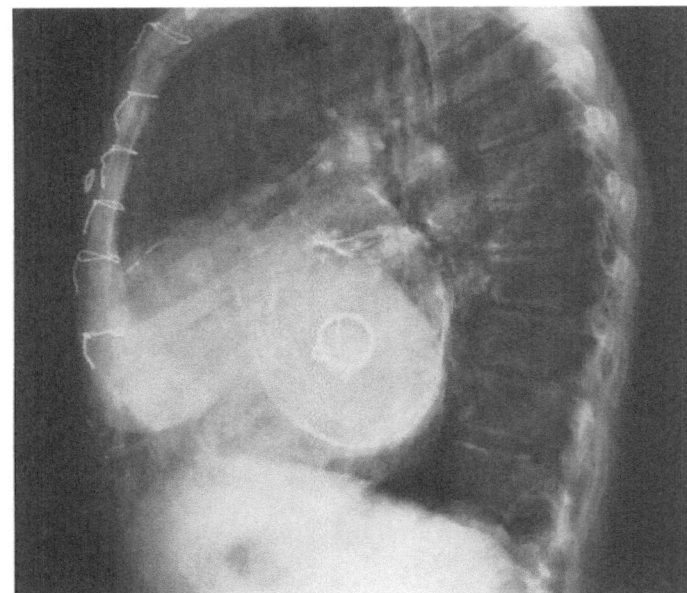

B

C

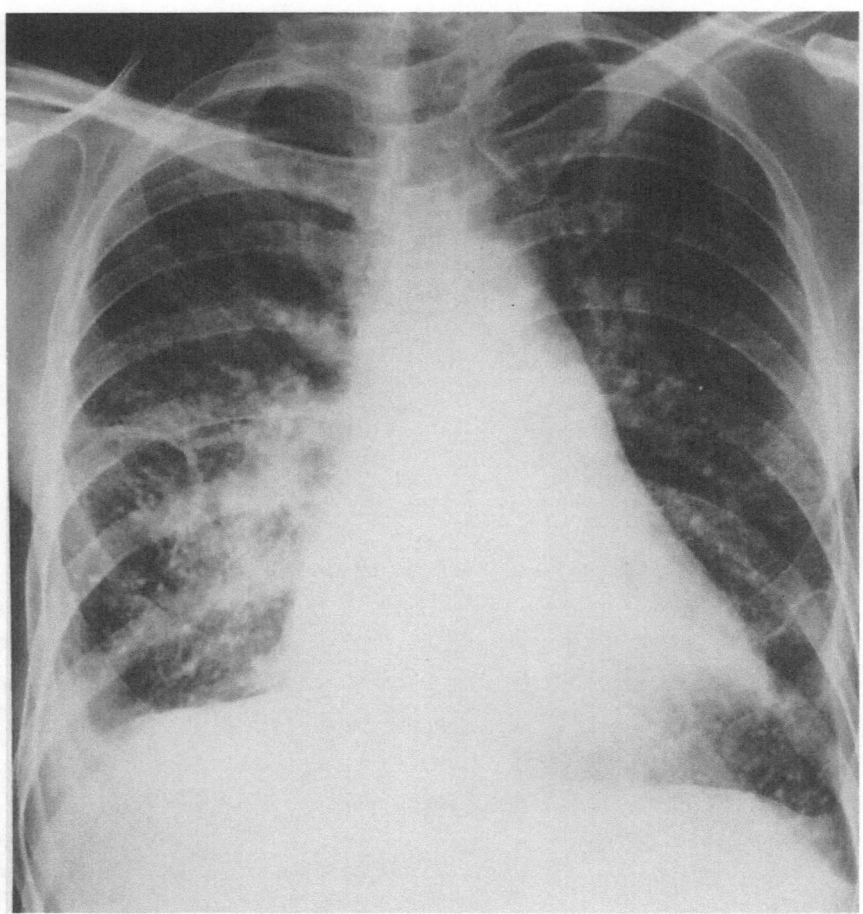

A

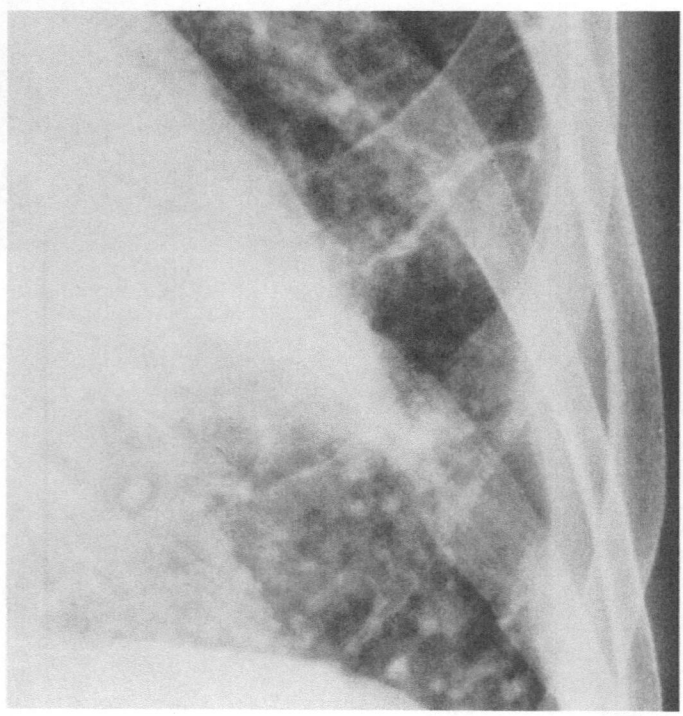

B

Fig. 5–33. *Hemosiderosis and pulmonary ossification in a man with severe mitral stenosis and a previous aortic valve replacement.* Ossific nodules associated with hemosiderosis are present in the pulmonary bases. Pulmonary vascular redistribution, hilar haze and right pleural effusion indicate moderate to severe pulmonary venous hypertension. In **B** (a coned-down view of the left lung base) the ossific nodules are better demonstrated.

Fig. 5–34. *Giant left atrium in a patient with pure mitral stenosis.* **A** PA view; **B** levophase of the pulmonary angiogram; **C** opacification of the right atrium. In **A** the typical "mitral heart" configuration is evident. The left atrium is huge and forms the right heart border. In **B** the giant left atrium is opacified (*arrows*). In **C** the right atrial cavity (*white arrows*) is enlarged but is within the borders of the giant left atrium. The catheter tip is at the junction of the superior vena cava and right atrium (*open arrows*).

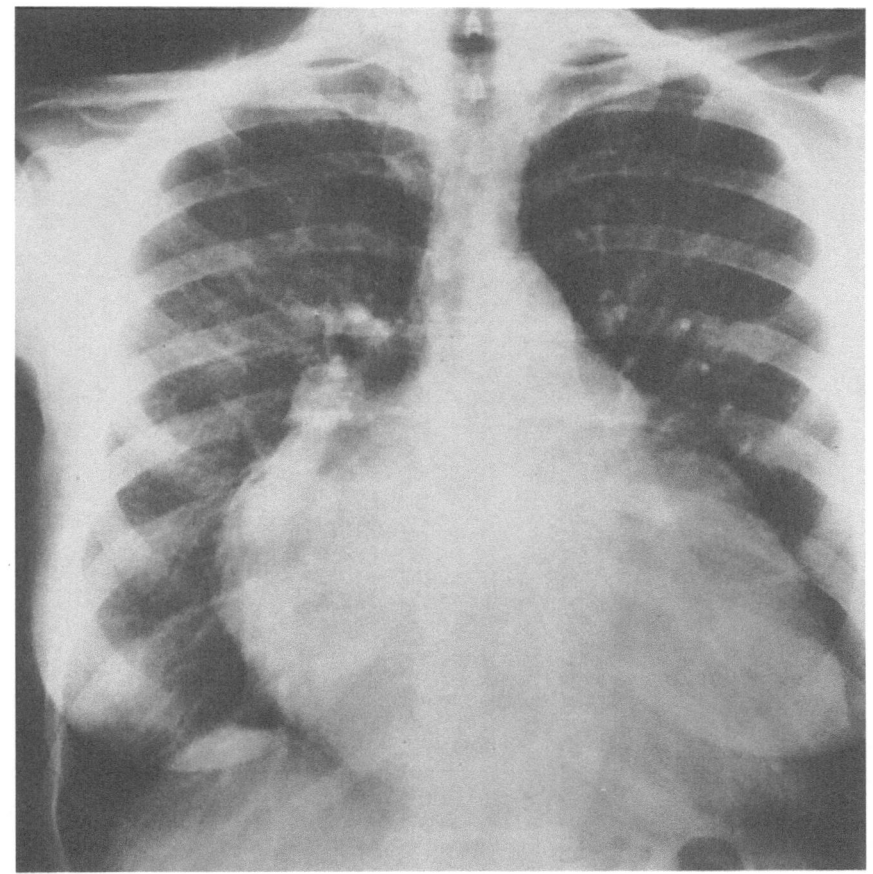

A

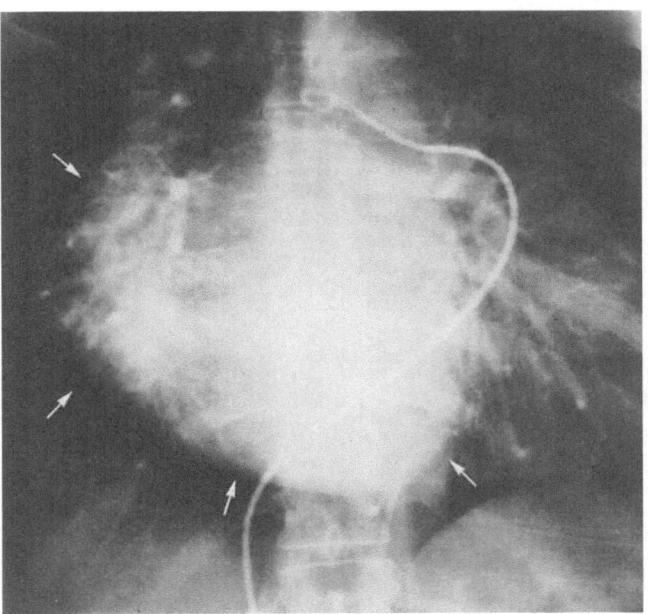

B

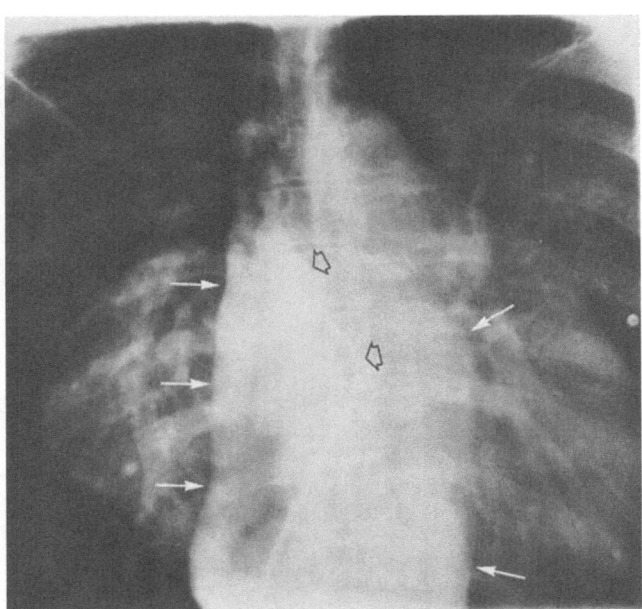

C

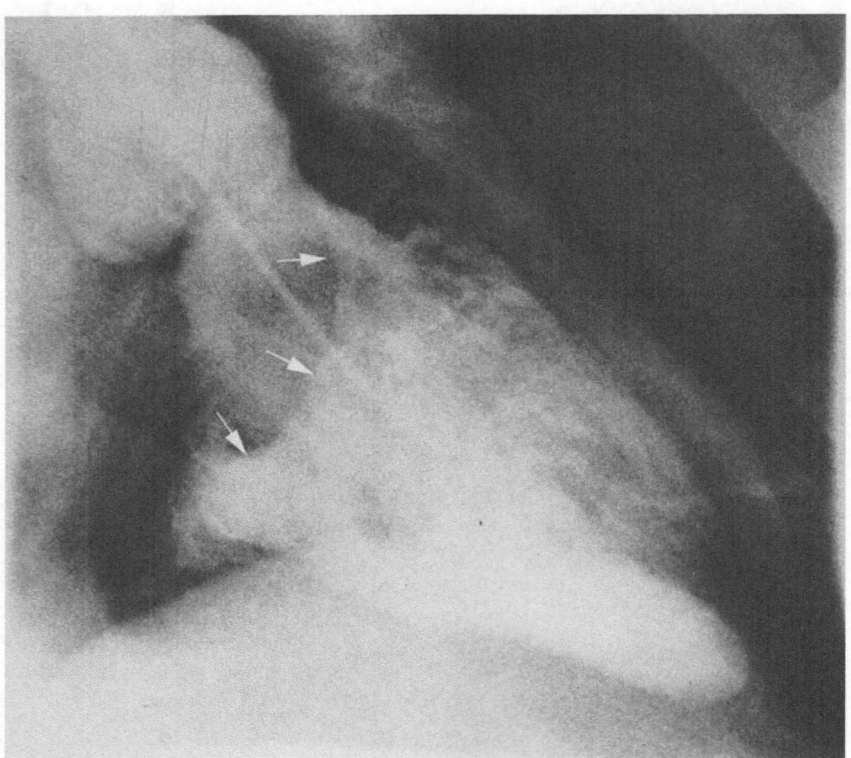

A

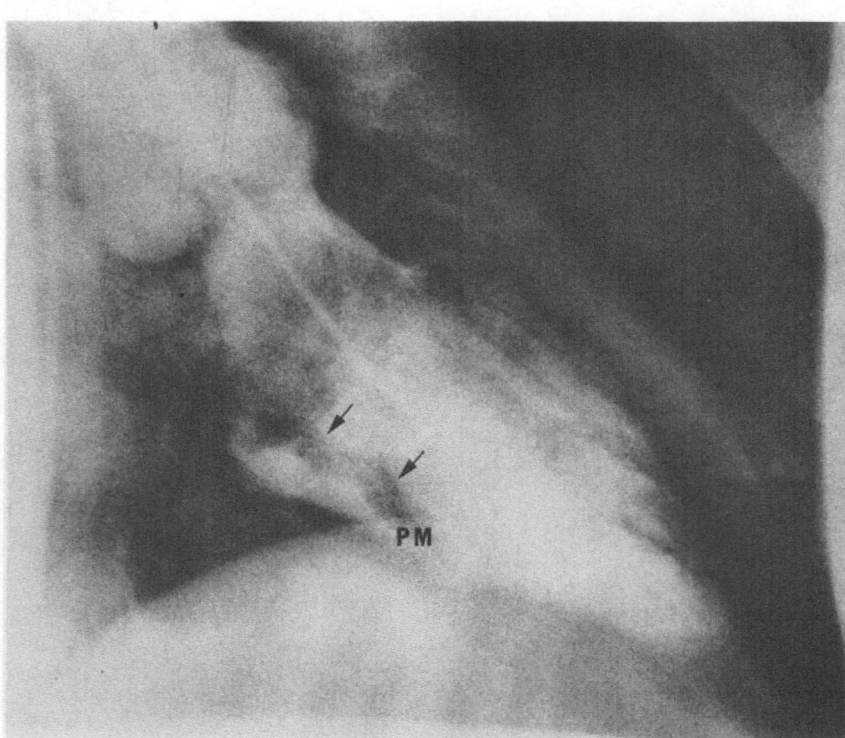

B

Fig. 5–35. *Cine angiogram in mitral stenosis.* **A** RAO view during diastole; **B** RAO view during systole. The mitral valve is domed during diastole (**A**) sharply outlining the posterior leaflet (*arrows*). Contrast material trapped in the subaortic curtain coats the ventricular surface of the anterior leaflet of the mitral valve. The diastolic wave of unopacified blood that normally rushes into the left ventricle is not present with mitral stenosis. Instead, the mitral valve remains sharply outlined during diastole. During systole (**B**) the papillary muscles (*PM*) are foreshortened, and the chordae tendineae are thickened and matted (*arrows*).

Fig. 5–36. *Retrodisplacement of the left ventricle secondary to right ventricular dilatation in a patient with mitral stenosis.* LAO views. **A** Diastole; **B** systole. The apex of the left ventricle is directed approximately toward 6:00 o'clock. (Normally the apex is directed toward 7:00 o'clock.) The degree of counterclockwise rotation corresponds to the extent of dilatation of the right ventricle. This type of rotation of the apex of the left ventricle as a criterion of right ventricular dilatation pertains only to the standard LAO view and not to any angulated views or the standard lateral views. On the standard lateral view the left ventricle is retrodisplaced, but its axis is relatively unchanged. Retrodisplacement of the left ventricle occurs with any condition (volume or pressure overload) that causes enlargement of the right ventricle in the presence of a relatively normal-sized left ventricle. In **A** the left ventricle is also rotated in its vertical axis so that the anterior leaflet of the mitral valve (*white arrows*) is superimposed on the ventricular septum. The bodies of the anterior papillary muscle and fused chordae tendineae (*black arrows*) are outlined in diastole. In **B** the posterior papillary muscle (*PM*) along with its fused foreshortened chordae tendineae (*arrows*) is demonstrated best during systole in this patient.

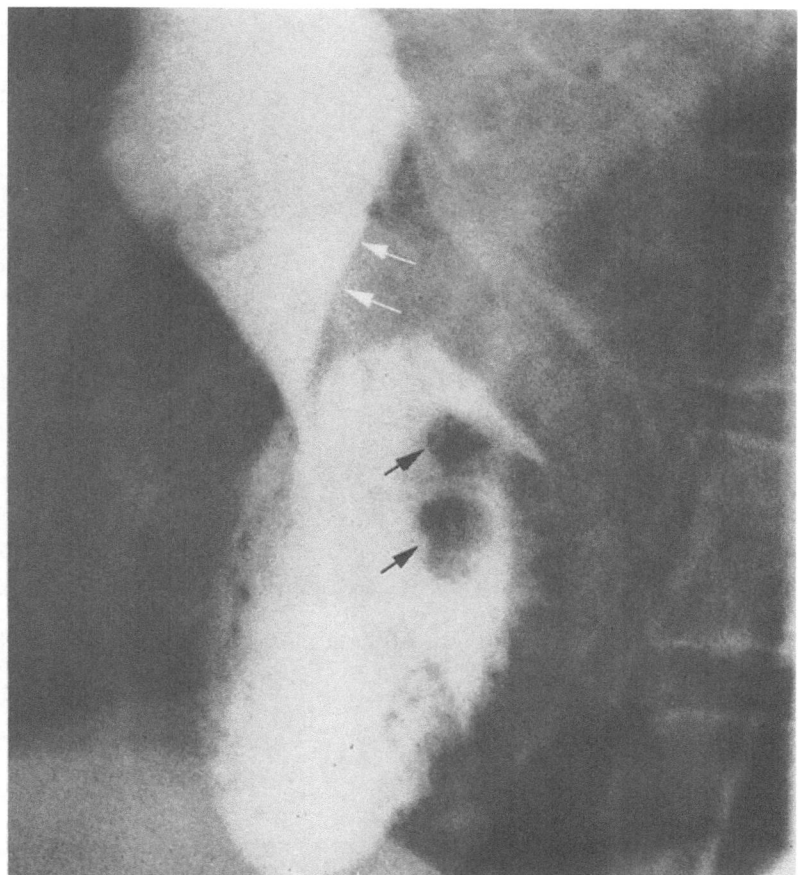

A

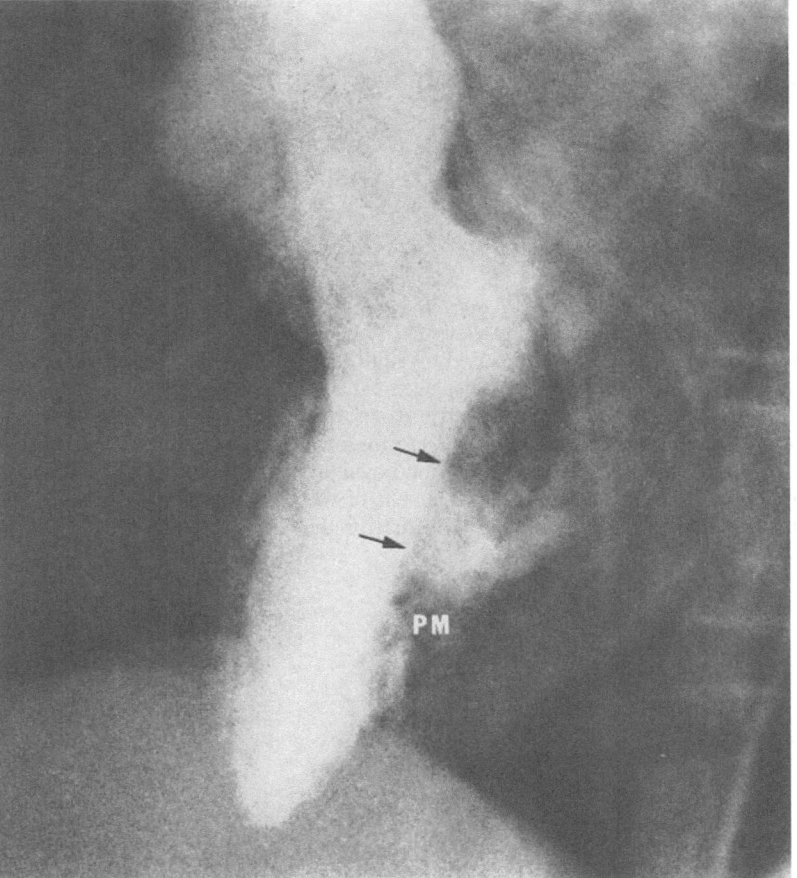

B

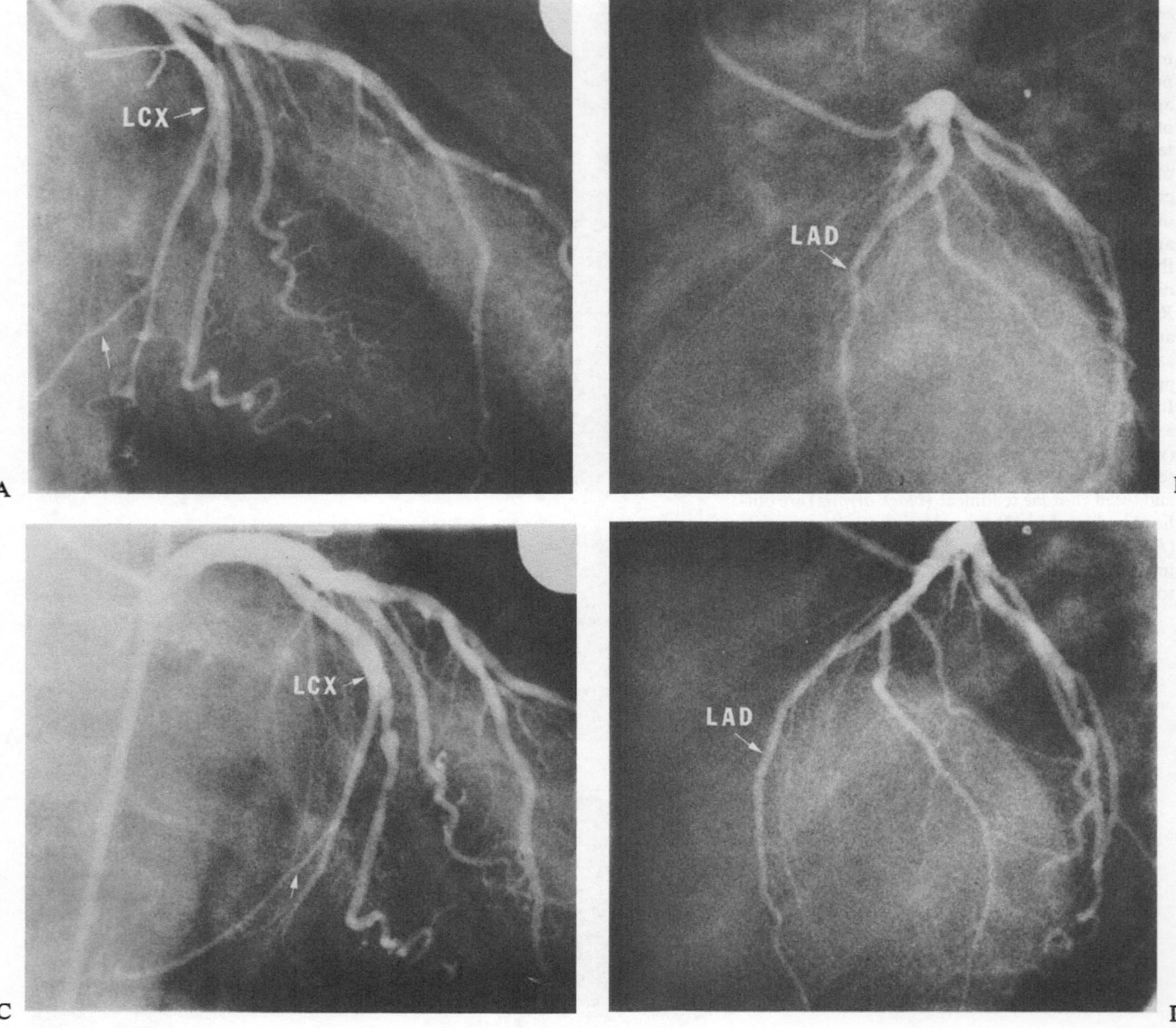

Fig. 5–37. *The appearance of the left coronary artery in mitral stenosis.* **A** RAO view; **B** LAO view; **C** PA view; **D** lateral view. The characteristic pattern is caused by right ventricular enlargement and hypertrophy, by retrodisplacement of the left ventricle and by enlargement of the left atrium. In the RAO and PA views, the left circumflex artery (*LCX*) forms a wide curve toward the apex of the left ventricle (anterior bowing, the opposite of the normal curve) because of enlargement of the left atrium. In the LAO and lateral views the left anterior descending artery (*LAD*) is retrodisplaced. This posterior displacement of the LAD corresponds to a similar retrodisplacement of the left ventricle caused by the dilated right ventricle. Compare with Fig. 5–36. Enlargement of the right ventricle also causes rotation of the heart around its vertical axis so that the LAD on the lateral view appears as if it were in the LAO projection. In **A** and **C** the left atrial circumflex artery is indicated by the *arrow*. This vessel is stretched to delineate the dilated left atrium.

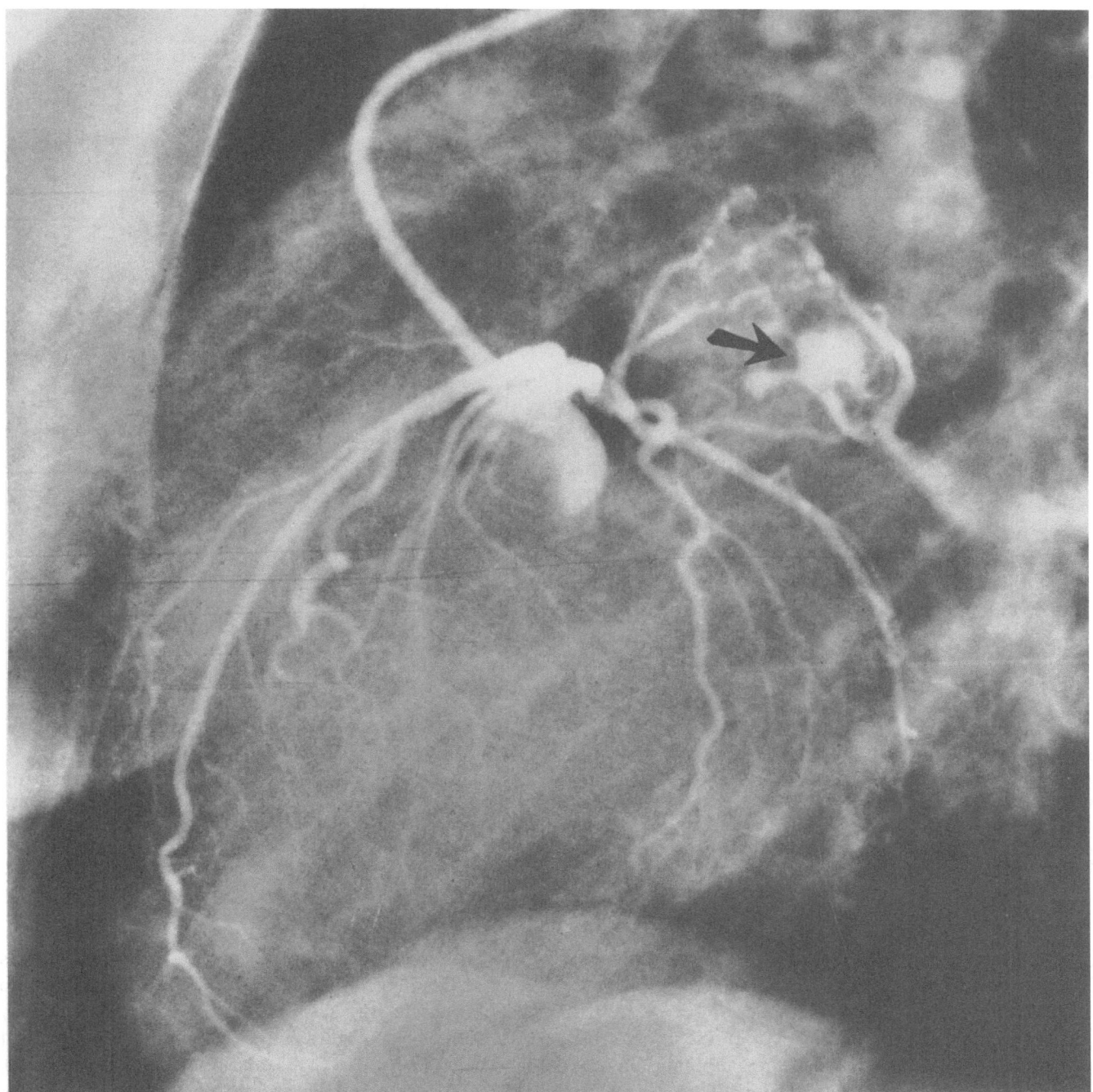

Fig. 5–38. *Neovascularity and direct intracavitary drainage into the left atrial appendage in a 63-year-old woman with mitral stenosis.* Lateral view of selective left coronary artery injection. Branches of the left atrial circumflex artery show numerous distal vessels (neovascularity) and direct drainage into the cavity of the left atrial appendage. The *arrow* points toward a momentary concentration or "puddle" of contrast medium within the left atrial appendage. This contrast material is quickly diluted and carried away by unopacified blood. No left atrial thrombus or neoplasm was observed at operation.

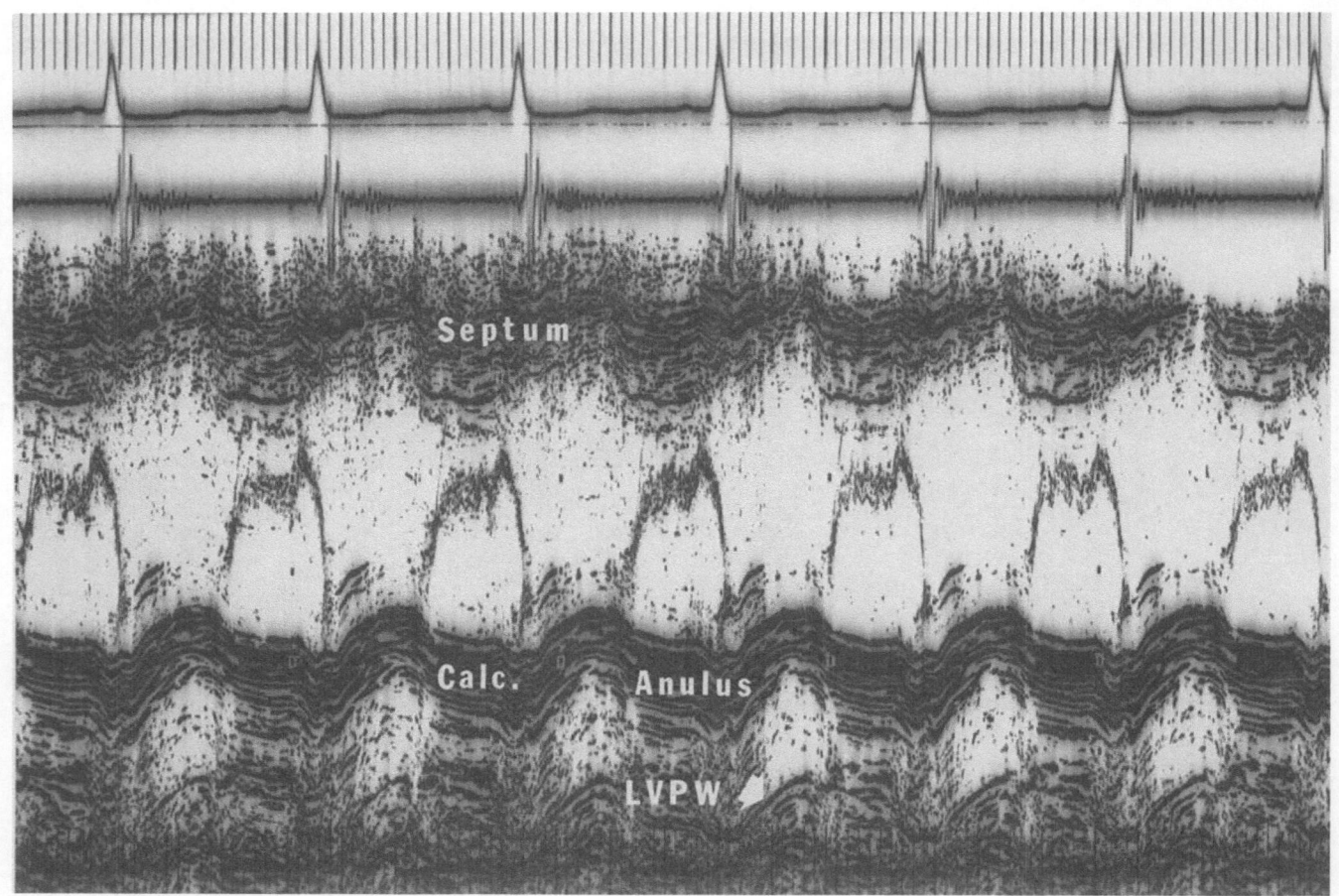

Fig. 5–39. *Calcification of the mitral anulus. M-mode echocardiogram in a patient without signs of mitral valve dysfunction. A dense band of echoes just posterior to the mitral valve (Calc. Anulus) obscures the posterior leaflet. The anterior leaflet of the mitral valve is not thickened and has a normal excursion. These findings militate against the diagnosis of mitral stenosis. (Diastolic* flutter of the anterior leaflet of the mitral valve may be due to aortic insufficiency.) The apparent echo-free space behind the calcified anulus caused by acoustic shadowing should not be mistaken for pericardial effusion. *Septum* = ventricular septum; *LVPW* = posterior wall of the left ventricle.

Dysfunction of the Mitral Valve Secondary to Calcification of the Mitral Anulus

Calcification of the mitral anulus is common in older persons and usually produces no signs or symptoms. On occasion it causes mitral valve dysfunction. If the leaflets are displaced, mitral insufficiency may result. If the calcium surrounds the MV it may reduce the size of its orifice and produce mitral stenosis. Calcium may also extend into the ventricular septum, producing left ventricular outflow tract obstruction and arrhythmias, including complete heart block.

Conditions that predispose toward or accelerate calcification of the mitral anulus are hypertension, aortic stenosis, possibly hypertrophic cardiomyopathy, hyperlipidemia, chronic hypercalcemia due to renal or parathyroid disease and abnormalities of connective tissue (e.g., Hurler syndrome, Marfan syndrome).

Clinical findings are those of mitral insufficiency, mitral stenosis or subaortic stenosis.

On M-mode echocardiography the calcium appears as a dense band just behind the MV, often extending into the LV muscle (Fig. 5–39). The LV posterior wall may be obscured by acoustic shadowing to produce an apparent echo-free space (not to be mistaken for pericardial effusion). The calcific density may also appear to extend into the LA as the echo beam is directed cephalad, beyond the LA–LV junction. The extension of the image is due to the intensity of the returning echoes, causing failure of lateral resolution.

The posterior mitral leaflet is often obscured; however, the anterior mitral leaflet is not thickened and usually has a normal E-F slope. These findings, if present, distinguish calcification of the mitral anulus from MV stenosis.

On 2-D echocardiography the calcified anulus may form a crescent at the atrioventricular junction in the short axis view (Fig. 5–40). The mitral leaflets move normally unless calcium restricts their motion. In severe cases with LV inflow obstruction, calcium deposits extend into the ventricular septum and between the aortic and mitral valves.

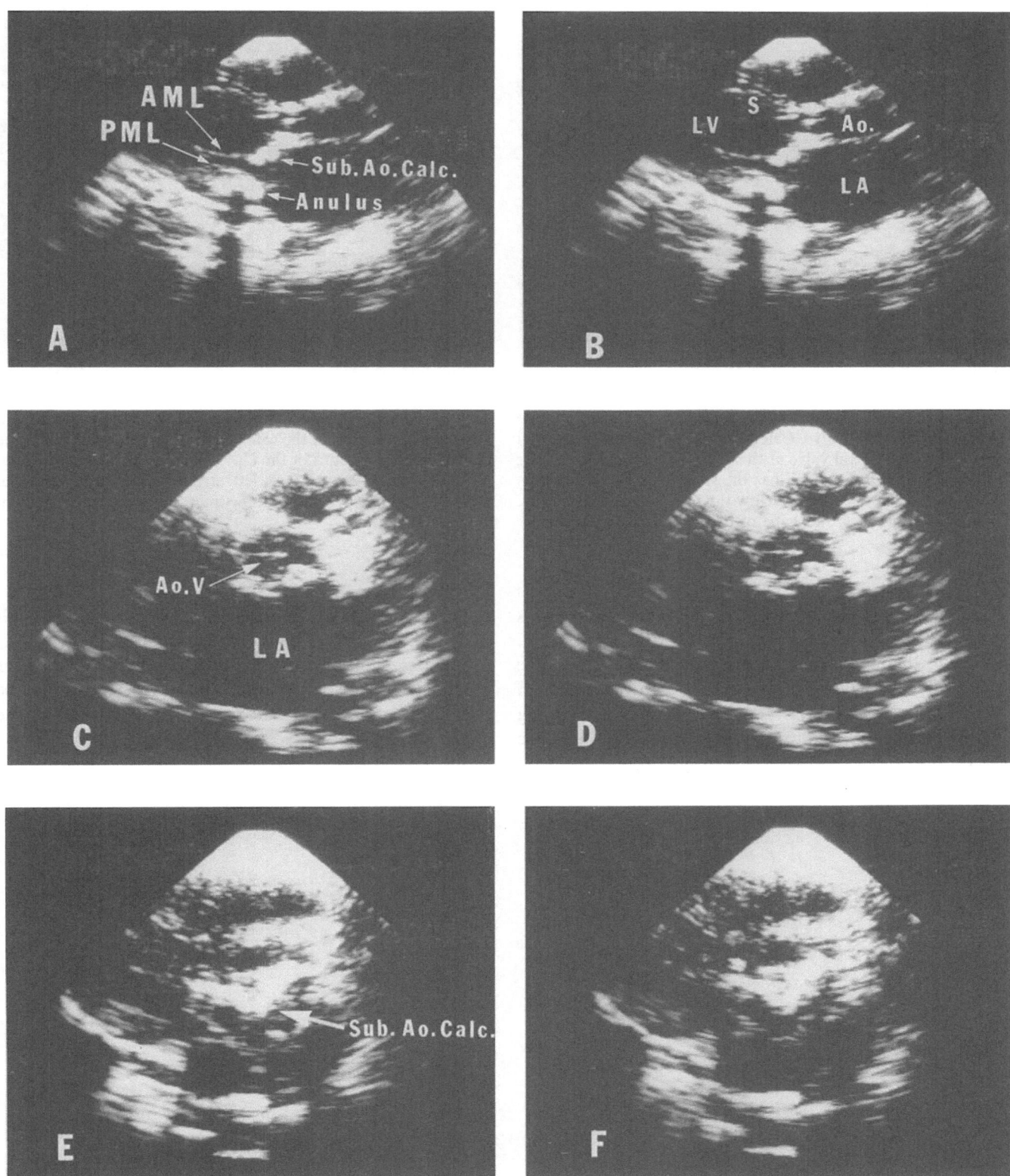

Fig. 5–40. *Two-dimensional echocardiogram in a 69-year-old woman with severe calcification of the mitral anulus causing mitral stenosis.* In this patient the calcium extends across the ventricular septum into the base of the anterior leaflet of the mitral valve to completely encircle the mitral orifice. **A** and **B** Long axis view of the left ventricle; **C** and **D** short axis view at the level of the aortic valve. **E–H** short axis views of the left ventricular outflow tract and mitral anulus. In **A** and **B** dense calcific masses are present within the mitral anulus and in the subaortic region (*Sub.*

Ao. Calc.). The orifice of the mitral valve is markedly narrowed. The anterior mitral leaflet (*AML*) and posterior mitral leaflet (*PML*) are displaced but are not thickened. Note acoustic shadowing behind the calcified mitral anulus. The left atrium (*LA*) is enlarged. In **C** and **D** the aortic orifice is not narrowed, and the aortic leaflet is not thickened. In **E** and **F** the transducer is aimed slightly below the aortic valve so that calcium is demonstrated within the base of the anterior mitral leaflet just below the aortic valve (*Sub. Ao. Calc.*). (*Continued*)

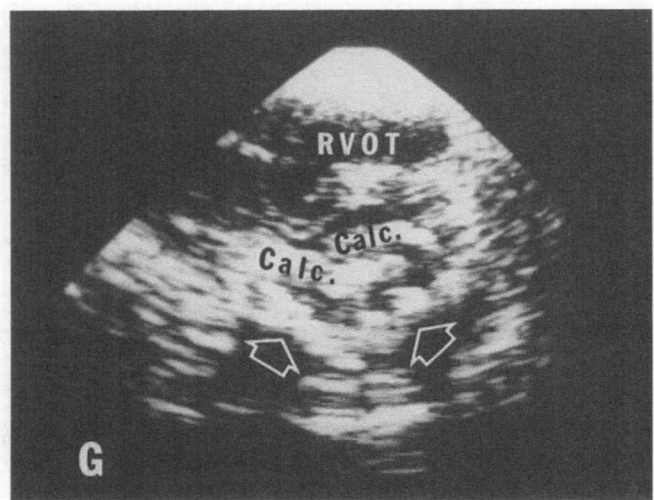

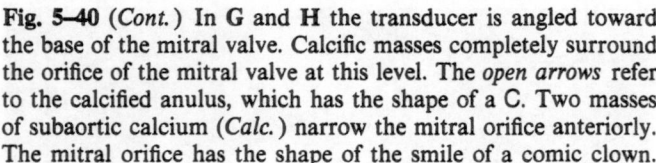

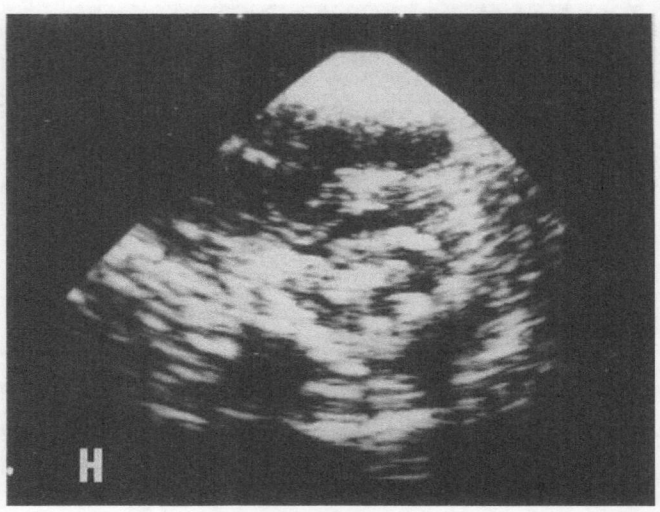

Fig. 5–40 (*Cont.*) In **G** and **H** the transducer is angled toward the base of the mitral valve. Calcific masses completely surround the orifice of the mitral valve at this level. The *open arrows* refer to the calcified anulus, which has the shape of a C. Two masses of subaortic calcium (*Calc.*) narrow the mitral orifice anteriorly. The mitral orifice has the shape of the smile of a comic clown.

This calcification pattern has been called the "O" configuration; however, in this patient the calcified mitral anulus had the shape of a "D" on plain films of the chest. See Fig. 5–42. *Ao.* = aorta; *Ao.V* = aortic valve; *LA* = left atrium; *LV* = left ventricle; *RVOT* = right ventricular outflow tract; *S* = ventricular septum.

On plain films or cine fluorography the calcium forms a C or J shape in the position of the mitral anulus (Fig. 5–41). On the lateral or LAO view the so-called O shape calcification of the mitral anulus may be observed if calcium extends across the base of the anterior mitral leaflet, closing the ring (Fig. 5–42). In the authors' case this has the shape of a D.

On angiography the mitral leaflets move normally, although the mitral orifice is reduced in size.

Medical and surgical treatment is similar to that for rheumatic MV disease. Replacement of the valve may be difficult because of associated disease and because of the localized calcification.

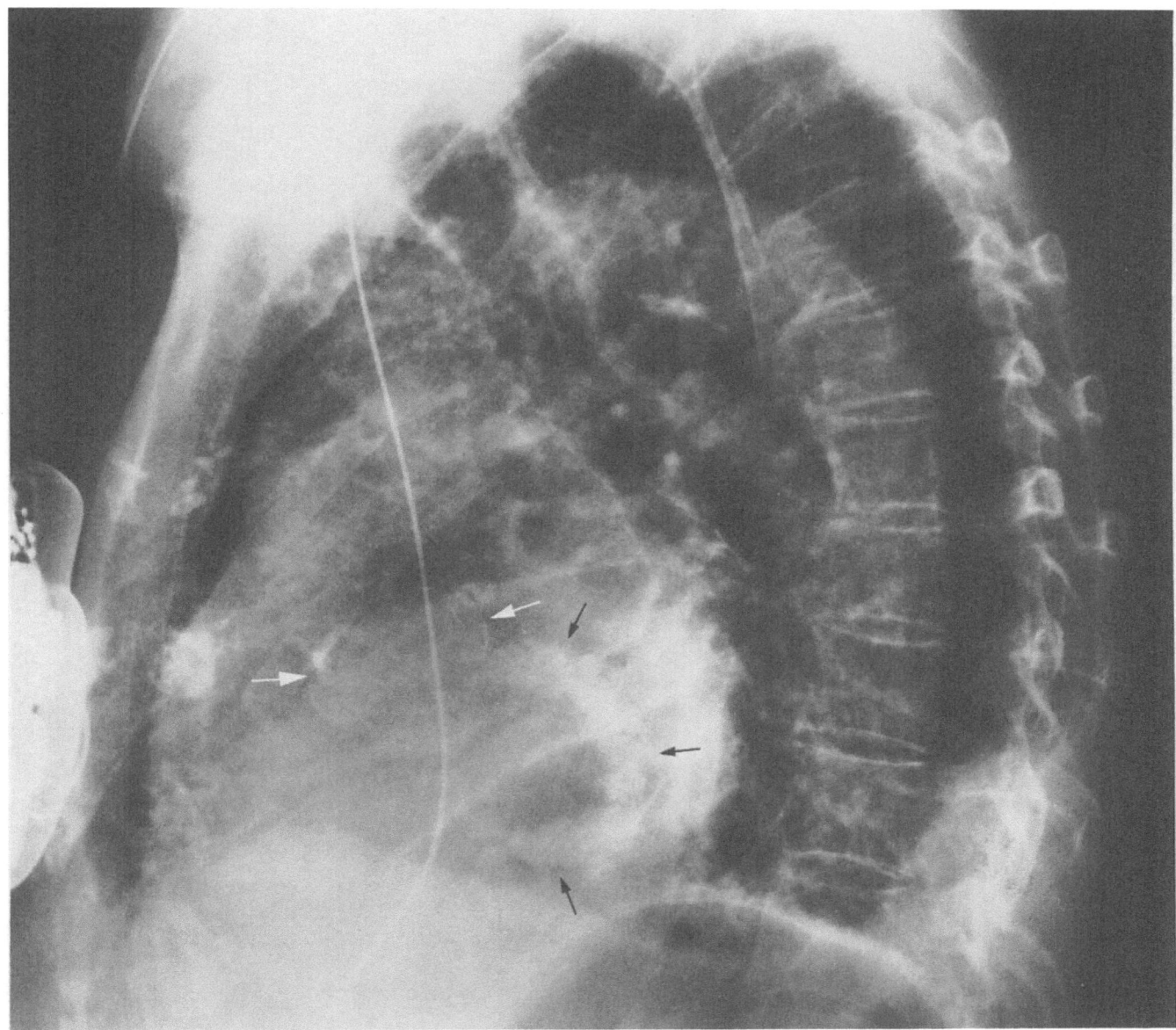

Fig. 5–41. *Calcification of the mitral anulus. Lateral roentgenogram of the chest in an asymptomatic 83-year-old woman.* The calcified mitral anulus forms a typical C shape (*black arrows*). Despite extensive calcification the mitral anulus did not interfere with the function of the mitral valve. The anterior mitral leaflet is not attached to the anulus. Superiorly it is in continuity with the aortic valve. Inferiorly it is attached to the posterior portion of the atrioventricular septum (see Fig. 7–34). Calcification of the aortic ring (*white arrows*) outlines the normal relationship between the aortic and mitral rings.

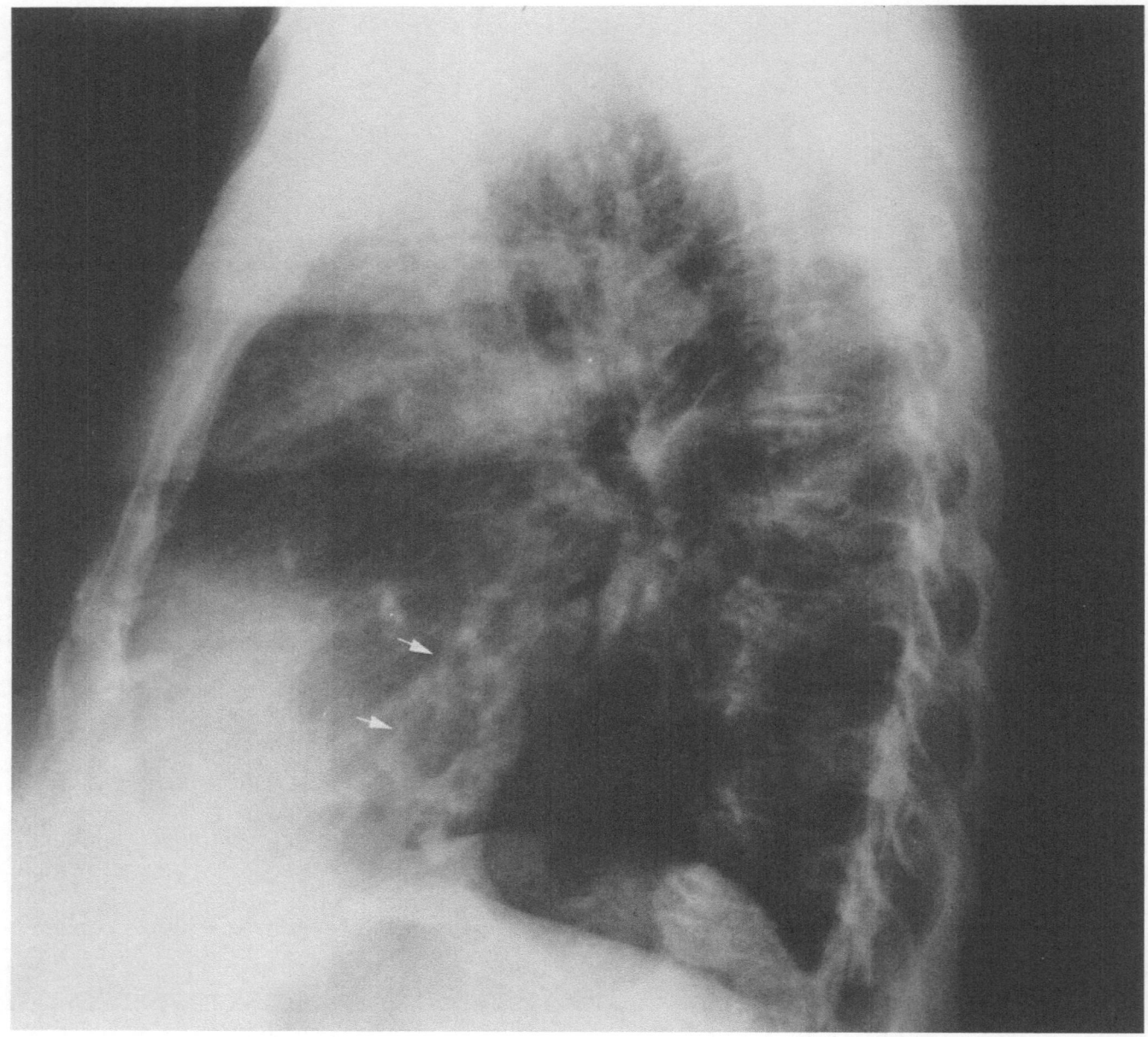

Fig. 5–42. *Calcification of the mitral anulus causing mitral stenosis in a 69-year-old woman.* The lateral roentgenogram of the chest demonstrates extensive calcification of the mitral anulus giving a C shaped appearance. Calcification extending across the ventricular aspect of the base of the anterior leaflet of the mitral valve forms a relatively straight line, completing the ring around the orifice of the mitral valve (*arrows*). On two-dimensional echocardiography (Fig. 5–40) and on left ventriculography the motion of the mitral leaflets was normal; however, heavy deposits of calcium narrowed the orifice.

Lutembacher Syndrome

This infrequently encountered syndrome consists of a combination of mitral stenosis and atrial septal defect, with the mitral stenosis almost always rheumatic in origin. The atrial septal defect allows the LA to decompress into the RA, creating a left-to-right shunt of variable size while reducing systemic blood flow. Symptoms of fatigue and dyspnea on exertion are prominent.

Plain films (Fig. 5–43) show a "mitral heart" with pulmonary overcirculation, which may be associated with pulmonary venous hypertension—an unusual combination in adults. The right side of the heart is enlarged. The LA will be enlarged if the atrial septal defect is small. Calcification of the mitral valve may be the only clue to the diagnosis of this entity on plain films. At cardiac catheterization the large atrial level shunt will be identified. Hemodynamic findings may be equivocal for mitral stenosis since the LA pressure may be normal or minimally elevated. Mitral stenosis will be diagnosed on left ventriculography or on left atrial injection.

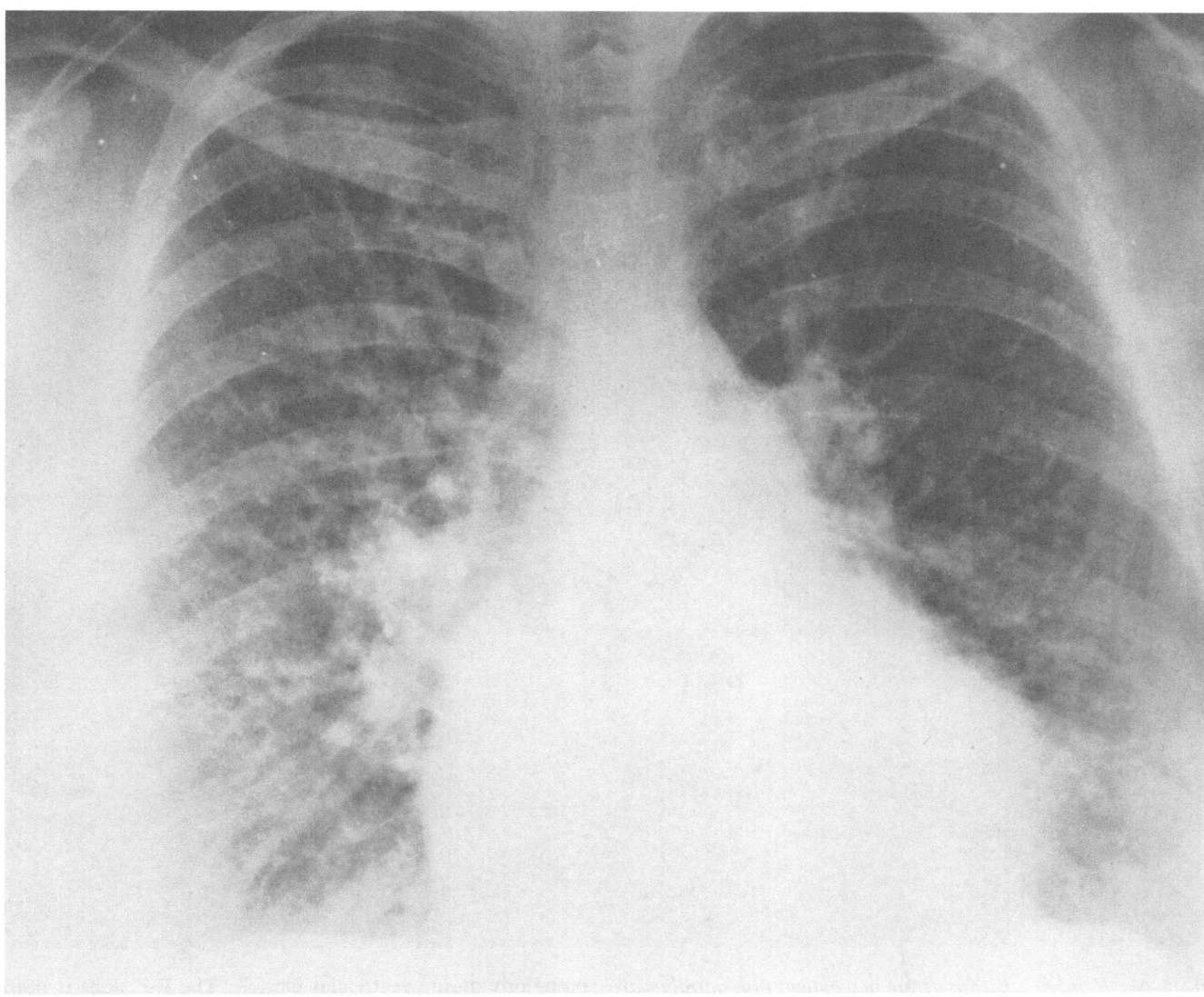

Fig. 5–43. *Lutembacher syndrome. Frontal plane roentgenogram of the chest after mitral commissurotomy.* Marked pulmonary overcirculation is present. The pulmonary arteries are dilated in both the basal and apical areas. The margins of the vessels are indistinct because of associated pulmonary venous hypertension. Both atria are enlarged. The left ventricle is normal in size. In summary, this roentgenogram shows the unusual combination of a "mitral heart" configuration with pulmonary overcirculation.

Mitral Insufficiency

Mitral insufficiency (MI) results from incomplete closure (inadequate coaptation) of the mitral valve. Scarring, shortening, rigidity and fixation of the mitral leaflets and chordae tendineae account for MI in rheumatic heart disease. Of course, insufficiency may be due to many other causes, such as rupture or dysfunction of the papillary muscles in ischemic heart disease; prolapse of the mitral valve secondary to either ischemic heart disease or myxomatous degeneration; bacterial endocarditis; rupture of chordae tendineae either due to infective endocarditis, spontaneous rupture or trauma; hypertrophic cardiomyopathy; and con-genital anomalies of the mitral valve apparatus (e.g., double mitral orifice, parachute mitral valves, cleft leaflets). Furthermore, functional MI may be the result of any condition that causes dilatation of the LV and mitral anulus (e.g., hypertension, aortic insufficiency, cardiomyopathy).

Clinical Features

Symptoms may be delayed for many years even with severe MI. Fatigue and dyspnea tend to begin imperceptibly and progress slowly unless a new attack of acute rheumatic fever or of bacterial endocarditis or rupture of the chordae tendineae supervenes. On physical examination in mild to moderate MI a hyperdynamic LV impulse is felt. A harsh

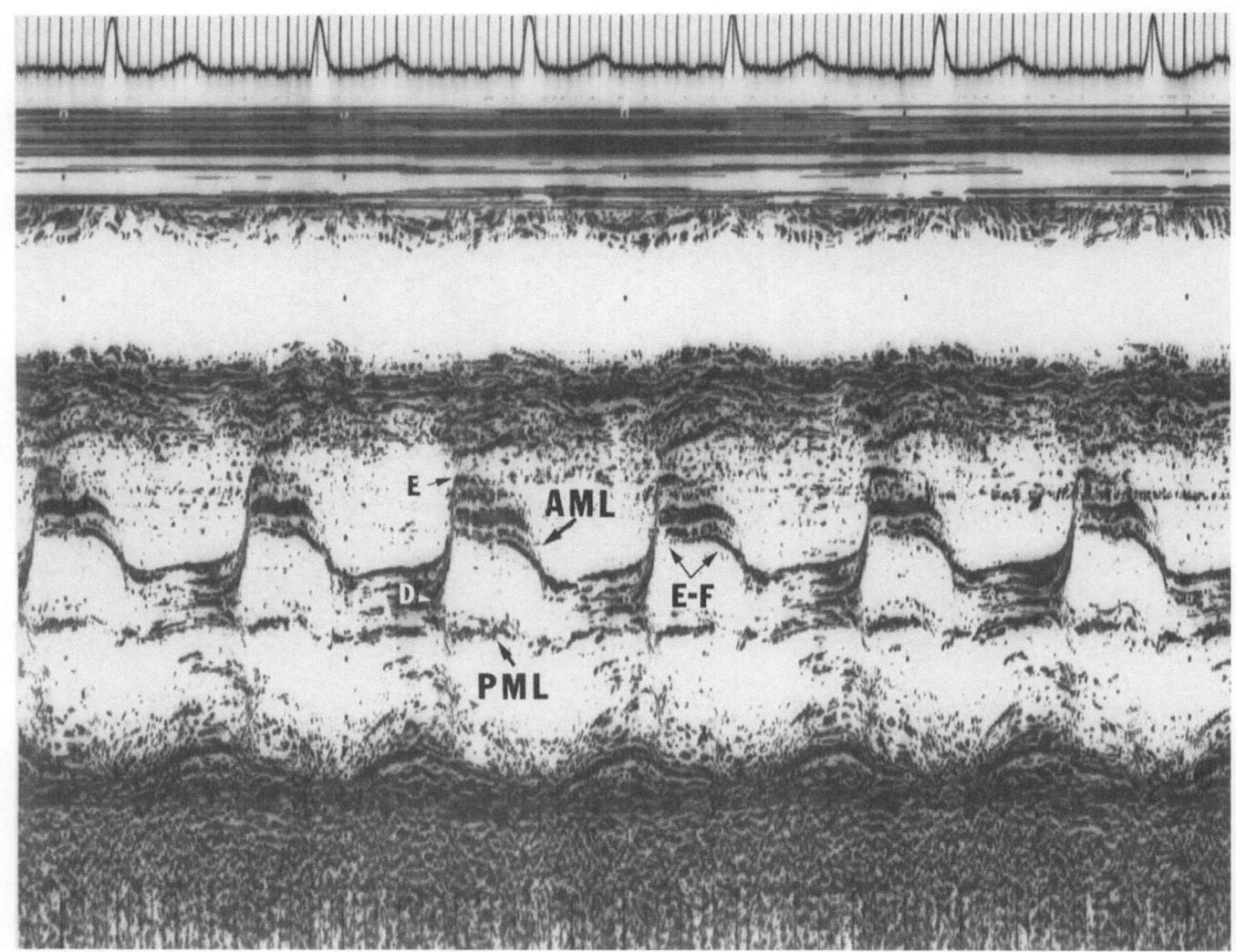

Fig. 5–44. *M-mode echocardiogram in a patient with mitral insufficiency secondary to rheumatic valvulitis.* The leaflets are thickened; however, the D-E excursion of the anterior leaflet (*AML*) is normal. The posterior leaflet of the mitral valve (*PML*) moves posteriorly during ventricular diastole. The E-F slope is nearly horizontal, suggesting mitral stenosis. Compare this tracing with those showing predominantly mitral stenosis (Fig. 5–27).

high-pitched pansystolic murmur is best heard at the apex, transmitting laterally toward the axilla. A thrill may be present as well, and an S$_3$ gallop may be heard.

With severe MI the apex impulse is diffuse and displaced laterally as a result of LV enlargement. A diastolic flow rumble indicates excessive flow into the LV, composed of pulmonary venous return plus regurgitant volume. Signs of right-sided overload are uncommon in MI. In addition, a mid systolic click or a late systolic murmur or both would indicate mitral valve prolapse. The electrocardiogram may show LA enlargement (p-mitrale) or atrial fibrillation. LV hypertrophy is common, while on occasion RV hypertrophy or even hypertrophy of both chambers occurs.

Echocardiography
Doppler echocardiography is used to distinguish regurgitant flow, and provides a rough estimate of severity. If structural changes of the mitral valve consistent with MI are present, these may be diagnosed by M-mode and 2-D echocardiography. Thus, thickening of the mitral valve associated with rheumatic valvulitis (Fig. 5–44), mitral valve prolapse (see Figs. 5–50 to 5–53), mitral vegetation (see Figs. 5–61 to 5–65) and flail mitral leaflet (see Fig. 5–66), can all be recognized. Calcification of the mitral anulus (Figs. 5–39 and 5–40), which may interfere with mitral valve function, is best assessed by 2-D echocardiography. In addition, LA size, LV size and LV function can also be evaluated.

Radiological (Plain Film) Features
Because of the increased work load (increased blood volume) caused by MI the LV may dilate, and the LA may enlarge. The degree of LA enlargement varies from mild to severe (giant LA) (Fig. 5–45). Varying degrees of pulmo-

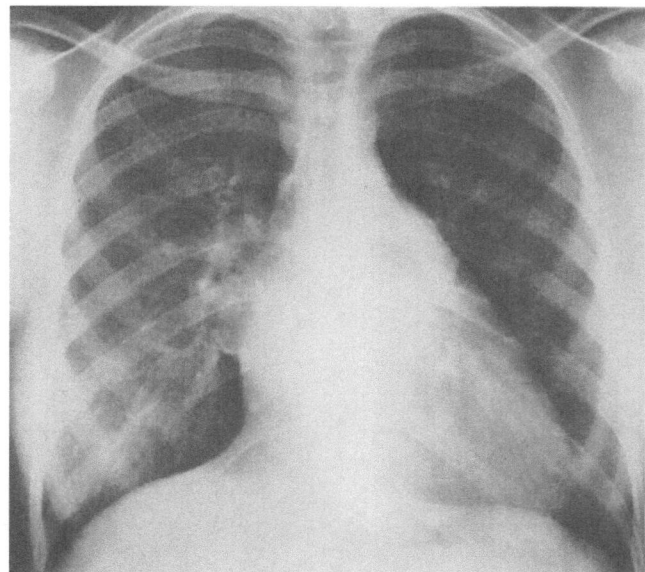

A

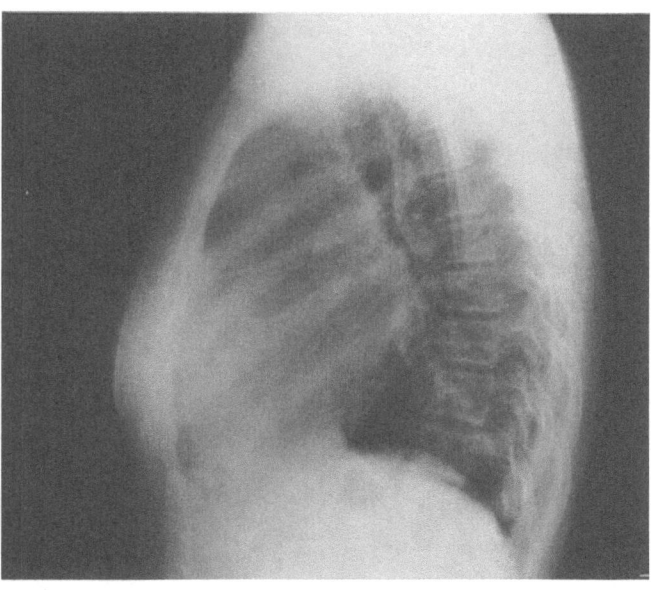

B

Fig. 5–45. *Mitral insufficiency in a 15-year-old girl with rheumatic mitral valve disease.* **A** PA chest roentgenogram; **B** lateral chest roentgenogram. The enlarged left atrium is border forming over the upper part of the convex portion of the right heart border, obliterating the clear space normally present between the right atrium and the pulmonary artery. Straightening of the left heart border is caused by enlargement of the left atrial appendage.

Left ventricular enlargement causes elongation of the left heart border so that the apex points downward. The aorta is inconspicuous. The pulmonary artery is mildly prominent. On the lateral view the enlarged left atrium displaces the left main bronchus posteriorly and superiorly. The retrosternal clear space is obliterated by the dilated right ventricular outflow tract.

nary venous hypertension may be present. Enlargement of the RV and RA occurs late in the disease (Fig. 5–46). Mitral valve calcification is unusual in pure MI.

Rarely, aneurysmal dilatation of the pulmonary veins occurs at the entrance to the LA (Fig. 5–47). The dilated vein or veins may simulate a paracardiac mass on the posteroanterior and lateral projections. Oblique views will demonstrate the area of aneurysmal dilatation at the entrance of the pulmonary veins into the LA. Angiography may be necessary for confirmation (Fig. 5–48).

Hemodynamics

The characteristic hemodynamic finding at cardiac catheterization is the demonstration of a large, early appearing (regurgitant) *v* wave in the pulmonary wedge tracing. The height of the *v* wave is determined by a combination of two factors: (1) the amount of regurgitant blood entering the LA during ventricular systole and (2) the compliance of the LA. With acute mitral insufficiency the LA is small and noncompliant, and the *v* wave is very large. With chronic MI and marked dilatation of the LA, the LA pressure wave may appear normal even in the presence of severe MI.

The LV end-diastolic pressure remains normal until late in the course. Cardiac output is also normal unless cardiac failure supervenes.

Contrast Studies

Selective cine biplane left ventriculography in the 30° RAO and 70° LAO projections is the procedure of choice (Fig. 5–49). The degree of MI (mild, moderate, severe) can be properly assessed during ventricular systole. Delayed emptying (prolonged opacification) due to repeated reopacification of the LA is another criterion used to assess the degree

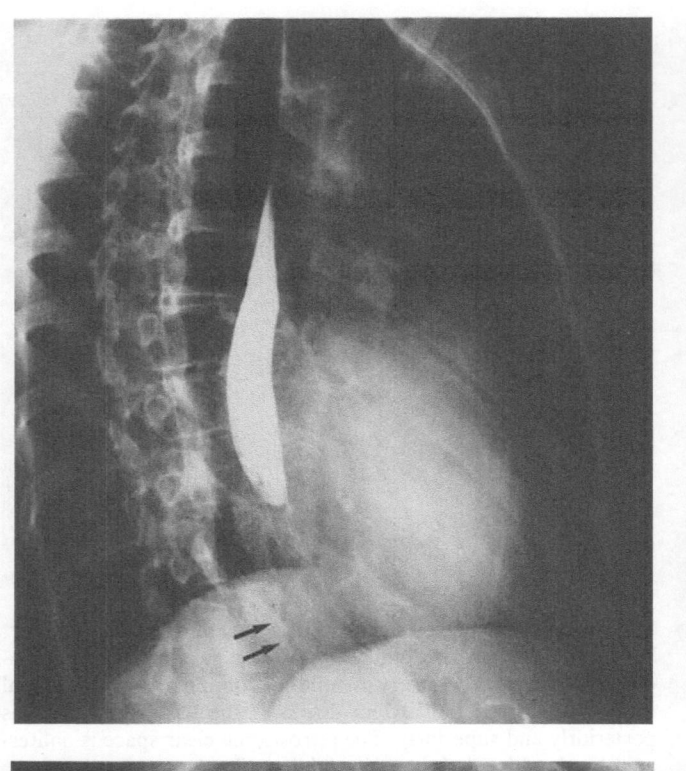

A

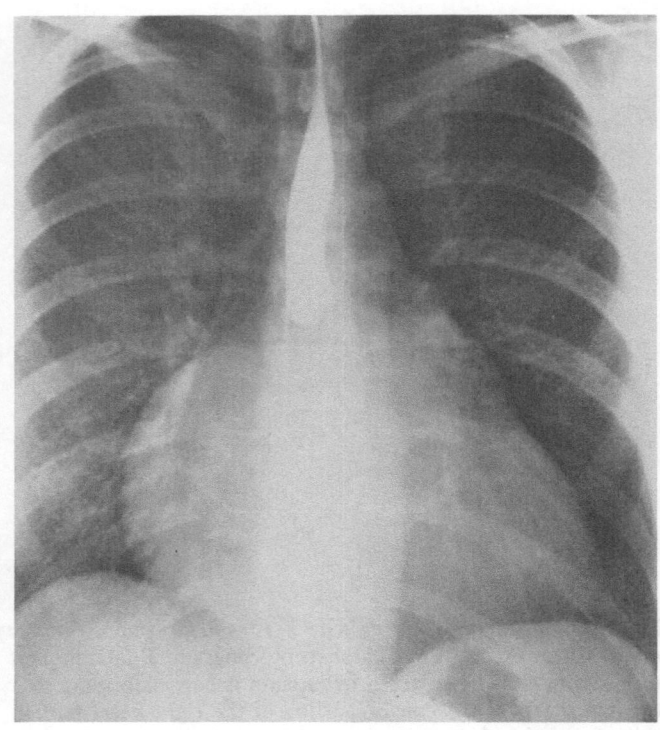

B

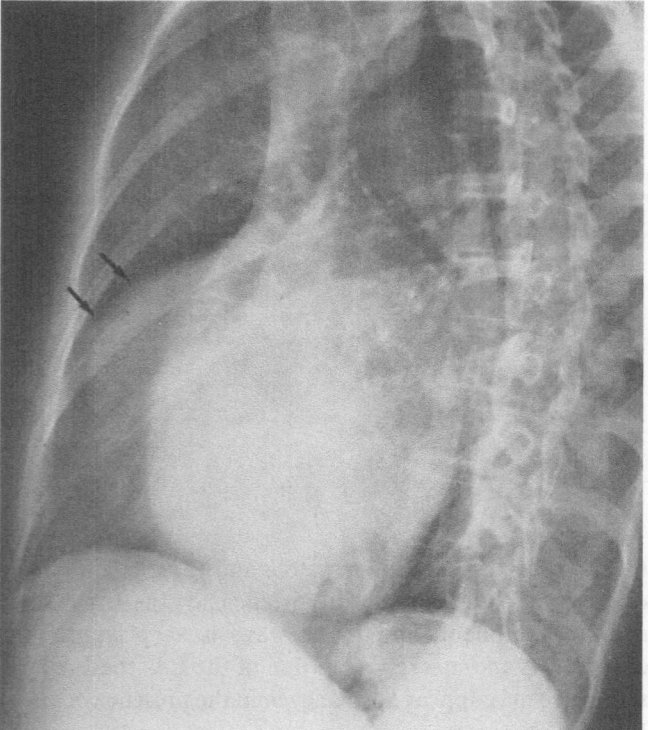

C

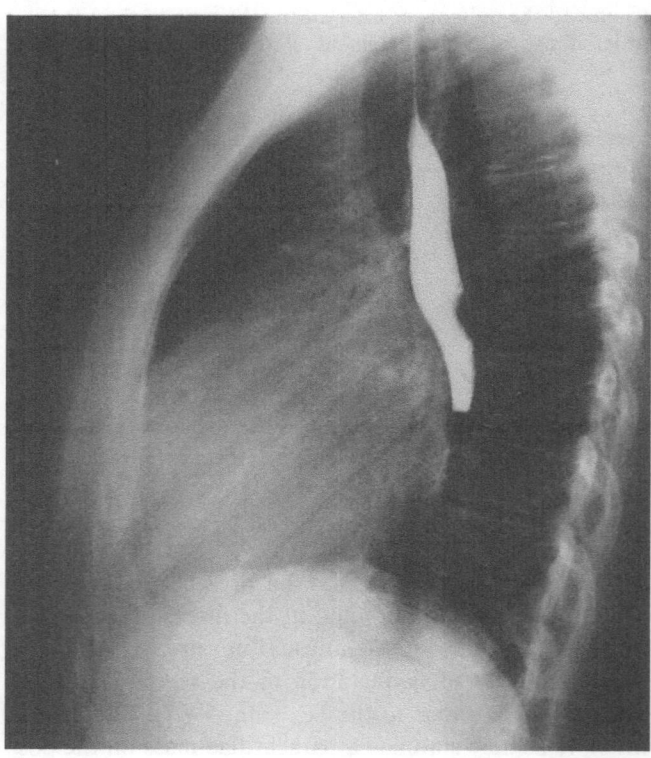

D

Fig. 5–46. *Severe mitral and tricuspid insufficiency in a 43-year-old woman with rheumatic heart disease.* **A** RAO view; **B** PA view; **C** LAO view; **D** lateral view. In addition to the classical findings of the "mitral heart" configuration, signs of right atrial enlargement in the absence of pulmonary venous hypertension indicate involvement of the tricuspid valve. In this patient enlargement of the left atrium is best demonstrated on the frontal plane (double density) and LAO views. The left atrial appendage forms a bump along the left heart border ("third mogul"). The left main-stem bronchus is elevated, particularly in the LAO view. On the RAO projection the left atrium does not indent the esophagus but appears to project posterior to it. This finding is explained by the left atrium having enlarged more laterally (toward the right) than posteriorly. Thus, the left atrium projects so far to the right of the esophagus that even on rotation into the RAO view a portion of the left atrium remains on the right side of the esophagus. Enlargement of the right atrium is also demonstrated on all views. It is border forming on the frontal plane view. On the RAO view it is below the left atrium (*arrows*). The shoulder configuration in the LAO view is the right atrial appendage (*arrows*), which is enlarged and also displaced by the enlarged right ventricle and right atrium. The left ventricle is mildly to moderately enlarged.

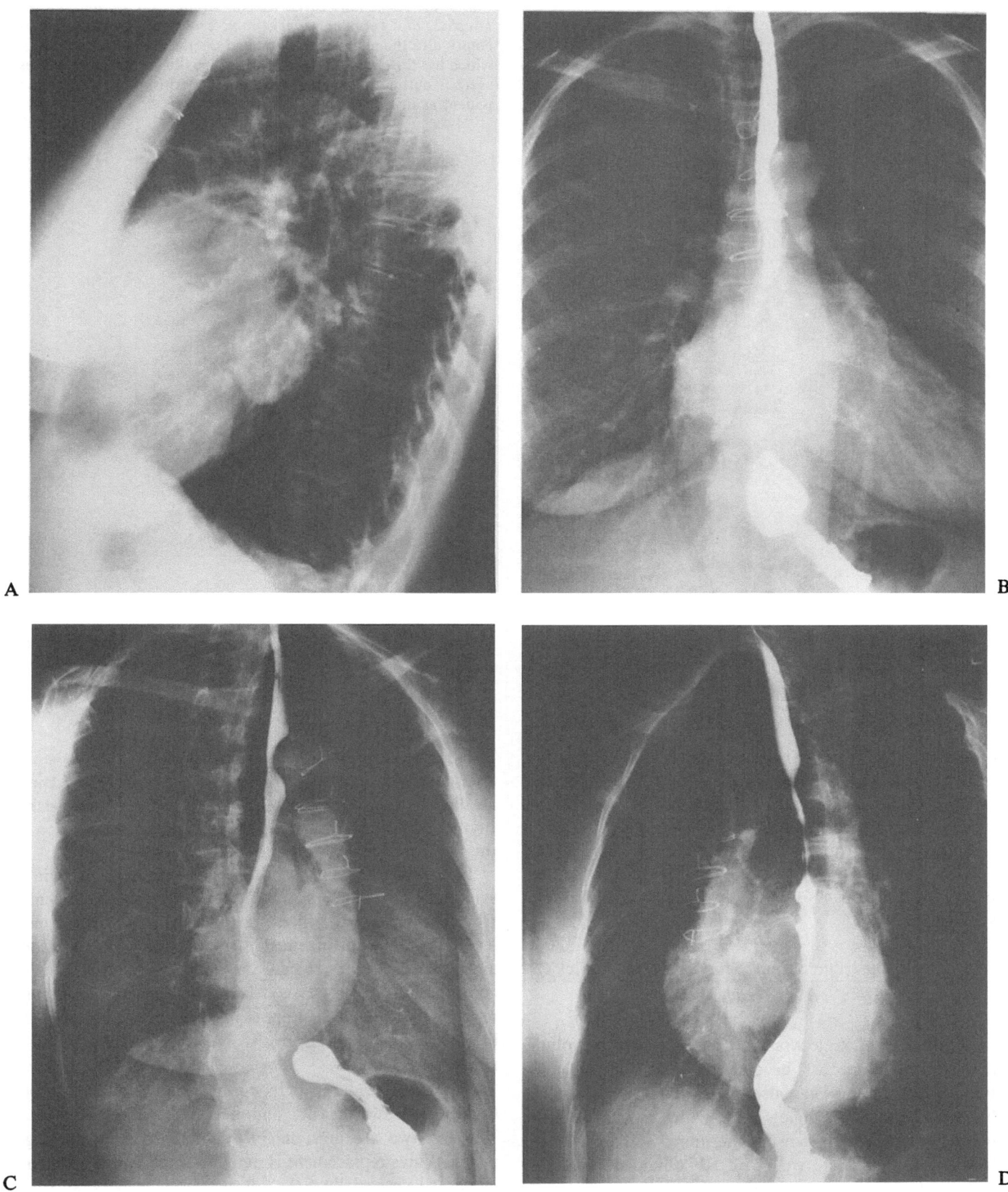

A

B

C

D

Fig. 5–47. *Pulmonary varix with severe mitral insufficiency.* **A** Lateral view; **B** PA view; **C** RAO view; **D** LAO view. The lateral view demonstrates a retrocardiac mass, which in the PA view is observed to be right sided. The right pulmonary veins converge toward the mass. The oblique films show that the mass rotates at the position of the confluence of the pulmonary veins. From these plain film findings the diagnosis of a varix of the pulmonary vein should be made. (See Fig. 5–48, for the angiogram from this patient.)

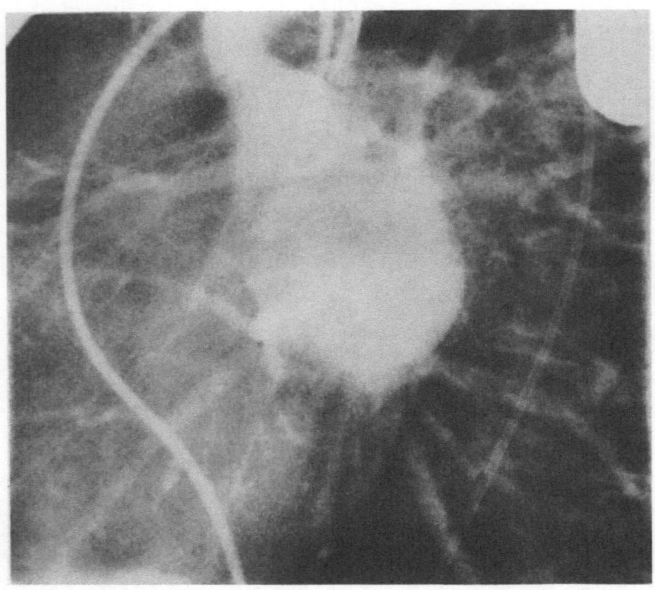

Fig. 5–48. *Pulmonary varix. Lateral 35-mm cine frame from the levophase of a pulmonary angiogram.* The right pulmonary veins empty into the aneurysmally dilated confluence of veins (varix), which has the shape of a pear. Soon after, the left atrium opacifies and the outlines of the varix are obliterated (not shown). (Same patient as in Fig. 5–47.)

of severity. Artifactual MI must be differentiated from true regurgitation. The former usually occurs during diastole and may be induced by the catheter position or by premature ventricular contractions (extrasystoles).

Quantitation of the severity of MI can be obtained by determining the LV regurgitant fraction (RF), which expresses the relationship between regurgitant flow and total ventricular flow:

$$RF = \frac{\text{angiographic output} - \text{forward output (Fick)}}{\text{angiographic output}}$$

In addition, the LV ejection fraction, end-diastolic volume and stroke volume can be determined angiographically. Regurgitant fractions can also be measured by gated equilibrium radionuclide angiography, which is a noninvasive method whose results can be determined serially and can be shown to correlate well with RF obtained at cardiac catheterization ($r = 0.85$). (See also Chapter 3, Cardiovascular Nuclear Medicine). Quantitation of valvular insufficiencies is important in the selection of patients for surgery.

Treatment

In asymptomatic patients, prevention of repeated attacks of rheumatic fever and bacterial endocarditis is essential.

In symptomatic individuals, rest, digitalis, diuretics and afterload reduction with vasodilators are of benefit. Atrial fibrillation may be controlled for a time with antiarrhythmic medications. With chronic severe dilatation of the LA, atrial fibrillation may become irreversible.

Indications for surgical treatment include disabling symptoms that no longer respond to medical treatment. Objective criteria are ill defined. Progressive cardiac enlargement or a fall in ejection fraction on serial nuclear angiographic studies signals the onset of myocardial decompensation. If surgery is delayed until severe symptoms or gross LV dilatation is present, the operative risk will be higher and the preoperative LV dysfunction may not regress after surgery.

Surgical procedures include mitral plication, the use of Carpentier-Edwards ring and mitral valve replacement. The first two are most likely to be successful in young people. Valve replacement is more often necessary in older individuals, especially if the mitral valve is heavily fibrosed or calcified.

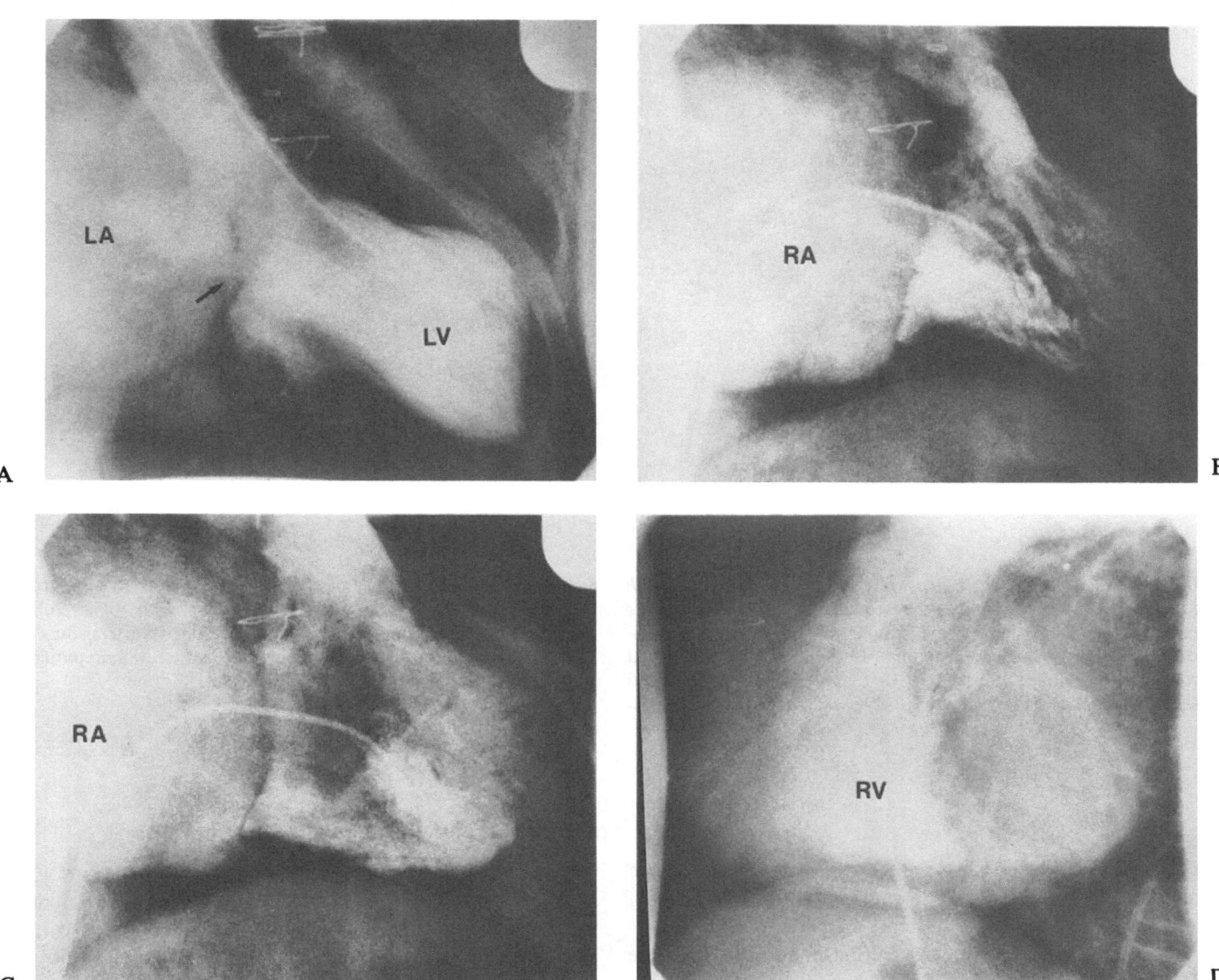

Fig. 5–49. *Severe mitral and tricuspid insufficiency. Cine angiograms in a woman with rheumatic heart disease.* **A** RAO view of the left ventriculogram during systole; **B** RAO view of the right ventriculogram during systole; **C** RAO view of the right ventriculogram during diastole; **D** LAO view of the right ventriculogram. In **A** the regurgitant jet (*arrow*) enters a dilated left atrium (*LA*). The jet indicates that the patient has a component of mitral stenosis along with the insufficiency. *LV* = left ventricle.

In **B** severe tricuspid insufficiency is demonstrated. The right atrium (*RA*) is markedly enlarged. In **C**, during diastole, right ventricular dilatation is demonstrated. In **D** the right atrium is border forming anteriorly and accounts for the shoulder configuration on the plain roentgenogram of the chest (compare with Fig. 5–46C). The right ventricle, although dilated, is not border forming.

Mitral Valve Prolapse

Mitral valve prolapse (MVP) is now recognized as one of the most common valvular abnormalities. In some of the older literature, overdiagnosis of mitral prolapse is apparent. Thus, in one report an incidence of almost 43% has been reported (Smith et al.). Strict adherence to criteria for angiographic diagnosis proposed by Spindola-Franco et al. has reduced the reported incidence to less than 5% of patients undergoing cardiac catheterization. This figure is somewhat lower than the reported incidence in the general population as ascertained by use of echocardiography.

Mitral prolapse has been identified as a familial characteristic, transmitted as an autosomal dominant. It occurs frequently in patients with Marfan disease and Ehlers-Danlos syndrome, both disorders of connective tissue. An increased incidence of MVP has also been reported by Pickering et al. in von Willebrand syndrome, raising the possibility that von Willebrand syndrome may be another form of mesenchymal dysplasia. Mitral prolapse has also been discovered in association with other disease states that apparently are not associated with any abnormality of connective tissue. These entities include periarteritis nodosa, myotonic dystrophy and Duchenne muscular dystro-

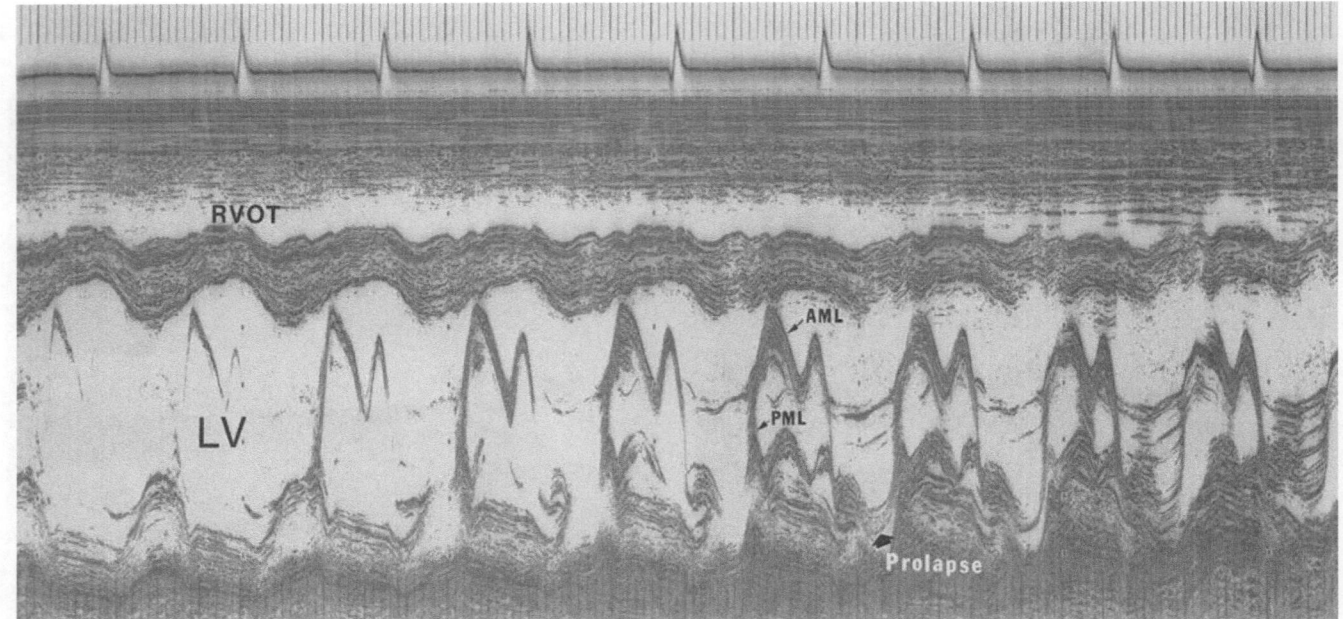

Fig. 5–50. *Prolapse of the mitral valve in an 11-year-old girl with Marfan syndrome. M-mode echocardiogram at the level of the mitral valve.* The first two beats demonstrate a dilated left ventricle (*LV*) with normal contractions. Both leaflets of the mitral valve, the anterior mitral leaflet (*AML*) and the posterior mitral leaflet, (*PML*) are thickened but pliable. The valve prolapses posteriorly throughout systole, and during the second half of systole the prolapse is more pronounced. On the last beat, pansystolic prolapse is present. Thus, by changing the angle of the transducer, varying patterns of prolapse can be demonstrated. (Same patient as Fig. 5–22.)

phy. Mitral prolapse is also associated with other cardiac disorders (e.g., secundum atrial septal defect, Ebstein anomaly).

Studies of catecholamine excretion in subjects with the MVP syndrome have indicated increased excretion in some of them. Cardiac biopsies have shown increased endocardial and intramyocardial fibrosis, nuclear chromatin clumping, intracellular edema and myocyte degeneration. These findings and the unexpectedly high incidence of MVP associated with idiopathic hypertrophic cardiomyopathy have led to a suspicion that the two entities may have a common predisposing factor.

The etiologic factor in prolapse of the mitral valve is usually myxomatous degeneration of the mitral valve, resulting in thickening and elongation of the leaflets and of the chordae tendineae. The aortic, pulmonary and tricuspid valves may also be affected, especially in cases of Marfan syndrome. Superimposed acute rheumatic fever and infective endocarditis may accelerate development of mitral insufficiency (MI). Rupture of the chordae tendineae may also occur and usually results in exacerbation of the degree of MI.

Ischemic heart disease and papillary muscle dysfunction may result in MI, but, in the authors' experience, does not by itself produce the classical findings of MVP.

Clinical Features

Most individuals with MVP are asymptomatic and remain without MI (or with a minimal amount) for many years, although a few show a tendency toward progressive mitral valve disease. Symptoms associated with MVP include nonspecific or atypical chest pain and palpitations. Symptomatic arrhythmias such as ventricular arrhythmias and supraventricular tachycardias may also occur. The development of cerebral emboli is also reported in individuals with MVP. These emboli may result from platelet aggregation and fibrin deposition on the exposed myxomatous tissue. Individuals with severe MI have symptoms similar to those occurring with other forms of MI. The failure to elicit a history of acute rheumatic fever in an individual with MI should arouse suspicion of the presence of MVP.

The characteristic physical feature in prolapse of the mitral valve is a mid-systolic or non-ejection click and a murmur that begins late in systole and continues until the second sound. In some patients multiple clicks may be present that sound superficial, as if produced outside the heart. The murmur may have an unusual whooping quality and may be modified with changes in posture or activity. Mitral prolapse may also present with a classical blowing apical murmur of MI. Some individuals with mitral prolapse will present with a gracile habitus, suggesting a form fruste of Marfan disease. The electrocardiogram is normal unless significant MI is present. Atrial or ventricular ar-

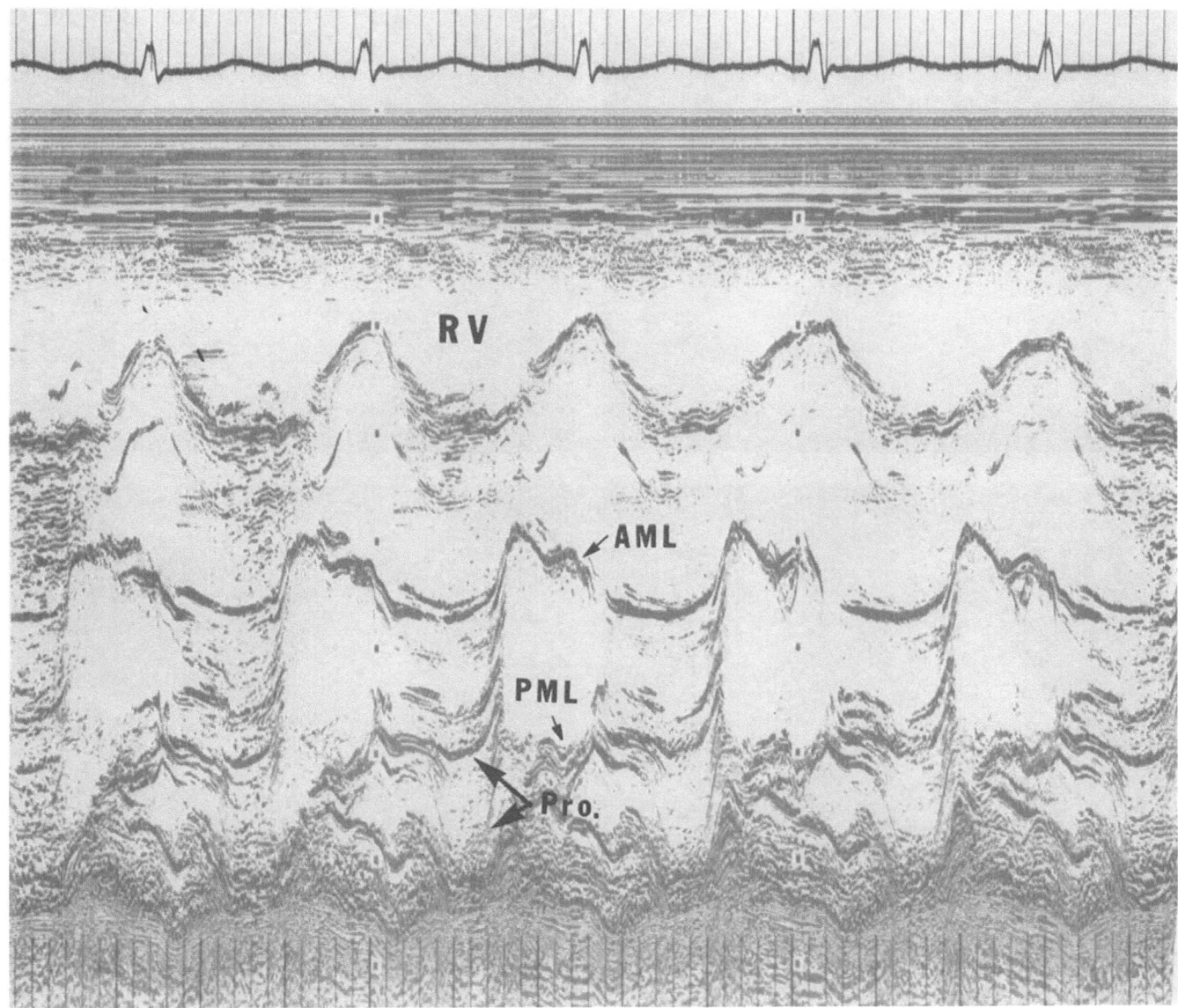

Fig. 5–51. *Prolapse of the mitral valve. M-mode echocardiogram.* In this patient without external features of Marfan syndrome the mitral valve leaflets are not thickened. Prolapse is virtually pansystolic. *AML*= anterior mitral leaflet; *PML* = posterior mitral leaflet; *Pro.* = prolapse; *RV* = right ventricle.

rhythmias may be apparent and the Wolff-Parkinson-White syndrome may coexist.

Echocardiography

Characteristic findings on M-mode echocardiography reflect the movement of the mitral leaflets superiorly and posteriorly into the LA cavity during ventricular systole. Posterior motion may involve a portion of the mitral valve or the entire valve, occurring as pansystolic prolapse or a late systolic prolapse (Figs. 5–50, 5–51). During diastole the excursion of the opening motion (D-E) may be greater than normal, reflecting excess mobility due to elongation of the structures. Ruptured chordae tendineae may be associated (see description in section on Infective Endocarditis). An artifactual pattern that resembles prolapse of the mitral valve occurs with pericardial effusion, when the heart rocks posteriorly during ventricular systole (see Fig. 9–3). In addition, a few normal individuals show slight posterior bowing of the mitral valves that gives the appearance of holosystolic prolapse. Some, but not all, of these false positive diagnoses will be eliminated if the transducer is directed perpendicular to the chest wall, rather than inferiorly and laterally at an oblique angle.

On 2-D echocardiography (Figs. 5–52A, 5–53A and B) the mitral valve may appear thickened, especially at its tip. Hypermobility and elongation of the leaflets may be evident during diastole (Figs. 5–53B). During systole the anterior leaflet may show an abnormal acute angle with the aortic root on the long axis view (Fig. 5–52C and D). With severe prolapse the convexity of one or both mitral valve leaflets is directed toward the LA instead of toward the ventricle on both long axis and four-chamber views.

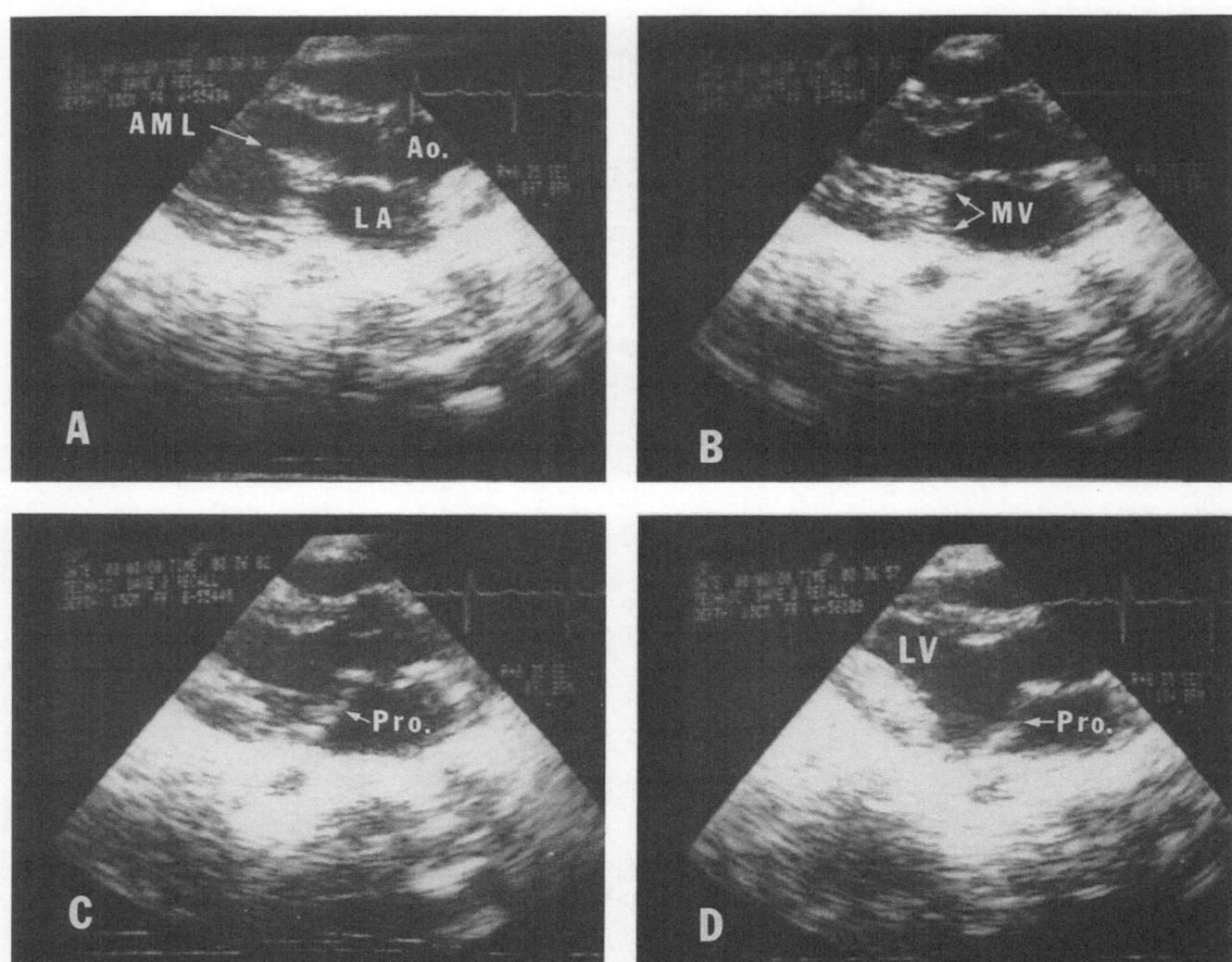

Fig. 5–52. *Prolapse of the mitral valve in a 12-year-old girl with Marfan syndrome. Long axis views of a two-dimensional echocardiogram.* **A** *diastole;* **B** *early systole;* **C** *and* **D** *mid to late systole from two slightly different angles.* During diastole (**A**) the mitral valve is thickened, but opens widely. During early systole (**B**) the mitral valve is closed; however, a normal angle is formed between the mitral valve (*MV*) and the root of the aorta. The mitral valve is convex toward the ventricular apex. Later during systole **C** and **D**) a sharp angle is formed between the root of the aorta and the anterior mitral leaflet as the mitral valve rotates toward the left atrium (rocking motion). The convexity of the mitral valve is now directed toward the left atrium. Note that the left ventricle (*LV*) in **D** has the shape of a ballerina's foot. This term has also been used to describe the angiogram of the left ventricle in the presence of prolapse of the mitral valve. Compare this with Fig. 5–60. *AML* = anterior mitral leaflet; *Ao.* = root of the aorta; *LA* = left atrium; *Pro.* = prolapse.

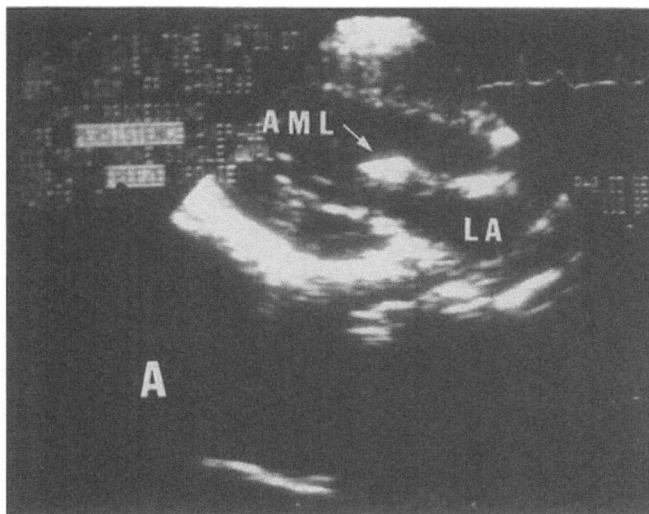

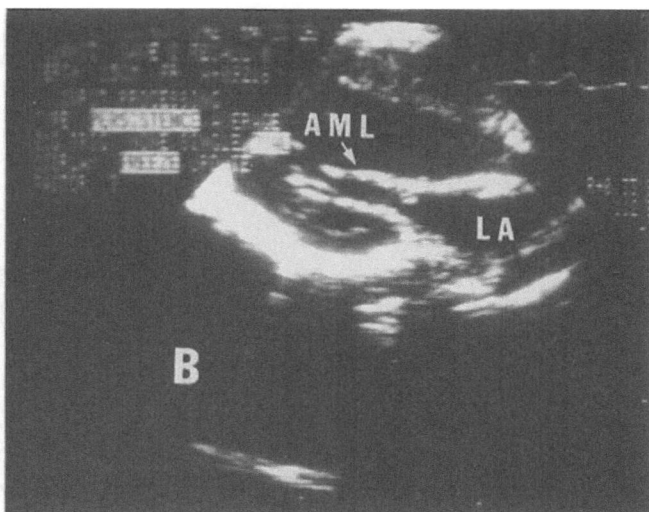

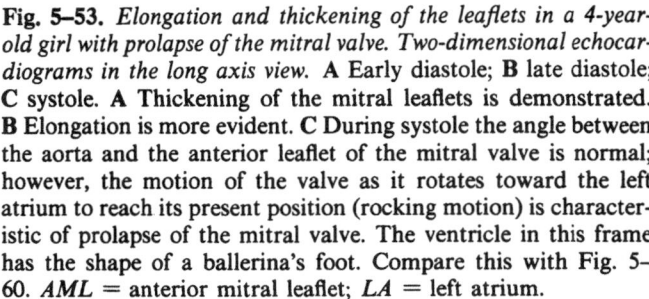

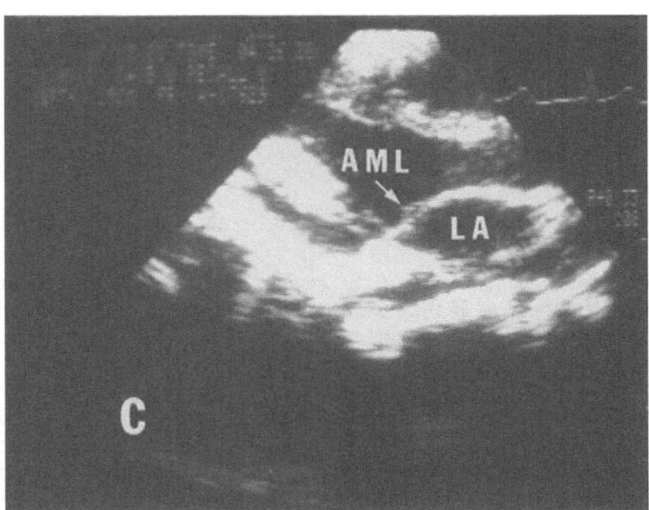

Fig. 5–53. *Elongation and thickening of the leaflets in a 4-year-old girl with prolapse of the mitral valve. Two-dimensional echocardiograms in the long axis view.* **A** Early diastole; **B** late diastole; **C** systole. **A** Thickening of the mitral leaflets is demonstrated. **B** Elongation is more evident. **C** During systole the angle between the aorta and the anterior leaflet of the mitral valve is normal; however, the motion of the valve as it rotates toward the left atrium to reach its present position (rocking motion) is characteristic of prolapse of the mitral valve. The ventricle in this frame has the shape of a ballerina's foot. Compare this with Fig. 5–60. *AML* = anterior mitral leaflet; *LA* = left atrium.

Associated findings on echocardiography may include LA dilatation or LV dysfunction or both. The aortic root may also be dilated, suggesting a generalized disorder of connective tissue.

Radiological (Plain Film) Features

The plain film may be normal or may show findings consistent with MI. The skeletal features of Marfan syndrome, Larsen syndrome, and the like may also be noted.

Contrast Studies

Angiographic diagnosis of MVP depends on an understanding of the angiographic anatomy of the normal mitral valve apparatus (see Figs. 4–35, 4–36)

The components of the mitral apparatus as demonstrated on left ventriculography include the mitral leaflets, the commissures, the chordae tendineae, the fulcrum, the ventricular fornix and the papillary muscles. The mitral valve has two leaflets: anterior (aortic) and posterior. The anterior leaflet has a larger surface area, but the posterior leaflet has a longer line of insertion (Fig. 5–54). Each leaflet has a rough zone along the free edge. This is the line of

coaptation and the line of insertion of the chordae tendineae. The middle of each leaflet is thinner (the clear zone). The base of the leaflets (the basal zone) is thick. The anterior leaflet is undivided and is roughly triangular. The posterior leaflet is divided into three "scallops" (Fig. 5–54). The scallops are named according to their position relative to the anterolateral and posteromedial commissures. The scallops are thus designated the anterolateral, posteromedial, and middle scallops, corresponding to descriptions at autopsy. In live subjects the axis of the heart is horizontal so that the mitral anulus is nearly vertical (sagittal). The anterior commissure is then superior, and the posterior commissure inferior.

On left ventriculography the line of insertion of the posterior leaflet is recognized on the RAO view in protodiastole, as the contrast material is trapped between the ventricular surface of the leaflet and the adjacent endocardium of the LV (see Fig. 4–35). The anterior leaflet is not visualized in the RAO projection because there is no narrow corner or recess behind the anterior leaflet where contrast material can form an interface (Fig. 4–35A, 4–35C). On the atrial side of the anterior leaflet is the orifice, with

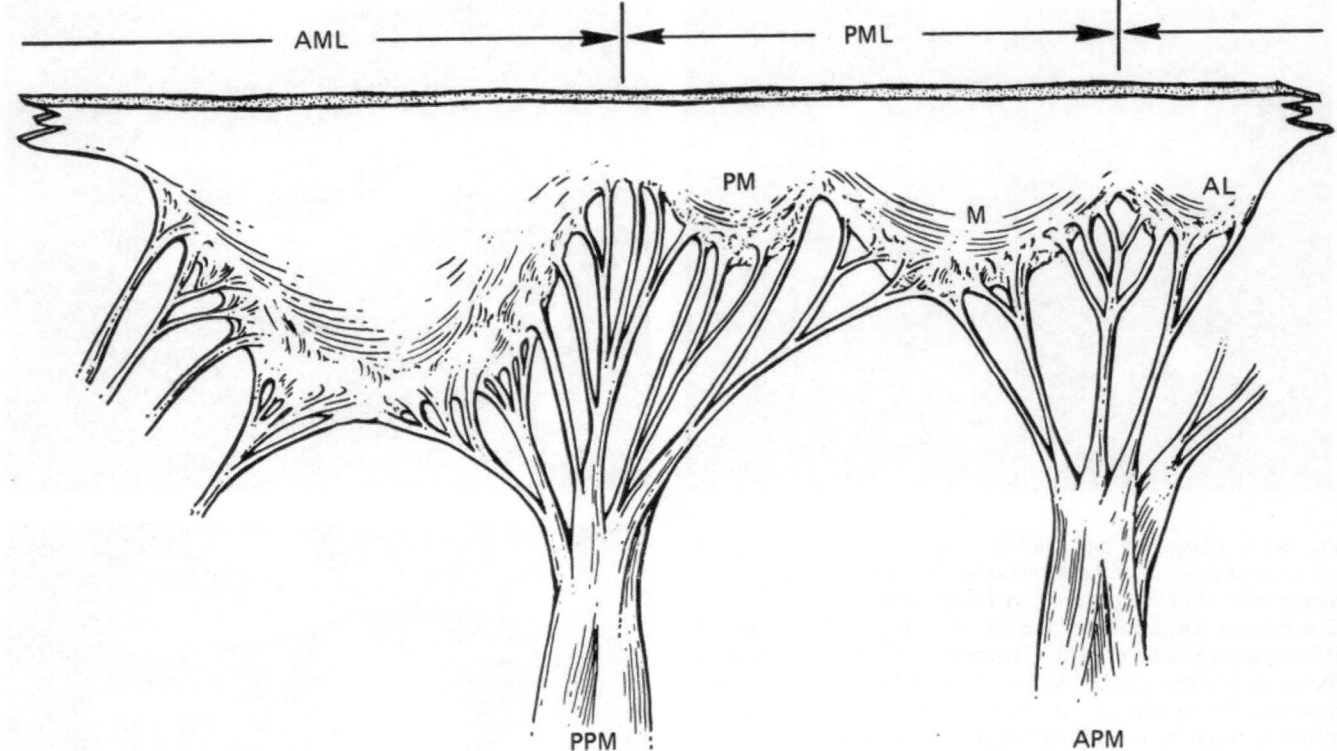

Fig. 5-54. *Components of the leaflets of the mitral valve.* The leaflets appear as if they were cut open along the anterolateral commissure. The surface area of the anterior leaflet of the mitral valve (*AML*) is greater than that of the posterior leaflet (*PML*); the length of the base of the posterior leaflet, however, is longer than that of the anterior leaflet. The anterior leaflet is not divided and is roughly triangular. The posterior leaflet is divided into three scallops designated posteromedial (*PM*), middle (*M*) and anterolateral (*AL*). Each leaflet has three zones that are demonstrated best on transillumination. Along the free edge is the "rough zone," which corresponds to the surface of coaptation of the valve during ventricular systole. The chordae tendineae attach in this area. The middle or clear zone is thin and translucent. The basal zone of the leaflet is normally thickened and opaque. Each papillary muscle contributes chordae tendineae to both leaflets. The posterior leaflet is attached to the mitral anulus and is semicircular on angiography in the frontal or RAO views. The anterior leaflet is in continuity with the root of the aorta, relating to the left and noncoronary cusps and is also attached to the ventricular septum, forming part of the posterior border of the atrioventricular septum (see Fig. 7-34). On angiography the anterior leaflet forms a nearly vertical line on the lateral or LAO view (see also Figs. 4-35 and 7-79). *PPM* = posterior papillary muscle; *APM* = anterior papillary muscle.

the LA behind it. On the ventricular side is the LV outflow tract. The anterior leaflet is demonstrated in the LAO view because it forms a sharp interface between the unopacified blood rushing into the LV and the opacified blood in the outflow tract (see Fig. 4-35C).

The scallops of the posterior leaflet may or may not be represented on the normal left ventriculogram by narrow radiolucent lines that separate them. The superior radiolucent line separates the anterolateral scallop from the middle scallop. The inferior lucent line separates the middle scallop from the posteromedial scallop. The posteromedial scallop extends around the lowermost point of the anulus (fulcrum) to meet the anterior leaflet of the mitral valve at the posteromedial commissure. The posteromedial scallop is outlined on both the RAO and LAO views and is the scallop most frequently involved in prolapse of the mitral valve. The other two scallops can also be recognized by their positions on the RAO and LAO view.

The mitral fulcrum is the point of attachment of the posterior mitral leaflet to the anulus fibrosus. This area is identified during protodiastole as contrast material is

trapped between the posterior leaflet of the mitral valve and the endocardium of the LV. For the purpose of diagnosing prolapse of the mitral valve, *fulcrum* refers to the lowermost point of attachment of the posterior mitral leaflet in the RAO view. The fornix of the LV is defined as that part of the LV between the insertion of the posterior mitral leaflet (fulcrum) and the base of the papillary muscles. As described by Spindola-Franco, four normal configurations of the mitral valve are distinguished by (1) the position of the fulcrum of the mitral valve (high or low) and (2) the shape of the fornix of the LV in the RAO projection (either notched or free of notching) (see Fig. 4-36).

Prolapse of the mitral valve is defined as paraanular displacement of one or both leaflets of the mitral valve beyond the level of the fulcrum. Thus the valve tissue must move not only posteriorly into the LA but also superiorly, inferiorly and laterally beyond the circumference of the mitral anulus. The posteromedial scallop is almost always involved in prolapse of the mitral valve; therefore identification of prolapse of this scallop is usually the best way to diagnose this entity. Prolapse of the posteromedial scallop

Fig. 5–55. *Prolapse of the mitral valve. Left ventricular angiogram in the RAO view.* The low fulcrum and absence of notching during diastole **(A)** make this a type I mitral valve configuration (see Fig. 4–36). During systole **(B)** the posteromedial scallop pivots posteriorly and inferiorly beyond the fulcrum, resulting in prolapse of the mitral valve (*Pro*). The left atrium (*LA*) is outlined because of mitral insufficiency. The term *fulcrum* refers to the point of attachment of the posterior mitral leaflet to the anulus. This corresponds to the lowermost point along the mitral anulus on the RAO view. The term *fornix* refers to that portion of the left ventricular wall between the fulcrum and the papillary muscle. *Ao* = aorta. Cohen MV, Shah PK, Spindola-Franco H (1979) Angiographic, echocardiographic correlation in mitral valve prolapse. Am Heart J 97:43–52. Copyright 1979. Reproduced by permission.

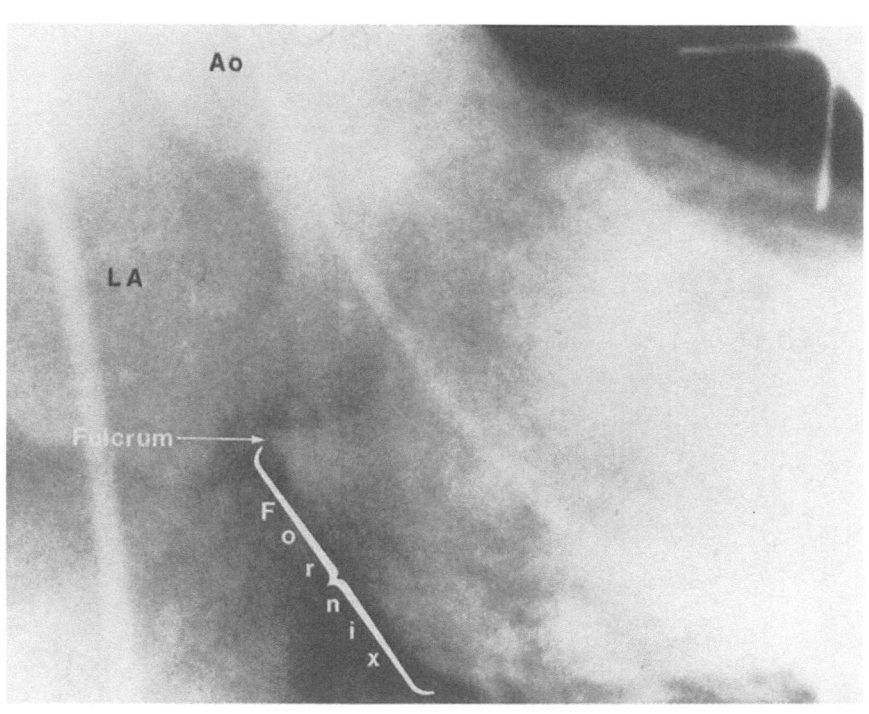

A

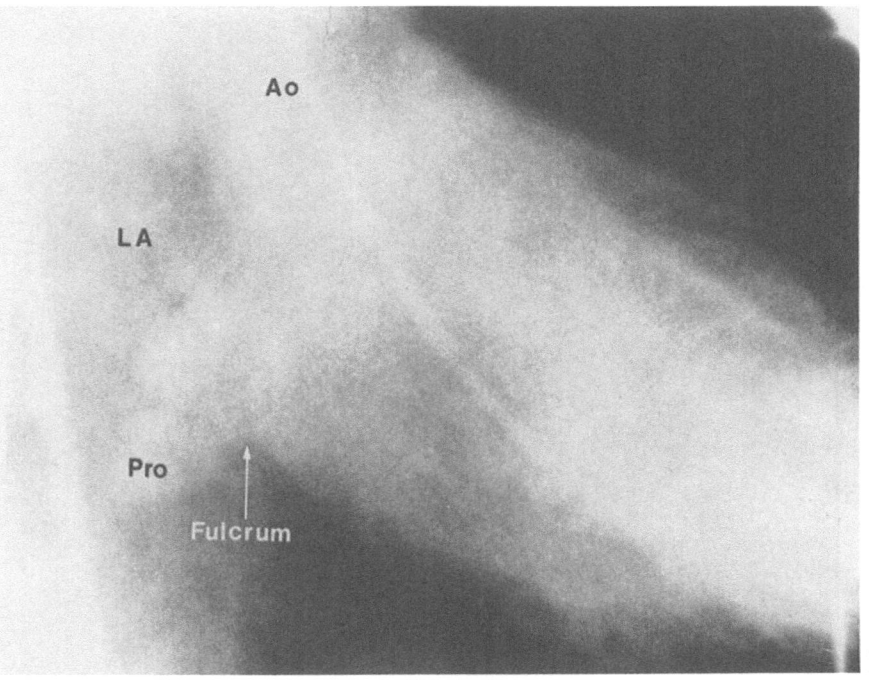

B

is demonstrated best in the RAO projection as a posterior and inferior displacement beyond the mitral fulcrum during ventricular systole (Fig. 5–55). Rarely, only the anterior leaflet (Fig. 5–56), the anterolateral scallop or the middle scallop (Fig. 5–57) is involved. Thus, recognition of prolapse of the individual scallops and of the anterior leaflet is necessary to avoid false negative diagnoses. Prolapse of the anterior leaflet is diagnosed when the leaflet projects superiorly beyond the border of the heart in the RAO view (Fig. 5–56). On the LAO view prolapse of this leaflet appears as a convexity protruding into the LA just below

the aortic valve. Prolapse of the anterolateral scallop may be difficult to separate from that of the anterior mitral leaflet. The anterolateral scallop should be posterior relative to the aortic valve in the LAO view. The middle scallop projects over the LV outflow tract in the RAO view (Fig. 5–57), appearing on the lateral or LAO view as a paraanular convexity projecting into the left atrium.

In type II configuration of the mitral valve (Fig. 5–58A, 5–59; see also Fig. 4–36) the fulcrum is low lying and the fornix is notched. This configuration is especially likely to be mistaken for mitral prolapse because of the

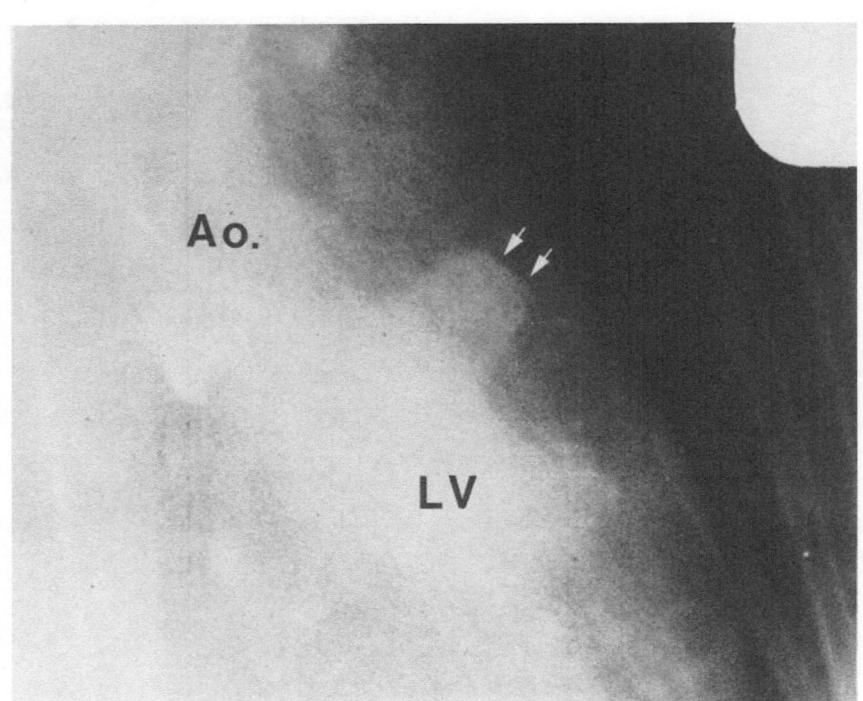

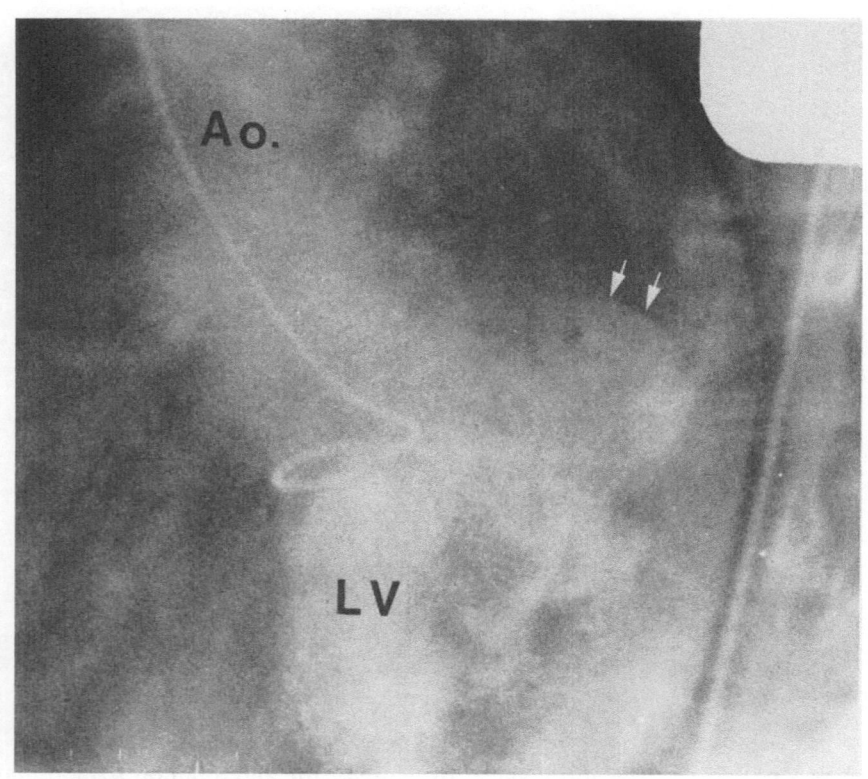

Fig. 5–56. *Prolapse of the anterior leaflet of the mitral valve. Left ventriculography in the RAO and LAO views,* **A** *and* **B** *respectively, during ventricular systole. The leaflet prolapses superiorly beyond the border of the heart in the RAO view. In the LAO view it projects into the left atrium just below the aortic valve.* Ao. *= root of aorta;* LV *= left ventricle.*

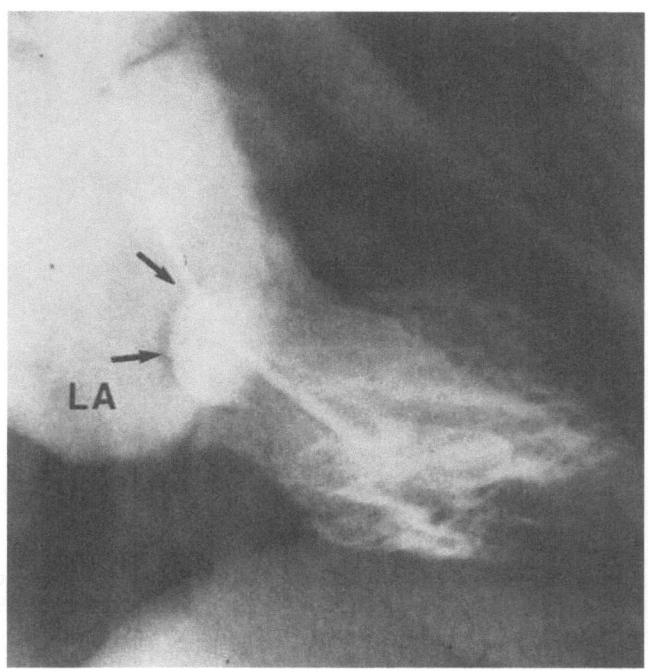

A

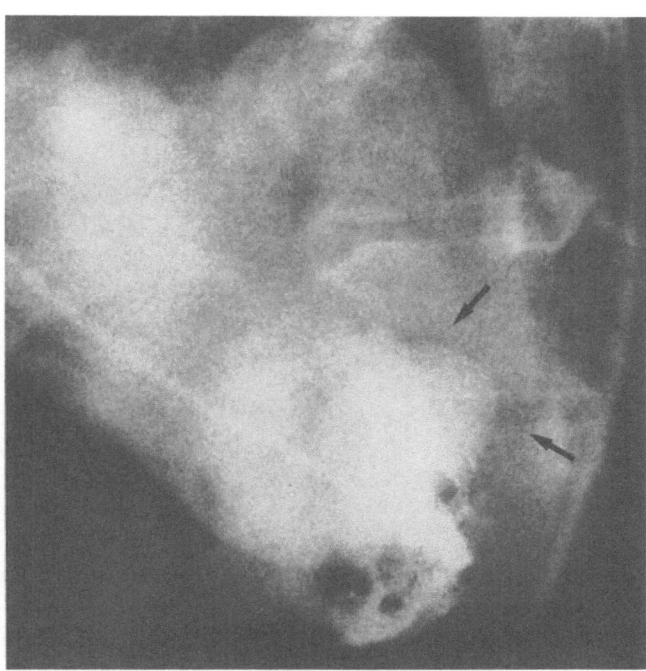

B

Fig. 5–57. *Isolated prolapse of the middle scallop of the mitral valve.* In **A,** the left ventriculogram in the RAO view, the middle scallop (*arrows*) prolapses across the left ventricular outflow tract into the left atrium (*LA*). On the LAO view (**B**) prolapse is

also observed. At surgery only the middle scallop prolapsed. This type of prolapse might be missed if one examines only for prolapse of the posteromedial scallop.

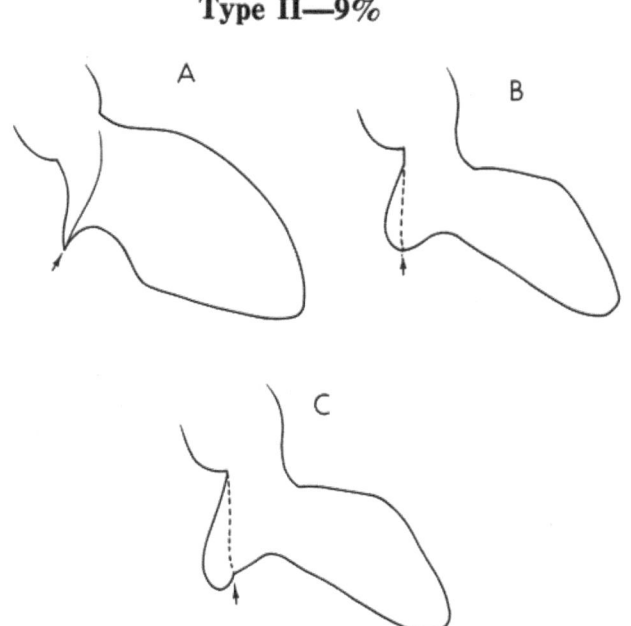

Type II—9%

◄ **Fig. 5–58.** *Type II configuration of the mitral valve with and without mitral valve prolapse.* **A** diastole; **B** systole without prolapse; **C** systole with prolapse. The arrows point to the fulcrum (see definition Fig. 5–55). This is an example of a type II configuration because the fulcrum is low and the fornix is notched. In **B** during ventricular systole the *dashed line* indicates the usual position of the mitral valve. In some patients the mitral valve may bulge during systole without inferior displacement, a normal variant designated pseudoprolapse. In **C** the mitral valve pivots posteriorly and inferiorly to the mitral fulcrum, resulting in prolapse of the mitral valve. Spindola-Franco H, et al (1980) Classification of the radiological morphology of the mitral valve. Differentiation between true and pseudoprolapse. Br Heart J 44:30–36. Copyright 1980. Reproduced by permission.

low position of the fulcrum. Normal systolic bulging of the mitral valve may cause further confusion. It is essential in these cases to identify the position of the fulcrum as the valve opens during diastole. If the leaflet does not pivot beyond and below the fulcrum of the mitral valve during systole then prolapse is not present. It is important in all four types of mitral valve not to diagnose mitral prolapse on the basis of mild posterior bulging of the mitral valve

leaflets (Fig. 5–58B), which constitutes a normal phenomenon occurring in up to 20% of normal persons and is designated *pseudoprolapse.*

Abnormalities of wall motion are found in up to 50% of patients with MVP. Global hypokinesis or localized wall motion abnormalities may be present. These are not limited to the posterior wall but may affect any segment. In a few cases the posteroinferior LV wall may bulge into the LV cavity during ventricular systole, forming a configuration in the RAO projection reminiscent of a ballerina's foot (Figs. 5–52D, 5–53C, 5–60).

Treatment

Treatment of symptomatic MI is the same as that described for MI with other types of mitral valve defects. If surgery is required, these valves are not likely to be amenable to

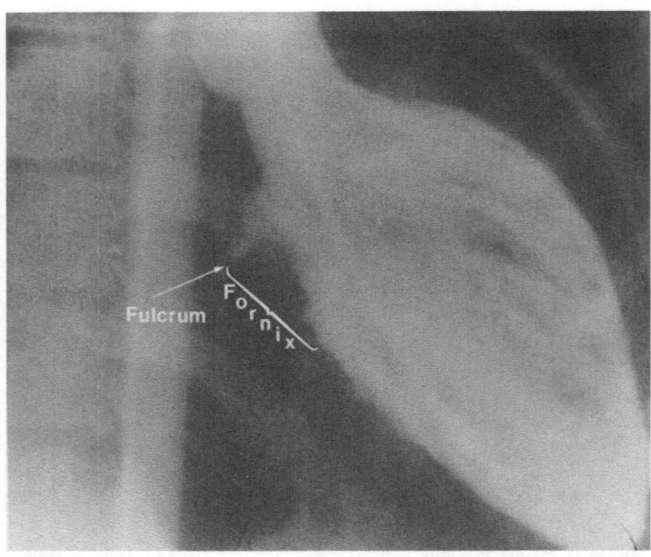

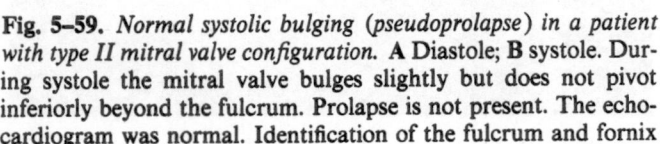

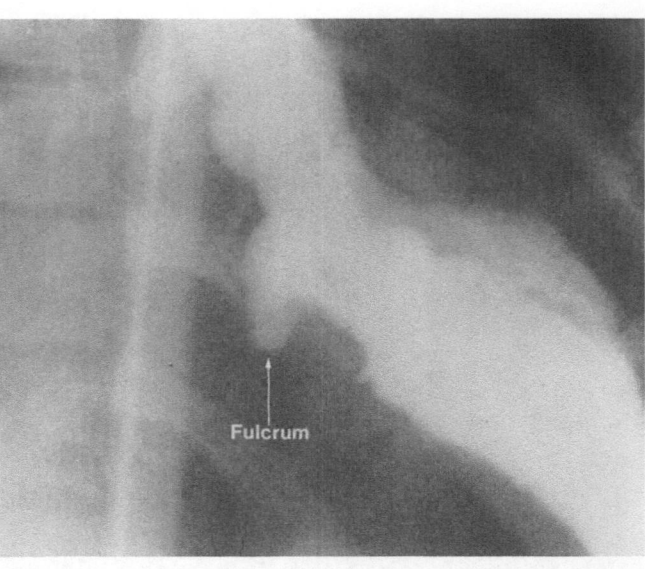

A   B

Fig. 5–59. *Normal systolic bulging (pseudoprolapse) in a patient with type II mitral valve configuration.* **A** Diastole; **B** systole. During systole the mitral valve bulges slightly but does not pivot inferiorly beyond the fulcrum. Prolapse is not present. The echocardiogram was normal. Identification of the fulcrum and fornix is essential to evaluate the presence or absence of prolapse of the mitral valve. Cohen MV, Shah PK, Spindola-Franco H (1979) Angiographic echocardiographic correlation in mitral valve prolapse. Am Heart J 97:43–52. Copyright 1979. Reproduced by permission.

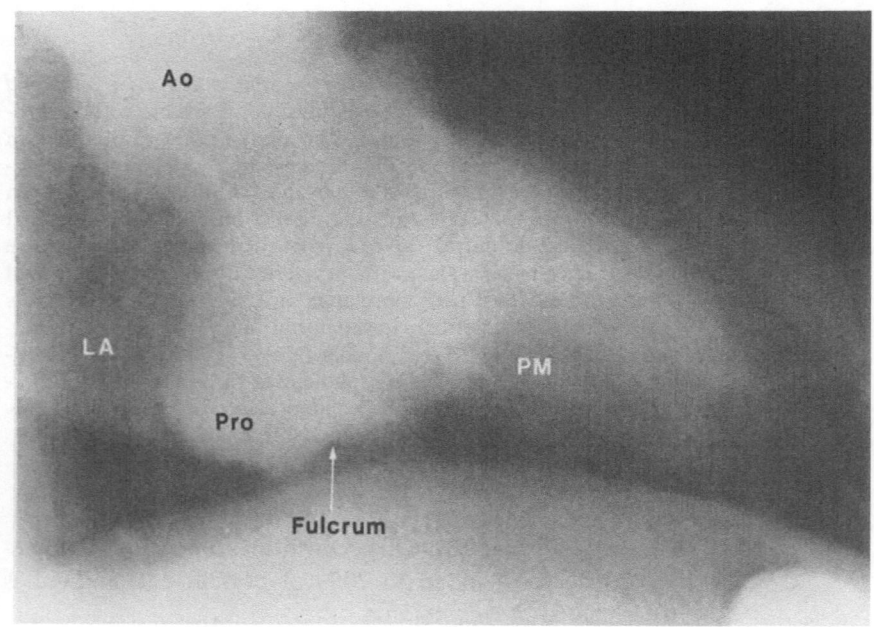

Fig. 5–60. *Mitral valve prolapse. Left ventriculogram in the RAO view during systole.* This case is an example of type I configuration of the mitral valve, so classified because the fulcrum is low and the fornix has no notching. The mitral valve (posteromedial scallop) pivots posteriorly and inferiorly beyond the fulcrum, resulting in mitral prolapse. The posteromedial papillary muscle (*PM*) bulges into the left ventricular cavity, again producing a configuration reminiscent of a ballerina's foot (compare with 2-D echocardiograms in Figs. 5–52D, 5–53C). *Ao* = aorta; *LA* = left atrium; *Pro* = prolapse. Cohen MV, Shah PK, Spindola-Franco H (1979) Angiographic echocardiographic correlation in mitral valve prolapse. Am Heart J 97:43–42. Copyright 1979. Reproduced by permission.

repair (anuloplasty), generally requiring replacement of the valve. Nonspecific chest pain associated with mitral prolapse is difficult to differentiate from angina pectoris. Beta blockers have been helpful in management. Antiplatelet drugs or anticoagulants have been suggested as prophylaxis for individuals with mitral prolapse who have had unexplained cerebral ischemic events. Arrhythmias (e.g., supra-ventricular tachycardia, ventricular extrasystoles) in patients with mitral prolapse are treated in the usual way (propranolol is the drug of choice). Mitral valve replacement has been suggested as a treatment for paroxysmal ventricular tachycardia refractory to medical management; however, insufficient numbers of patients are reported to evaluate results.

Infective Endocarditis

Infective endocarditis (IE) is separated into two syndromes on the basis of the rate of progression of symptoms. Subacute bacterial endocarditis (SBE) is generally caused by organisms of relatively low virulence (e.g., *Streptococcus viridans, Staphylococcus epidermidis*) and may present with subtle manifestations and a chronic course. Acute bacterial endocarditis (ABE), on the other hand, tends to be caused by virulent organisms such as *Staphylococcus aureus,* presenting with severe systemic manifestations (e.g., high fever) and often progressing rapidly to destruction of the valve and congestive heart failure. SBE occurs on valves that have been previously damaged or are congenitally deformed. Rheumatic valves and bicuspid aortic valves are the most common underlying conditions. Other cardiac abnormalities (e.g., mitral prolapse, hypertrophic cardiomyopathy, valvar prostheses) also predispose toward bacterial implantation. With congenital heart defects the infection often occurs within the chamber that receives a jet or shunt. As an example, with ventricular septal defect the vegetation often occurs within the right ventricular cavity (the jet lesion) or on the tricuspid valve. With ductus arteriosus or aorta-to-pulmonary artery anastomosis the vegetation tends to occur within the pulmonary artery near the opening of the ductus or anastomosis.

Transient bacteremia has been recognized particularly after dental, urological and gynecological procedures and after other types of surgery as well. These procedures have also been known to precede the onset of SBE. Intravenous catheters, chronic infections and immunological deficiency also may predispose toward infection of the heart. Individuals known to have valvar defects and congenital heart defects are now given antibiotics just prior to dental and surgical procedures as prophylaxis against SBE. ABE is often encountered in drug addicts using intravenous injections but may occur in others as well, involving normal valves including right-sided valves. In one series (Hubbel et al.) all four heart valves were affected with about equal frequency.

Yeasts and fungi also cause cardiac infection in addicts, in immunosuppressed individuals and in those with prosthetic heart valves. Vegetations caused by fungi may be large and friable, resulting in embolic complications.

The major hemodynamic alteration occurring with infection of the aortic valve is aortic regurgitation. This sequela may be caused by necrosis and loss of valvar substance, prolapse secondary to erosion of a cusp near its commissural attachment, or by large vegetations that interfere with valvular function. Extension into the ventricular septum and myocardium may result in formation of an abscess (subaortic or ring abscess). As a result, arrhythmias, including complete heart block, may develop. Rarely aneurysm or perforation of the septum results. Infective involvement of the wall of the aorta above the valve may produce mycotic aneurysms, which may rupture into the pericardium, mediastinum or into any cardiac chamber. Involvement of the mitral valve may result in mitral regurgitation secondary to perforation of the leaflets or rupture of the chordae tendineae. Abscess of the mitral anulus is uncommon.

Infection of the tricuspid and pulmonary valves results in valvular insufficiency, septic pulmonary emboli and multiple pulmonary abscesses, which may lead to pulmonary failure. With involvement of the pulmonic and tricuspid valves, cardiac symptoms and signs are often less prominent than are the pulmonary and systemic effects of septicemia.

Clinical Features

New or changing murmurs of valvular insufficiency may not be evident with SBE. The stigmata of IE are malaise, fever, weight loss, splenomegaly, petechiae, subungual hemorrhages (splinter hemorrhages), Osler nodes and Janeway lesions. Ocular signs include Roth spots and other types of hemorrhages and exudates. ABE is more likely to present with a heart murmur than is SBE. The valvular disorder may be rapidly progressive, and congestive heart failure may develop.

Radiological (Plain Film) Features

Plain films reflect the hemodynamic alterations. The radiological features of left ventricular and left atrial enlargement and congestive heart failure may be observed. Mycotic aneurysm may be suggested by a widened mediastinum or a bulge of the ascending aorta. With acute rupture of the ventricular septum or sinus of Valsalva, signs of pulmonary venous hypertension (congestive heart failure) overshadow signs of left-to-right shunt. Acute mitral insufficiency generally results in pulmonary edema. The heart is often enlarged, but it may be normal in size.

Echocardiography

Echocardiography in patients with IE who have no clinical signs of valvar damage may show evidence of cardiac infection in only one-third to one-half of cases. If signs of valvar damage are present, echocardiographic studies are more likely to be positive. A combined approach using M-mode and 2-D echocardiography is recommended in studying these patients. Sessile lesions and involvement of right-sided valves is better recognized on 2-D echocardiography, whereas small pedunculated masses and involvement of the mitral valve may be better demonstrated on M-mode. In endocarditis of the aortic valve M-mode echocardiography reveals signs of aortic insufficiency (Fig. 5–18, A–C). The LV may be enlarged and hyperkinetic. Flutter of the mitral valve, decreased mitral excursion and early closure of the mitral valve (Fig. 5–19) may be evident. An infected aortic valve often is thickened, with a "shaggy" appearance during diastole and a normal excursion during systole (Fig. 5–61). Valves thickened by other processes tend not to produce a shaggy appearance and generally have a limited excursion during systole. If pedunculated vegetations are attached to the aortic valve they may be observed in the aortic root during systole and in the LV outflow tract dur-

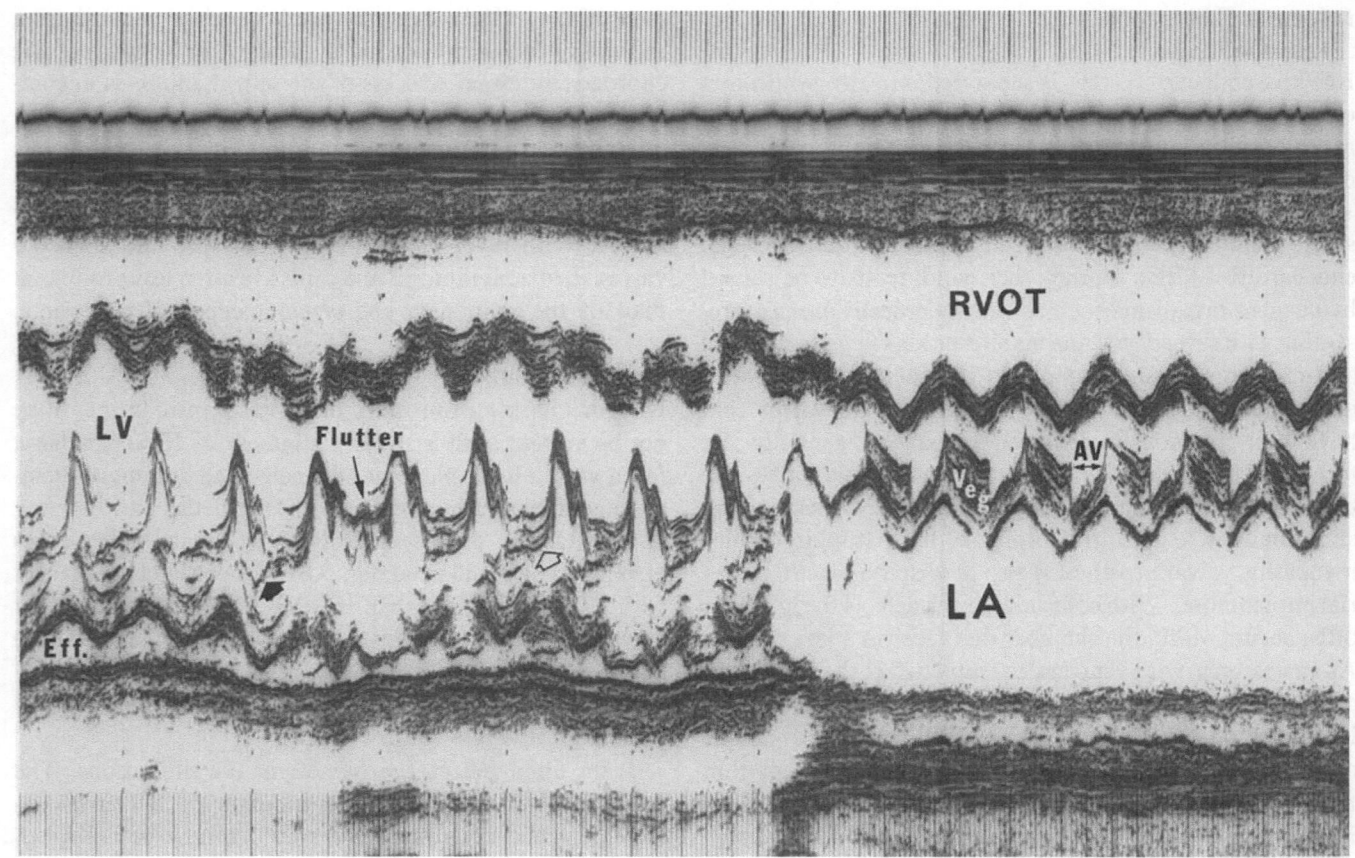

Fig. 5–61. *Infective endocarditis. M-mode echocardiogram showing an arc scan from the left ventricle to the aortic valve.* The aortic valve *(AV)* is thickened by the vegetation *(Veg)*, but its excursion is normal. (Valvar thickening due to other causes usually results in limitation of excursion.) During systole fine flutter of the aortic valve gives a slightly shaggy appearance. The left ventricle *(LV)* and left atrium *(LA)* are enlarged. A pericardial effusion *(Eff.)* is present. Systolic flutter of the mitral valve, chaotic motion of the posterior leaflet *(solid arrow)* and mitral prolapse *(open arrow)* are consistent with ruptured chordae tendineae. Note also the pleural effusion, which extends behind the left atrium. *RVOT* = right ventricular outflow tract.

ing diastole. On 2-D echocardiography, fine mitral flutter is not as easily recognized as with M-mode. Thickening of the aortic valve may be identified, and the motion of the valve can be observed (Fig. 5–61). A flail aortic valve is best demonstrated on 2-D echocardiography. The size and motion of a vegetation are also best demonstrated on 2-D echocardiology. Vegetation that does not move may be difficult or impossible to differentiate from thickening of the aortic valve due to other causes. A double density or outpouching of the aortic root suggests subaortic abscess or aneurysm of the sinus of Valsalva (see also Fig. 5–71C and D). Doppler echocardiography confirms the presence of aortic regurgitation, showing reversed flow in the LV outflow tract during diastole (Fig. 2–42C). The additional Doppler finding of reversed flow in the aortic arch or descending aorta throughout diastole indicates that aortic insufficiency is hemodynamically significant.

The M-mode echocardiogram in infection of the mitral valve may reveal only signs of mitral insufficiency (e.g., dilated LA, hyperkinetic LV). Signs of valvar thickening or destruction may also be present. The thickening of the mitral valve may be nonspecific or may present a shaggy appearance, similar to that observed with aortic valve involvement (Fig. 5–62). If a vegetation on the mitral valve is pedunculated it may appear on M-mode as a fine line moving anteriorly behind the anterior mitral leaflet as the valve opens (Fig. 5–63). If the vegetation is large it may appear as a mass behind the mitral valve, which moves into the orifice during diastole and into the LA during systole (Fig. 5–64). The appearance may be the same as that of a pedunculated tumor. 2-D echocardiography (Fig. 5–65) confirms these findings and demonstrates the attachment of the vegetation to the mitral leaflet rather than the LA wall, as would occur with a pedunculated tumor.

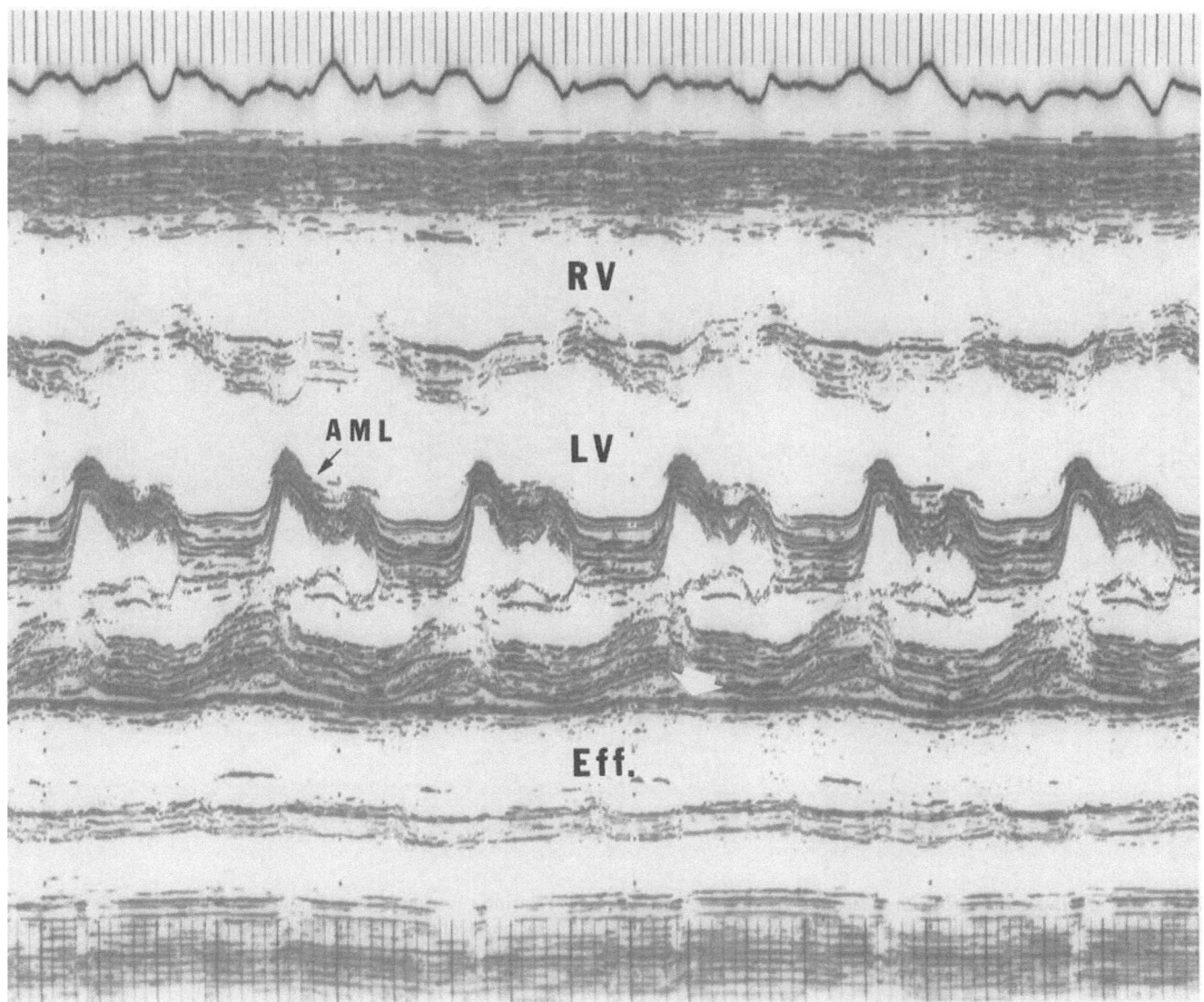

Fig. 5–62. *Infective endocarditis. M-mode echocardiogram at the level of the mitral valve.* The anterior leaflet of the mitral valve (*AML*) is thickened and has a "shaggy" appearance caused by flutter of the leaflet during diastole. The flutter may be indistinguishable from that produced by aortic insufficiency. A large, probably pleural, effusion (*Eff.*) is present behind the heart—pleural because the pericardium (*white arrow*) lies close to the posterior wall of the left ventricle (*LV*). *RV* = right ventricle.

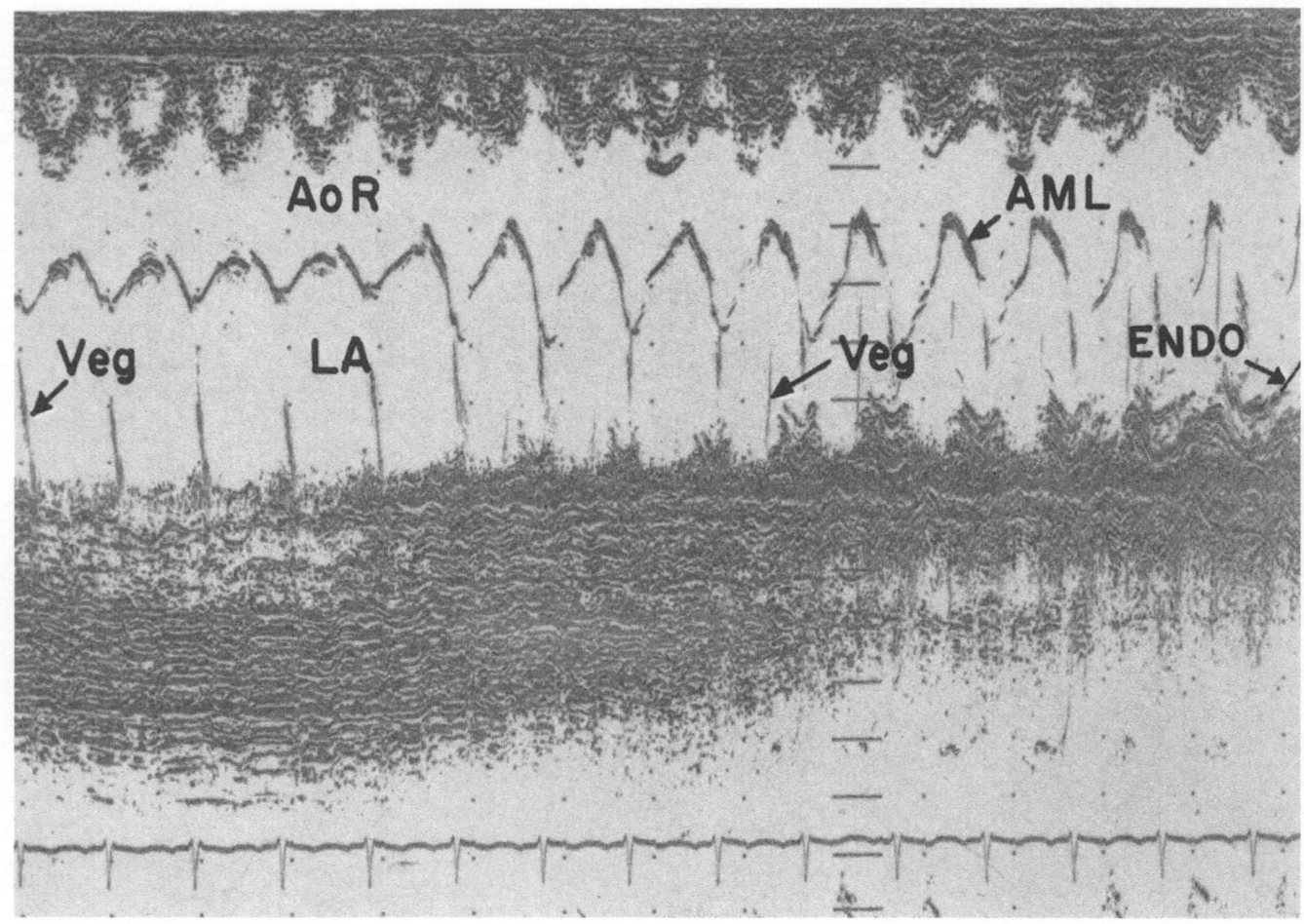

Fig. 5–63. *Infective endocarditis in a teenage girl with fever and mitral insufficiency.* M-mode arc scan from the aortic root (*AoR*) to the left ventricle. A small pedunculated vegetation (*Veg*) appears as a fine line that moves posteriorly into the left atrium (*LA*) during ventricular systole and then moves anteriorly behind the anterior leaflet of the mitral valve (*AML*) during diastole. *Endo*= endocardium of the left ventricle. (Same patient as Fig. 5–64.)

Destruction of the mitral valve apparatus results in ruptured chordae tendineae and flail mitral leaflet (Fig. 5–66). In such instances the M-mode echocardiogram may simulate prolapse of the mitral valve or may show extension of the flail leaflet into the LA during systole. Other signs of flail mitral leaflet on M-mode echocardiography are a coarse chaotic motion of the flail leaflet during diastole and fine flutter of the mitral valve during systole. The 2-D echocardiogram may also demonstrate extension of the flail leaflet into the LA. With ruptured chordae tendineae the tip of the mitral leaflet is sometimes observed to be pointing backward into the LA. This finding may help to distinguish ruptured chordae tendineae from prolapse of the mitral valve. Doppler echocardiography identifies reversed flow behind the mitral valve during ventricular systole (Fig. 2–47C). Vegetations on the tricuspid valve present in similar fashion to those on the mitral valve.

Again a shaggy appearance is characteristic (Fig. 5–67). The vegetation may appear as a fine line behind the tricuspid valve or may suggest a mass density that moves between the RA and the RV cavity. 2-D echocardiography will confirm the appearance of the mass attached to the tricuspid valve (Fig. 5–68). Again, pedunculated tumors and clots usually cannot be distinguished from vegetation. Demonstration of attachment to a leaflet of the tricuspid valve would be evidence in favor of vegetation, although a clot may become entangled in chordae tendineae and produce a similar appearance. Again, Doppler echocardiography may be helpful in recognizing tricuspid insufficiency.

Echocardiographic identification of vegetation on the pulmonary valve has also been reported. Flutter of the tricuspid valve may result if insufficiency of the pulmonic valve is present. A Doppler examination will identify pulmonary insufficiency.

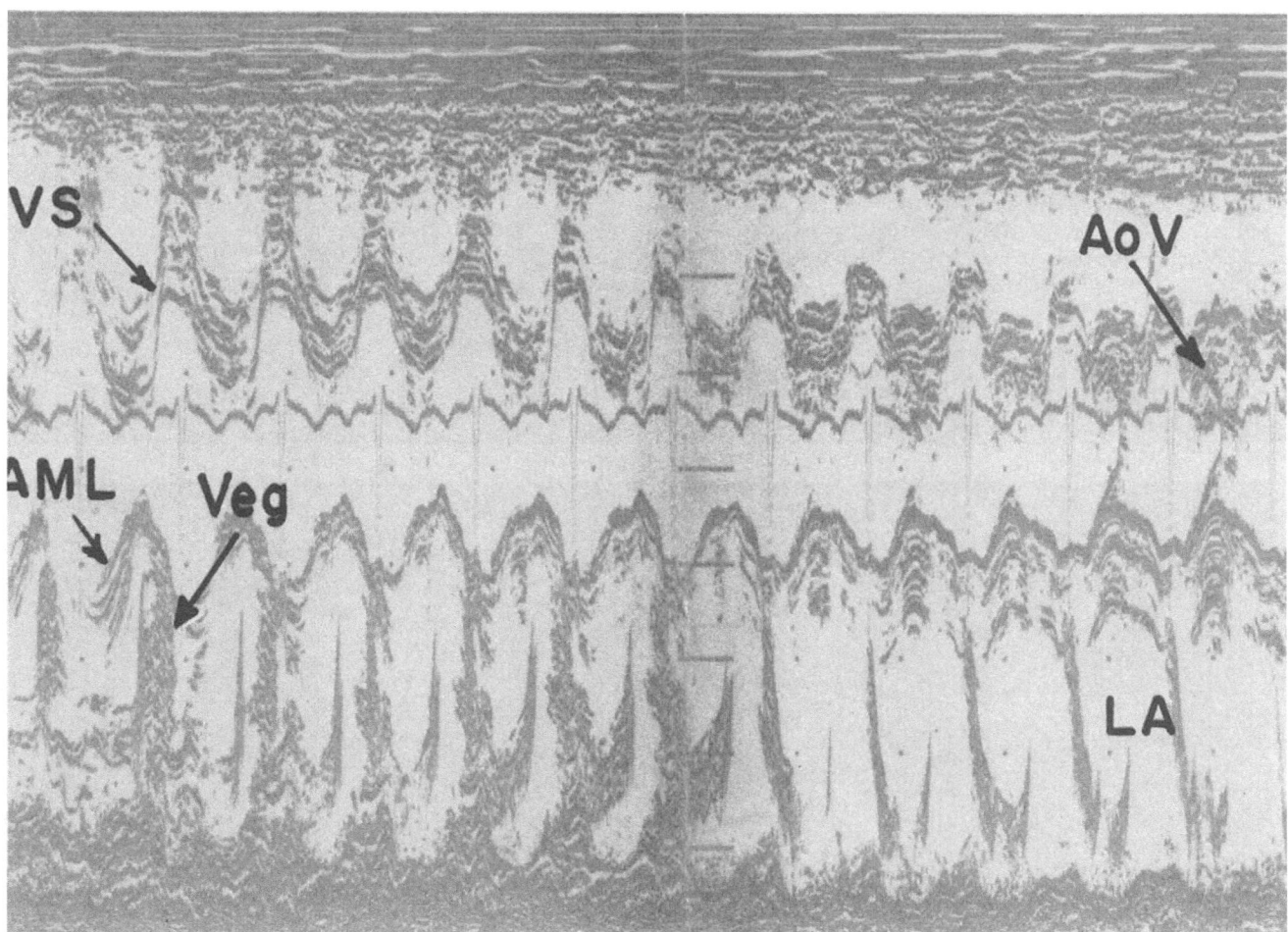

Fig. 5–64. *Infective endocarditis. M-mode arc scan from the mitral valve to the aortic valve in the patient in Fig. 5–63 (10 days later). The vegetation (Veg) is now larger, but its motion is the same as in Fig. 5–63. During diastole the vegetation appears as a mass* behind the mitral valve, while during ventricular systole it extends into the left atrium *(LA). AML* = anterior mitral leaflet; *AoV* = aortic valve; *VS* = ventricular septum.

Radiological (Plain Film) Features

Plain films may reveal the hemodynamic changes associated with disease of the aortic or mitral valve (usually insufficiency). Ruptured chordae tendineae will result in heart failure—pulmonary venous hypertension—with normal to slightly increased heart size. Plain films with acute left-to-right shunts also demonstrate heart failure rather than pulmonary overcirculation.

Endocarditis of the right side of the heart produces septic pulmonary emboli and multiple nodular or segmental (flame-shaped) pulmonary infiltrates bilaterally that may form cavities (Fig. 5–69). The RA and RV may be enlarged.

Contrast Studies

Although echocardiography is able to define the changes in the valves, complications, especially around the root of the aorta, are best delineated by aortography. A qualitative assessment of severity of aortic insufficiency is obtained and at the same time the status of the leaflets is assessed (Fig. 5–70). A central jet indicates deformity and thickening of the leaflets. Perforation of a leaflet may be reflected in a jet through the affected leaflet. If the eccentric jet through the aortic valve impinges on the mitral valve the anterior leaflet of the mitral valve may perforate secondarily resulting in mitral insufficiency. A subaortic abscess presents on aortography as a collection of contrast material in a pocket, usually in the interventricular septum just below the aortic valve (Fig. 5–71), with the mouth in the sinus of Valsalva. The abscess may communicate with the LV, RV, RA, or rarely the LA. Mycotic aneurysms of the outflow tract of the LV, sinus of Valsalva, aortic root and ascending aorta may be demonstrated. Involvement of the membranous septum may result in aneurysm or perforation into the RV or RA.

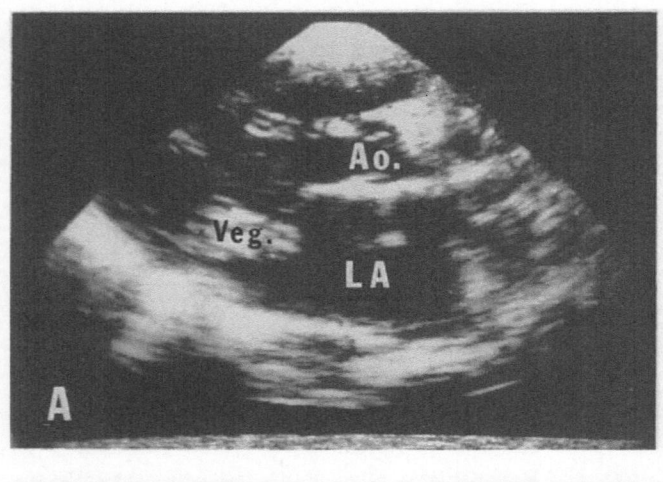

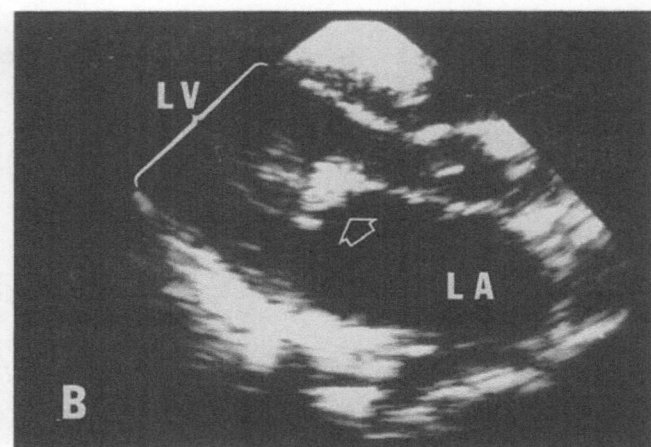

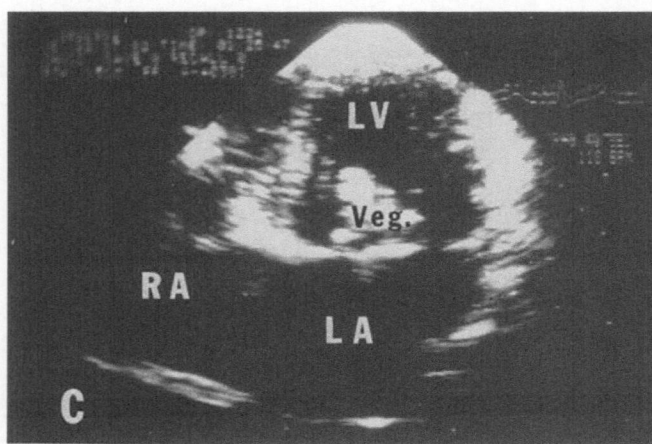

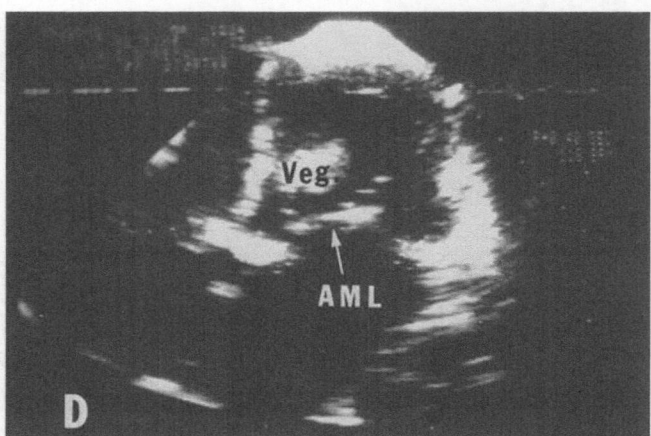

Fig. 5–65. *Infective endocarditis. Two-dimensional echocardiograms in a 24-year-old woman show a pedunculated mass attached to the anterior leaflet of the mitral valve.* **A** Long axis of the left ventricle, systole; **B** long axis, diastole; **C** apex four-chamber view, systole; **D** apex four-chamber view, diastole. In the long axis view during systole (**A**) the vegetation (*Veg.*) presents as a mass near the papillary muscle. During diastole (**B**) the mass (*open arrow*) swings anteriorly at the tip of the anterior leaflet of the mitral valve. The left atrium (*LA*) is enlarged. In the apex four-chamber view (**C** and **D**) the vegetation abuts the mitral leaflet in systole (**C**) and pivots into the left ventricle during diastole (**D**). *Ao.* = aorta; *LV* = left ventricle; *RA* = right atrium; *AML* = anterior mitral leaflet. (A left ventriculogram from this patient is shown in Fig. 5–72.)

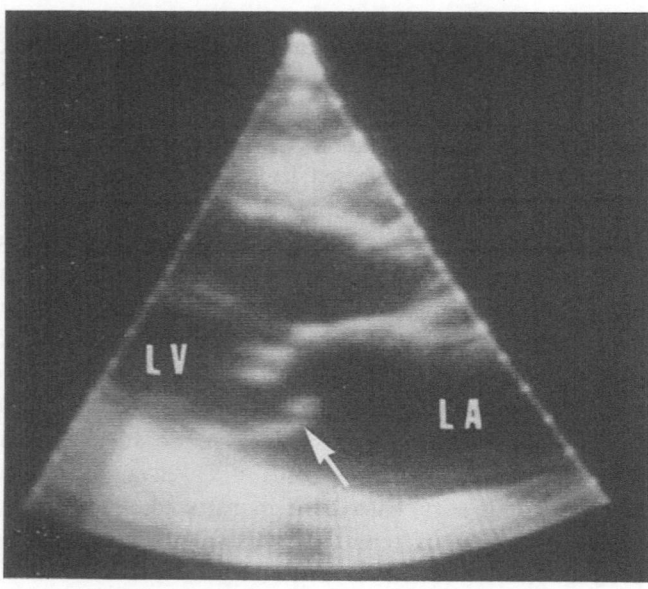

Fig. 5–66. *Flail mitral leaflet in a patient with infective endocarditis.* A two-dimensional echocardiogram in the long axis view demonstrates the posterior mitral leaflet (*arrow*) floating into the left atrial cavity during ventricular systole. *LV* = left ventricle; *LA* = left atrium. Courtesy of Mark Strom, M.D., Bronx, N.Y.

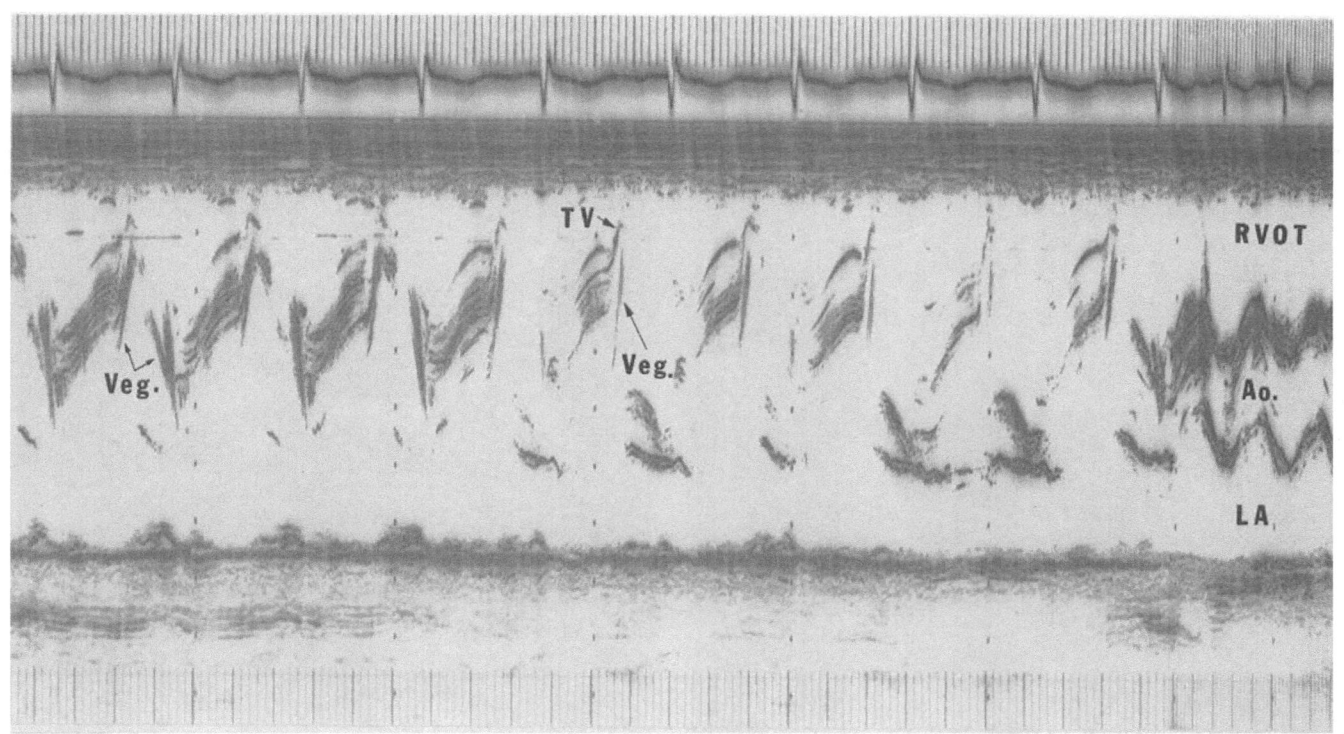

A

Fig. 5–67. *Infective endocarditis in a 10-year-old girl with a small ventricular septal defect, fever and positive blood cultures.* The M-mode arc scan (**A**) from the tricuspid valve (*TV*) to the right ventricular outflow tract (*RVOT*) demonstrates the vegetation (*Veg.*), which presents in some beats as a linear density and in other beats as a mass behind the tricuspid valve. **B** shows the vegetation (*Veg.*) as a "shaggy" density during diastole. (Other views from this patient are shown in Fig. 5–68.) *Ao.* = aorta; *LA* = left atrium.

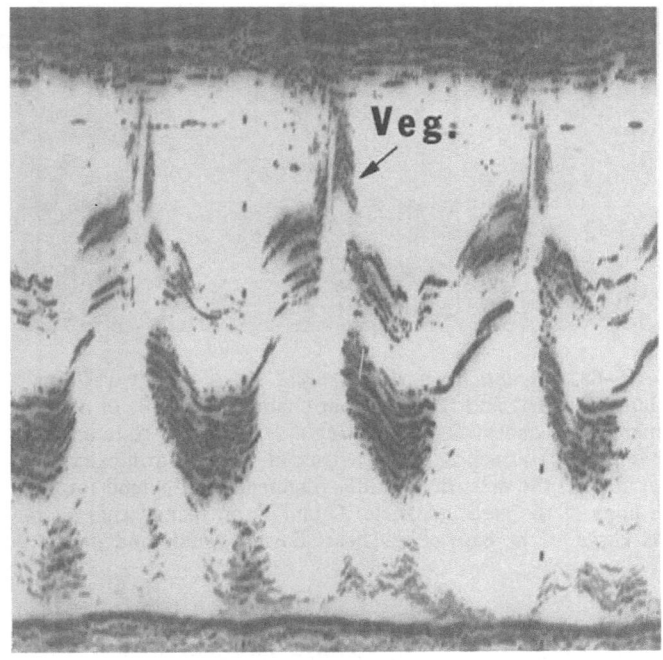

B

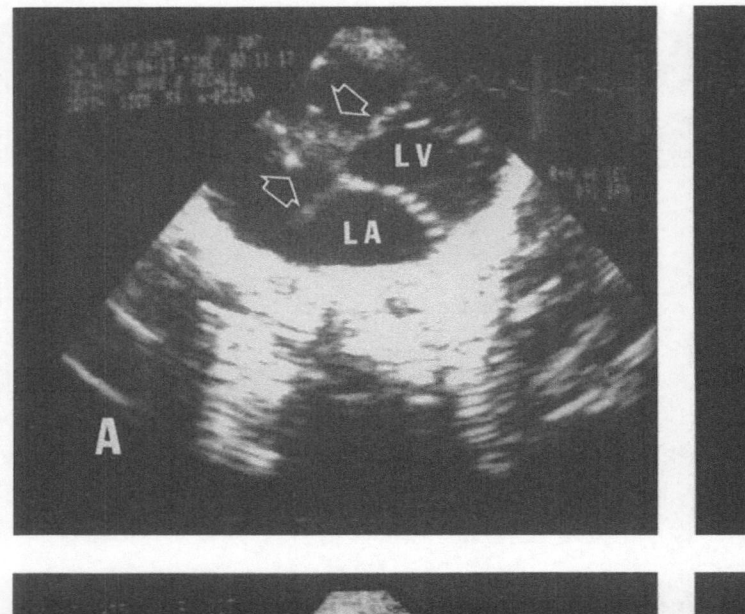
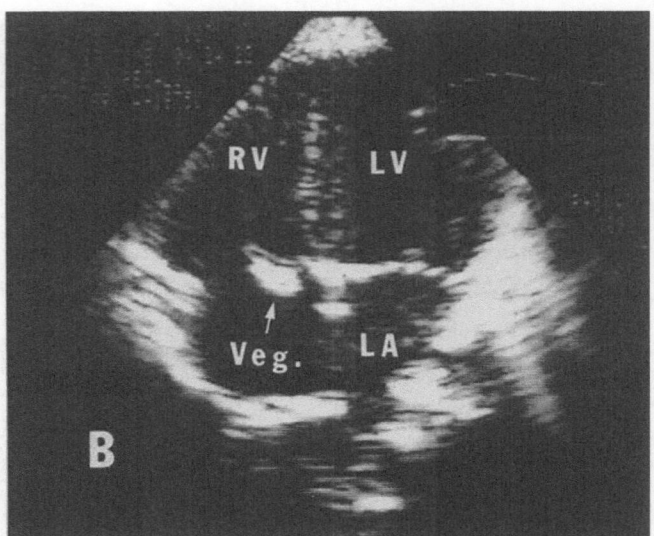
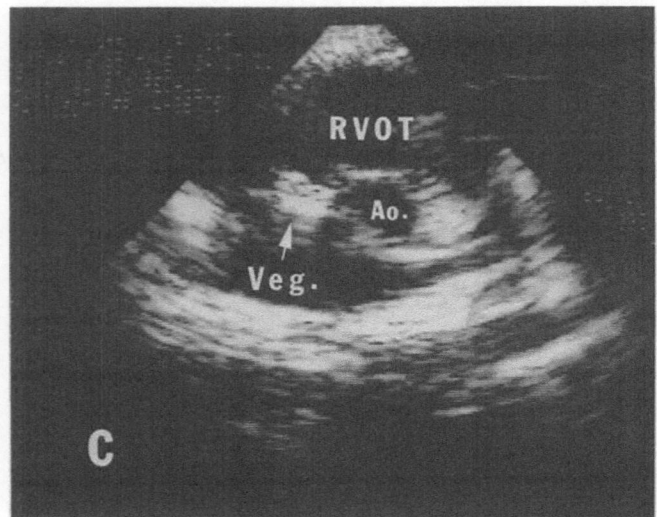
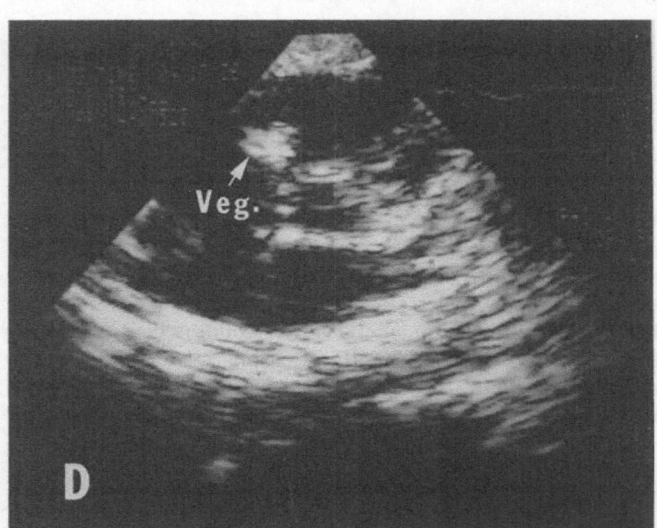

Fig. 5–68. *Vegetation on the tricuspid valve.* The parasternal oblique view (**A**) and the apex four-chamber view (**B**) of a two-dimensional echocardiogram during systole demonstrate a mass (*open arrows*) attached to the tricuspid valve. During diastole (not shown) the mass divides into fragments that extend toward the apex of the right ventricle. **C** and **D** are parasternal short axis views at the base of the heart during systole and diastole respectively. During systole (**C**) the vegetation is superimposed on the tricuspid valve. During diastole (**D**) the tricuspid valve and its vegetation swing into the right ventricular outflow tract (*RVOT*). (Other views of this patient are shown in Fig. 5–67.) *LA* = left atrium; *LV* = left ventricle; *Veg* = vegetation; *RV* = right ventricle; *Ao.* = aortic root.

Vegetations are not often demonstrated by angiography. Left ventriculography is avoided in patients with aortic valve infection for fear of dislodging friable infected tissue. Most patients who undergo catheterization with aortic valve involvement have severe aortic insufficiency so that the LV is opacified at the time of aortography. Patients with isolated mitral valve involvement require left ventriculography (Fig. 5–72).

Contrast studies have little to add in instances of IE involving the right side of the heart. Clinical findings, M-mode and 2-D echocardiograms with Doppler studies, and plain films are usually adequate for diagnosis and management.

Treatment

Treatment consists of high doses of antibiotics specific for the organism identified or suspected on the basis of clinical presentation. If heart failure becomes unmanageable, surgical replacement of the aortic or mitral valve during the active stage of infection is necessary, even though the risk is high. The tricuspid or pulmonary valve may be removed without prosthetic replacement as insufficiency of either is tolerated without severe cardiac decompensation. Surgical repair of complications such as perforation of the sinus of Valsalva or ventricular septum is performed at the same time. Postoperative paravalvular leaks are not infrequent after valve replacement during active infection. Recurrence of infection is frequent in narcotic addicts.

Fig. 5–69. *Septic emboli in infective endocarditis of the tricuspid valve.* Multiple, large, cavitations (abscesses) are demonstrated in the lungs. At surgery, a vegetation was removed from the tricuspid valve.

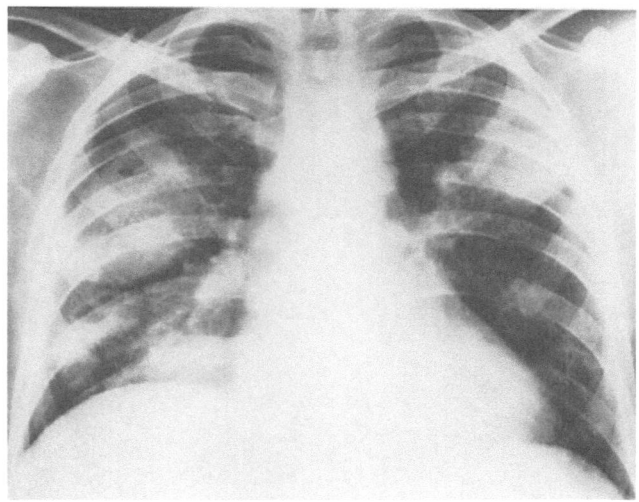

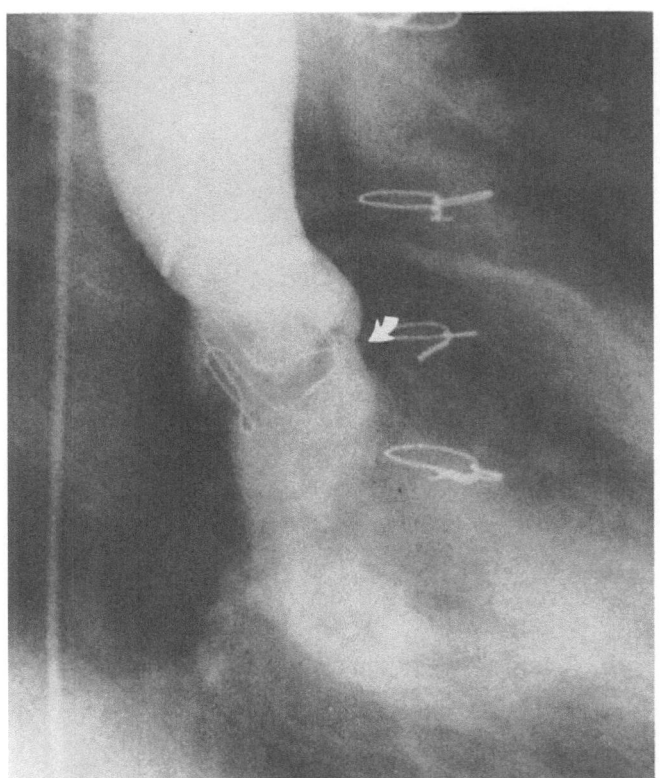

A

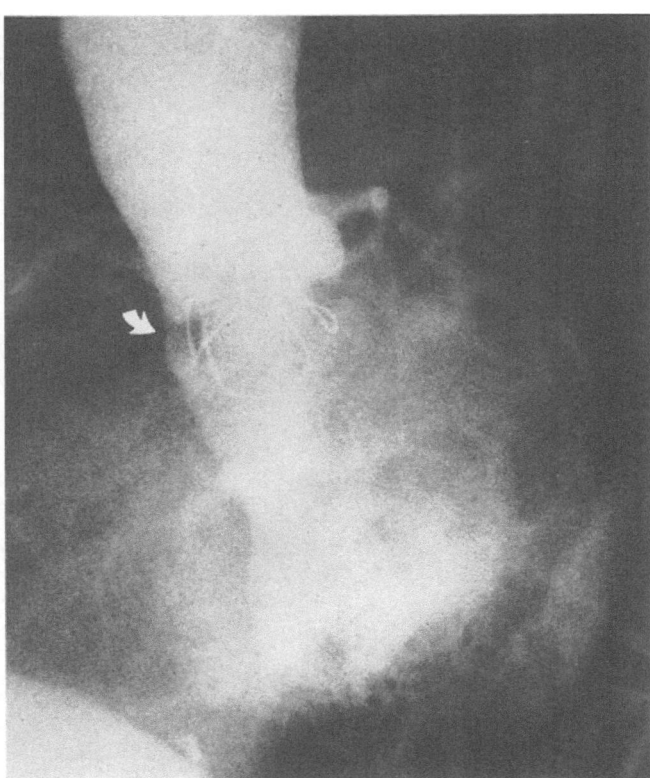

B

Fig. 5–70. *Paravalvular leak in a patient with infective endocarditis.* The RAO view **(A)**, and the LAO view **(B)** of the aortogram illustrate severe aortic insufficiency in a man with a porcine het-erograft aortic prosthesis. In addition to the central regurgitant jet, contrast material between the wire strut of the prosthesis and the wall of the aorta (*arrow*) indicates a paravalvular leak.

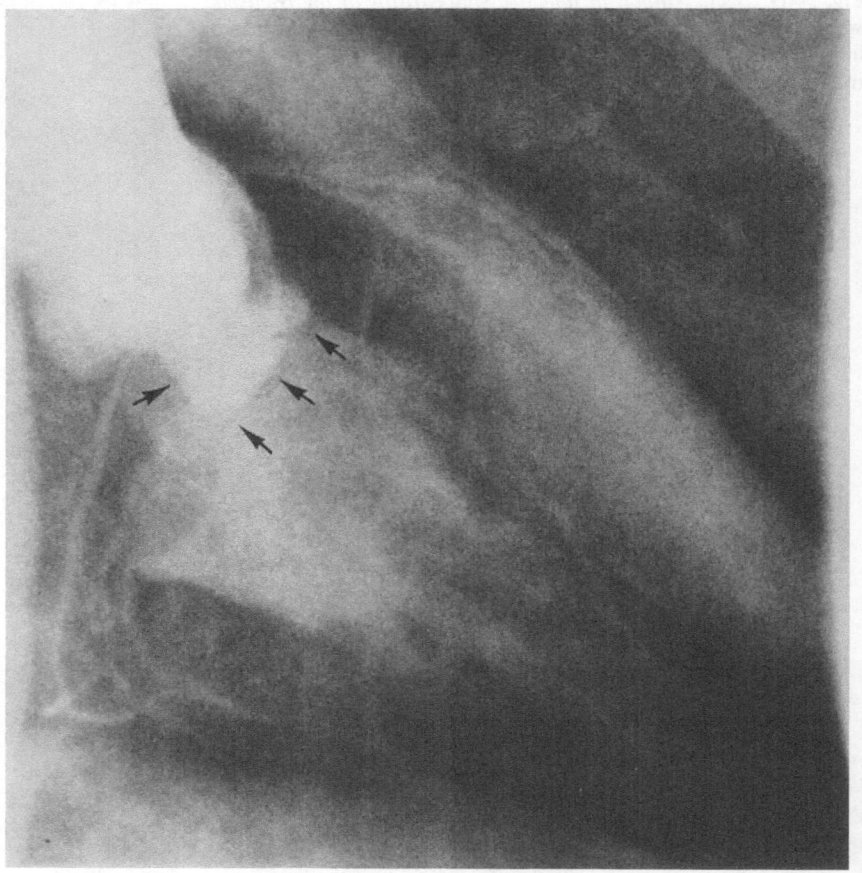

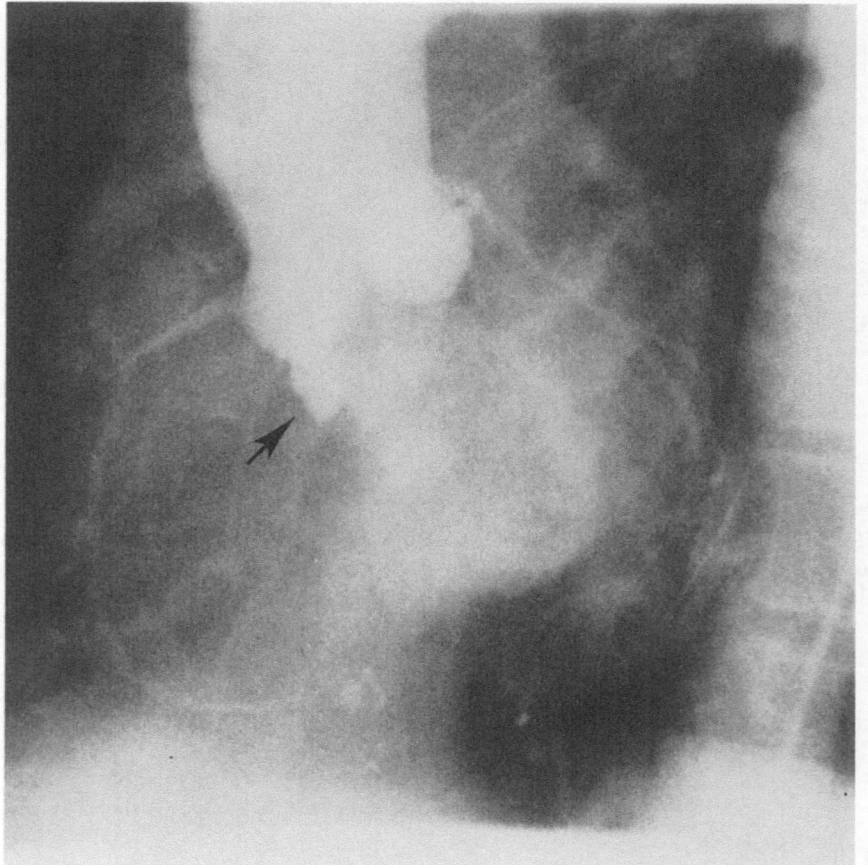

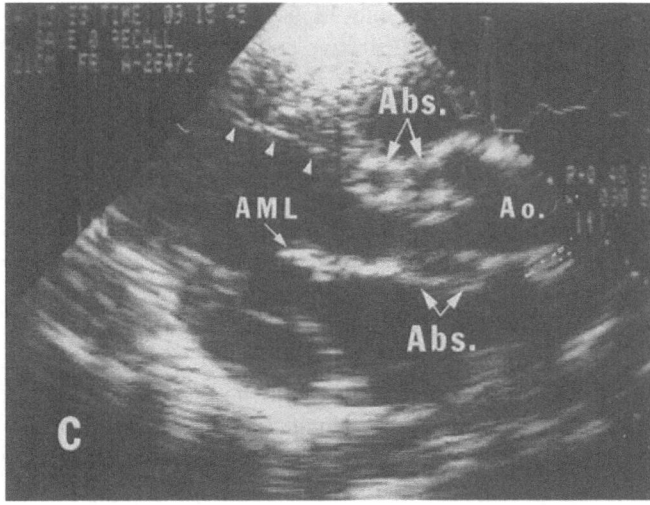

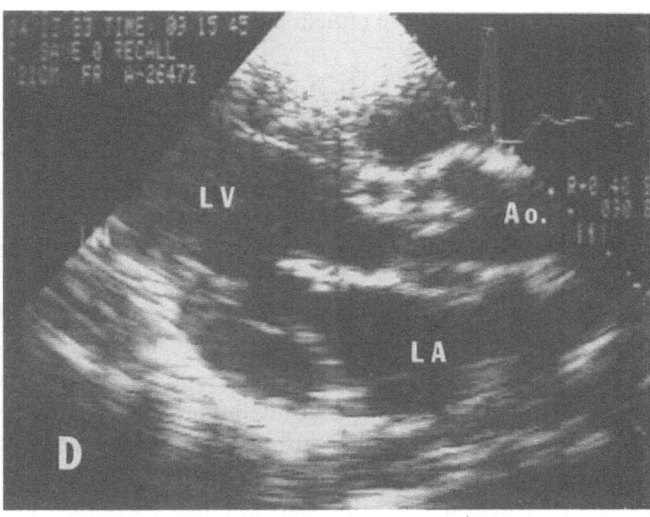

Fig. 5–71. *Subaortic abscess in a patient with infective endocarditis.* The RAO view (**A**) and the LAO view (**B**) of a cine aortogram demonstrate contrast material in the left ventricle, secondary to aortic regurgitation. In addition, contrast material collects in a pocket in the ventricular septum below the anterior (right) semilunar sinus (*arrows*). The mouth of the pocket is in the sinus of Valsalva. On cine aortography the abscess was found to communicate by way of a small perforation (not shown) into the left ventricular chamber. **C** and **D** are parasternal long axis views of the two-dimensional echocardiogram in the same patient. They show an echo-free space within the ventricular septum just below the aortic valve and in the base of the anterior leaflet of the mitral valve (*Abs.*). These represent the subaortic abscess. *Ao.* = aortic root; *AML* = anterior leaflet of the mitral valve; *LA* = left atrium; *LV* = left ventricle; *arrowheads* = left side of ventricular septum.

Fig. 5–72. *Vegetation on the mitral valve in a patient with infective endocarditis.* The RAO view of a left ventriculogram shows a globular filling defect near the mitral valve (*Veg.*). The left atrium (*LA*) is opacified because of mitral regurgitation. (2-D echocardiograms from this patient are shown in Fig. 5–65.)

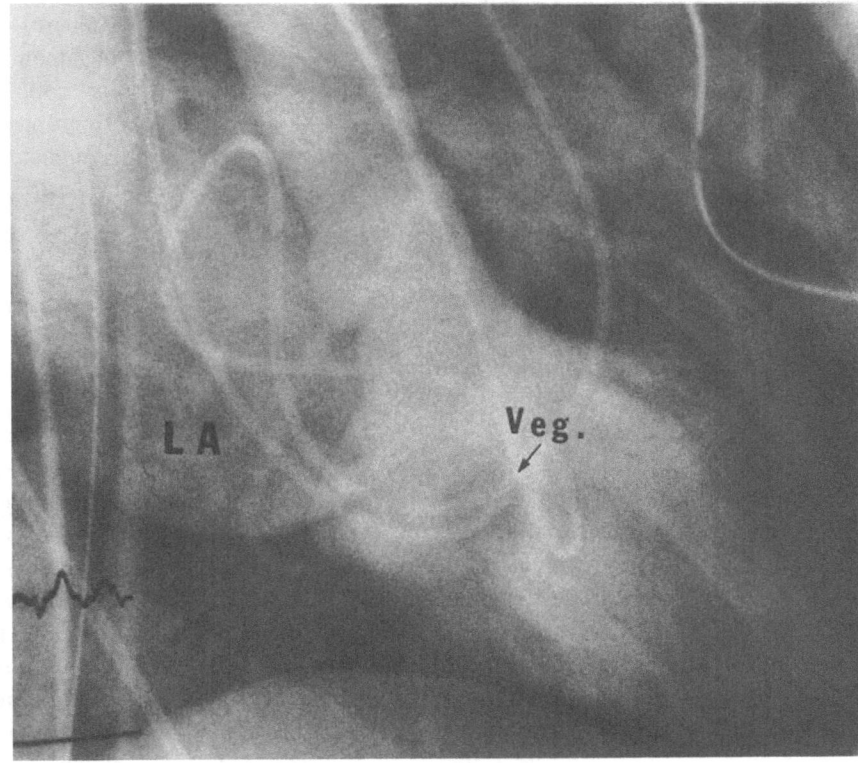

Aortic Arteritis Syndromes: Takayasu Arteritis and Giant Cell Arteritis

These entities represent inflammatory processes involving the intima and media of the aorta and its branches. Takayasu arteritis shows a preponderance for young Orientals. Giant cell arteritis is more likely to occur in middle-aged Caucasians. Both disorders, however, have a worldwide distribution.

The acute phase of the disorders may be accompanied by systemic symptoms and signs (e.g., fever, malaise, arthritis). The basic pathological lesion of giant cell arteritis is characterized by granulomatous inflammation of the media of small- to medium-caliber arteries, especially those of the head and neck. Occlusion of the vessels can produce blindness, cerebral ischemia, paresthesias, Raynaud phenomena, claudication of arms or legs, and great vessel steal syndromes. The predominant pathologic process in Takayasu arteritis is marked intimal proliferation and fibrosis with fibrous scarring and degeneration of the elastic fibers leading to obliteration of the brachiocephalic vessels and/or the abdominal aorta. Round cell infiltration is a relatively minor feature. On occasion the pulmonary arteries are involved, causing pulmonary hypertension. Both Takayasu and giant cell arteritis may result in dilatation of the aorta and aortic anulus with separation of the commissures causing aortic valvular insufficiency (Fig. 5–26). Death may result from intramural hematoma (dissecting aneurysm) of the aorta.

Ankylosing Spondylitis

The cardiovascular lesion of ankylosing spondylitis occurs in about 12% of cases, usually more than 15 years after the onset of the arthritis symptoms. An inflammatory process involves the aortic wall immediately above the sinuses of Valsalva. Dense adventitial scar tissue forms a fibrous ridge below the base of the aortic valve and extends into the base of the mitral valve as well. The aortic cusps, as a result, may become thickened and shortened, producing aortic insufficiency, which may be progressive and severe. Rarely the mitral valve becomes insufficient but almost always to a mild degree. The fibrous scar may extend into the ventricular septum to produce arrhythmias and abnormalities of conduction.

Rheumatoid Arthritis, the Reiter Syndrome, and Relapsing Polychondritis

About 5%–10% of patients with rheumatoid arthritis, Reiter syndrome or relapsing polychondritis develop an inflammation of the root of the aorta. The elastic tissue is destroyed, and progressive dilatation or aneurysm of the aorta ensues. As in other forms of aortitis, aortic insufficiency may result. Other diseases that may be associated with aortitis are systemic lupus erythematosus, scleroderma, psoriasis and ulcerative colitis.

Syphilitic Aortitis

This infective disorder is now rarely encountered. The latent period after the primary stage of infection is usually between 10 and 25 years. The ascending aorta is most commonly involved, although the leaflets of the aortic valve and the ostia of the coronary arteries may also be affected. The hallmark of the disease is an aneurysm of the ascending aorta caused by inflammation in the media of the aorta. Occlusive endarteritis of the vasa vasorum occurs during the acute phase, with perivascular cuffing by plasma cells and lymphocytes. Giant cells and microgummas may also be observed on histological sections. These changes are followed by scarring and weakening of the wall of the aorta. Luetic aneurysms of the ascending aorta are usually saccular but may be fusiform. They may reach huge proportions without rupturing and may cause symptoms by compressing or eroding surrounding structures (e.g., sternum, ribs) causing cough, dysphagia and stridor.

Aortic insufficiency, usually progressive, may be caused by dilatation of the aortic ring and separation of the leaflets.

Clinical features include a tambour sound of aortic closure and other findings of aortic insufficiency (e.g., diastolic murmur, increased cardiac impulse, bounding pulses). If the coronary ostia are involved, angina may be a prominent feature.

Plain chest roentgenograms demonstrate features of aortic insufficiency and often an aneurysm of the ascending aorta containing a thin layer of calcium within the wall of the aneurysm. In the absence of an aneurysm a thin layer of calcium in the wall of the ascending aorta is usually atherosclerotic but may also be due to a syphilitic process.

Aortography demonstrates dilatation of the ascending aorta. An aneurysm of the ascending aorta and aortic insufficiency are frequent. The coronary ostia may be narrowed.

Aortic Insufficiency Secondary to Systemic Hypertension

About 10% of patients with systemic hypertension have a basal diastolic decrescendo murmur, suggesting mild aortic insufficiency (AI). Rarely, marked aortic dilatation and severe aortic regurgitation result. Intraoperative and postmortem examinations of such patients have demonstrated no degenerative changes of the aortic root or of the aortic valve that could account for the severity of the AI. The AI may be due to dilatation of the aortic root and anulus, resulting in failure of the leaflets to coapt.

Plain films may be normal or may show signs of congestive heart failure. A dilated aortic root is not always evident. The LV may or may not be enlarged. Echocardiograms demonstrate the dilated aortic root, dilated LV and mitral flutter.

On aortography the degree of aortic regurgitation is quantitated, and other causes for AI are excluded. Surgery is indicated for individuals with severe AI and congestive heart failure which does not improve with control of hypertension.

Bibliography

Aortic Stenosis

Clawson BJ (1940) Rheumatic heart disease; analysis of 796 cases. Am Heart J 20:454–474

Fowles RE, Martin RP, Abrams JM, Schapiro JN, French JW, Popp RL (1979) Two-dimensional echocardiographic features of bicuspid aortic valve. Chest 75:434–440

Gaasch WH (1979) Left ventricular radius to wall thickness ratio. Am J Cardiol 43:1189–1194

Gorlin R, Gorlin G (1951) Hydraulic formula for calculation of stenotic mitral valves, other cardiac valves and central circulatory shunts. Am Heart J 41:1–29

Gorlin R, McMillan IKR, Medd WE, Matthews MB, Daley R (1955) Dynamics of the circulation in aortic valvular disease. Am J Med 18:855–870

Gross L, Friedberg CK (1936) Lesions of the cardiac valves in rheumatic fever. Am J Pathol 12:469–494

Hancock EW (1959) Differentiation of valvar and subvalvar aortic stenosis. Circulation 20:709

Klatte EC, Tampas JP, Campbell JA, Lurie PR (1962) The roentgenographic manifestations of aortic stenosis and aortic valvar insufficiency. Am J Roentgenol 88:57–69

Love JW, Jahnke EJ, Zacharies D, Davidson WA, Kidder WR, Luan LL (1980) Calcific aortic stenosis and gastrointestinal bleeding (letter). N Engl J Med 302:968

Nanda NC, Gramiak R, Manning J, Mahoney EB, Lipchik EO, Deweese JA (1974) Echocardiographic recognition of the congenital bicuspid aortic valve. Circulation 49:870–875

Radford DJ, Bloom KR, Izukawa T, Moes CAF, Rowe RD (1976) Echocardiographic assessment of bicuspid aortic valves. Angiographic and pathologic correlates. Circulation 53:80–85

Rahimtoola SH (1983) Valvular heart disease: A perspective. J Am Coll Cardiol 1:199–215

Roberts WC (1970) Anatomically isolated aortic valvular disease. The case against its being of rheumatic etiology. Am J Med 49:151–159

Roberts WC (1970) The structure of the aortic valve in clinically isolated aortic stenosis. An autopsy study of 162 patients over 15 years of age. Circulation 42:91–97

Weaver GA, Arquin PL, Davis JS, Ramsey WH (1980) More on aortic stenosis and gastrointestinal bleeding (letter). N Engl J Med 303:584

Bicuspid Aortic Valve

Fenoglio Jr. JJ, McAllister HA, Jr. DeCastro CM, Davia JE, Cheitlin MD (1977) Congenital bicuspid aortic valve after age 20. Am J Cardiol 39:164–169

Fowles RE, Martin RP, Abrams JM, Schapiro JN, French JW, Popp RL (1979) Two-dimensional echocardiographic features of bicuspid aortic valve. Chest 75:434–440

Friedberg CK (1966) Diseases of the heart, 3rd ed. Saunders, Philadelphia, p.1130

Johnson AD, Detwiler JH, Higgins CB (1978) Left coronary artery anatomy in patients with bicuspid aortic valves. Br Heart J 40:489–493

Roberts WC, Elliot LP (1968) Lesions complicating the congenitally bicuspid aortic valve. Anatomic and radiographic features. Radiol Clin North Am 6:409–421

Schlant C (1971) Calcific aortic stenosis. Am J Cardiol 27:581–583

Spindola-Franco H, Fish BG, Dachman A, Grose R, Attai L (1982) Recognition of bicuspid aortic valve by plain film calcification pattern. AJR 139:867–872

Waller BF, Carter JB, Williams Jr. HJ, Wang W, Edwards JE (1973) Bicuspid aortic valve. Comparison of congenital and acquired types. Circulation 48:1140–1150

Aortic Insufficiency

Baron MG (1971) Angiocardiographic evaluation of valvular insufficiency. Circulation 43:599–605

Brandenburg RO, Tajik AJ, Edwards WD, Reeder GS, Shub C, Seward JB (1983) Accuracy of 2-dimensional echocardiographic diagnosis of congenitally bicuspid aortic valve: echocardiographic–anatomic correlation in 115 patients. Am J Cardiol 51:1469–1473

Bulkey BH, Roberts WC (1973) Ankylosing spondylitis and aortic regurgitation. Description of the characteristic cardiovascular lesion from study of eight necropsy patients. Circulation 48:1014–1027

Buchbinder NA, Roberts WC (1972) Left-sided valvular active endocarditis. Am J Med 53:20–35

Carson NAJ, Dent CE, Field CMB, Gaull GE (1965) Homocystinuria. Clinical and pathological review of ten cases. J Pediatr 66:565–783

Case Records of the Massachusetts General Hospital. Case 21 (1979) Aneurysmal dilatation of the aorta with aortic regurgitation. N Engl J Med 300:1204–1209

Criscitiello MG, Ronan JA, Besterman EMM, Schoenwetter W (1965) Cardiovascular abnormalities in osteogenesis imperfecta. Circulation 31:255–262

Croft CH, Lipscomb K, Mathis K, Firth BG, Nicod P, Tilson G, Winniford MD, Hillis LD (1984) Limitations of qualitative angiographic grading in aortic or mitral regurgitation. Am J Cardiol 53:1593–1598

Fenichel NM (1950) Artheriosclerotic aortic insufficiency. Am Heart J 40:117–124

Gelfand ML, Kantor T (1969) Cogan's syndrome associated with cardiovascular manifestations. Circulation 40(suppl 3):87

Henry WL, Bonow RO, Borer JS, Ware JH, Kent KM, Redwood DR, McIntosh CL, Morrow AG, Epstein SE (1980) Observations on the optimum time for operative intervention for aortic regurgitation. I. Evaluation of the results of aortic valve replacement in symptomatic patients. Circulation 61:471–483

Honig HS, Weintraub AM, Gomes NM, Hufnagel CA, Roberts

WC (1977) Severe aortic regurgitation secondary to idiopathic aortitis. Am J Med 63:623–633

Imaizumi T, Orita Y, Koiwaya Y, Hirata T, Nakamura M (1982) Utility of two-dimensional echocardiography in the differential diagnosis of the etiology of aortic regurgitation. Am Heart J 103:887–896

McKusick VA (1965) The genetic mucopolysaccharidoses (editorial). Circulation 31:1–4

O'Rourke RA, Crawford MH (1980) Timing of valve replacement in patients with chronic aortic regurgitation (editorial). Circulation 61:493–495

Payne DD, DeWeese, Mahoney EB, Murphy GW (1974) Surgical treatment of traumatic rupture of the normal aortic valve. Ann Thorac Surg 17:223–229.

Sandler H, Dodge HT, Hay RE, Rackley CE (1963) Quantitation of valvular insufficiency in man by angiocardiography. Am Heart J 65:501–513

Spindola-Franco H, Fish BG, Dachman A, Grose R, Attai L (1982) Recognition of bicuspid aortic valve by plain film calcification. AJR 139:867–872

Swensson RE, Linnebur AC, Paster SB (1975) Striking aortic root dilatation in a patient with the Larsen syndrome. J Pediatr 86:914–915

Tatsuno K, Konno S, Ando M, Sakakibara S (1973) Pathogenetic mechanisms of prolapsing aortic valve and aortic regurgitation associated with ventricular septal defect. Anatomical, angiographic, and surgical considerations. Circulation 48:1028–1037

Toone EC, Jr., Pierce EL, Hennigar GR (1959) Aortitis and aortic regurgitation associated with rheumatoid spondylitis. Am J Med 26:255–263

Marfan Syndrome

Bachhuber TE, Lalich JJ (1954) Production of dissecting aneurysms in rats fed Lathyrus odoratus. Science 120:712–713

Boucek RJ, Noble NL, Gunja-Smith Z, Butler WT (1981) The Marfan syndrome: A deficiency in chemically stable collagen cross-links. N Engl J Med 305:988–991

Carson NAJ, Dent CE, Field CMB, Gaull GE (1965) Homocystinuria: Clinical and pathological review of ten cases. J Pediatr 66:565–583

Criscitiello MG, Ronan JA, Besterman EMM, Schoenwetter W (1965) Cardiovascular abnormalities in osteogenesis imperfecta. Circulation 31:255–262

Freiden J, Hurwith ES, Leader E (1962) Ruptured aortic cusp associated with heritable disorder of connective tissue. Am J Med 33:615–618

Gallotti R, Ross DN (1980) The Marfan syndrome: Surgical technique and follow-up in 50 patients. Ann Thorac Surg 29:428–433

James TN, Frame B, Schatz IJ (1964) Pathology of cardiac conduction system in Marfan's syndrome. Arch Intern Med 114:339–343

Kiel EA, Frias JL, Victorica BE (1983) Cardiovascular manifestations in the Larsen syndrome. Pediatrics 71:942–946

McDonald GR, Schaff HV, Pyeritz RE, McKusick VA, Gott VL (1981) Surgical management of patients with Marfan's syndrome and dilatation of the ascending aorta. J Thorac Cardiovasc Surg 81:180–186

McKusick VA (1955) The cardiovascular aspects of Marfan's syndrome: A heritable disorder of connective tissue. Circulation 11:321–342

McKusick VA (1965) The genetic mucopolysaccharidoses. Circulation 31:1–4

Pyeritz RE (1981) Maternal and fetal complications of pregnancy in the Marfan syndrome. Am J Med 71:784–790

Pyeritz RE, McKusick VA (1981) Basic defects in the Marfan syndrome (editorial). N Engl J Med 305:1011–1012

Scheie HG, Hambrick GW JR., Barness LA (1962) A newly recognized forme fruste of Hurler's disease (gargoylism). Am J Opthalmol 53:753–769

Sloper JC, Storey G (1953) Aneurysms of the ascending aorta due to medial degeneration associated with arachnodactyly (Marfan's disease). J Clin Pathol 6:299–303

Spangler RD, Nora JJ, Lortscher RH, Wolfe RW, Okin JT (1976) Echocardiography in Marfan's syndrome. Chest 69:72–78

Mitral Valve Disease

Amplatz K (1962) The roentgenographic diagnosis of mitral and aortic valvular disease. Am Heart J 64:556–566

De Sanctis RW, Dean DC, Bland EF (1964) Extreme left atrial enlargement; some characteristic features. Circulation 29:14–23

Figley MM (1964) Angiocardiography in valvular heart disease: Morphologic and volumetric considerations. Radiol Clin North Am 11:409–423

Gorlin R, Gorlin SG (1951) Determination of valve area. Am Heart J 41:1–29

Kennedy JW, Yarnall SR, Murray JA, Figley MM (1970) Quantitative angiocardiography. IV. Relationships of left atrial and ventricular pressure and volume in mitral valve disease. Circulation 41:817–824

Lewis BM, Gorlin R, Houssay HEJ, Heynes FW, Dexter L (1952) Mitral valve area and symptoms related to its reduction. Am Heart J 43:2–26

Melhem RE, Dunbar JD, Booth RW (1961) The "B" lines of Kerley and left atrial size in mitral valve disease. Their correlation with the mean left atrial pressure as measured by left atrial puncture. Radiology 76:65–69

Shapiro JH, Jacobson HG, Rubinstein BM, Popple MH, Schwedel JB (1963) Calcifications of the heart. Thomas, Springfield, Ill

Van Houten FX, Adams DF, Abrams HL (1974) Radiology of valvular heart disease. In: Sonnenblick EH and Lesh M (eds): Valvular heart disease. Grune & Stratton, New York

Mitral Stenosis

Abernathy WS, Willis PW III (1973) Thromboembolic complications of rheumatic heart disease. Cardiovasc Clin 5(2):31

Akins CW, Korklin JK, Block PC, Buckley MJ, Austein WG (1978) Pre-operative evaluation of subvalvular fibrosis in mitral stenosis. A predictive factor in conservative vs. replacement surgical therapy. Circulation 60:71–76

Cohen MV, Gorlin R (1972) Modified orifice equation for the calculation of mitral valve area. Am Heart J 84:839–840

Edler I (1956) Ultrasound-cardiogram in mitral valvular disease. Acta Chir Scand 111:230–231

Effert S (1967) Pre- and postoperative evaluation of mitral stenosis by ultrasound. Am J Cardiol 19:59–65

Esposito MJ (1955) Focal pulmonary hemosiderosis in rheumatic heart disease. Am J Roentgenol 73:351–365

Ferguson FC, Kobilak RE, Deitrick JE (1944) Varices of bronchial veins as source of hemoptysis in mitral stenosis. Am Heart J 28:445–456

Fleischner FG, Reiner L (1954) Linear x-ray shadows in acquired pulmonary hemosiderosis and congestion. N Engl J Med 250:900–905

Fleming HA, Robinson CLN (1957) Pulmonary ossification with cardiac calcification in mitral valve disease. Br Heart J 19:532–538

Galloway RW, Epstein EJ, Coulshed N (1961) Pulmonary ossific nodules in mitral valve disease. Br Heart J 23:297–307

Hatle L, Angelsen B, Tromsdal A (1979) Noninvasive assessment of atrioventricular pressure half-time by Doppler ultrasound. Circulation 60:1096–1104

Henry WL, Morganroth J, Pearlman AS, Clark CE, Redwood DR, Itscoitz SB, Epstein SE (1976) Relation between echocardiographically determined left atrial size and atrial fibrillation. Circulation 53:273–279

Lane EJ, Whalen JP (1969) A new sign of left atrial enlargement. Posterior displacement of the left bronchial tree. Radiology 93:279–284

Martin RP, Rakowski H, Kleiman JH, Beaver W, London E, Popp RL (1979) Reliability and reproducibility of two dimensional echocardiographic measurement of the stenotic mitral valve orifice area. Am J Cardiol 43:560–568

Mullin EM Jr, Glancy DL, Higgs LM, Epstein SE, Morrow AG (1972) Current results of operation for mitral stenosis. Clinical and hemodynamic assessments in 124 consecutive patients treated by closed commissurotomy, open commissurotomy, or valve replacement. Circulation 46:298–308

Nichol PM, Gilbert BW, Kisslo JA (1977) Two-dimensional echocardiographic assessment of mitral stenosis. Circulation 55:120–128

Parker BM, Friedenberg MJ, Templeton AW, Burford TH (1965) Preoperative angiocardiographic diagnosis of left atrial thrombi in mitral stenosis. N Engl J Med 273:136–140

Reichek N, Shelburne JC, Perloff JK (1973) Clinical aspects of rheumatic valvular disease. Prog Cardiovasc Dis 15:491–535

Taylor HE, Strong GF (1955) Pulmonary hemosiderosis in mitral stenosis. Ann Intern Med 42:26–35

Wood P (1954) An appreciation of mitral stenosis. I. Clinical features. Br Med J 1:1051–1063

Wood P (1954) An appreciation of mitral stenosis. II. Investigations and results. Br Med J 1:1113–1124

Mitral Valve Dysfunction Secondary to Calcification of Mitral Anulus

D'Cruz IA, Cohen HC, Prabhu R, Bisla V, Glick G (1977) Clinical manifestations of mitral anulus calcification with emphasis on its echocardiographic features. Am Heart J 94:367–377

DePace NL, Rohrer AH, Kotler MN, Brezin JH, Parry WR (1981) Rapidly progressing, massive mitral anular calcification. Occurrence in a patient with chronic renal failure. Arch Intern Med 141:1663–1665

Hakki A, Iskandrian AS (1980) Obstruction to left ventricular inflow secondary to combined mitral anular calcification and idiopathic hypertrophic subaortic stenosis. Cathet Cardiovasc Diagn 6:191–196

Korn D, DeSanctis RW, Sell S (1962) Massive calcification of the mitral anulus. A clinicopathological study of fourteen cases. N Engl J Med 267:900–909

Osterberger LE, Goldstein S, Khaja F, Lakier JB (1981) Functional mitral stenosis in patients with massive mitral anular calcification. Circulation 64:472–476

Roberts WC, Waller BF (1981) Mitral valve "anular" calcium

forming a complete circle or "O" configuration: Clinical and necropsy observations. Am Heart J 101:619–621

Lutembacher's Syndrome

Espino-Vela J (1959) Malformaciones cardiovasculares congenitas. Instituto Nacional de cardiologia de Mexico, pp 125–134

Espino-Vela J (1959) Rheumatic heart disease associated with atrial septal defect: Clinical and pathological study of 12 cases of Lutembacher's syndrome. Am Heart J 57:185–202

Lutembacher R (1916) De la stenose mitrale avec communication interauriculaire. Arch Mal Coeur 9:237

Muller WH Jr, Littlefield JB, Beckwith JR (1966) Surgical treatment of Lutembacher's syndrome. J Thorac Cardiovasc Surg 51:66–70

Nadas AS, Alimurung MM (1953) Apical diastolic murmurs in congenital heart disease. The rarity of Lutembacher's syndrome. Am Heart J 43:691–706 Am Heart J 43:691–706

Steinbrunn W, Cohn KE, Seizer A (1970) Atrial septal defect associated with mitral stenosis. The Lutembacher syndrome revisited. Am J Med 48:295–302

Mitral Insufficiency

Abbasi AS, Allen MW, DeCristafaro D, Ungar I (1980) Detection and estimation of the degree of mitral regurgitation by range-gated pulsed Doppler echocardiography. Circulation 61:143–147

Braunwald E, Awe WC (1963) The syndrome of severe mitral regurgitation with normal left atrial pressure. Circulation 27:29–35

Braunwald E (1969) Mitral regurgitation: Physiologic, clinical, and surgical considerations. N Engl J Med 281:425–433

Burgess J, Clark R, Kamigaki M, Cohn K (1973) Echocardiographic findings in different types of mitral regurgitation. Circulation 48:97–106

Cohn LH (1978) Surgical treatment of valvular heart disease. Am J Surg 135:444–451

Dashkoff N, Karacuschansky M, Come PC, Fortuin NJ (1977) Echocardiographic features of mitral anulus calcification. Am Heart J 94:585–592

Fennell WH (1982) Afterload reduction in the therapy of heart failure. Tex Heart Inst J 9:61–69

Fowler NO, Van Der Bel-Kahn JM (1979) Indications for surgical replacement of the mitral valve with particular reference to common and uncommon causes of mitral regurgitation. Am J Cardiol 44:148–157

Hsu I, Kelser GA, Shefferman MM (1976) Pulmonary varix regression after mitral valve replacement. Am J Cardiol 37:928–932

Kay JH, Zubiate P, Mendez MA, Vanstrom N, Yokayama T (1978) Mitral valve repair for significant mitral insufficiency. Am Heart J 93:253–262

Miyatake K, Nimura Y, Sakakibara H, Kinoshita N, Okamoto M, Nagata S, Kawazoe K, Fujita T (1982) Localization and direction of mitral regurgitant flow in mitral orifices studied with combined use of ultrasonic pulsed Doppler technique and two-dimensional echocardiography. Br Heart J 48:449–458

Priest EA, Finlayson JK, Short DS (1962) The x-ray manifestations in the heart and lungs of mitral regurgitation. Prog Cardiovasc Dis 5:219–229

Roberts WC, Braunwald E, Morrow AG (1966) Mitral regurgitation secondary to ruptured chordae tendineae. Circulation 33:58–70

Salomon NW, Stinson EB, Griepp RB, Shumway NE (1977) Patient related risk factor as predictors of results following isolated mitral valve replacement. Ann Thorac Surg 24:519–530

Sandler S, Dodge HT, Hay RE, Rackley C (1963) Quantitation of valvular insufficiency in man by angiocardiography. Am Heart J 65:501–513

Schott OR, Kotler MN, Parry WR, Segal BL (1977) Mitral annular calcification. Clinical and echocardiographic correlations. Arch Intern Med 137:1143–1150

Schuler G, Peterson KL, Johnson A, Francis G, Dennish G, Utley J, Daily PO, Ashburn W, Ross J., Jr (1979) Temporal response of left ventricular performance in mitral valve surgery. Circulation 59:1218–1231

Selzer A, Katayama F (1972) Mitral regurgitation: Clinical patterns, pathophysiology and natural history. Medicine 51:337–366

Sorensen SG, O'Rourke RA, Chandhuri TK (1980) Noninvasive quantitation of valvular regurgitation by gated equilibrium radionuclide angiography. Circulation 62:1089–1098

Spencer FC (1979) Acquired heart disease. In: Schwartz SI, Shires GT, Spencer FC, Storer EH, (eds): Principles of surgery, 2nd edn. McGraw Hill, New York, p 813

Sweatman T, Selzer A, Kamagaki M, Cohn K (1972) Echocardiographic diagnosis of mitral regurgitation due to ruptured chordae tendineae. Circulation 46:580–586

Wann LS, Feigenbaum H, Weyman AE, Dillon JC (1978) Cross-sectional echocardiographic detection of rheumatic mitral regurgitation. Am J Cardiol 41:1258–1263

Wexler L, Silverman JF, DeBusk RF, Harrison DC (1971) Angiographic features of rheumatic and nonrheumatic mitral regurgitation. Circulation 44:1080–1086

Yoran C, Yellin EL, Becker RM, Gabbay S, Frater RWM, Sonnenblick EH (1979) Mechanism of reduction of mitral regurgitation with vasodilator therapy. Am J Cardiol 43:773–777

Mitral Valve Prolapse

Barlow JB, Pocock WA (1979) MItral valve prolapse, the specific billowing mitral leaflet syndrome, or an insignificant nonejection systolic click. Am Heart J 97:277–285

Boudoulas H, Reynolds JC, Mazzaferri E, Wooley CF (1980) Metabolic studies in mitral valve prolapse syndrome. Circulation 61:1200–1205

Brock RC (1952) The surgical and pathological anatomy of the mitral valve. Br Heart J 14:489–513

Cabin HS, Roberts WC (1981) Ebstein's anomaly of the tricuspid valve and prolapse of the mitral valve. Am Heart J 101:177–180

Chiechi MA, Lees WM, Thompson R (1956) Functional anatomy of the normal mitral valve. J Thorac Surg 32:378–398

Child JS, Cabeen WR Jr., Roberts NK (1978) Mitral valve prolapse complicated by ruptured chordae tendineae. West J Med 129:160–163

Coghlan HC, Phares P, Cowley M, Copley D, James TN (1979) Dysautonomia in mitral valve prolapse. Am J Med 67:236–244

Cohen MV, Shah PK, Spindola-Franco H (1979) Angiographic-echocardiographic correlation in mitral valve prolapse. Am Heart J 97:43–52

Corrigall D, Bolen J, Hancock EW, Popp RL (1977) Mitral valve prolapse and infective endocarditis. Am J Med 63:215–222

Crawford MH (1977) Mitral valve prolapse due to coronary artery disease. Am J Med 62:447–451

Darsee JR, Mikolich R, Nicoloff NB, Lesser LE (1979) Prevalence of mitral valve prolapse in presumably healthy young men. Circulation 59:619–622

DeMaria AN, Neumann A, Lee G, Mason DT (1977) Echocardiographic identification of the mitral valve prolapse syndrome. Am J Med 62:819–829

Gardin JM, Talano JV, Stephanides L, Fizzano J, Lesch M (1981) Systolic anterior motion in the absence of asymmetric septal hypertrophy. A buckling phenomenon of the chordae tendineae. Circulation 63:181–187

Gulotta SJ, Gulco L, Padmanabhan V, Miller S (1974) The syndrome of systolic click, murmur, and mitral valve prolapse—a cardiomyopathy? Circulation 49:717–728

Jaffe AS, Geltman EM, Rodey GE, Uitto J (1981) Mitral valve prolapse: A consistent manifestation of type IV Ehlers-Danlos syndrome. The pathogenetic role of the abnormal production of type III collagen. Circulation 64:121–125

Jeresaty RM (1975) Mitral valve prolapse-click syndrome in atrial septal defect (editorial). Chest 67:132–133

Kay JH, Krohn BG, Zubiate P, Hoffman RL (1979) Surgical correction of severe mitral prolapse without mitral insufficiency but with pronounced cardiac arrhythmias. J Thorac Cardiovasc Surg 78:259–268

Kiel EA, Frias JL, Victorica BE (1983) Cardiovascular manifestations in the Larsen syndrome. Pediatrics 71:942–946

King BD, Clark MA, Baba N, Kilman JW, Wooley CF (1982) "Myxomatous" mitral valves: Collagen dissolution as the primary defect. Circulation 66:288–296

Kostuk WJ, Boughner DR, Barnett HJM, Silver MD (1977) Strokes: A complication of mitral-leaflet prolapse? Lancet 2:313–316

Markiewicz W, Popp RL (1978) Effect of transducer placement on echocardiographic mitral valve motion. Am Heart J 96:555–556

Markiewicz W, Stoner J, London E, Hunt SA, Popp RL (1976) Mitral valve prolapse in one hundred presumably healthy young females. Circulation 53:464–473

Miller SW, Spindola-Franco H (1974) Systolic prolapse of the mitral valve. Contemp Surg 5:100–104

Pickering NJ, Brody JI, Barrett MJ (1981) Von Willebrand syndromes and mitral-valve prolapse. Linked mesenchymal dysplasias. N Engl J Med 305:131–134

Ranganathan N, Lam JHC, Wigle ED, Silver MD (1970) Morphology of the human mitral valve. Circulation 41:459–467

Ranganathan N, Silver MD, Robinson TI, Wilson JK (1976) Idiopathic prolapsed mitral leaflet syndrome: Angiographic-clinical correlations. Circulation 54:707–716

Rippe JM, Sloss LJ, Angoff G, Alpert JS (1979) Mitral valve prolapse in adults with congenital heart disease. Am Heart J 97:561–573

Sahn DJ, Wood J, Allen HD, Peoples W, Goldberg SJ (1977) Echocardiographic spectrum of mitral valve motion in children with and without mitral valve prolapse: The nature of false positive diagnosis. Am J Cardiol 39:422–431

Sanyal SK, Leung RKF, Tierney RC, Gilmartin R, Pitner S (1979) Mitral valve prolapse syndrome in children with Duchenne's progressive muscular dystrophy. Pediatrics 63:116–123

Schutte JE, Gaffney FA, Blend L, Blomqvist CG (1981) Distinctive anthropometric characteristics of women with mitral valve prolapse. Am J Med 71:533–538

Smith ER, Fraser DB, Purdy JW, Anderson RN (1977) Angiographic diagnosis of mitral valve prolapse: Correlation with echocardiography. Am J Cardiol 40:165–170

Somerville J, Kaku S, Saravally O (1978) Prolapsed mitral cusps in atrial septal defect. An erroneous radiological interpretation. Br Heart J 40:58–63

Spindola-Franco H, Björk L, Adams DF, Abrams HL (1980) Classification of the radiological morphology of the mitral valve. Differentiation between true and pseudoprolapse. Br Heart J 44:30–36

Spindola-Franco H, Björk L, Miller S (1974) Prolapse of the mitral valve: Description of two new angiocardiographic signs and an analysis of the mitral apparatus. Proceedings of the VII World Congress of Cardiology. Buenos Aires, Argentina. Sept. 1–7

Spindola-Franco H, Björk L, Miller S, Adams DF (1974) Prolapse of the mitral valve: Analysis of variations of the normal mitral valve apparatus and a description of two new angiographic signs. Circulation 50(suppl 3):207

Spindola-Franco H, Shah PK, Cohen MV (1978) Mitral valve prolapse: An angiographic and echocardiographic study. International Congress Series no. 470. In: Hayase S, Murao S (eds). Proceedings of the VIII World Congress of Cardiology, Tokyo. Sept. 17–23. Exerpta Medica, Amsterdam.

Tempo CP-Bon, Ronan JA Jr, de Leon AC Jr, Twiss HL (1975) Radiographic appearance of the thorax in systolic click-late systolic murmur syndrome. Am J Cardiol 36:27–31

Tutassaura H, Gerein AN, Miyagishima RT (1976) Mucoid degeneration of the mitral valve. Clinical review, surgical management, and results. Am J Surg 132:276–281

Udoshi MB, Shah A, Fisher VJ, Dolgin M (1981) Incidence of mitral valve prolapse in subjects with thoracic skeletal abnormalities—A prospective study. Am Heart J 97:303–311

Walsh PN, Kansu TA, Corbett JJ, Savino PJ, Goldburgh WP, Schatz NJ (1981) Platelets, thromboembolism and mitral valve prolapse. Circulation 63:552–559

Weiss AN, Mimbs JW, Ludbrook PA, Sobel BE (1975) Echocardiographic detection of mitral valve prolapse. Exclusion of false positive diagnosis and determination of inheritance. Circulation 52:1091–1096

Winkle RA, Lopes MG, Fitzgerald JW, Goodman DJ, Schroeder JS, Harrison DC (1975) Arrhythmias in patients with mitral valve prolapse. Circulation 52:73–81

Winkle RA, Lopes MG, Popp RL, Hancock EW (1976) Life-threatening arrhythmias in the mitral valve prolapse syndrome. Am J Med 60:961–967

Winters SJ, Schreiner B, Griggs RC, Rowley P, Nanda NC (1976) Familial mitral valve prolapse and myotonic dystrophy. Ann Intern Med 85:19–22

Infective Endocarditis

Arnett EN, Roberts WC (1976) Valve ring abscess in active infective endocarditis. Frequency, location, and clues to clinical diagnosis from the study of 95 necropsy patients. Circulation 54:140–145

Berger M, Gallerstein PE, Benhuri P, Balla R, Goldberg E (1981) Evaluation of aortic valve endocarditis by two-dimensional echocardiography. Chest 80:61–67

Buchbinder NA, Roberts WC (1972) Left-sided valvular active infective endocarditis. A study of forty-five necropsy patients. Am J Med 53:20–35

Child JS, Skorton DJ, Taylor RD, Krivokapich J, Abbasi A, Wong M, Shah PD (1979) M mode and cross-sectional echocardiographic features of flail posterior mitral leaflets. Am J Cardiol 44:1383–1390

Come PC, Isaacs RE, Riley MF (1982) Diagnostic accuracy of M-mode echocardiography in active infective endocarditis and prognostic implications of ultrasound-detectable vegetations. Am Heart J 103:839–847

Hubbell G, Cheitlin MD, Rapaport G (1981) Presentation, management, and follow-up evaluation of infective endocarditis in drug addicts. Am Heart J 102:85–94

Lerner PI, Weinstein L (1966) Infective endocarditis in the antibiotic era. N Engl J Med 274:199–206, 259–266, 388–393

Melvin ET, Berger M, Lutzker LG, Goldberg E, Mildvan D (1981) Noninvasive methods for detection of valve vegetations in infective endocarditis. Am J Cardiol 47:271–278

Meyer JF, Frank MJ, Goldberg S, Cheng TO (1977) Systolic mitral flutter, an echocardiographic clue to the diagnosis of ruptured chordae tendineae. Am Heart J 94:3–8

Mildvan D, Goldberg E, Berger M, Altchek MR, Lukban SB (1977) Diagnosis and successful management of septal myocardial abscess: A complication of bacterial endocarditis. Case report. Am J Med Sci 274:311–316

Mintz GS, Kotler MN, Segal BL, Parry WR (1979) Comparison of two-dimensional and m-mode echocardiography in the evaluation of patients with infective endocarditis. Am J Cardiol 43:738–744

Nishimura T, Takahashi M, Osakada G, Yasunaga K, Kawai C, Kotoura H, Konishi Y, Tatsuta N (1978) Two-dimensional echocardiographic findings in ruptured chordae tendineae of the mitral valve. J Cardiogr 8:589

Nolan CM, Kane JJ, Grunow WA (1981) Infective endocarditis and mitral prolapse. A comparison with other types of endocarditis. Arch Intern Med 141:447–450

Prager RL, Maples MD, Hammon JW Jr, Friesinger GC, Bender HW Jr (1981) Early operative intervention in aortic bacterial endocarditis. Ann Thorac Surg 32:347–350

Roberts WC, Buchbinder NA (1972) Right-sided valvular infective endocarditis. A clinicopathologic study of 12 necropsy patients. Am J Med 53:7–19

Roberts WC, Buchbinder NA (1977) Healed left-sided infective endocarditis: A clinicopathologic study of 59 patients. Am J Cardiol 40:876–888

Sheikh MU, Covarrubias EA, Ali N, Lee WR, Sheikh NM, Roberts WC (1981) M-mode echocardiographic observations during and after healing of active bacterial endocarditis limited to the mitral valve. Am Heart J 101:37–45

Sheikh MU, Covarrubias EA, Ali N, Sheikh NM, Lee WR, Roberts WC (1981) M-mode echocardiographic observations in active bacterial endocarditis limited to the aortic valve. Am Heart J 101:66–75

Stafford A, Wann LS, Dillon JC, Weyman AE, Feigenbaum H (1979) Serial echocardiographic appearance of healing bacterial vegetations. Am J Cardiol 44:754–760

Sze KC, Nanda NC, Gramiak R (1978) Systolic flutter of the mitral valve. Am Heart J 96:157–162

Thell R, Martin FH, Edwards JE (1975) Bacterial endocarditis in subjects 60 years of age and older. Circulation 51:174–182

Todd EP, Hubbard SG, Teok JV, Utley JR, Jones MR, Vine DL, Cole JS (1980) Repair of mycotic aneurysms of the aorta involving the aortic valve. Ann Thorac Surg 30:160–163

Aortic Arteritis Syndromes

Austen WG, Blennerhassett JB (1965) Giant-cell aortitis causing an aneurysm of the ascending aorta and aortic regurgitation. N Engl J Med 272:80–83

Honig HS, Weintraub AM, Gomes MN, Hufnagel CA, Roberts WC (1977) Severe aortic regurgitation secondary to idiopathic aortitis. Am J Med 63:623–633

Ishikawa K (1978) Natural history and classification of occlusive thromboaortopathy (Takayasu's disease). Circulation 57:27–35

Klein RG, Hunder GG, Stanson AW, Sheps SG (1975) Large artery involvement in giant cell (temporal) arteritis. Ann Intern Med 83:806–812

Lande A, LaPorta A (1976) Takayasu arteritis. An arteriographic-pathological correlation. Arch Pathol Lab Med 100:437–440

Lupi-Herrera E, Sanchez-Torres G, Marcushamer J, Mispireta J, Horwitz S, Vela JE (1977) Takaysau's arteritis. Clinical study of 107 cases. Am Heart J 93:94–103

Paulley JW, Hughes JP (1960) Giant-cell arteritis, or arteritis of the aged. Br Med J 2:1562–1567

Scully RE, Mark EJ, McNeely BU (1981) Case 51. Takayasu's arteritis involving axillary arteries. N Engl J Med 25:1519–1524

Ankylosing Spondylitis

Bulkley BH, Roberts WC (1973) Ankylosing spondylitis and aortic regurgitation. Description of the characteristic cardiovascular lesion from study of eighty necropsy patients. Circulation 48:1014–1027

Davidson P, Baggenstoss AH, Slocumb CH, Daugherty GW (1963) Cardiac and aortic lesions in rheumatoid spondylitis. Proc Staff Meet Mayo Clin 38:427–435

Lande A, Berkman GM (1976) Aortitis. Pathologic, clinical and arteriographic review. Radiol Clin North Am 14:219–240

Newman JH, Cooney LM (1980) Cardiac abnormalities associated with rheumatoid arthritis: Aortic insufficiency requiring valve replacement. J Rheumatol 7:375–378

Rheumatoid Arthritis, Reiter Syndrome and Relapsing Polychondritis

Csonka W, Litchfield W, Oates JK, Wilcox RR (1961) Cardiac lesions in Reiter's disease. Br Med J 1:243–247

Paloheimo JA (1967) Obstructive arteritis of Takayasu's type. Acta Med Scand suppl 468, pp 7–45

Paulus HE, Pearson CM, Pitts W Jr (1972) Aortic insufficiency in five patients with Reiter's syndrome. A detailed clinical and pathologic study. Am J Med 53:464–472

Pearson CM, Kroening R, Verity MA, Getzen HJ (1967) Aortic insufficiency and aortic aneurysm in relapsing polychondritis. Trans Assoc Am Physicians 80:71–90

Roth LM, Kissane JM (1964) Panaortitis and aortic valvulitis in progressive systemic sclerosis (scleroderma). Am J Clin Pathol 41:287–296

Zvaifler NJ, Weintraub AM (1963) Aortitis and aortic insufficiency in the chronic rheumatic disorders—A reappraisal. Arthritis Rheum 6:241–245

Syphilitic Aortitis

Cornell HS (1973) The roentgenographic diagnosis of the disease of the thoracic aorta. Thomas, Springfield, Ill

Heggtveit HA (1964) Syphilitic aortitis. A clinicopathologic autopsy study of 100 cases, 1950 to 1960. Circulation 29:346–355

Merten CW, Finby N, Steinberg I (1956) The antemortem diagnosis of syphilitic aneurysm of the aortic sinuses. Report of nine cases. Am J Med 20:345–360

Aortic Insufficiency Secondary To Systemic Hypertension

Waller BF, Roberts WC (1982) Severe aortic regurgitation secondary to systemic hypertension (without aortic dissection). Cardiovasc Rev Rep 3:1504–1518

Waller BF, Zoltick JM, Rosen JH, Katz NM, Gomes MN, Fletcher RD, Wallace RB, Roberts WC (1982) Severe aortic regurgitation from systemic hypertension (without aortic dissection) requiring aortic valve replacement: Analysis of 4 patients. Am J Cardiol 49:473–477

6 Cardiomyopathies

Cardiomyopathy is the term used to describe a heterogenous spectrum of disorders of the myocardium. If the cause can be identified, it may be found that it involves the heart exclusively, or it may be part of a systemic disorder. In many instances no etiology can be determined. These comprise the idiopathic group.

In a report of the WHO-ISFC task force the idiopathic cardiomyopathies are divided into three groups:

1) Dilated, also called congestive.

2) Hypertrophic, formerly called idiopathic hypertrophic cardiomyopathy, idiopathic hypertrophic subaortic stenosis, asymmetrical septal hypertrophy, and so on.

3) Restrictive, also known as obliterative, including endomyocardial fibrosis and Löffler's endocarditis.

The authors have added a fourth group, arrhythmogenic right ventricular dysplasia, which has recently been described by Fontaine et al., and Uhl anomaly, which mainly affects the right ventricle.

Fowler, Giles and McGuire have each classified the secondary cardiomyopathies according to their etiology. Table 6–1 is a compilation of their data as well as information from other sources. Most secondary cardiomyopathies are of the dilated type. Even those initially presenting as hypertrophic may deteriorate into a dilated form.

Congestive Cardiomyopathy

Dilated or congestive cardiomyopathy is characterized by impaired ventricular performance. Right and left ventricular volumes are increased, and ejection fractions are reduced. Increased ventricular filling pressure is reflected as high right atrial, left atrial, and pulmonary venous pressure. Mitral insufficiency may occur late in the disorder because of dilatation of the mitral anulus or papillary muscle dysfunction. Mural thrombi may occur, which may or may not produce embolic complications. This form of cardio-

myopathy may be due to many of the causes listed in table 6–1. Some are reversible or preventable. The diagnosis of idiopathic dilated cardiomyopathy is one of exclusion.

Clinical Features

The symptoms of congestive cardiomyopathy are those of left ventricular failure (e.g., fatigue, dyspnea on exertion, orthopnea), which may progress slowly or rapidly.

On physical examination a precordial prominence, a diffuse cardiac impulse and often a gallop rhythm are present. P_2 may be accentuated. A murmur of mitral insufficiency may be detected. Jugular venous distention and hepatomegaly would indicate systemic venous hypertension. Pulses and peripheral perfusion may be decreased. Edema may be present. The electrocardiogram commonly shows sinus tachycardia and ST-T wave changes. Arrhythmias are also quite common and left or right bundle-branch block may be noted. Abnormal Q waves may be observed, even without infarction.

Echocardiography

The echocardiogram shows dilatation and decreased contractions of the left ventricle (LV) (Fig. 6–1). The septum and LV wall may be normal, increased, or decreased in thickness. The left atrium (LA) is usually dilated as well. The motion of the mitral valve may reflect the high diastolic pressure (Fig. 6–2). Right ventricular (RV) and right atrial (RA) enlargement occur late. Pericardial effusion may be present (Fig. 6–3). Mural thrombi may be seen on 2-D echocardiography (Fig. 6–4). Major abnormalities of the valves and anomalous origin of the left coronary artery from the pulmonary artery are excluded by echocardiography. Doppler echocardiography aids in recognition of mitral insufficiency or tricuspid insufficiency due to ventricular dilatation, or pulmonary insufficiency secondary to pulmonary hypertension. Some centers have also applied

Table 6–1. Classification of Cardiomyopathies

I. Idiopathic cardiomyopathies

  A. Dilated

  B. Hypertrophic

  C. Restrictive

  D. Arrhythmogenic right ventricular dysplasia; Uhl anomaly

II. Secondary cardiomyopathies (associated with known systemic disease)

  A. Ischemic

  B. Hypertensive

  C. Valvular cardiomyopathies

  D. Infective (e.g., viral, bacterial, fungal, rickettsial, protozoal)

    1. Viral
      Coxsackie virus infection
      Echovirus infection
      Adenovirus infection
      Influenza
      Varicella
      Poliomyelitis
      Mumps
      Rabies
      Hepatitis
      Epstein-Barr virus infection
      Rubella
      Rubeola
      Cytomegalovirus infection
      Arbovirus infection
      Variola
      Vaccinia
      Yellow Fever
      Herpes simplex infection
      Respiratory Syncytial virus infection
      Mycoplasma pneumoniae infection
      Psittacosis

    2. Bacterial
      Staphylococcal infection
      Streptococcal infection
      Meningococcal infection
      Tuberculosis
      Salmonellal infection
      Diphtheria
      Actinomycosis
      Brucellosis
      Clostridial infection
      Syphilis
      Leptospirosis (Weil's disease)
      Relapsing fever
      Lyme disease (*I. dammini spirochetosis*)

    3. Fungal
      Aspergillosis
      Blastomycosis
      Cryptococcosis
      Candidiasis
      Coccidioidomycosis
      Histoplasmosis

    4. Rickettsial
      Coxiella infection (Q fever)
      Scrub typhus
      Rocky mountain spotted fever

    5. Protozoal
      Trypanosomiasis (Chagas' disease)
      Malaria
      Toxoplasmosis
      Amebic infections

    6. Metazoal
      Schistosomiasis
      Fluke disease
      Trichinosis
      Filariasis
      Cysticercosis
      Echinococcus disease (Hydatid cyst)
      Visceral larva migrans

    7. Probably infective (Whipple disease)

  E. Metabolic

    1. Endocrine
      Hyperthyroidism
      Hypothyroidism
      Hypoparathyroidism
      Hyperparathyroidism
      Acromegaly
      Diabetes mellitus
      Cushing Syndrome
      Pheochromocytoma
      Nesidioblastosis

    2. Electrolyte disturbance
      Potassium
      Phosphate
      Magnesium
      Multiple electrolyte imbalance (e.g., uremia)

    3. Nutritional
      Beriberi (thiamine)
      Pellagra
      Scurvy
      Hypervitaminosis D
      Kwashiorkor
      Starvation

    4. Inborn errors of metabolism
      Glycogen storage disease (Pompe disease)
      Hurler syndrome
      Refsum syndrome
      Niemann-Pick disease
      Hand-Schüller-Christian disease
      Fabry disease
      Morquio-Ullrich syndrome
      Sickle cell disease
      Gaucher disease
      Carnitine deficiency
      Mitochondrial-lipid deposition cardiomyopathies

  F. Immunologic
    1. Postvaccinial
    2. Serum sickness
    3. Urticaria
    4. Transplant rejection
    5. Giant cell myocarditis
    6. Acute rheumatic fever

  G. Toxic
    1. Alcohol
    2. Cobalt
    3. Cadmium
    4. Doxorubicin
    5. Cyclophosphamide
    6. Bleomycin
    7. Anesthetic gases
    8. Antimony
    9. Emetine
    10. Isoprenaline
    11. Carbon monoxide
    12. Lead
    13. Chloroquine
    14. Lithium
    15. Hydrocarbons
    16. Phosphorus
    17. Mercury
    18. Reserpine
    19. Corticosteroids
    20. Paracetamol

  H. Connective Tissue Disorders
    1. Systemic lupus erythematosus
    2. Polyarteritis nodosa
    3. Rheumatoid arthritis
    4. Scleroderma, dermatomyositis
    5. Polymyositis
    6. Acute rheumatic fever

  I. Infiltrative
    1. Amyloidosis
      Immunocytic dyscrasia
      Idiopathic
    2. Carcinomatosis with cardiomyopathy
    3. Hemochromatosis
    4. Glycogen storage disease
    5. Sarcoidosis

  J. Associated with generalized neuromuscular disease
    1. Progressive muscular dystrophy
    2. Myotonic dystrophy
    3. Friedreich ataxia

Table 6–1 (*Continued*)

K. Hematologic disorders
  1. Sickle cell disease
  2. Polycythemia vera
  3. Thrombotic thrombocyto-
     penic purpura
  4. Leukemia

L. Hypersensitivity
  1. Methyldopa
  2. Penicillin
  3. Sulfonamide
  4. Tetracycline
  5. Phenindione

6. Phenylbutazone
7. Antituberculous drugs
   (paraaminosalicylic acid,
   streptomycin)

M. Neoplastic
  1. Carcinomatosis with car-
     diomyopathy
  2. Leiomyofibroma
  3. Lymphoma
  4. Myxoma
  5. Rhabdomyoma, rhabdomyo-
     sarcoma

N. Physical agents
  1. Heat stroke
  2. Hypothermia
  3. Radiation

O. Miscellaneous
  1. Postpartum cardiomyopathy
  2. Insect sting
  3. Snake bite
  4. Obesity
  5. Anorexia nervosa
  6. Endocardial fibroelastosis

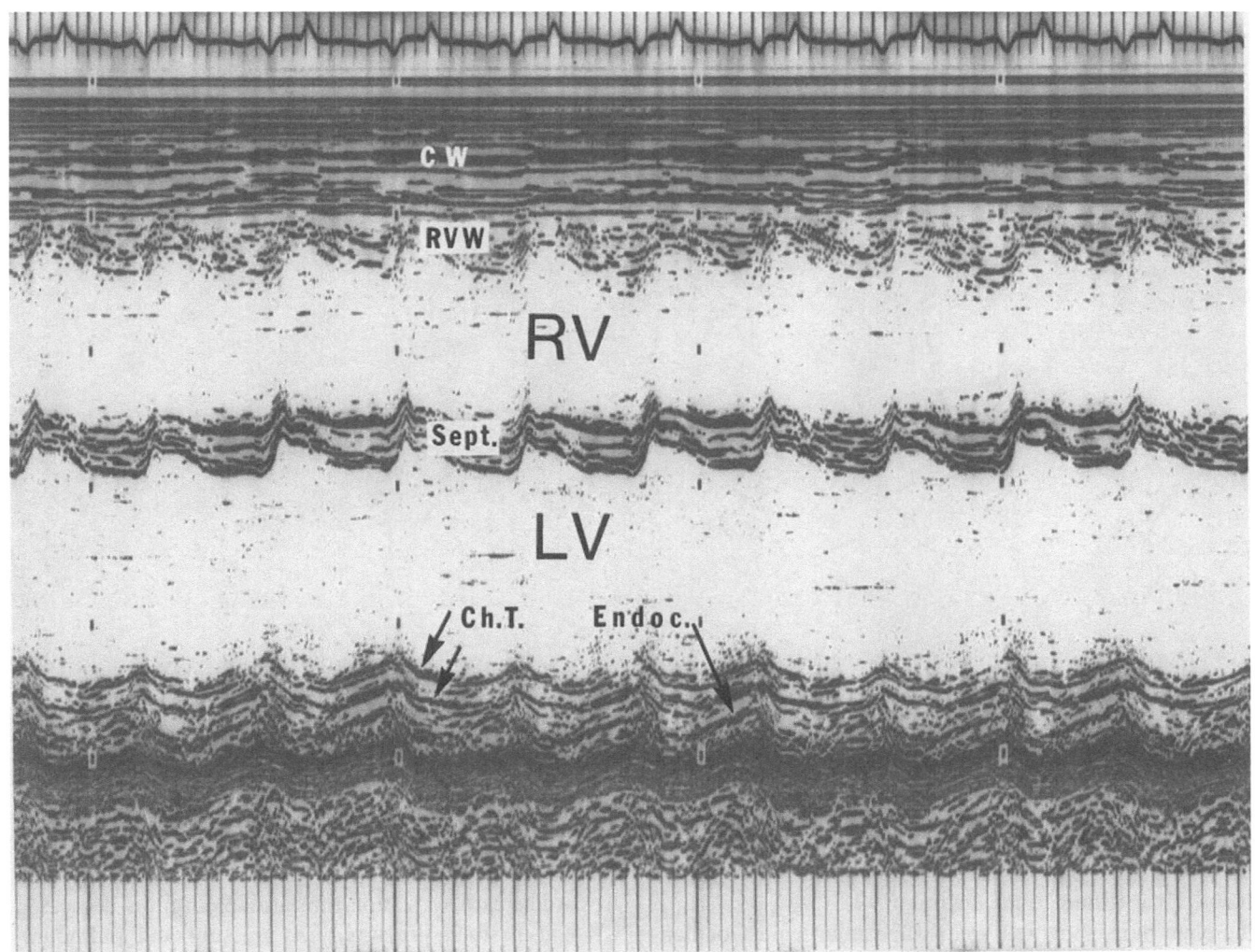

Fig. 6–1. *Dilated cardiomyopathy. M-mode echocardiogram in an infant with severe congestive heart failure.* The left ventricle contracts poorly while the right ventricle is dilated. The left ventricular wall, septum and right ventricular free wall are of normal thickness. *LV* = left ventricle; *RV* = right ventricle; *CW* = chest wall; *RVW* = right ventricular free wall; *Sept.* = septum; *Ch.T.* = chordae tendineae; *Endoc.* = endocardium;

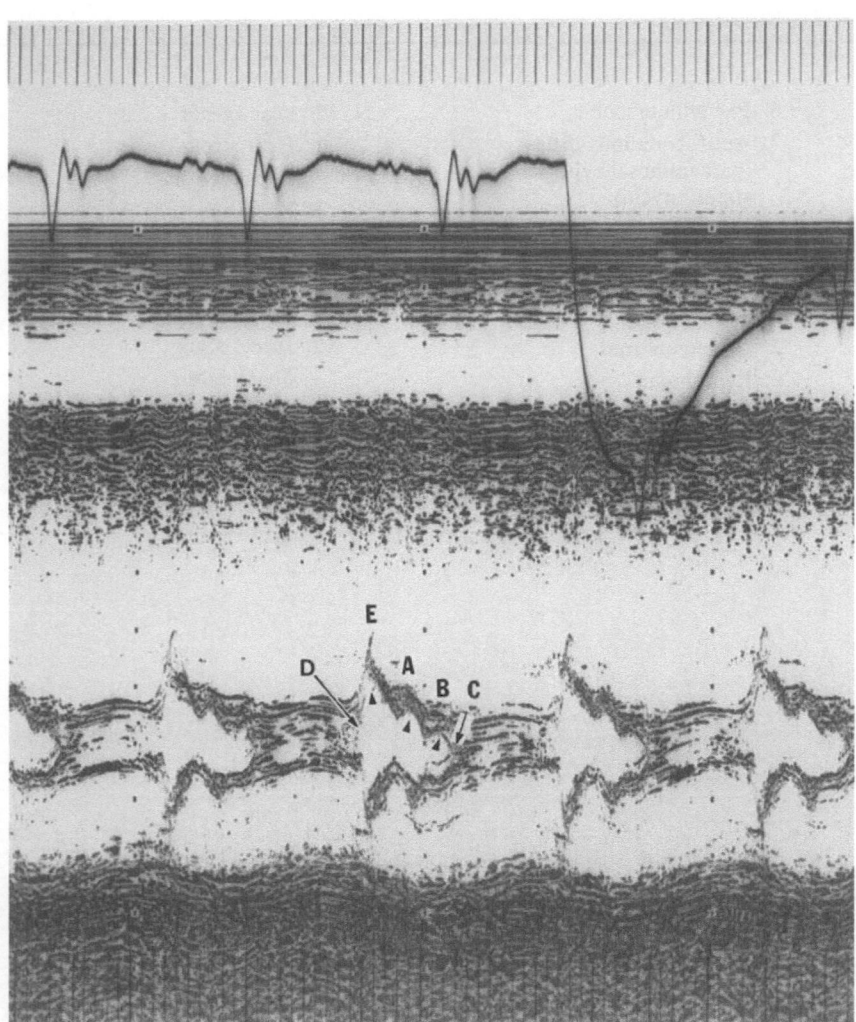

Fig. 6–2. *Dilated cardiomyopathy. M-mode echocardiogram.* The mitral valve opening is restricted and closure is delayed. D = opening of mitral valve; E = peak of mitral valve opening motion; F = approximate end of the rapid filling phase of the left ventricle (not labeled); A = atrial contraction; B = onset of ventricular contraction; C = mitral closure. (Normally B and C are superimposed, and no "bump" is present at B).

Doppler to the measurement of cardiac output in order to study the course of the disease or to evaluate the effect of medical treatment.

Radiological (Plain Film) Features

The plain films show left ventricular enlargement or non-specific cardiomegaly (Figs. 6–5, 6–6). Pulmonary venous hypertension may or may not be evident. Pulmonary edema, pleural effusion or both are usually late findings. The differential diagnosis of this constellation of findings includes ischemic cardiomyopathy, primary and secondary congestive cardiomyopathy and pericardial effusion. Pericardial effusion is easily ruled out by echocardiography.

Hemodynamics

At cardiac catheterization the cardiac output is decreased. LV end-diastolic pressure, LA pressure and pulmonary venous wedge pressure are elevated. In severe cases the pulmonary artery pressure is also elevated.

Contrast Studies

Ventriculography shows a dilated left ventricle with global

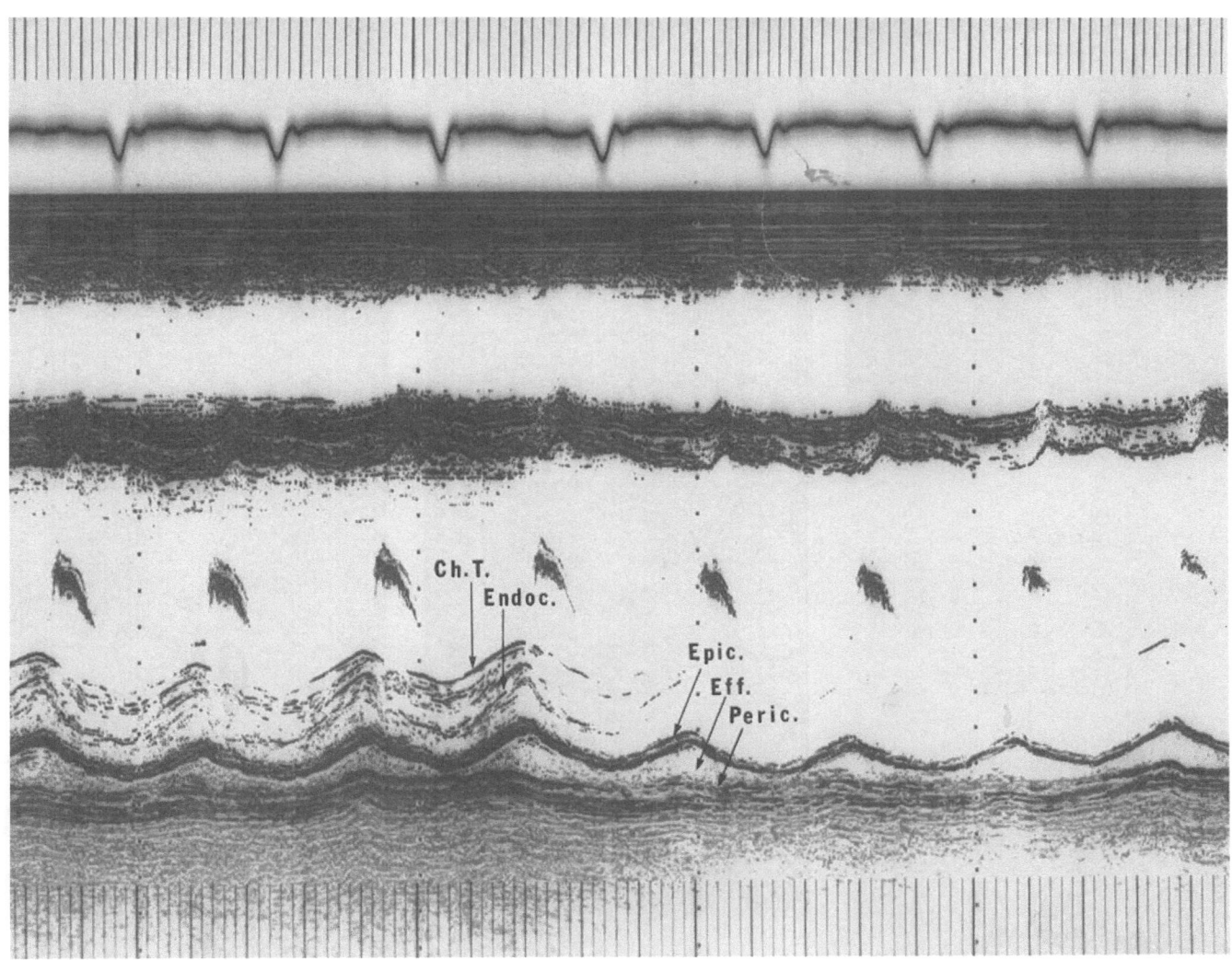

Fig. 6–3. *Dilated cardiomyopathy. M-mode echocardiogram in an adult.* The diameters of the ventricles are increased, and left ventricular contractions are reduced. On reduction of gain a poste-rior pericardial effusion becomes evident. *Ch.T.* = chordae tendineae; *Endoc.* = endocardium; *Epic.* = epicardium; *Eff.* = effusion; *Peric.* = pericardium.

hypokinesis (Fig 6–7). End-systolic and end-diastolic volumes are increased while ejection fraction and stroke volume are diminished. Mitral insufficiency may be present. Coronary arteriography shows normal but dilated coronary arteries (Fig. 6–8). In contrast, with ischemic cardiomyopathy the coronary arteries are stenosed or occluded and the LV shows focal or segmental wall motion abnormalities. In late stages ischemic hearts also show global hypokinesis.

Treatment

Medical treatment for idiopathic dilated cardiomyopathy

includes digitalis, diuretics, afterload reducers and antiarrhythmic agents. Some centers are evaluating the use of antiinflammatory agents monitored by serial ventriculography and heart biopsy in patients found to have myocarditis on initial biopsy. Heart transplantation constitutes a radical treatment that is carried out in a few centers.

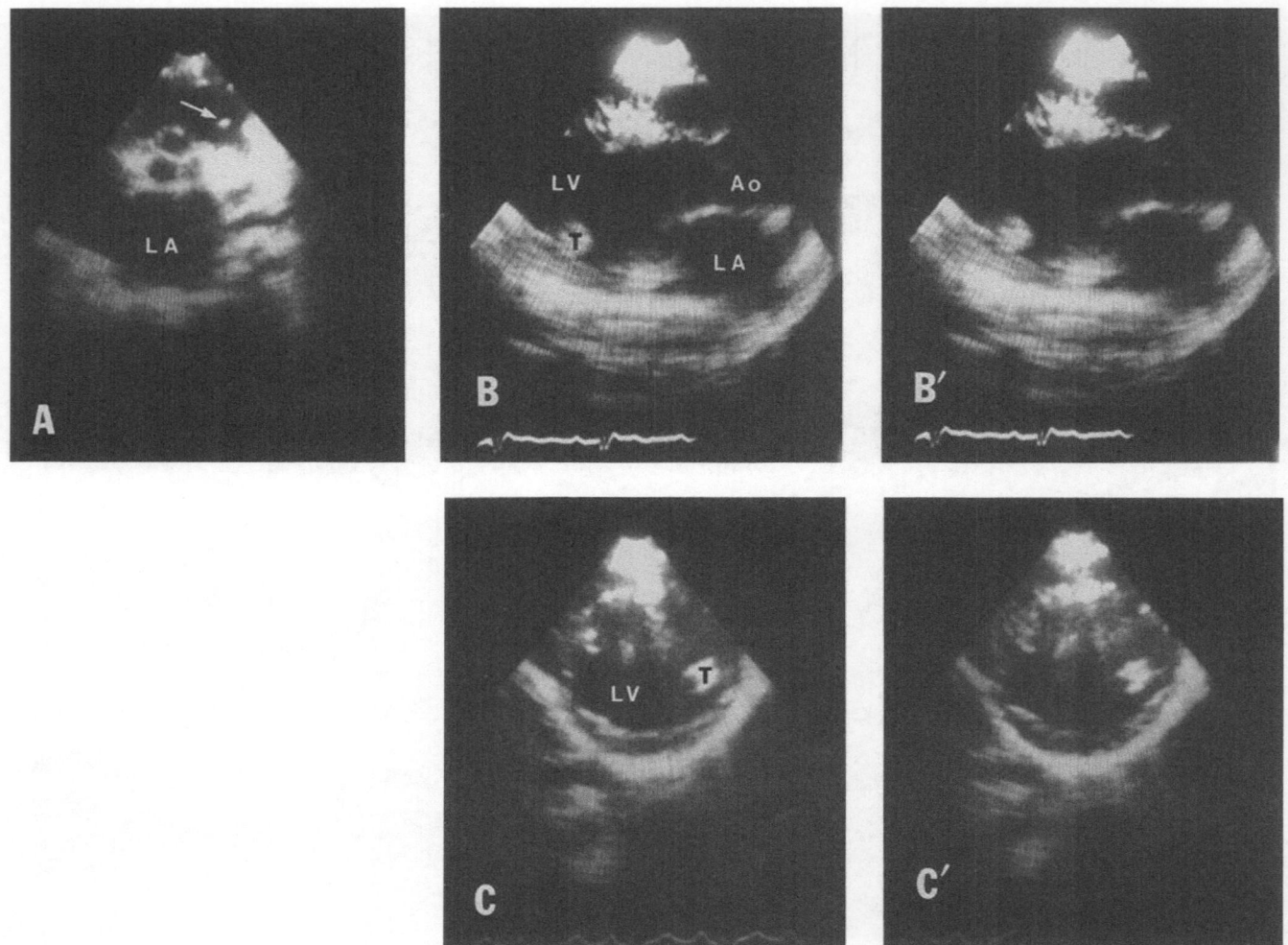

Fig. 6–4. *Two-dimensional echocardiography in an adolescent male with dilated cardiomyopathy and a mural thrombus.* In **A**, a short axis view at the level of the aortic valve (identified by a "Mercedes Benz sign"), the left atrium (*LA*) is dilated. The pulmonary valve is indicated by an arrow. **B** A long axis view shows the left ventricle (*LV*) and left atrium (*LA*) to be dilated. A thrombus (*T*) is identified in the area of the posterior papillary muscle. **B'** is the same view without labels. In **C** a short axis view of the left ventricle (*LV*) below the papillary muscles, the thrombus (*T*) is again demonstrated. The inner curved line posteriorly represents endocardium, while the gray crescent outside the endocardium is the myocardium, and the bright outer semicircle is the pericardium. The left ventricular free wall is not thickened. **C'** is the same view without labels. *Ao* = aorta.

Hypertrophic Cardiomyopathy

Hypertrophic cardiomyopathy (HCM) is also known as idiopathic hypertrophic subaortic stenosis (IHSS), obstructive cardiomyopathy, and asymmetrical septal hypertrophy (ASH). HCM is characterized by disproportionate hypertrophy of the ventricular septum in the region forming the outflow tract of the LV. This abnormality may cause LV outflow tract obstruction and mitral regurgitation. The cause of hypertrophic cardiomyopathy is not known, but it may be a disorder of the effects of or production of catecholamines or anomalies of neural crest tissue. It is usually genetically transmitted as an autosomal-dominant trait. Although HLA-A and HLA-B have not been found to correlate with inheritance of HCM, one group in Japan has discovered an association of a HLA-DR locus with HCM. Microscopical examinations have demonstrated a disordered myocardial architecture (hypertrophied, maloriented cells with bizarre shapes and disarray of myofibrils and myofilaments).

Hypertrophic cardiomyopathy has been described in association with congenital cardiac defects (endocardial cushion defects, pulmonic stenosis, postpulmonary artery banding, discrete subaortic stenosis) or acquired heart disease (aortic valvular disease, coronary artery disease) and anomalies of neural crest tissue (pheochromocytoma, tuberous sclerosis, neurofibromatosis). Cardiomyopathic lentiginosis or Leopard syndrome (sensorineural deafness, genital hypoplasia and psychic and somatic infantilism) is a less well known associated neuroectodermal disorder. Abnormali-

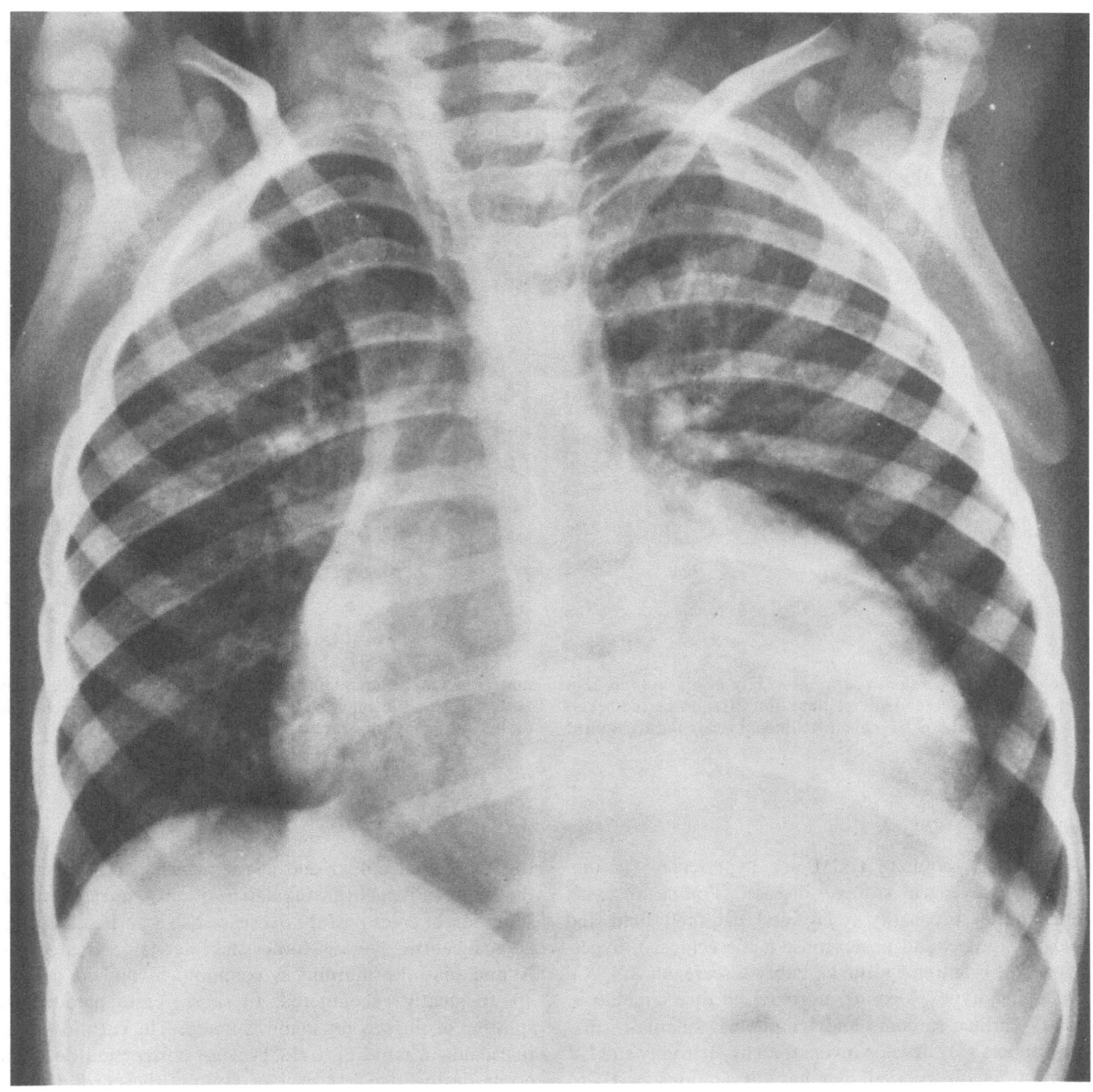

Fig. 6–5. *Dilated cardiomyopathy. Frontal-plane chest roentgenogram in a 2-year-old boy.* This view demonstrates generalized cardiomegaly with the left ventricle predominating. Observe pulmonary vascular redistribution, bilateral perivascular haze and mild blunting of the left costophrenic angle, consistent with moderate pulmonary venous hypertension.

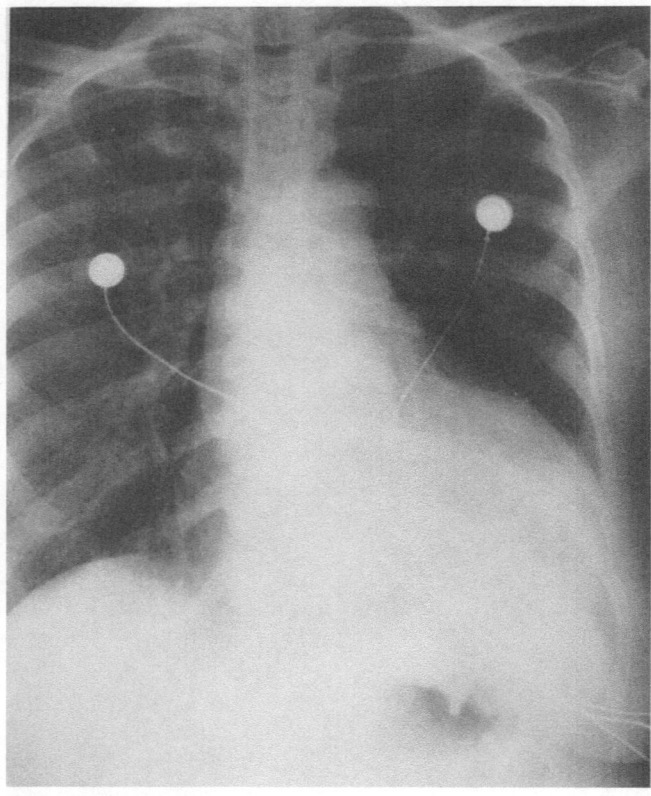

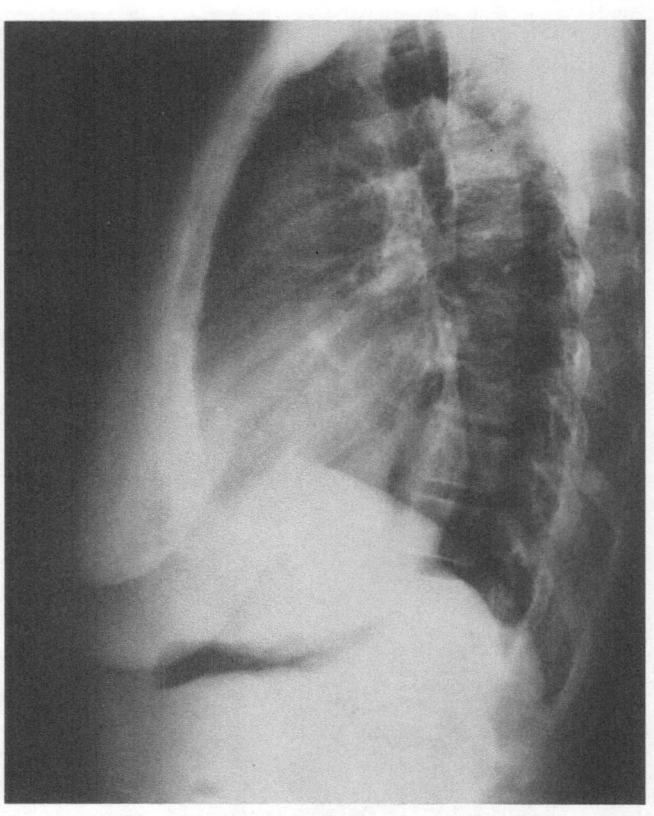

A   B

Fig. 6–6. *Dilated cardiomyopathy in a 52-year-old woman.* The frontal plane film (**A**) and lateral plane film (**B**) show cardiomegaly with left ventricular enlargement. Pulmonary vasculature is unre-markable. On the lateral film the left ventricle projects excessively posteriorly to the inferior vena cava, while the gastric bubble outlines the diaphragmatic wall of the left ventricle.

ties that may simulate HCM are hypertensive cardio-myopathy, glycogen storage disease (Pompe disease), mitochondrial myopathy (congenital cataract, lipid and glycogen storage, and postexercise lactic acidosis), hyperthyroidism, Friedreich's ataxia, Fabry disease, 46 XX, XY Turner phenotype (Noonan syndrome), cardiac sarcoidosis, primary cardiac sarcoma and lymphoma. Infants of diabetic mothers may develop myocardial hypertrophy and LV outflow tract obstruction that has the features of HCM but resolves during the first year of life. Infants with hyperinsulinemia due to nesidioblastosis have the same clinical features as do infants of diabetic mothers, including thickening of the ventricular septum. In infants of diabetic mothers, these features resolve gradually after birth, whereas in infants with nesidioblastosis they do not.

Clinical Features

The natural history of HCM is variable. It is usually characterized by a relatively benign course and slow progression; however, premature death is not uncommon. Such deaths are usually sudden, but they may occur in the setting of chronic, progressive congestive heart failure.

The usual symptoms are fatigue, dizziness, dyspnea, angina and syncope. On physical examination a double precordial impulse is noted. A systolic murmur heard along the left sternal border and at the apex is accentuated by the Valsalva maneuver, inhalation of amyl nitrate and assumption of erect posture. Absence of an aortic click suggests subaortic stenosis rather than aortic valve stenosis. A mid diastolic murmur is common. S_3 and S_4 gallops are frequently encountered. In severe cases paradoxical splitting of the second sound is noted. The carotid pulsations show a rapid upstroke because obstruction does not occur during the first part of systole, the carotid pulse contour has a rapid early peak followed by a notch (spike and dome configuration) characteristic of obstructive HCM. This contour is different from the slowly rising upstroke seen in patients with fixed subvalvular or valvular stenosis. The electrocardiogram shows LA hypertrophy, LV hypertrophy, LV strain, ST-segment and T-wave abnormalities and deep left-sided Q waves (septal hypertrophy).

Echocardiography (Figs. 6–9 to 6–15)

The most frequent and characteristic echocardiographic finding in HCM is a disproportionately thickened ventricular septum (Figs. 6–9, 6–10, 6–12, 6–13). In some cases with obstruction and in many cases without obstruction (concentric form) the LV free wall is also thickened (Fig. 6–12). Because of the variability among cases, the ratio of septum to wall thickness is not a diagnostic marker

Fig. 6–7. *Dilated cardiomyopathy (endocardial fibroelastosis)* in a 2-month-old male infant. Levophase of a pulmonary angiogram. **A** Ventricular diastole; **B** ventricular systole. Virtually no change is observed in ventricular size or in opacification whereas the change in the size of the left atrium is obvious. The left atrium refills with contrast material during ventricular systole (mitral insufficiency). The coronary arteries were found to be normal, thus excluding anomalous origin of the left coronary artery, which produces similar clinical and ventriculographic findings.

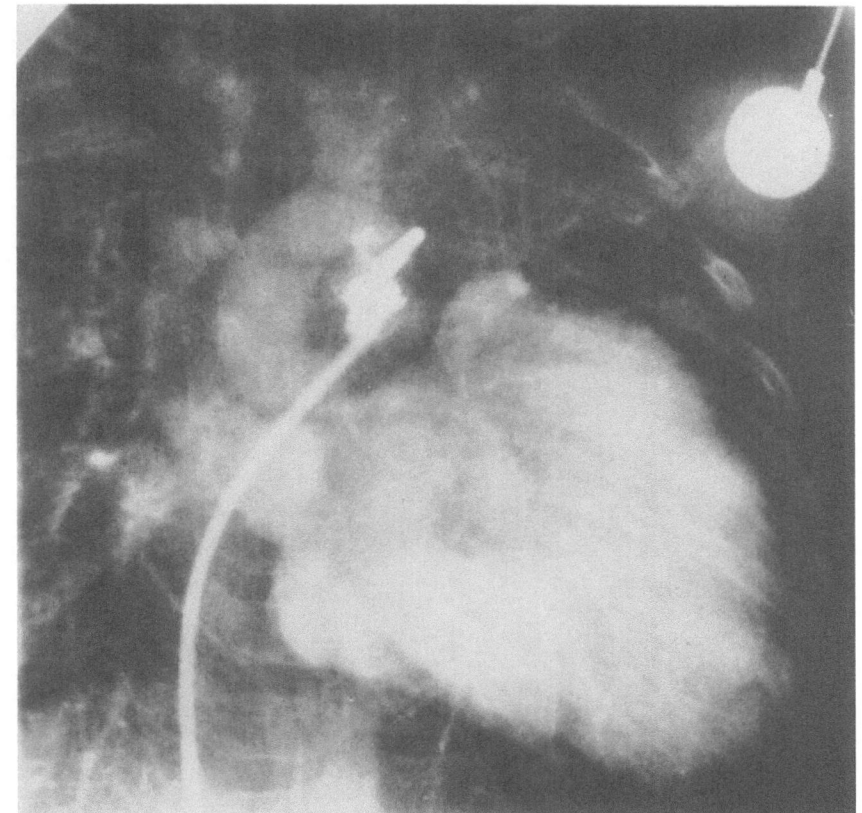

A

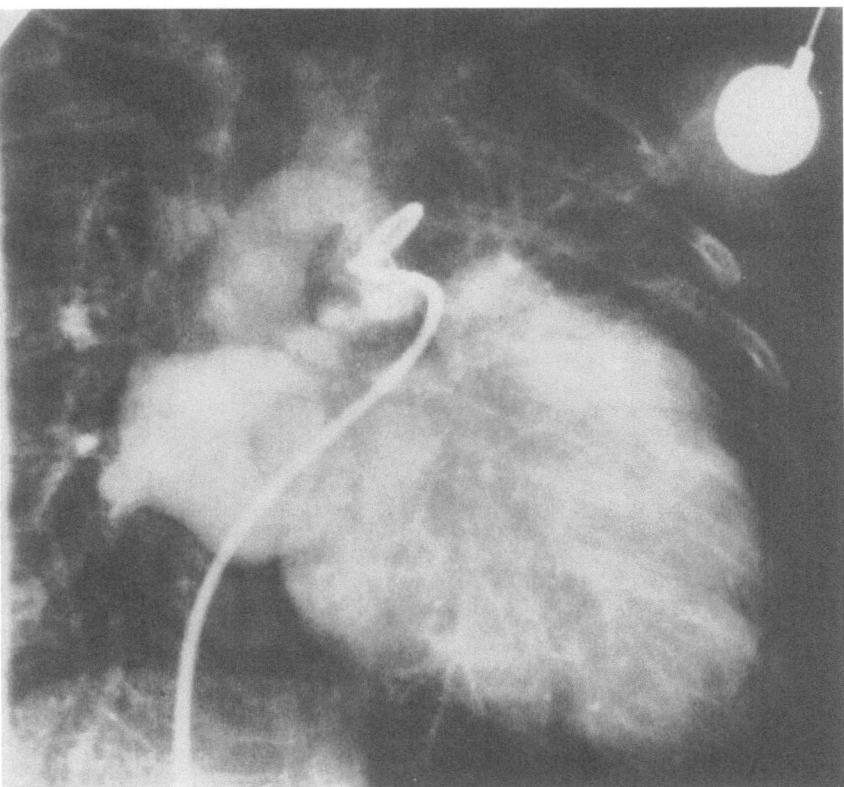

B

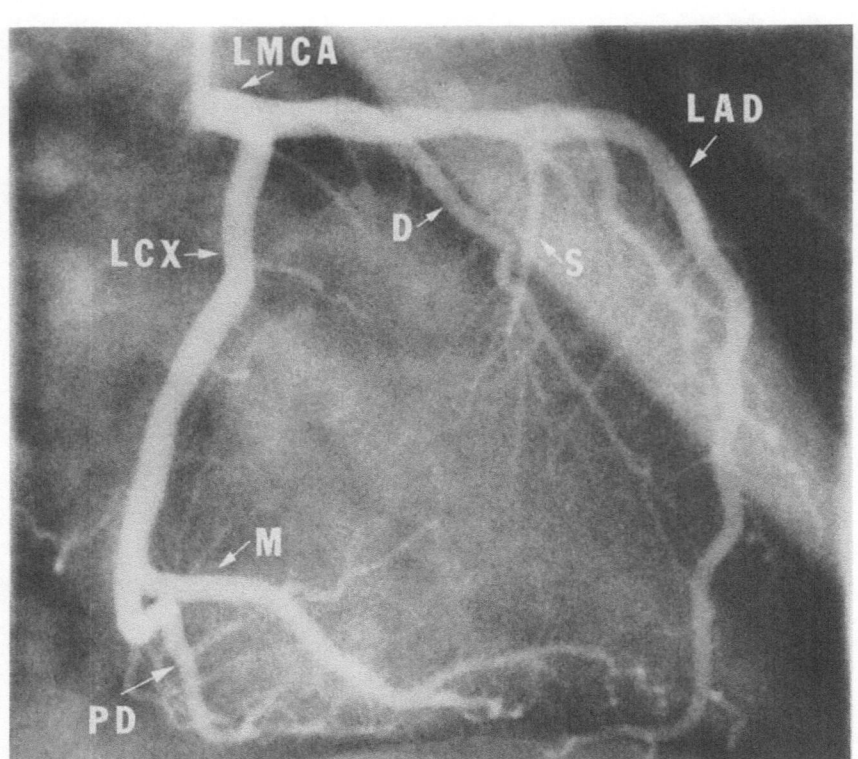

A

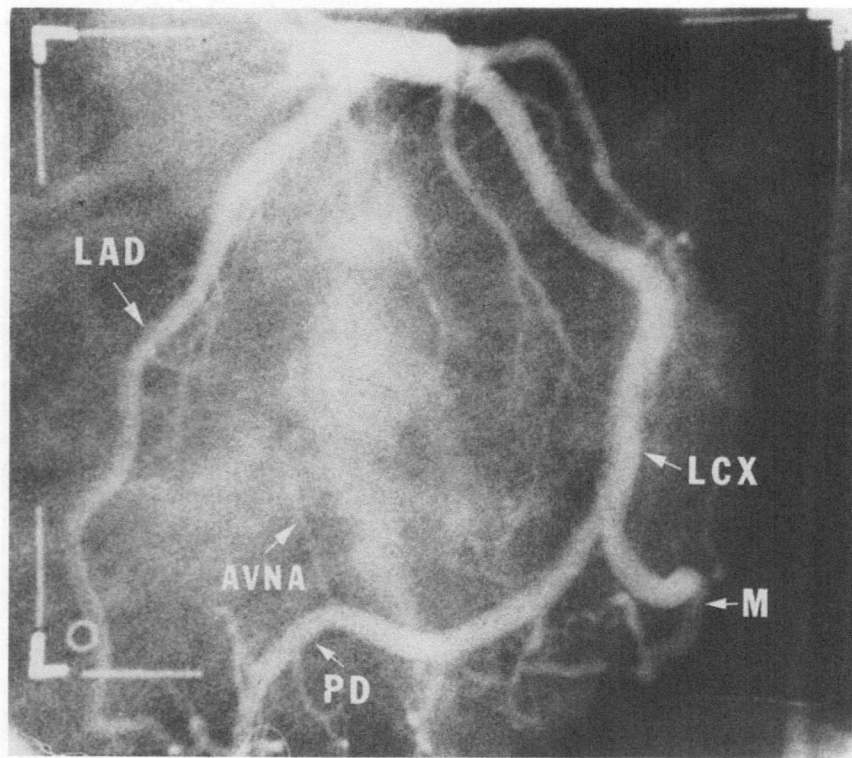

B

Fig. 6–8. *Coronary arteries in dilated cardiomyopathy.* **A** RAO view and **B** LAO view during a selective left coronary artery injection. The coronary arteries are dilated and stretched. In this instance the left coronary artery is dominant. The posterior descending artery (*PD*) is the branch distal to the atrioventricular node artery (*AVNA*). Subjectively, the velocity of the coronary blood flow appears more rapid than normal; a hand injection requires more force for optimal visualization of the coronary arteries. *LMCA* = left main coronary artery; *LAD* = left anterior descending artery; *LCX* = left circumflex artery; *D* = diagonal artery; *M* = marginal artery; *S* = septal artery. Note: This is an excellent example of a dominant left coronary artery (see Chapter 4).

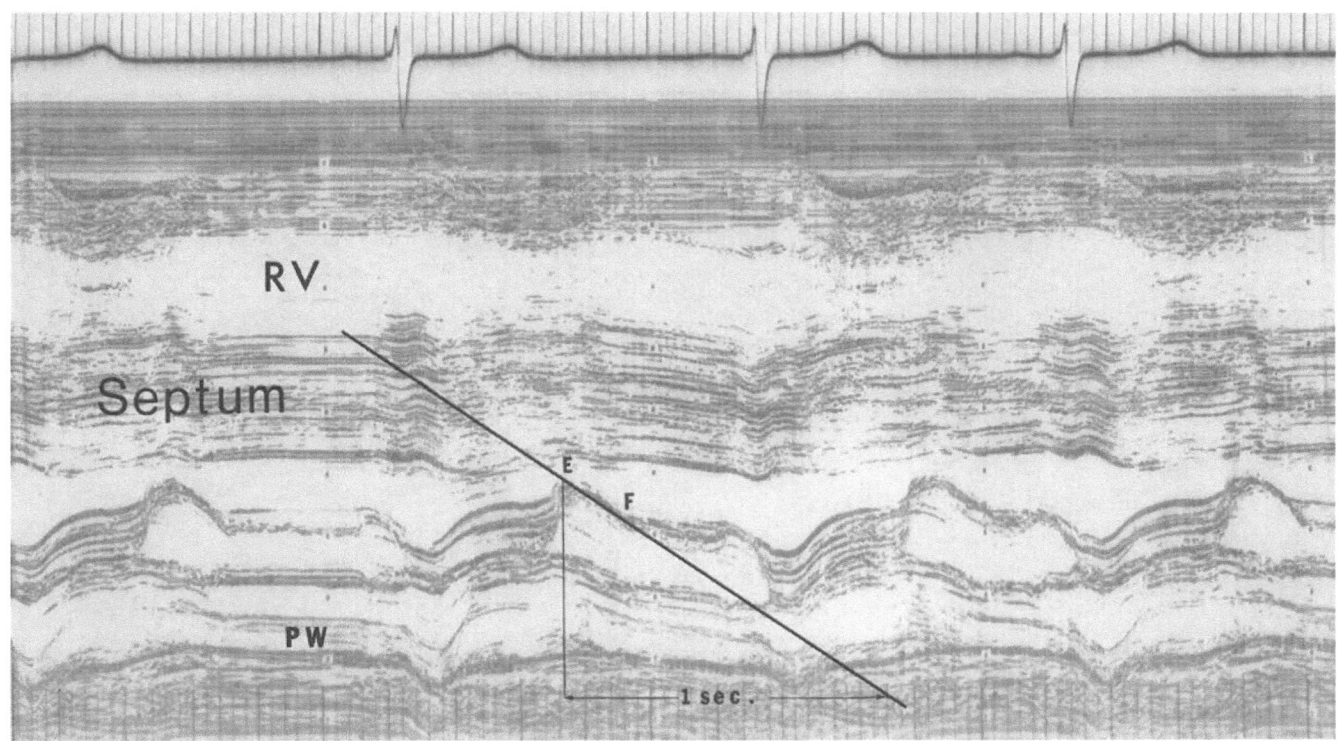

Fig. 6–9. *M-mode echocardiogram in a teenage male with hypertrophic cardiomyopathy.* The septum is disproportionately thickened. The E-F slope of the mitral valve is 35 mm/sec (normal > 60 mm/sec), a feature consistent with slow filling secondary to decreased left ventricular compliance. *RV* = right ventricle; *PW* = posterior wall of the left ventricle.

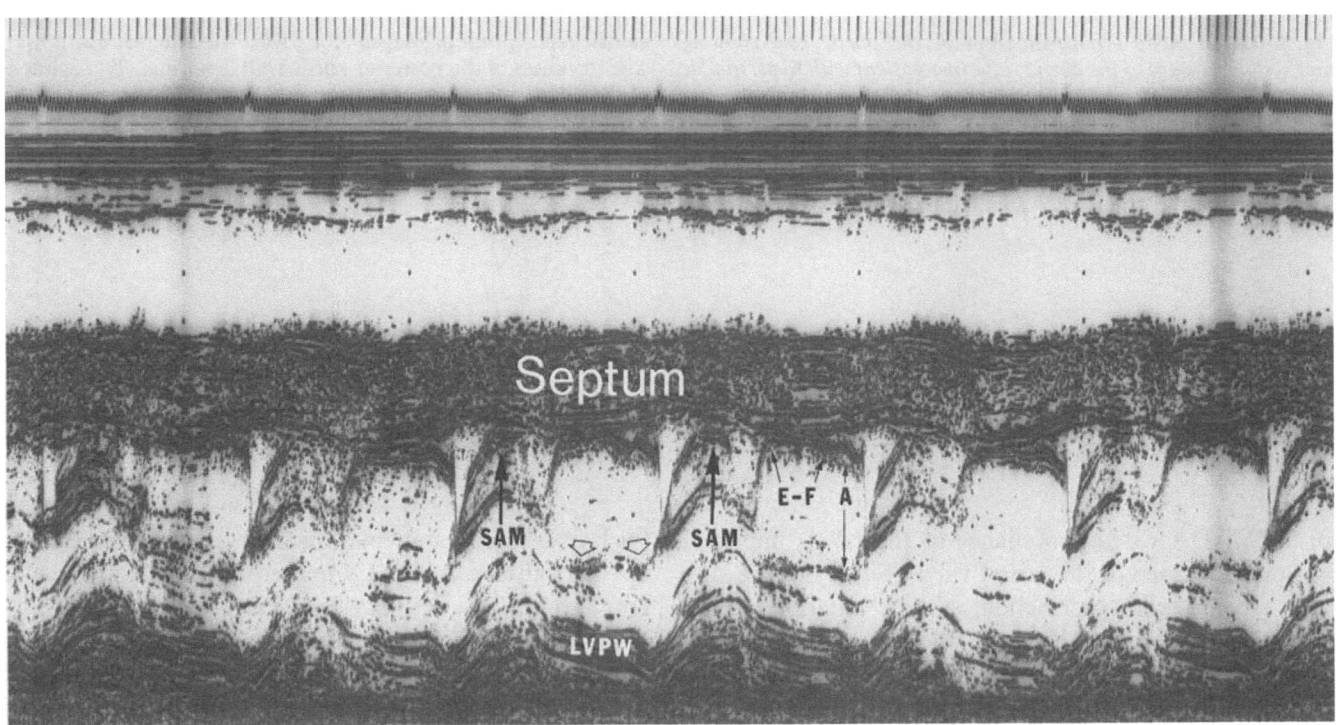

Fig. 6–10. *M-mode echocardiogram in an adult with hypertrophic cardiomyopathy.* The septum is disproportionately thickened as compared to the left ventricular posterior wall (*LVPW*). Systolic anterior motion (*SAM*) of the anterior leaflet of the mitral valve is evident during ventricular systole. The markedly decreased E-F slope of the mitral valve during diastole is consistent with slow left ventricular filling (decreased left ventricular compliance). This finding is not indicative of mitral stenosis because (1) the posterior leaflet (*open arrows*) of the mitral valve moves posteriorly away from the anterior leaflet during ventricular diastole and (2) the atrial "kick" (*A*) is evident on both the anterior and posterior leaflets. (Courtesy of Naftali Neuberger M.D., Brooklyn, N.Y.)

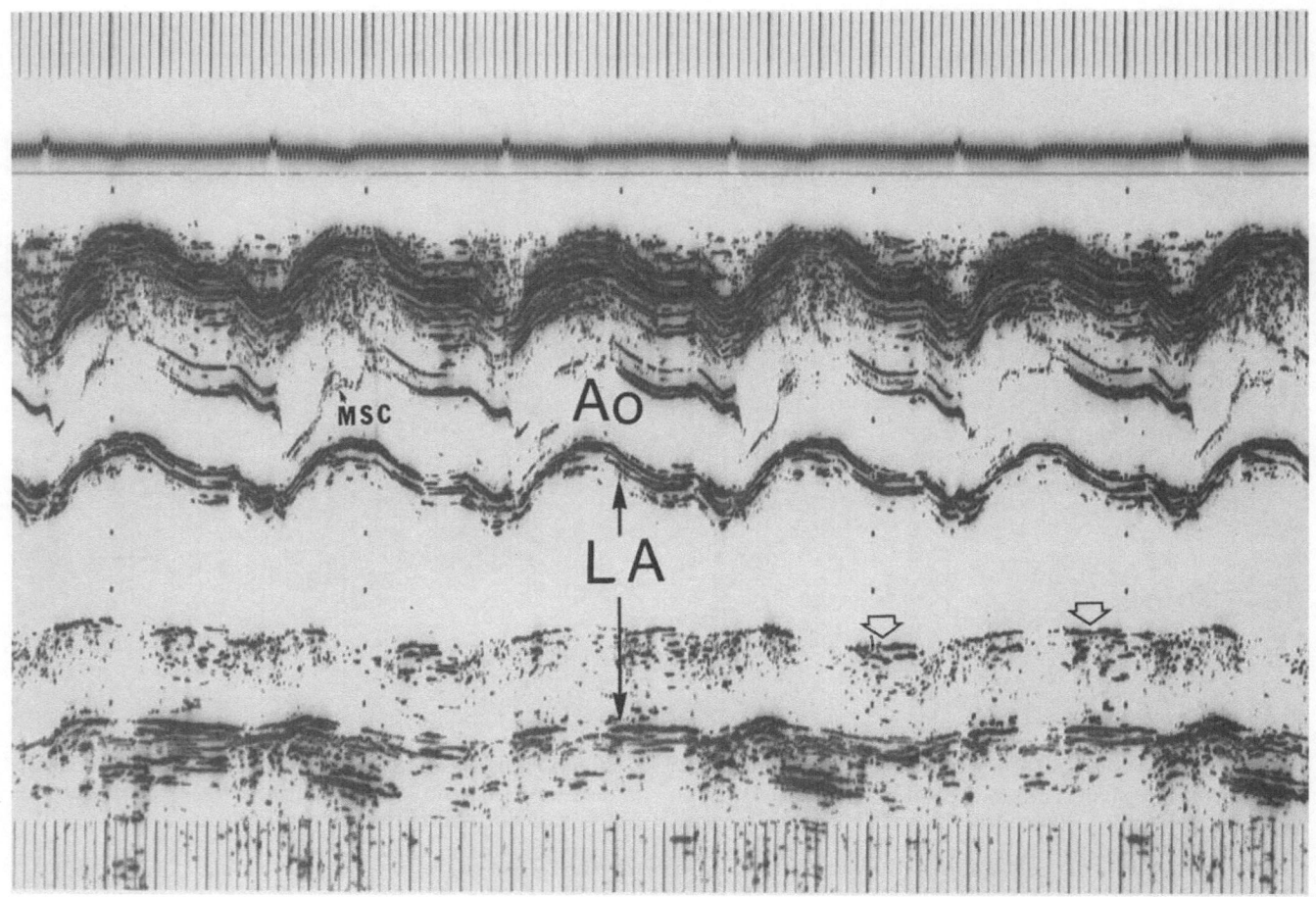

Fig. 6–11. *M-mode echocardiogram of the aortic root showing mid systolic closure of the aortic valve in a patient with hypertrophic cardiomyopathy.* Mid systolic closure (*MSC*) occurs in patients with left ventricular outflow tract obstruction. This echogram is from the patient in Figure 6–10. The anterior wall of the aortic root (*Ao*) appears thickened, probably because of slight inferior angulation of the transducer so that the summit of the thick ventricular septum is imaged along with the anterior aortic wall. The thickness of the posterior aortic wall is normal. The diameter of the left atrium (*LA*) is increased. The echoes observed within the left atrium (*open arrows*) have been explained as originating from the openings of the pulmonary veins as they enter the left atrium. (Courtesy of Naftali Neuberger M.D., Brooklyn, N.Y.)

for HCM. Decreased compliance of the LV is indicated by slow E-F slope of the mitral valve (Fig. 6–9).

In patients with obstruction, systolic anterior motion (SAM) of the anterior leaflet of the mitral valve is also observed (Figs. 6–10, 6–13). SAM may be induced by the Valsalva maneuver or by amyl nitrite in patients without this finding at rest. SAM does not correlate with the severity of obstruction.

The aortic valve echogram in HCM with obstruction reveals mid systolic closure, indicating mid systolic narrowing of the LV outflow tract and abrupt reduction in ejection velocity (Fig. 6–11).

None of the findings detailed in the foregoing is specific for HCM. Inordinate septal thickness may also be encountered in individuals with LV hypertrophy from other causes and also in those with RV hypertrophy.

SAM has been observed in numerous other conditions, including aortic valve stenosis, aortic regurgitation, discrete and tunnel subaortic stenosis, Friedreich ataxia, ischemic heart disease, hypertensive heart disease and in infants with D-transposition of the great vessels and LV outflow tract obstruction.

Infants of diabetic mothers may show all the features of HCM at birth (Fig. 6–14), but during the first year of life the echocardiographic findings disappear. Infants with type II glycogen storage disease (Pompe disease) and those

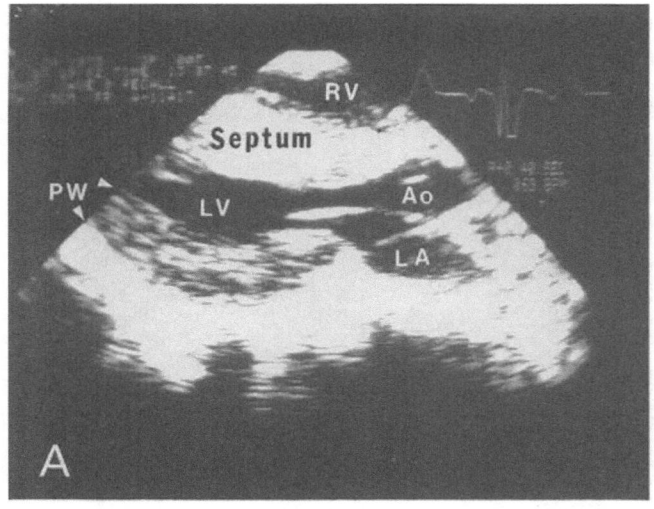
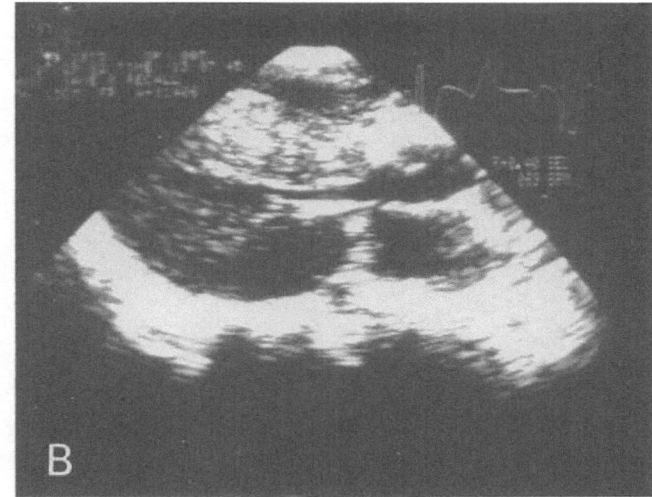
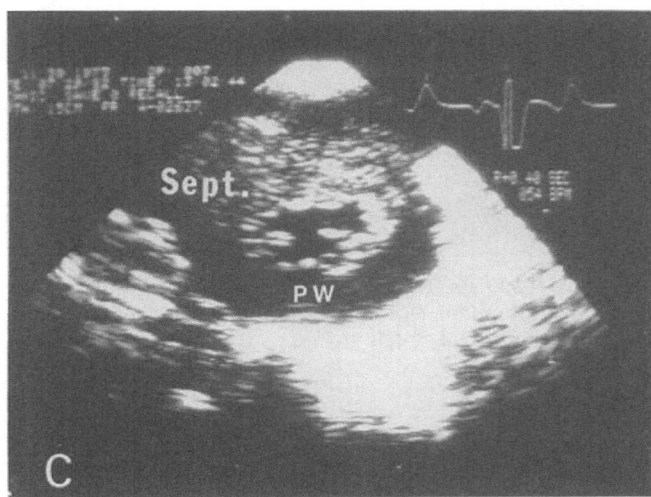
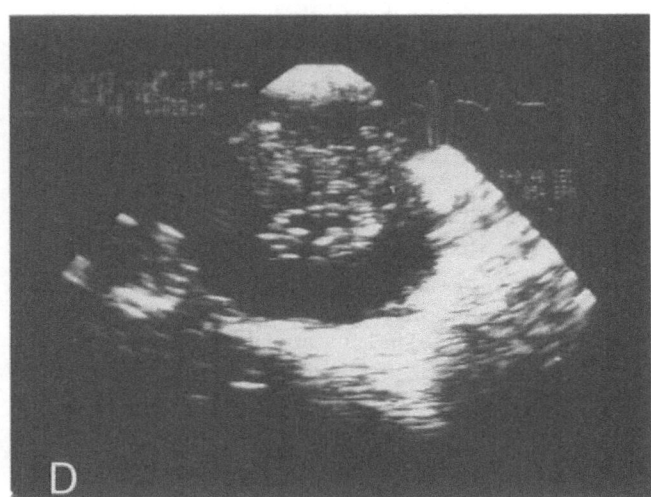

Fig. 6–12. *Two-dimensional echocardiogram in an 8-year-old boy with hypertrophic cardiomyopathy.* **A** Long axis, diastole; **B** long axis, systole; **C** short axis, diastole; **D** short axis, systole. The septum (*Sept.*) and the left ventricular posterior wall (*PW*) are both thickened. Cavitary obliteration occurs during ventricular systole. *RV* = right ventricle; *Ao* = aorta; *LA* = left atrium; *LV* = left ventricle.

with mitochondrial myopathy (Fig. 6–15) also show very thick ventricular free wall and septum as well as slow E-F slope due to poor LV compliance. (See also Fig. 6–19.)

Doppler echocardiography shows a high velocity jet inside the LV corresponding to the area of stenosis. The direction of this jet is similar to the direction of mitral insufficiency; and therefore these two hemodynamic disturbances can not easily be distinguished.

Radiological (Plain Film) Features
The heart is usually normal in size. If the heart is enlarged the LV (Figs. 6–16, 6–17A) and LA are most prominent. If the compliance of the LV is poor or if there is mitral insufficiency, pulmonary venous hypertension will be present. The absence of dilatation of the ascending aorta in these cases may help to distinguish them from valvar aortic stenosis.

Hemodynamics
At catheterization the intraventricular gradient can be altered by increasing or decreasing arterial pressure, myocardial contractility or ventricular volume. Thus, the outflow gradient can be reduced (or abolished) by phenylephrine, squatting, hand grip and propranolol and increased by nitroglycerin, amyl nitrite, Valsalva maneuver, post-extrasystolic contraction (Fig. 6–17B), isoproterenol and digitalis. Provocative interventional techniques are particularly im-

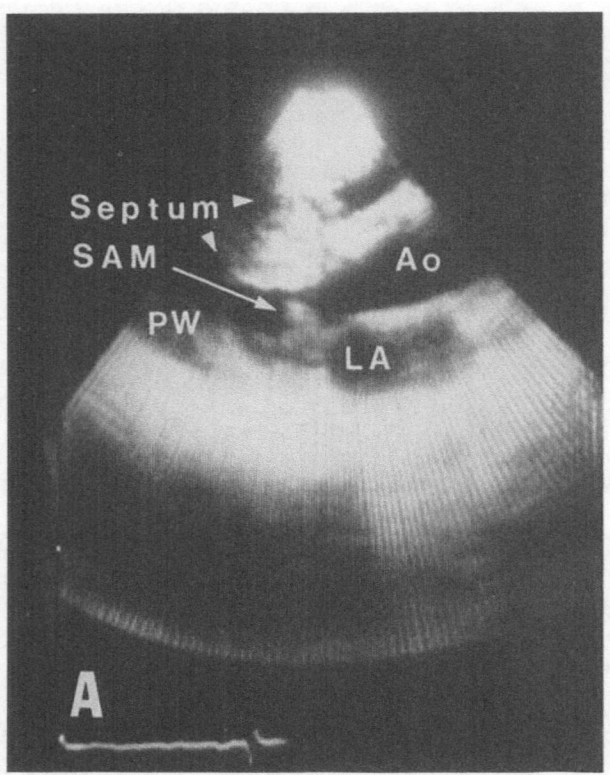
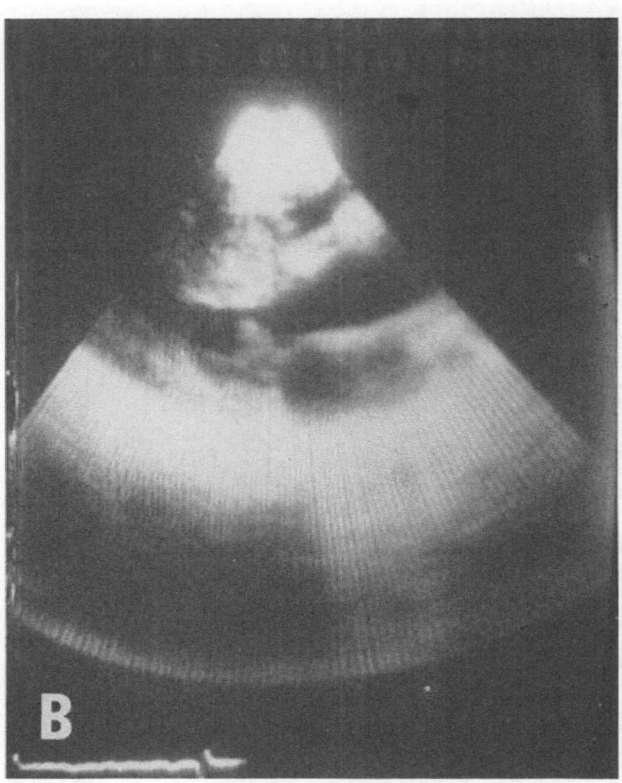

Fig. 6–13. *Two-dimensional echocardiogram in a young adult with hypertrophic cardiomyopathy.* **A** with labels; **B** without labels. The septum is thickened. The left ventricular posterior wall (*PW*) is of normal thickness. This frame, obtained in mid systole, shows systolic anterior motion (*SAM*) of the anterior leaflet of the mitral valve. *Ao* = aorta; *LA* = left atrium.

portant in identifying patients with HCM who have no resting outflow gradient. Isoproterenol infusion, Valsalva maneuver and the post-premature ventricular contraction response are commonly used. The abnormal response of the arterial pulse pressure after an extrasystole is considered characteristic of HCM. In normal individuals an increase in the arterial pulse pressure occurs in the beat after the extrasystole; whereas in patients with HCM the pulse pressure of the post extrasystolic beat is decreased or unchanged (Fig. 6–17B).

Additional hemodynamic features in HCM include elevation of the LV end-diastolic pressure and LA pressure.

Contrast Studies

Ventriculography (Fig. 6–18) reveals marked LV hypertrophy with prominent papillary muscles, asymmetrical hypertrophy of the ventricular septum, a hyperkinetic ventricle, cavitary obliteration and, finally, an increase in the calculated ejection fraction. The ventriculographic findings in mitochondrial myopathy are similar (Fig. 6–19).

If systolic obstruction is present at the outflow tract of the LV, it occurs at the point where the free edge of the anterior leaflet of the mitral valve is opposed to the

Fig. 6–14. *M-mode echocardiogram in a newborn infant of a diabetic mother showing the features of hypertrophic cardiomyopathy.* In panel A the ventricular septum is disproportionately thickened. The right ventricular cavity is represented by a slit between the RV wall (*RVW*) and the septum. The left ventricular posterior wall (*PW*) is also thicker than normal. The mitral valve E-F slope is decreased. Systolic anterior motion (*SAM*) of the anterior leaflet of the mitral valve is evident. The septum is relatively nonreflective, especially the anterior half. This finding may be due to abnormal orientation of muscle fibers such that more are parallel to the echo beam or due to abnormal tissue composition. Panel B reveals mid systolic closure (*MSC*) of the aortic valve. A follow-up echocardiogram of this subject at age 6 months was normal. *LV* = left ventricle; *RVOT* = right ventricular outflow tract; *Ao* = aortic root; *LA* = left atrium.

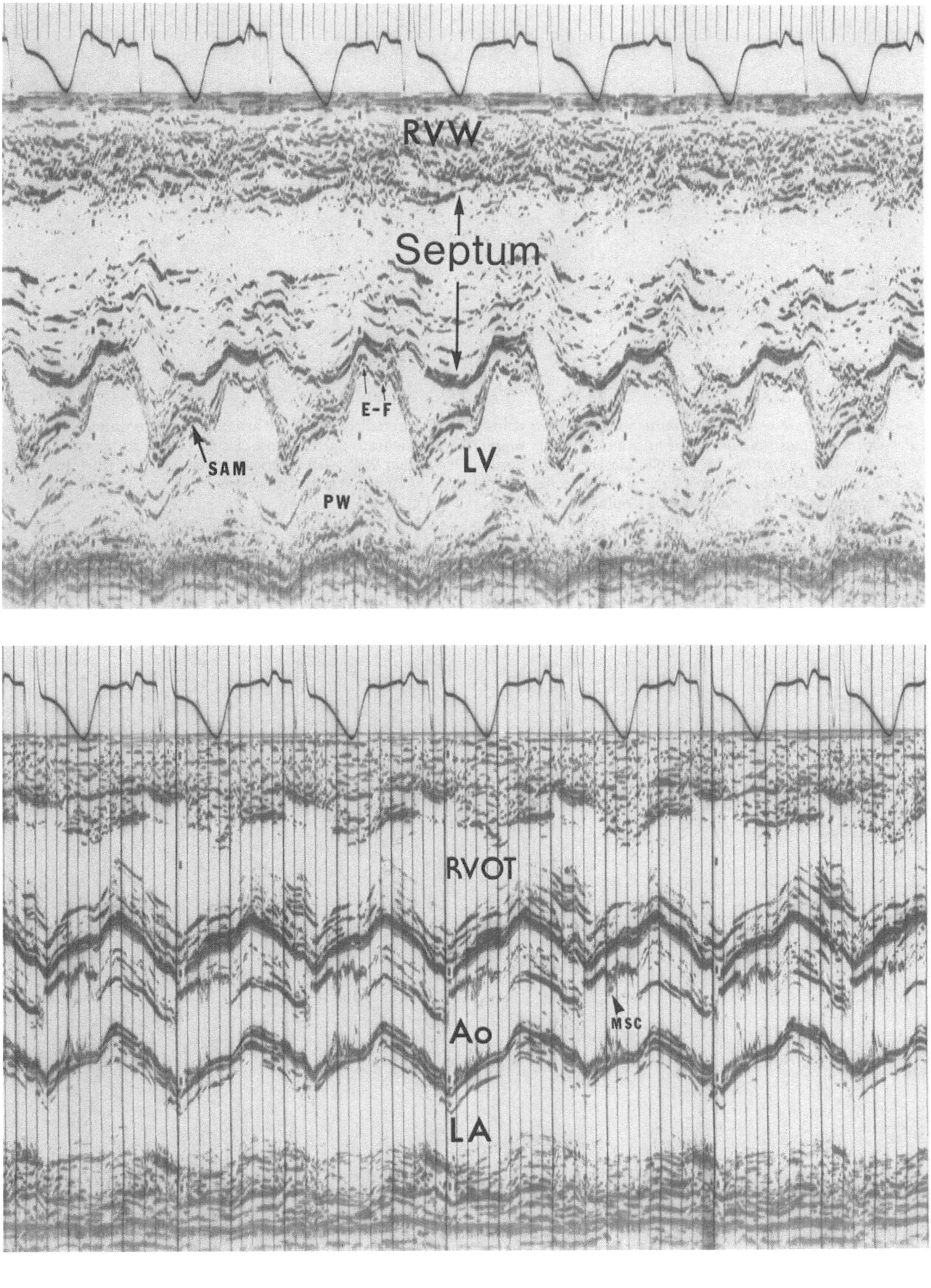

RVW

Septum

E-F

SAM

PW

LV

A

RVOT

Ao

MSC

LA

B

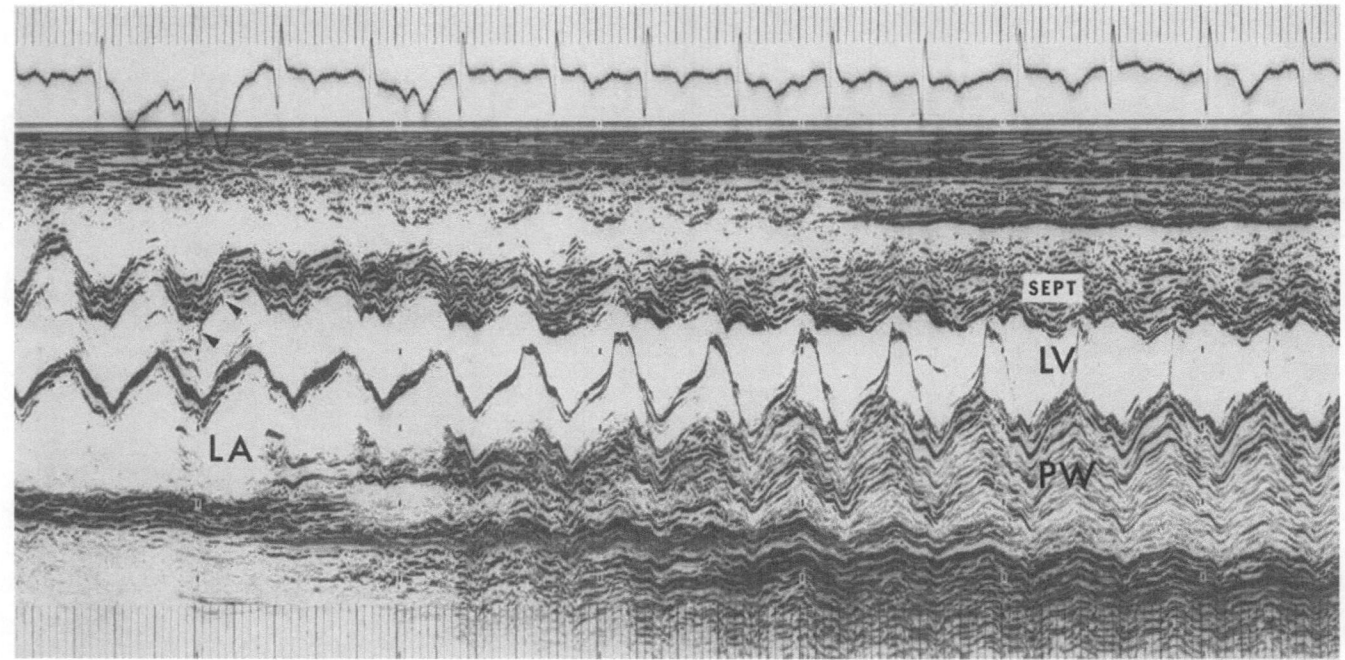

Fig. 6–15. *M-mode arc-scan from the aortic valve to the left ventricle, demonstrating massively thickened myocardium in an infant with mitochondrial myopathy.* Midsystolic closure of the aortic valve and systolic anterior motion of the anterior leaflet of the mitral valve are not evident. Nevertheless, a mild intraventricular pressure gradient was found at cardiac catheterization. The *arrowheads* indicate opening and closing of the aortic valve. *LA* = left atrium; *PW* = left ventricular posterior wall; *LV* = left ventricle; *SEPT* = ventricular septum. For the left ventriculogram see Fig. 6–19.

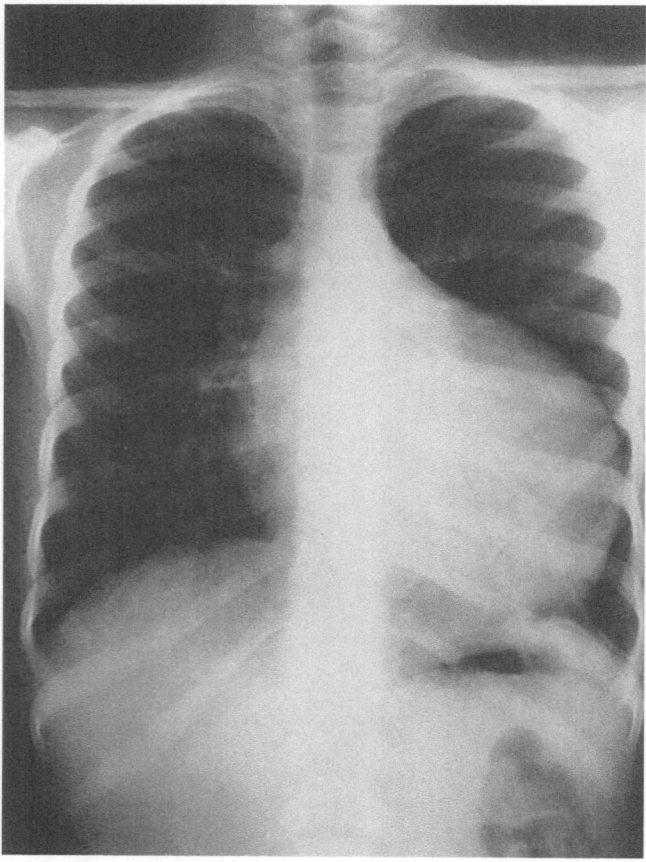

A

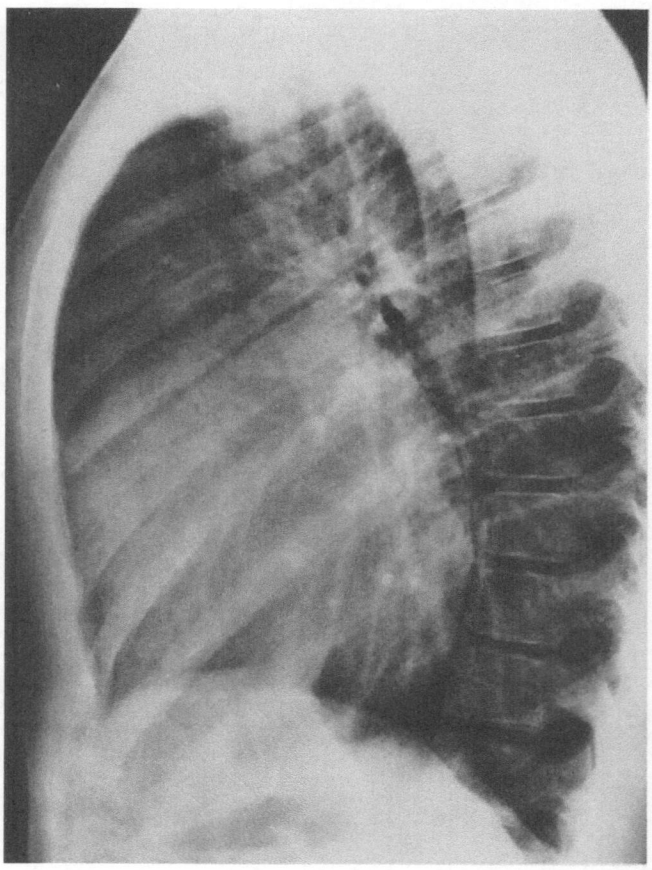

B

Fig. 6–16. *PA and lateral chest roentgenograms in an 8-year-old boy with hypertrophic cardiomyopathy, showing marked left ventricular enlargement with rounding and elevation of the apex of the heart on PA film.* On the lateral film the left ventricle projects excessively behind the inferior vena cava. Rounding of the left heart border on the frontal-plane view **(A)** as well as obliteration of the retrosternal clear space on the lateral film **(B)** suggest right ventricular enlargement. However, the left ventricular angiogram showed that the left ventricular enlargement was responsible for the plain film findings. Even though a double density is present within the cardiac silhouette, the left atrium is not enlarged. The pulmonary vascularity is normal.

Fig. 6–17. *Hypertrophic cardiomyopathy.* **A** PA chest roentgenogram in a 22-year-old man with hypertrophic cardiomyopathy. In contrast to Fig. 6–16, this film shows the typical appearance of left ventricular enlargement (elongation of the left heart border and projection of the cardiac apex below the left hemidiaphragm). Absence of dilatation of the ascending aorta favors subaortic stenosis rather than aortic valvular disease. The ventriculogram from this patient is found in Fig. 6–18. **B** Dynamic obstruction of the left ventricular outflow tract in a 15-year-old boy with hypertrophic cardiomyopathy (HCM). Pressure tracings in the left ventricle (*LV*) and the brachial artery (*BA*) demonstrate a marked pressure difference between the LV and the BA (peak systolic gradient = 75 mm Hg). After a premature ventricular contraction the left ventricular systolic pressure rises markedly, while the systolic pressure and the pulse pressure in the brachial artery do not rise. Augmentation of the intraventricular pressure gradient is a result of post extrasystolic potentiation of cardiac contractility. This phenomenon is characteristic of HCM.

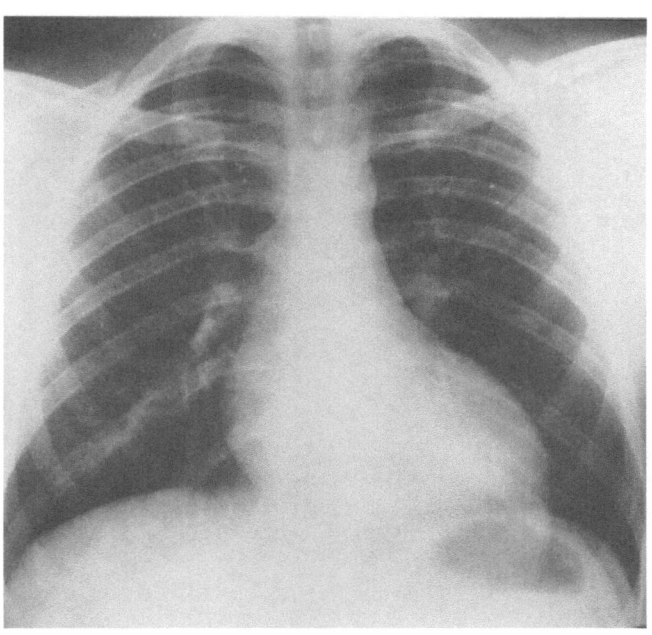

A

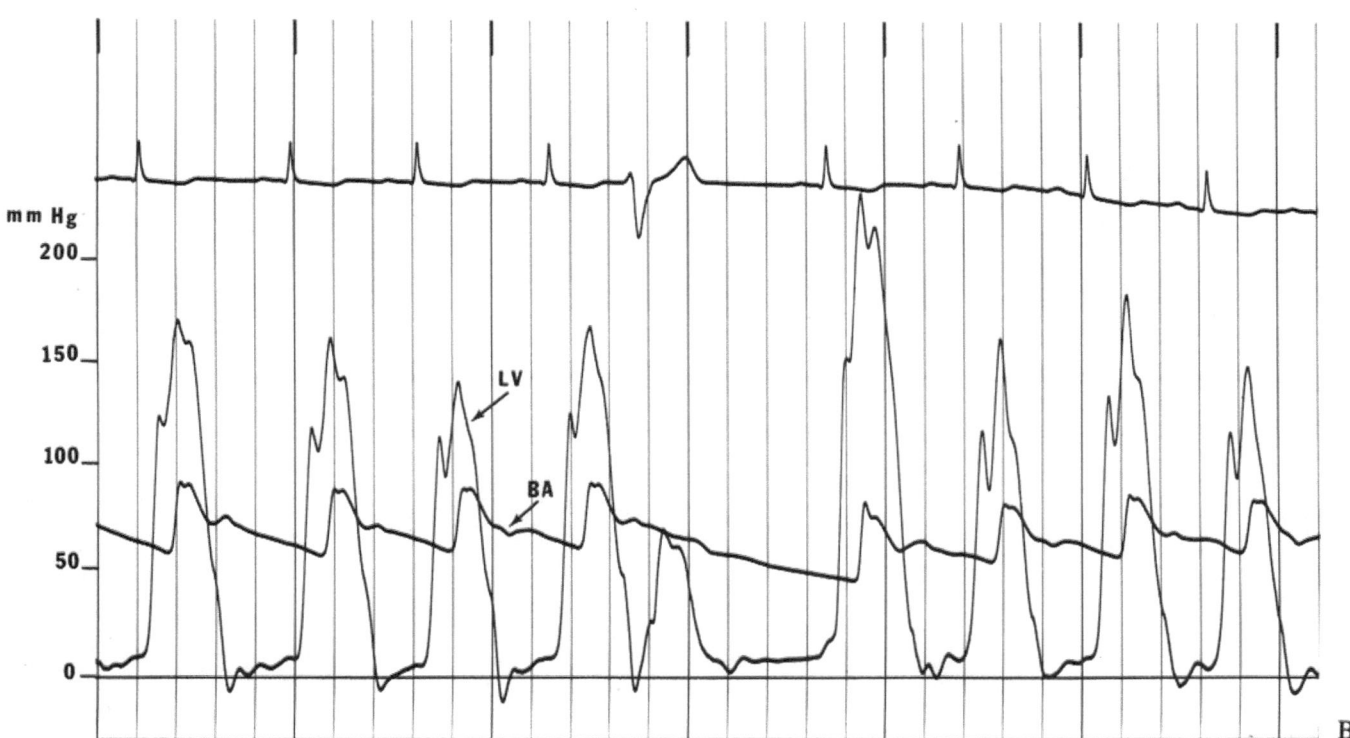

B

interventricular septum. This abnormal systolic apposition of the anterior leaflet of the mitral valve may be demonstrated by angiography and echocardiography. The normal systolic motion of the mitral valve leaflets is restricted by the septal thickening that causes angulation of the LV and displacement of the papillary muscles from their usual alignment, producing abnormal traction on the chordae tendineae and mitral leaflets. Restriction of the posterior motion of the mitral leaflets also impairs their coaptation and may result in mitral insufficiency.

Biventricular Angiography for the Assessment of HCM Biventricular angiography is a useful method for assessing the thickness of the septum in HCM (Figs. 6–20 and 6–21). The triangular shape of the ventricular septum observed on the LAO projection of a biventricular angiogram (Fig. 6–20C) has been regarded as specific for HCM. However, the authors have observed this finding in individuals with HCM, in those with normal ventricles (Fig. 6–22C) and in patients with hypertrophy from other causes. Biventricular angiography in the RAO view tends

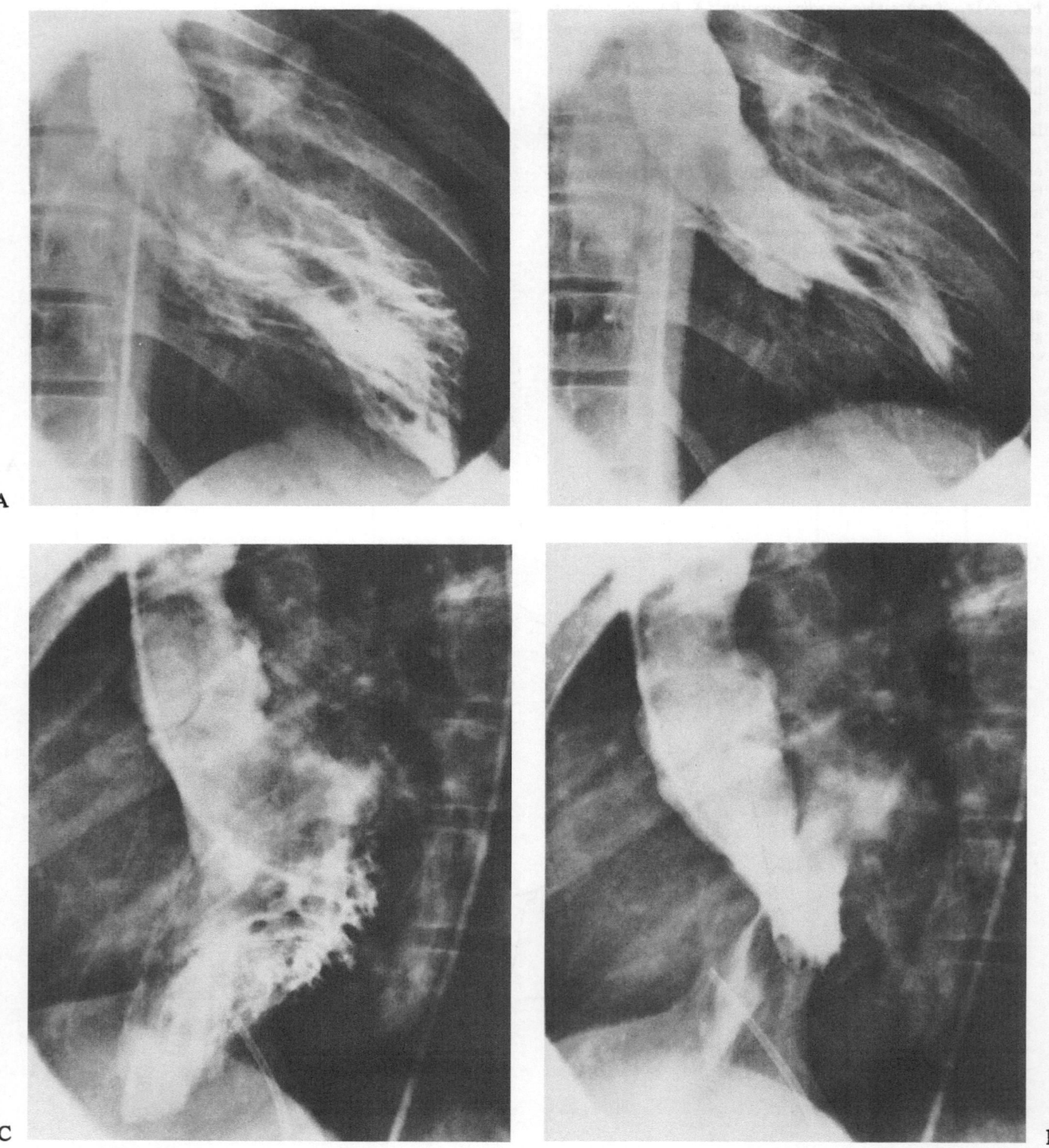

Fig. 6–18. *Left ventriculogram in a 22-year-old man with hyper-trophic cardiomyopathy.* **A** and **B** RAO views; **C** and **D** LAO views. Left ventricular hypertrophy is indicated by the marked thickening of the left ventricular wall and by the coarse trabecula-tions (feathery appearance) observed during diastole (**A** and **C**). During systole (**B** and **D**) the hypertrophied papillary muscles come into apposition (the "kissing" effect), thus closing off the ventricular sinus (cavitary obliteration). The left ventricular cavity is normal in size during diastole. Mild mitral insufficiency occurs during systole. This ventriculogram is from the patient in Fig. 6–17A.

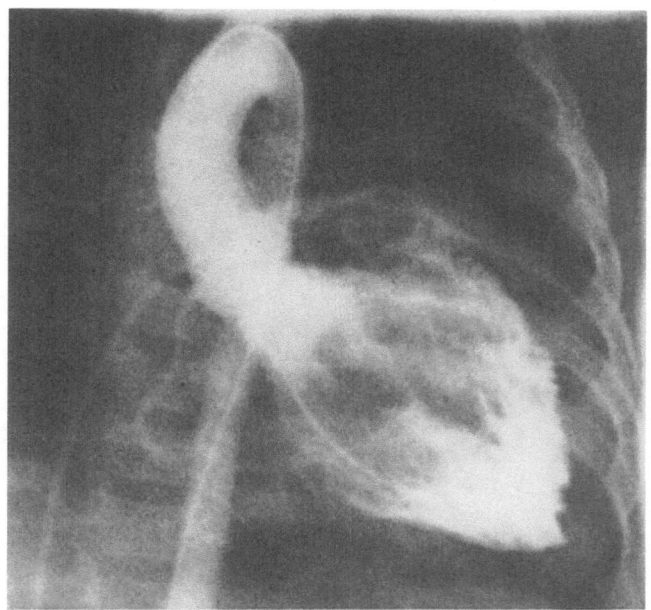

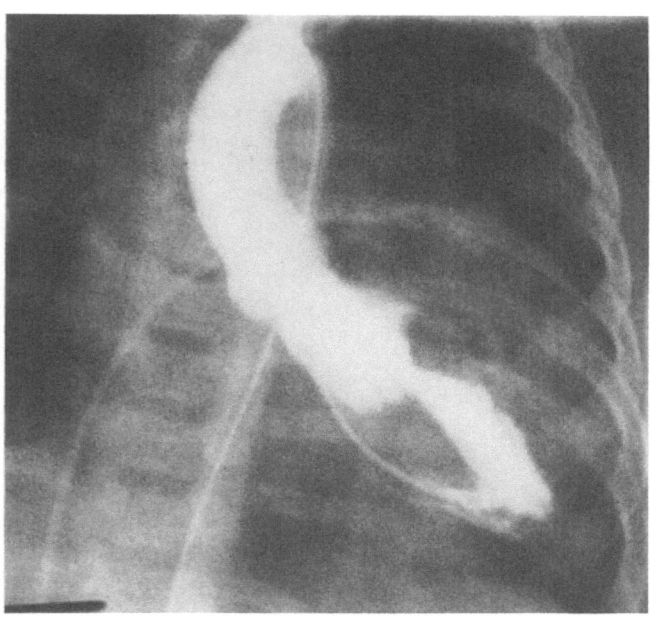

Fig. 6–19. *Frontal projections of a left ventriculogram in an infant with mitochondrial myopathy mimicking hypertrophic cardiomyopathy.* **A** Diastole; **B** systole. The ventricular cavity is normal in size during diastole. Hypertrophied muscle walls and papillary muscles are apparent during diastole. Cavitary obliteration occurs during systole. This ventriculogram is from the patient in Fig. 6–15.

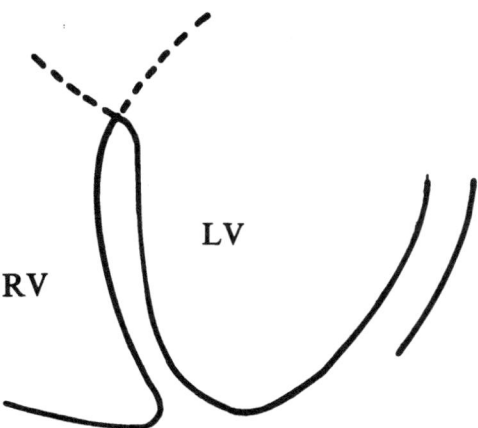

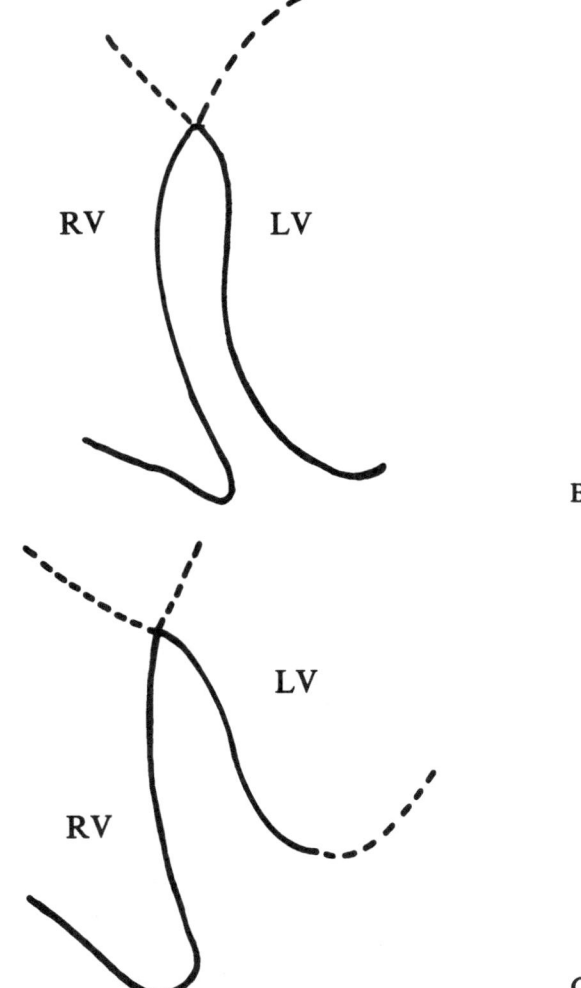

Fig. 6–20. *Appearance of the ventricular septum during biventricular angiography in the LAO view.* **A** represents the normal configuration; **B** represents hypertrophy from causes other than hypertrophic cardiomyopathy (HCM), and **C** represents the triangular appearance that some consider diagnostic for HCM. The authors have found configuration **B** in patients with HCM and configuration **C** in normal individuals and in patients with left ventricular hypertrophy from other causes. *RV* = right ventricle; *LV* = left ventricle.

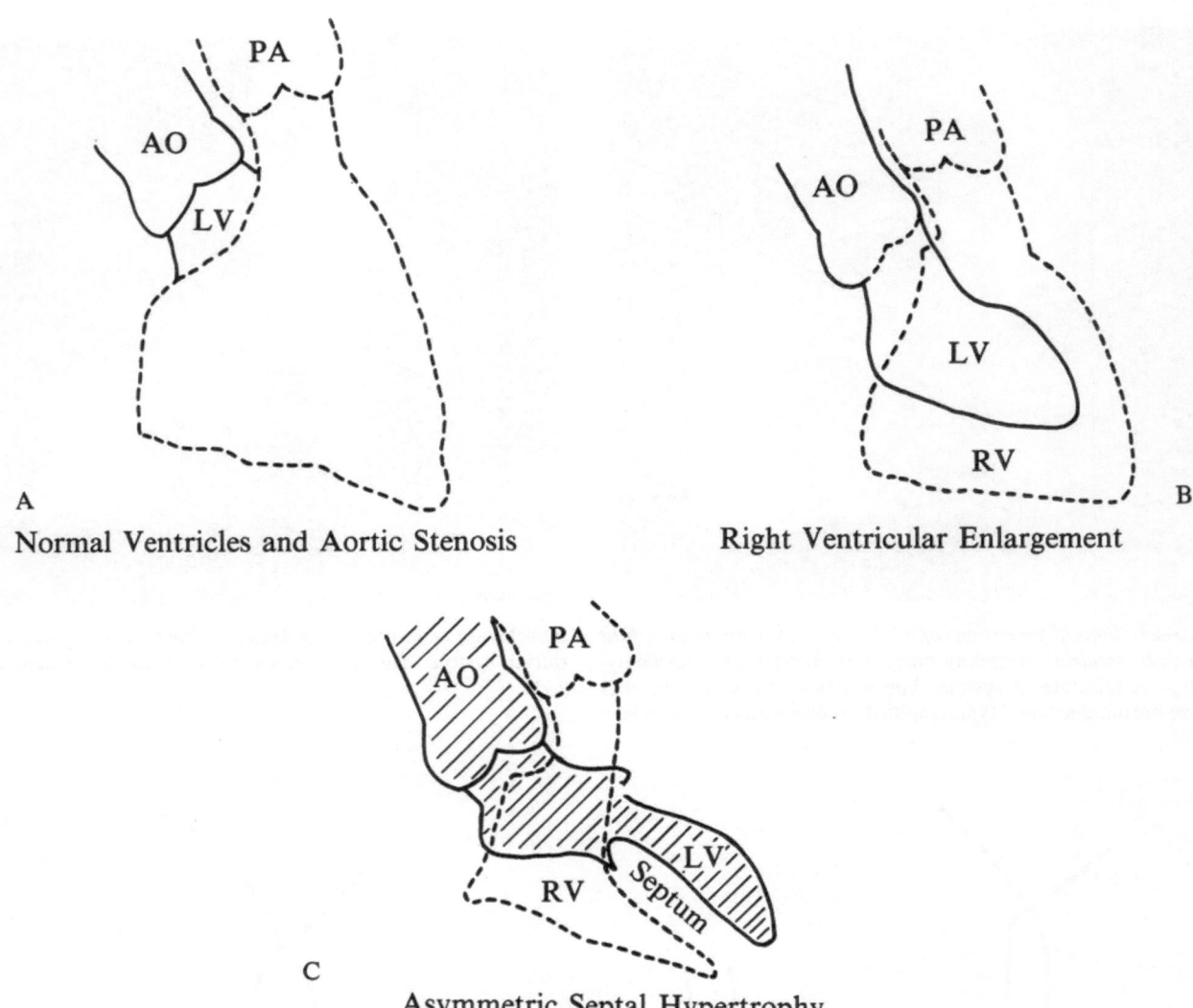

A

Normal Ventricles and Aortic Stenosis

B

Right Ventricular Enlargement

C

Asymmetric Septal Hypertrophy

Fig. 6–21. *Ventricular morphology observed on biventricular angiography in the RAO view.* In normal hearts (A) the ventricles are superimposed during systole and diastole except for the outflow tracts. In right ventricular dilatation (B) the left ventricle projects within the silhouette of the right ventricle. In hypertrophic cardiomyopathy (C) the ventricles separate during ventricular systole so that the ventricular septum is sharply outlined. *PA* = pulmonary artery; *LV* = left ventricle; *RV* = right ventricle; *AO* = aorta.

to identify individuals with HCM. Three patterns were observed in a study by the authors (Figs. 6–21 to 6–23): (1) In patients with normal ventricles or with LVH or RVH, complete overlap of the ventricles during systole made it impossible to differentiate the chambers (Fig. 6–22A and B). (2) In individuals with RV enlargement, the LV can be identified through the enlarged RV, which completely encompasses the LV cavity. (3) In patients with HCM, both ventricular chambers are seen to move away from each other during systole, permitting visualization of the interventricular septum (Fig. 6–23B). This separation of ventricular cavities and visualization of the interventricu-

lar septum during systole in the RAO view is considered by the authors to be characteristic of HCM.

Green et al. have reported that the caudocranial LAO view provides excellent definition of the ventricular septum and LV free wall. SAM of the mitral valve was also demonstrated on this projection.

Coronary arteriography in individuals with HCM ordinarily does not demonstrate any intrinsic coronary artery disease. However, the vessels are usually dilated and tortuous in severe cases (Fig. 6–24). Neovascularity of the ventricular septum has been observed by the authors.

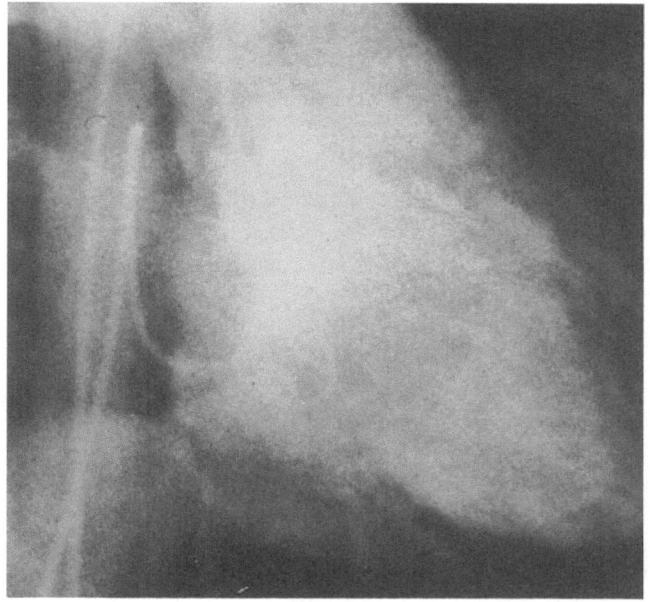

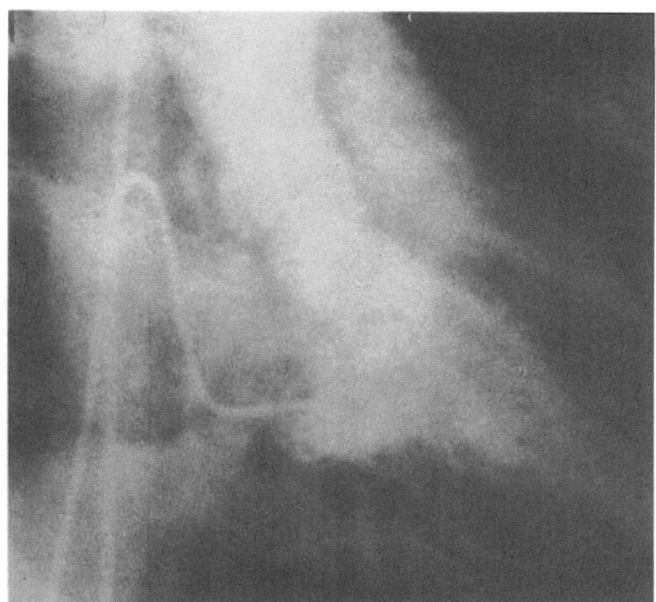

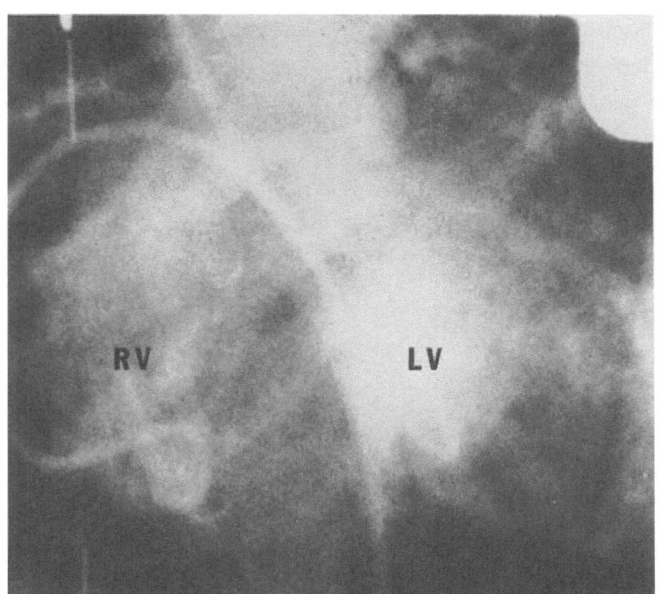

Fig. 6–22. *Biventricular angiogram in patient with normal ventricles.* RAO views during **A** diastole and **B** systole; **C** LAO view during ventricular systole. In **A** and **B** the ventricles overlap and cannot be distinguished except for the outflow tracts. In **C** the septum is triangular. *RV* = right ventricle; *LV* = left ventricle.

Treatment

Medical treatment consists of administration of beta adrenergic blockers (e.g., propranolol), which reduce the rate of cardiac contraction. Thus, functional obstruction of the LV outflow tract may be reduced as well as tension of the LV wall. Verapamil is beneficial in some patients, perhaps by improving the diastolic filling rate. However, this drug causes deleterious, and at times fatal, effects in a small percentage of patients, possibly due to peripheral vasodilatation. Cardiac inotropic agents (e.g., digoxin, isoproterenol), are contraindicated. Diuretics are avoided since they may reduce LV volume, thus increasing the degree of LV outflow tract obstruction. Atrial fibrillation is treated without delay because of the need for the atrial contribution to myocardial filling in HCM.

Surgical treatment usually involves removal of septal muscle tissue. A transaortic approach is the method of choice. Complications include complete heart block and the creation of an interventricular septal defect. Even though the outflow gradient is often reduced, arrhythmias are still common, and sudden death may occur.

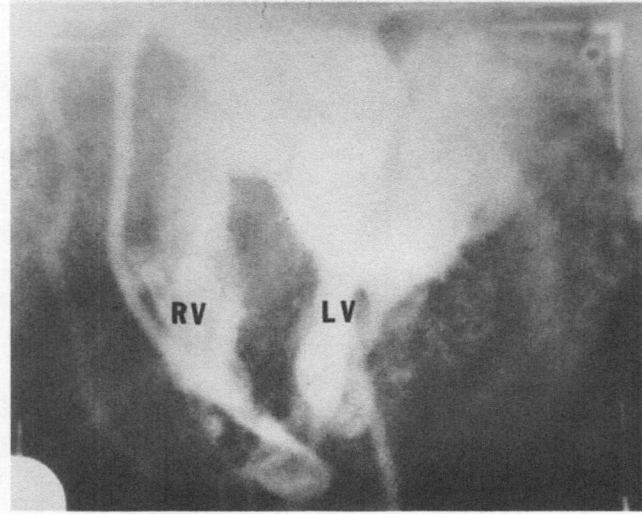
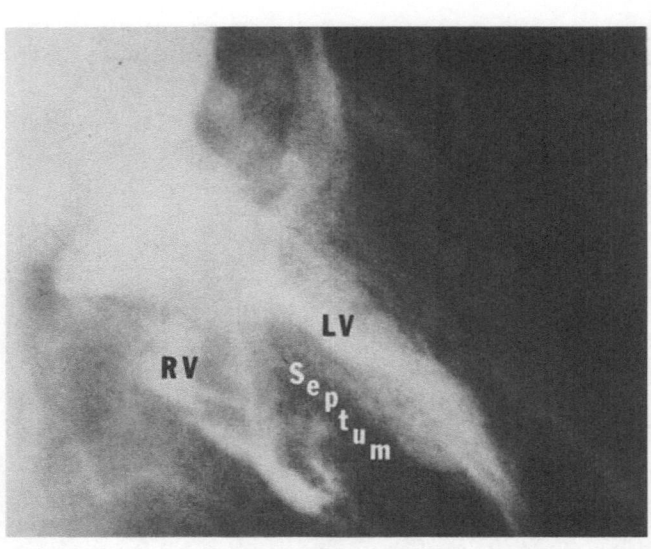

Fig. 6–23. *Biventricular angiogram during ventricular systole in hypertrophic cardiomyopathy.* **A** LAO view; **B** RAO view. **A** The septum is thickened but does not show a triangular configuration.

B The ventricles have rotated so that the ventricular septum is sharply outlined between the ventricular cavities. Compare with Fig. 6–22B. *LV* = left ventricle; *RV* = right ventricle.

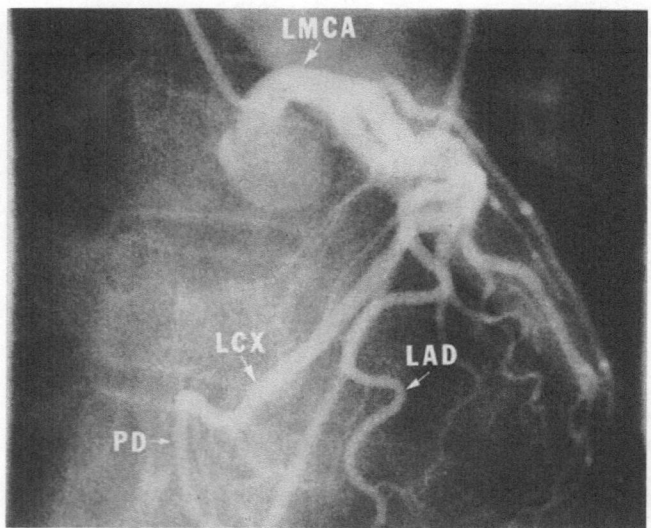
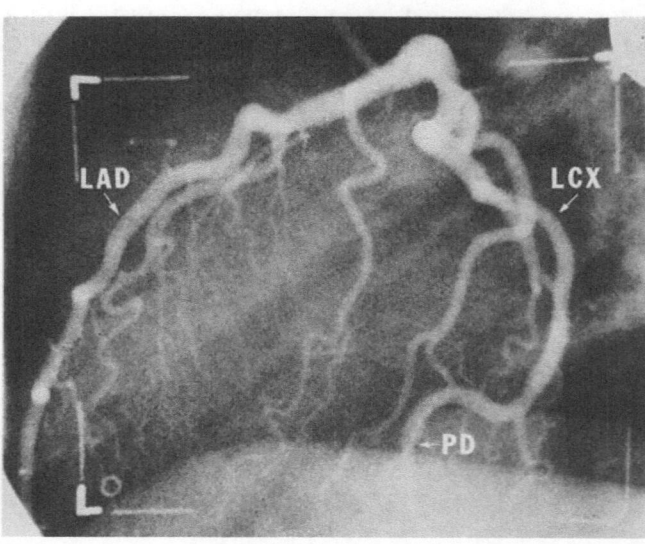

Fig. 6–24. *Coronary arteries in hypertrophic cardiomyopathy.* **A** Frontal view and **B** lateral view during a selective left coronary artery injection. The vessels are dilated and tortuous. In some cases neovascularity is evident in the septum. Compare with Fig.

6–8. *LMCA* =left main coronary artery; *LAD* = left anterior descending artery; *LCX* = left circumflex artery; *PD* = posterior descending artery.

Restrictive Cardiomyopathy

Restrictive cardiomyopathy may be caused by fibrosis of the endocardium or by an infiltrative process that impairs diastolic function. The most severe form of restrictive cardiomyopathy is caused by endomyocardial fibrosis (EMF). Becker disease, Davies disease, Jamaican myocarditis and the Löffler hypereosinophilic syndrome probably represent a spectrum of the same disorder culminating in EMF. Thrombotic endocarditis (endocardial synechiae), which occurs rarely after mitral valve replacement, also may progress to EMF. Infiltrative diseases that may produce similar

hemodynamic alterations include sarcoidosis, amyloidosis, and hemochromatosis-hemosiderosis.

The restrictive presentation is due to a rigid myocardium that fails to relax in diastole. Constrictive pericarditis or pericardial or myocardial neoplasm also limits cardiac filling and therefore may present with similar features. See chapter 9 for a comparison between constrictive pericarditis and restrictive cardiomyopathy.

Plain films in restrictive cardiomyopathy show no consistent characteristic features. The heart may be normal in size or even markedly enlarged. Signs of pulmonary venous hypertension may be present. The characteristic

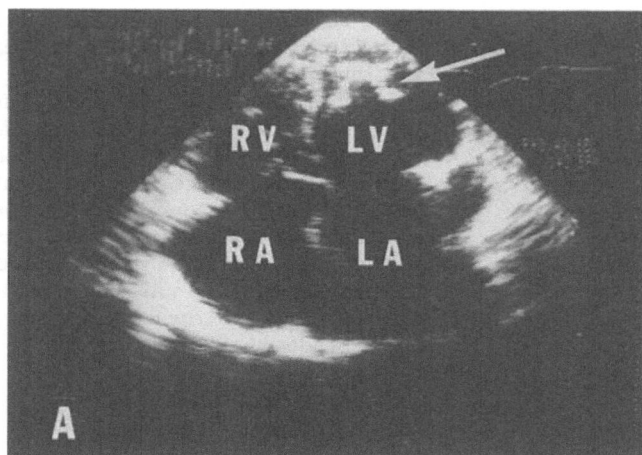
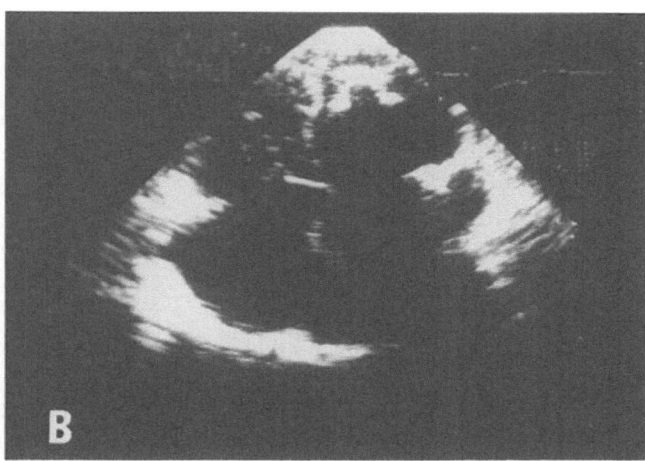

Fig. 6–25. *Intraventricular calcification in a patient with endomyo-cardial fibrosis.* Apex four-chamber view of a 2-D echocardio-gram. **A** with labels; **B** without labels. The apex of the left ventricle (*LV*) is filled by a V-shaped calcific density (*arrow*), corresponding to the V-shaped calcification noted on the plain films (Fig. 6–

26). The mitral valve prosthesis is not visualized, probably because of shadowing behind the calcified mass. A calcific density in the left ventricle may also represent a calcified thrombus, tumor or fibrous tissue. *RV* = right ventricle; *LA* = left atrium; *RA* = right atrium.

hemodynamic feature of restrictive cardiomyopathy is an early diastolic dip and late plateau, reflected in the pressure waves of the affected atrium and ventricle. The end-dia-stolic pressure is elevated. On ventriculography the ventri-cle may fail to relax in diastole. The ejection fraction is also reduced, but the ejection rate may be relatively normal. Ventriculography may also show insufficiency of the mitral or tricuspid valve. The coronary arteries are normal. Differ-entiation of restrictive cardiomyopathy from constrictive pericarditis may be difficult or even impossible at times so that the distinction can be made only at thoracotomy.

Endomyocardial Fibrosis

Endomyocardial fibrosis (EMF) is a major form of heart disease among young Africans, first described by Davies in 1948. Löffler observed extremely elevated eosinophil counts in the blood in patients with acute endomyocardial necrosis; in some of these the disease progressed to early death. Others developed endomyocardial thrombus fol-lowed by hyaline fibrosis of the endocardium. Andy et al. confirmed that eosinophilia preceded the onset of chronic EMF by many months. These studies suggest that the eosinophilic endocarditis described by Löffler and the EMF of Davies may be acute and chronic forms of a single disease. A similar disorder has been described by Becker in light-skinned Europeans and Americans, although eo-sinophilia was not present. The etiology is not known. Mi-crofilaria are suspected to cause eosinophilia in Löffler en-docarditis, but other possible causes are schistosomes and various viral organisms.

EMF is characterized by thickening and fibrosis of the endocardium of either or both ventricles. The inflow tract, apex, papillary muscles and chordae tendineae are predomi-

nantly affected. In some cases the apex is completely filled by a mass of fibrous tissue and thrombus, while the outflow tracts are relatively spared. The fibrotic layer may be as much as 10 mm thick in the RV and 20 mm thick in the LV. Septa of fibrous tissue may extend into the rela-tively normal myocardium. The hemodynamic abnormali-ties resulting from EMF are (1) decreased ventricular com-pliance, (2) mitral or tricuspid valvar insufficiency and (3) partial obliteration of either or both ventricular chambers by the mass of fibrous tissue.

Clinical Features
Progressive fatigue, dyspnea on exercise, edema and ascites are frequently encountered. Pulmonary and systemic em-bolization are known to occur in the European form of the disease but are uncommon in the African form. Death due to LV failure or arrhythmia usually occurs 3 to 4 years after the onset of symptoms.

Signs of right or left heart failure will be predominant, depending on the degree and extent of involvement of either ventricle. Murmurs of mitral or tricuspid insufficiency or both and gallop rhythms are prominent features on physical examination. The electrocardiogram may be normal or may show ventricular hypertrophy or T-wave changes.

Echocardiography
The echocardiogram shows intense echoes associated with involvement of the endocardium of the RV free wall, both sides of the ventricular septum and the LV free wall. Obliteration of the apex of the RV or LV may be recognized on 2-D echocardiography (Fig. 6–25). The motion of the ventricular septum may be paradoxical. One or both atria may be dilated. The presence of pericardial effusion is easily documented if present.

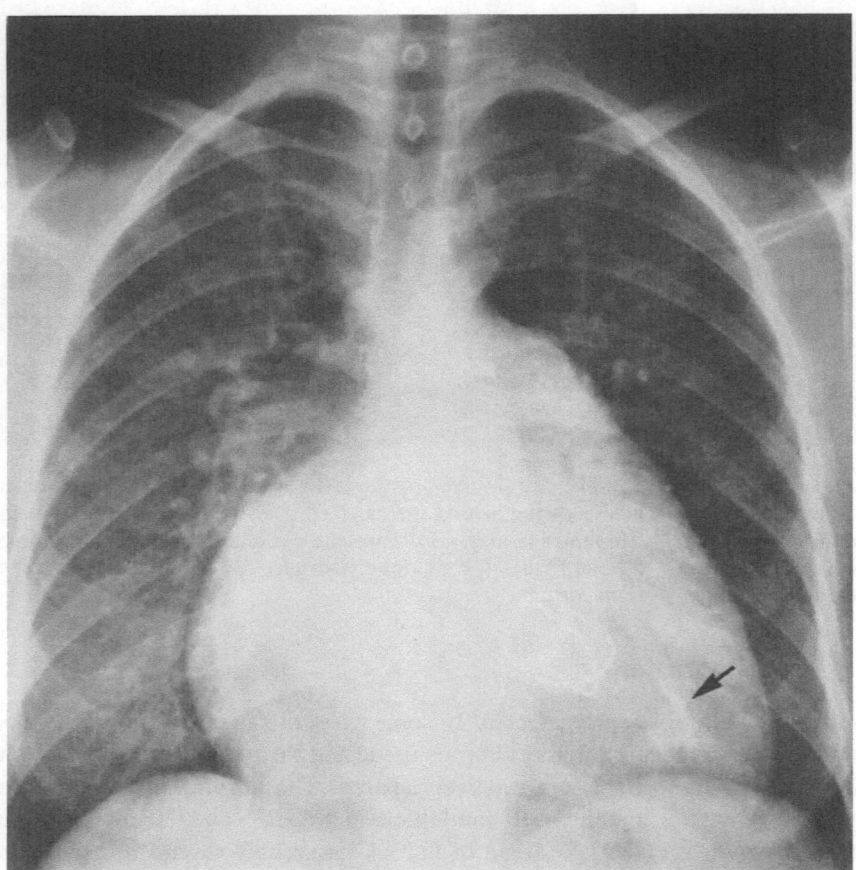

A

Fig. 6–26. *Endomyocardial fibrosis in a 46-year-old woman.* **A** PA view and **B** lateral view showing typical "mitral heart" configuration. The left atrium, right ventricle and right atrium are enlarged. The pulmonary artery is dilated. The aorta is inconspicuous. Pulmonary vascular redistribution with mild interstitial changes is consistent with moderate pulmonary venous hypertension. Intraventricular calcification (*arrow*) in a patient with a prosthetic mitral valve might indicate thrombosis and intracavitary synechiae or calcified endomyocardial fibrosis.

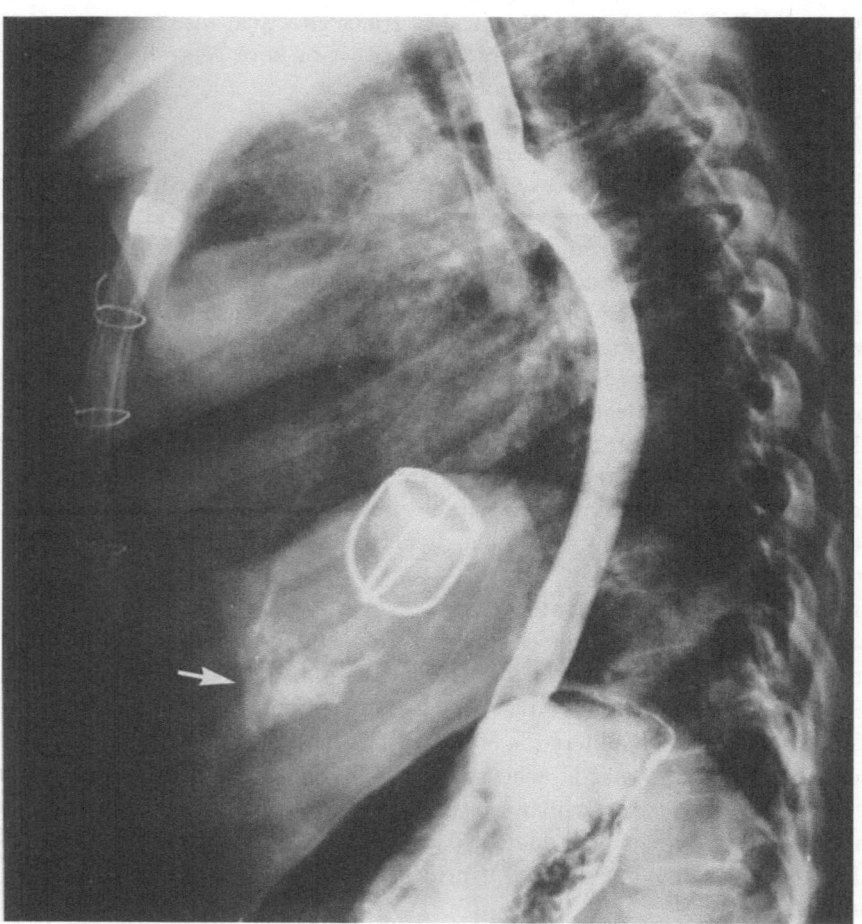

B

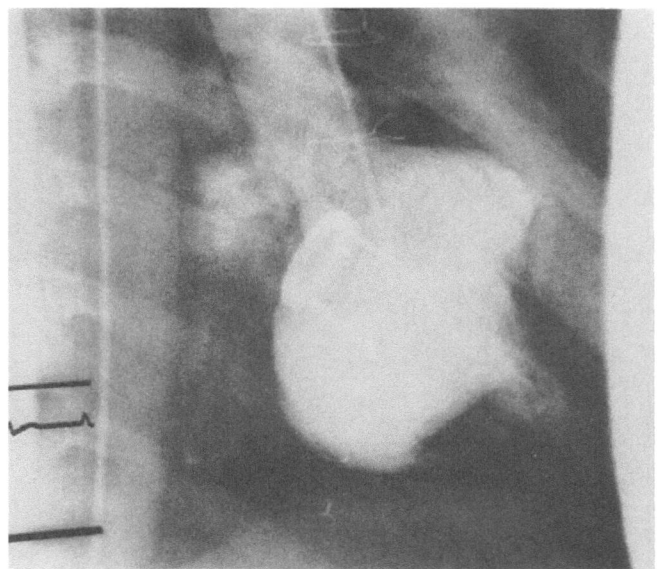

A

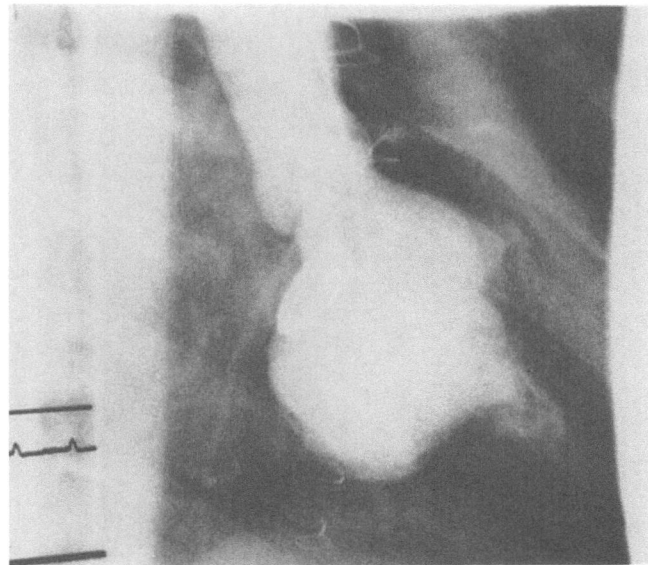

B

Radiological (Plain Film) Features

With predominantly left-sided EMF the findings are similar to those of pure mitral stenosis (enlargement of the LA, RV, RA and pulmonary venous hypertension) (Fig. 6–26). Even though mitral insufficiency is prominent on physical examination, the left ventricle is not enlarged because of restriction to dilatation by the fibrotic tissue lining the LV cavity.

With EMF of the RV, the RA is enlarged, as are the superior and inferior venae cavae. Hepatomegaly is also evident. The diaphragms may be elevated by abdominal ascites. The lungs may show undercirculation. In either type (right or left ventricular involvement) diffuse intracavitary calcification may be observed (Fig. 6–26). This type of calcification differs from the linear calcification of the endocardium associated with ischemic heart disease (Fig. 4–41).

Hemodynamics

In cases with predominantly RV involvement the RA pressure is elevated. The RV diastolic pressure is also elevated. An early diastolic dip in the pressure wave of the RV (the "dip-plateau" configuration) is apparent in this disease as well as in constrictive pericarditis (Fig. 9–9).

In cases of LV involvement the diastolic dip-plateau wave form is noted in the LV. The LV end-diastolic pressure, pulmonary capillary wedge pressure, pulmonary artery pressure and the RV systolic pressure are elevated. The RV diastolic pressure and the RA pressures may be normal.

Contrast Studies (Fig. 6–27)

The characteristic findings in advanced cases of EMF of the LV are amputation or obliteration of the LV apex by the fibrous mass. The fornix, or subvalvular region, may

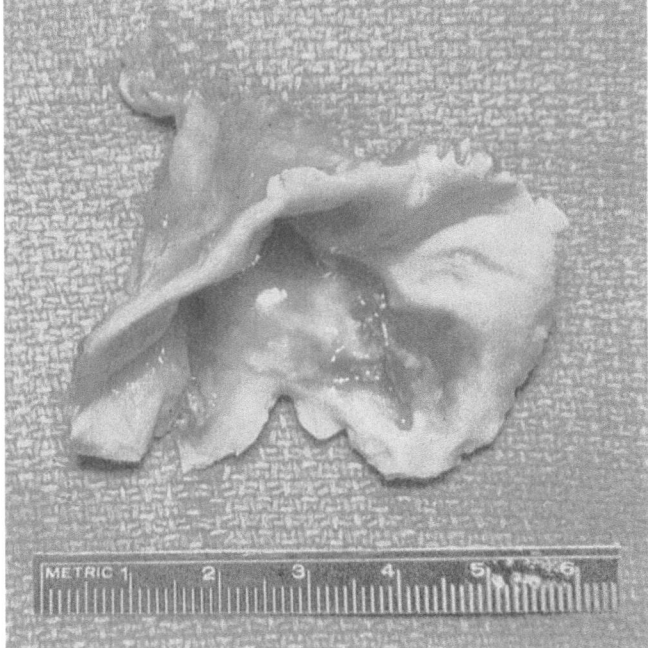

C

Fig. 6–27. *Endomyocardial fibrosis.* Left ventricular angiogram (A diastole; B systole) and surgical specimen (C). The apex of the left ventricle is obliterated by a mass of fibrous tissue. Only the outflow tract dilates during diastole. The distance between the papillary muscles is the same during systole and diastole, indicating adiastole of the ventricular chamber. The mitral valve prosthesis had been placed approximately 10 years previously. The patient died about 2 weeks after myocardial decortication (C). The diagnosis of endomyocardial fibrosis was confirmed at autopsy. Angiographically these findings are characteristic for endomyocardial fibrosis; however, similar findings may be encountered rarely after mitral valve replacement secondary to apical thrombosis and synechiae. A neoplasm may also produce similar findings. Coronary arteriography will reveal neovascularity if the tumor is vascular. This angiogram is from the patient in Fig. 6–25 and Fig. 6–26. (Surgical specimen courtesy of George Robinson, M.D., Bronx, N.Y.).

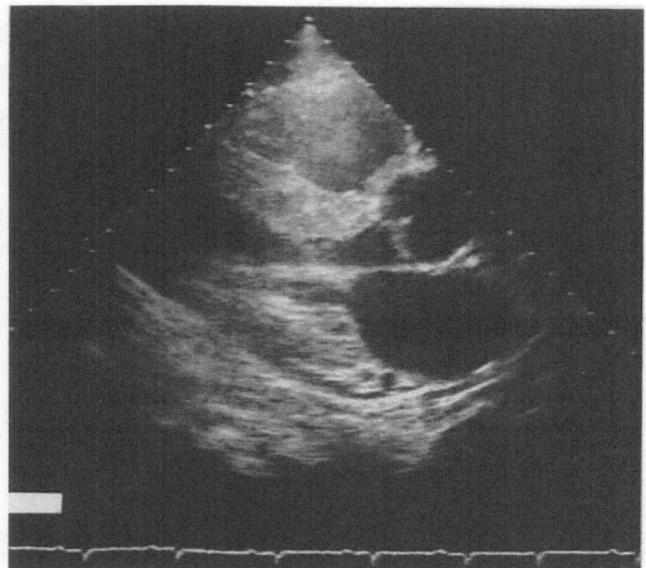

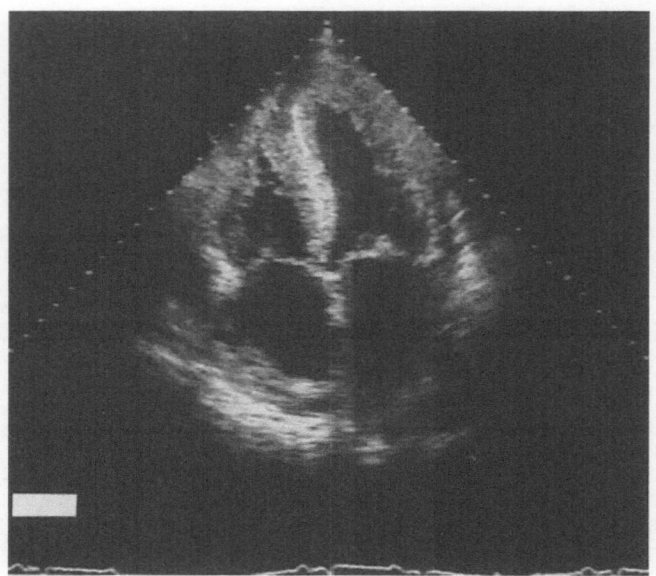

A

B

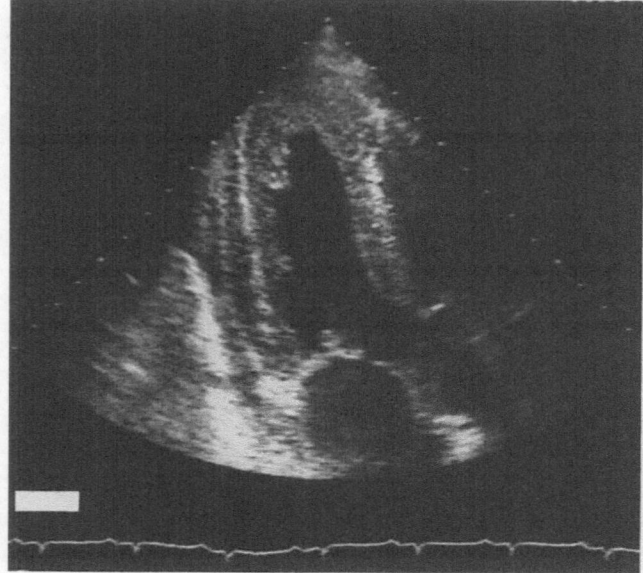

C

Fig. 6–28. *Two-dimensional echocardiograms in a patient with amyloidosis proven at autopsy.* **A** Parasternal long-axis view; **B** apex four-chamber view; **C** apex two-chamber view. The ventricular septum is thickened. Speckling of the myocardium is conspicuous. In the apical views a linear pattern of increased echo density is noted in the ventricular septum. (Courtesy of Dr. Balendu C. Vasavada, and Dr. Howard Friedman, Brooklyn, N.Y.).

also be involved. The papillary muscles are held in close apposition by the dense fibrous tissue, resulting in adiastole, or absence of ventricular dilatation during diastole. The outflow tract is usually the only part of the ventricle that dilates. Severe mitral insufficiency and LA enlargement are characteristic. In EMF of the RV, cavitary obliteration with adiastole, tricuspid insufficiency and RA enlargement are associated. The coronary arteries are normal with both types. Absence of neovascularity militates against a diagnosis of suspected intracardiac tumor.

Treatment
Medical treatment includes rest and diuretics. Anticoagulants may prevent embolization in the European form of the disease. Surgical treatment consists of excision of the massive fibrotic endocardium and papillary muscles (Fig. 6–27C). The atrioventricular valve in the predominantly affected ventricle is replaced. The other atrioventricular valve is preserved, if possible.

Infiltrative Cardiomyopathies

Amyloidosis, sarcoidosis and hemochromatosis produce deposits within the muscle of the heart. Each may present as a dilated cardiomyopathy if contractile function is predominantly impaired or as a restrictive cardiomyopathy if ventricular compliance is the dominant abnormality.

Amyloid and sarcoid infiltration will cause a stippled or "sparkling" appearance of the myocardium on 2-D echocardiography (Fig. 6–28). Evaluation of wall thickness, systolic ejection rate and diastolic filling rate by echocardiography and nuclear angiography will help to elucidate the hemodynamics.

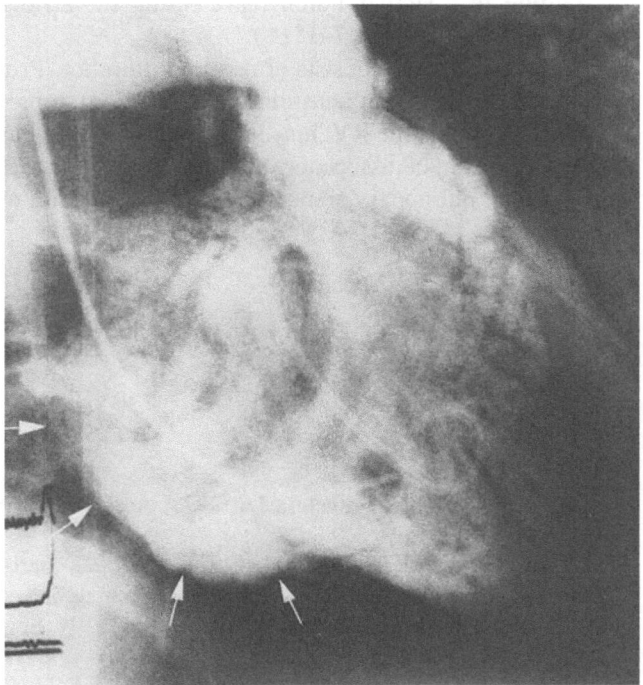
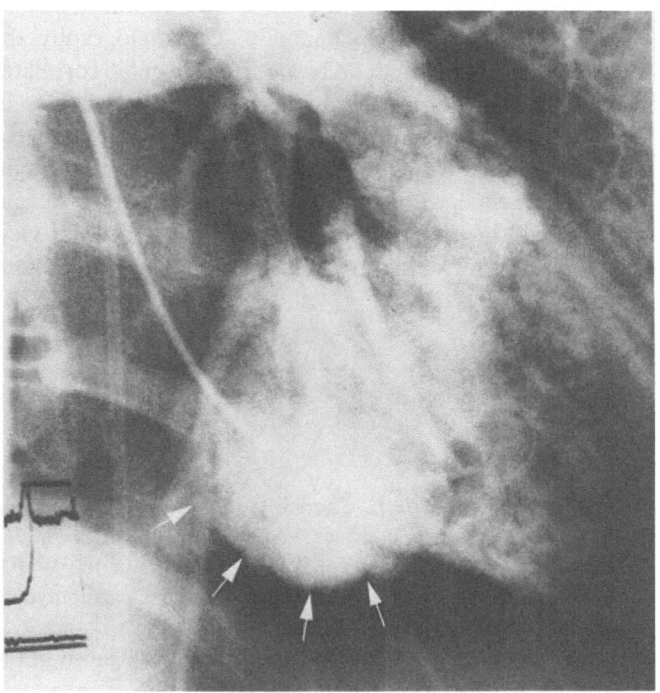

A   B

Fig. 6–29. *Right ventriculogram in a patient with arrhythmogenic right ventricular dysplasia.* **A** Diastole, **B** systole. A localized aneurysm in the inflow portion of the right ventricular wall (*arrows*) becomes especially prominent during systole. The trabeculations in the wall of the aneurysm indicate the presence of myocardium. Thus, partial Uhl anomaly is excluded. The coronary arteries were normal on selective coronary arteriography. At operation subepicardial fatty infiltration was found.

Arrhythmogenic Right Ventricular Dysplasia

This entity, consisting of a specific cardiomyopathy generally limited to the RV, was first described by Fontaine in 1976. The entity is characterized by global dilatation or focal aneurysms of the RV free wall. At surgery, excess subepicardial fat is observed over the RV, together with adipose and fibrous tissue between the muscle cells of the affected myocardium. The process may extend into the adjacent ventricular septum and LV wall.

Affected individuals present with ventricular premature beats, left bundle-branch block or paroxysms of ventricular tachycardia singly or in a combination.

The plain films may show RV dilatation or a localized bulge in the outflow tract. On M-mode echocardiography the RV may be enlarged, 2-D echocardiography may reveal areas of hypokinesis or outpouching of the RV wall. Right ventriculography (Fig. 6–29) shows localized wall motion abnormalities or aneurysms of the free wall in the inflow portion, apex, or outflow tract. Trabeculations in the wall of such aneurysms indicate the presence of myocardium, thus differentiating these abnormalities from examples of partial Uhl anomaly. The coronary arteries are normal on selective angiography.

Surgery is indicated if arrhythmias are refractory to treatment. Epicardial mapping during induced ventricular tachycardia at the time of surgery shows that the abnormal activation arises over the area of abnormal myocardium. Incisions are made in the wall of the RV to interrupt the course of the abnormal activation. A radical approach consists of complete excision and reimplantation of the RV wall, while preserving the coronary artery supply.

Uhl Anomaly

Uhl anomaly or the "parchment right ventricle" of Osler consists of hypoplasia or aplasia of the entire RV myocardium. The epicardium and endocardium of the wall of the RV lie adjacent to each other with no intervening cardiac muscle. The myocardium of the septum is normal, but at the junction of the septum and the RV wall the myocardium ends abruptly. The coronary arteries are normal. The RA and RV are markedly dilated. A right-to-left shunt may occur at the atrial level and may be accompanied by cyanosis.

The electrocardiogram shows RA and LV hypertrophy. On plain films Uhl anomaly may simulate Ebstein anomaly, cardiomyopathy, pericardial effusion, congenital tricuspid insufficiency with short chordae tendineae or idiopathic dilatation of the RA. M-mode echocardiographic findings are similar to those associated with Ebstein anomaly. The RV is dilated, the tricuspid valve closes later than normal (normally, tricuspid closure occurs no later than 0.03 seconds after mitral closure). A relatively normal position of the tricuspid valve in instances of the Uhl anomaly tends to differentiate that disorder from the Ebstein anomaly. On 2-D echocardiography in instances of Uhl anomaly the tricuspid valve is attached normally and not displaced distally as in the Ebstein anomaly. On angiography the RV is dilated and akinetic. Absence of trabeculae correlates with the absence of myocardium within the RV free wall. The attachment of the tricuspid valve is at the atrioventricular groove, while in Ebstein anomaly the tricuspid valve is attached within the RV cavity, causing a second notch along the diaphragmatic surface on the frontal view of the right ventriculogram. This second notch is present in addition to a similar notch representing the atrioventricular groove (see Fig. 7–151C).

Medical treatment consists of rest and diuretics. Procedures such as the Glenn anastomosis or the Fontan procedure, which bypass the RV, may improve pulmonary blood flow. Correction of associated abnormalities (e.g., atrial septal defect, pulmonary stenosis, pulmonary atresia) may be necessary.

Bibliography

General References

Bradenburg RO, Chazov E, Cherian G, Falase AO, Grosgogeat Y, Kawai C, Joogen F, Judez VM, Orinius E, Goodwin JF, Olsen EGJ, Oakley CM, Pisa Z (1981) Report of the WHO-ISFC task force on definition and classification of cardiomyopathies. Circulation 64:437A–438A

Fowler NO (1964) Classification and differential diagnosis of the myocardiopathies. Prog Cardiovasc Dis 7:1–16

Giles TD (1981) Cardiomyopathy: A spectrum of disease. Cardiol Ser Baylor Coll Med 4:6–36

Goodwin JF (1972) Clarification of the cardiomyopathies. Mod Concepts Cardiovasc Dis 41:41–46

Goodwin JF, Gordon H, Hollman A, Bishop MB (1961) Clinical aspects of cardiomyopathy. Br Med J 1:5219–5230

Harris LC, Nghiem ZX (1972) Cardiomyopathies in infants and children. Prog Cardiovasc Dis 15:255–287

McGuire J (1969) The cardiomyopathies (primary myocardial disease, myocardosis, idiopathic cardiac hypertrophy, myocardiopathy, cardiopathy, idiopathic cardiomyopathy). Semin Roentgenol 4:299–310

Dilated Cardiomyopathy

Corya BC, Feigenbaum H, Rasmussen S, Black MJ (1974) Echocardiographic features of congestive cardiomyopathy compared with normal subjects and patients with coronary artery disease. Circulation 49:1153–1159

Elkayam U, Gardin JM, Berkley R, Hughes CA, Henry WL (1983) The use of Doppler flow velocity measurement to assess the hemodynamic response to vasodilators in patient with heart failure. Circulation 67:377–383

Fenoglio JT, Ursell PC, Kellog CF, Drusin RE, Weiss MB (1983) Diagnosis and classification of myocarditis by endomyocardial biopsy. N Engl J Med 308:12–18

Fuster V, Gersch BJ, Guiliani ER, Tajik AJ, Brandenburg RO, Frye RL (1981) The natural history of idioathic dilated cardiomyopathy. Am J Cardiol 47:525–531

Hassell LA, Fowles RE, Stinson EB (1981) Patients with congestive cardiomyopathy as cardiac transplant recipients. Indications for and results of cardiac transplantation and comparison with patients with coronary artery disease. Am J Cardiol 47:1205–1209

Hill CA, Harle TS, Gaston W (1968) Cardiomyopathy: A review of 59 patients with emphasis on the plain chest roentgenogram. Am J Roentgenol 104:433–439

James TN (1983) Myocarditis and cardiomyopathy. N Engl J Med 308:39–41

Pierpont GL, Cohn JN, Franciosa JA (1978) Arch Intern Med 138:1847–1850

Steere AC, Grodzicki RL, Kornblatt AN, Craft JE, Barbour AG, Burgdorfer W, Schmid GP, Johnson E, Malawista SE (1983) The spirochetal etiology of Lyme disease. N Engl J Med 308:733–740

Tripp ME, Katcher ML, Peters HA, Gilbert EF, Arya S, Hodach RJ, Shug AL (1981) Systemic carnitive deficiency presenting as familial endocardial fibroelastosis: a treatable cardiomyopathy. N Engl J Med 305:385–390

Waber LJ, Valle D, Neill C, DiMauro S, Shug A (1982) Carnitive deficiency presenting as familial cardiomyopathy: a treatable defect in carnitive transport. J Pediatr 101:700–705

Hypertrophic Cardiomyopathy

Awdeh MR, Erwin S, Young JM, Nunn S (1978) Systolic anterior motion of the mitral valve caused by sarcoid involving the septum. South Med J 71:969–971

Blaufuss AH, Laks MM, Garner D, Ishimoto BM, Criley JM (1979) Production of ventricular hypertrophy simulating idiopathic hypertropic subaortic stenosis (IHSS) by subhypertensive infusion of norepinephrine (NE) in the conscious dog. Clin Res 23:77A

Boughner DR, Schuld RL, Persuad JA (1975) Hypertrophic obstructive cardiomyopathy. Assessment by echocardiographic and Doppler ultrasound techniques. Br Heart J 37:917–923

Breitweser JA, Meyer RA, Sperling MA, Tsang RC, Kaplan S (1980) Cardiac septal hypertrophy in hyperinsulinemic infants. J Pediatr 96:535–539

Brockenbrough EC, Braunwald E, Morrow AG (1961) A hemodynamic technic for the detection of hypertropic subaortic stenosis. Circulation 23:189–194

Cabin HS, Costello RM, Vasudevan G, Maron BJ, Roberts WC (1981) Cardiac lymphoma mimicking hypertrophic cardiomyopathy. Am Heart J 102:466–468

Clark CE, Henry WL, Epstein SE (1973) Familial prevalence and genetic transmission of idiopathic hypertrophic subaortic stenosis. N Engl J Med 289:709–714

Colucci WS, Lorell BH, Schoen FJ, Warhol MJ, Grossman W (1982) Hypertrophic obstructive cardiomyopathy due to Fabry's disease. N Engl J Med 307:926–928

Come PC, Bulkley BH, Goodman ZD, Hutchins GM, Pitt BM, Fortuin NJ (1977) Hypercontractile states simulating hypertrophic cardiomyopathy. Circulation 55:901–908

Darsee JR (1981) The hypertrophic heart syndromes: A glance at the chromosome. Am Heart J 101:124–126

Dinsmore RE, Sanders CA, Harthorne JW (1966) Mitral regurgitation in idiopathic hypertrophic subaortic stenosis. N Engl J Med 275:1225–1228

Doi Yl, McKenna WJ, Gehrke J, Oakley CM, Goodwin JF (1980) M-mode echocardiography in hypertrophic cardiomyopathy: Diagnostic criteria and prediction of obstruction. Am J Cardiol 45:6–14

Ferraus VJ, Morrow AG, Roberts WC (1972) Myocardial ultrastructure in idiopathic hypertrophic subaortic stenosis. A study of operatively excised left ventricular outflow tract muscle in 14 patients. Circulation 45:769–792

Green CE, Elliot LP, Coghlan HC (1981) Improved cineangiographic evaluation of hypertrophic cardiomyopathy by caudocranial left anterior oblique view. Am Heart J 102:1015–1021

Henry WL, Clark CE, Epstein SE (1973) Asymmetric septal hypertrophy (ASH): The unifying link in the IHSS disease spectrum: Observations regarding its pathogenesis, pathophysiology, and course. Circulation 47:827–832

Isner JM, Falcone MW, Virmani R, Roberts WC (1979) Cardiac sarcoma causing "ASH" and simulating coronary heart disease. Am J Med 66:1025–1030

Maron BJ, Epstein SE (1980) Hypertrophic cardiomyopathy. Recent observations regarding the specificity of three hallmarks of the disease: Asymmetric septal hypertrophy, septal disorganization and systolic anterior motion of the anterior mitral leaflet. Am J Cardiol 45:141–154

Matsumori A, Kawai C, Wakabayashi A, Terasaki PI, Park MS, Sakurami T, Veno Y (1981) HLA-DRW4 antigen linkage in patients with hypertrophic obstructive cardiomyopathy. Am Heart J 101:14–16

Popp RL, Harrison CD (1969) Ultrasound in the diagnosis and evaluation of therapy of idiopathic hypertrophic subaortic stenosis. Circulation 40:905–914

Redwood DR, Scherer JL, Epstein SE (1974) Biventricular cine angiography in the evaluation of patients with asymmetric septal hypertrophy. Circulation 49:1116–1121

St. John Sutton MG, Tajik AJ, Gurliani ER, Gordon H, Daniel WP (1981) Hypertrophic obstructive cardiomyopathy and lentiginosis: A little known neural ectodermal syndrome. Am J Cardiol 47:214–217

Sanderson JE, Gibson DG, Brown DJ, Goodwin JF (1977) Left ventricular filling in hypertrophic cardiomyopathy. An angiographic study. Br Heart J 39:661–670

Sengers RCA, ter Haar JMF, Trijbels JL, Willems JL, Daniels O, Stradhouders AM (1975) Congenital cataract and mitochondrial myopathy of skeletal and heart muscle associated with lactic aridosis after exercise. The Journal of Pediatrics 86:873–880

Shah PM, Gramiak R, Kramer DH (1969) Ultrasound localization of left ventricular outflow obstruction in hypertrophic obstructive cardiomyopathy. Circulation 40:3–11

Shub C, Williamson MD, Tajik AJ (1981) Dynamic left ventricular outflow tract obstruction associated with pheochromocytoma. Am Heart J 102:286–290

Simon AL, Ross J Jr., Gault JH (1967) Angiographic anatomy of the left ventricle and mitral valve in idiopathic hypertrophic subaortic stenosis. Circulation 36:852–867

Spindola-Franco H, Codini MA, Nivatpumin T (1976) Biplane, biventricular angiography for the assessment of idopathic hypertrophic subaortic stenosis. Circulation 54:41

Way GL, Wolfe RR, Eshaghpour E, Bender RL, Jaffe RB, Rutenberg HD (1979) The natural history of hypertrophic cardiomyopathy in infants of diabetic mothers. J Pediatr 95:1020–1025

Restrictive Cardiomyopathy

Burch GE, DePasquale NP (1970) Recognition and prevention of cardiomyopathy. Subcommittee on cardiomyopathy. Circulation 42:A47–A53

Fine G (1968) Neoplasms of the pericardium and heart. In: Gould SE (ed) Pathology of the heart and blood vessels, 3rd edn. Thomas, Springfield, Ill, pp 851–883

Hall SW Jr, Theologides A, From AHL, Gobel FL, Fortuny IE, Lawrence CJ, Edwards JE (1977) Hypereosinophilic syndrome with biventricular involvement. Circulation 55:217–222

Hansen AT, Eskildsen P, Gorzsche H (1951) Pressure curves from the right auricle and the right ventricle in chronic constrictive pericarditis. Circulation 3:881–888

Hill KR, Still WJS, McKinney B (1967) Jamaican cardiomyopathy. Br Heart J 29:594–601

Hirschmann JV (1978) Pericardial constriction. Am Heart J 96:110–122

Meaney E, Shabetai R, Bhargava V, Shearer M, Weidner C, Mangiardi LM, Smalling R, Peterson K (1976) Cardiac amyloidosis, constrictive pericarditis and restrictive cardiomyopathy. Am J Cardiol 38:547–556

Tyberg TI, Goodyer AVN, Hurst VW, Alexander J, Langou RA (1981) Left ventricular filling in differentiating restrictive amyloid cardiomyopathy and constrictive pericarditis. Am J Cardiol 47:791–796

Endomyocardial Fibrosis

Andy JJ, Bishara FF, Soyinka OO (1981) Relation of severe eosinophilia and microfilariasis to chronic African endomyocardial fibrosis. Br Heart J 45:672–680

Becker BJP, Chatgidakis CB, van Lingen B (1964) Cardiovascular collagenosis with parietal endocardial thrombosis. A clinicopathologic study of forty cases. Circulation 7:315–356

Chew CYC, Ziady GM, Raphael MJ, Nellen M, Oakley CM (1977) Primary restrictive cardiomyopathy: Non-tropical endomyocardial fibrosis and hypereosinophilic heart disease. Br Heart J 39:399–413

Davies JNP (1948) Endocardial fibrosis in Africans. East African Med J 25:10–14

Davies JNP, Coles RM (1960) Some considerations regarding obscure disease affecting the mural endocardium. Am Heart J 59:600–631

Dubost C, Prigent C, Gerbaux A, Maurice P, Passelecq, J Rulliere R, Carpentier A, Deloche A (1981) Surgical treatment of constrictive fibrous endocarditis. J Thorac Cardiovasc Surg 82:585–591

Hess OM, Turina M, Senning A, Goebel NH, Scholer Y, Krayenbuehe HP (1978) Br Heart J 40:406–415

James CF, Hutchins GM (1980) Congestive heart failure secondary to diffuse organized biventricular mural thrombus following mitral valve replacement. Chest 72:338–340

Metras D, Coulibaly O, Ouattera K, Chauvet J, Ekra A, Longechaud A, Bertrand E, Castaneda AR (1982) Endomyocardial fibrosis. J Thorac Cardiovasc Surg 83:52–64

Roberts WC, Leigler DG, Carbone PP (1969) Endomyocardial disease and eosinophilia. A clinical and pathologic spectrum. Am J Med 46:28–42

Shillingbard JP, Somers K (1961) Clinical and hemodynamic patterns in endomyocardial fibrosis. Br Heart J 33:433–436

Infiltrative Cardiomyopathies (Amyloidosis, Sarcoidosis and Hemochromatosis)

Arnett EN, Neinhuis AW, Henry WL, Ferrans VJ, Redwood DR, Roberts WC (1975) Massive myocardial hemosiderosis: A structure-function conference at the National Heart and Lung Institute. Am Heart J 90:777–787

Borer JS, Henry WL, Epstein SE (1977) Echocardiographic observations in patients with systemic infiltrative disease involving the heart. Am J Cardiol 39:184–188

Chew C, Ziady GM, Raphael MJ, Oakley CM (1975) The functional defect in amyloid heart disease. The "stiff heart" syndrome. Am J Cardiol 36:438–444

Silverman KJ, Hutchins GM, Bulkley BH (1978) Cardiac sarcoid: A clinicopathologic study of 84 unselected patients with systemic sarcoidosis. Circulation 58:1204–1211

Siqueira-Filho AG, Cunha CLP, Tajik AJ, Seward JB, Schattenberg T, Giuliani ER (1981) M-mode and two-dimensional echocardiographic features in cardiac amyloidosis. Circulation 63:188–196

Arrythmogenic Right Ventricular Dysplasia

Baron A, Nanda NC, Falkoff M, Barold SS, Gallagher JJ (1982) Two-dimensional echocardiographic detection of arrhythmogenic right ventricular dysplasia. Am Heart J 103:1066–1067

Dungan WT, Garson A Jr, Gillette PC (1981) Arrhythmogenic right ventricular dysplasia: A cause of ventricular tachycardia in children with apparently normal hearts. Am Heart J 102:745–750

Fontaine G, Guiraudon G, Frank R, Vedel J, Grosgogeat Y, Cabrol C, Facquet J (1977) Stimulation studies and epicardial mapping in ventricular tachycardia: Study of mechanisms and selection for surgery. In Kulbertus HE (ed.): Reentrant arrhythmias. Lancaster, MTP Press Ltd, p. 344

Guiraudon G, Fontaine G, Frank R, Leandri R, Barra J, Cabrol C (1981) Surgical treatment of ventricular tachycardia guided by ventricular mapping in 23 patients without coronary artery disease. Ann Thorac Surg 32:439–450

Guiraudon GM, Klein GJ, Gulamhusein SS, Painvin GA, Del Campo C, Gonzales JC, Ko PT (1983) Total disconnection of the right ventricular free wall: Surgical treatment of right ventricular tachycardia associated with right ventricular dysplasia. Circulation 67:463–470

Uhl HSM (1952) A previously undescribed congenital malformation of the heart. Almost total absence of the myocardium of the right ventricle. Bull Johns Hopkins Hosp 91:197–209

Uhl Anomaly

Arcilla RA, Gasul BM (1961) Congenital aplasia or marked hypoplasia of the myocardium of the right ventricle (Uhl's anomaly) J Pediatr 58:381–388

Asayama J, Matsuura T, Endo N, Matsukubo H, Furukawa K (1977) Idiopathic enlargement of the right atrium. Am J Cardiol 40:620–623

Barritt DW, Urich H (1956) Congenital tricuspid incompetence. Br Heart J 18:133–136

Cote M, Davignon A, Fouron J (1973) Congenital hypoplasia of right ventricular myocardial (Uhl's anomaly) associated with pulmonary atresia in a newborn. Am J Cardiol 31:658–661

French JW, Baum D, Popp R (1975) Echocardiographic findings in the Uhl's anomaly. Am J Cardiol 36:349–353

Perrin EV, Mehrizi A (1965) Isolated free-wall hypoplasia of the right ventricle. Am J Dis Child 109:558–566

Segall HN (1950) Parchment Heart (Osler). Am Heart J 40:948–950

Sheldon WC, Johnson DC, Favaloro RG (1969) Idiopathic enlargement of the right atrium. Am J Cardiol 23:278–284

Uhl HSM (1952) Previously undescribed congenital malformation of the heart: Almost total absence of myocardium of the right ventricle. Bull Johns Hopkins Hosp 91:197–205

Zuberbuhler JR, Blank E (1970) Hypoplasia of right ventricular myocardium. Am J Roentgenol 110:491–496

7 Congenital Heart Disease

Hugo Spindola-Franco, Bernard G. Fish,
and Robert Eisenberg,

The classification of heart disease in children presents some practical difficulties. In general usage; the term *congenital* has come to mean those structural abnormalities of the heart due to faulty embryogenesis, regardless of etiology. Some congenital heart diseases thus designated may not be detectable until later in childhood; some may not be detected until adulthood; and some may not become clinically apparent at any time. Conversely, infective heart disorders may be acquired in utero and thus be present at birth. The traditional approach is to classify heart disease in children as congenital or acquired, regardless of the presence or absence of disease at birth. In general, that approach will be followed in this work.

In the underdeveloped nations of the world, rheumatic heart disease, the most common form of acquired heart disease, is still the predominant problem. In the developed nations the use of penicillin for the treatment and prophylaxis of streptococcal infections has reduced the incidence of rheumatic heart disease dramatically. As a result, congenital heart defects are more commonly encountered than infective heart disease.

Etiology of Congenital Heart Defects

Factors that predispose toward congenital heart defects may be toxic, metabolic, infective or hereditary. Toxic agents demonstrated to be associated with heart defects include alcohol and various drugs (e.g., dilantin, thalidomide). Maternal diabetes also has been shown to be related to an increased incidence of congenital heart defects. Maternal lupus erythematosus is associated with congenital heart block. Rubella is known to produce peripheral pulmonic stenosis as well as intracardiac defects. Many types of heart disorders have been shown to have a Mendelian inheritance pattern in some family groups; atrial septal defect, ventricular septal defect, mitral valve prolapse and hypertrophic cardiomyopathy are examples. Inherited syndromes, such as Noonan Syndrome, Holt-Oram syndrome and Ellis van Creveld Syndrome may also be associated with heart defects. Most of the chromosomal defects include congenital heart disease. Turner syndrome, Down syndrome, trisomy 13–15 (Bartholin-Patau syndrome) and trisomy 17–18 (trisomy E) are most common. These factors are mentioned in the descriptions of the entities below.

Incidence of Congenital Heart Defects

The incidence of congenital heart disease is in the area of 7/1000 live births. The incidence of individual malformations is difficult to assess and varies appreciably with age. Studies by Mitchell et al. and by Ober et al. provide considerable data on the incidence in the newborn period. Spontaneous closure of ventricular septal defects on the one hand and death of some babies with complex cardiac lesions at the other extreme significantly change the incidence and relative frequency of individual lesions during the first year of life. In the newborn the most common causes of early difficulty (heart failure or cyanosis or both) are hypoplastic left heart syndrome, transposition of the great arteries, pulmonary atresia with intact ventricular septum, atrioventricularis communis (A-V communis, atrioventricular canal), tetralogy of Fallot, ventricular septal defect, total anomalous pulmonary venous return, truncus arteriosus, cardiomyopathy (e.g., endocardial fibroelastosis, anomalous origin of the left coronary artery, transient left ventricular dysfunction), and patent ductus arteriosus (premature infants). The most common acyanotic lesions present in childhood, in approximate order of frequency, are ventricular septal defect, patent ductus arteriosus, coarctation of the aorta, isolated pulmonic valvar stenosis, aortic valvar stenosis and atrial septal defect. The only common cyanotic lesion in children is tetralogy of Fallot and its variants.

On occasion, children survive with unoperated transposition of the great arteries, tricuspid atresia, single ventricle, persistent truncus arteriosus, A-V communis and pulmonary atresia.

Classification of Congenital Heart Defects

Congenital heart disease may be classified in many ways. However, giving primary consideration to the radiological presentation, a classification conceived by the authors appears rational, functional and practical (Table 7-1).

The authors have separated the cardiac disorders into six groups. The first four are defined by the hemodynamic abnormalities that are common to each group. The final two, abnormalities of the great vessels and abnormalities of visceroatrial situs, relate to the anatomy of the disorder. Many lesions have a variable presentation, depending on severity and the presence or absence of associated defects. As an example, uncomplicated tricuspid atresia occurs as a form of obstruction to the right side of the heart with cyanosis and decreased pulmonary vascularity. When transposition of the great vessels is also present, pulmonic stenosis is usually less severe, and pulmonary vascularity may be increased as with admixture lesions. Atresia of the mitral valve is classified as a left-sided obstructive lesion, but affected infants may have cyanosis and pulmonary overcirculation suggesting also an admixture lesion.

Terminology Used Frequently to Describe Congenital Heart Defects

Definitions of the hemodynamic abnormalities (e.g., left-to-right shunt, right heart obstruction) are included, with a brief presentation of hemodynamic data used to quantitate the severity of the lesions. Terms used to describe cardiac malpositions and abnormalities of visceroatrial situs are described briefly here and in detail in the appropriate section.

Situs and Atrioventricular Connections

Situs refers to the position of the viscera and the atria within the body. *Situs solitus* is normal and indicates that the right atrium is on the right and the left atrium is on the left. The situs of the lungs corresponds to the situs of the heart (thoracic situs). The liver, stomach and spleen are usually concordant, the liver being on the right and the stomach and spleen being on the left (abdominal situs solitus). A mirror-image of thoracic and abdominal situs solitus is called *situs inversus*. Rare cases are reported in which the thoracic situs is different from the abdominal situs (thoracoabdominal discordance). When one refers to the thoracic situs one refers only to the position of the atria. The ventricles may or may not be concordant with their respective atria. Normal connections are called *atrio-*

Table 7-1. Classification of Congenital Heart Defects

1. *Systemic-to-pulmonary communications*
   (L → R shunts)
   Increased pulmonary blood flow without cyanosis
2. *Admixture lesions*
   Transposition complexes, truncus arteriosus and total anomalous pulmonary venous return
   Increased pulmonary blood flow with cyanosis
3. *Right heart obstruction*
   Valvular, subvalvular, extracardiac with or without secondary R → L shunt
   Normal to decreased pulmonary blood flow (with or without cyanosis)
4. *Left heart obstruction*
   Valvular, subvalvular (discrete; muscular), extracardiac
   Normal pulmonary vasculature or pulmonary venous hypertension pattern without cyanosis (Infants may be cyanotic)
5. *Abnormalities of the great vessels* (*rings, slings, etc.*)
   Pulmonary vasculature normal unless associated with circulatory disturbances
6. *Cardiac malpositions and abnormalities of visceroatrial situs*
   Pulmonary vasculature variable
   Specific entities are predictable on the basis of other plain film findings

ventricular concordance, whereas reversed connections are called *atrioventricular discordance.* Situs solitus with atrioventricular concordance means that the right atrium is on the right and connects with the right ventricle. In situs solitus with atrioventricular discordance the right-sided right atrium connects to a left ventricle. Atrioventricular discordance is also called *ventricular inversion.* The atrioventricular valves follow their respective ventricles; thus the anatomical left ventricle carries a mitral valve, while the anatomical right ventricle has a tricuspid valve.

Left and Right Heart

The left heart in situs solitus normally includes the pulmonary veins, the left atrium, the left ventricle and the aorta. If the ventricles are inverted the anatomical right ventricle is on the left side, becoming part of the physiological left heart. The right heart normally includes the superior and inferior vena cava, right atrium, right ventricle and pulmonary arteries. Again, whichever ventricle is in the position to receive systemic venous (unoxygenated) blood and to pump the blood into the lungs is part of the physiological right heart or pulmonary circuit. The chambers that carry pulmonary venous blood (oxygenated blood) and pump into the aorta constitute the physiological left heart or systemic circulation. In situs inversus the structures are reversed. The physiological left heart (pulmonary veins, left atrium, left ventricle, aorta) is on the right, and the right heart (great veins, right atrium, right ventricle, pulmonary artery) is on the left. In situs inversus with ventricular inversion the anatomical left ventricle becomes part of the right heart, and the anatomical right ventricle becomes part of the left heart.

Right Heart Obstruction

According to the definitions just recorded, right heart obstruction might involve the pulmonary arteries (isolated or multiple pulmonic branch stenosis), the main pulmonary artery (supravalvar pulmonic stenosis), the pulmonary valve, (valvar pulmonic stenosis), the right ventricular outflow tract (infundibular pulmonic stenosis or atresia), the right ventricle (anomalous muscle bundle), the tricuspid valve (tricuspid stenosis or atresia) or the right atrium (neoplasms).

Table 7–5, in Section 3 of this chapter, is a list of the entities causing right heart obstruction. Hemodynamically these result in elevation of pressure proximal to the obstruction. If obstruction is severe and a communication exists between the right and left heart (e.g., ventricular septal defect, foramen ovale), a right-to-left shunt occurs, allowing blood to bypass the lungs. It is readily apparent that obstruction to the right side of the heart may thus result in pulmonary undercirculation and cyanosis.

Left Heart Obstruction

Obstruction of the left side of the heart may involve the aortic arch (coarctation of the aorta), ascending aorta (supravalvar aortic stenosis), aortic valve (valvar aortic stenosis), left ventricular outflow tract (membranous or muscular subaortic stenosis), left ventricle (endocardial fibroelastosis), mitral valve (mitral stenosis, parachute mitral valve), left atrium (cor triatriatum), or the pulmonary veins (pulmonary venous thrombosis, stenosis, or atresia). Table 7–7, in Section 4, is a list of entities causing left heart obstruction. Physiological consequences of severe left heart obstruction are reduction in systemic blood flow and development of pulmonary venous hypertension. During infancy high pressure in the left atrium may stretch the foramen ovale so that a left-to-right shunt results.

Left-to-Right Shunt

Left-to-right shunt indicates flow of blood from the left heart into the right heart. Left-to-right shunts result in pulmonary venous blood (oxygenated blood) returning to the pulmonary circulation. Thus pulmonary blood flow is augmented (pulmonary overcirculation). If a communication exists between chambers of the left and the right heart at the same level, blood flows from the left heart into the right heart because the pressures are normally higher in the left heart. The shunt will be reversed only if an additional abnormality (e.g., pulmonic stenosis or high pulmonary resistance) is associated.

A left-to-right shunt can be found at the atrial level (e.g., atrial septal defects, anomalous pulmonary venous return), the ventricular level (ventricular septal defect, coronary arteriovenous fistula), the great vessel level (patent ductus arteriosus, aorticopulmonary window) or in the periphery (arteriovenous malformations). Table 7–3, in Section 1, is a list of entities causing left-to-right shunt.

In situs solitus the left heart is on the left, the right heart is on the right, and a left-to-right shunt is directed from the left side of the body to the right side of the body. Thus, in this instance a physiological left-to-right shunt is also an anatomical left-to-right shunt. In situs inversus the left heart is on the right side of the body; in this situation a shunt from the left heart to the right heart is an anatomical right-to-left shunt, although the shunt behaves physiologically as if it were left to right. It is important to distinguish the concept of a physiological left-to-right shunt from that of an anatomical left-to-right shunt. The direction of flow of the shunt, apparent on angiography, has different physiological consequences that depend upon the situs.

A left-to-right shunt is identified at catheterization by the appearance of oxygenated blood in a chamber where it is not expected to be (an "oxygen step-up"). As an example, if on sampling in the right atrium the oxygen saturation is found to be 70% and saturation in the right ventricle is 80%, a left-to-right shunt at the ventricular level is strongly suspected. The differential diagnosis of this oxygen step-up includes ventricular septal defect, coronary arteriovenous fistula, or ruptured sinus of Valsalva communicating with the right ventricle. An ostium primum atrial septal defect may also produce an oxygen step-up in the right ventricle because it is so close to the tricuspid valve that oxygenated blood may stream directly from the left atrium into the right ventricle without mixing in the right atrium. Left-to-right shunts at other levels are indicated by oxygen step-up in the right atrium or pulmonary artery. Of course, once a step-up develops it will be carried over into the subsequent chambers. As an example, given a left-to-right shunt at the atrial level, the oxygen step-up will be detected in the right atrium and carried over to the right ventricle and pulmonary artery. If a second shunt is present a further step-up may be encountered.

Normal oxygen saturations and normal intracardiac pressures are listed in Table 7–2, along with minimum oxygen step-ups that would indicate left-to-right shunts. Note that a small oxygen step-up normally occurs between the superior vena cava and the right atrium; thus a step-up of 12% is required to identify a shunt at the atrial level. Smaller oxygen step-ups are required to diagnose shunts at the ventricular and great vessel level. See below for quantitation of left-to-right shunts.

Right-to-Left Shunt

A right-to-left shunt indicates flow from the right heart into the left heart, resulting in desaturation of the systemic circulation. For a right-to-left shunt to occur a communication between the two sides must be present as well as an additional disorder (e.g., tricuspid atresia, pulmonic stenosis, increase of pulmonary resistance). As an example, blood flows from left to right through an uncomplicated ventricular septal defect; however, if pulmonic stenosis or increased pulmonary vascular resistance is also present, blood will flow from right to left through the ventricular septal defect. Right-to-left shunts can occur at other levels as well. They

Table 7-2. Normal Intracardiac Pressures and Oxygen Saturations

	Infants	Children	Adults	O₂ Sat (%)	Minimum Step-Up
Superior vena cava				65–75	
Inverior vena cava				65–80	
Right atrium	a wave = 3–6 v wave = 2–4 mean = 0–4	a = 3–7 v = 2–5 m = 2–5	a = 2–10 v = 2–10 m = 0–8	65–80	RA { 8–10% Sat† 6–7% Sat‡ 1.9 Vol% O₂ content†
Right ventricle	$\frac{15-25}{1-5}$	$\frac{15-30}{2-5}$	$\frac{15-30}{0-8}$	63–75	RV { 6–8% Sat† 4–5% Sat‡ 0.9 Vol% O₂ content†
Pulmonary artery*	$\frac{15-25}{10-16}$ (12–20)	$\frac{15-30}{5-10}$ (10–20)	$\frac{15-30}{4-12}$ (9–16)	63–75	PA { 3% Sat† 0.5 Vol% O₂ content†
Pulmonary wedge (Left atrium)	a = 3–5 v = 4–7 m = 3–6	a = 3–7 v = 3–15 m = 5–10	a = 3–15 v = 3–15 m = 1–12	97–100	Desaturation 94% or lower
Left ventricle	$\frac{65-80}{0-5}$	$\frac{80-110}{5-12}$	$\frac{90-140}{3-12}$	97–100	94% or lower
Aorta*	$\frac{65-80}{45-60}$ (60–65)	$\frac{80-110}{65-75}$ (70–80)	$\frac{90-140}{60-90}$ (70–105)	97–100	94% or lower

* $\frac{\text{Systolic}}{\text{Diastolic}}$ (mean) † One set of data ‡ Two sets of data

are identified in the catheterization laboratory by desaturation of the chamber into which the shunt occurs and of subsequent chambers as well.

Bidirectional Shunts

Bidirectional shunting is frequently observed if a ventricular septal defect is associated with moderate pulmonic stenosis. During cardiac catheterization, sampling will reveal an oxygen step-up in the right side of the heart as well as systemic desaturation. Bidirectional shunting can occur at other levels as well if the pressures are equal on the two sides of a defect. Bidirectional shunting is present at the atrial level in transposition of the great vessels with atrial septal defect and at the great vessel level in aorticopulmonary window with high pulmonary resistance.

Venous Admixture

An admixture lesion is one in which mixing of systemic and pulmonary venous blood occurs, because all the blood flows through a single chamber. Transposition complexes, truncus arteriosus, single ventricle, atrioventricularis (A-V) communis, double-outlet right ventricle, total anomalous pulmonary venous drainage and criss-cross heart are included in this group. Because of mixing of the two venous streams, desaturation of the arterial circulation occurs along with pulmonary overcirculation. The oxygen saturation of the systemic circulation is determined by the relative amount of pulmonary and systemic venous return. If pulmonary blood flow is unobstructed the oxygen saturation will be high and clinical cyanosis may not be visible. Nevertheless, blood studies will demonstrate desaturation. On the other hand, if pulmonic stenosis or elevation of pulmo-

nary resistance reduces pulmonary blood flow, then the oxygen saturation will be low and cyanosis evident.

Uncomplicated Dextrotransposition of the Great Vessels

Dextrotransposition of the great vessels (D-TGA) is considered to be an admixture lesion because it occurs with cyanosis in combination with pulmonary overcirculation. Nevertheless the hemodynamics are unique because of the abnormal connections. Consequently the concepts of left heart, right heart, left-to-right shunt, and right-to-left shunt require some explanation.

With D-TGA the two sides of the heart are connected in parallel so that pulmonary venous blood returns to the left atrium and is pumped back to the lungs by the left ventricle (physiologic left-to-right shunt). The systemic venous blood returns to the right atrium and right ventricle and is recirculated to the body (physiologic right-to-left shunt). The two streams might be termed systemic circulation and pulmonary circulation. The right heart (right atrium and right ventricle) is part of the systemic circulation, while the left heart (left atrium and left ventricle) is part of the pulmonary circulation. Under these circumstances blood flowing from the right atrium into the left atrium through an atrial septal defect constitutes an anatomic right-to-left shunt, which augments pulmonary blood flow. Conversely, blood that flows from the left atrium to the right atrium defines an anatomical left-to-right shunt, which returns oxygenated blood to the systemic circuit. In these instances the concept of effective pulmonary blood flow is very important. Effective pulmonary blood flow may be defined as the unoxygenated blood that crosses from the systemic circulation into the pulmonary circulation to enter the lungs. An equal and opposite left-to-right shunt must coexist so that oxygenated blood is returned to the systemic circuit. If this bidirectional shunt is small (poor mixing) the patient will be severely cyanotic and acidotic. If the shunt is adequate, oxygen supply to the systemic circulation allows activity and growth.

Quantitation of Blood Flow, Size of the Shunt and Vascular Resistance

Systemic and pulmonary blood flow are calculated by means of the Fick equation: Cardiac output ($\dot{Q}s$) is equal to the amount of oxygen consumed per unit time by the subject ($\dot{V}O_2$), divided by the amount of oxygen extracted from each liter of blood.

$$\text{(I)} \quad \dot{Q}s \text{ (liters/min)} = \frac{\dot{V}O_2 \text{ (ml } O_2/\text{min)}}{Ca_{O_2} - Cv_{O_2} \text{ (ml } O_2/\text{liter)}}$$

where Ca_{O_2} = oxygen content of arterial blood and Cv_{O_2} = oxygen content of mixed venous blood. Mixed venous blood is obtained from the pulmonary artery in individuals without left-to-right shunts. In those with left-to-right shunts systemic venous blood is sampled in the chamber proximal to the shunt.

Similarly pulmonary blood flow ($\dot{Q}p$) is calculated by the formula:

$$\text{(II)} \qquad \dot{Q}p = \frac{\dot{V}O_2}{Cpv_{O_2} - Cpa_{O_2}}$$

where Cpv_{O_2} = pulmonary venous oxygen content and Cpa_{O_2} = pulmonary artery oxygen content. Normally, pulmonary blood flow ($\dot{Q}p$) is equal to systemic blood flow.

If a left-to-right shunt is present the oxygen step-up will raise pulmonary artery O_2 content and narrow the pulmonary arteriovenous difference. The calculated pulmonary blood flow will then be greater than the systemic blood flow by the amount of the left-to-right shunt.

$$\text{(III)} \qquad \dot{Q}L \rightarrow R = \dot{Q}p - \dot{Q}s$$

For description of complex defects with bidirectional shunting a concept designated effective pulmonary blood flow ($\dot{Q}ep$) is used to define the amount of mixed venous blood that eventually reaches the lungs to be oxygenated.

Effective pulmonary blood flow is calculated by this formula:

$$\text{(IV)} \qquad \dot{Q}ep = \frac{\dot{V}O_2}{Cpv_{O_2} - Cmv_{O_2}}$$

where Cpv_{O_2} = O_2 content of pulmonary venous blood and Cmv_{O_2} = O_2 content of mixed systemic venous blood.

Resistance

This term is defined as the ratio of driving pressure to blood flow:

$$R = \frac{P}{F}$$

where R = resistance, P = mean driving pressure (or pressure difference across the system) and F = flow rate. Depending upon the units used, resistance may be expressed in Wood units (WU = mmHg $\div$ liters/min) or as absolute resistance units (dyne/cm^2 $\div$ cm^3/sec) or dyne $\cdot$ sec $\cdot$ cm^{-5}. WU are converted to absolute resistance units (ARU) by multiplying by a factor of 80.

$$WU \times 80 = ARU$$

Calculations for the various representations of vascular resistance follow:

$$Rp = \frac{(\overline{PA} - \overline{LA})}{\dot{Q}p}$$

$$Rpt = \frac{\overline{PA}}{\dot{Q}p}$$

$$Rs = \frac{\overline{SA} - \overline{RA}}{\dot{Q}s}$$

$$Rst = \frac{\overline{SA}}{\dot{Q}s}$$

$$\frac{Rp}{Rs} = \frac{\dot{Q}s}{\overline{SA}} \times \frac{\overline{PA}}{\dot{Q}p} = \frac{\dot{Q}s}{\dot{Q}p} \times \frac{\overline{PA}}{\overline{SA}}$$

Where Rp = pulmonary artery resistance (also called pulmonary vascular resistance); Rpt = total pulmonary resistance; Rs = systemic arterial resistance (also called systemic vascular resistance); Rst = total systemic resistance; $\overline{PA}$ = mean pulmonary artery pressure; $\overline{LA}$ = mean left atrial pressure; $\overline{SA}$ = mean systemic arterial pressure; $\overline{RA}$ = mean right atrial pressure; and Rp/Rs = resistance ratio.

Both flow and resistance can be normalized to body surface area so that results obtained for different-sized children and adults can be compared. This is done by dividing $\dot{Q}s$ and $\dot{Q}p$ by the body surface area (BSA) in square meters (M^2). The data obtained are often called indexes (e.g., $\dot{Q}s$/BSA = cardiac index, $\dot{Q}p$/BSA = indexed pulmonary blood flow, Rs/BSA = systemic resistance index). A normal total systemic resistance in an adult is about 1130 $\pm$ 178 dyne $\cdot$ sec $\cdot$ cm^{-5} ARU (18 $\pm$ 2 WU). Normal total pulmonary resistance is approximately 205 $\pm$ 51 ARU (2.6 $\pm$ .7WU), and normal pulmonary artery resistance is 67 $\pm$ 23 ARU (0.8 $\pm$ 0.3 WU). The resistance ratio (Rpt/Rst) should be less than 0.25. Pulmonary artery resistance is considered to be increased mildly when pulmonary artery resistance is greater than one third of systemic arterial resistance or >4–5 WU. Pulmonary artery resistance is severely increased when it is greater than 950 ARU (12 WU) or two thirds to three fourths of systemic resistance.

Another method of evaluating shunts is consideration of the ratio of pulmonary to systemic blood flow, or $\dot{Q}p/\dot{Q}s$. The formula for $\dot{Q}p/\dot{Q}s$ appears complicated, but can be simplified as follows:

$$\text{(V)} \qquad \frac{\dot{Q}p}{\dot{Q}s} = \frac{\dot{V}_{O_2}}{C_{pv_{O_2}} - C_{pa_{O_2}}} \times \frac{Csa_{O_2} - Cmv_{O_2}}{\dot{V}_{O_2}}$$

If $\dot{V}_{O_2}$ is canceled:

$$\text{(VI)} \qquad \frac{\dot{Q}p}{\dot{Q}s} = \frac{Csa_{O_2} - Cmv_{O_2}}{C_{pv_{O_2}} - C_{pa_{O_2}}}$$

In this equation O_2 saturations can be substituted for O_2 content. Thus this formula is useful in laboratories where micro O_2 contents may not be easily available, or if oxygen consumption has not been measured. Note that the factors of equation V include the Fick calculation of pulmonary blood flow (equation II) and the reciprocal of the Fick calculation of systemic blood flow (equation I):

$$\text{(VII)} \qquad \frac{\dot{Q}p}{\dot{Q}s} = \frac{\text{Sat } O_2 \text{ sa} - \text{Sat } O_2 \text{ mv}}{\text{Sat } O_2 pv - \text{Sat } O_2 \text{ pa}}$$

Where Sat O_2 sa = arterial O_2 saturation; Sat O_2 mv = mixed venous O_2 saturation; Sat O_2 pv = pulmonary vein O_2 saturation and Sat O_2 pa = pulmonary artery O_2 saturation.

A shunt that results in a pulmonary–systemic flow ratio of 1.5:1 or less is considered a small shunt. A ratio of 2:1 is designated a moderate shunt, and above 2.5:1 the shunt is large. On the other hand, pulmonary flow–systemic flow ratios less than 1:1 indicate the presence of a right-to-left shunt. On plain films a shunt less than 1.5:1 is difficult to recognize. Above $\dot{Q}p:\dot{Q}s = 1.8:1$, pulmonary overcirculation is evident on plain films. $\dot{Q}p:\dot{Q}s$ greater than 2:1 causes pulmonary overcirculation and enlargement of the cardiac chambers. The anatomical level of the shunt is then assessed by examining the size of the left atrium, left ventricle and aorta. If the shunt is at the atrial level the left atrium will be decompressed and thus will not be prominent. Instead, the right atrium, right ventricle and pulmonary artery are enlarged, while the aorta is normal or small. In the presence of a ventricular level shunt the left atrium will be enlarged by the excess pulmonary venous return and will be prominent on plain films. The left ventricle, right ventricle and pulmonary artery may also be enlarged, while the aorta is normal or small. If the shunt is at the great-vessel level (e.g., patent ductus arteriosus [PDA]) the shunted blood passes through the left atrium, left ventricle and ascending aorta. Thus these left-sided chambers may all be prominent. Although the size of the aorta is stressed as an important sign in the

differentiation of PDA from VSD, it is often unreliable, especially in infants and young children. In addition, LA enlargement may not always be evident on plain films of the chest in patients with VSD or PDA.

Indicator-Dilution Method

Indocyanine green dye is an indicator used in quantitating cardiac output and in identifying shunts. The dye is sensed by drawing blood through the cardiac catheter past a cuvette with one sensor that is sensitive to the color of the dye and one sensitive to the color of hemoglobin. The relative intensity of the two colors is used to calculate the concentration of dye in the blood. The area under the curve of concentration versus time can be used to quantitate cardiac output. The shape of the curve can be used to identify shunts if the injection site and the sampling site are known. As an example, if green dye is injected into the superior vena cava during sampling in the pulmonary artery, the dye should appear in the pulmonary artery about 7 seconds later, reach a peak and decline logarithmically. About 12 seconds later the dye should reappear, after circulating through the body and returning through the heart (Fig. 7–1).

If a left-to-right shunt is present, the dye will be carried back to the right side of the heart immediately after it flows through the lungs. The recirculated dye will then be carried out to the pulmonary artery and will appear as a deflection on the logarithmic downward slope of the curve of concentration. This phenomenon is called early recirculation or early reappearance of green dye. The height of the secondary peak can be used to estimate the size of the shunt. Other combinations of site of injection and site of sampling are used to localize shunts. In the presence of a right-to-left shunt the green dye will be carried from the right side of the heart almost immediately into the left side, without traversing the lungs. If the injection is in a vein and the site of sampling is in the arterial circulation, a peak of concentration will be noted before the onset of the normal curve—designated early appearance. Again, the height of the peak can be used to estimate the size of the right-to-left shunt.

Hydrogen Electrode

The hydrogen electrode is also used to identify left-to-right shunts. If hydrogen gas is breathed by the subject it will be absorbed into the pulmonary venous blood. If a platinum electrode is in the right side of the heart during the inhalation a voltage will be produced if the hydrogen is carried into the right side by a left-to-right shunt. The location of the shunt is determined by moving the electrode from chamber to chamber during successive inhalations. The most proximal chamber in which a change in voltage occurs is considered to be the one into which the left-to-right shunt flows. Although the hydrogen electrode is very sensitive to shunts, its use is limited because of its inability to

Fig. 7–1. *A normal green dye curve, curves observed with left-to-right shunts and curves observed with right-to-left shunts.* These curves are made by drawing blood from an artery after injection of green dye into a vein. The *arrows* mark the time of injection and the normal appearance time. The concentration curve normally reaches a peak 6–10 seconds after its appearance and then descends logarithmically. After about 12–14 seconds a recirculation curve interrupts the downslope of the initial curve. With a left-to-right shunt early recirculation occurs, causing a bump on the downslope of the curve before the normal recirculation curve (early recirculation). This is because of the blood that immediately reenters the pulmonary circulation without circulating through the systemic bed. In patients with large left-to-right shunt the downslope of the curve is entirely displaced, remaining higher than normal throughout, and never developing a logarithmic descent. Valvar insufficiency also tends to spread out the curve so that cardiac output and shunts can not be reliably detected in face of insufficiency. A right-to-left shunt is indicated by early appearance of the green dye producing a bump on the buildup slope. This bump is caused by venous blood that bypasses the lungs.

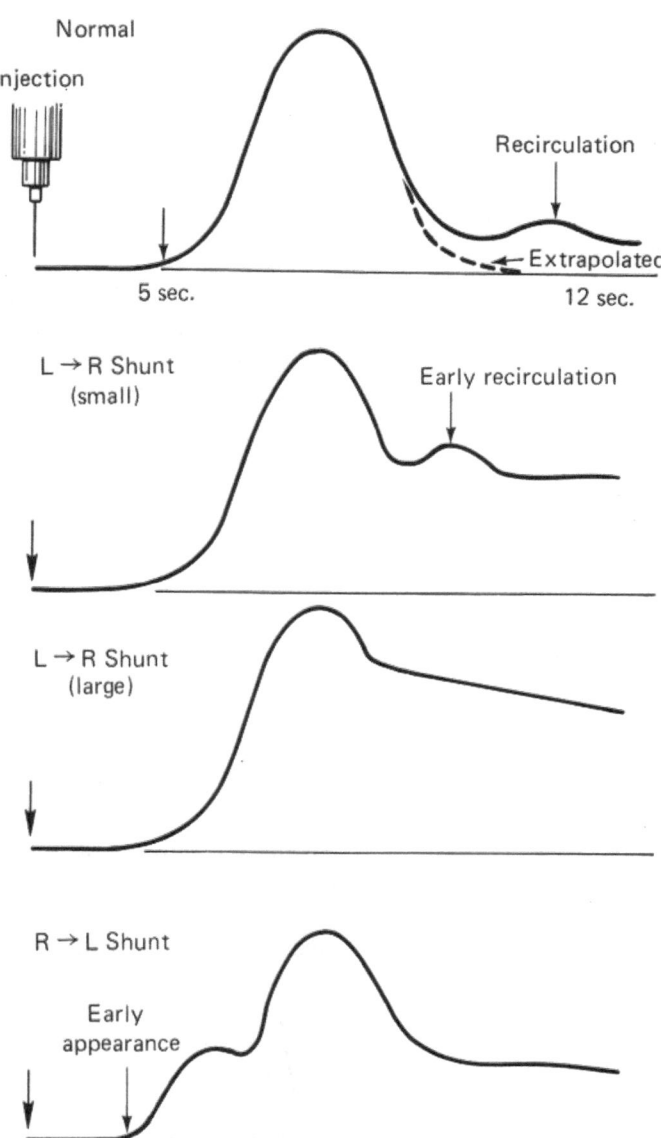

quantitate shunts and because of the flammability of hydrogen gas.

Angiocardiography for Recognition of Shunts.
Contrast studies are definitive in establishing the location of shunts. The injection is made into the chamber from which the shunt flows. The size of the shunt can be roughly estimated by comparing the relative density of the contrast medium in the receiving chamber.

Bibliography

Congenital Heart Disease
Barratt-Boyes BG, Wood EH (1958) Cardiac output and related measurements and pressure values in the right heart and associated vessels, together with an analysis of the hemodynamic response to the inhalation of high oxygen mixtures in healthy subjects. J Lab Clin Med 51:72–90

Butler LJ, Snodgrass AJAI, France NE, Sinclair L, Russell A (1965) No. E (16–18) trisomy syndrome: Analysis of 13 cases. Arch Dis Child 40:600–611

Dubois D, Dubois EF (1916) A height-weight formula to estimate the surface area of man. Proc Soc Exp Biol NY 13:77–78

Keith JD, Rowe RD, Vlad P (1978) Heart disease in infancy and childhood, 3rd edn. New York, MacMillan, pp 3–13

Mitchell SC, Korones SB, Berendes HW (1971) Congenital heart disease in 56,109 births. Incidence and natural history. Circulation 43:323–332

Ober WB, Moore TE (1955) Congenital cardiac malformations in the neonatal period. An autopsy study. N Engl J Med 253:272–275

Patau K, Smith DW, Therman E, Inhorn SL, Wagner HP (1960) Multiple congenital anomaly caused by an extra chromosome. Lancet 1:790–793

Rowe RD, Cleary TE (1960) Congenital cardiac malformation in the newborn period; frequency in a children's hospital. Can Med Assoc J 83:299–302

Rudolph AM (1974) Cardiac catherization and angiography. In Congenital Diseases of the Heart. Chicago, Yearbook Medical Publishers, pp 49–167

Warburg M, Mikkelsen M (1963) A case of 13–15 trisomy or Bartholin-Patau's syndrome. Acta Ophthalmol 41:321–334

Wilkinson JL, Acerete F (1973) Terminological pitfalls in congenital heart disease. Reappraisal of some confusing terms, with an account of a simplified system of basic nomenclature. Br Heart J 35:1116–1177

Young D (1980) Pathophysiology of congenital heart disease. In: Anesthetic considerations for pediatric cardiac surgery. Anesthesiol Clin 18:5–26

Chapter 7, Section I
Systemic-to-Pulmonary Communications

Systemic-to-pulmonary communications represent cardiac lesions that result in left-to-right shunts at the atrial, ventricular or great vessel level (Table 7–3). Atrial level shunts are defects that cause return of pulmonary venous blood to the right atrium or systemic veins. Total anomalous pulmonary venous return, an admixture lesion, is also included here because of its embryological similarity to partial anomalous pulmonary venous return. Defects such as ruptured sinus of Valsalva into a cardiac chamber and coronary arteriovenous fistulas may cause shunts at any level of the heart and are included here as well.

Atrial Level Communications

Atrial Septal Defect

Atrial septal defect (ASD) is a common congenital heart lesion with an approximate incidence of 10%. ASD is the most frequent congenital shunt in adults. [Parenthetically, a bicuspid aortic valve is the most common congenital heart lesion in adults. Ventricular septal defect (VSD) is the most common heart disorder in children, but is uncommon in adults. The reason may be a high incidence of spontaneous closure of VSD in childhood.]

The various types of ASD are classified according to their location: (1) fossa ovalis defects (ostium secundum ASD), (2) endocardial cushion defect (ostium primum ASD), (3) superior caval defect (sinus venosus ASD), (4) common atrium, (5) inferior caval ASD, and (6) coronary sinus ASD. ASD may be associated with other left-to-right shunts (e.g., VSD, patent ductus arteriosus, double-outlet right ventricle without pulmonic stenosis), right-sided obstructive lesions (e.g., pulmonary atresia, tricuspid atresia, tricuspid stenosis, Ebstein malformation, tetralogy of Fallot), left heart obstruction (e.g., coarctation of aorta, hypoplastic left heart syndrome, left ventricular fibroelastosis), and transposition complexes. ASD is virtually always present in cases of partial or total anomalous pulmonary venous drainage. The association of mitral stenosis and ASD is called Lutembacher's syndrome (described with mitral stenosis).

ASD may occur as a familial defect with or without one of the following recognizable syndromes:
• The Upper Limb–Cardiovascular Complex. This complex comprises the association of cardiovascular malformations (generally septal defects) and bony anomalies (most frequently of the thumb and the radius). The Holt-Oram syndrome, Duane syndrome and ventriculoradial dysplasia are considered a part of this complex.
• Holt-Oram Syndrome (Figs. 7–2 to 7–4). This syndrome

Table 7–3. Systemic-to-Pulmonary Communications
Left-to-Right Shunts
Increased Pulmonary Blood Flow Without Cyanosis

1. Atrial level communications
   Atrial septal defect
       Ostium secundum
       Ostium primum
       Sinus venosus
   Partial anomalous pulmonary venous return with ASD
   Scimitar syndrome
   Rupture of sinus of Valsalva into right atrium
   Left ventricular–right atrial communication
   Coronary arteriovenous fistula into right atrium or coronary sinus
   Other, uncommon, types of ASD
2. Ventricular level communications
   Isolated ventricular septal defect
       Infracristal
       Supracristal
       Muscular
       Inlet
   Ventricular septal defect with aortic insufficiency
   Endocardial cushion type of ventricular septal defect (including some inlet VSDs)
   Levotransposition of the great arteries with ventricular septal defect without pulmonic stenosis
   Double-outlet right ventricle with subaortic ventricular septal defect without pulmonic stenosis
   Coronary arteriovenous fistula into right ventricle
   Rupture of sinus of Valsalva into right ventricle
3. Great vessel level communications
   Patent ductus arteriosus
   Aorticopulmonary window
   Ductus arteriosus sling
   Anomalous origin of either coronary artery from the pulmonary artery*

* These defects are classified here as left-to-right shunts; however, their behavior reflects myocardial ischemia rather than a left-to-right shunt.

consists of familial ASD, cardiac arrhythmias, and malformations of the hand (one or both thumbs). The syndrome is transmitted in an autosomal dominant inheritance pattern. The cardiac lesion is usually a secundum ASD, but VSD or patent ductus arteriosus or both have been described. The thumb may be short, hypoplastic or absent (Fig. 7–2); it may possess an accessory phalanx (triphalangism), with the distal phalanx turning inward. The thumb is nonapposable and resembles the other fingers (Fig. 7–3). Other bony anomalies include phocomelia, hypoplasia of the bones of the shoulder and pectoral musculature (Fig. 7–4), hemivertebra, spina bifida, scoliosis and Sprengel deformity. The radius may be hypoplastic or joined to the ulna. The thenar eminence may be hypoplastic. The karyotypes are normal.

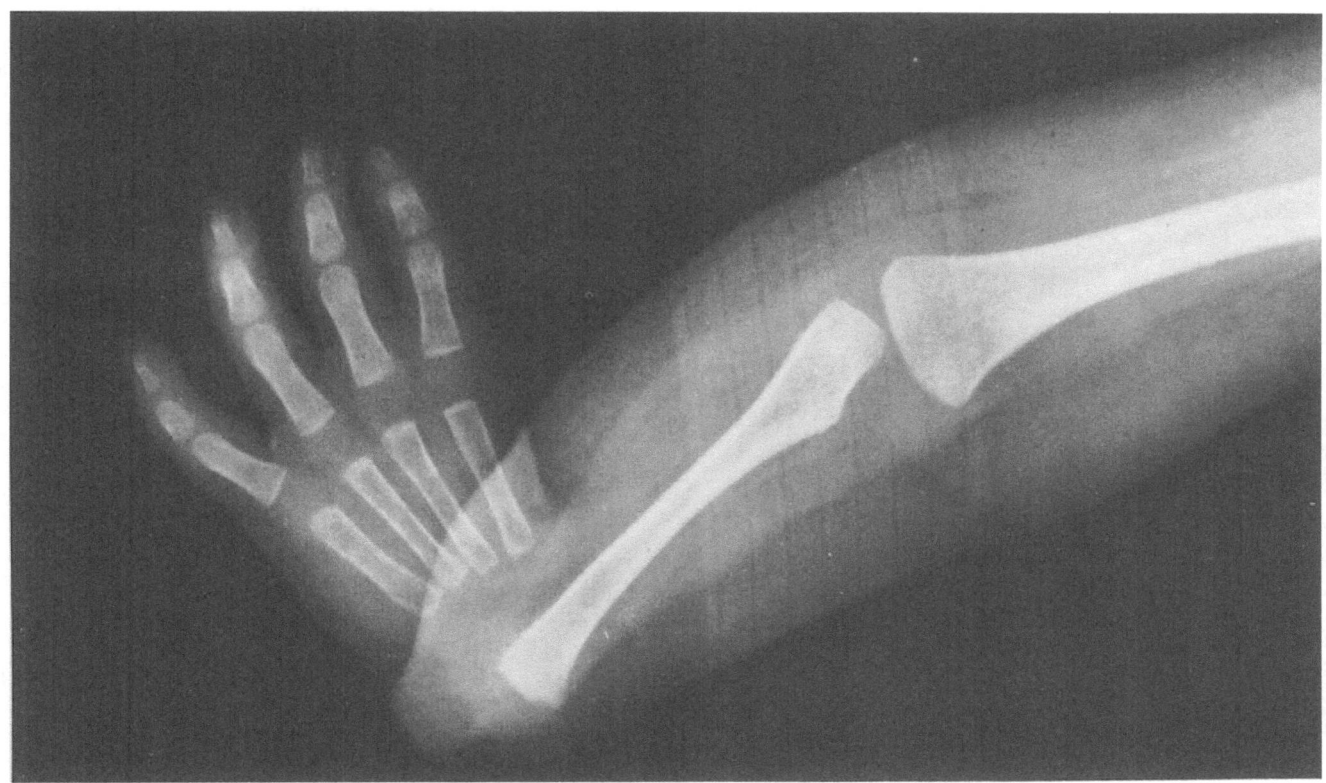

Fig. 7-2. *Absence of the thumb in Holt-Oram syndrome.* The radius and carpal bones are also absent. Radial deviation of the hand is noted. Both siblings, the father and the paternal grandfather had atrial septal defects. This baby had an atrial septal defect and a patent ductus arteriosus.

• Duane Syndrome. In this congenital ocular anomaly, abnormal function of the lateral recti muscles results in congenital deficiency of ocular abduction, impairment of adduction, retraction and superior or inferior deviation of the globe on abduction and narrowing of the palpebral fissure on adduction. In addition, these patients may exhibit the cardiac and skeletal features of the Holt-Oram syndrome.

• Ventriculoradial Dysplasia. This syndrome is characterized by absence or hypoplasia of the radius and VSD. Patients may also have abnormalities of the thumb similar to those associated with the Holt-Oram syndrome.

• Ellis van Creveld Syndrome. Occurring in Amish (Mennonite) kindreds, this syndrome includes polydactyly, abnormalities of the carpal and metacarpal bones and absence of the atrial septum (common atrium), with or without a cleft mitral valve.

• Pierre Robin Syndrome. This syndrome includes micrognathia, cleft palate and glossoptosis. One variety also exhibits clubfoot, ASD and persistence of the left superior vena cava; this type may be inherited as an X-linked recessive gene. Karyotypes are normal.

Anatomical Types of Atrial Septal Defect. *Fossa Ovalis ASD* (Ostium Secundum Defect). This entity is the most

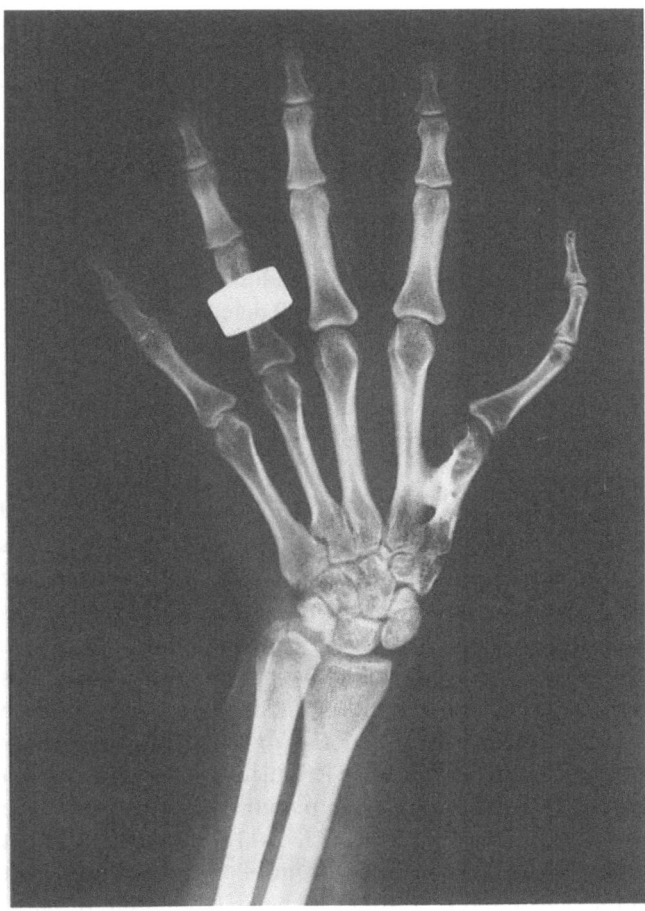

Fig. 7-3. *Triphalangism of the thumb in Holt-Oram syndrome.* The thumb has an accessory phalanx and turns inward. It is nonapposable and resembles the other fingers. This patient had a secundum atrial septal defect.

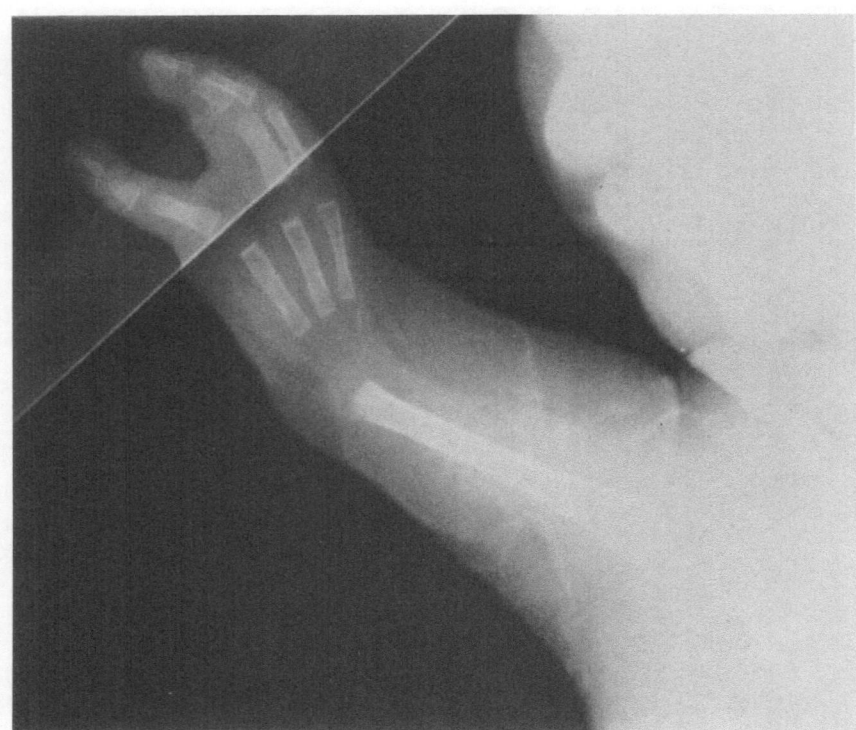

Fig. 7–4. *Phocomelia in Holt-Oram syndrome.* This 1-year-old boy had an atrial septal defect and multiple muscular ventricular septal defects.

common form of ASD and is the type most frequently associated with other heart defects and with the syndromes described before. ASD at the fossa ovalis may result from (1) an enlarged or stretched foramen ovale, (2) a short valve of the foramen ovale causing enlargement of the ostium secundum, (3) fenestration in the valve of the foramen ovale, (4) absence of the valve of the foramen ovale (common atrium), and (5) herniation or aneurysm (or both) of the free edge of the valve of the foramen ovale with associated incompetence. A short valve of the foramen ovale is by far the most common form of secundum ASD. Second in frequency is the fenestrated or perforated ASD. The other forms of ostium secundum ASD are rare.

Inferior Caval ASD. This unusual defect overrides the inferior vena cava, which thus drains directly into both atria. The pulmonary veins also empty into both atria. The eustachian valve tends to be attached to the anulus ovalis. A large Chiari network may obscure the lower pole of the defect.

Sinus Venosus ASD (also known as Superior Caval ASD or High ASD). The defect is independent of the fossa ovalis and is located high in the interatrial septum, underlying the orifice of the superior vena cava (SVC). The defect is often accompanied by partial anomalous pulmonary venous return. The right superior pulmonary vein usually drains into the SVC, the middle pulmonary vein empties into the right atrium (RA) and the right inferior pulmonary vein opens normally into the left atrium (LA). On occasion the right middle or inferior pulmonary veins may open into the SVC (see Figs. 7–10C, 7–11D). A persistent left SVC may be present. The ostium of the SVC is adjacent to the defect and may straddle the atrial septum, draining

into both atria. If straddling is marked, cyanosis may be evident. Even in patients without clinical cyanosis a right-to-left shunt may be detected at cardiac catheterization.

Coronary Sinus ASD. This abnormality is rare, apparently occurring only as part of a developmental complex. The complex includes ASD, persistent left SVC terminating in the left atrium and absence of the coronary sinus. The coronary veins drain individually into the corresponding atria. A right-to-left shunt is part of the disorder and generally results in cyanosis. A left-to-right shunt through the ASD is also present.

Persistent Left Superior Vena Cava. A true persistent left SVC (persistent left anterior cardinal vein) drains into the coronary sinus and RA through the vein of Marshall (Fig. 7–5). A persistent left SVC draining into the coronary sinus is a benign and not uncommon anomaly in the absence of other defects. However, when the left SVC drains directly into the LA, cyanosis may develop because of the resulting right-to-left shunt; this anomaly is rare and is usually associated with other cardiac malformations (e.g., ASD, common atrium, endocardial cushion defect, absence of coronary sinus, and situs ambiguus especially polysplenia). Rarely the right SVC may be absent. When this occurs the persistent left SVC and right innominate vein form a mirror image of the normal venous system. This defect is one of the numerous anomalies of venous connections that can occur with abnormalities of visceroatrial situs. Rarely, a persistent left SVC may drain into the left pulmonary veins.

Ostium Primum ASD. This disorder forms part of a group of anomalies called endocardial cushion defects (ECDs), ranging from the simplest form (ostium primum defect)

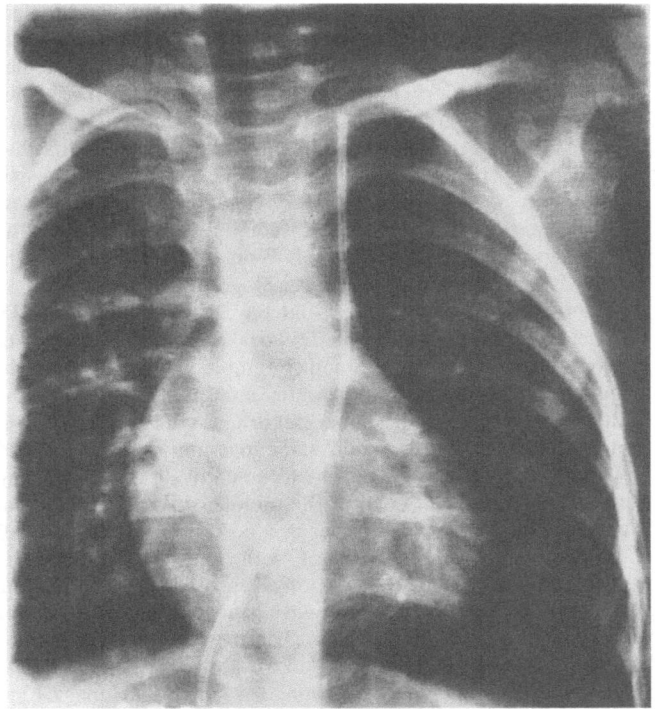

A

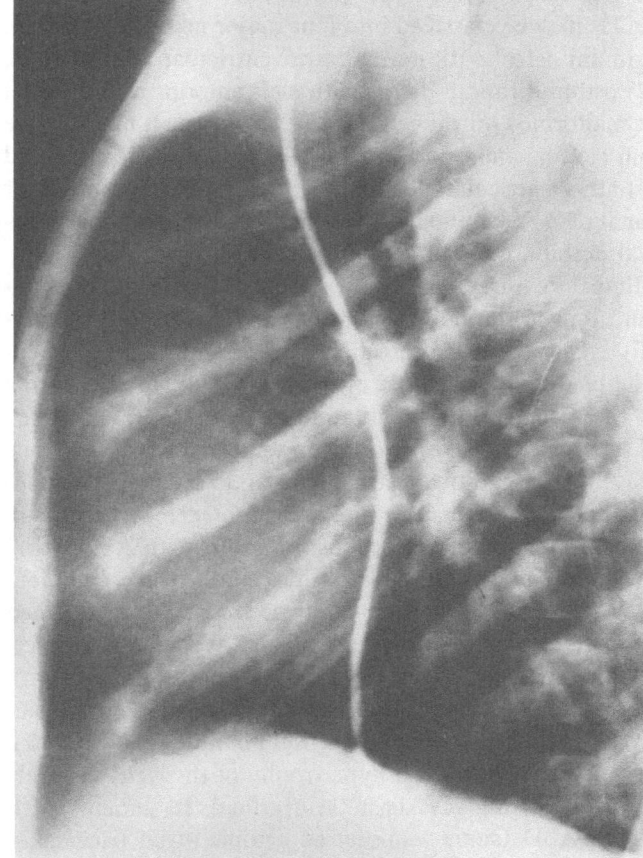

B

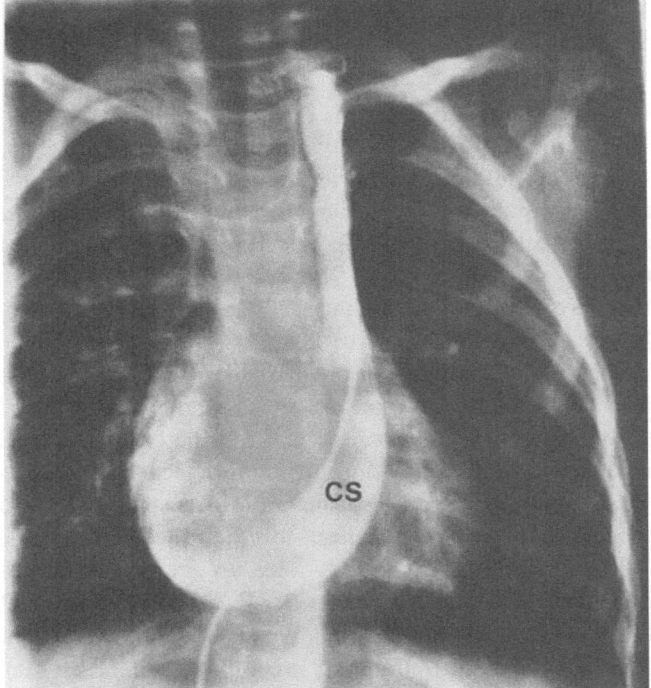

C

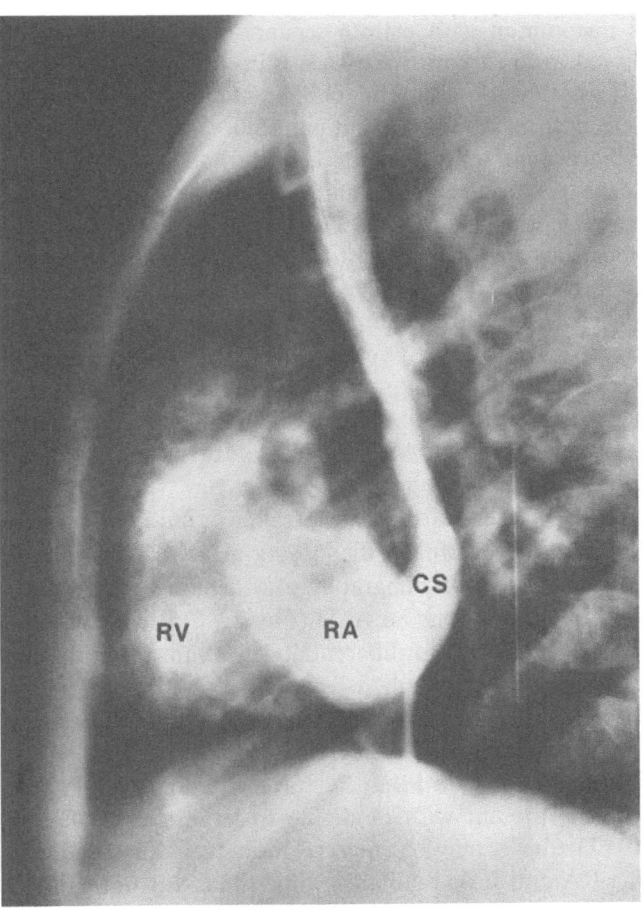

D

Fig. 7–5. *Persistent left superior vena cava.* Position of a catheter in a persistent left superior vena cava in the frontal view (**A**) and the lateral view (**B**) and the angiographic appearance in the frontal view (**C**) and the lateral view (**D**). The catheter traverses the inferior vena cava, right atrium, coronary sinus (*CS*) and persistent left superior vena cava. The coronary sinus and left superior vena cava are posterior structures on the lateral view. Injection in the left superior vena cava shows drainage into the right atrium via the coronary sinus. On the lateral view the right ventricle (*RV*) is opacified. Persistent left superior vena cava was an associated finding in this patient with tetralogy of Fallot and trisomy 22. *RA* = right atrium.

to the most severe type (atrioventricularis communis). ECDs may be classified into four major groups: (1) ostium primum defect with normal atrioventricular (A-V) valves; (2) ostium primum defect with cleft anterior mitral leaflet or malformed mitral valve; (3) ECD with cleft mitral valve and cleft or malformed tricuspid valve (septal leaflet); and (4) atrioventricularis communis (common atrioventricular canal or A-V communis). (See also description of endocardial cushion defects.)

Clinical Features Children with ASD of the ostium secundum type are usually asymptomatic. The diagnosis generally is suspected by detection of a murmur. A right ventricular heave, a systolic ejection murmur, fixed splitting of the second heart sound, and a diastolic "flow rumble" of the tricuspid valve are often present. On occasion, infants may have congestive heart failure and recurrent pneumonia. Some children show intolerance to exercise and a tendency to respiratory infections. In adults with ASD, atrial dysrhythmias and right-sided heart failure are common. Cyanosis may develop in adults secondary to right-sided heart failure or increased pulmonary vascular resistance.

The usual electrocardiographic findings in patients with an ostium secundum ASD consist of an RsR' in V_1 and broad S wave in V_6 (incomplete right bundle-branch block), right axis deviation and hypertrophy of the right ventricle (RV), indicating RV diastolic overload. In patients with a high ASD (sinus venosus) an ectopic atrial pacemaker (abnormal P wave axis) may occur. Left axis deviation of the QRS complex (counterclockwise frontal vector loop) is uncommon with ostium secundum defects, but is observed in most patients with ostium primum ASD. Thus, left axis deviation is useful in differentiating ostium primum defects from ostium secundum ASD.

Echocardiography M-mode echocardiography shows evidence of RV enlargement and paradoxical or asynchronous septal motion (Fig. 7–6). These findings are not specific, since they may occur with other conditions such as pulmonic or tricuspid insufficiency, anomalous pulmonary venous drainage, Ebstein anomaly, congenital absence of the pericardium, congestive cardiomyopathy and type B Wolff-Parkinson-White syndrome. Two-dimensional echocardiography from the subxiphoid window is most sensitive in detecting secundum ASD because the atrial septum is perpendicular to the echo beam in this view (Fig. 7–6B and C). Contrast echocardiography (saline or indocyanine green dye) may be helpful in diagnosing a large ASD (Fig. 7–7). Doppler echocardiography also demonstrates the left-to-right shunt across an ASD (Fig. 2–48). Echocardiography is very useful in differentiating ostium primum ASD from ostium secundum defects (Figs. 7–8 and 7–9) (see description of echocardiographic findings in the section, Endocardial Cushion Defects).

Radiological (Plain Film) Features Pulmonary overcirculation is present with moderate to large shunts (Fig. 7–10). The heart may be enlarged in its transverse diameter. The RA and RV are dilated while the LA is not enlarged except in rare instances in which mitral valve disease coex-

Fig. 7–6. *Echocardiography in patients with ASD.* **A** Paradoxical motion of the ventricular septum and right ventricular enlargement in a patient with an atrial septal defect. The ventricular septum moves anteriorly during ventricular systole (*arrow*) rather than posteriorly. Paradoxical motion of the ventricular septum occurs with atrial septal defect and with other abnormalities that cause right ventricular volume overload (pulmonary or tricuspid regurgitation or both) or pulmonary hypertension. Paradoxical septal motion may also occur with congestive cardiomyopathy, left bundle-branch block and type B Wolff-Parkinson-White syndrome. **B** Two-dimensional echocardiography from a location medial to the apex in a 6-year-old boy with secundum ASD. The defect is in the middle of the atrial septum in the area of the foramen ovale (*arrow*). Doppler sample volume in the right atrium near the defect demonstrates continuous flow into the right atrium (left-to-right shunt) (see Fig. 2–48). **C** Two-dimensional echocardiogram from the same location in a one-year-old boy with sinus venosus ASD. The foramen ovale is intact, being represented by a bright echo in the middle of the atrial septum. The defect (*arrow*) is far superior and posterior next to the wall of the atrium. A frequent finding with sinus venosus ASD is partial anomalous pulmonary venous return of part or all of the right lung to the superior vena cava. In addition the superior vena cava may override the interatrial septum to a greater or lesser extent, sometimes resulting in a right-to-left shunt. RV = right ventricle; RA = right atrium; LA = left atrium; LV = left ventricle; AML = anterior leaflet of the mitral valve. (Frame B courtesy of Henry Issenberg, M.D., Bronx, New York.)

ists. The pulmonary artery is dilated, but the aorta is normal or small. If pulmonary vascular obstruction develops the central pulmonary arteries dilate considerably and the interlobar pulmonary arteries taper abruptly (pruned-tree appearance) (see Fig. 1–22). The RV dilates even further on such occasions.

Hemodynamics The catheter easily crosses the atrial septum. The position of the catheter as it crosses may help in identifying the location of the defect. With fossa ovalis defects the catheter crosses at the midpoint of the atrial septum; in sinus venosus defects the catheter crosses high in the atrium; and in ostium primum defects the crossing of the catheter occurs just above the tricuspid valve, and the catheter may even appear to enter the left ventricle (LV) directly from the RA. A "step-up" in oxygen saturation is usually detected within the RA, but may occur at the SVC-RA junction in sinus venosus defect with right partial anomalous pulmonary venous return (PAPVR). Additional step-ups within the innominate vein, SVC or inferior vena cava (IVC) would suggest other forms of PAPVR. In ostium primum defects, and in a few secundum defects, the step-up may appear to occur in the RV because of streaming from a low ASD directly into the RV. Calculations of the size of the shunt, may be difficult, since no chamber contains mixed venous blood. The level of SVC O_2 saturation may be used, or a weighted average of SVC and IVC (SVC × 2 + IVC). In spite of large left-to-right shunts the pressures in the RV and main pulmonary artery (MPA) usually are normal in children. In adults, pressures in the RV and MPA may be elevated, and the shunt may be bidirectional or right to left. With ostium primum ASD

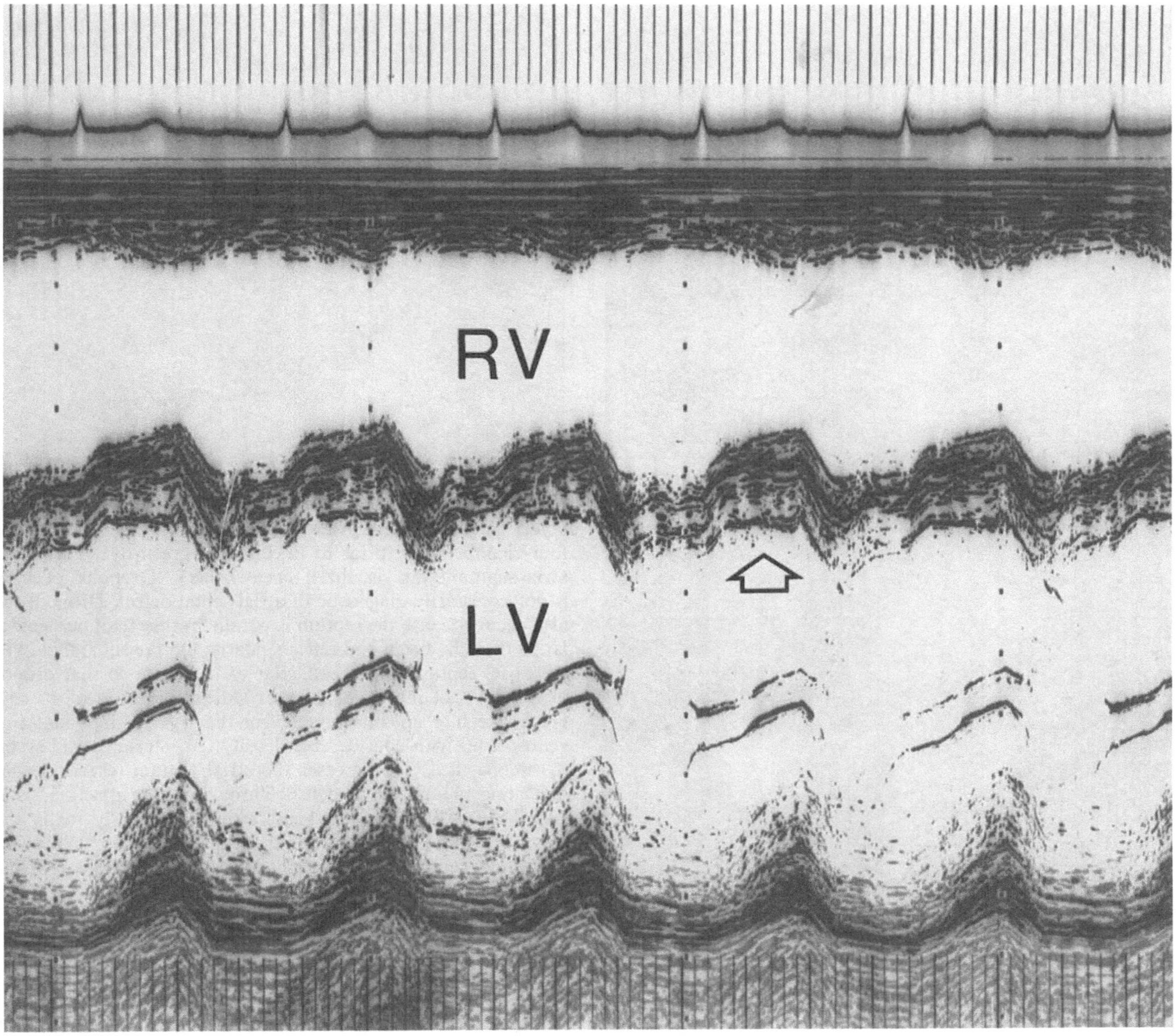

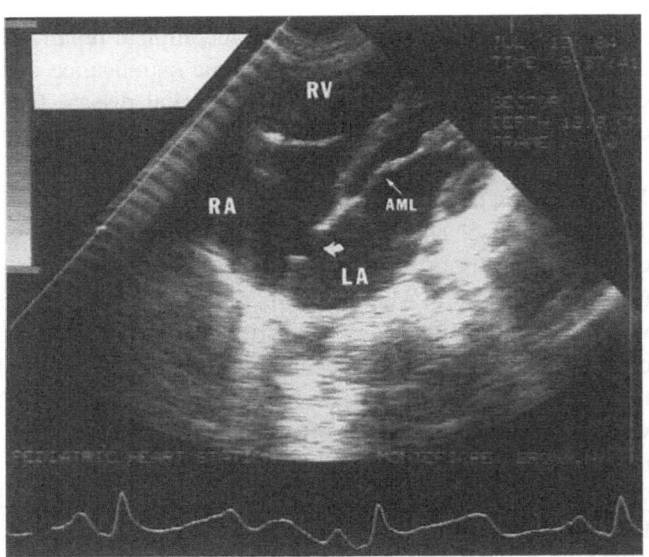

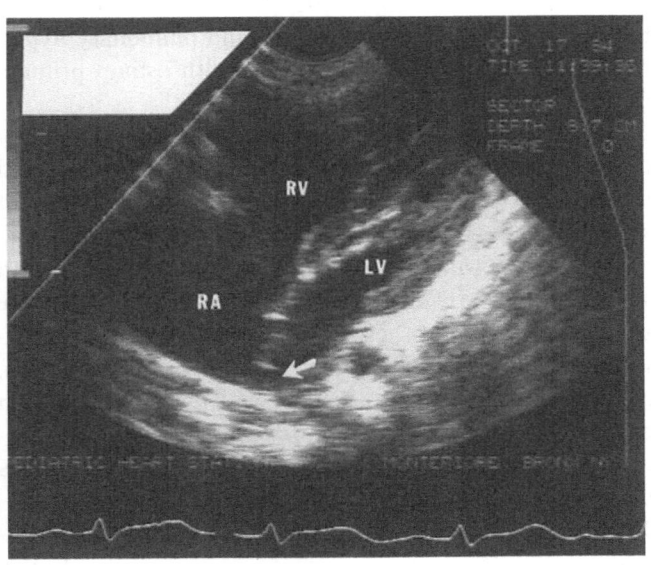

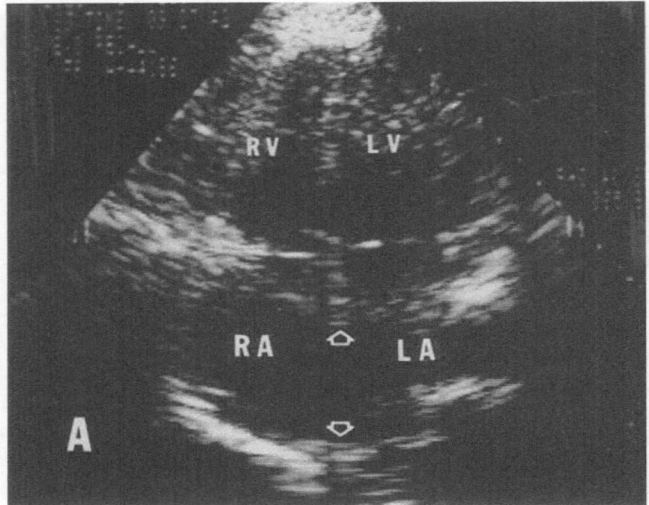

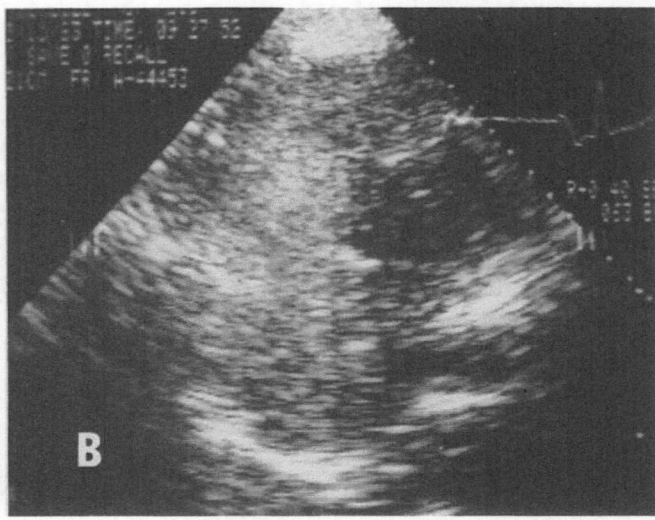

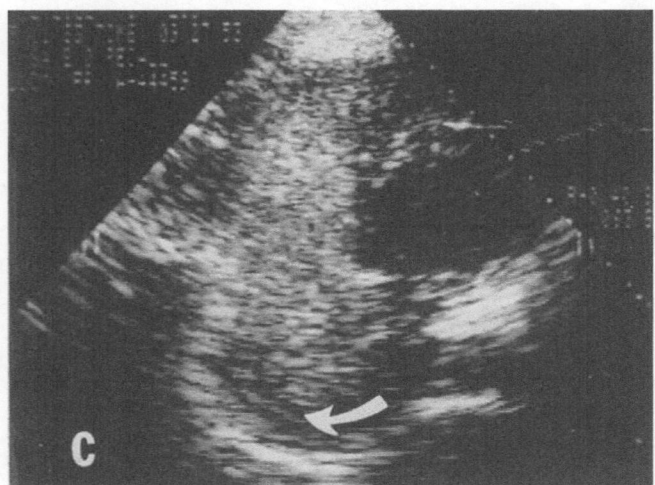

Fig. 7–7. *Contrast echocardiogram in a patient with atrial septal defect.* A four-chamber view is best for this study. A is the apex four-chamber view prior to injection of green dye. Part of the atrial septum is not visualized (*open arrows*). "Dropout" of echoes is not necessarily diagnostic of atrial septal defect. Dropout may also occur because the septum is parallel rather than perpendicular to the echo beam and reflects poorly. On the subxiphoid view the atrial septum is perpendicular to the beam so that dropout of echoes is of more significance. During injection of 10 cc of green dye into an antecubital vein the right atrium and right ventricle fill with considerable density (**B**). During atrial systole (**C**) unopacified blood crosses the atrial septum (*curved arrow*), indicating an atrial septal defect. Throughout the injection, which lasts about 5 seconds, the right atrium repeatedly refills with contrast medium and then is partly deopacified. *LA* = left atrium; *LV* = left ventricle; *RA* = right atrium; *RV* = right ventricle.

and mitral insufficiency the regurgitant flow through the mitral valve is directed across the ASD, adding to the volume load on the right side (LV-to-RA shunt). Thus the shunt is likely to be very large, and pulmonary hypertension is more likely in individuals with ostium primum defects.

Contrast Studies The levophase of the pulmonary angiogram or right ventriculogram (Fig. 7–11) is diagnostic and is helpful in estimating the size of the atrial left-to-right shunt. With secundum ASD, both atria opacify simultaneously. The SVC and IVC may opacify later by reflux. With sinus venosus ASD and PAPVR, the SVC opacifies before the RA. If present, other forms of PAPVR can be recognized readily. On the LAO view with axial angulation, an injection directly into the LA will reveal the position of the ASD. Left ventriculography is important for recognition and evaluation of suspected ECDs. This subject is discussed in the section, Endocardial Cushion Defects.

Treatment Surgical closure of an ASD is indicated in infants and children who are symptomatic (rare). Elective surgery is indicated in asymptomatic children and adults if the shunt is greater than 1.5:1. The surgical mortality

is under 1%, and the results are usually excellent. The size of the heart usually returns to normal following surgery. A persistently enlarged heart may be secondary to (1) residual defect or defects due to incomplete repair, (2) persistent arrhythmias of hemodynamic significance as a complication of surgery and (3) myocardial disease (cardiomyopathy of volume loading).

Endocardial Cushion Defects

The spectrum of endocardial cushion defects (ECDs) includes (1) ostium primum ASD without cleft mitral valve; (2) ostium primum ASD with cleft mitral valve with or without mitral insufficiency; (3) ostium primum ASD with cleft mitral valve and involvement of the septal leaflet of the tricuspid valve; (4) endocardial cushion type of VSD with atrioventricular (A-V) valve abnormality; (5) atrioventricularis communis (also known as A-V communis, atrioventricular canal or A-V canal). Some authors (Titus and Rastelli) also include inlet VSD as a form of ECD. They call it ventricular septal defect of the AV canal type.

The partial or incomplete form of ECD usually consists of an ostium primum ASD and a cleft mitral valve. In

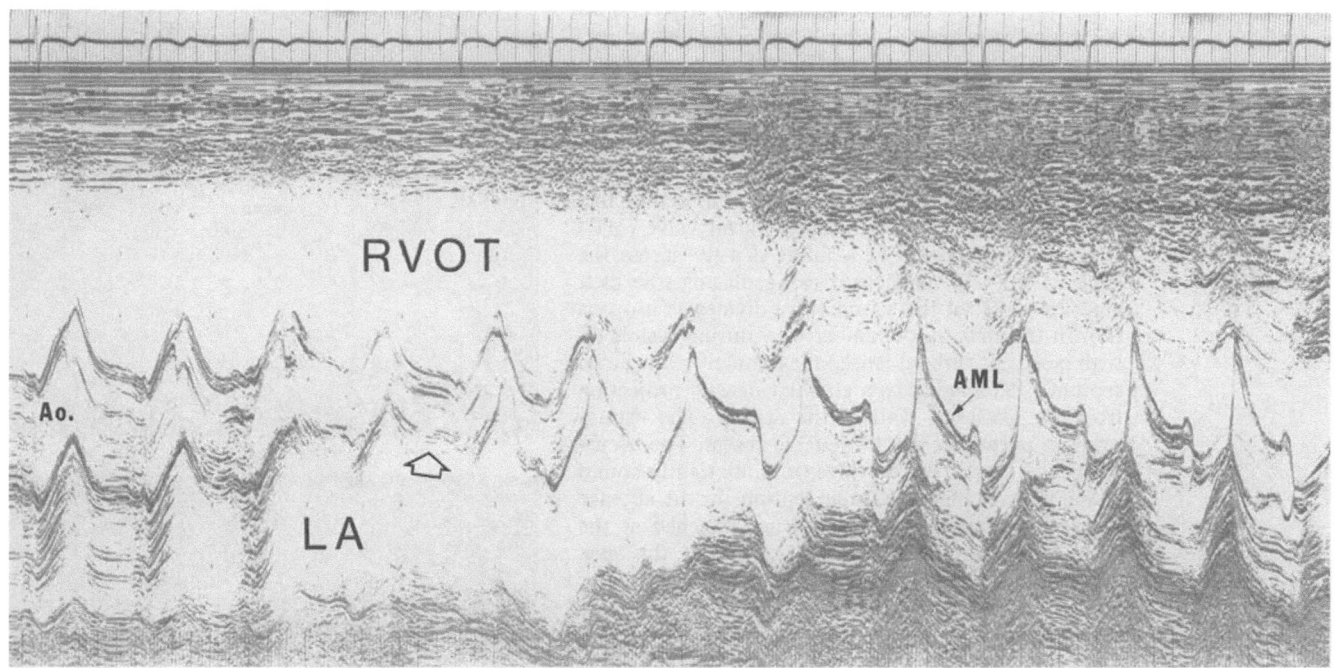

Fig. 7–8. *Ostium primum atrial septal defect.* The arc scan from the aorta to the mitral valve shows an abnormal anterior position (*open arrow*) of the anterior leaflet of the mitral valve (*AML*) relative to the aortic root and ventricular septum. The anterior position of the anterior leaflet of the mitral valve results in narrowing of the left ventricular outflow tract, which is equivalent to the "gooseneck" deformity observed on angiography with ostium primum atrial septal defect (Fig. 7–16). The anterior mitral leaflet abuts against the ventricular septum during early diastole, but does not cross the ventricular septum. In patients with atrioventricularis communis (A-V communis) the mitral valve appears to cross the ventricular septum in the area of the ventricular septal defect (Fig. 7–12). *Ao.* = aorta; *LA* = left atrium; *RVOT* = right ventricular outflow tract.

these defects, even though that portion of the ventricular septum contributed by the A-V canal is absent, the mitral and tricuspid valves are bound to the summit or crest of the muscular septum so that no interventricular communication is present. The hemodynamics are those of ASD. If the mitral valve is incompetent the jet will be directed across the ASD into the RA, thus adding to the volume load in the RV (LV-to-RA shunt).

Some authors use the term *intermediate form of A-V canal* to describe an ostium primum defect in which the cleft in the mitral leaflet extends across the top of the ventricular septum, leaving a small unguarded space. A left-to-right shunt may or may not be present in this area; however, if surgery is undertaken it may be necessary to alter the operation in order not to bind the mitral valve to the ventricular septum.

The A-V canal type of VSD (also called sinus VSD or inlet VSD) is uncommon. This type differs from the membranous VSD in that the aortic valve does not form one of its boundaries. It occurs more posteriorly than the membranous VSD, just below and in front of the A-V valves. The membranous septum forms the anterior superior border of the defect and separates it from the aortic valve. The A-V valves may be normal or may show findings similar to those occurring with A-V canal. A straddling tricuspid valve may be associated.

The complete form of A-V canal (A-V communis) is common. In this defect the inferior portion of the atrial septum and the superior portion of the ventricular septum are absent. The mitral and tricuspid valves are represented by a primitive common A-V orifice, which is guarded by anterior and posterior leaflets, and two lateral leaflets. This valve may or may not be competent. Rastelli et al. described three fairly distinct patterns of attachment of the anterior leaflet of the common A-V valve. In type A the anterior leaflet is divided into right and left segments and is attached to both sides of the ventricular septum by chordae tendineae. In type B the anterior leaflet is also divided but is not attached to the ventricular septum. Instead it is attached by chordae tendineae to an anomalous papillary muscle in the right ventricle. In type C, the anterior leaflet is not divided and floats freely, having no chordal attachments to the ventricular septum. The anterior leaflet may be attached to the walls of the ventricles or to anterior papillary muscles of each ventricle.

Some cases of A-V communis will show a relatively hypoplastic LV or RV. Complete repair will be impossible if either ventricle is too small.

Incidence and Associated Disorders In children who are otherwise normal ECDs are uncommon. Complete A-V canal occurs in Down syndrome as frequently as does VSD. Thus A-V canal is either the most frequent or second most frequent disorder identified in children with Down syndrome. ECDs are often observed in cases of asplenia and polysplenia. With asplenia, A-V communis is often associated with severe intracardiac defects such as pulmonary

Fig. 7–9. *Ostium primum atrial septal defect.* This is a two-dimensional echocardiogram in the long axis (**A** and **B**), short axis (**C** and **D**), and apex four-chamber views (**E,E′** and **F**). In the long axis view during systole (**A**), the anterior leaflet of the mitral valve (*AML*) is in its closed position and appears thickened. During diastole (**B**) the anterior leaflet of the mitral valve abuts against the ventricular septum. In the short axis view (**C**) during systole, the mitral valve (*MV*) is closed and appears as a linear density across the back of the left ventricle. During diastole the cleft anterior leaflet of the mitral valve divides as it opens (**D**). In the apex four-chamber view during systole (**E** with labels; **E′** without labels) the remnant of the atrial septum (*AS*) appears as a globular density projecting from the posterior wall of the atrium. The ostium primum portion of the AS (*OP*) is absent. The tricuspid valve (*tv*) and mitral valve (*mv*) are tightly bound to the peak of the ventricular septum. In the absence of a membranous septum, both are attached at the same level, forming a line convex toward the apex of the heart. During diastole (*F*) the atrioventricular valves are open. Again the attachment of the atrioventricular valves to the peak of the ventricular septum (*Sept.*) militates against a ventricular septal defect.

Ao. = aorta; LA = left atrium.

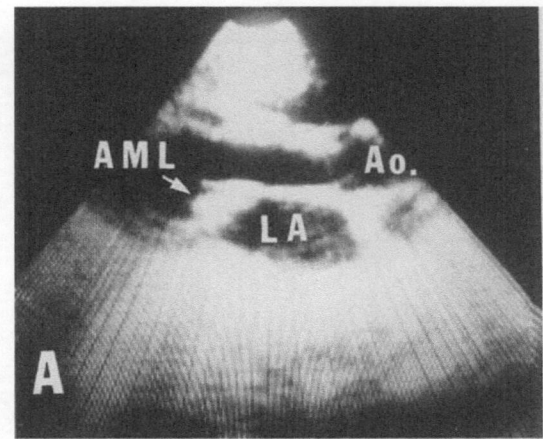

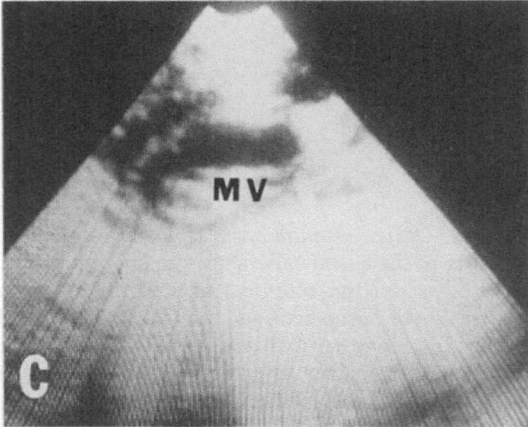

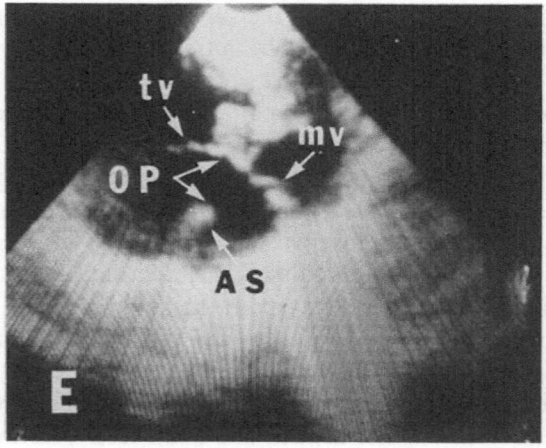

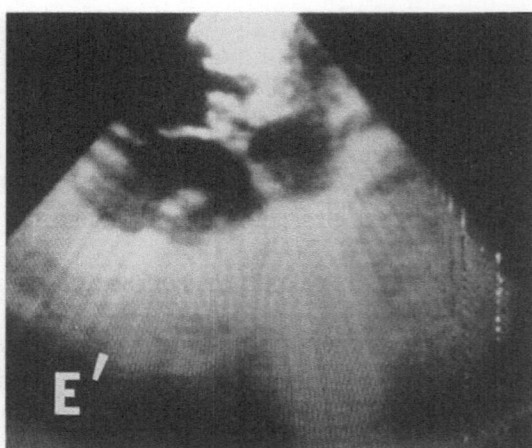

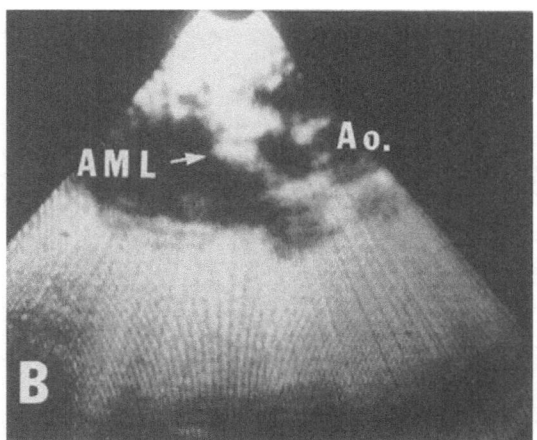

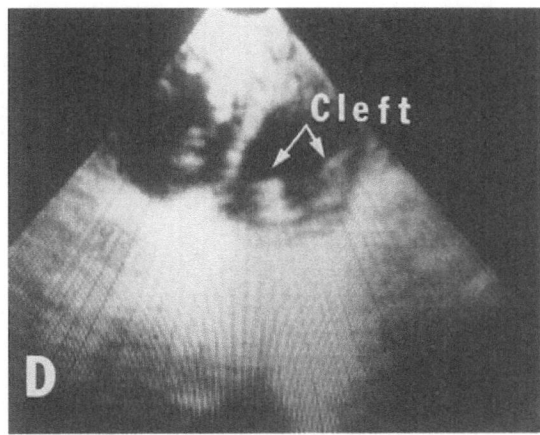

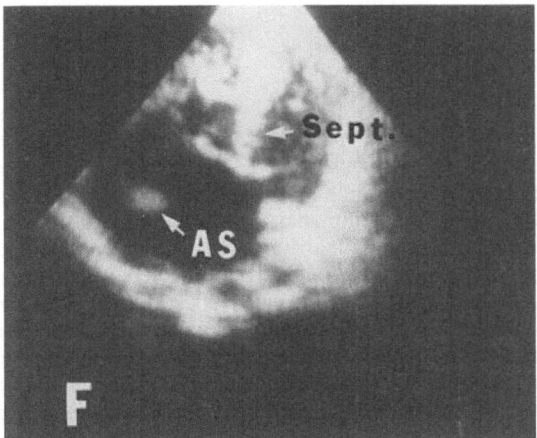

atresia and single ventricle. In polysplenia, ostium primum ASD is most common, although complex abnormalities also occur. The Ellis van Creveld syndrome in Amish families can include ASD or common atrium. (Common atrium is considered by some authors to be a form of ECD.) Other intracardiac defects that may be associated with ECD are ostium secundum ASD, pulmonic stenosis or atresia, patent ductus arteriosus, tetralogy of Fallot, double-outlet RV, and persistence of the left superior vena cava (SVC). Subaortic obstruction may occur in complete A-V canal and in ostium primum ASD because of tethering of the anterior leaflet to the ventricular septum or because of a discrete subaortic diaphragm.

Clinical Features Some individuals with ostium primum ASD have clinical features similar to those associated with ostium secundum ASD. More often, the patient with an ostium primum defect has a very large left-to-right shunt and congestive heart failure. This is especially true if mitral insufficiency (LV-to-RA shunt) is associated. This shunt is designated obligatory because it is not dependent on pulmonary vascular resistance.

On physical examination a right ventricular heave or combined heave is apparent. With significant mitral insufficiency an apical thrill is felt. On auscultation a pulmonary ejection murmur, a widely split second sound, and a tricuspid flow rumble are heard; a gallop may or may not be present. A pansystolic murmur of mitral or tricuspid insufficiency may be present.

With A-V communis, heart failure usually occurs in early infancy because of the large left-to-right shunt. If A-V valve insufficiency is also severe, the heart failure will be difficult or impossible to manage. A bidirectional shunt is usually present; however, the baby will not be obviously cyanotic unless there is associated pulmonic stenosis or elevation in pulmonary vascular resistance. The characteristic electrocardiogram for all types of ECD shows a superior QRS axis (superior counterclockwise frontal vector loop) and an RsR' in lead V_1 (incomplete right bundle-branch block). A prolonged PR interval may also be present. The conduction defects may progress to complete right bundle-branch block or complete heart block or both.

Echocardiography On M-mode, the characteristic feature of ostium primum ASD is the apparent anterior position of the mitral valve relative to that of the aortic root (Fig. 7–8). The mitral valve appears to be attached in the middle of the aortic root instead of to the posterior wall as in normal persons. During diastole the mitral valve is observed to press closely against the ventricular septum. This relatively anterior position of the mitral leaflet may be the echocardiographic equivalent of the "gooseneck" deformity noted on LV angiography. Multiple mitral echoes and some vibrations may result in a shaggy appearance to the mitral leaflets. On scanning through the LV outflow tract the D-E (opening) motion of tricuspid and mitral valves may be present on the same tracing. The motion of the tricuspid valve occurs in front of the ventricular septum, and the mitral motion occurs posteriorly behind the ventricular

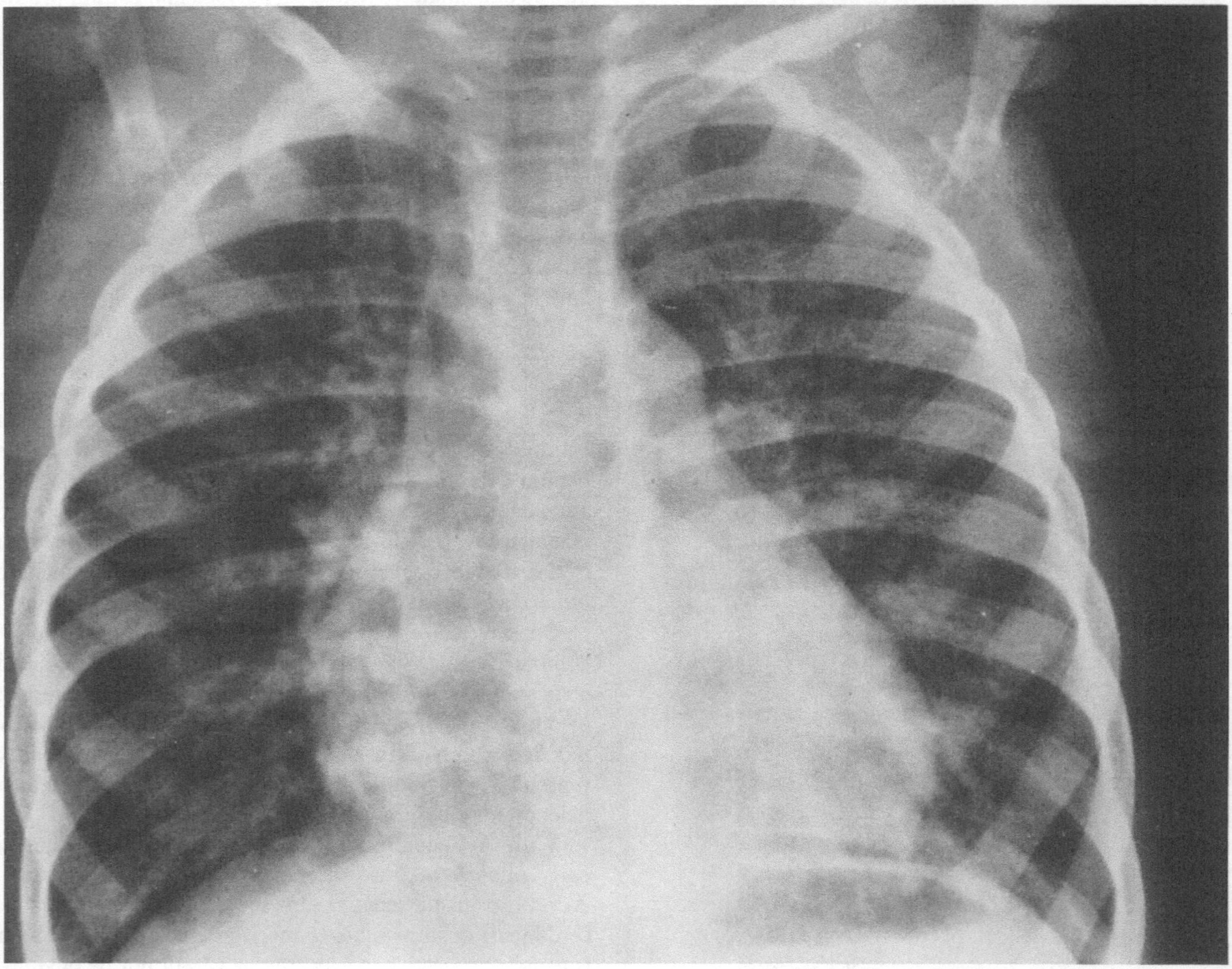

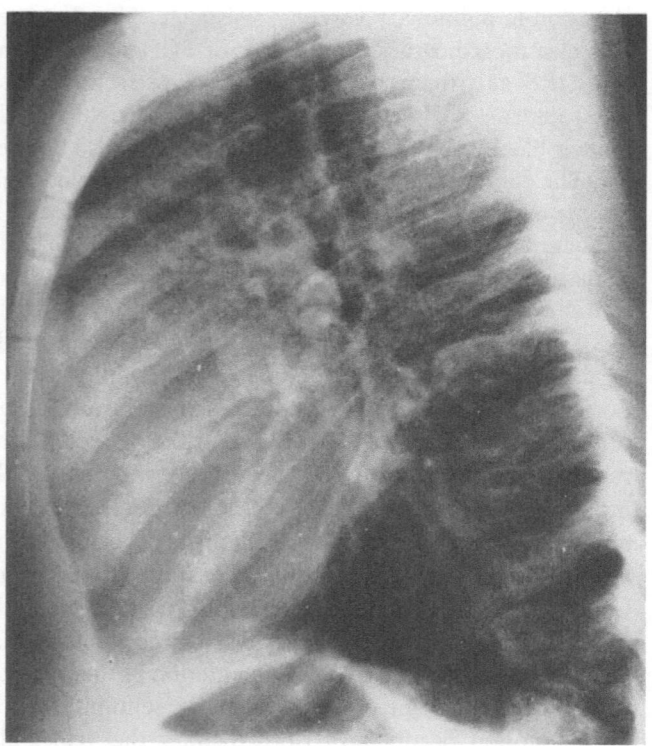

A

B

Fig. 7–10. *Atrial septal defect.* **A** and **B** are frontal and lateral plain chest roentgenograms in a 1-year-old girl with ostium secundum atrial septal defect. Pulmonary overcirculation is present. The heart is enlarged. The right atrium, right ventricle and pulmonary artery are enlarged. The left atrium and left ventricle are not enlarged, and the aorta is inconspicuous. These plain film findings may be encountered with other shunts at the atrial level (e.g., other forms of atrial septal defect, including ostium primum atrial septal defect, left ventricular-to-right atrial communication, coronary arteriovenous fistula to the right atrium, aneurysm of the sinus of Valsalva opening into the right atrium, partial anomalous pulmonary venous return). Frame **C** is a frontal chest film obtained from a 4-year-old boy with sinus venosus atrial septal defect and anomalous pulmonary venous return from the right lung. The curvilinear density within the cardiac silhouette on the right (*arrow*) represents the confluence of the right pulmonary veins as they enter the posterior wall of the superior vena cava at its junction with the right atrium (see also Fig. 7–11D).

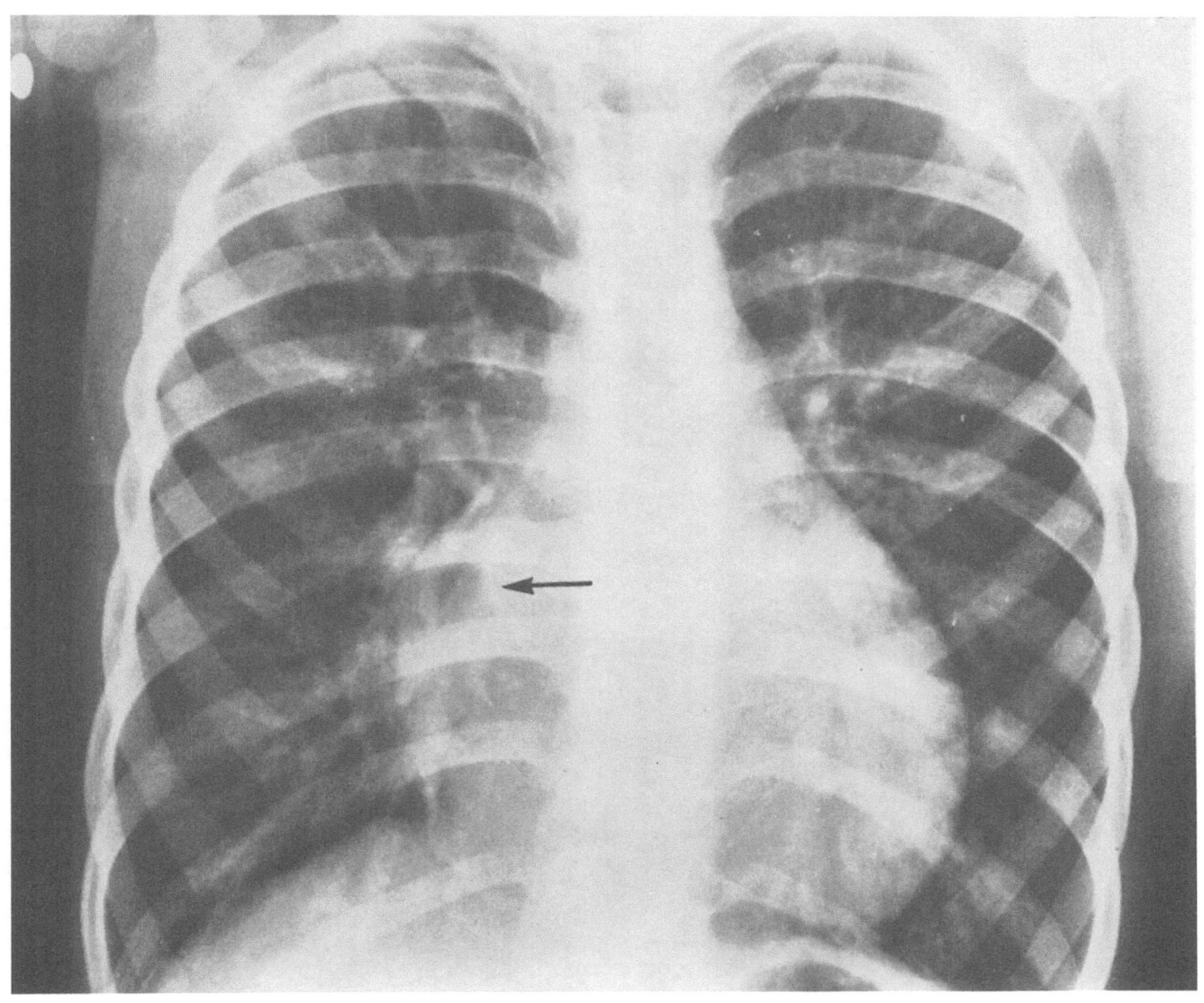

C

septum. On close inspection the two lines will be discontinuous in all views in cases of ostium primum ASD. In A-V communis the mitral and tricuspid echoes will continue across the ventricular septum in some scanning angles (Fig. 7–12).

As with ostium secundum ASD, the M-mode echocardiogram in ostium primum ASD may show dilatation of the RV and paradoxical motion of the ventricular septum. With severe mitral insufficiency and with A-V communis, both ventricles are dilated; thus, the septum may be stationary or may move normally toward the LV during ventricular systole.

The 2-D echocardiogram is very useful in distinguishing the different types of ECDs. The remnant of the atrial septum projects into the atrial cavity posteriorly on the parasternal short axis view and on the apex four-chamber view (Fig. 7–9E and E'). The arch of the A-V valves is convex toward the ventricular apex. On the apex four-chamber view, both A-V valves insert at the same level on the summit or crest of the ventricular septum (Fig. 7–9E and F). The cleft in the mitral valve is observed on the short axis view of the LV cavity (Fig. 7–9D). In ostium primum ASD the A-V valves are tightly bound to the top of the ventricular septum (Fig. 7–9E and F), whereas with the complete forms a space may be identified between the A-V valves and the top of the ventricular septum (Fig. 7–13). In some instances this space may not be obvious so that the echocardiographic distinction between partial and complete A-V canal is not always apparent. In type A, A-V communis, the chordae tendineae attach to the top of the ventricular septum. In type B the chordae appear to join and descend into the RV. In type C (free floating) no chordae are identified below the middle of the anterior leaflet. Echocardiography in VSD of the A-V canal type demonstrates findings of membranous VSD (e.g., LA enlargment, hyperkinetic LV). In addition, 2-D echocardiography may show a VSD posteriorly between the A-V valves on the apex four-chamber view and a cleft mitral valve

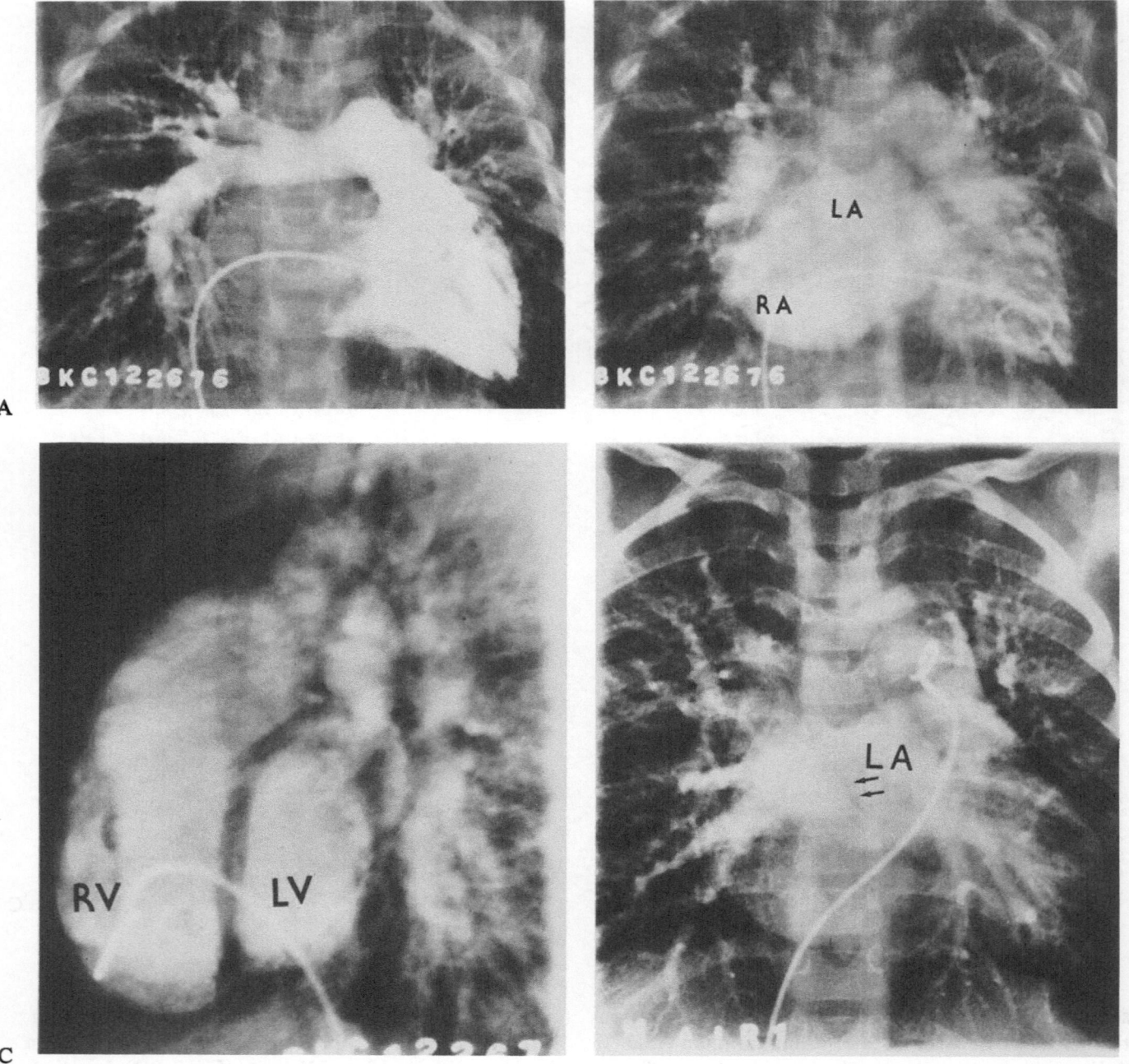

Fig. 7–11. *Atrial septal defect.* **A,B** and **C** Films from a right ventriculogram in a 1-year-old infant with ostium secundum atrial septal defect (same patient as Fig. 7–10A and B). Frame **D** is a film from the levophase in a boy with sinus venosus atrial septal defect (same patient as Fig. 7–10C). In **A** the dilated right ventricle is responsible for the straightening or slight convexity of the left heart border observed on the frontal plain film. The pulmonary arteries and peripheral branches are dilated (pulmonary overcirculation). In **B,** the levophase, the left atrium (*LA*) and right atrium (*RA*) are opacified equally, and the interface that normally separates them is obliterated. In **C,** the lateral view of the levophase, the right and left ventricles are opacified equally. The left ventricle is retrodisplaced and rotated by the enlarged right ventricle so that the ventricular septum is clearly outlined in the lateral view. The dilated right ventricular outflow tract accounts for obliteration of the retrosternal clear space on the lateral chest roentgenogram. Frame **D,** a film from the levophase in a patient with sinus venosus atrial septal defect, reveals the confluence of the right pulmonary veins as they join the superior vena cava at its entrance into the right atrium. Contrast material flows across the high atrial septal defect. The lucent line (*arrows*) below the atrial septal defect represents the top of the interatrial septum. *RV* = right ventricle; *LV* = left ventricle.

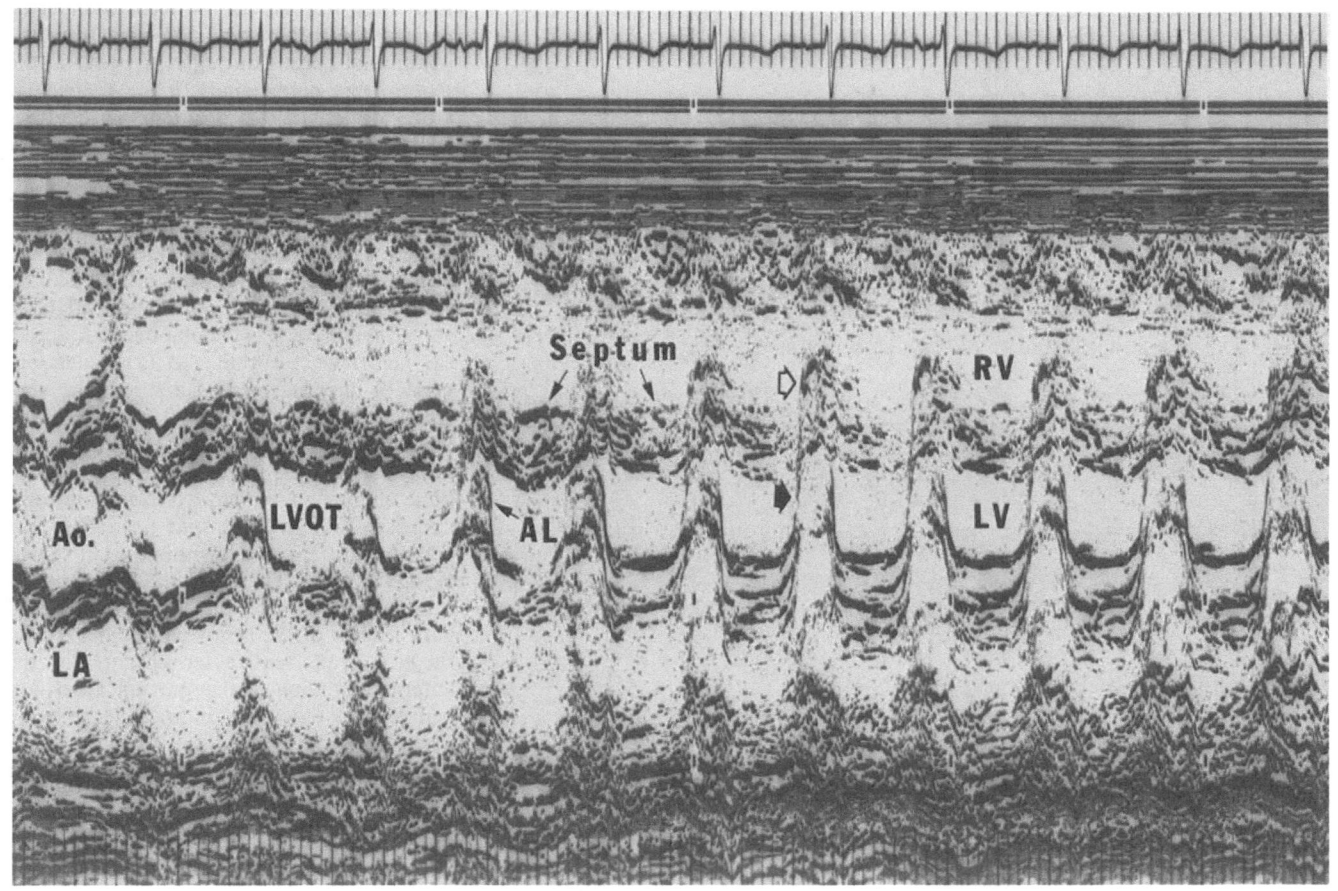

A

Fig. 7–12. *Atrioventricularis communis (A-V communis).* A M-mode arc scan from the aortic root (*Ao.*) to the left ventricle (*LV*) shows the anterior leaflet of the common A-V valve (*AL*) projecting into the left ventricular outflow tract (*LVOT*) during diastole. Further toward the apex the A-V valve appears to cross the ventricular septum during diastole (*arrows*). The anterior leaflet of the atrioventricular valve extends from the left ventricle across the peak of the ventricular septum into the right ventricle, opening superiorly and anteriorly. The echo beam encounters the left side of the atrioventricular valve initially (*closed arrow*). As the valve opens further, the right side of the leaflet, anterior to the septum (*open arrow*), comes into view. Multiple echoes lend a shaggy appearance to the atrioventricular valve. *LA* = left atrium; *RV* = right ventricle. (*Continued*)

on LV short axis view. The atrial septum is intact. The A-V valves may or may not arch down into the ventricular cavities.

Radiological (Plain Film) Features The findings are determined by the size and level of the shunt. The potential hemodynamic disturbances that may be reflected on plain films are:

1) Atrial level left-to-right shunt
2) Ventricular level left-to-right shunt
3) Mitral or tricuspid insufficiency
4) LV-to-RA shunt
5) Pulmonary hypertension, secondary to high pulmonary blood flow or to high pulmonary resistance
6) Pulmonic stenosis or atresia
7) Congestive heart failure
8) Combinations of the above (Figs. 7–14, 7–15)

Associated anomalies may alter the hemodynamics so that plain film findings may not be diagnostic. Clinical data such as left axis deviation or presence of trisomy 21 (Down syndrome) are helpful. For instance, if the plain film findings are those of ASD the clinical finding of left axis deviation should lead to consideration of an ostium primum ASD rather than an ostium secundum defect.

Hemodynamics On cardiac catheterization a characteristic finding is the ability to move the catheter freely from the RA directly into the LV, presumably without passing through the LA. The catheter passes from the RA to LA just above the diaphragm in the absence of the septum primum.

In individuals with ostium primum ASD a left-to-right atrial level shunt is identified by O_2 saturation studies. Frequently the oxygen step-up is sensed in the RV rather than in the RA because the shunted blood streams directly across the atrial defect and into the RV. If mitral insufficiency is present the regurgitant jet will be directed across the ASD, adding to the right-sided volume load (LV-to-RA shunt). Thus pulmonary blood flow may be markedly elevated and pulmonary hypertension may be present. The LV-to-RA shunt is obligatory because it consists of shunting from the high-pressure LV into the low-pressure RA. Therefore this shunt is not limited by changes in pulmonary resistance.

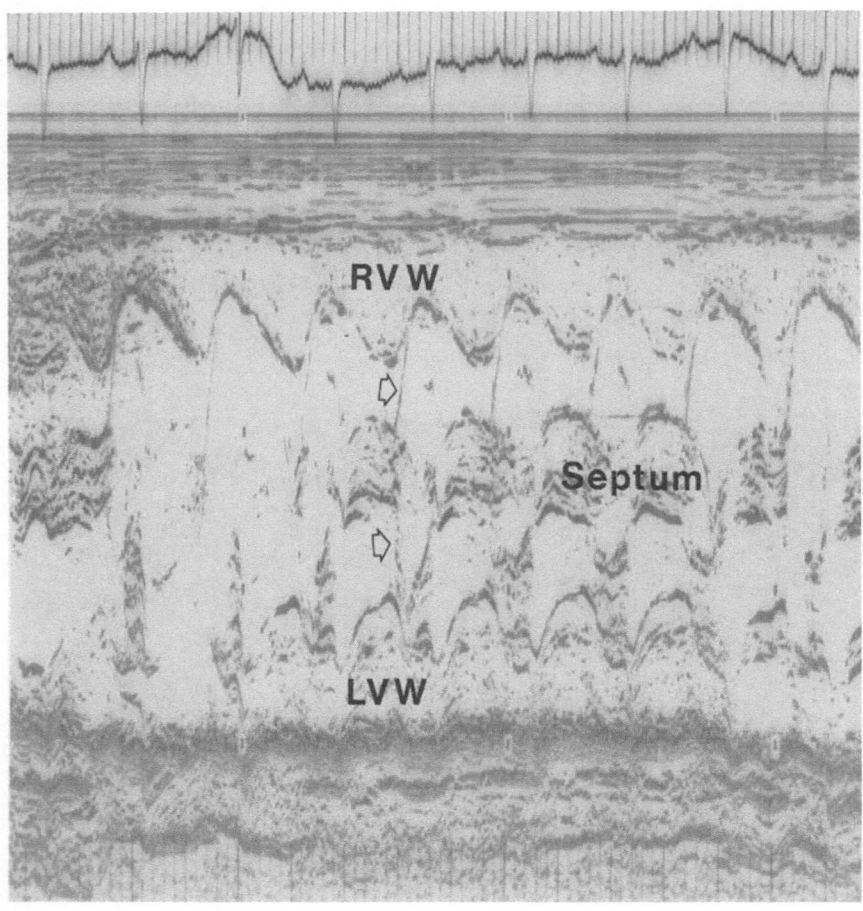

B

Fig. 7–12 (*Cont.*). In **B,** from a different patient, the transducer is directed from the left sternal border through the break in the septum that corresponds to the ventricular septal defect. In this position the atrioventricular valve (*open arrows*) opens anteriorly and posteriorly away from the ventricular septum during diastole. This motion is characteristic of A-V communis. Note that this pattern is reminiscent of straddling of the atrioventricular valve. In other defects, straddling of the atrioventricular valve involves two factors: (1) anular override across the ventricular septum and (2) malattachment of chordae tendineae across the ventricular septum. With A-V communis the anulus of the common atrioventricular valve always crosses the top of the ventricular septum, similar to anular override; however, chordae from the tricuspid portion of the valve only rarely attach within the left ventricle or vice versa. Therefore in A-V communis this pattern may be due to attachment of both leaflets of the atrioventricular valve to the peak of the ventricular septum, with the anterior common leaflet moving anteriorly and the posterior common leaflet moving posteriorly during diastole.

RVW = right ventricular wall; *LVW* = left ventricular wall.

Fig. 7–13. *Two-dimensional echocardiogram in type A atrioventricularis communis (A-V communis)—anterior common leaflet attached to the ventricular septum.* **A,** Long axis view of the left ventricle during systole; **B,** long axis view of the left ventricle during diastole; **C,** apex four-chamber view during systole; **D** and **E,** subxiphoid four-chamber view during systole and diastole respectively. In **A** multiple echoes occur in the vicinity of the closed atrioventricular valve (*arrow*). During diastole (**B**) the left portion of the anterior leaflet of the common atrioventricular valve (*arrow*) is pressed tightly against the ventricular septum as in ostium primum atrial septal defect (see fig. 7–9). The ventricular septal defect is not demonstrated here. In the four-chamber views (**C** to **E**) the remnant of the atrial septum protrudes from the back wall of the heart, partially separating the two atria. The ostium primum atrial septal defect (*arrow* in **C′**) occurs just above the common atrioventricular valve. In these same views during systole the chordal attachments between the anterior common leaflet and the peak of the ventricular septum are evident. The ventricular septal defect (*arrow* in **C′**) consists of the spaces between the chordae tendineae. During diastole (**E**) the anterior common leaflet swings toward the apex draping over the peak of the ventricular septum (*conjoined arrows*). The lateral leaflets are indicated by two small separate arrows.

The four chamber views are the keys to differentiation of type A, B, and C of A-V communis.

Ao. = aortic root; *LV* = left ventricle; *LA* = left atrium; *RV* = right ventricle; *RVOT* = right ventricular outflow tract.

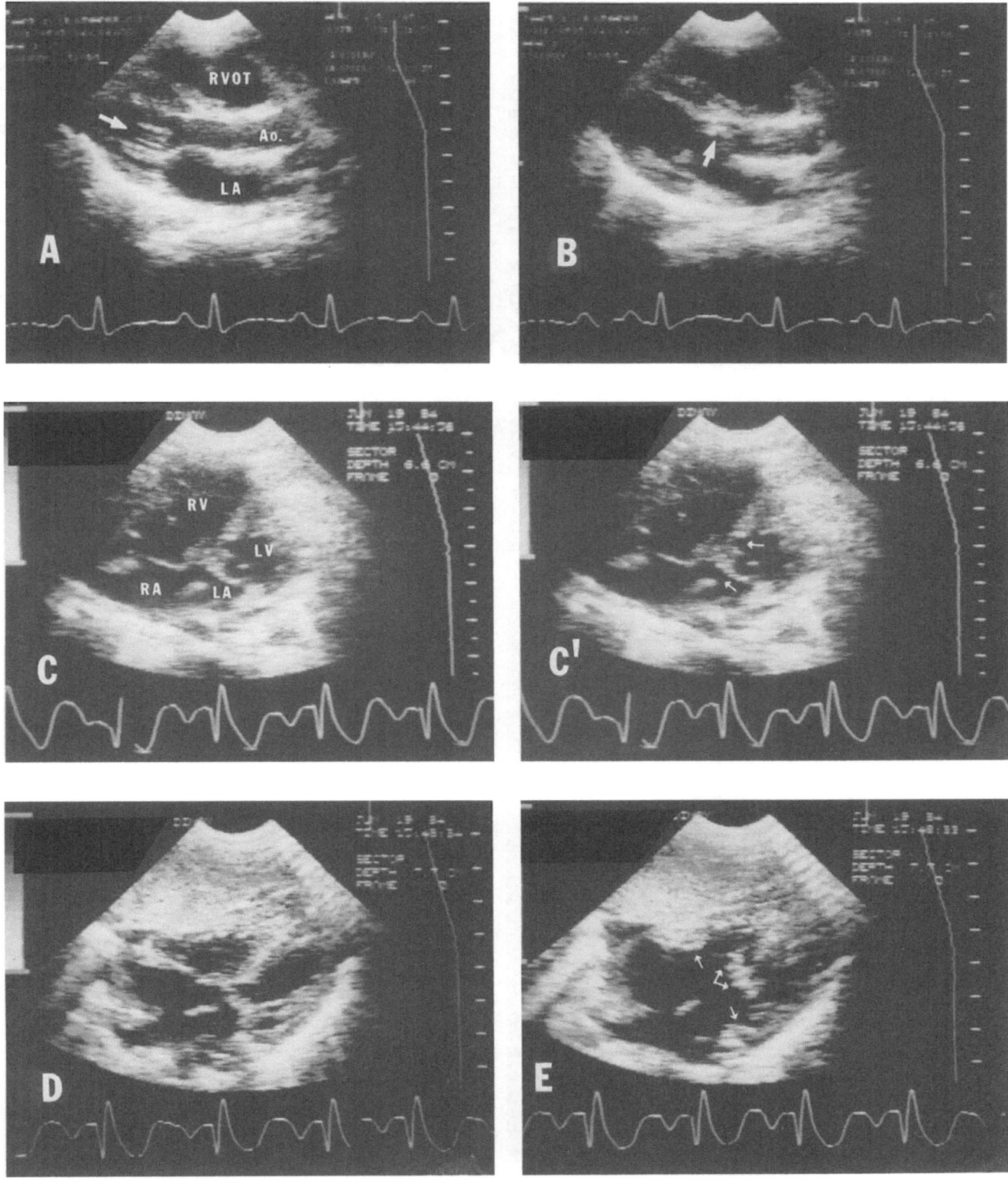

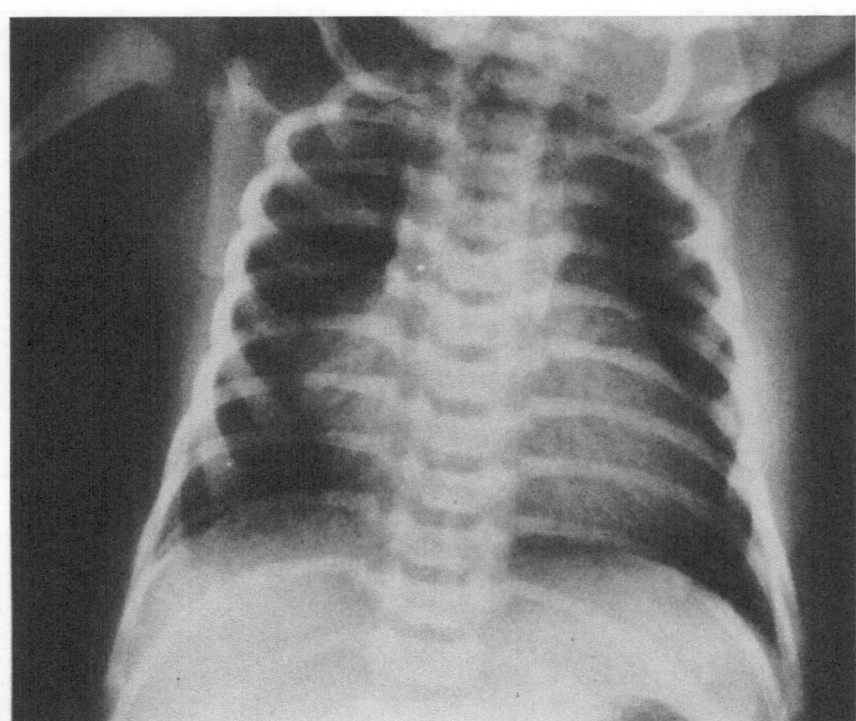

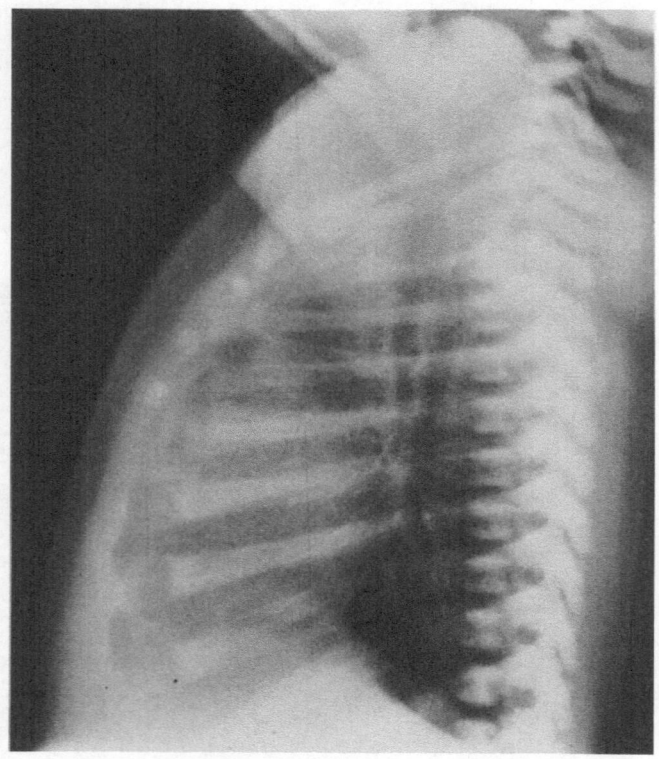

Fig. 7–14. *A-V communis with high pulmonary resistance in a 1-week-old girl with cyanosis.* Bilateral pulmonary undercirculation is present, together with biventricular enlargement and right atrial enlargement. As pulmonary resistance decreased, the cyanosis resolved, and the baby developed pulmonary overcirculation and congestive heart failure.

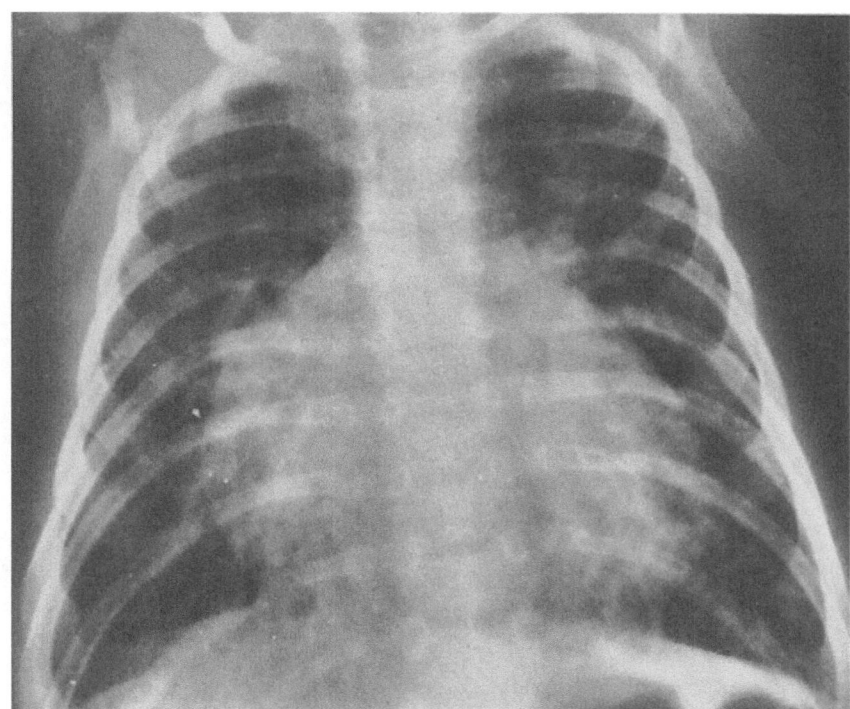

A

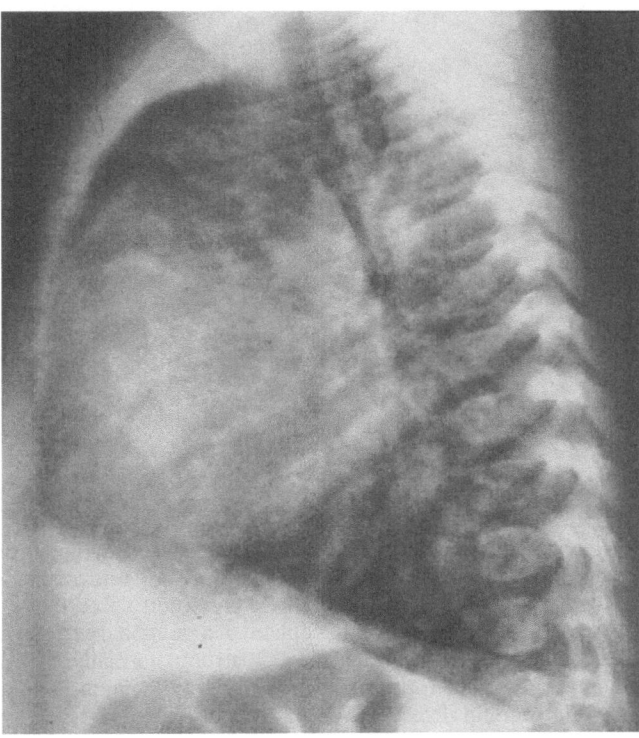

B

Fig. 7–15. *A-V communis without increase in pulmonary resistance.* Frontal (**A**) and lateral (**B**) chest roentgenograms in a 3-month-old girl with Down syndrome. Pulmonary overcirculation and four-chamber enlargement (globular heart) are present. The history, the left axis deviation on the electrocardiogram and these plain film findings constitute strong evidence for A-V communis.

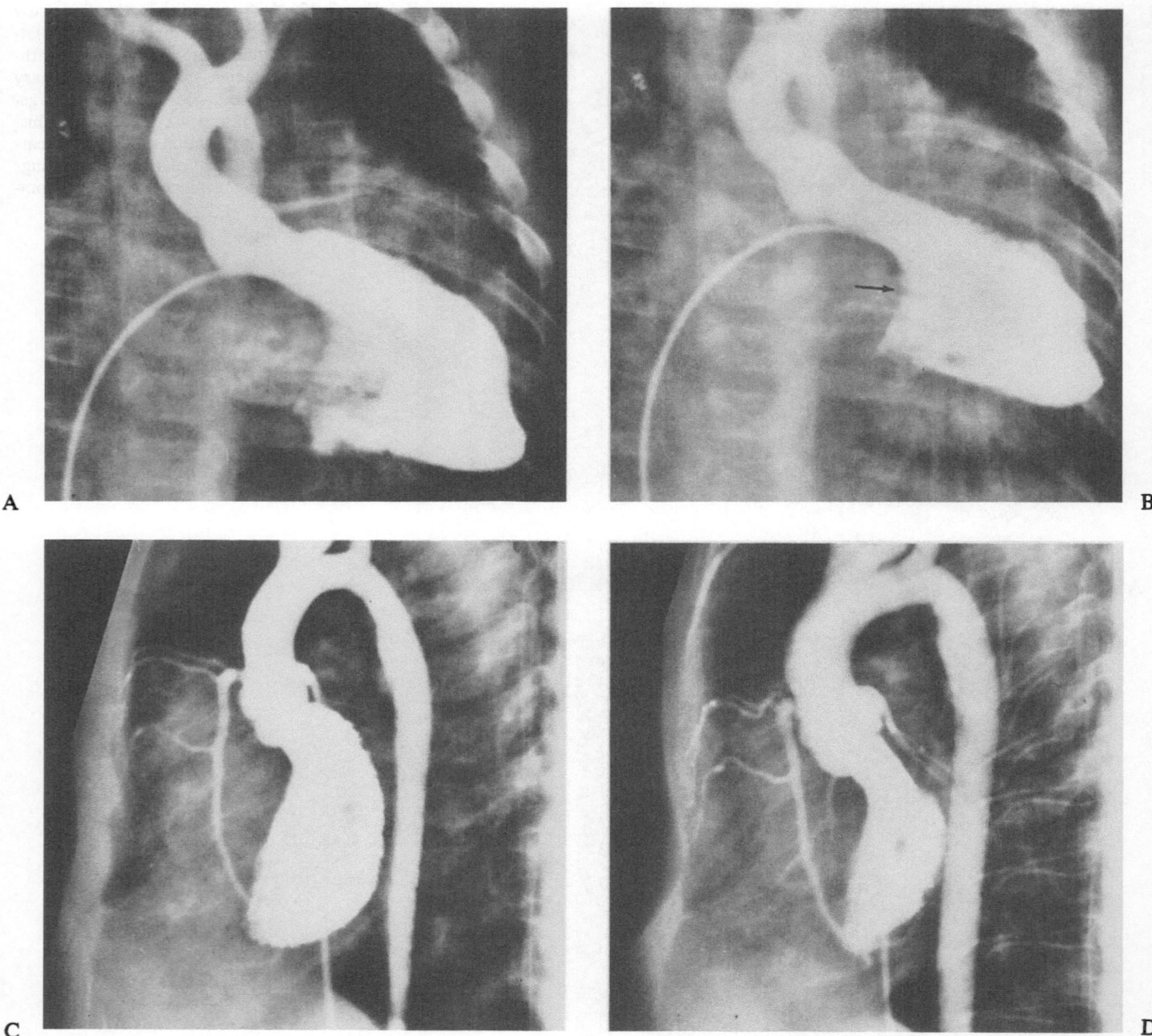

Fig. 7–16. *Endocardial cushion defect (Ostium primum atrial septal defect) in a 5-month-old boy with Down syndrome.* Left ventriculogram in the frontal view in diastole (**A**) and systole (**B**) and in the lateral view in diastole (**C**) and systole (**D**). **E** is a frame from the levophase of a pulmonary arteriogram. In **A** and **B** the "gooseneck" deformity of the left ventricle is apparent. The cleft in the mitral valve appears as a nonopaque notch (*arrow*). The serrations represent the tertiary chordae tendineae which attach the anterior leaflet of the mitral valve to the ventricular septum. In the lateral view (**C** and **D**) no ventricular level shunt is identified. The left ventricle is retrodisplaced by the enlarged right ventricle. In **E** (levophase of a pulmonary angiogram) the pulmonary veins enter the left atrium normally. A jet of contrast medium (*arrows*), low in the atrial septum defines an ostium primum defect.

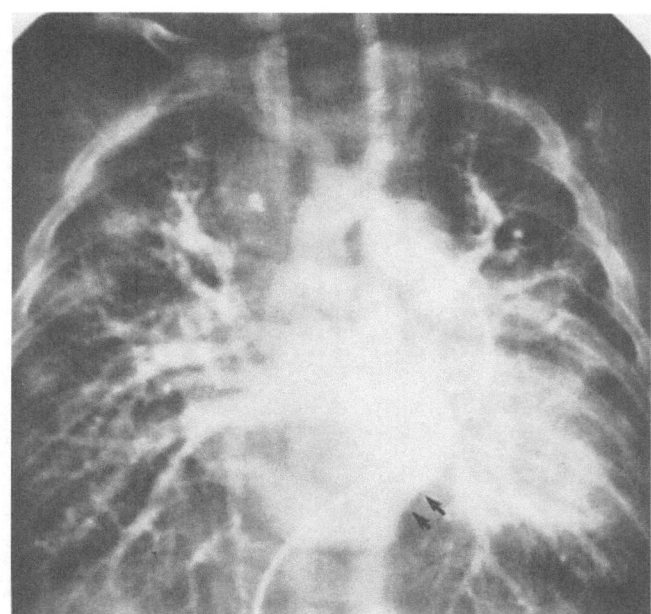

E

lar view (four-chamber view) is very helpful in imaging the LV outflow tract. In addition, the A-V valve and its attachments are often demonstrated better in this view than on other projections. Mitral insufficiency is usually present and is directed through the ASD toward the RA. A ventricular level shunt is usually directed anteriorly into the RV cavity and is therefore best observed on lateral or LAO views. Separate streams of blood may be directed toward the RA and toward the RV. Simultaneous filling of the RV and RA suggests combined mitral insufficiency and VSD, whereas sequential filling of the RA and then the RV is consistent with mitral insufficiency (LV-to-RA shunt). In A-V canal type A (divided anterior leaflet attached to the septum) (Figs. 7–18, 7–19) the ventricular shunt passes under the anterior mitral leaflet and is divided into multiple jets by the chordae tendineae. In type C (undivided anterior leaflet) (Fig. 7–17) the anterior leaflet appears on lateral, LAO and angulated views as an arch

With A-V communis, shunting occurs at the atrial as well as the ventricular level. Insufficiency of the A-V valve may add to the volume load. Bidirectional shunting may occur with or without increase in pulmonary resistance. The pressures in the atria are equal, as are those in the ventricles. Coarctation of the aorta, patent ductus arteriosus, pulmonic stenosis or pulmonary atresia may complicate the hemodynamics.

Contrast Studies The characteristic angiographic finding in all forms of ECD, except isolated VSD of the A-V canal type, is the gooseneck deformity of the LV outflow tract (Fig. 7–16). This is best observed in the frontal and RAO views, appearing as a "scooping out" of the right border of the LV silhouette. The deformity is produced by the abnormal attachment of the left A-V valve to the crest of the shortened ventricular septum. Scallops or serrations are formed by the attachments of the chordae tendineae. The cleft of the mitral leaflet is a nonopaque notch pointing into the LV during systole. During diastole the anterior leaflet opens and is sharply delineated by the contrast medium in the LV outflow tract above it and the unopacified blood entering the LV below it. The LV outflow tract appears narrow during systole and even more so during diastole. The atrioventricular septum, which normally forms part of the right border of the LV silhouette on frontal and RAO views, is not present in ECDs (for comparison with normal see Fig. 4–35A and B). On the lateral and LAO views during diastole the attachment of the superior segment of the cleft anterior leaflet of the mitral valve (or the anterior leaflet in A-V communis) is represented by a nearly horizontal curved line below the aortic valve, delineated by the contrast material above it and the unopacified blood below it (Fig. 7–17). Conversely, the normal attachment of the anterior mitral leaflet is a vertical line in continuity with the aortic valve (see Figs. 4–35C and 7–79A).

The LAO view with cranial angulation or hepatoclavicu-

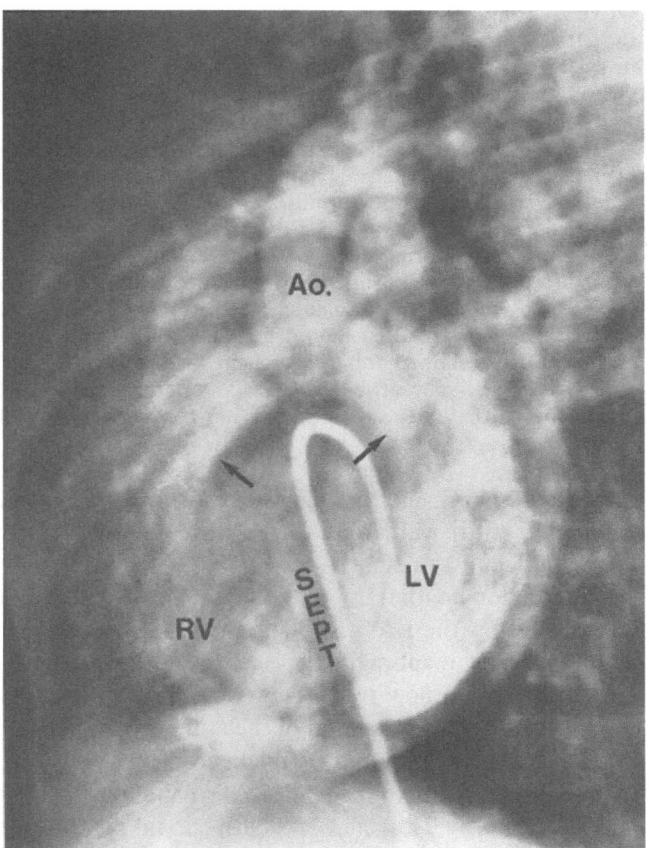

Fig. 7–17. *A-V communis type C of Rastelli (undivided, free floating anterior leaflet).* On the lateral view of the left ventriculogram the anterior leaflet of the common atrioventricular valve appears as a curved horizontal line below the aorta (*Ao.*). The leaflet (*arrows*) extends across the ventricular septum (*SEPT*) from the left ventricle (*LV*) into the right ventricle (*RV*), being delineated by contrast material above and unopacified blood entering the ventricles below. If the anterior leaflet were divided or attached, the curved line would be indented in the middle to form two arches. (The catheter enters the right atrium from the inferior vena cava, crosses the atrial septum into the left atrium, and its tip lies in the apex of the left ventricle.)

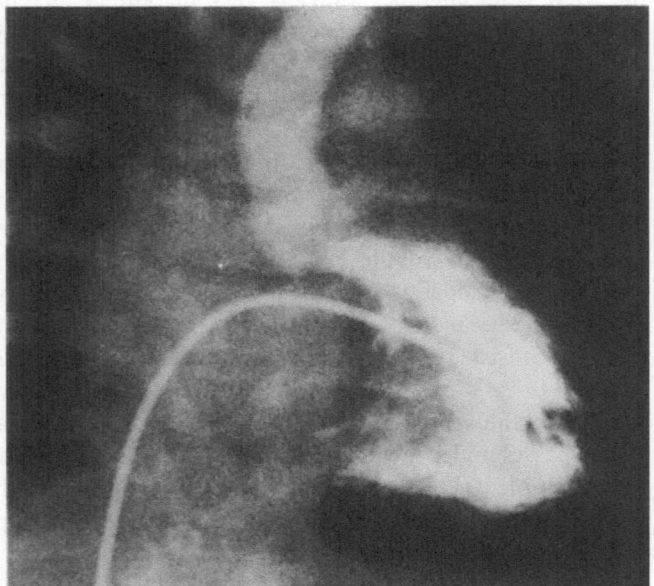

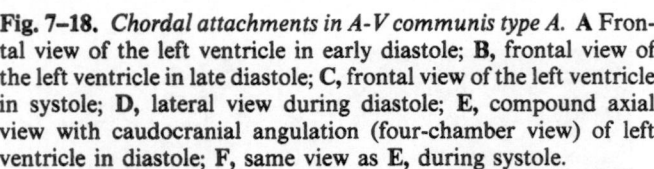

A

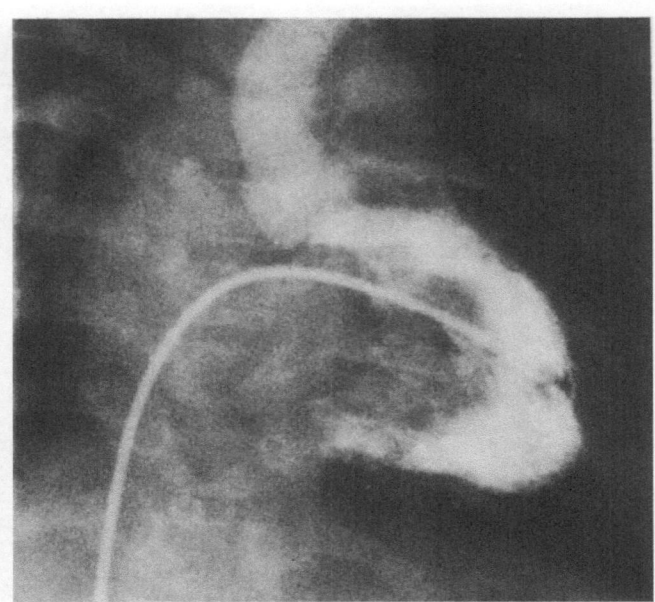

B

Fig. 7–18. *Chordal attachments in A-V communis type A.* **A** Frontal view of the left ventricle in early diastole; **B,** frontal view of the left ventricle in late diastole; **C,** frontal view of the left ventricle in systole; **D,** lateral view during diastole; **E,** compound axial view with caudocranial angulation (four-chamber view) of left ventricle in diastole; **F,** same view as **E,** during systole.

The standard frontal and lateral views demonstrate the findings of endocardial cushion defect, but may not be sufficient to differentiate the various types of deformities of the atrioventricular valve in A-V communis. In **A** and **B** a typical "gooseneck" deformity is demonstrated. During systole (**C**) the "cleft" (*arrow*) of the left half of the common atrioventricular valve is noted. These two radiological features are not specific for identification of any one type of endocardial cushion defect. The lateral view during diastole (**D**) also shows findings consistent with endocardial cushion defect. The atrioventricular valve (anterior common leaflet) opens toward the observer, forming a horizontal line below the

aortic valve. Contrast medium is trapped within the left ventricular outflow tract above the atrioventricular valve while unopacified blood fills the left ventricle below the valve. During systole (not illustrated) the right atrium and right ventricle opacified simultaneously.

It was not possible to determine the type of A-V communis from these studies. The compound axial LAO view with cranial tilt (hepatoclavicular view) (**E** and **F**) was necessary in further delineating anatomical detail. In **F** the anterior common leaflet is bound to the peak of the ventricular septum, so that contrast material passing from the left ventricle to the right ventricle is forced through multiple small channels formed by the chordae tendineae, the leaflets and the septum. During diastole (**E**) the gooseneck is formed by the abnormal opening motion of the anterior leaflet of the atrioventricular valve. Unopacified blood enters below the leaflet, while contrast agent remains within the left ventricular outflow tract above the anterior common leaflet.

that extends horizontally below the aortic valve, encompassing the entire width of the A-V orifice. The attachments may be difficult to define.

Obstruction to the LV outflow tract is often demonstrated best on the LAO angulated (cranial) view. A discrete subaortic diaphragm appears as a radiolucent line across the LV outflow tract. Tethering of a leaflet is indicated by restriction of motion of the anterior mitral leaflet; the leaflet may or may not be thickened.

A VSD of the inlet type (called A-V canal type by Neufeld et al. and by Titus and Rastelli), should be differentiated from an endocardial cushion type of VSD with involvement of the mitral and tricuspid valves. With the former, no gooseneck deformity is evident since this defect involves only the inlet portion of the ventricular septum and does not deform the tricuspid or mitral valve (Fig. 7–20). On angiography this defect appears some distance below the crista supraventricularis and membranous septum. In contrast, a typical gooseneck deformity is observed with a VSD of the endocardial cushion type with cleft mitral and tricuspid valves. This VSD is located just below the crista supraventricularis (Fig. 7–21).

Treatment Ostium primum ASD and common atrium may be managed medically during infancy. These abnormalities are repaired by patching the atrial defect. The severity of mitral valve insufficiency significantly influences outcome. On occasion the mitral valve must be replaced at the time of initial surgery, or thereafter.

Complete A-V canal often results in severe congestive heart failure. Banding of the main pulmonary artery (MPA) may or may not be successful, as it controls only the ventricular level shunt and not the atrial shunt. If A-V valve insufficiency is severe, then MPA banding is unlikely to be of benefit. Complete repair in infants with severe A-V valve insufficiency is also unlikely to succeed. The A-V valve is often found to be poorly formed in these infants and may be dysplastic. If the infant survives to the age of 1 year then definitive repair may be undertaken. Factors that influence the outcome are (1) severity of A-V valve insufficiency, (2) relative size of the ventricles and (3) pulmonary vascular resistance.

Postoperative findings include (1) residual mitral insufficiency, (2) residual VSD, (3) complete heart block, (4) persistent pulmonary hypertension and (5) problems associ-

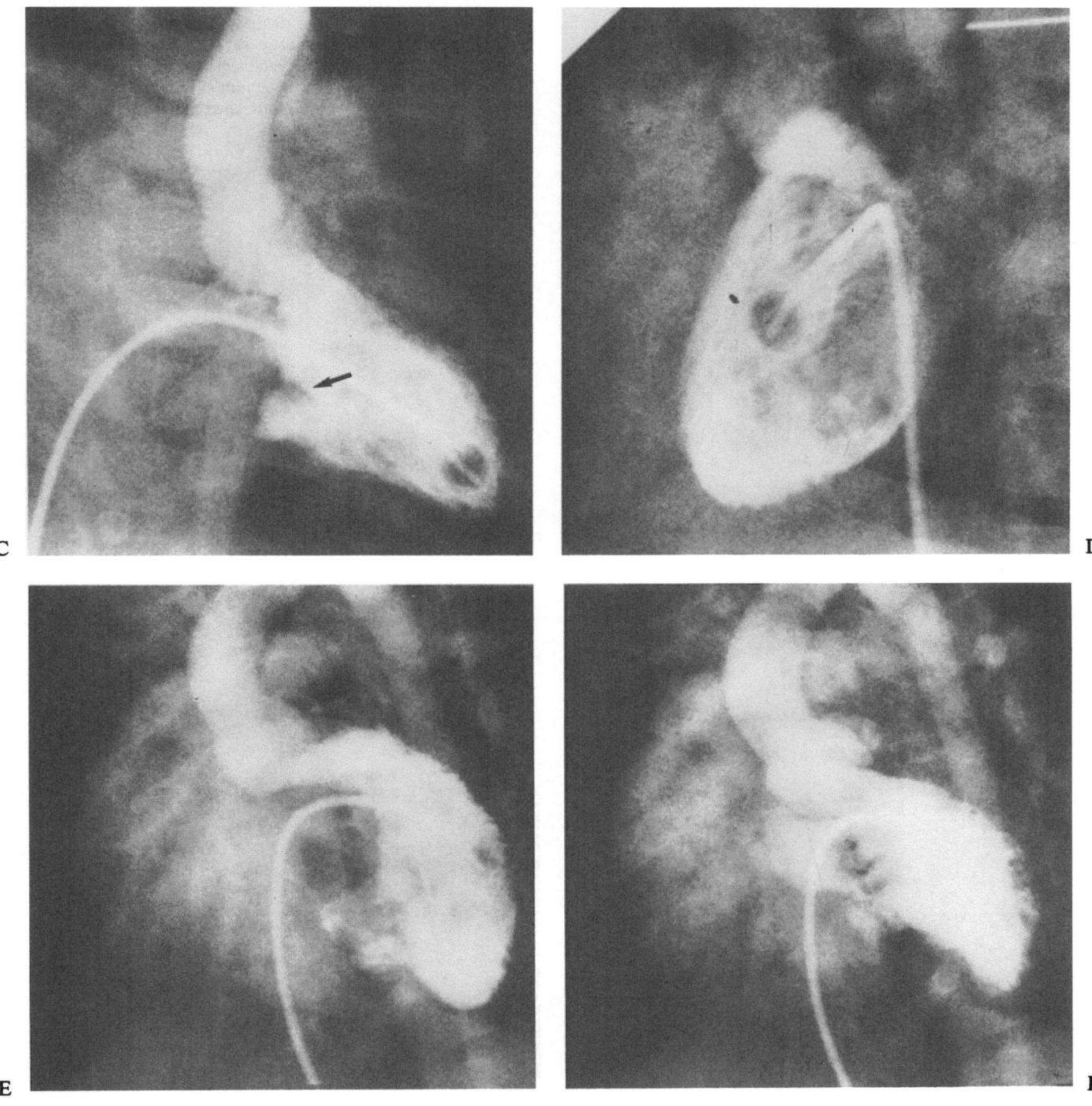

C

D

E

F

ated with a prosthetic valve if used as part of the repair.

Anomalous Pulmonary Venous Return

In this developmental malformation the pulmonary veins enter the RA (or its tributaries) instead of the LA. Two forms are recognized—partial and total—depending on the number of the anomalous pulmonary veins. Partial anomalous pulmonary venous return (PAPVR) consists of a group of acyanotic defects that may cause mild symptoms or may not cause any symptoms. The radiological findings are similar to those of ASD. Total anomalous pulmonary venous return (TAPVR) is closely related embryologically,

but is an admixture lesion in which the newborn has cyanosis and severe cardiac symptoms. The radiological features are variable, depending on the presence or absence of pulmonary venous obstruction.

Partial Anomalous Pulmonary Venous Return   This uncommon disorder (0.4%–0.7% of postmortem studies) generally involves one lung or a part of a lung. The right lung is more frequently involved than the left.

PAPVR of the right lung takes two forms. Commonly the anomalous veins join either the superior vena cava (SVC) or the RA, or both. A high ASD (sinus venosus) is usually present. The second type of anomalous connec-

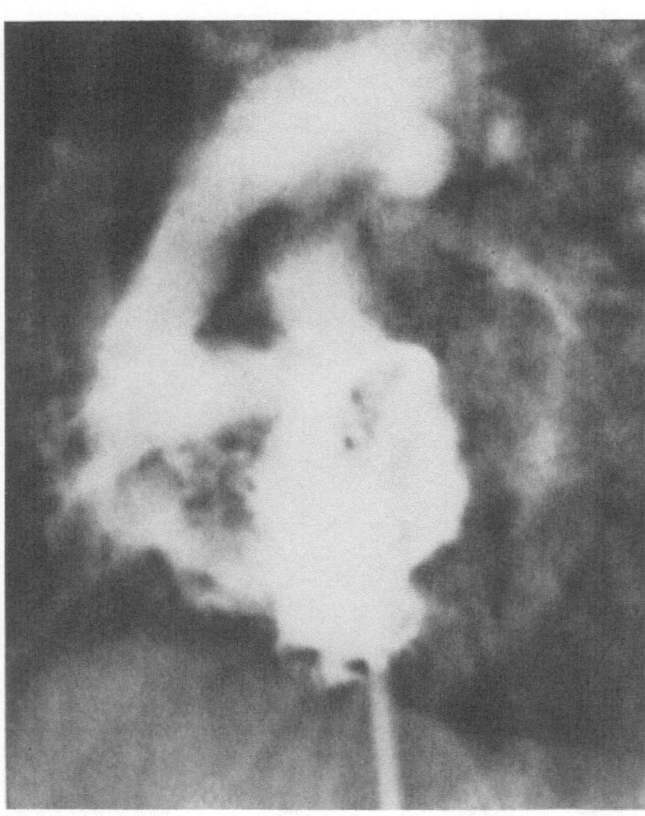

Fig. 7–19. *Chordal attachment in A-V communis type A.* A lateral view of a left ventriculogram delineates a funnel-shaped jet of contrast medium below the aortic valve. The shape of the jet suggests that the ventricular septal defect is restricted in size because the anterior leaflet of the common atrioventricular valve is bound to the septum (septally attached anterior leaflet).

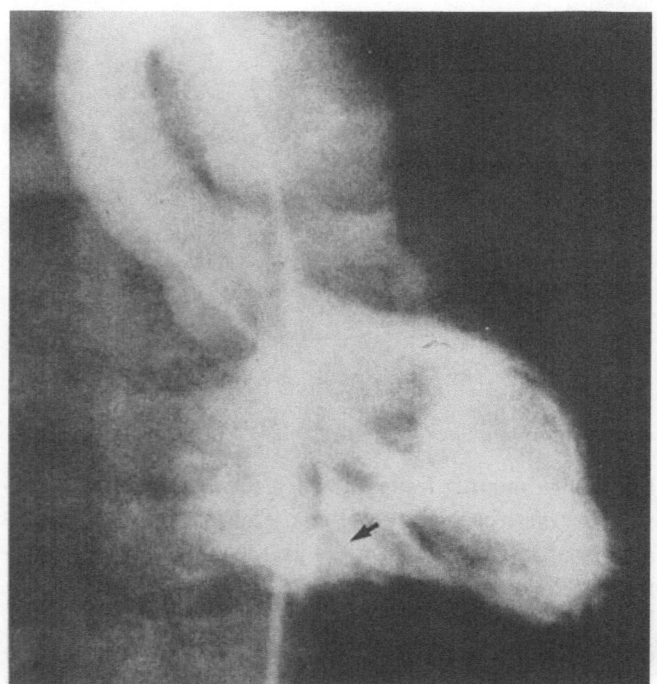

A

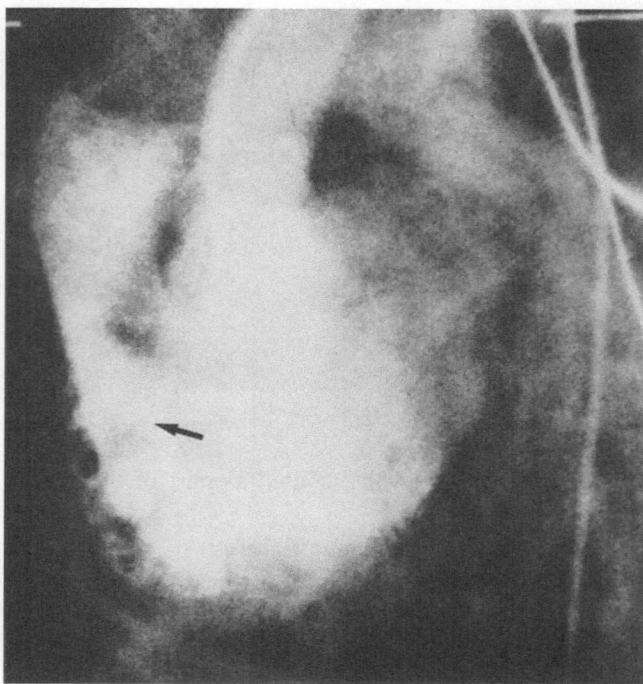

B

Fig. 7–20. *Inlet type of ventricular septal defect.* This is designated by Neufeld et al. and by Titus and Rastelli as a ventricular septal defect of the atrioventricular canal type. No gooseneck deformity is present on the frontal view (A). The jet of contrast medium representing the ventricular septal defect (*arrow*) is located some distance below the crista supraventricularis and adjacent to the tricuspid valve on the frontal view. On the lateral view (B) the membranous septum is intact, and the shunt (*arrow*) is inferior (posterior) to it.

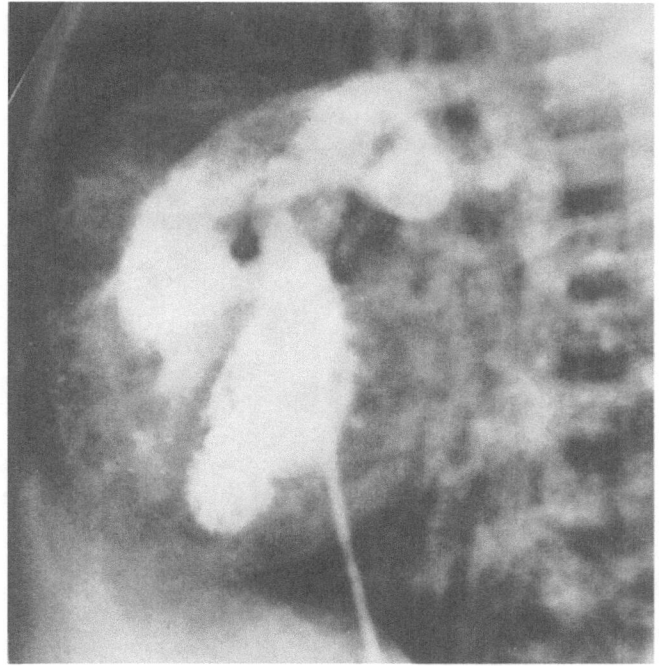

A

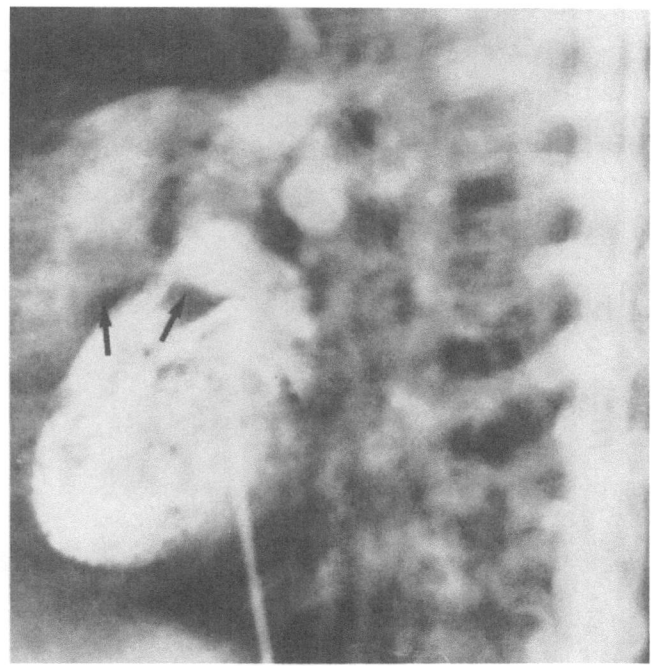

B

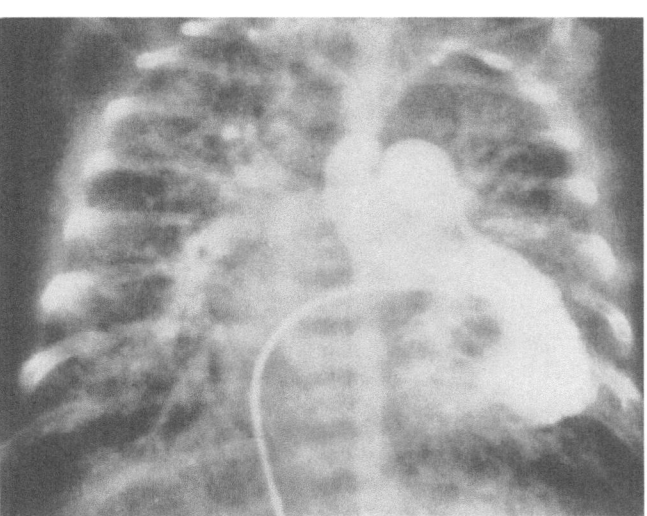

C

Fig. 7–21. *Ventricular septal defect of the endocardial cushion type.* A left ventricular angiogram in a 1-month-old infant with a ventricular level communication without an atrial septal defect. **A** Lateral view during systole; **B** lateral view during diastole; **C** frontal view during diastole. During systole (**A**) the ventricular septal defect is visualized immediately below the crista supraventricularis. During diastole (**B**) the curved horizontal line representing the open atrioventricular valve extends across the ventricular septum (*arrows*). The valve is outlined by contrast medium above it and unopacified blood below it. In the frontal view (**C**) a typical gooseneck deformity is demonstrated.

tion involves all or part of the right lung, the anomalous veins forming a common vessel that perforates the diaphragm to join the inferior vena cava (IVC) (scimitar syndrome, vena cava bronchovascular syndrome).

Anomalous return of the left lung may involve the entire left lung or only the left upper lobe. The anomalous veins from the left lung often enter a left-sided vertical vein that drains into the left innominate vein. The "vertical vein" probably represents a remnant of a persistent left SVC that has lost its connection with the coronary sinus. On occasion the anomalous veins drain into a persistent left SVC or directly into the coronary sinus (CS). An ASD at the fossa ovalis is usually associated.

PAPVR is usually asymptomatic if the amount of shunt is small. In the presence of a large left-to-right shunt the clinical picture is indistinguishable from that of ASD. In the absence of associated ASD the second sound will be widely split, but will vary with respiration. This feature

is unusual, since only occasional individuals with PAPVR have an isolated defect. The ECG findings are also similar to those associated with secundum ASD. The M-mode echocardiographic findings are similar to those with ASD (Fig. 7–6). On 2-D echocardiography, absence of normal pulmonary venous connections from one lung should lead one to the suspicion that partial anomalous pulmonary venous connection is present. Findings on plain films in individuals with PAPVR are indistinguishable from those of ASD, except in cases of drainage of the right lung into the IVC (scimitar syndrome) and total unilateral anomalous pulmonary venous drainage of the left lung. These lesions are discussed subsequently. The hemodynamics are similar to those with ASD except that an O_2 step-up will be present at the site of the anomalous connection. Injection of contrast material into the main pulmonary artery usually demonstrates the anomalous connections. In a few instances, selective injection into one pulmonary artery or

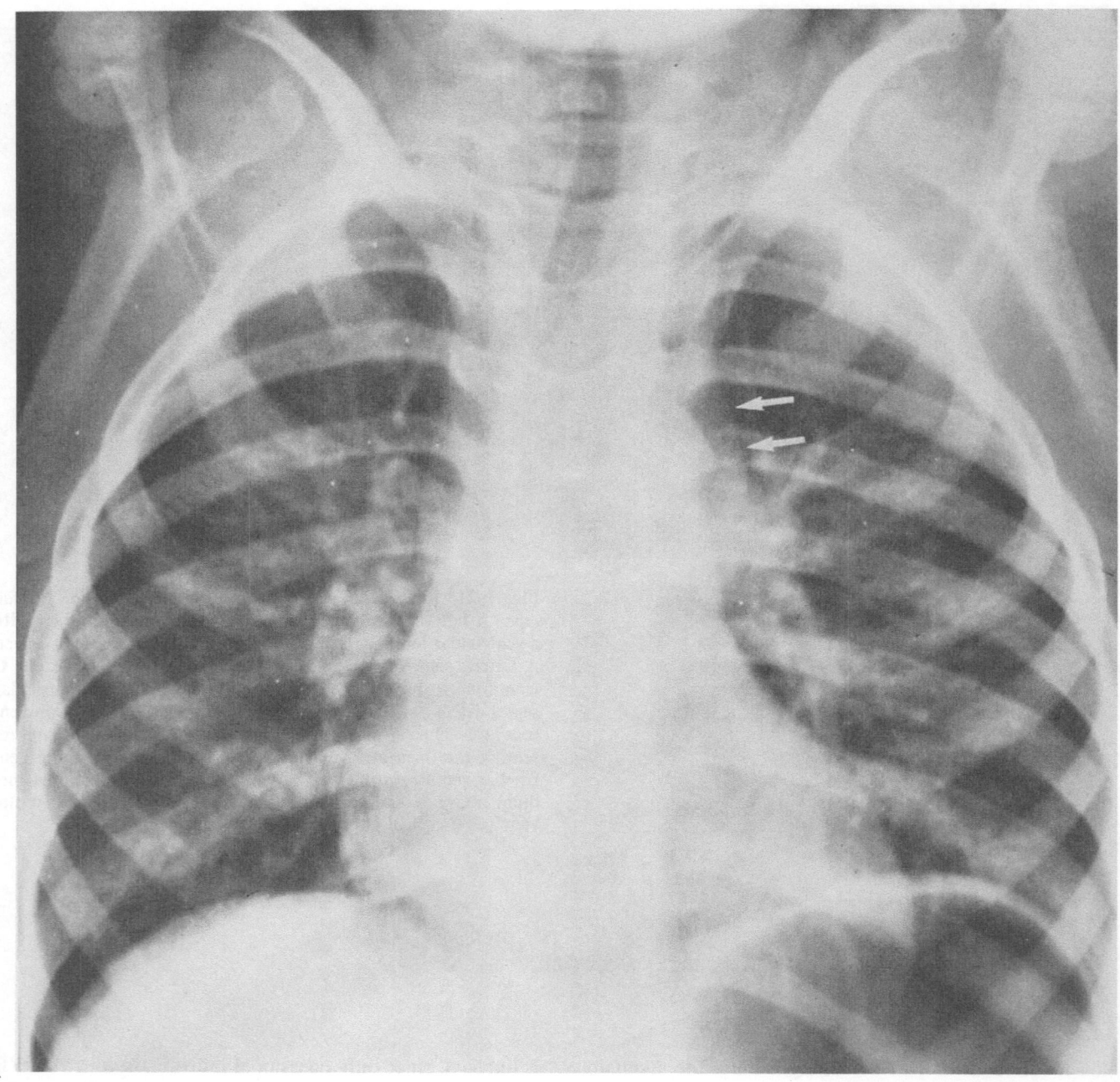

Fig. 7–22. *Total unilateral anomalous pulmonary venous return of the left lung in a 3-year-old acyanotic girl.* The frontal (**A**) and lateral (**B**) chest roentgenograms demonstrate pulmonary overcirculation. The superior mediastinum is widened by the enlarged superior vena cava on the right and by the vertical vein that forms a distinct structure on the left side lateral to the aorta

directly into the anomalous veins is necessary to confirm the diagnosis. Surgery for anomalous right pulmonary venous return is part of the repair of ASD. A patch is used to redirect the pulmonary venous blood and close the ASD. Surgery for anomalous left pulmonary venous connection via a common trunk (the vertical vein) involves anastomosis of the venous trunk to the wall of the LA and ligation of the vein near its site of drainage into the innominate vein. If the left lung drains into the CS the repair requires excision of the roof of the CS and closure of the ASD so that the pulmonary venous blood returns with CS drainage

into the LA. This operation will result in mild hypoxemia; however, the passage of emboli to the systemic circulation and other complications associated with right-to-left shunts do not occur.

Total Unilateral Anomalous Pulmonary Venous Return of the Left Lung In this unusual anomaly the entire left lung drains into a vertical vein, which in turn joins the left innominate vein, ultimately draining through the SVC into the RA. The findings on plain films of the chest are similar to those in TAPVR of the supracardiac type (in a patient without cyanosis) (Fig. 7–22). Widening of the superior

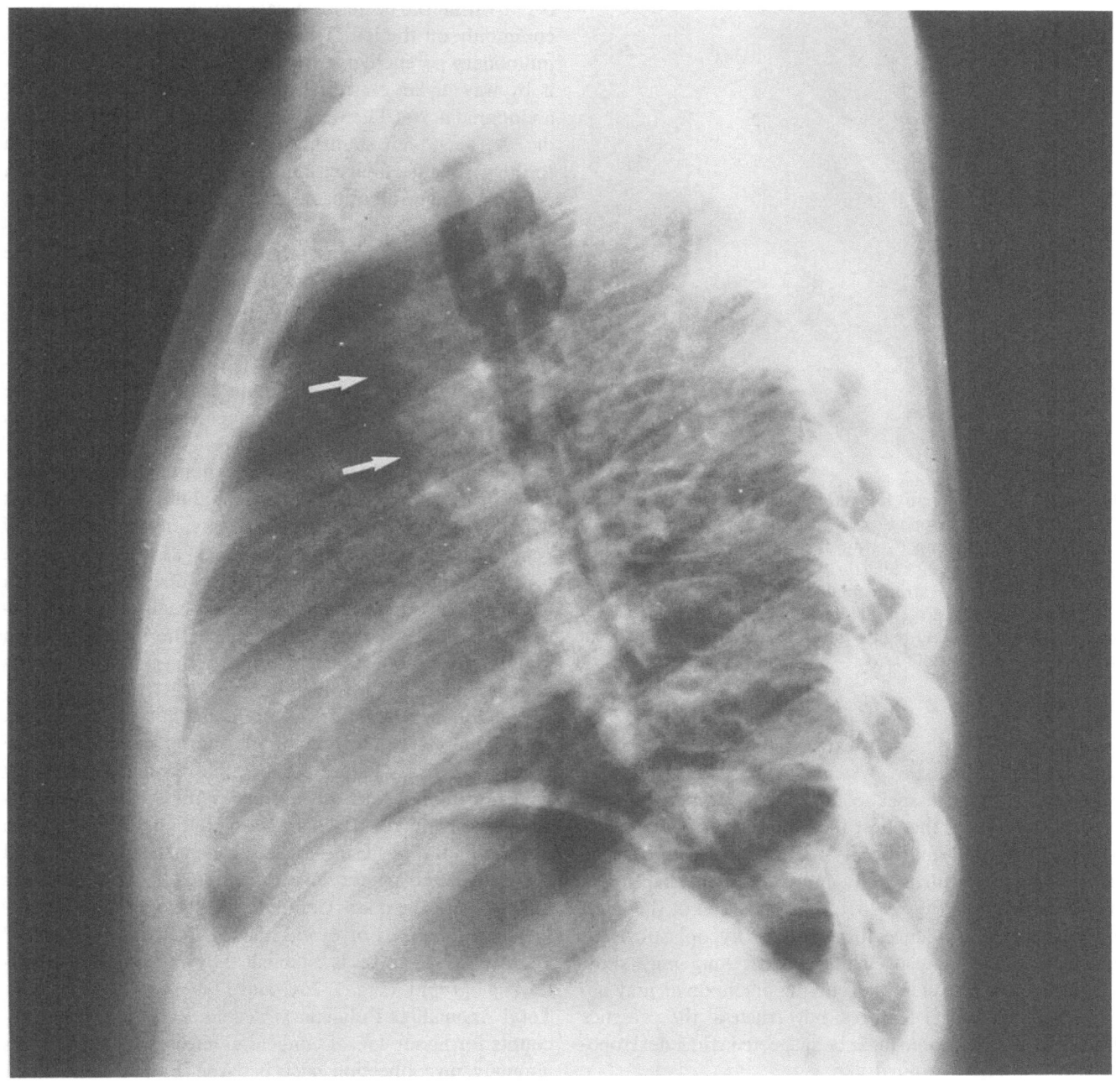

B

and the pulmonary artery (*arrows*). On the lateral view the vertical vein and the dilated superior vena cava form an apparent mass anterior to the trachea (*arrows*). The appearance of the cardiovas-cular silhouette is grossly similar to the snowman configuration associated with total anomalous pulmonary venous return of the supracardiac type. (Patient in Fig. 7–23).

mediastinum is caused by the vertical vein on the left and the dilated SVC on the right. In addition, as in TAPVR, the vertical vein and the dilated SVC create a "mass" density anterior to the trachea on the lateral film of the chest. The widening and mass effect are less prominent than those associated with TAPVR. Although total unilateral anomalous pulmonary venous return of the left lung is almost invariably associated with ASD a few reports refer to individuals in whom this anomaly was an isolated lesion (Fig. 7–23).

Scimitar Syndrome Anomalous pulmonary venous drain-age of the right lung into the IVC presents a unique appear-ance on plain films of the chest (Fig. 7–24A). The right lower and middle lobes drain downward via a common trunk, which joins the IVC at its junction with the RA (just above or just below the diaphragm) (Fig. 7–24B). The vein of the right upper pulmonary segment may or may not drain with the others. If the vein of the right upper lobe is separate it may drain normally into the LA or abnormally into the SVC or azygos vein. In patients with this type of anomalous pulmonary venous connection the right lung is usually hypoplastic, and the heart is shifted

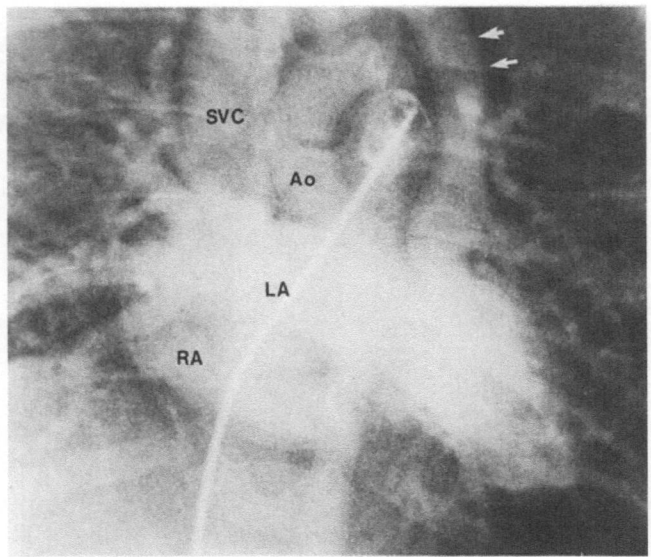

Fig. 7–23. *Total unilateral anomalous pulmonary venous return of the left lung.* The levophase of a pulmonary angiogram reveals drainage of the left lung by way of a vertical vein (*arrows*) to the left innominate vein which in turn drains into the superior vena cava (*SVC*). No atrial septal defect was identified either at angiography or at surgery. The right pulmonary veins empty into the left atrium (*LA*), while the right atrium (*RA*) fills from the SVC. *Ao* = ascending aorta.

into the right hemithorax (dextroposition). A pulmonary sequestration, supplied by systemic vessels from below the diaphragm, may be associated. An ASD is often present.

On plain films of the chest the pulmonary venous trunk forms a gently curving density to the right of the heart, which gradually widens as it approaches the diaphragm (the scimitar sign) (Fig. 7–24). Dextroposition of the heart and radiological evidence for a mildly hypoplastic right lung are usually evident, while the left lung may show overcirculation. Frequently occurring pneumonias may obscure the radiological features; nevertheless, the presence of the scimitar syndrome must be suspected when dextroposition of the heart is noted.

Pulmonary Sequestration Pulmonary sequestration is a relatively common pulmonary malformation that occurs as a solid or cystic mass in the lung or outside the lung. The entity consists of normal lung constituents (e.g., smooth muscle, bronchial epithelium, cartilage), but lacks the branching structure of normal airways. In most instances, pulmonary sequestration lacks communication with the adjacent pulmonary parenchyma. The vascular supply for sequestration arises from the systemic circulation; venous return may be to the pulmonary veins, the azygos vein, or the IVC. Some sequestrations are attached to the esophagus or stomach by way of ligaments or abnormal bronchi. Two distinct entities—intralobar and extralobar sequestrations—are recognized; however, many examples fail to fit the standard descriptions because of an atypical vascular supply or gastrointestinal connections.

Intrapulmonary (or intralobar) sequestrations usually

occur within the posterior basal segments of the lung, more commonly on the left. The mass is surrounded by normal pulmonary parenchyma. Blood supply to the sequestration is by way of large arterial branches from the thoracic or abdominal aorta. The veins drain into the pulmonary veins or LA (left-to-left shunt). Attachment or communication to the gastrointestinal system is not observed. Presentation is usually the result of bacterial infection later in childhood or adult life.

In contrast, extralobar sequestration occurs outside the lung, and may occur below the diaphragm. The mass is invested with its own pleura. The arterial supply is by way of small local arterial branches, while the veins drain into the caval or azygos system (left-to-right shunt). Extralobar sequestrations may communicate with or may be attached to the stomach or esophagus via a patent bronchus or a fibrotic strand.

Included in the group of malformations designated as sequestration are instances of a normal pulmonary segment with abnormal systemic arterial supply, normal pulmonary venous drainage and normal bronchus, as well as a normal lobe or lung with normal arterial connections but with the bronchus originating from the esophagus. Scimitar syndrome is also considered by some authors to be a form of pulmonary sequestration because of the abnormal venous connections of the involved lung.

Pulmonary sequestrations in infancy may be associated with pulmonary infection or, if arterial connections are large, with heart failure. Older children and adults may have infection or loud murmurs over the area of sequestration. The plain roentgenograms of the chest demonstrate a mass in the posterior basal segments (Fig. 7–25A and B), more often on the left. Pneumonia or bronchiectasis may obscure the mass. Computerized tomography will delineate a lobulated or cystic mass as well as the "feeder" vessels. The diagnosis is established by aortography or digital angiography (Fig. 7–25C and D).

Total Anomalous Pulmonary Venous Return TAPVR accounts for about 1% of congenital cardiac lesions. In this anomaly, no connection exists between the pulmonary veins and the LA, since all the pulmonary veins enter the RA, either directly or by way of the SVC, vertical vein, coronary sinus (CS), portal vein or ductus venosus. The systemic circuit is supplied with blood by way of a right-to-left (obligatory) shunt through an interatrial communication (ASD or patent foramen ovale). Darling et al. classified TAPVR into four types, according to the site of emptying of the pulmonary venous blood into the systemic venous system: (1) supracardiac, (2) cardiac, (3) infracardiac (infradiaphragmatic) and (4) combinations of these. In type 1 (supracardiac) the pulmonary veins form a confluence behind the heart (common pulmonary vein), which connects directly to the SVC or, more commonly, to a vertical vein that drains through the left innominate vein into the SVC. In type 2 (cardiac) the pulmonary veins drain directly into the RA or into the CS. In type 3 (infracardiac) the pulmonary veins converge behind the heart to form a common

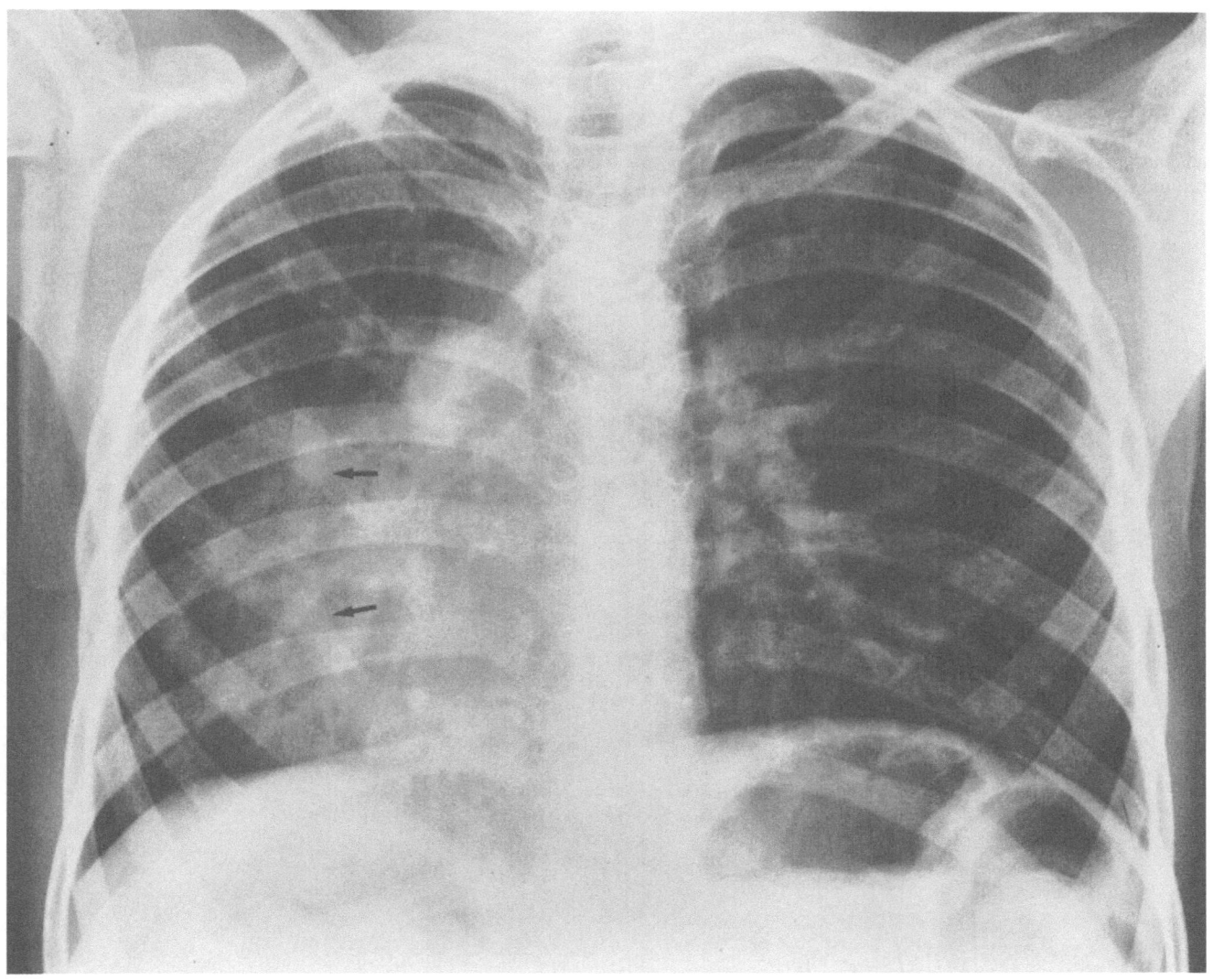

A

Fig. 7–24. *Scimitar syndrome.* The frontal chest roentgenogram (A) demonstrates the typical curvilinear density (*arrows*) in the right hemithorax formed by the anomalous pulmonary venous trunk as it descends to join the inferior vena cava at its junction with the right atrium. Because of marked dextroposition of the heart, the vein projects through the heart rather than being paracardiac as in other cases. (*Continued*)

pulmonary vein that descends through the diaphragm to join the portal system or the ductus venosus.

Pulmonary venous obstruction (PVO) invariably occurs in type 3 (infracardiac), because of diversion of pulmonary venous return through the hepatic sinusoids after spontaneous closure of the ductus venosus. PVO may also occur with type 1, as a result of compression of the vertical vein by the trachea and esophagus, and in type 2, because of compression of the arteries and veins of the left lower lobe by the enlarged and rotated heart. PVO may also be due to intrinsic narrowing of the common pulmonary vein.

Disorders commonly associated with TAPVR are patent ductus arteriosus, VSD, coarctation of the aorta and other anomalies of the aortic arch. TAPVR is frequently part of the situs indeterminus complexes (asplenia, polysplenia, anisosplenia) and is accompanied by such major intracardiac malformations as atrioventricularis communis and single ventricle (see section on abnormalities of visceroatrial situs).

Clinical Features The clinical (and radiological) features may reflect pulmonary venous hypertension and inadequate pulmonary blood flow due to pulmonary venous obstruction (mostly with type 3 TAPVR) or pulmonary artery hypertension due to a large left-to-right shunt (usually with types 1, 2, or 4). Some infants will be in extremis with a large left-to-right shunt along with pulmonary venous obstruction.

In patients without PVO, cyanosis is mild and may be hardly apparent at rest. Congestive heart failure is the dominant feature on presentation. The cardiac impulse is right ventricular and hyperkinetic. The first heart sound is loud and the second sound is loud and widely split with no respiratory variations. A grade 2–3/6 systolic ejection murmur is usually heard at the upper left sternal border; it is due to increased pulmonary blood flow across the pulmonary valve. A gallop and middiastolic rumble are often heard. The electrocardiogram shows RV and RA hypertrophy. In the presence of PVO the clinical manifestations

Fig. 7–24 (*Cont.*). The levophase of a pulmonary angiogram (**B**) demonstrates drainage of the right upper and right middle lobes into the common pulmonary trunk, while the right lower lobe vein (*arrows*) drains separately into the left atrium. Note the position and rotation of the left ventricle (dextroposition and dextrorotation). (*Continued*)

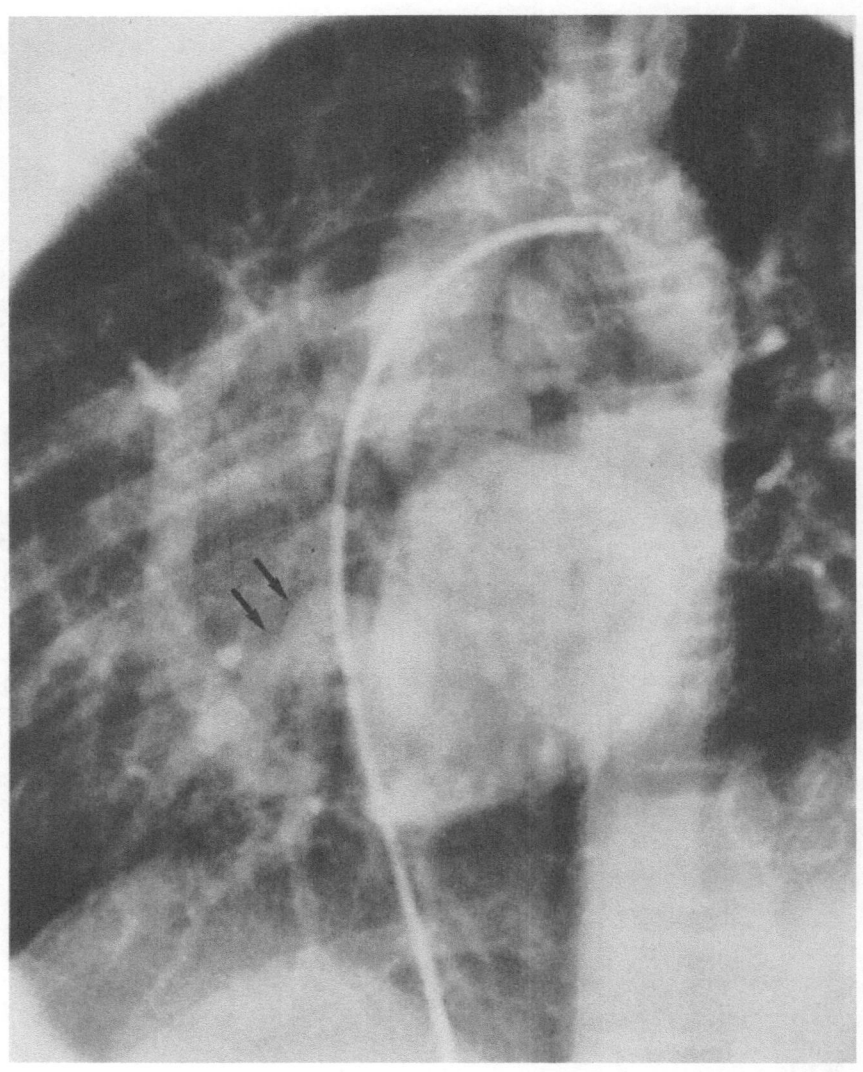

B

are more severe and begin earlier, usually within the first week of life. Respiratory distress and cyanosis may be prominent. No murmurs will be heard if pulmonary flow is severely obstructed.

Echocardiography The RV and main pulmonary artery are markedly dilated. Signs of pulmonary hypertension are present (e.g., long RV pre-ejection period, short RV ejection time, absence of pulmonary "a" kick, midsystolic closure of the pulmonary valve). The LV may be displaced posteriorly so that only careful search demonstrates its presence. If a common pulmonary vein is present behind the heart it may be represented by an echo-free space behind the LA on M-mode. This finding is not diagnostic since the aorta and other mediastinal structures may produce the same appearance. On 2-D echocardiography the common pulmonary vein may be visualized, and scanning may reveal its entry point into the right side of the heart. Massive dilatation of the CS is strong evidence for TAPVR to that structure (Sahn et al.) (Fig. 7–26). Cross sections of the LA in numerous planes do not demonstrate any pulmonary veins draining normally.

Radiological (Plain Film) Features On plain films of the chest, pulmonary overcirculation is the predominant pattern in patients with types 1 and 2 (Figs. 7–27A and B, 7–28, 7–29A and B). Pulmonary venous hypertension (PVH, congestive heart failure pattern) is invariably present in type 3 (Fig. 7–30). A mixed (overcirculation and PVH) pattern is often observed in cases of type 2 with drainage into the CS. A curious finding in patients with TAPVR to the CS is underperfusion of the left lower lobe due to compression of the local arteries and veins (Fig. 7–29A). On occasion a PVH pattern is present in instances of type 1 in which the vertical vein is compressed (obstructed) between the pulmonary artery and the left main bronchus. The vertical vein is usually anterior to these structures and therefore unobstructed.

The heart is enlarged in types 1 and 2. The RA, RV and pulmonary trunk are dilated. The LV, LA and aorta are inconspicuous.

Cardiomegaly and widening of the superior mediastinum result in a "figure-of-eight," "snowman" or "cottage-loaf" configuration in patients with type 1 (Figs. 7–27,

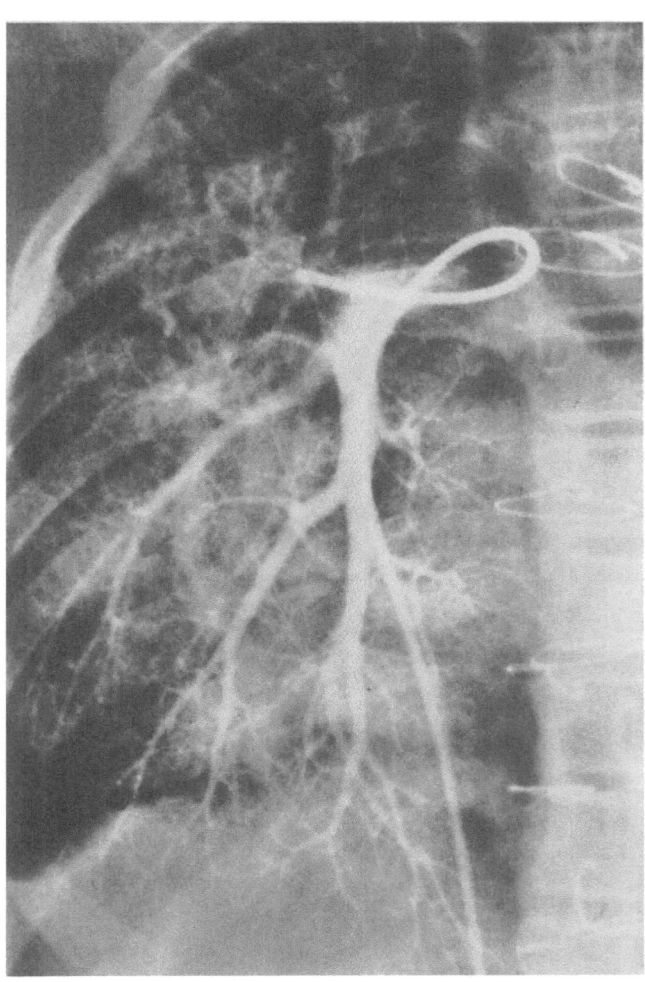

Fig. 7-24 (*Cont.*): Injection of contrast material into the right pulmonary artery (**C**) shows hypoplasia of this vessel. The intense capillary phase appearing simultaneously with intense opacification of the right pulmonary artery indicates slow washout of the contrast medium (prolonged transit time), consistent with high pulmonary resistance.

C

7–28). Widening of the superior mediastinum is due to dilatation of the vertical vein on the left side, and of the SVC on the right (Fig. 7–27C). Dilatation of these veins produces a "mass" effect anterior to the trachea on the lateral view (Fig. 7–27B and D). This finding aids in differentiating TAPVR of the supracardiac type from truncus arteriosus. Truncus arteriosus may widen the superior mediastinum on the frontal projection, but no mass effect is present on the lateral view.

With rare cases of type 1, in which the common pulmonary vein drains directly into the SVC, unilateral (right-sided) widening of the superior mediastinum is noted. Rarely the confluence of the pulmonary veins, or "common pulmonary vein," may be intrapulmonary instead of mediastinal. The course and location of this intrapulmonary channel differ from those of the scimitar syndrome (PAPVR of the right lung to the IVC).

In patients with type 2 TAPVR to the coronary sinus the dilated CS may simulate LA enlargement on the lateral film (Fig. 7–29B).

In patients with type 3 the heart tends to be normal in size (Fig. 7–30A and B). The combination of severe PVH and a normal heart size in a cyanotic infant is highly suggestive of TAPVR type 3. Of course, other entities deserve consideration, including the hypoplastic left heart syndrome, severe coarctation of the aorta, cor triatriatum, stenosis of pulmonary veins and the idiopathic respiratory distress syndrome of the newborn.

Hemodynamics The classic features of TAPVR are (1) high O_2 concentration in the common pulmonary vein if it can be entered, (2) equal O_2 saturation in all other chambers of the heart, (3) elevated pulmonary pressure, sometimes greater than systemic in patients with pulmonary venous obstruction. Pulmonary flow is massively increased in patients without pulmonary venous obstruction, but it may be markedly reduced if the pulmonary veins are obstructed. In some instances the ASD or foramen ovale is restrictive so that flow to the left side of the heart is inadequate.

Contrast Studies The levophase of injections of contrast medium in the RV (Fig. 7–27C) or in the pulmonary artery (Figs. 7–29C and D, and 7–30C) demonstrates the type

Fig. 7–25. *Pulmonary sequestration in a 2-month-old boy.* Frontal (**A**) and lateral (**B**) chest roentgenograms demonstrate a mass in the posterior basal segment of the right lung. Pulmonary overcirculation and pulmonary venous hypertension are present. Frontal films from an aortogram during the arterial phase (**C**) and the venous phase (**D**) reveal arterial supply by way of a large vessel from the abdominal aorta. Three large veins drain into the left atrium. Opacification of the right ventricle and pulmonary artery occurred because of simultaneous drainage into the inferior vena cava from the area of sequestration and because of an associated atrial septal defect.

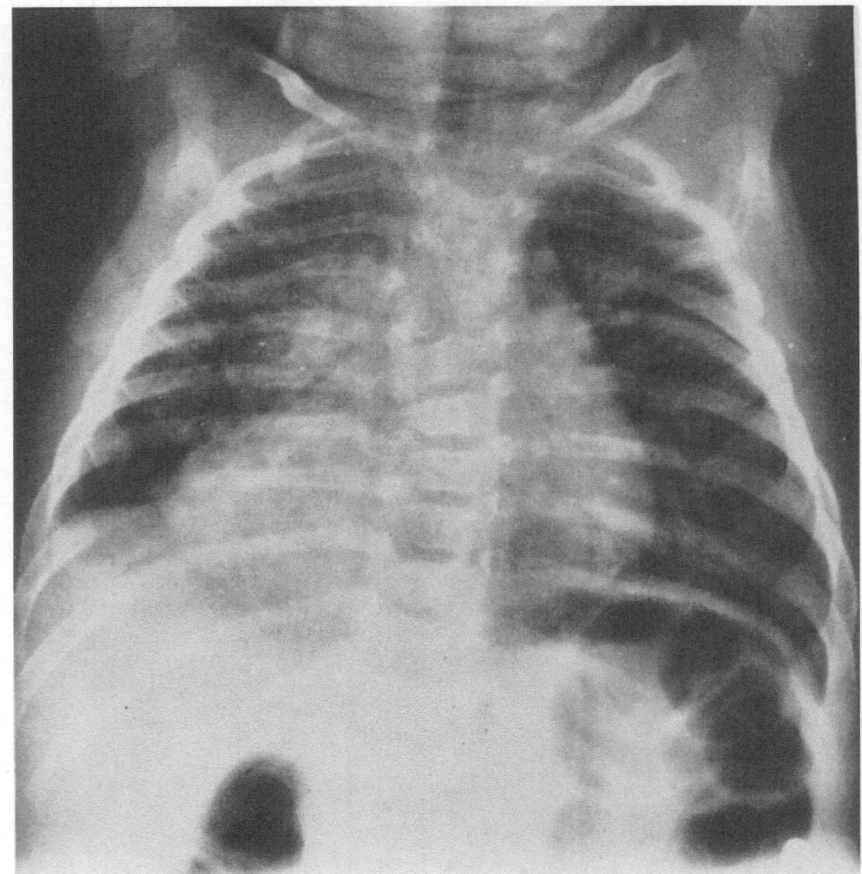

A

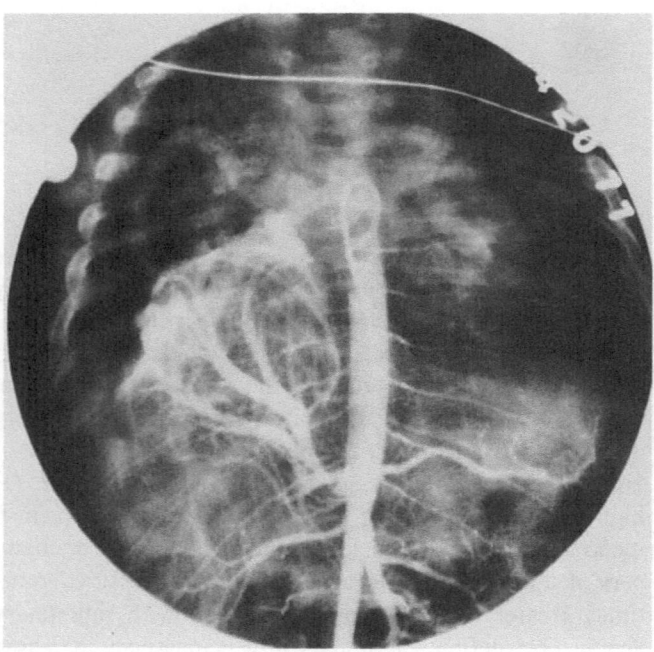

C

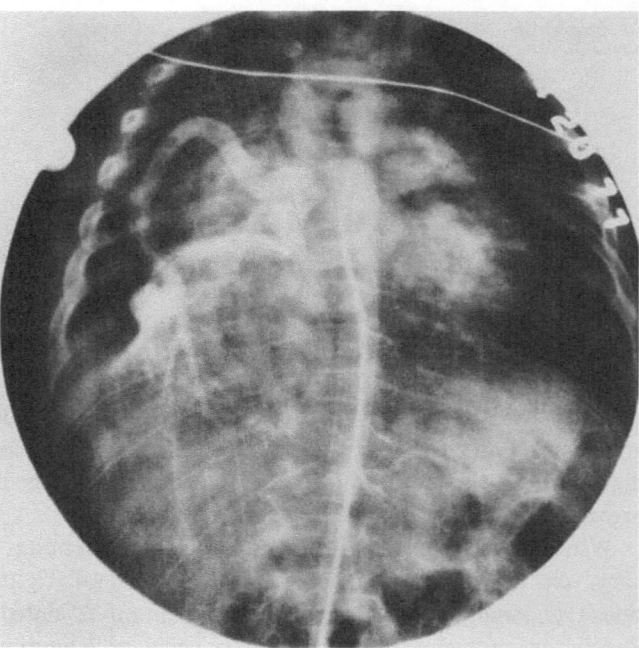

D

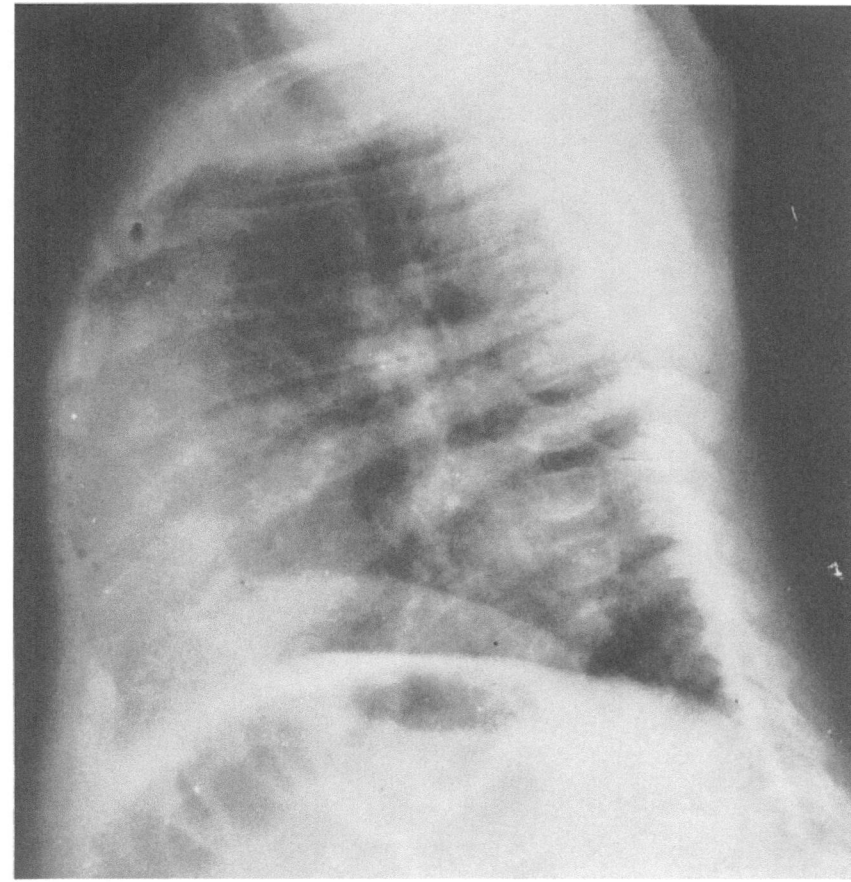

B

of TAPVR and the site of obstruction, if any. Left ventriculography reveals the size of the LV and aorta (which are usually small) and any associated abnormalities, if present. **Treatment** No palliative procedure is available for infants with TAPVR. Medical management may be of temporary benefit for some infants without pulmonary venous obstruction. In most instances, complete repair in infancy is necessary. The use of deep hypothermia and circulatory arrest has produced a dramatic improvement in results. Repair of the infradiaphragmatic type is the most difficult. It requires lifting the apex of the heart for construction of an anastomosis between the common pulmonary vein and the back wall of the LA. TAPVR to the coronary sinus is repaired by unroofing the coronary ostium so that it opens into the LA. The ASD is then closed (Figs. 7–29E and F). The supradiaphragmatic type is repaired by anastomosis of the common pulmonary vein to the LA (Fig. 7–28). Mixed types require combinations of these approaches. In neonates a functionally closed ductus arteriosus may reopen during or shortly after operation for TAPVR. Consequently the ductus is usually ligated at the time of surgery,

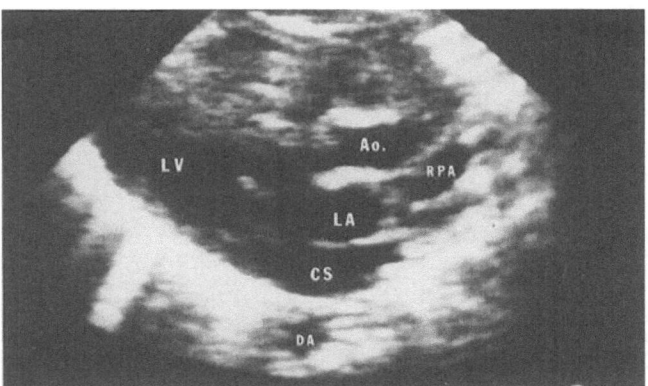

Fig. 7–26. *Two-dimensional echocardiography in total anomalous pulmonary venous return to the coronary sinus.* An accesory chamber behind the heart is noted. In this case it represents the coronary sinus (*CS*) which is dilated by the pulmonary venous flow entering it. In TAPVR of the supracardiac type the confluence of pulmonary veins occurs in a similar location behind the left atrium, but empties into a vertical vein which connects to the innominate vein and thence into the superior vena cava. *LA* = left atrium; *LV* = left ventricle; *Ao.* = aortic root; *RPA* = right pulmonary artery; *DA* = descending aorta. (Courtesy of Henry Issenberg, M.D., Bronx, New York.)

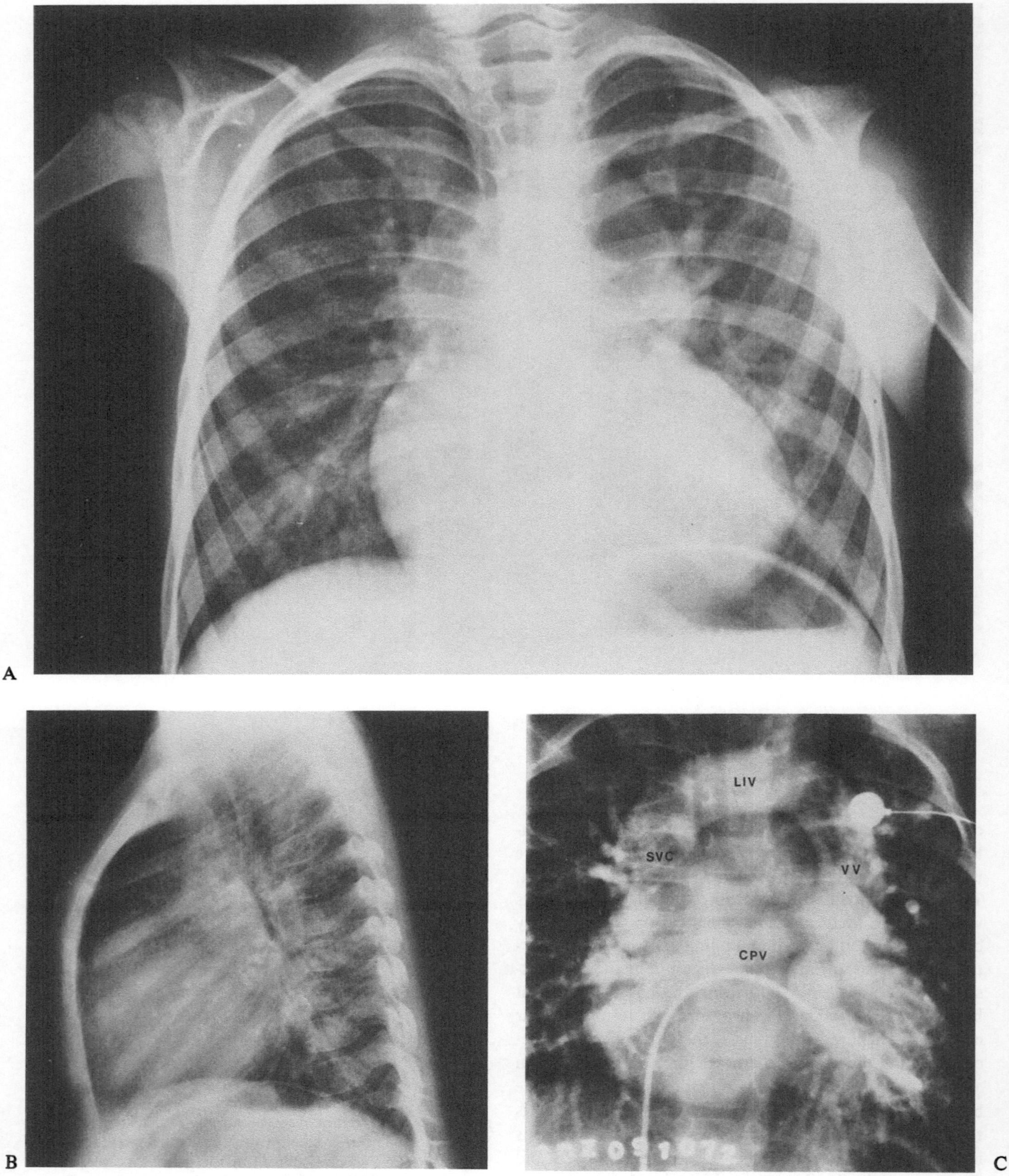

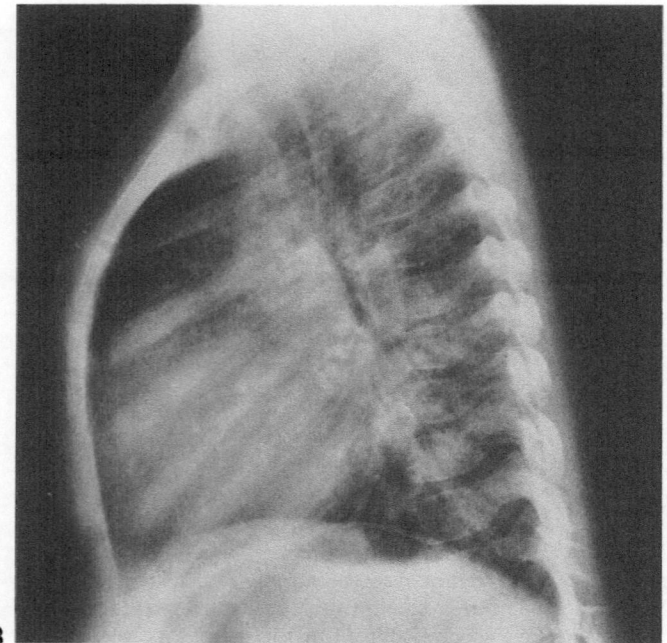

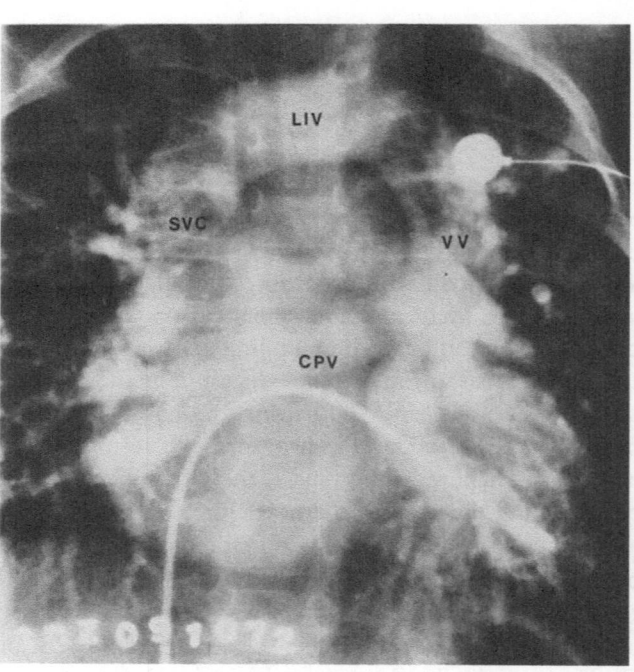

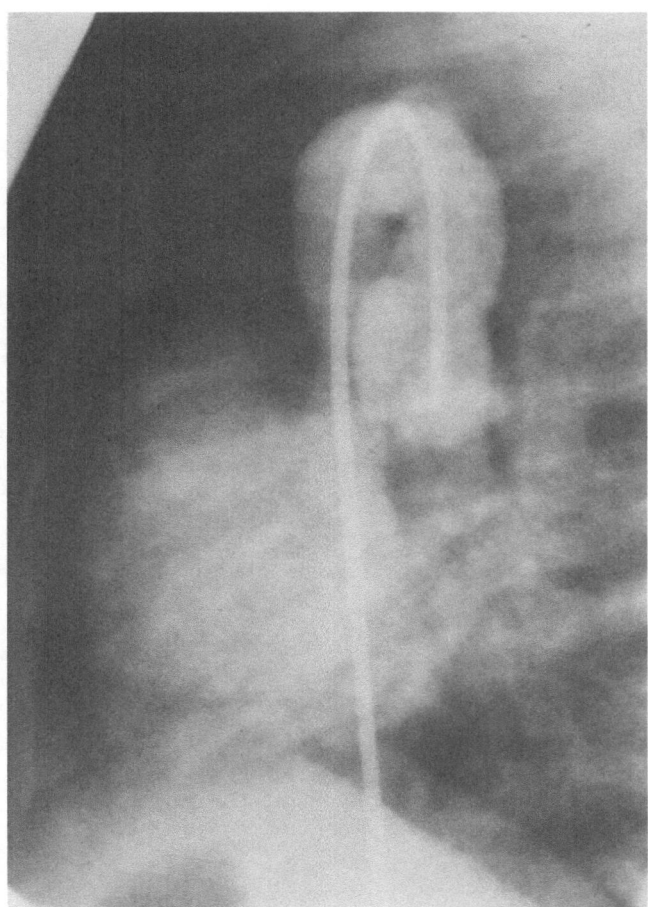

D

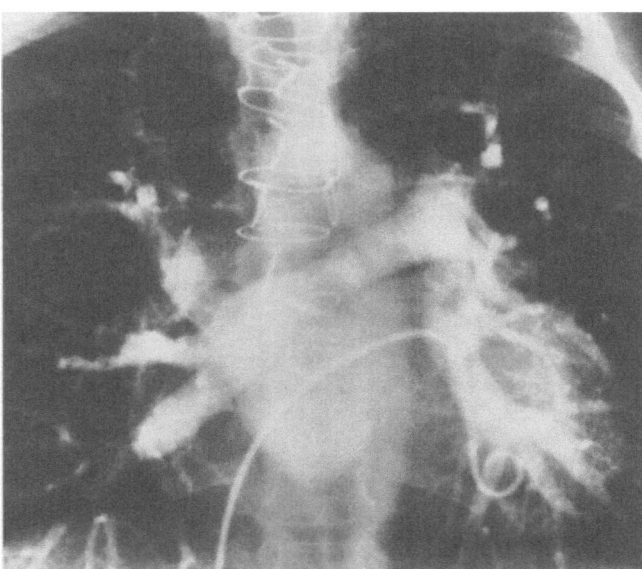

Fig. 7-28. *Total anomalous pulmonary venous return to the superior vena cava (type 1, supracardiac).* Postoperative angiogram of the patient in Fig. 7-27 shows the common pulmonary vein to be anastomosed to the back of the left atrium. The vertical vein has been closed, achieving normal pulmonary venous drainage. The superior mediastinum now appears normal.

◀ **Fig. 7-27.** *Total anomalous pulmonary venous return to the superior vena cava (type 1, supracardiac).* **A** PA and **B** lateral chest roentgenograms; **C** frontal film of the levophase of a right ventriculogram; **D** lateral film of selective injection into the vertical vein (the vertical vein was catheterized in retrograde fashion via the SVC). On the frontal plain film, pulmonary overcirculation and a typical "snowman" configuration are evident. Widening of the superior mediastinum forms the top of the snowman and the heart forms the bottom of the snowman. The widening of the mediastinum is caused by dilatation of the vertical vein on the left and the superior vena cava on the right. The apparent mass anterior to the trachea in the lateral film is also caused by the anomalous veins. On the angiogram, pulmonary veins join to form a common pulmonary vein (*CPV*), behind the heart. This vein in turn drains into the vertical vein (*VV*), which joins the left innominate vein (*LIV*). The innominate vein drains into the superior vena cava (*SVC*). The right atrium is enlarged. On the lateral view (**D**) the vertical vein and the superior vena cava are anterior to the trachea, accounting for the mass in the lateral chest roentgenogram.

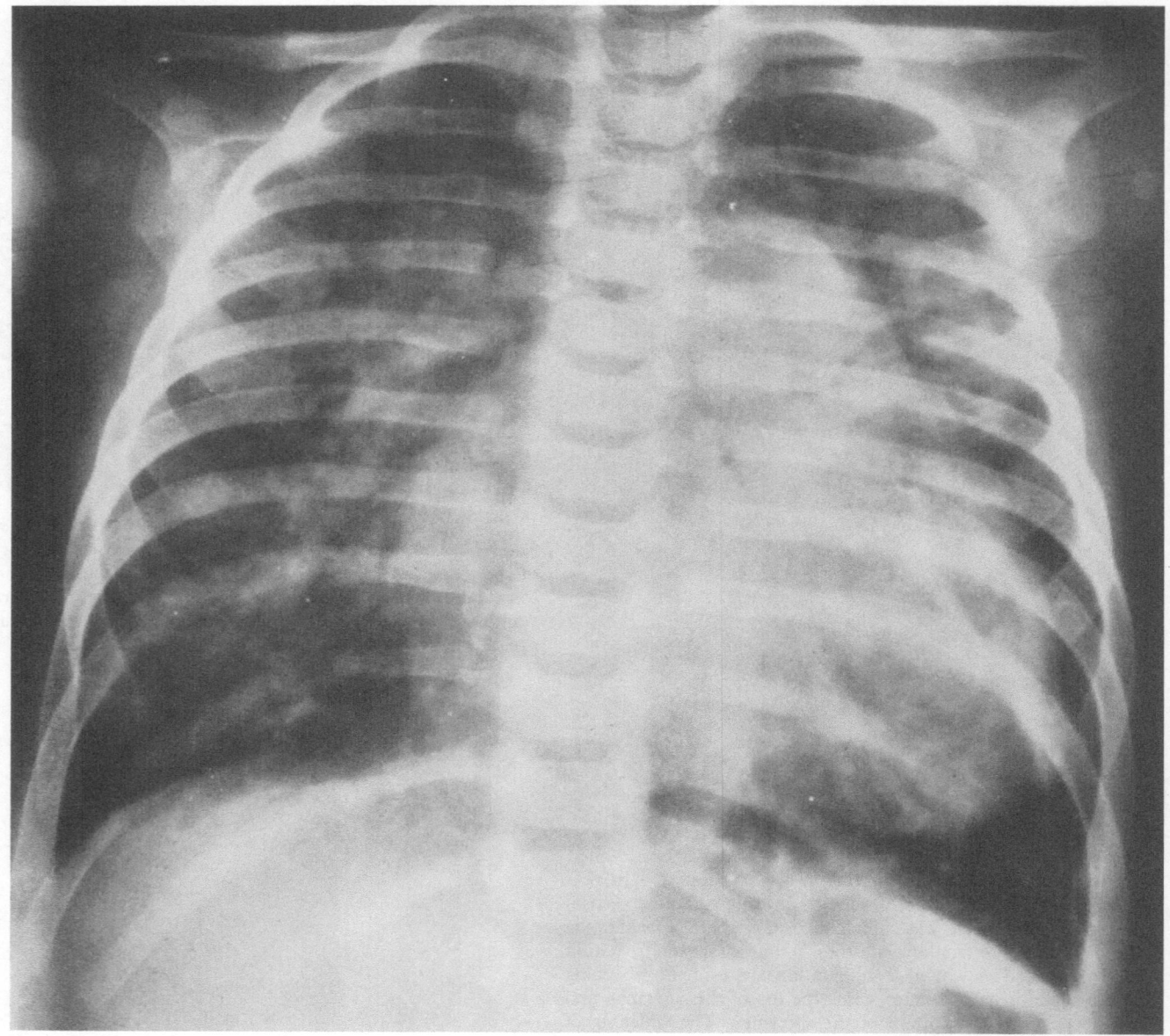

A

Fig. 7–29. *Total anomalous pulmonary venous drainage to the coronary sinus (type 2 of Darling) in a 1-year-old girl.* **A** frontal and **B** lateral plain chest roentgenograms; **C** frontal film of a pulmonary angiogram; **D** film from the levophase of the same pulmonary angiogram; **E** and **F** early and late frames from a pulmonary angiogram after surgical correction.

In **A**, prominent pulmonary overcirculation is evident. The pulmonary vessels are dilated but indistinct, indicating superimposed pulmonary venous hypertension. The perfusion to the left lower lobe is decreased, because of compression of the pulmonary arteries and veins by the heart (see *arrows,* panel **C**). Marked cardiomegaly is noted with enlargement of the right atrium, right ventricle and pulmonary artery. The aorta is inconspicuous. The left atrium is not enlarged, while enlargement of the right ventricle and pulmonary artery causes a slight convexity of the left heart border.

On the làteral film **(B)**, elevation and retrodisplacement of the left atrium by the dilated chambers of the right side of the heart and coronary sinus simulate left atrial enlargement. The left ventricle is also retrodisplaced by the large right ventricle. Obliteration of the retrosternal clear space is not readily apparent on the lateral plain film in this patient. *(Continued)*

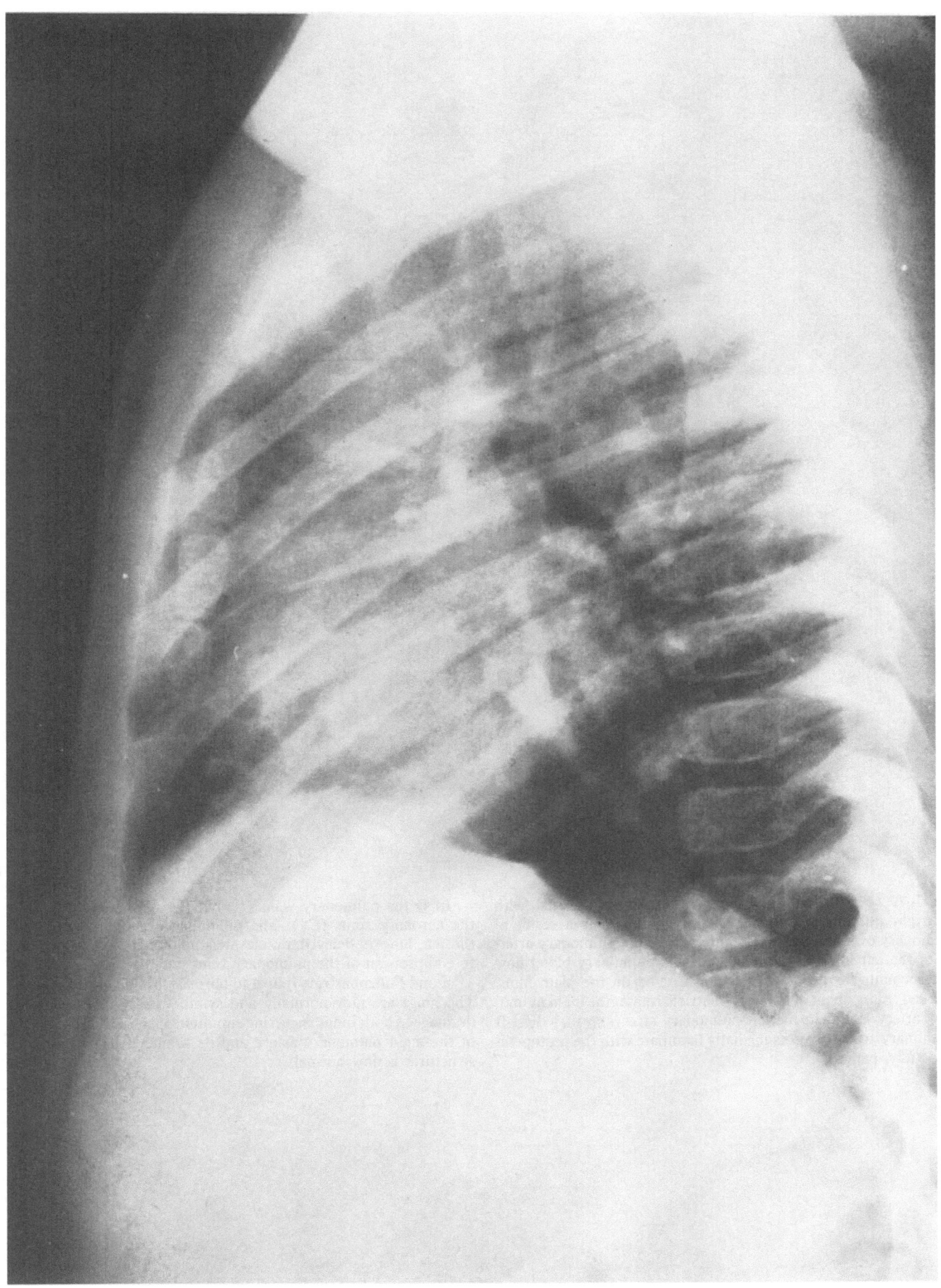

B

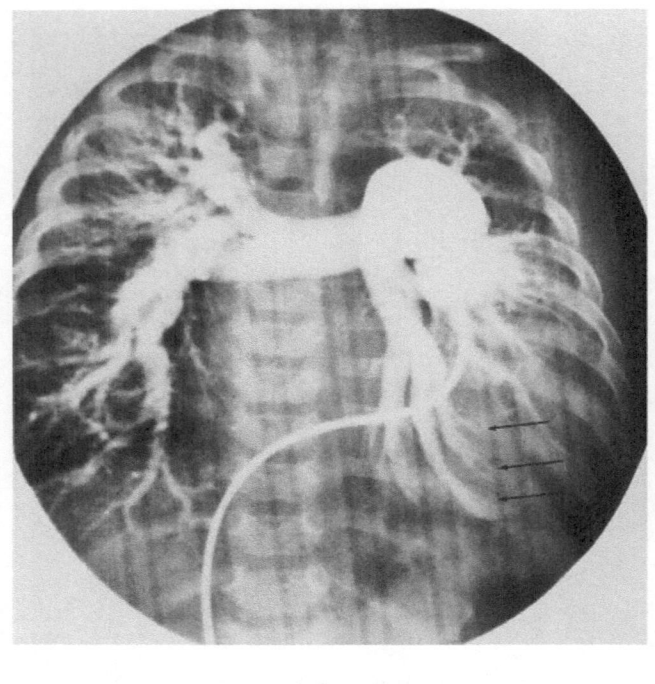

C

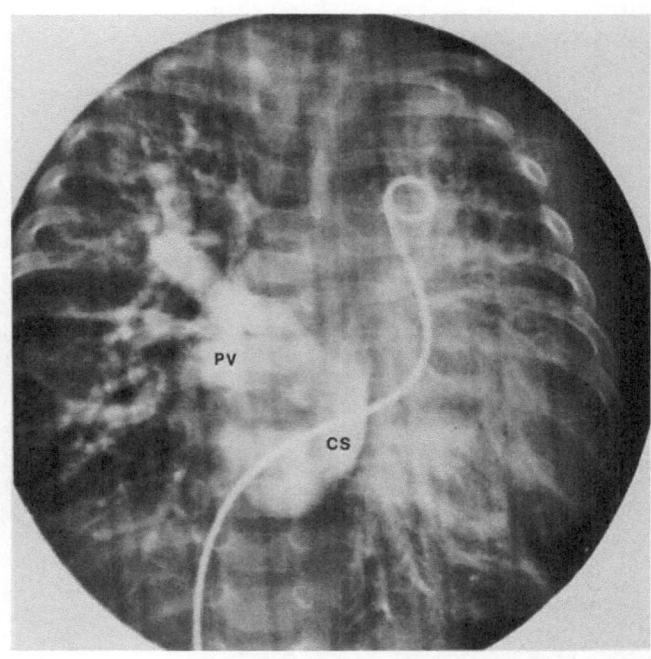

D

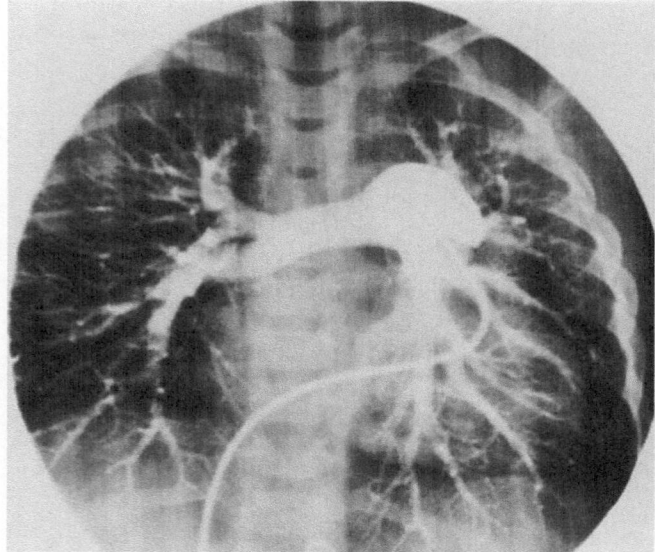

E

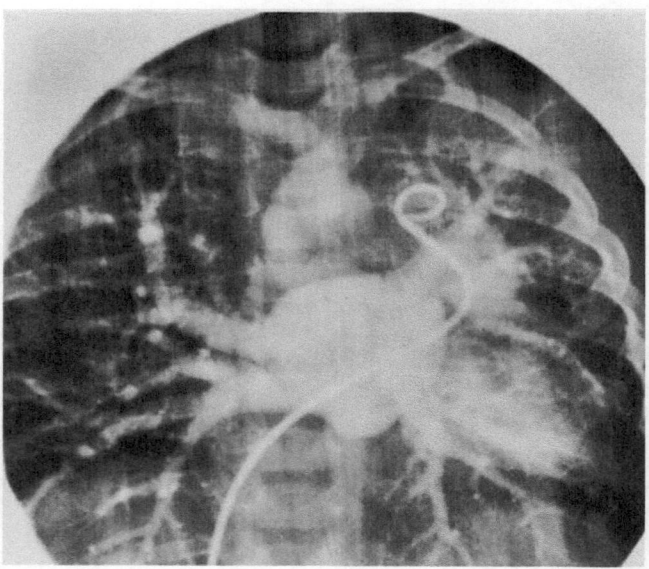

F

Fig. 7–29 (*Cont.*). In **C** the pulmonary arteries are dilated, with the right pulmonary branches slightly tortuous as a result of pulmonary overcirculation. Compression of the pulmonary arteries of the left lower lobe (*arrows*) delays pulmonary blood flow and accounts for decreased perfusion noted on the plain films. Marked enlargement of the right ventricle rotates the main pulmonary artery lateral to the left pulmonary artery, so that the left pulmonary artery projects medially (compare with the postoperative study, panel **E**).

In **D** the pulmonary veins (*PV*) of the right lung drain into the coronary sinus (*CS*). The pulmonary venous return from the left lung is delayed by elevated pulmonary resistance due to compression of the pulmonary veins and arteries.

E and **F** demonstrate return to normal physiological function. The lungs are now normally and symmetrically perfused, with drainage of both lungs occurring simultaneously. The relationship of the main pulmonary artery and its branches to surrounding structures is now normal.

Fig. 7–30. *Total anomalous pulmonary venous return below the diaphragm (type 3 of Darling), with obstruction to pulmonary venous return in a cyanotic infant.* **A** and **B** frontal and lateral plain chest roentgenograms. **C** 35-mm cine frame from the levophase of a pulmonary angiogram. The pulmonary vessels are normal in size, but they are indistinct because of perivascular edema—a finding consistent with severe pulmonary venous hypertension. The cardiovascular silhouette is normal in size. The differential diagnosis on the basis of these films includes idiopathic respiratory distress syndrome, cor triatriatum, pulmonary vein stenosis and various forms of the hypoplastic left heart syndrome (e.g., coarctation of the aorta, mitral atresia, aortic atresia). In **C** the pulmonary veins converge behind the heart, forming the common pulmonary vein, which descends below the diaphragm to join the portal vein. The common pulmonary vein is not obstructed. Obstruction of pulmonary venous drainage occurs because pulmonary venous blood is diverted through the hepatic sinusoids after closure of the ductus venosus.

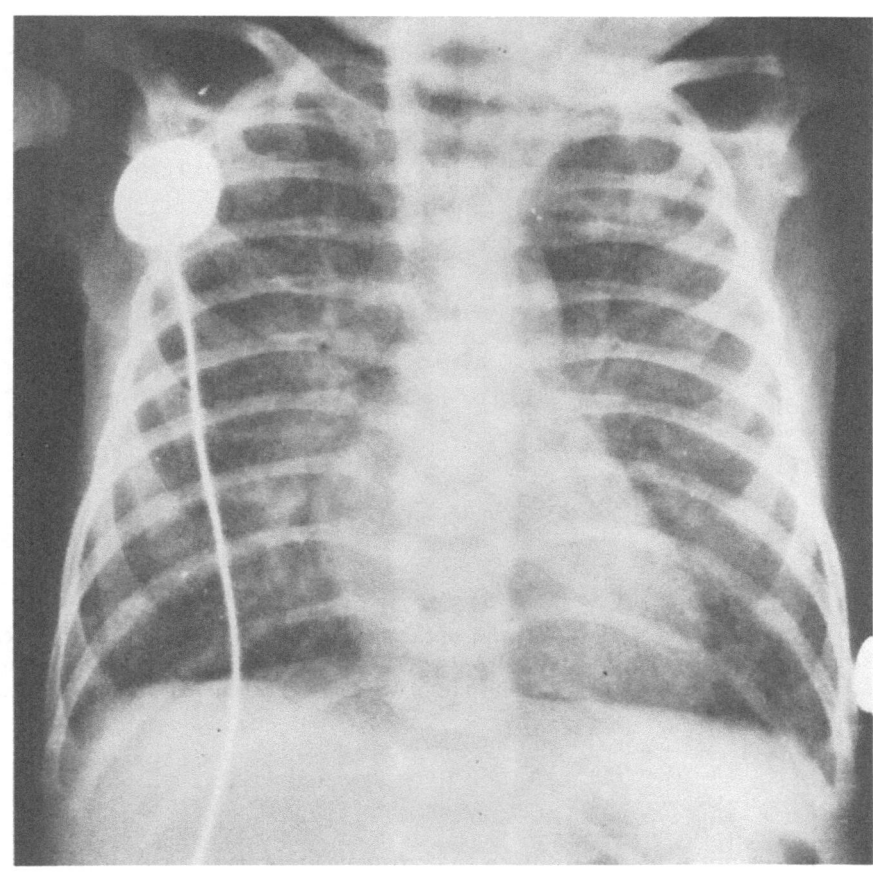

A

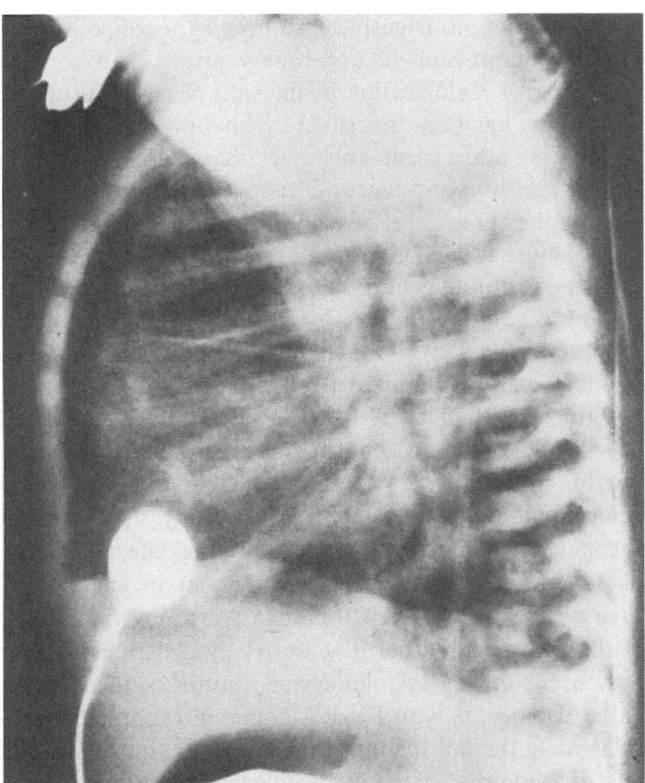

B

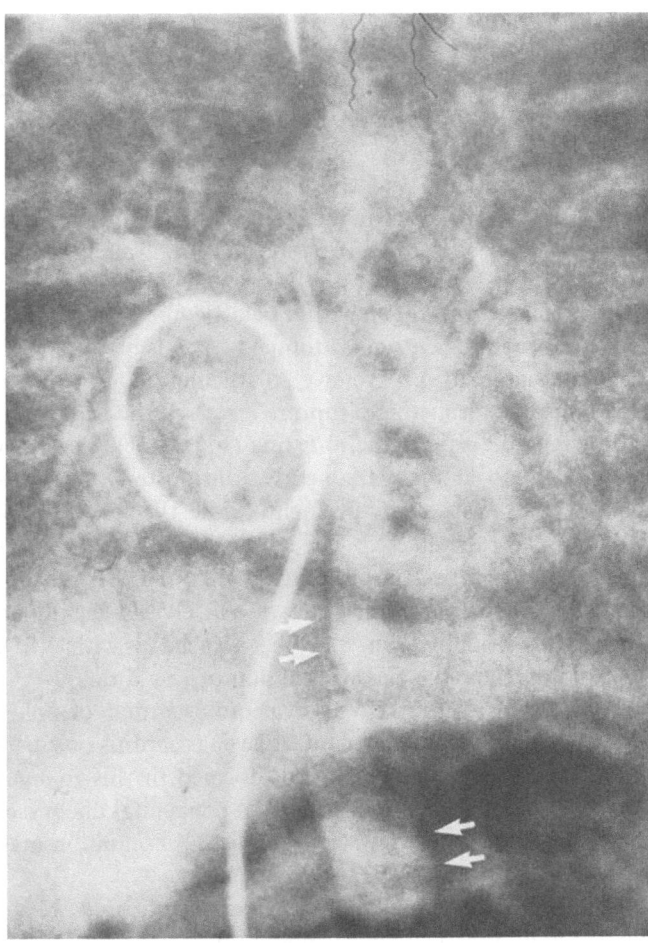

C

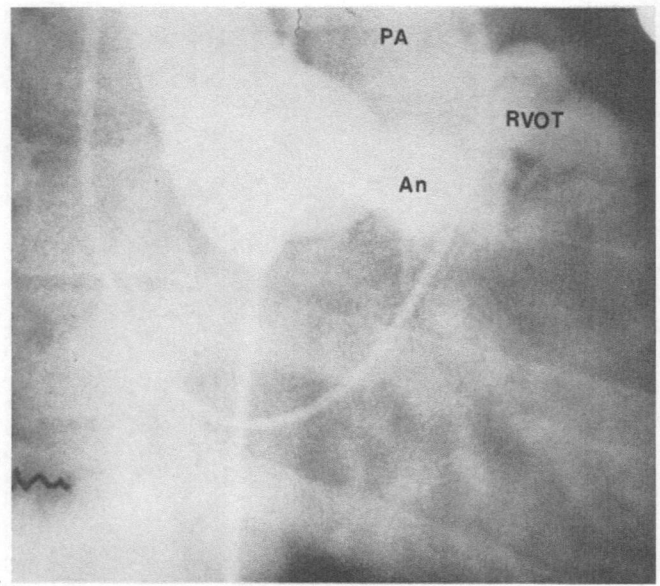

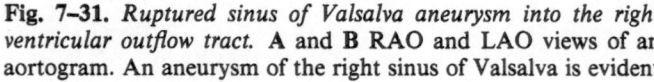

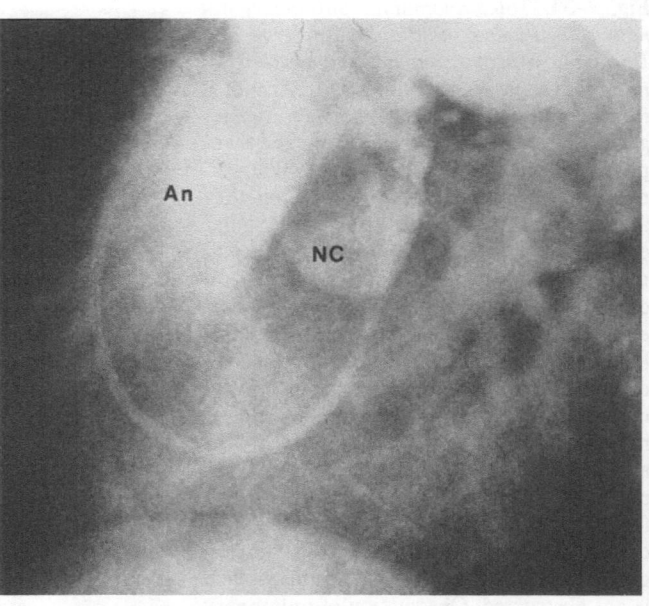

Fig. 7–31. *Ruptured sinus of Valsalva aneurysm into the right ventricular outflow tract.* **A** and **B** RAO and LAO views of an aortogram. An aneurysm of the right sinus of Valsalva is evident (*An*). The right ventricular outflow tract (*RVOT*) and pulmonary artery (*PA*) are opacified secondary to the large shunt through the ruptured anterior cusp. *NC* = noncoronary sinus of Valsalva.

whether or not it has been shown to be patent at cardiac catheterization.

Postoperative complications include persistent obstruction to pulmonary venous drainage secondary to narrowing of the anastomsis or kinking of a pulmonary vein, and dehiscence of the repair of the ASD.

Rupture of Sinus of Valsalva into a Cardiac Chamber
Discontinuity between the media of the aorta and the anulus fibrosus of the aortic valve results in an aneurysm of a sinus of Valsalva. The wall of the aneurysm is composed only of collagenous tissue without elastic fibers, in contrast to the aortico-left ventricular tunnel, which is invested with elastic tissue. With progressive enlargement, an aneurysm of a sinus of Valsalva may rupture into a cardiac chamber, producing an aorticocameral fistula (Fig. 7–31). The right sinus is involved most frequently, the posterior sinus is next in frequency of involvement, while the left sinus of Valsalva is rarely affected. The aneurysm usually ruptures into the RV or RA. Rupture into the LA or LV is uncommon. An aneurysm of the sinus of Valsalva is usually an isolated abnormality, but may be associated with VSD, bicuspid aortic valve and coarctation of the aorta.

Rupture of a sinus of Valsalva into a cardiac chamber may also occur secondary to infective endocarditis or tuberculosis. An aorticocameral fistula formed in this manner may be difficult to distinguish from a congenital aneurysm that has ruptured. Review of the clinical presentation may be helpful.

The presence of an unruptured aneurysm may be an incidental finding on angiocardiography or autopsy. Rarely an unruptured aneurysm may protrude into a cardiac chamber, producing various disorders (e.g., RV outflow tract obstruction, tricuspid insufficiency, cardiac ischemia due to compression of a coronary artery, and complete heart block). Calcification of the wall of large unruptured aneurysms has been described by Shapiro et al.

Rupture into a cardiac chamber characteristically occurs during the third and fourth decades. If the resulting shunt is large the acute onset of pain in the chest and congestive heart failure is encountered. Physical examination demonstrates a continuous murmur, a hyperdynamic cardiac impulse and bounding pulses. Electrocardiography may show T wave changes, while later changes consistent with the overload pattern imposed by the defect are apparent. In addition, heart block is relatively common. On M-mode echocardiography an abnormal structure may be observed moving within the LV outflow tract or the RV outflow tract. Two-dimensional echocardiography may delineate the aneurysm and its opening into the affected cardiac chamber. Some findings are reminiscent of aneurysm of the right coronary artery or coronary arteriovenous fistula. If the fistula enters the RA, flutter of the tricuspid valve may occur during systole (systolic flutter of the tricuspid valve also occurs with LV-RA communication). If the fistula enters the LV the mitral valve flutters during diastole as it does with aortic valve insufficiency.

On plain roentgenograms of the chest during acute rupture of an aneurysm of the sinus of Valsalva, the predominant finding will be pulmonary venous hypertension rather than pulmonary overcirculation. The heart is enlarged, but the cardiac configuration is nonspecific in appearance. Car-

Fig. 7–32. *Defects of the membranous septum, including left ventricular–right atrial communication.* Perry et al. have classified defects of the membranous interventricular septum (IVS) into five types: (*A*) a defect in the membranous interventricular septum and perforation of the tricuspid valve (TV) with adherence of the TV to the septal defect; (*B*) a defect in the membranous interventricular septum below the TV without perforation of the TV (this type represents a membranous interventricular septal defect, the most common form of interventricular septal defect); (*C*) perforation of the TV without a septal defect; (*D*) a defect of the membranous interventricular septum with perforation of the TV without adherence of the TV to the interventricular septum and (*E*) a defect in the atrioventricular portion of the membranous interventricular septum with a normal TV. Only the first and last are left ventricular–right atrial communications inasmuch as they allow blood to shunt directly from the left ventricle into the right atrium. Perry EL, Burchell HB, Edwards JE (1949) Congenital communication between the left ventricle and the right atrium: Coexisting ventricular septal defect and double tricuspid orifice. Proc Staff Meet Mayo Clin 24:198–206.

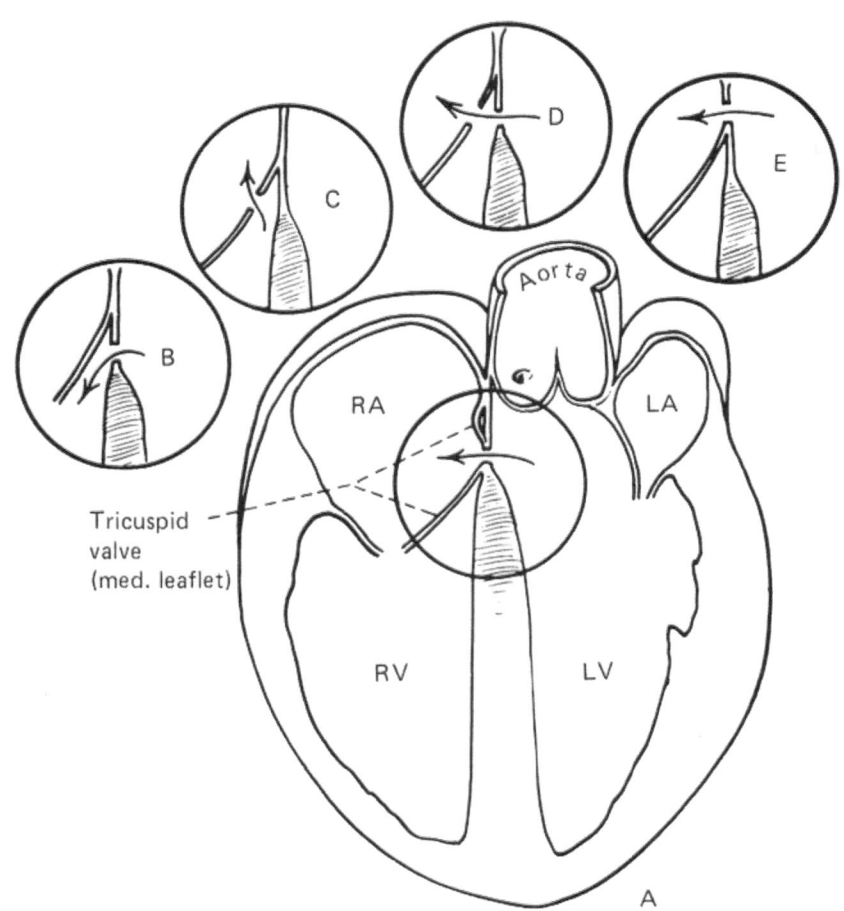

diac catheterization demonstrates an oxygen "step-up" in the cardiac chamber into which the rupture occurred. The diagnosis is made by aortography (Fig. 7–31).

At surgery the defect is usually closed from within the aortic root, but in some instances the best surgical approach is through the involved chamber.

Left Ventricular–Right Atrial Communication

LV-RA comunication is a rare lesion. Autopsies demonstrate an incidence of 0.08% of all congenital heart defects (Laurichesse et al.). In order to understand the anatomy of LV-RA communication it is necessary to study the membranous portion of the ventricular septum (Figs. 7–32, 7–33, 7–34). Laurichesse et al. and Baron et al. have provided understanding of the position and relationships of the membranous septum, showing that the tricuspid valve divides the membranous septum into an anterior portion (the membranous interventricular septum) and a posterior portion (the atrioventricular septum) (Figs. 7–33, 7–34). A defect in the membranous interventricular septum is the most common form of interventricular septal defect (IVSD) consisting of a communication between the two ventricles, whereas a defect in the atrioventricular septum allows communication directly from the LV to the RA. Perry, Burchell and Edwards have classified defects of the

membranous septum into five types (Fig. 7–32). (1) a defect in the membranous interventricular septum and perforation of the tricuspid valve with adherence of the tricuspid valve to the septal defect; (2) a membranous interventricular septal defect without perforation of the tricuspid valve; (3) perforation of the tricuspid valve without a septal defect; (4) a defect of the membranous interventricular septum with perforation of the tricuspid valve, without adherence of the tricuspid valve to the ventricular septum and (5) a defect in the atrioventricular portion of the membranous septum with a normal tricuspid valve. Only the first and the last defects represent true LV-RA communications inasmuch as they allow blood to shunt directly from the LV into the RA. An IVSD with perforation of a nonadherent tricuspid valve is not a direct LV-RA communication, although some blood may pass from the LV to the RA because of the direction of the jet. The anatomical features of a LV-RA communication differ considerably from those in the LV-RA shunt associated with endocardial cushion defect (ECD). The membranous ventricular septum is absent or deficient in ECD, and the mitral and tricuspid valves are abnormal. The LV-RA shunt in ECD results from mitral regurgitation (through the cleft) that is directed across the atrial septal defect into the right atrium.

The findings on auscultation with LV-RA communica-

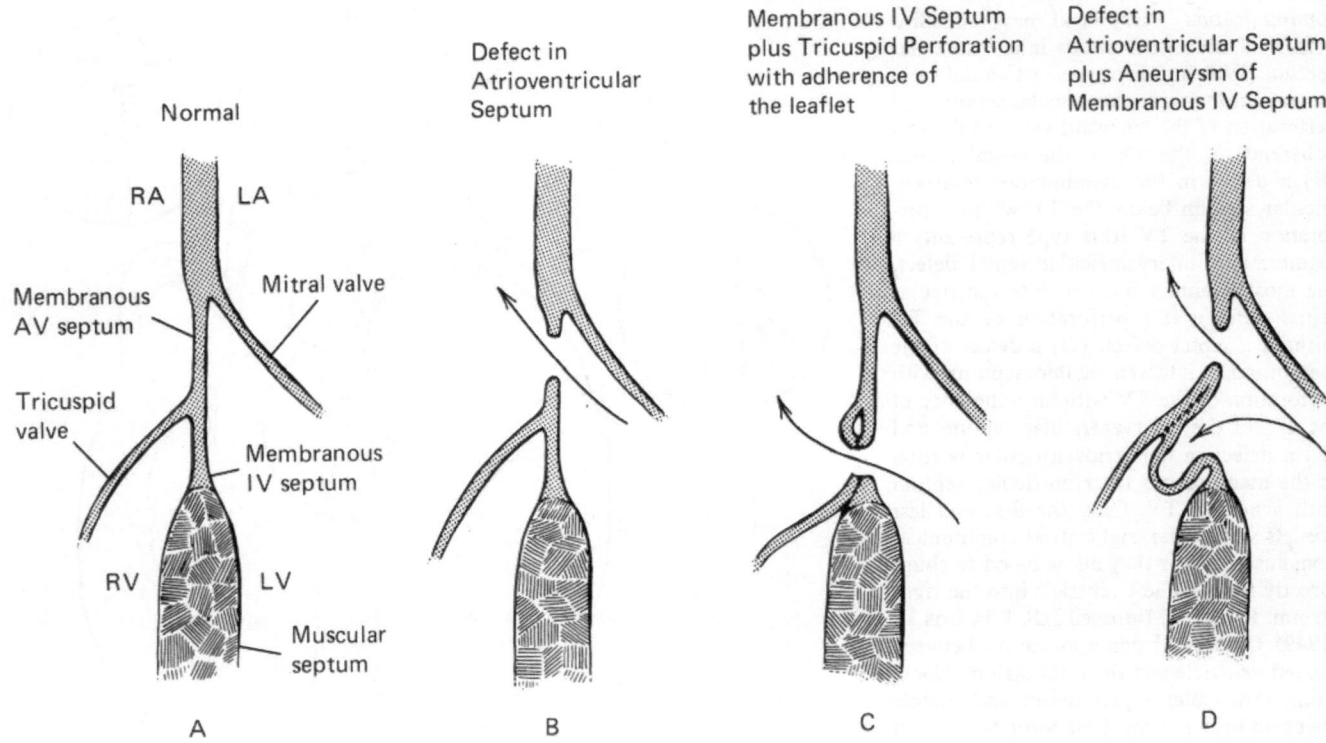

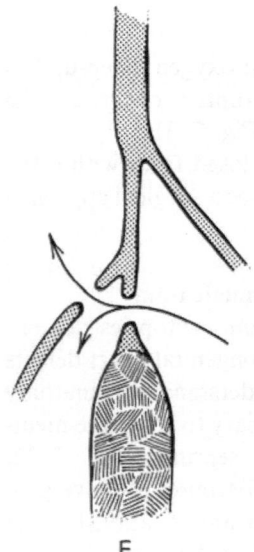

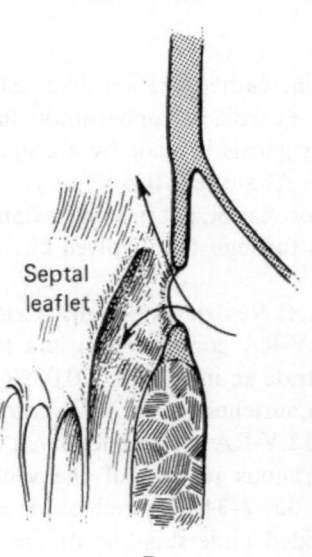

Fig. 7–33. *The normal membranous septum and left ventricular–right atrial communications.*

A represents the two portions of the membranous septum. The membranous septum is divided into two portions by the insertion of the septal leaflet of the tricuspid valve. The atrioventricular portion of the membranous septum (*AV Septum*) is above the tricuspid valve, while the interventricular portion of the membranous septum (*IV Septum*) is below it.

B and C are the usual forms of left ventricular–right atrial communication. In B a defect is present in the AV Septum, allowing blood to flow from the left ventricle to the right atrium. In C the defect is in the membranous IV Septum; however, the tricuspid valve is adherent and perforated, again allowing direct communication from left ventricle to right atrium.

D is a case described by the authors and illustrated in this section (Figs. 7–35 and 7–36). In this case a typical defect in the AV Septum is associated with an aneurysm of the membranous IV Septum.

E represents a defect in the membranous IV Septum associated with a perforated tricuspid valve that is not adherent to the defect. This defect does not represent a left ventricular–right atrial communication, but is, in fact, a membranous ventricular septal defect. Nevertheless, the right atrium receives blood directly from the left ventricle if the jet through the interventricular septal defect is directed toward the perforation in the tricuspid valve.

F represents a defect in the membranous IV Septum with a wide commissure between the septal and anterior leaflets of the tricuspid valve (another form of interventricular septal defect with tricuspid insufficiency). This again is not a true left ventricular–right atrial communication although the right atrium receives blood directly from the left ventricle.

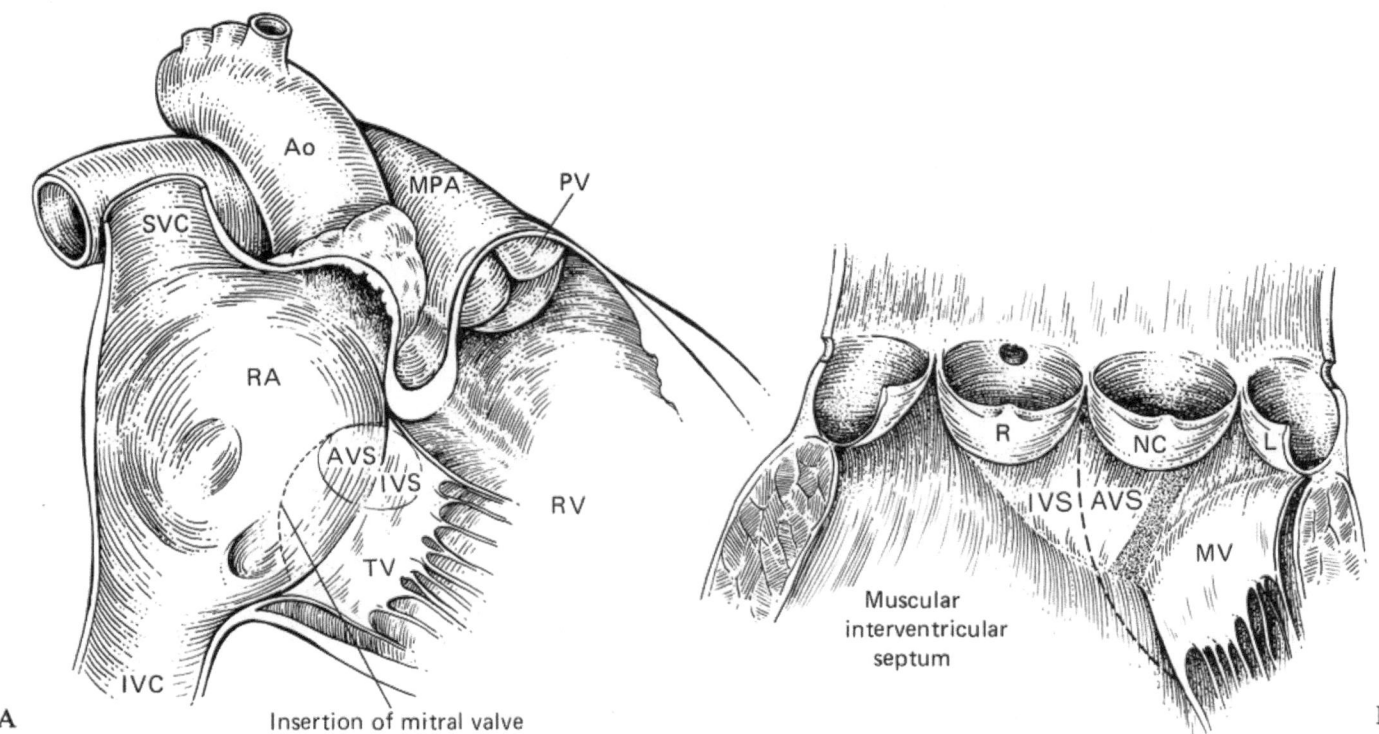

A

B

Fig. 7–34. *The two portions of the membranous septum and their relationship to the mitral, tricuspid and aortic valves.*

Panel **A** shows the right side of the septum. The ellipse represents the membranous septum. The septal leaflet of the tricuspid valve (*TV*) crosses the membranous septum, dividing it into two segments. That portion of the membranous septum anterior (inferior) to the TV is the interventricular portion of the membranous septum (*IVS*), while the segment posterior (superior) to the TV is the atrioventricular portion of the membranous septum (*AVS*). The insertion of the mitral valve (*MV*) is slightly posterior to the membranous septum.

B delineates the basal portion of the ventricular septum as observed from the left ventricular side. The membranous septum

forms a triangle bounded superiorly by the aortic valve and inferiorly by the muscular septum. Posteriorly the right fibrous trigone separates the membranous septum from the mitral valve. The *dashed line* represents the attachment of the TV on the other side. Note that a portion of the muscular septum is also included in the atrioventricular septum. *Ao* = aorta; *MPA* = main pulmonary artery; *PV* = pulmonic valve; *SVC* = superior vena cava; *RA* = right atrium; *TV* = tricuspid valve; *RV* = right ventricle; *IVC* = inferior vena cava; *R* = right sinus of Valsalva; *NC* = non coronary sinus of Valsalva; *L* = left sinus of Valsalva. After Baron MG, Wolf BS, Grishman A, Van Mierop LHS (1964) Aneurysm of the membranous septum. Am J Roentgenol 91:1303–1313.

tion are reminiscent of VSD. A thrill and a pansystolic murmur are present at the left sternal border. The second sound is normally split; a third sound or flow rumble is heard. The electrocardiogram characteristically shows an rsR' pattern in lead V$_1$ usually with a normal QRS axis. In patients with large shunts right atrial enlargement may be evident on the electrocardiogram.

The plain films demonstrate pulmonary overcirculation. Prominence of the RA, RV and pulmonary artery are present. The LA and LV may be mildly enlarged or may be normal in size. The aortic arch may be relatively inconspicuous. Thus the findings on plain films are reminiscent of ASD rather than VSD (Fig. 7–35). A ball-like or globular configuration has also been described (Kramer and Abrams).

On echocardiography the tricuspid valve flutters during systole—a finding not specific for LV-RA communication, since it also occurs with rupture of an aneurysm of a sinus of Valsalva into the RV. Doppler echocardiography identi-

fies a distinct jet into the right atrium. This finding does not differentiate LV-RA communication from VSD with tricuspid insufficiency (see Fig. 2–46).

Cardiac catheterization demonstrates an oxygen step-up in the RA. If the defect is VSD plus tricuspid perforation, then an additional step-up may be present in the ventricle. Left ventriculography is the optimum method of diagnosing LV-RA communications. Contrast material from the LV opacifies the RA and subsequently the RV and pulmonary arteries (Fig. 7–36). An aneurysm of the membranous ventricular septum may be demonstrated. A "gooseneck" deformity is not present.

Surgery is indicated for large left-to-right shunts, but repair of small shunts may also be recommended to lower the risk of bacterial endocarditis. Surgical mortality is low. The defect is closed by way of an atrial incision.

Congenital Coronary Arteriovenous Fistulas

A coronary arteriovenous fistula represents an abnormal

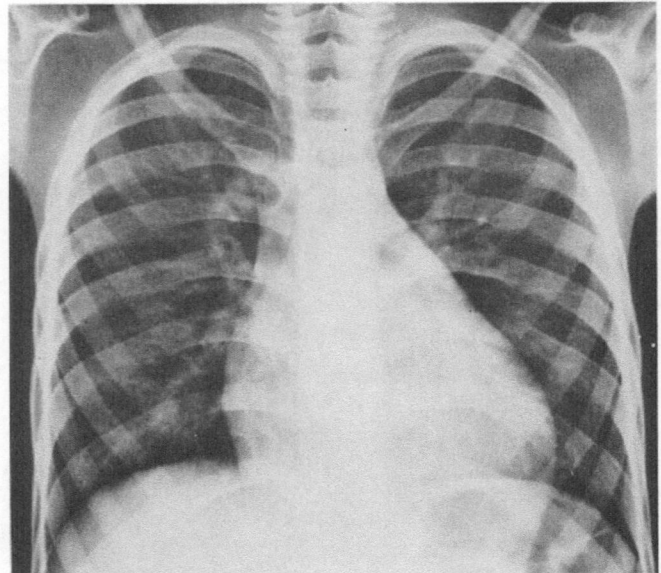

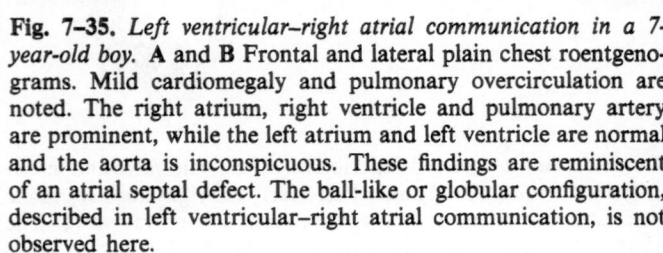

A

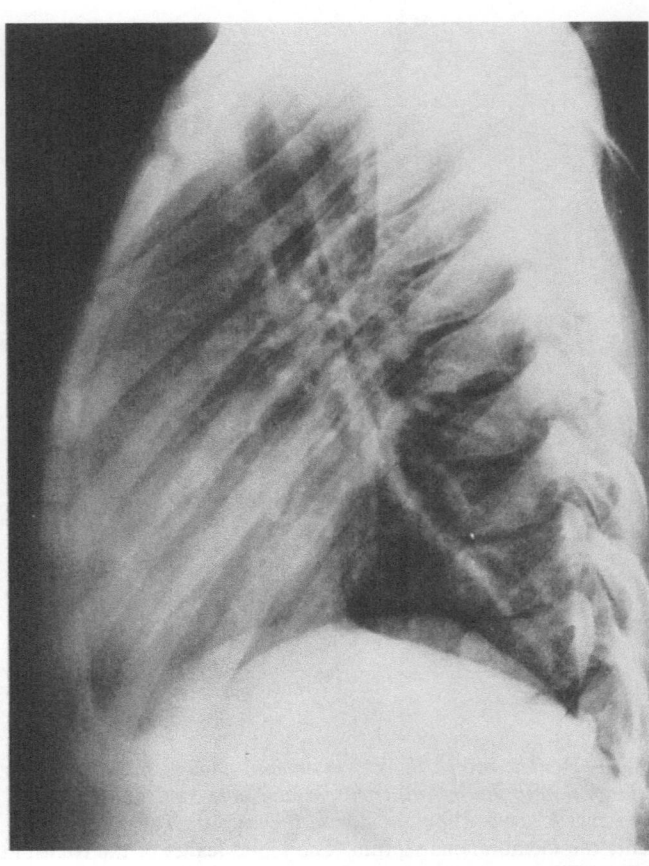

B

Fig. 7–35. *Left ventricular–right atrial communication in a 7-year-old boy.* **A** and **B** Frontal and lateral plain chest roentgenograms. Mild cardiomegaly and pulmonary overcirculation are noted. The right atrium, right ventricle and pulmonary artery are prominent, while the left atrium and left ventricle are normal and the aorta is inconspicuous. These findings are reminiscent of an atrial septal defect. The ball-like or globular configuration, described in left ventricular–right atrial communication, is not observed here.

communication from a coronary artery that may enter any cardiac chamber, a pulmonary artery, the coronary sinus, or the superior vena cava. The origins of the coronary arteries are normal. Either coronary artery may be involved, rarely both are affected. The general order of frequency of the receiving chamber or vessel, as reported by Ogden is the RV, RA, pulmonary artery, coronary sinus, coronary veins, LA and LV. Communication with the LA and LV is uncommon; even less common is a connection into the superior vena cava or a pulmonary vein. The fistulous connection may be single or multiple and may occur anywhere along the course of the coronary vessel. The coronary artery will be dilated and tortuous if the shunt is large. Aneurysms may occur in the affected artery proximal to the fistulous connection.

The embryogenesis has been attributed to persistence of the connections between the coronary capillaries and the trabecular chambers present in the embryo. Some fistulas into a pulmonary artery may originate from an acces-

sory conus artery that arises from the left or right coronary artery. Electrocardiographic, plain film and hemodynamic findings are determined by the size of the shunt and the site of drainage of the fistulous connection.

Clinical Features Most patients are asymptomatic, the most prominent clinical finding, however, is a continuous murmur. Infants with large shunts may have congestive heart failure. In these infants the murmur may not be characteristic. Affected adults may have angina, which may or may not be attributable to the anomaly. It is important to differentiate arteriovenous fistula from patent ductus arteriosus (PDA) because the surgical approach for correction of the two disorders is different. Murmurs with coronary arteriovenous fistula are generally heard only over the front of the chest, whereas a murmur associated with PDA is often transmitted to the back. In addition, a murmur due to an arteriovenous fistula is likely to sound less harsh than that attributed to PDA.

If the shunt is large the cardiac findings will be deter-

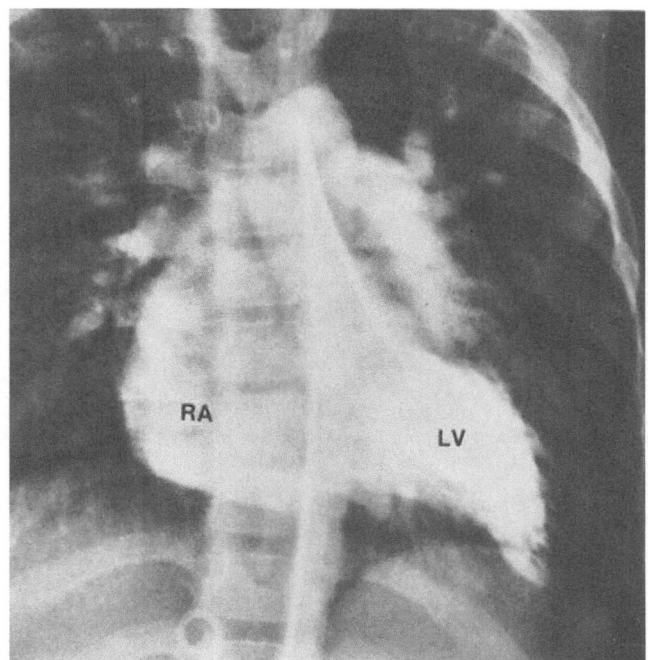

A

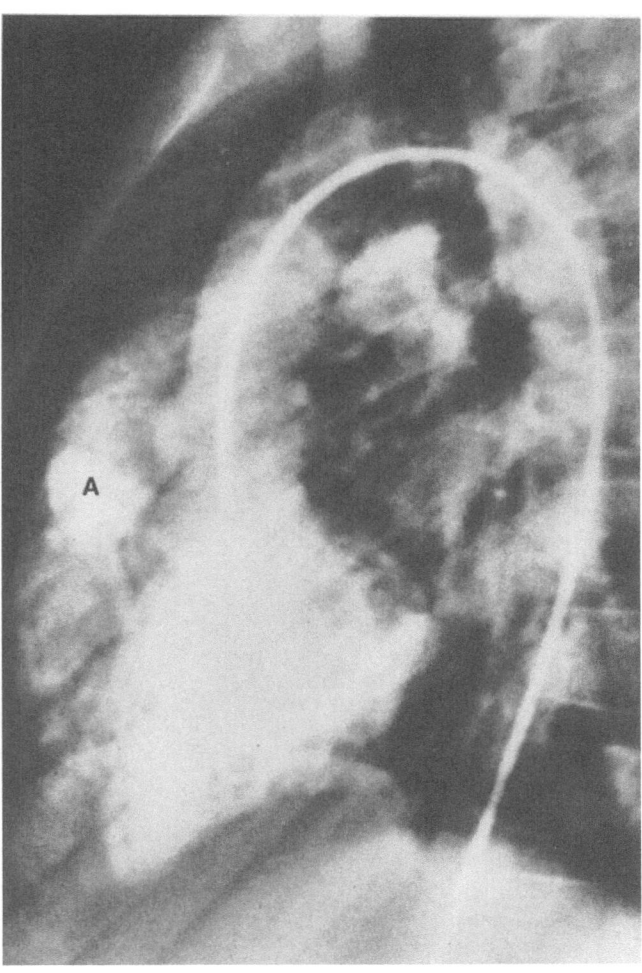

B

Fig. 7–36. *Left ventricular–right atrial communication.* **A** and **B** Frontal and lateral films of a left ventriculogram. In the frontal film, blood from the left ventricle (*LV*) opacifies the right atrium (*RA*), and subsequently the right ventricle and pulmonary artery. In the lateral film a large aneurysm (*A*) of the membranous interventricular septum fills with contrast medium during ventricular systole, but does not communicate with the right ventricle. Opacification of the right ventricle occurs late, after the right atrium has filled. Thus an interventricular septal defect with tricuspid insufficiency is excluded.

mined by the site of drainage. A combined RV and LV heave is felt in the presence of drainage into the right side of the heart. A LV heave is found with drainage into the left side of the heart. The pulses may be increased in amplitude. The electrocardiogram may be normal or may reflect the enlargement of the individual chambers affected by the site of drainage.

Echocardiography Dilatation of a heart chamber depends on the site of drainage. The ostium of the affected coronary artery may be enlarged, and its course may be followed for a variable distance because of the large size of its lumen. Doppler echocardiography may identify the site of drainage of the fistula.

Radiological (Plain Film) Features If the shunt is large, overcirculation will be present. In instances of drainage into the superior vena cava, coronary sinus or RA the plain film of the chest will be reminiscent of an ASD. The dilatation of the RA, RV and pulmonary artery tends to obscure the enlargement of the left-sided heart chambers.

If the fistula drains into the RV the radiological pattern will mimic a VSD (biventricular and LA enlargement). Drainage into a pulmonary artery will produce enlargement of the main pulmonary artery, LA and LV, similar to a PDA. With drainage into the LA, this chamber may become massively dilated. A fistula into the LV will simulate aortic insufficiency, aortico-left ventricular tunnel or ruptured sinus of Valsalva.

One specific radiological feature that should suggest a coronary arteriovenous fistula is a bulge or bump on either the left or right border of the heart. This finding is especially likely in cases of fistula between the left circumflex artery and the coronary sinus. In such instances the bump is in the left A-V groove (Fig. 7–37). Rarely the affected coronary arteries become calcified, so that their tortuous course may be outlined on plain film.

Hemodynamics An oxygen step-up occurs at the site of drainage if the shunt is significant, however, the shunt is seldom large enough to produce changes in pressures.

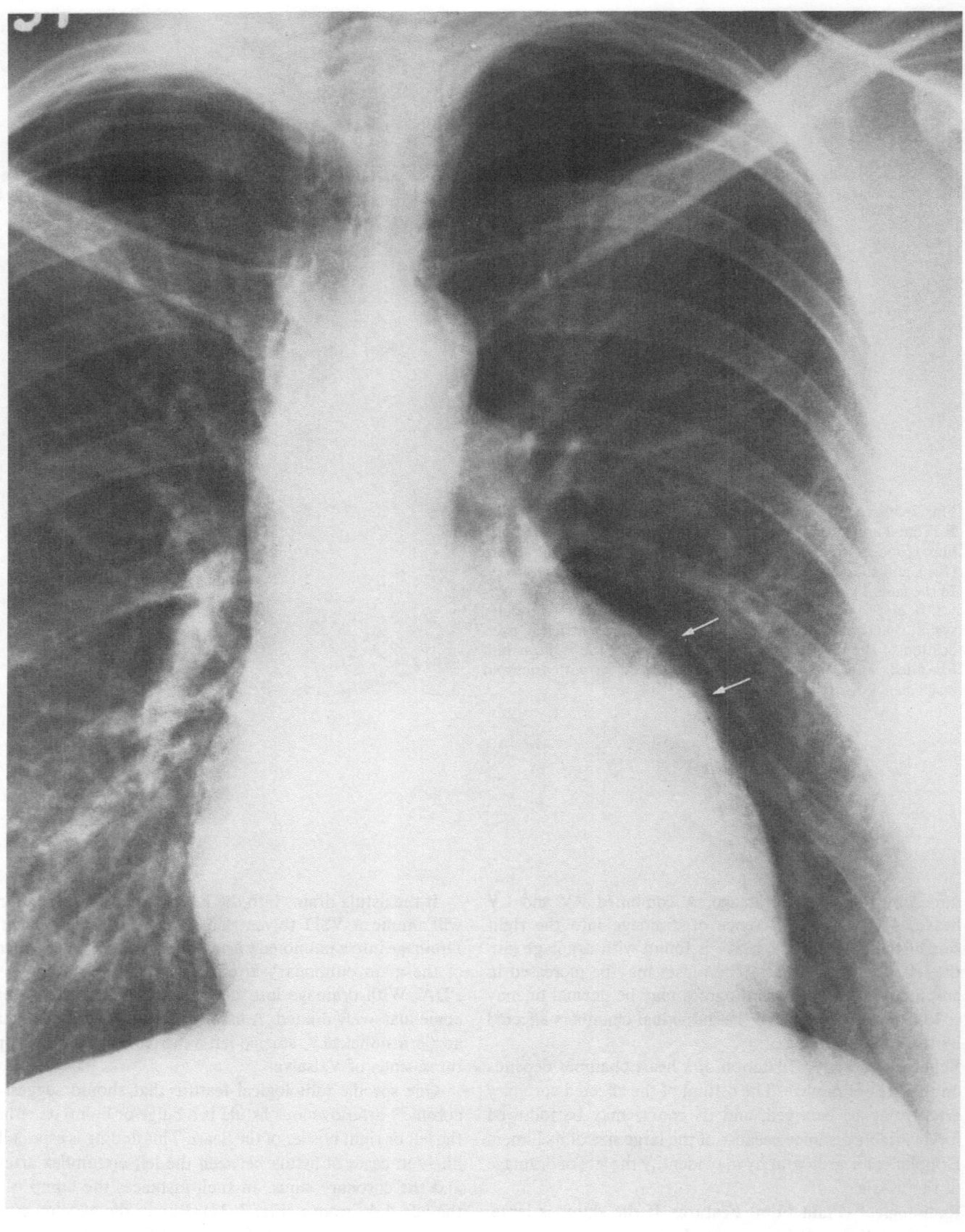

A

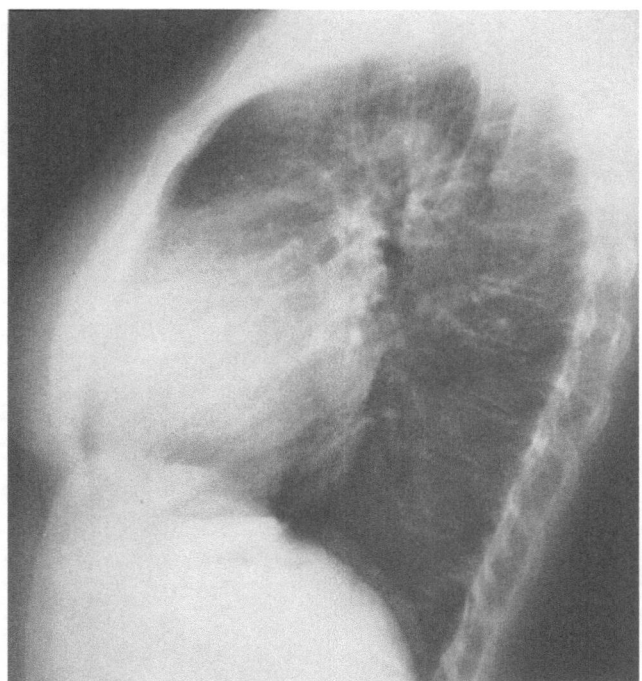

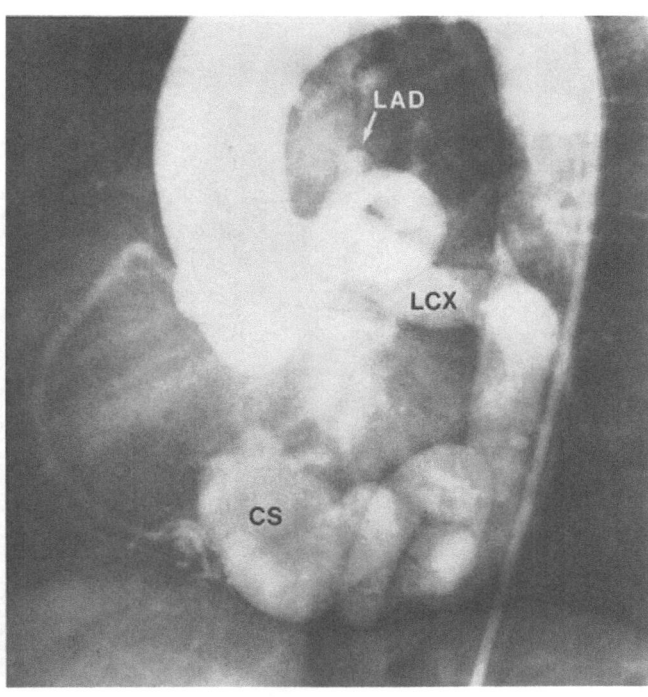

B

C

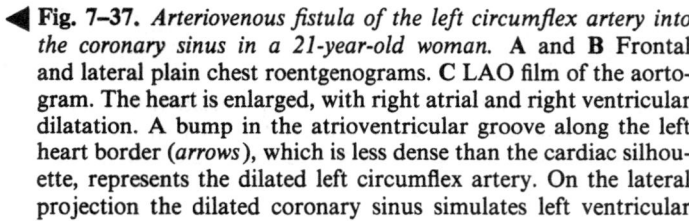

Fig. 7–37. *Arteriovenous fistula of the left circumflex artery into the coronary sinus in a 21-year-old woman.* **A** and **B** Frontal and lateral plain chest roentgenograms. **C** LAO film of the aortogram. The heart is enlarged, with right atrial and right ventricular dilatation. A bump in the atrioventricular groove along the left heart border (*arrows*), which is less dense than the cardiac silhouette, represents the dilated left circumflex artery. On the lateral projection the dilated coronary sinus simulates left ventricular enlargement. A bump in this location and a dilated coronary sinus in a patient with a continuous murmur are highly suggestive of this type of coronary arteriovenous fistula.

The aortogram (**C**) demonstrates the markedly dilated and tortuous left circumflex artery (*LCX*), which connects to the coronary sinus (*CS*). Only the origin of the left anterior descending coronary artery (*LAD*) is opacified in this study. The LAD was outlined on cine aortography.

Contrast Studies Left ventriculography, aortography (Fig. 7–37C) and selective coronary arteriography generally opacify the anomaly. All three are often necessary to fully delineate the origin, course and termination of a coronary arteriovenous fistula.

Experience with infants with large shunts involving the right coronary artery has shown that left ventriculography often produces better opacification than aortography because a more optimum volume of contast medium is injected into the LV by means of a pressure injector and because mixing is more complete (Fig. 7–38). If the left coronary artery is involved then aortography and selective coronary arteriography will be more accurate than left ventriculography. With left ventriculography in instances of left coronary artery involvement, contrast in the LV will be superimposed on the fistulous artery, preventing definition of the course and drainage.

An incidental finding in patients with severe mitral stenosis is fistulous connection between a branch of the left circumflex artery and the LA appendage. Most such fistulous connections end in a network of fistulous tracts. The shunt generally is small. Such communications are thought by some investigators to be due to erosion of the endocardium by thrombus; others have considered these to represent neovascularity, associated with an organized thrombus in the LA appendage. The authors have observed these communications with and without atrial thrombi (Fig. 5–38), and have also observed similar fistulas in the RA and RA appendage in patients with mitral stenosis and pulmonary hypertension. Thus the cause of these fistulous communications is unclear.

Treatment Repair is recommended in large coronary arteriovenous fistulas because of congestive heart failure. Although the role of surgery in small defects is not well defined, some are repaired to prevent bacterial endocarditis, acute myocardial infarction or rupture of a coronary artery aneurysm. A single communication may be ligated from outside the heart, while multiple entry sites are closed from inside the chamber during cardiopulmonary bypass.

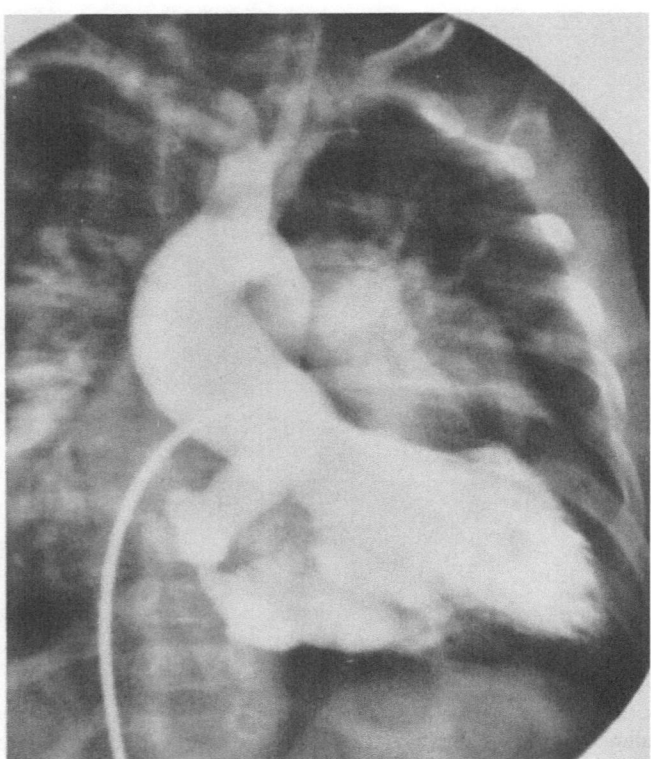
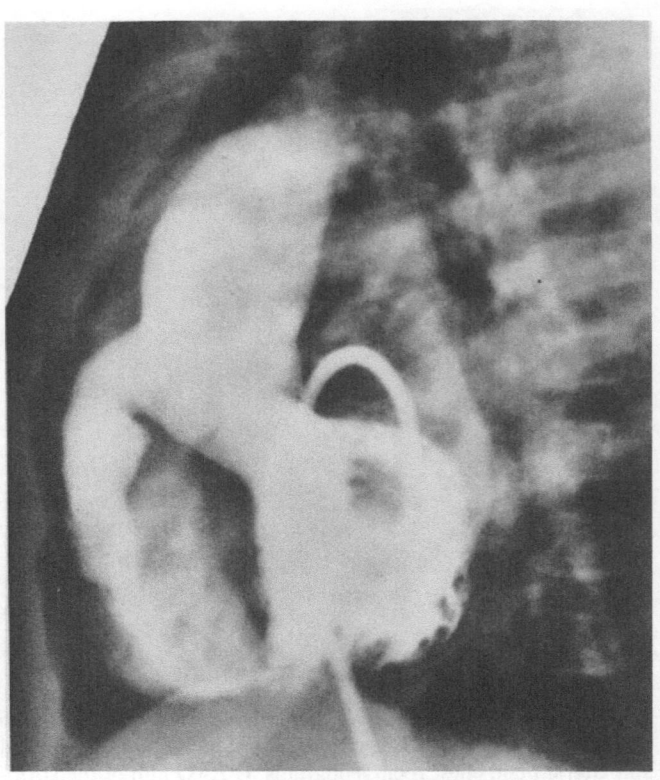

A
B

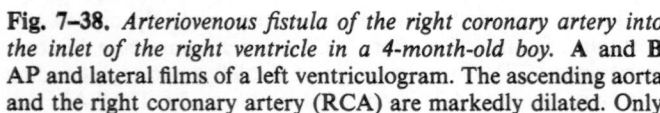

Fig. 7–38. *Arteriovenous fistula of the right coronary artery into the inlet of the right ventricle in a 4-month-old boy.* **A** and **B** AP and lateral films of a left ventriculogram. The ascending aorta and the right coronary artery (RCA) are markedly dilated. Only a single fistulous tract is demonstrated. Opacification is excellent because of mixing of contrast medium in the left ventricle. Selective injections into the RCA were diluted immediately by unopacified blood, so that opacification was less than optimal.

Ventricular Level Communications

The plain film findings with ventricular level communications are the same regardless of its location in the ventricular septum. The predominant radiological features are biventricular enlargement, left atrial enlargement, prominence of the pulmonary artery, a normal or small (inconspicuous) aorta, and pulmonary overcirculation. Isolated ventricular septal defect (VSD) is the most common cause of left to right shunt at the ventricular level. Other defects that may produce a similar radiological appearance are listed in Table 7–3. A similar radiographic picture may also occur with some potentially cyanotic lesions (e.g., A-V communis, double-outlet right ventricle with subaortic VSD, and single ventricle) while cyanosis may not be clinically evident. In addition, many instances of shunts at the great vessel level do not cause obvious enlargement of the aorta, and therefore cannot be distinguished on the basis of plain films alone. Therefore, all these defects must be considered as well in interpretation of chest roentgenograms. Clinical data are of assistance in some instances.

Discussed in this section is isolated VSD and VSD with aortic insufficiency. VSD occurring with other valvular defects or complex cyanotic defects will be discussed in those sections.

Isolated Ventricular Septal Defect

Ventricular septal defect (VSD) is the most common congenital heart malformation, with an incidence of approximately 20%–30% of all congenital heart abnormalities. The defect is usually located in the membranous septum (infracristal, subaortic), but it may occur in the infundibular septum (supracristal, subpulmonic), in the inlet portion of the septum (inlet VSD) or in the trabecular septum (muscular) (Fig. 7–39). The term *perimembranous* has been used by Soto et al. to designate defects that are contiguous with the central fibrous body but may extend into the subaortic region, the inlet region, or the trabecular septum. Used in this way the term was meant to connote a specific relationship of the conduction system posterior and inferior to this group of defects. The authors prefer the term *membranous* and describe extensions of the defects according to the area involved. VSDs vary in size from a few millimeters to complete absence of the septum. Most are small. Spontaneous closure occurs frequently. VSD may be associated with atrial septal defect, patent ductus arteriosus, coarctation of the aorta or discrete diaphragmatic subaortic stenosis. The defect also may be part of complex heart malformations such as tetralogy of Fallot, transpositions, truncus arteriosus, tricuspid atresia and endocardial cushion defects, or associated with noncardiac defects such as

Fig. 7–39. *The components of the ventricular septum from the right ventricular side.* The muscular septum consists of three components, the inlet and infundibular portions are smooth, whereas the apical portion is trabeculated. The trabecular septum is the location of muscular ventricular septal defects ("swiss cheese" type), and the infundibular septum is the area where supracristal (subpulmonic, conal, or bulbar) ventricular septal defects occur. The membranous septum is posterior and inferior to the crista supraventricularis and extends across the anulus of the tricuspid valve (*TV*) into the right atrium. The membranous septum is limited posteriorly by the right fibrous trigone and the anterior leaflet of the mitral valve, and superiorly by the aortic valve. The muscular (trabecular) septum is below. The septal leaflet of the TV transects the membranous septum, dividing it into two portions—the interventricular and the atrioventricular. The interventricular portion is commonly referred to as the membranous septum and is the site where most ventricular septal defects occur. Membranous ventricular septal defects are also called infracristal, subaortic and high ventricular septal defects. The bundle of His courses approximately 2–3 mm below the inferior border of the membranous septum. *MPA* = main pulmonary artery. (For further information concerning the relationships of the membranous septum see Figs. 7–32 to 7–34.)

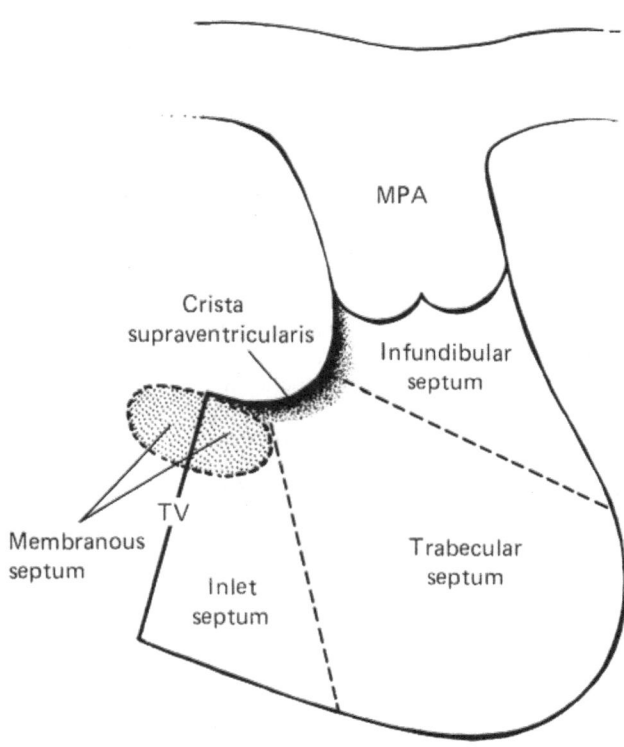

tracheoesophageal fistula and renal anomalies. In addition, VSD may be a feature of some chromosomal syndromes (e.g., Down syndrome, trisomy D, trisomy E, cri du chat syndrome) and heritable disorders (Apert syndrome, Beckwith-Wiedemann syndrome, Conradi-Hünermann syndrome).

Clinical Features The clinical findings, including the age of presentation, are determined by the size of the defect. Individuals with small defects are asymptomatic. A harsh pansystolic murmur is heard at the third to fourth left intercostal space. A thrill may or may not be palpated. The cardiac impulse is normal. No sign of cardiac overload is present on electrocardiograms or roentgenograms of the chest. The maladie de Roger (tiny VSD with inordinately loud murmur) is included in this group of defects.

Moderate-sized defects may be noted early in life with mild tachypnea or later with dyspnea on exertion. In addition to the pansystolic murmur and thrill at the fourth left intercostal space, the second sound may be accentuated and a third sound or diastolic flow rumble may be heard at the apex (secondary to high flow across the mitral valve). The electrocardiogram shows LV hypertrophy and, on occasion, biventricular hypertrophy.

In infants with congestive heart failure due to a large VSD the murmur may be soft and may be an ejection murmur rather than pansystolic initially. A marked combined heave, a loud second sound and gallop rhythm are the predominant cardiac findings. Signs of systemic and pulmonary venous congestion (hepatomegaly, tachypnea) and decreased systemic perfusion (cool extremities, thready pulses) are also evident. Impaired growth and repeated pulmonary infections complicate the course.

Natural History of Isolated Ventricular Septal Defect In patients with untreated VSD the clinical course may be divided into four groups with the development of (1) spontaneous closure, (2) Eisenmenger syndrome, (3) infective endocarditis, and (4) infundibular stenosis with persistence of the VSD (acquired tetralogy of Fallot, "Gasul phenomenon").

The mechanisms for spontaneous closure include: (1) fibrous ingrowth with or without formation of aneurysm of the membranous septum; (2) adherence of the septal leaflet of the tricuspid valve to the rim of the defect, on occasion associated with perforation of the tricuspid leaflet (VSD and tricuspid insufficiency or LV-RA communication); and (3) prolapse of an aortic cusp into the VSD. The last-named entity usually involves supracristal defects with deficient support of the aortic valve and results in aortic regurgitation.

Eisenmenger syndrome occurs if a large VSD with pul-

Fig. 7–40. *Ventricular septal defect with a large left-to-right shunt in a 3 month old infant.* **A** M-mode echocardiogram through the right ventricular outflow tract (*RVOT*), aortic root (*Ao.*) and left atrium (*LA*), which is enlarged. **B** is a view through the right ventricle (*RV*) and left ventricle (*LV*). The left ventricle is large for a baby of this age, and the shortening fraction is 40%, which is in excess of normal. The diameter of the right ventricle is relatively small; perhaps the right ventricle is displaced away from the echo beam by the dilated left ventricle. These findings also occur with patent ductus arteriosus.

Ventricular septal defects are not generally demonstrated on M-mode unless overriding of the aorta or malalignment of the ventricular septum is present.

IVS = interventricular septum; *PW* = posterior wall of the left ventricle.

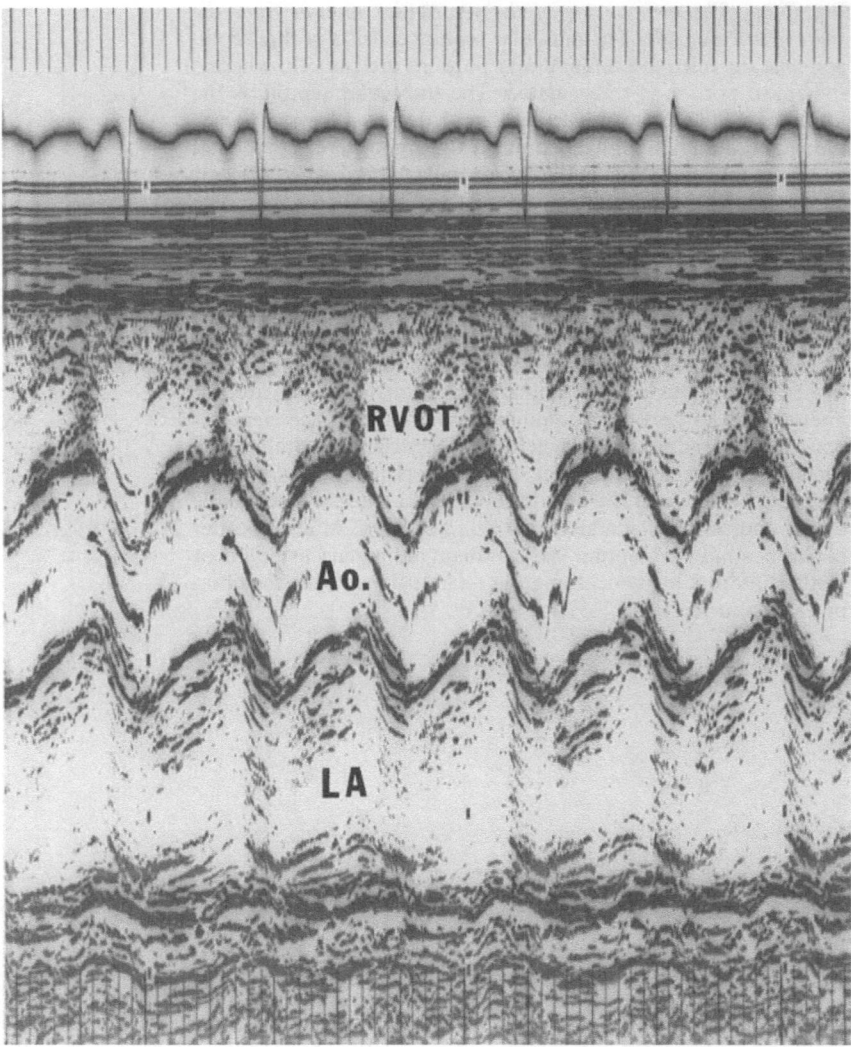

A

monary hypertension is left untreated. The syndrome consists of changes in the pulmonary arteries that tend to narrow the small vessels and restrict blood flow through the lungs, thus limiting and eventually reversing the left-to-right shunt. According to Heath and Edwards the vascular changes begin with medial hypertrophy and then progress to fibrosis of the medial musculature and thickening of the intima, which further narrows and obliterates the lumina of the arterioles. Thereafter, atherosclerosis and chronic thromboemboli develop within the vessels. Later developments include saccular aneurysms of the arterioles, which may rupture into the alveoli to produce hemoptysis.

Irreversible hypertensive changes may begin by the age of 12 to 18 months if pulmonary pressure remains near systemic pressure. Thereafter, even if pulmonary pressure is reduced by palliation or repair of the VSD, the vascular changes may progress. If repair is carried out in children

with advanced vascular disease, the RV may fail, with death ensuing rapidly. Prevention of Eisenmenger syndrome by operation in infancy is necessary if long-term survival is to be expected.

RV outflow tract obstruction may be acquired before or, rarely, after spontaneous or surgical closure of VSD. Histological studies of resected infundibular muscle in two patients demonstrated abnormal shape and orientation of cardiac muscle cells resembling the histological changes in idiopathic hypertrophic subaortic stenosis (IHSS).

Infective endocarditis may develop before or after surgical repair. In unoperated patients with VSD the vegetation characteristically forms inside the free wall of the RV cavity, opposite the VSD. This is also the location of a fibrous thickening of the endocardium that is presumed to be caused by shunted blood striking the wall of the heart (the jet lesion).

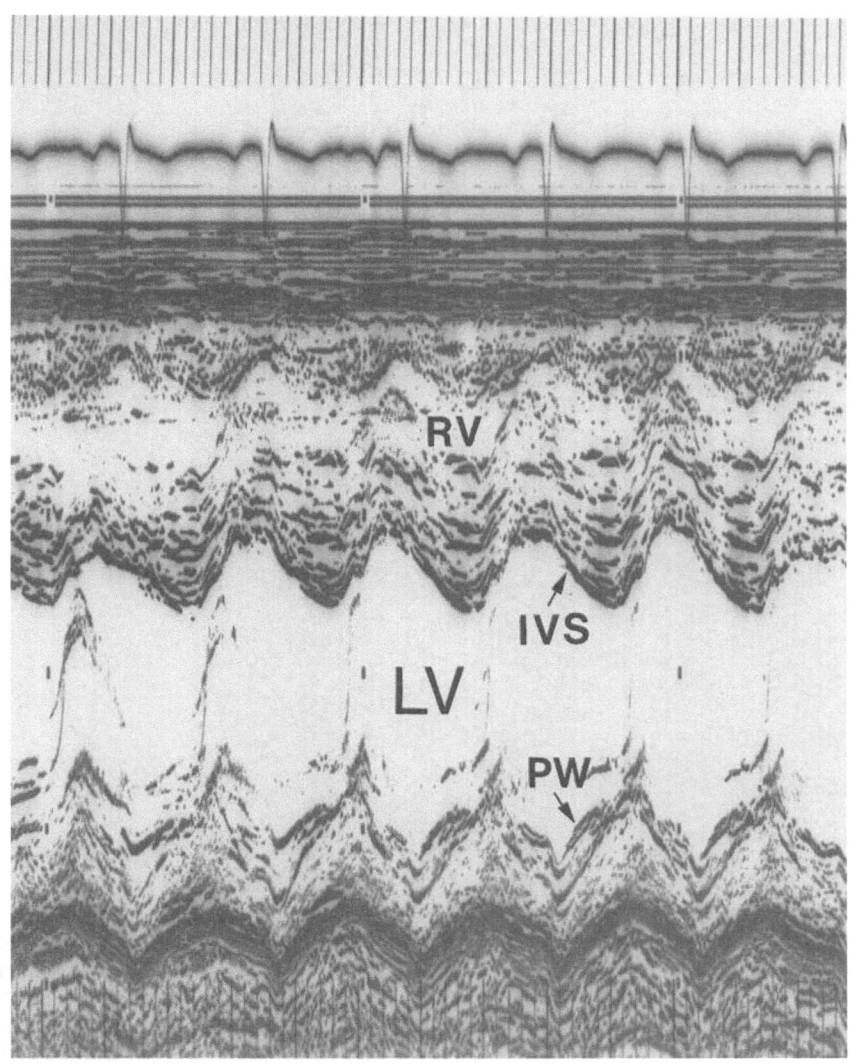

RV

IVS

LV

PW

B

Echocardiography M-mode echocardiography is used to evaluate the extent of cardiac overload in patients with left-to-right shunts in infancy. A dilated LA and a hypercontractile LV are identified with both VSD and patent ductus arteriosus (PDA) (Fig. 7–40).

Comparison of systolic time intervals of the pulmonary valve and the aortic valve by M-mode is helpful in estimating pulmonary artery pressure (Fig. 7–41).

Except for malalignment VSDs (Fig. 7–42) and VSDs associated with Tetralogy of Fallot (see Fig. 2–16), isolated VSDs are not imaged by M-mode echocardiography. On the other hand, most moderate- to large-sized defects, and aneurysms of the membranous septum, can be imaged by 2-D echocardiography (Figs. 7–43, 7–44, 7–45). Left-to-right shunts through small defects are identified by use of saline or green dye as contrast agent. The technique requires injection into the LA or LV. This technique might be useful when injection of a radiopaque medium is contra-indicated or in postoperative patients with a catheter in the LA.

Ultrasound imaging of right-to-left shunts, on the other hand, requires injection in a systemic vein. Thus, ultrasound is an effective method of identifying the level of right-to-left shunts in patients with reversed shunts secondary to pulmonic stenosis or high pulmonary resistance.

Doppler echocardiography appears to be useful in detection of VSDs because of its ability to assess abnormal cardiac flow patterns. The left-to-right shunt is often best recognized from the parasternal window in either the short-axis or long-axis view (Fig. 2–46). The Doppler sample volume is scanned across the RV outflow tract to detect a jet toward the transducer adjacent to the membranous septum. The velocity of the jet allows an estimate of the pressure difference between the ventricles. In patients with muscular defects the jet may be identified by placing the sample volume elsewhere in the right ventricle near the

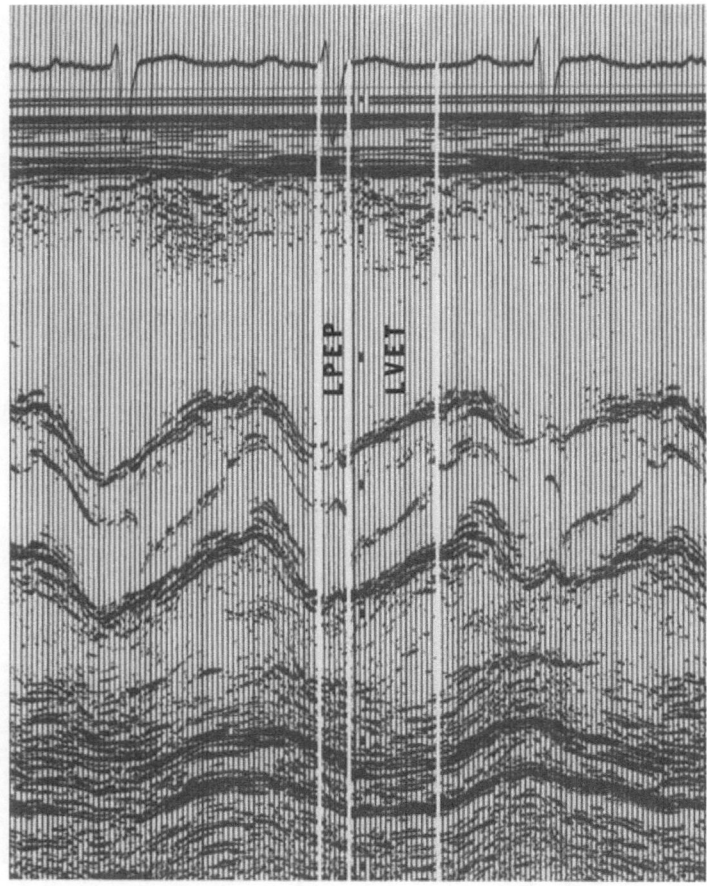

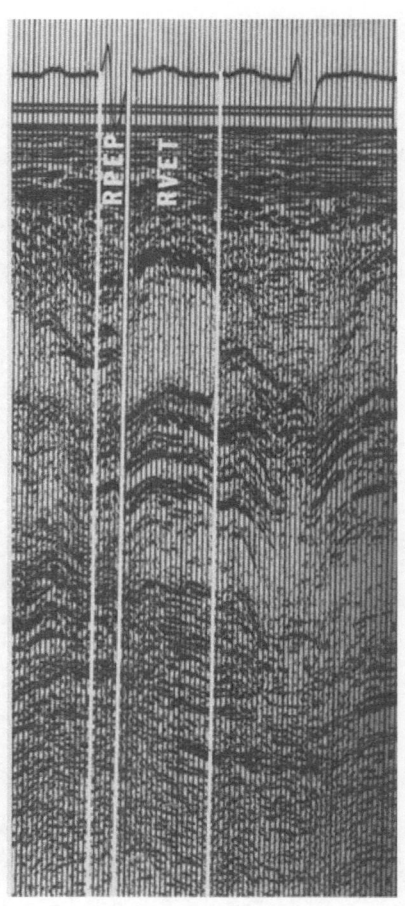

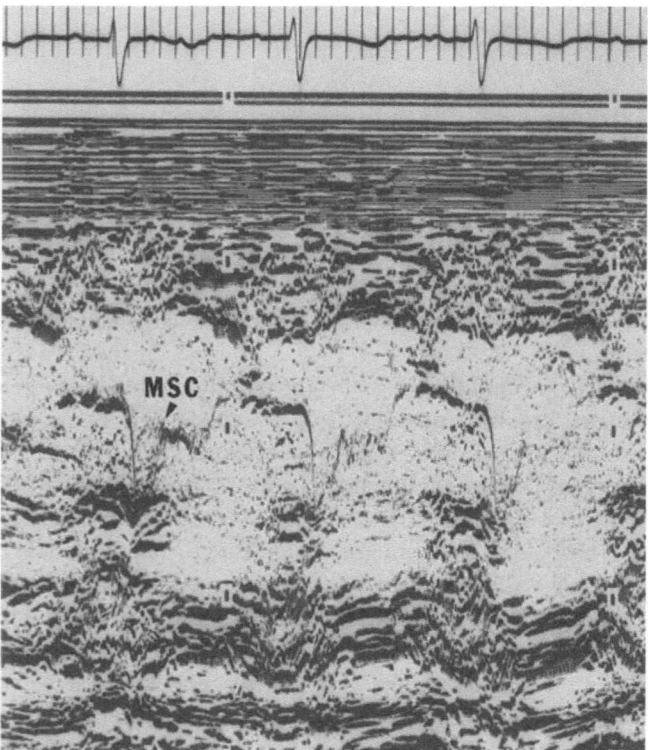

Fig. 7–41. *Ventricular septal defect with pulmonary hypertension.* **A** and **B** are M-mode echocardiograms through the aortic and pulmonary valves. The time lines are 10 msec apart. The aortic or left ventricular preejection period (*LPEP*) is 50 msec. The left ventricular ejection time (*LVET*) is 170 msec. The pulmonary or right ventricular preejection period (*RPEP*) is also 50 msec, and the right ventricular ejection time (*RVET*) is 180 msec. The systolic time intervals of the two semilunar valves are nearly identical. Thus equal pressures in the aorta and pulmonary artery are predicted. At cardiac catheterization the pulmonary artery pressure was at systemic level.

Frame C is an M-mode echocardiogram through the pulmonary valve from another infant with pulmonary hypertension. Mid systolic closure (*MSC*) and absence of the atrial kick are signs of pulmonary hypertension.

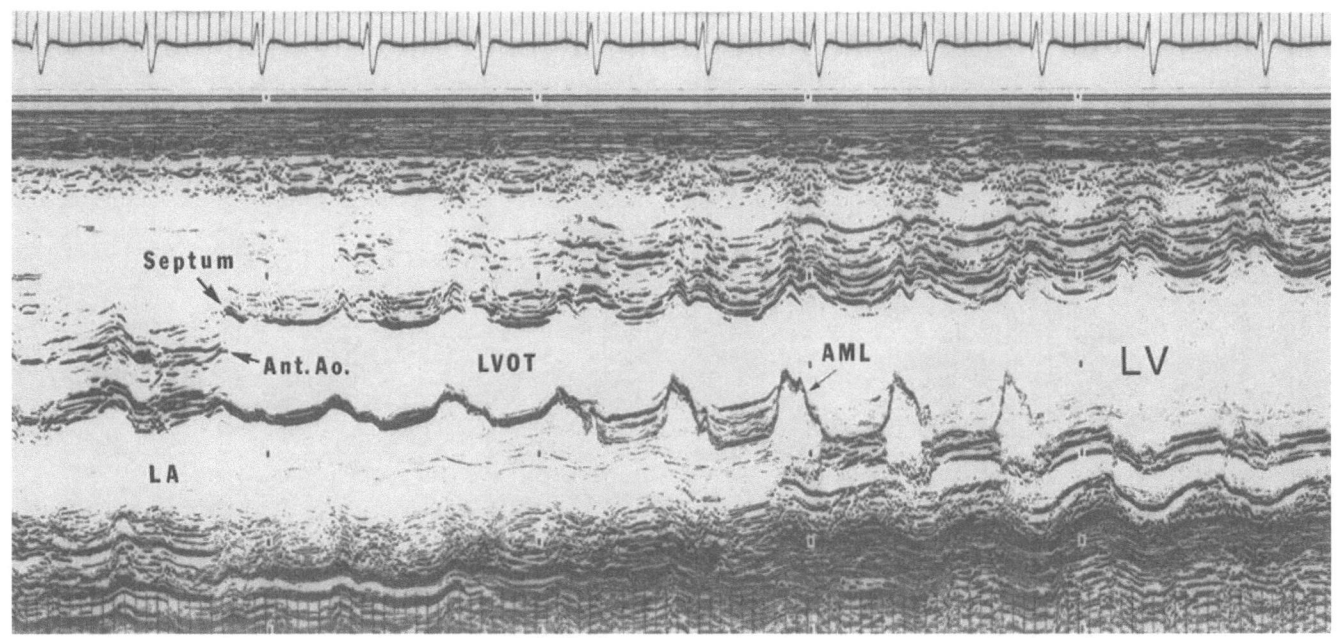

Fig. 7–42. *"Conoventricular malalignment" in an infant with ventricular septal defect and subaortic stenosis.* The left ventricular outflow tract (*LVOT*) is narrowed by the conal septum, which is deviated toward the left. This M-mode arc scan reveals a break between the anterior wall of the aortic root (*Ant. Ao.*) and the ventricular septum (*Septum*). Echoes from the displaced conal muscle are probably mixed with the echoes of the anterior aortic root. At autopsy, conus tissue was observed inside the left ventricle, forming the upper margin of the ventricular septal defect.

LA = left atrium; *AML* = anterior leaflet of the mitral valve; *LV* = left ventricle.

ventricular septum, or even within the ventricular septum at sites of suspected defects.

Radiological (Plain Film) Features With small shunts and normal pulmonary pressure plain films of the chest are normal. With moderate or large shunts the pulmonary vascularity is increased Fig. 7–46, the degree of overcirculation depending on the size of the VSD and the pulmonary vascular resistance. Superimposition of congestive heart failure and pneumonia is frequently encountered with large shunts.

The size of the heart may be normal, but often the heart is enlarged with moderate or large shunts. The LV, RV and LA are dilated. The pulmonary artery is prominent, while the aorta is small or normal in size. A reduction in the size of the heart and the degree of overcirculation may be observed on serial roentgenograms in patients with a closing VSD. Such patients should be distinguished from those who develop high pulmonary arterial resistance and a right-to-left shunt (Eisenmenger syndrome). In the Eisenmenger group the films of the chest often show markedly dilated central pulmonary vessels, with abrupt decrease in caliber of the interlobar pulmonary arteries (pruned-tree appearance) (see Fig. 1–22). In long-standing cases aneurysmal dilatation of the main pulmonary artery may be present. Rarely, calcification of the pulmonary arteries may be noted.

Hemodynamics An oxygen saturation step-up at the ventricular level is observed in most cases of VSD. The size of the step-up correlates with the size of the left-to-right shunt. The left-to-right shunt and the ratio of pulmonary to systemic blood flow can be calculated from the oxygen consumption and the oxygen concentration in the blood of the chambers proximal and distal to the shunt (see section on Hemodynamics in the Introduction to this chapter). If the defect is small the shunt may be detectable only by hydrogen electrode. In patients with a large VSD the oxygen step-up may also be small or undetectable if the pulmonary resistance is high or if pulmonary stenosis is present.

Pressures in the RV and pulmonary arteries (PA) are normal with small defects. With moderate-sized defects, RV and PA pressures may be normal or moderately elevated. With large defects, pressures in the RV and PA will approach or equal those in the LV and aorta. RV pressure will also be elevated in the presence of pulmonic stenosis. In such instances the PA pressure will be normal or low. In cases with RV pressure at or near systemic level, with or without infundibular stenosis, the shunt may be bidirectional or right to left.

Contrast Studies Biplane (frontal-lateral, LAO-RAO) and compound axial left ventriculography delineates the size

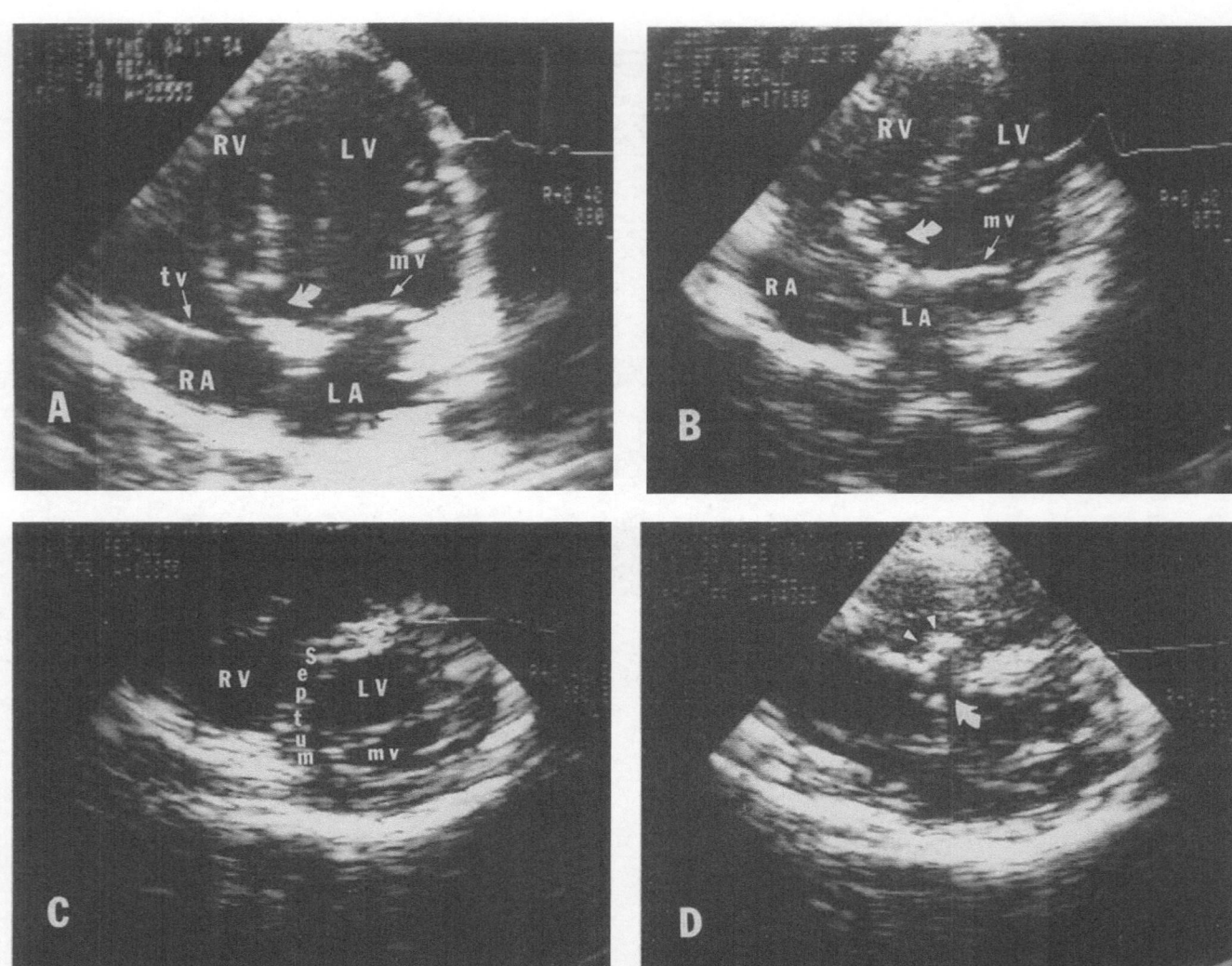

Fig. 7–43. *Aneurysm of the membranous septum in a 10-year-old boy.* The four-chamber view of the two-dimensional echocardiogram (**A**) demonstrates an aneurysm (*curved arrow*) at the superior border of the ventricular septum next to the central fibrous body. The parasternal oblique view (**B**) also identifies the membranous aneurysm. A short axis view of the left ventricle just below the aortic valve during diastole (**C**) demonstrates the left ventricle (*LV*) and mitral leaflets. During systole (**D**) the ventricular septal aneurysm is evident. The *curved arrow* inside the left ventricle points toward the opening of the ventricular septal defect, while the *arrowheads* point toward the aneurysm. **E** and **F** are M-mode echocardiograms through the right ventricle at the level of the membranous septum, just below the aortic valve and slightly toward the patient's right side. In **E** the motion of the tricuspid valve is present (*tv*). During systole the aneurysm (*Aneur.*) bulges anteriorly. **F** is a magnified image showing the motion of the aneurysm (*Memb. Aneurysm*) into the right ventricle (*RV*). *mv* = mitral valve.

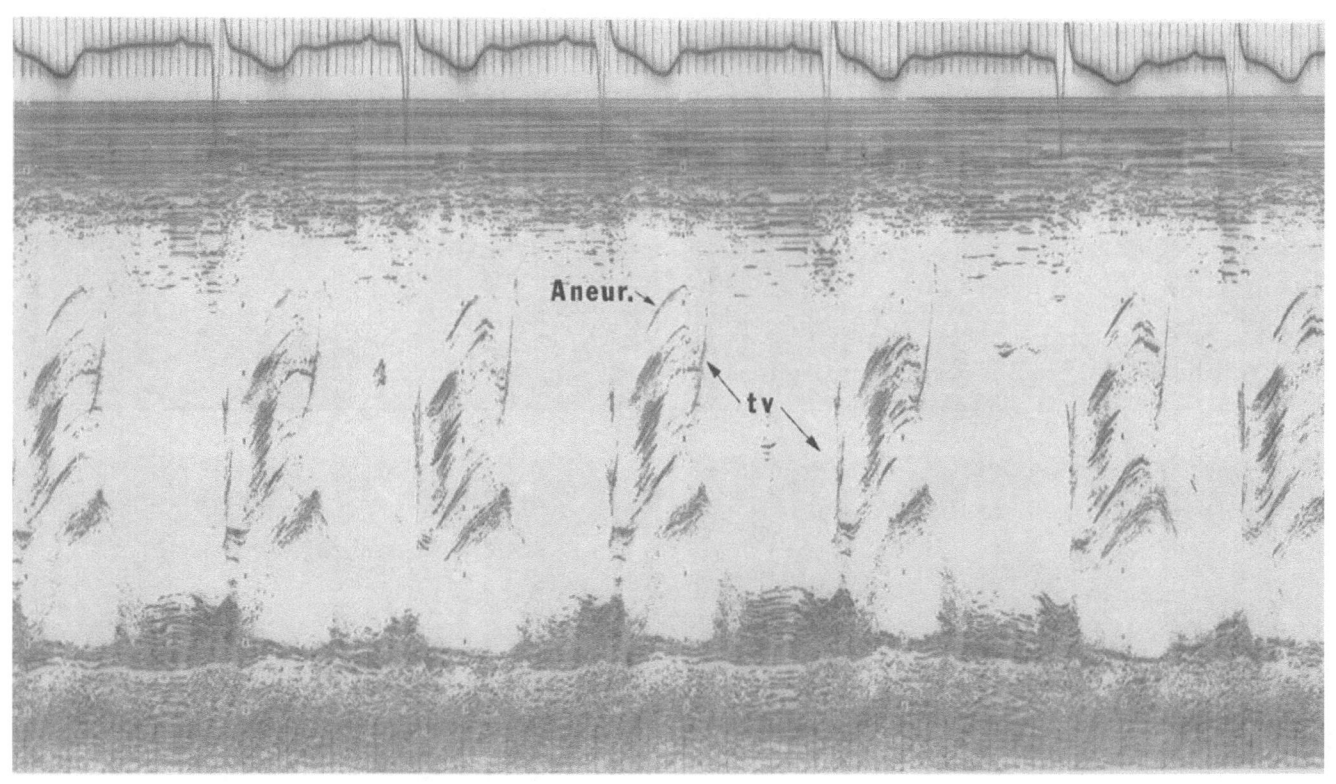

E

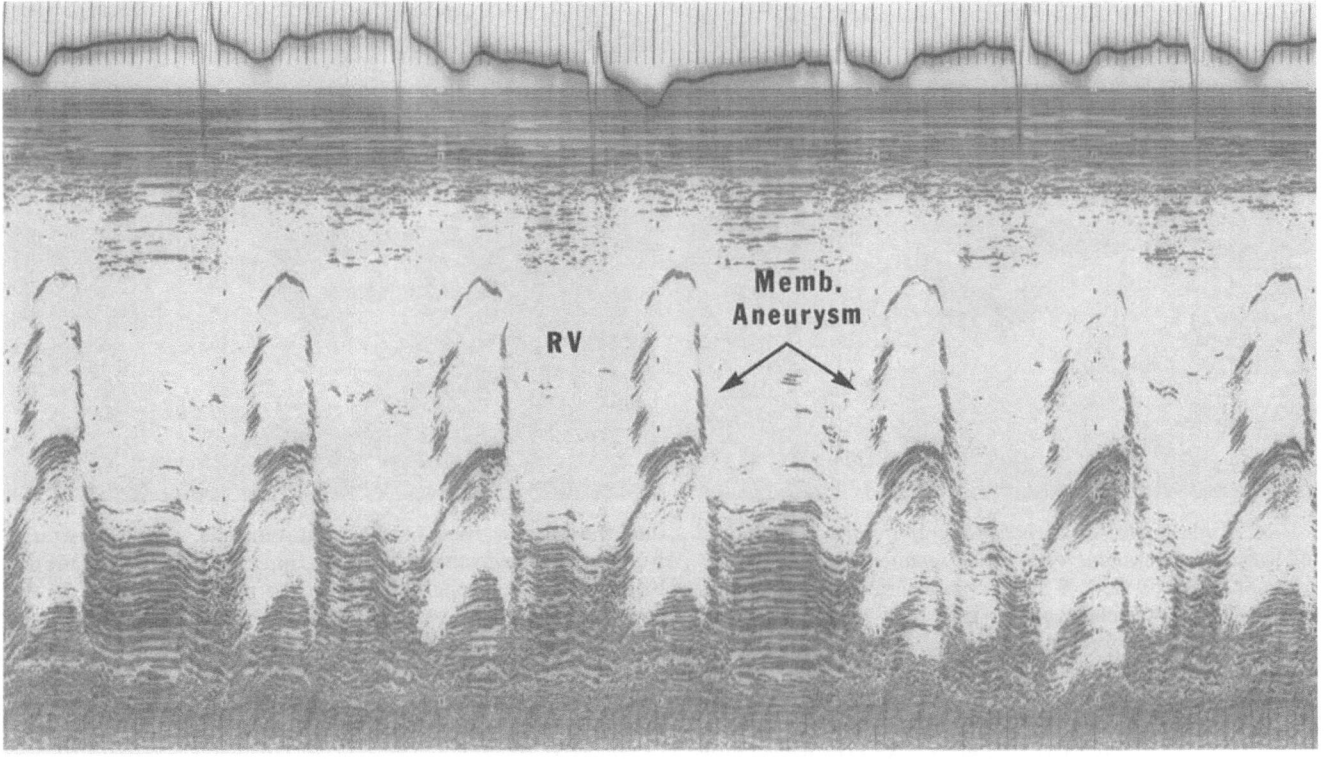

F

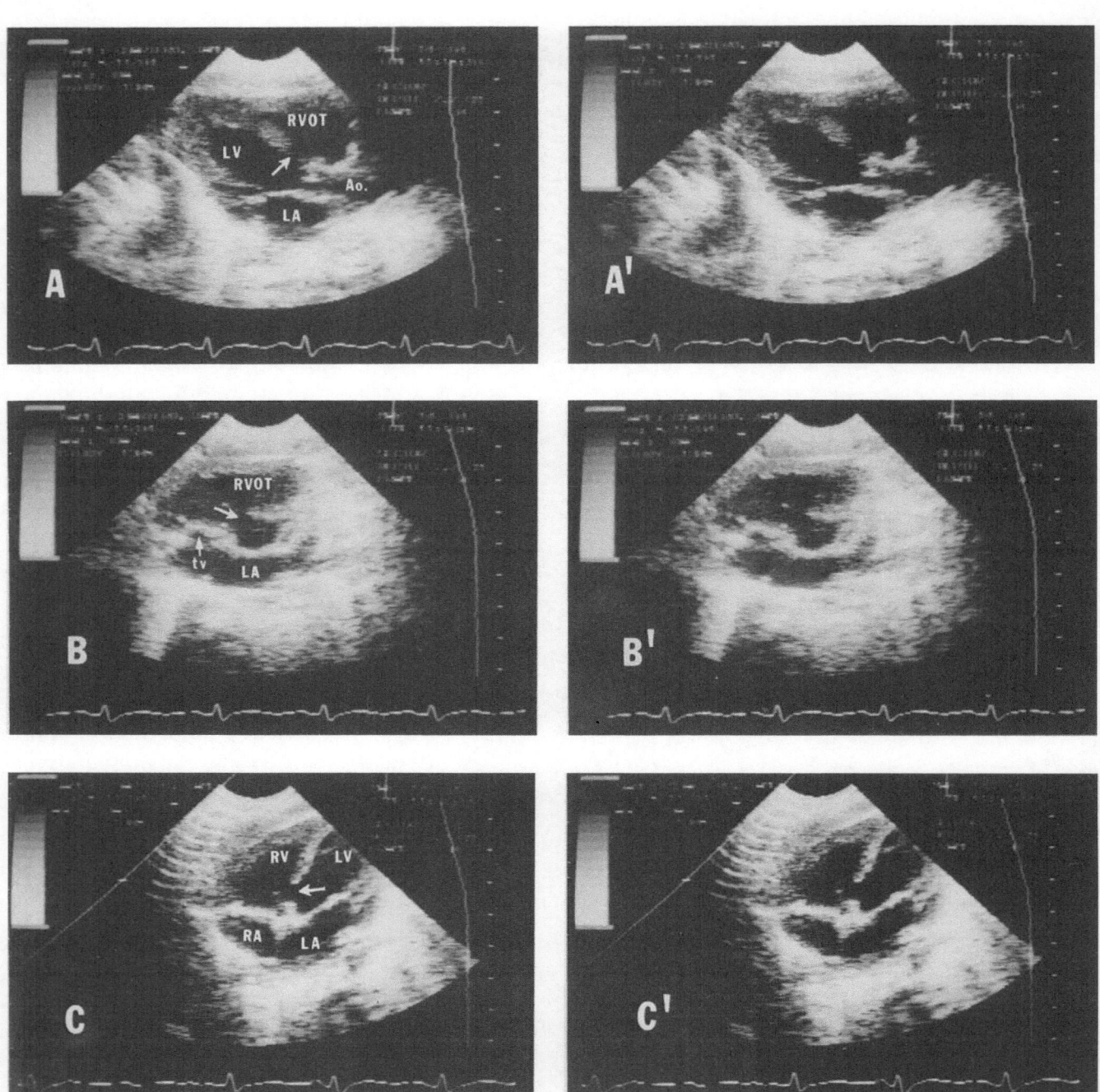

Fig. 7–44. *Two-dimensional echocardiography in a 1-month-old infant with a membranous ventricular septal defect.* **A** and **A'** Parasternal long axis view; **B** and **B'** parasternal short axis view across the left ventricular outflow tract just below the aortic valve; **C** and **C'** apex four-chamber view. In **A** the ventricular septal defect results in a lack of echoes (*arrow*) just beneath the aortic valve. In **B** the defect (*arrow*) is next to the tricuspid valve (*tv*) and immediately below the commissure between the noncoronary and the right coronary cusp. Compare **B** here with the same view in a patient with a supracristal ventricular septal defect (Fig. 7–51B). A supracristal ventricular septal defect opens into the outflow tract of the right ventricle, and is separated from the tricuspid valve by the conus muscle, occurring anteriorly, below the right coronary cusp near the pulmonary valve. In the apex four-chamber view (**C** and **C'**) the ventricular septal defect is at the top of the ventricular septum. Dropout of echoes of the atrial septum in this view does not necessarily represent a defect in the atrial septum, but may occur because the atrial septum is parallel to the echo beam, reflecting poorly.

Ao. = aorta; *LA* = left atrium; *LV* = left ventricle; *RV* = right ventricle; *RVOT* = right ventricular outflow tract.

Fig. 7–45. *Muscular ventricular septal defect.* Apex four-chamber view of a two-dimensional echocardiogram in a 30-year-old woman. The defect (vsd) is in the trabeculated portion of the septum. *LA* = left atrium; *LV* = left ventricle; *RA* = right atrium; *RV* = right ventricle; *mv* = mitral valve; *tv* = tricuspid valve; *p veins* = pulmonary veins. Courtesy of Mark Stern, M.D.

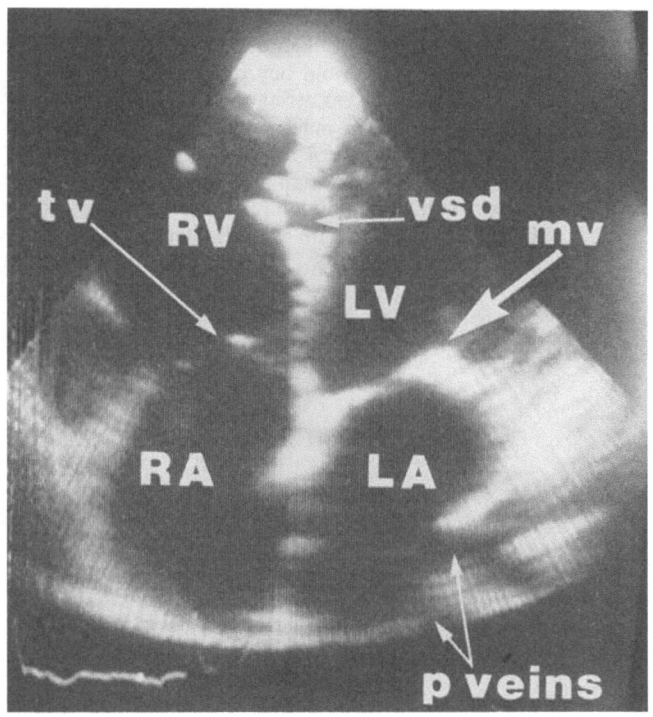

and location of the defect (infracristal, Figs. 7–47 and 7–48; supracristal, Fig. 7–49; muscular or trabecular, Fig. 7–50; and inlet septum, Fig. 7–20). Left ventriculography is also useful in the evaluation of associated abnormalities such as aneurysm of the membranous septum (Fig. 7–48), LV-RA communication, subaortic stenosis and coarctation of the aorta. A right ventriculogram may be necessary to delineate the RV outflow tract. An aortogram will reveal an associated prolapsing aortic cusp or patent ductus arteriosus.

Treatment The principal indications for primary repair of a large VSD in the first year of life are intractable congestive heart failure, failure to thrive and increasing pulmonary vascular resistance. Primary repair is considered superior to two-stage repair, which consists of initial PA banding followed by intracardiac repair and debanding of the pulmonary artery. The combined mortality of the two-stage repair is considerably higher than mortality of primary intracardiac repair. Furthermore, in some instances, heart failure persists because of inadequate pulmonary artery banding. In others, patients may develop a right-to-left shunt and cyanosis if the band is too tight. Narrowing of the PA at its bifurcation may present serious difficulties at the time of debanding.

For patients with an infracristal VSD (subaortic) a transatrial surgical approach is preferred. For a muscular VSD, right ventriculotomy is the procedure of choice, while a transpulmonary incision is considered the appropriate surgical approach for a supracristal VSD.

Repair of a VSD is indicated in children beyond infancy

if a large left-to-right shunt persists ($\dot{Q}p/\dot{Q}s$ greater than 2/1) or if pulmonary resistance remains increased. Severely increased pulmonary resistance (Eisenmenger syndrome) is a contraindication to surgical closure of a VSD.

Ventricular Septal Defect with Aortic Insufficiency

Aortic insufficiency (AI) is an unusual abnormality associated with VSD. In some cases one or two aortic cusps prolapse into the defect. Two concepts have evolved to explain prolapse of the aortic cusps: (1) Inadequate support of the structures of the aortic valve due to deficiency of conal musculature (this deficiency has been associated mainly with supracristal VSD; however, it has also been described in infracristal defects). (2) Congenital abnormality of the sinus of Valsalva (this occurs more often with infracristal VSD).

Healed bacterial endocarditis has been suspected in cases of VSD with AI without prolapse of an aortic cusp. In other such cases the aortic valve has been found to be bicuspid or myxomatous. The aortic valve has been known to prolapse in such a way as to reduce the shunt or completely seal the defect. Nevertheless, the defect remains large and may be found at surgery in patients operated on for isolated AI. The AI is progressive in VSD and AI, and may continue to progress even after the VSD is closed.

Clinically, patients with VSD and AI have a VSD with the added finding of a diastolic decrescendo murmur of AI along the left sternal border. In some individuals the AI murmur is not heard, even though significant regurgita-

Fig. 7–46. *Ventricular septal defect.* **A** and **B** are PA and lateral plain chest roentgenograms in a 7-month-old boy demonstrating cardiomegaly with left atrial and biventricular enlargement. The main pulmonary artery is enlarged and the aorta is inconspicuous. Pulmonary overcirculation is present. **C** and **D** are frontal and lateral projections in a 10-year-old boy also with a ventricular septal defect and a significant left-to-right shunt. The findings are similar; however, biventricular enlargement is better defined in the older child.

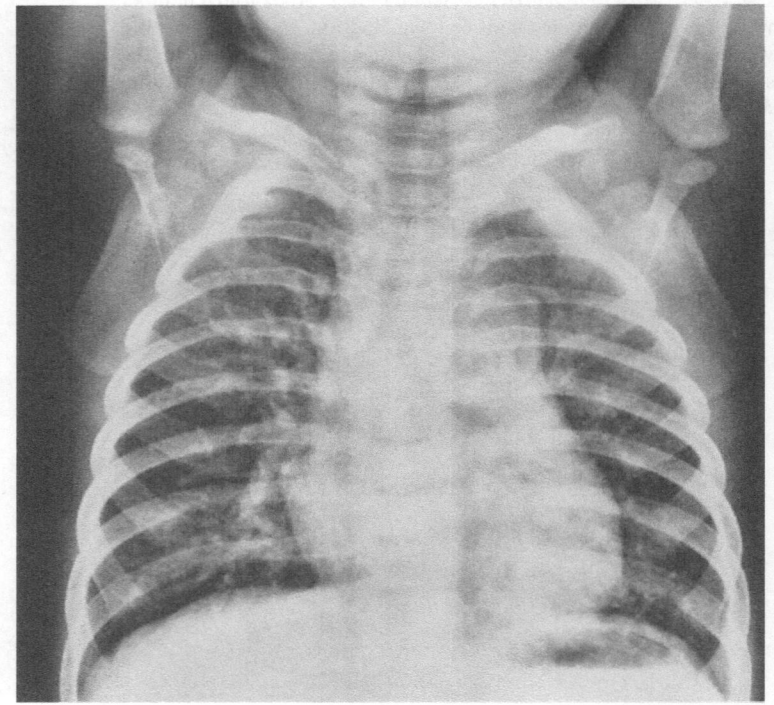

A

B

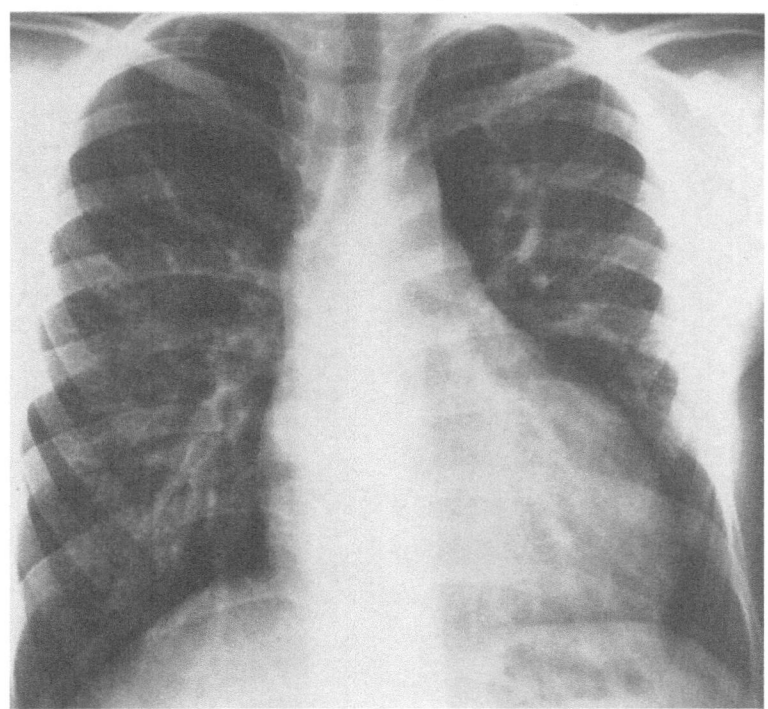

C

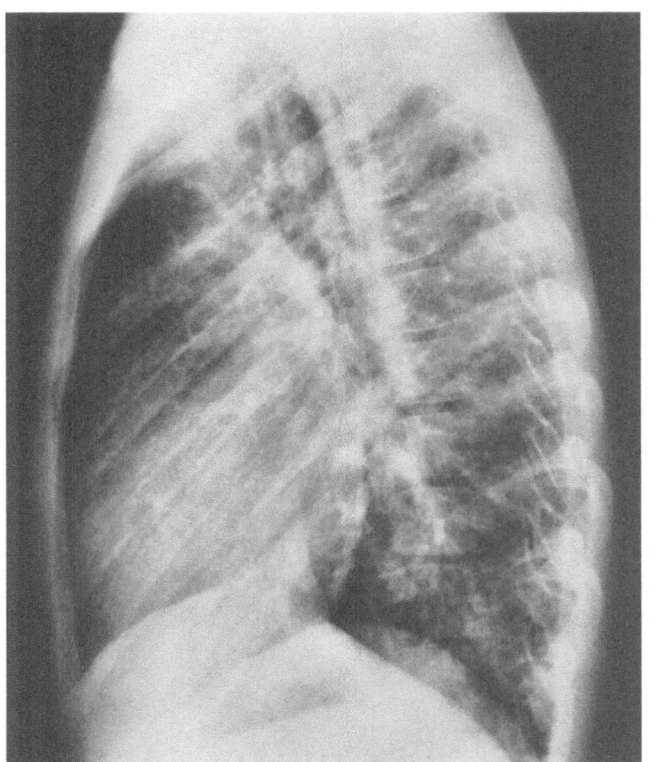

D

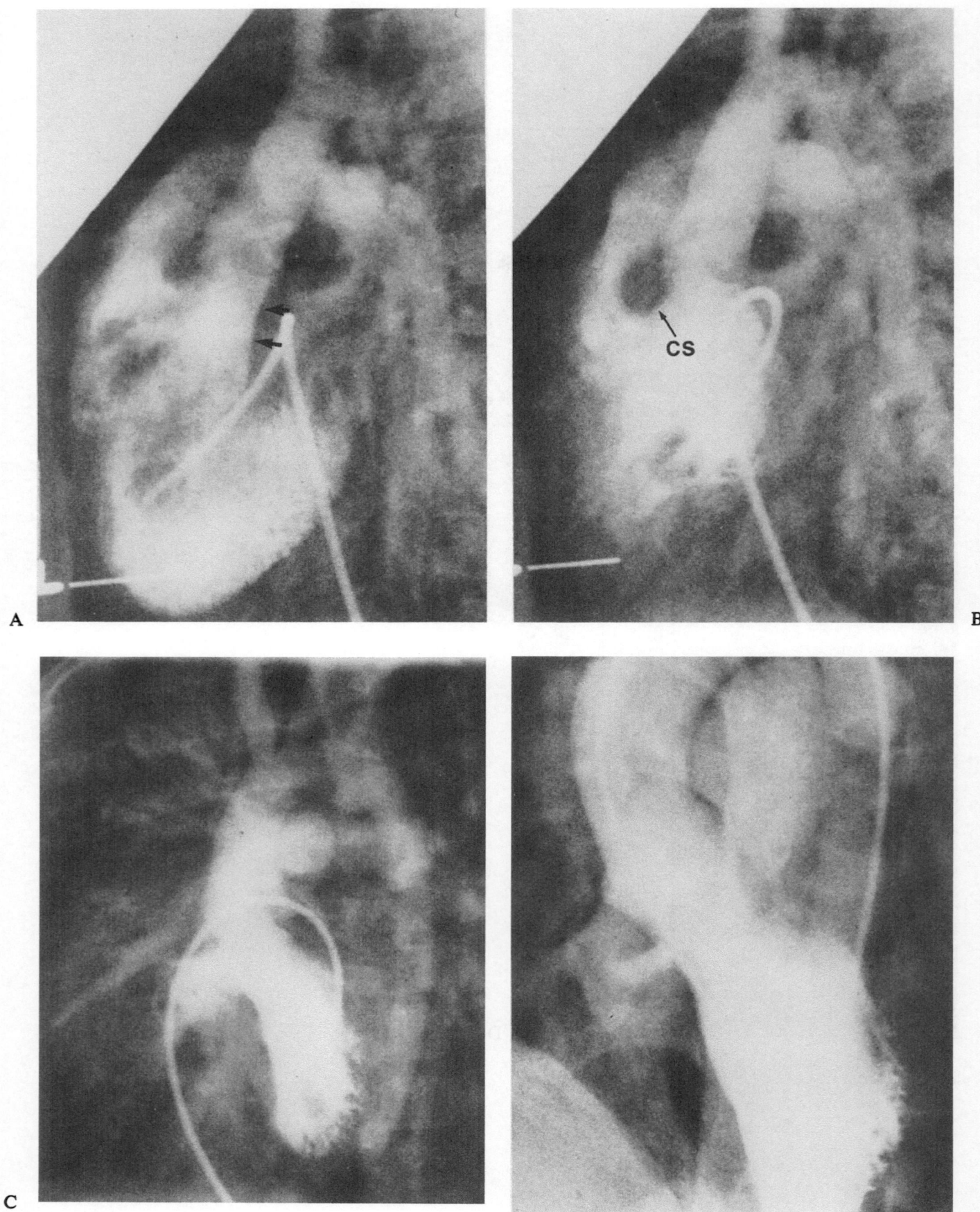

Fig. 7–47. *Large infracristal ventricular septal defect in a 9-month-old girl (A–C) and Maladie de Roger (small ventricular septal defect) in a different patient (D).* **A** and **B** are diastolic and systolic frames of the lateral projection of a left ventriculogram. **C** is an LAO view with cranial angulation of a second left ventriculogram. Both views indicate a large ventricular septal defect below the crista supraventricularis (*CS*). On the lateral view the right ventricular outflow tract narrows during systole, but is not obstructed (dynamic infundibulum). The axial view (**C**) also defines the location of the defect and excludes additional muscular defects. The *arrows* in frame **A** indicate the anterior leaflet of the mitral valve, which is in fibrous continuity with the aortic valve. **D** LAO view with caudocranial tilt demonstrates a small defect in the membranous septum, with a discrete jet of contrast medium. This view outlines the ventricular septum in its entirety and is especially useful for determining the location of ventricular septal defects and also for assessing associated abnormalities of the left ventricular outflow tract and mitral valve.

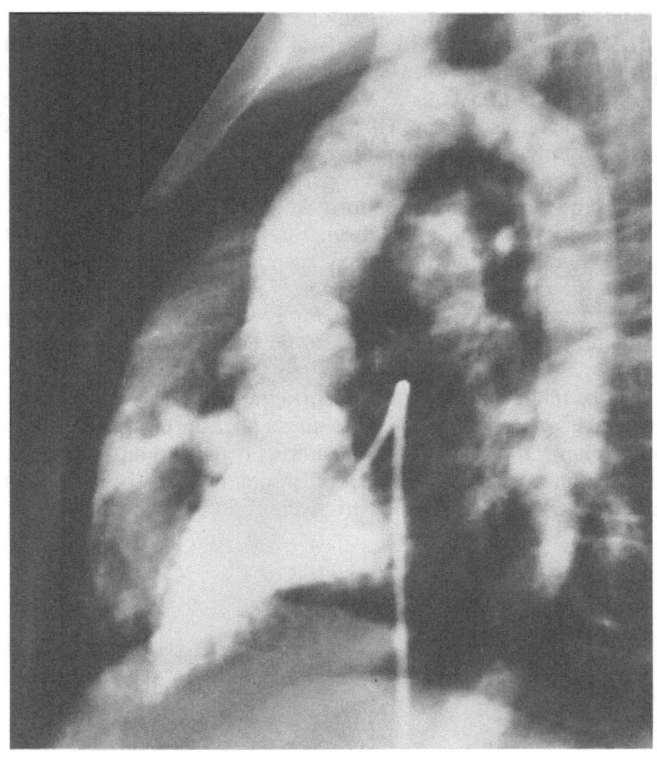

A

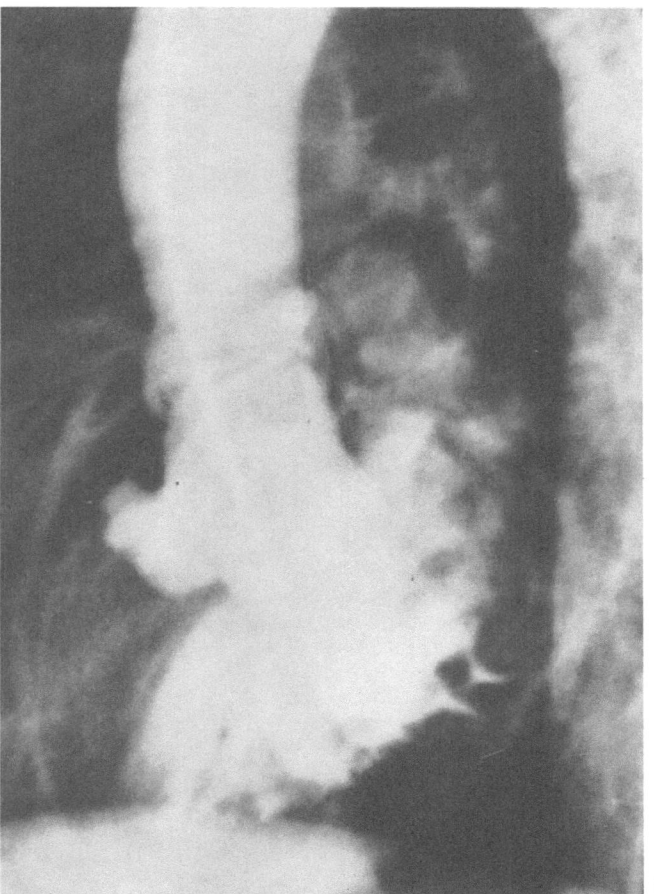

B

Fig. 7–48. *Two patients with aneurysm of the membranous septum.* **A** is from a 6-year-old girl who had a large VSD (proven at cardiac catheterization) and congestive heart failure during infancy. **B** is from a 13-year-old boy with valvar aortic stenosis, in whom the aneurysm was an incidental finding. The lateral view of each left ventriculogram shows an outpouching of the membranous septum. In **A** a residual shunt (small VSD) remains. In **B** no VSD is evident. These examples demonstrate one mechanism of spontaneous closure of membranous ventricular septal defects.

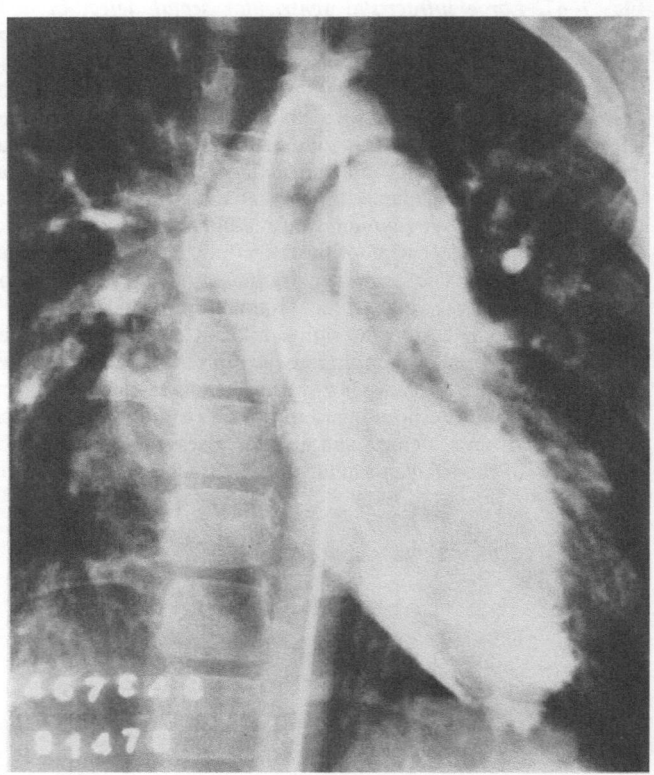

A

Fig. 7–49. *Supracristal ventricular septal defect.* Injection into the left ventricle demonstrates a left-to-right shunt at the ventricular level.

A Frontal view during systole; **B** lateral view during systole; **C** lateral view during early diastole; **D** lateral view late in diastole. The right ventricular outflow tract opacifies densely while the apex and inflow tract remain unopacified. These findings are appreciated on the frontal and lateral projections. On the lateral projection during systole (**B**) the crista supraventricularis is partly obscured by contrast medium and appears below the defect. These changes may also occur with infracristal defects if the shunt is directed upward, obscuring the crista supraventricularis and filling the right ventricular outflow tract. On the lateral projection the contrast agent flows inferiorly from the right ventricular outflow tract toward the apex during diastole (**C** and **D**). The LAO projection with cranial tilt may demonstrate a jet through or above the crista supraventricularis. If a supracristal ventricular septal defect is diagnosed, aortography is mandatory, since such patients often have a prolapsed aortic cusp and aortic insufficiency.

E lateral projection of the aortogram in the same patient. The right (anterior) semilunar sinus is slightly deformed due to its prolapse into the VSD, and aortic regurgitation is present. The column of regurgitant blood is not uniform because it is diluted by unopacified blood from the right ventricle.

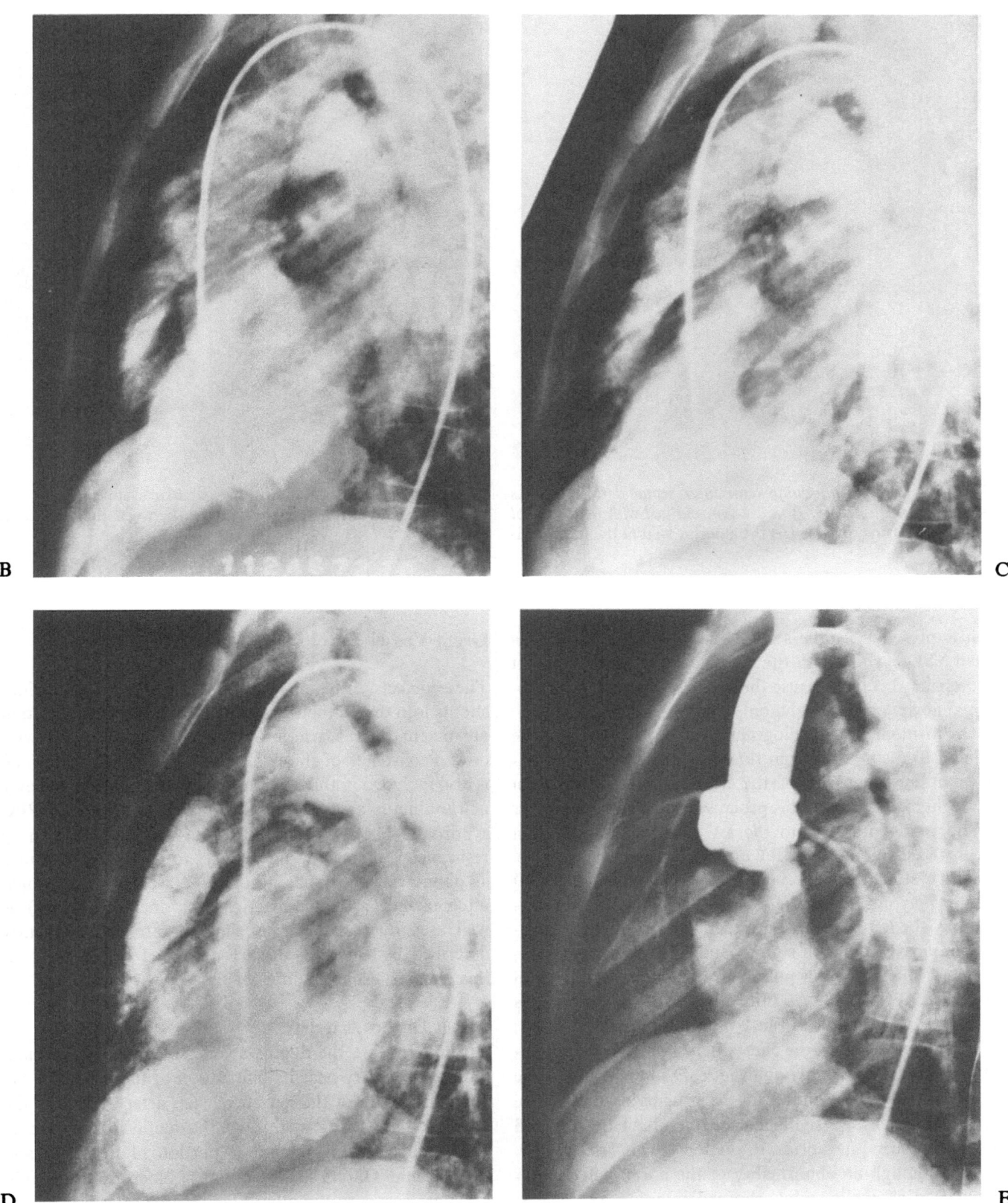

B

C

D

E

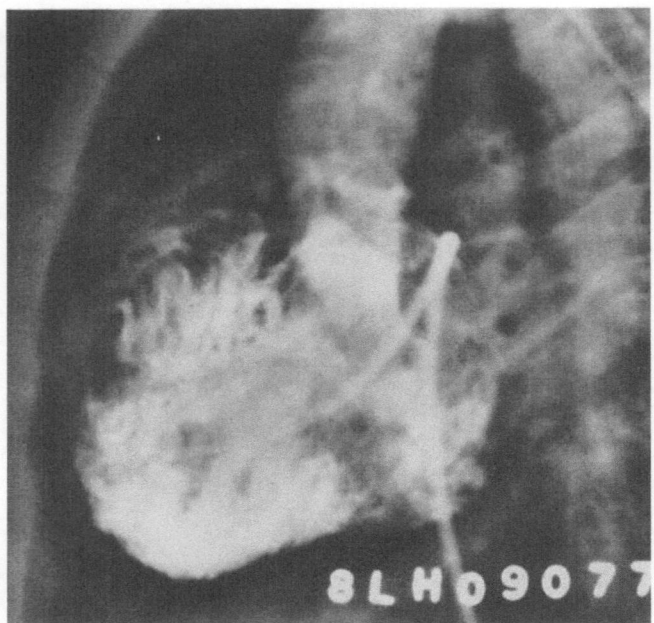
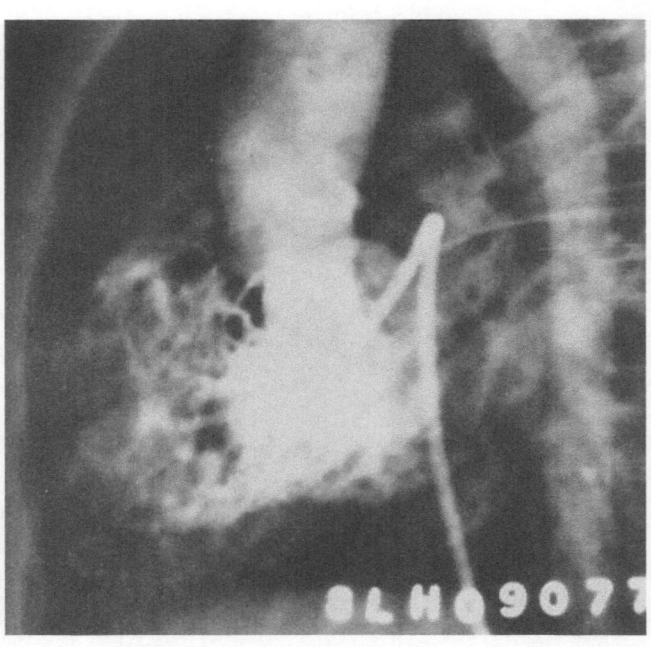

Fig. 7–50. *Multiple muscular ventricular septal defects ("Swiss cheese" ventricular septum) in a 1-year-old girl with fetal alcohol syndrome. During diastole (A) the anterior wall of the left ventri-* cle is irregular (shaggy). During ventricular systole (B) contrast material passes through many crevices between the trabeculae carnae.

tion is present. In others the findings may be those of a small VSD even though the defect is large. This apparent discrepancy occurs because the shunt is limited by the prolapsed aortic cusp. Rarely, only a murmur of AI is heard.

On M-mode echocardiography the appearance may be difficult to distinguish from that of a dilated sinus of Valsalva or an aneurysm of the membranous septum. On 2-D echocardiography the prolapsed cusp may curve far inferior and anterior into the LV outflow tract or even across the septum into the RV outflow tract during diastole. During systole the portion of the cusp that covers the VSD may or may not move (Fig. 7–51). On Doppler echocardiography the left-to-right shunt tends to be directed superiorly in individuals with supracristal VSD and may be detected primarily in the pulmonary artery rather than in the RV outflow tract. Additionally, aortic insufficiency is found on examination of the LV outflow tract.

Roentgenograms of the chest often show normal pulmonary vasculature even though the VSD may be large. The size of the shunt is limited by the prolapsed aortic cusp. In the presence of a significant degree of AI the LV and often the ascending aorta are dilated (Figs. 7–52, 7–53).

Even though an abnormality of the aortic valve is not recognized clinically or by echocardiography, AI must be suspected in any case of supracristal VSD, and aortography should be performed in search of the prolapsed leaflet (Figs. 7–49E and 7–53).

The VSD is repaired if the shunt is large or if AI is severe. At surgery the aortic valve must be repaired or replaced at the time of closure of the VSD. If significant AI remains after surgery, intractable LV failure may ensue.

Great-Vessel Level Communications

These defects, listed in Table 7–3, result in left-to-right shunts into the pulmonary artery. Discussed in this section are patent ductus arteriosus and aorticopulmonary window. Persistence of the fetal circulation (PFC syndrome) is also included in this section, because physiologic patency of the ductus arteriosus is an important feature of PFC syndrome. The shunt is right to left while the pulmonary resistance is increased, but reverses to a left-to-right shunt as pulmonary resistance decreases. Vascular rings (which often include a ductus arteriosus or ductus ligament) as well as a ductus arteriosus sling (a rare entity recently described by Binet et al.) are described in section 5 of this chapter, Abnormalities of the Great Arteries.

Patent Ductus Arteriosus

During fetal life the ductus arteriosus connects the main pulmonary artery near its bifurcation to the aorta just beyond the origin of the left subclavian artery. Most of the blood from the RV flows through the ductus to the descending aorta supplying the lower portion of the body and the placenta. Only a small amount of blood from the right ventricle passes to the lungs. The ductus arteriosus closes functionally soon after birth (muscular contraction). Anatomical closure (intimal proliferation and fibrosis) follows.

Patent ductus arteriosus (PDA) in term babies more than 1 week of age is abnormal. In premature babies PDA is considered a physiological phenomenon that relates to immaturity of the ductal muscle rather than a congenital defect. Factors in addition to prematurity that tend to pro-

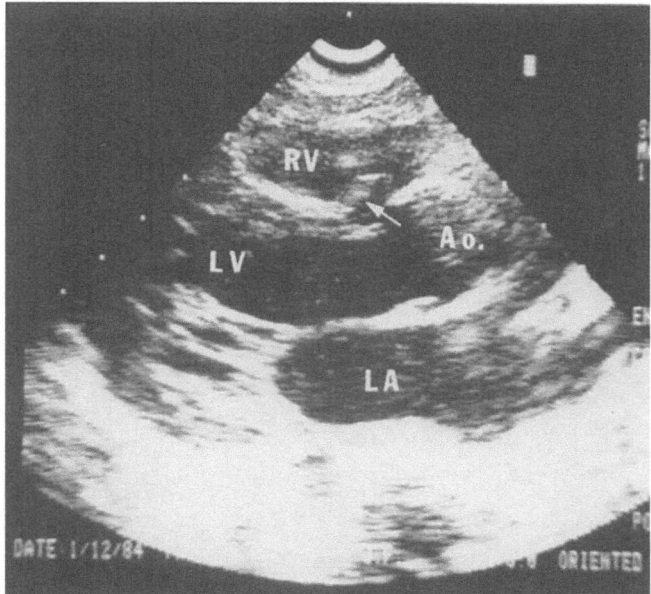

A

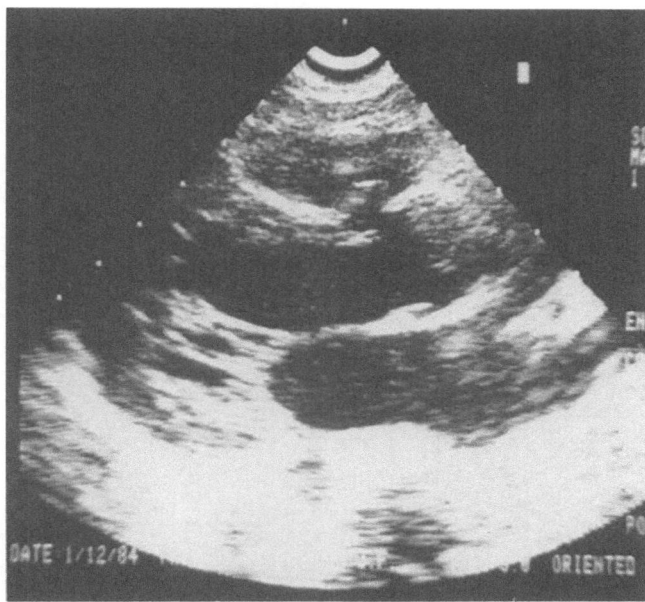

A'

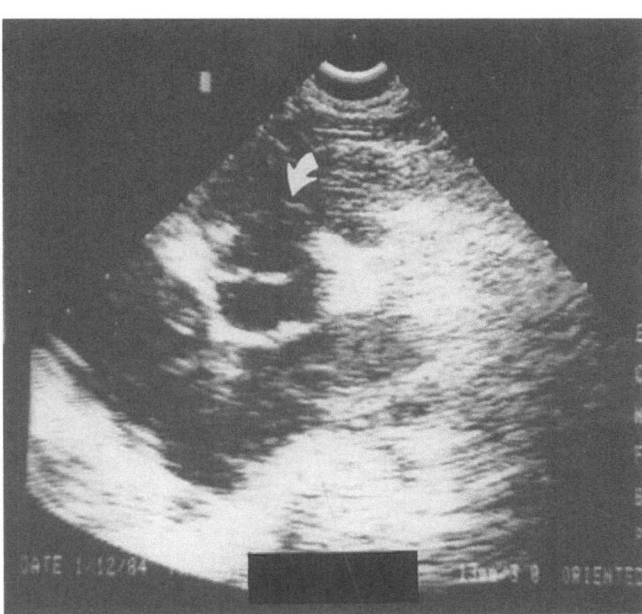

B

Fig. 7–51. *Two-dimensional echocardiograms in a patient with a supracristal ventricular septal defect and aortic insufficiency.* **A** and **A'** are parasternal long axis views, and **B** is a parasternal short axis view just below the aortic valve. In **A** the ventricular septal defect is adjacent to the right coronary cusp, and a portion of the cusp protrudes through the defect *(arrow)*. The arrow passes through the ventricular septal defect. In **B** the ventricular septal defect results in drop-out of echoes of a portion of the ventricular septum anteriorly just below the right coronary cusp. The ventricular septal defect is separated from the tricuspid valve by conus muscle. Here also the right coronary cusp is delineated faintly *(arrow)* as it protrudes through the defect into the right ventricular outflow tract. Compare this picture with the same view of a membranous ventricular septal defect (Fig. 7–44B). A membranous ventricular septal defect is next to the tricuspid valve immediately below the noncoronary cusp.

Ao. = aorta; *LV* = left ventricle; *RV* = right ventricle; *LA* = left atrium.

mote patency of the ductus are pulmonary disease and perinatal stress, which result in hypoxia and acidosis. During delivery and in stressed neonates, pulmonary resistance remains high and flow through the ductus is right to left (persistance of fetal circulatory pathways, PFC). If the ductus remains patent as pulmonary resistance decreases after birth, flow through the ductus reverses so that a left-to-right shunt occurs. This results in volume overload in the pulmonary circulation and the left side of the heart. A large left-to-right shunt causes dilatation of the pulmonary arteries (pulmonary overcirculation) and enlargement of the LA, LV and aorta.

Congestive heart failure (CHF) secondary to PDA often complicates the course in infants. In premature infants, CHF occurs during the first few days of life, usually at the same time as idiopathic respiratory distress syndrome (IRDS). In infants born with PDA at term, pulmonary resistance remains increased for a time, and onset of CHF is delayed.

In older children a small to moderate PDA usually causes a typical continuous (machinery) murmur. If the PDA is large, high flow and pulmonary hypertension may lead to fixed changes of pulmonary arterioles, representing Eisenmenger physiology.

Associated Defects Coarctation of the aorta and VSD often occur in association with PDA. Aortic and pulmonic stenosis are less common. PDA often forms a part of complex heart defects (e.g., transpositions, tricuspid atresia, pulmonary atresia, hypoplastic left-heart syndrome, preductal coarctation of the aorta, interruption of the aortic arch). A right aortic arch is associated rarely with PDA; if so, the PDA is often left sided and forms a vascular ring. A right-sided PDA in association with a right aortic arch is very rare. In tetralogy of Fallot with a right arch and

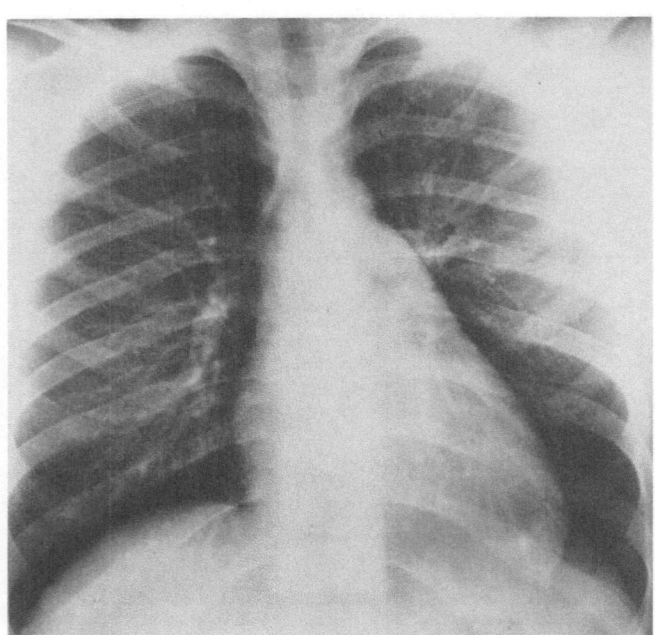

Fig. 7–52. *Ventricular septal defect and aortic insufficiency.* Frontal plain chest radiograph in a 10-year-old boy who had a previous history of ventricular septal defect with only a residual murmur of aortic insufficiency (same patient as in Fig. 7–53). The pulmonary vasculature is normal. The left heart border is elongated, and the apex projects below the left hemidiaphragm, indicating left ventricular enlargement. The ascending aorta is slightly enlarged. These features, in the context of the history, suggest a ventricular septal defect with a prolapsing aortic cusp.

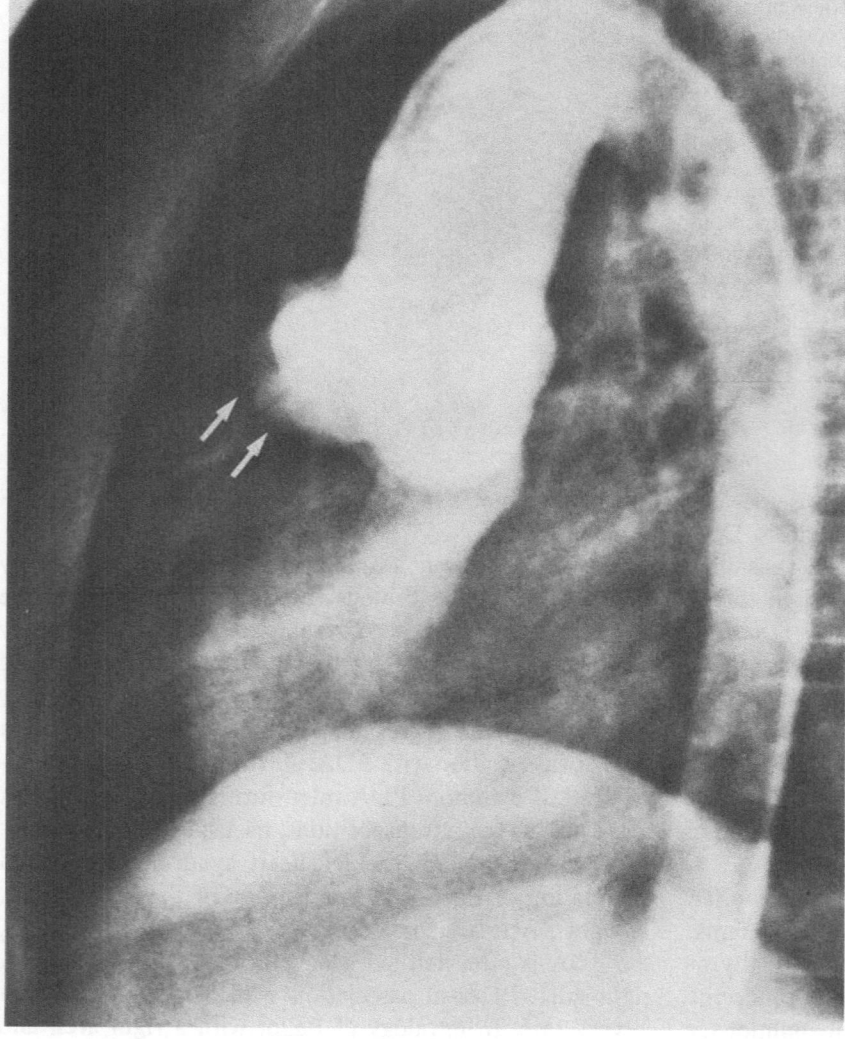

Fig. 7–53. *Ventricular septal defect and aortic insufficiency.* Lateral view of the aortogram in the patient in Fig. 7–52 demonstrates aortic insufficiency. The right (anterior) cusp protrudes through the ventricular septal defect, obliterating the defect. The prolapsed cusp (*arrows*) produces a separate density, simulating a fourth semilunar sinus or bilobed semilunar cusp.

PDA, the ductus is left sided and extends between the left-sided innominate artery (mirror-image branching) and the left pulmonary artery. Another rare lesion associated with PDA is an anomalous origin of one pulmonary artery from the ascending aorta (hemitruncus). (See also section 5 of this chapter, Abnormalities of the Great Vessels).

Clinical Features The description of clinical features is divided into three sections to reflect the three distinct presentations of PDA—in premature infants, in infants born at term and in older children and adults.

PDA in Premature Infants Patency of the ductus arteriosus in premature infants is considered to be a physiological phenomenon associated with an inadequate reponse of the muscle layer of the ductus to oxygen. In addition, the muscle layer of the pulmonary arterioles (media) is poorly developed so that pulmonary resistance decreases almost immediately at birth. Onset of CHF secondary to a left-to-right shunt is usually within the first few days of life, often simultaneous with idiopathic respiratory distress syndrome (IRDS), which is also common in premature babies. The respiratory symptoms secondary to CHF may be indistinguishable from the respiratory symptoms of IRDS. A murmur may or may not be present. A presumptive diagnosis of PDA in association with IRDS is made by the findings of a hyperkinetic cardiac impulse and bounding peripheral pulses, and by a large heart on plain films of the chest. Echocardiography with Doppler studies is especially useful in this age group as the clinical findings may not be obvious (Fig. 7-54; also see Fig. 2-50). A description of echocardiographic findings follows clinical features of PDA in children and adults below.

PDA in Infants Born at Term Patency of the ductus arteriosus in term babies, especially beyond a few days of life, is no longer considered a simple physiological phenomenon. The cause of persistent patency is unknown and is being studied actively; however, no single specific mechanism has been recognized. Babies with rubella embryopathy and those born at high altitudes have a greater than normal tendency toward PDA. Isolated PDA accounts for about 10% of all congenital heart defects, but PDA also may occur in combination with almost every other congenital heart defect. In contrast to its effects on premature infants who develop heart failure very early, a widely patent ductus may produce a large left-to-right shunt and CHF some time after the neonatal period in term babies (characteristically at age 6–12 weeks). The murmur of PDA in infants differs from that occurring in older children, being heard usually only in systole. The murmur may be heard predominantly in the front in infants rather than in the back as it is in older children. As in other age groups, a large left-to-right shunt through a PDA results in bounding pulses, a dynamic cardiac impulse and sometimes in CHF.

PDA in Children and Adults In older children and adults a continuous, machinery, murmur is heard beneath the left clavicle and over the left side of the back. A moderate left-to-right shunt is associated with a LV heave. A large PDA with pulmonary hypertension usually produces a bi-ventricular heave. Bounding pulses are characteristic of PDA with large left-to-right shunt, but also may occur with other disorders such as arteriovenous fistulas and aortic regurgitation.

Long-term high pulmonary blood flow and pulmonary hypertension may lead to the Eisenmenger physiology in older children and adults with PDA. The continuous murmur is absent. In its place may be the descrescendo murmur typical of pulmonary valve insufficiency. The second sound is loud, and a right ventricular heave is present. Differential cyanosis may be evident. Thus the left hand and both feet may be cyanotic, whereas the right hand and head are relatively acyanotic.

Echocardiography Echocardiography in infants with moderate to large PDA usually demonstrates LA enlargement (increased LA/Ao ratio) and a hyperkinetic LV (Fig. 7-54). In addition to LA/Ao ratio greater than 1.3/1 (Fig. 7-54) Johnson et al. have suggested the use of the ratio of the pre-ejection period to the left ventricular ejection time (LPEP/LVET $\leq$ 0.24) as a positive finding for the presence of PDA in premature infants, based on the finding that LPEP is short in these babies. Heitz et al. reported a reversal of the ratio of LPEP/RPEP (LPEP/RPEP < 1). Again, LPEP is shortened because diastolic pressure is less than normal. Additionally, the RPEP may be increased because of an elevation in pulmonary pressure and resistance. Systolic time intervals are especially useful in premature infants who are on respirators with fluid restriction so that the LA may not be dilated. On Doppler echocardiography continuous flow is detected in the pulmonary artery as well as reversal of flow in the abdominal aorta throughout diastole (see Fig. 2-50). In children and adults with small PDA continuous flow into the pulmonary artery recognized by Doppler examination may be the only echocardiographic finding. Echocardiography can identify other defects such as VSD, truncus arteriosus and aorticopulmonary window, which may have clinical features similar to PDA. Recognition of a coarctation of the aorta in an infant with signs of PDA will allow appropriate repair at the time of ductal ligation.

Radiological (Plain Film) Features Cardiomegaly is present with moderate to large shunts. The LA and LV are enlarged. Dilatation of the aorta proximal to the PDA may be helpful in distinguishing PDA from VSD (Fig. 7-55), but in infants the ascending aorta is often not discernible on roentgenograms of the chest, and therefore it cannot be used to distinguish PDA in this age group. In older children and adults a dilated aorta is a meaningful sign if present. The pulmonary trunk and pulmonary arteries are dilated (pulmonary overcirculation). Aneurysm and calcification of the ductal wall may occur in adults (Fig. 7-56). The ductus may occasionally be aneurysmal in infants as well.

Aneurysmal dilatation of the ductus may also occur in the presence of a ductus arteriosus that is not patent. If a ductal aneurysm is suspected on plain films, angiography is indicated to establish the diagnosis, since aneurysms

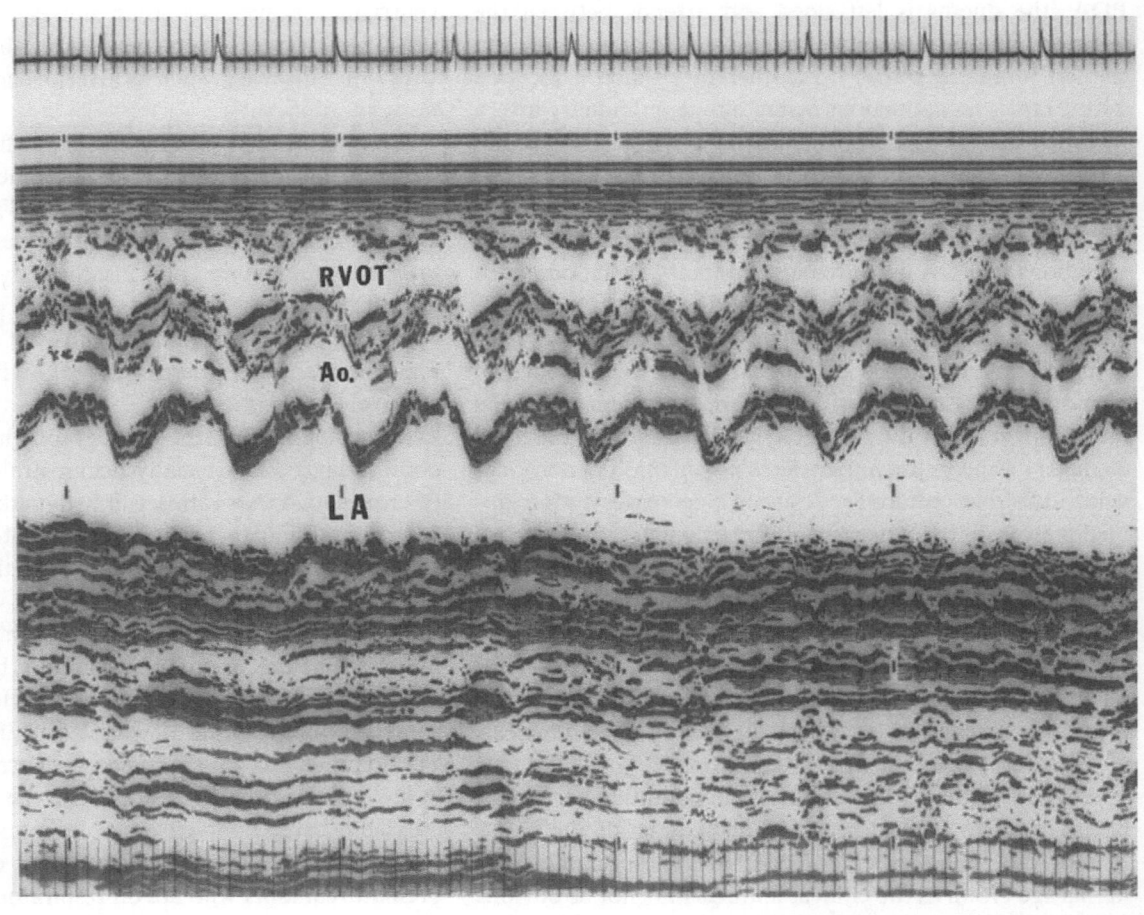

A

Fig. 7–54. *Patent ductus arteriosus in a 1-week-old premature infant weighing 1200 g.*

A The M-mode echocardiogram through the root of the aorta (*Ao.*) and left atrium (*LA*) shows a large diameter of the left atrium compared to that of the aorta. Using the leading edges of the aorta and left atrium, the LA/Ao. ratio is 1.5:1 (normal <1.3:1).

B The tracing through the left ventricle (*LV*) and right ventricle (*RV*) shows a large diastolic dimension with a large shortening fraction (40%), indicating a volume overloaded left ventricle. In C, the same view from a different patient, fluttering of both leaflets of the mitral valve probably indicates high flow across the valve during diastole.

RVOT = outflow tract of the right ventricle; *AML* = anterior leaflet of the mitral valve; *PML* = posterior leaflet of the mitral valve.

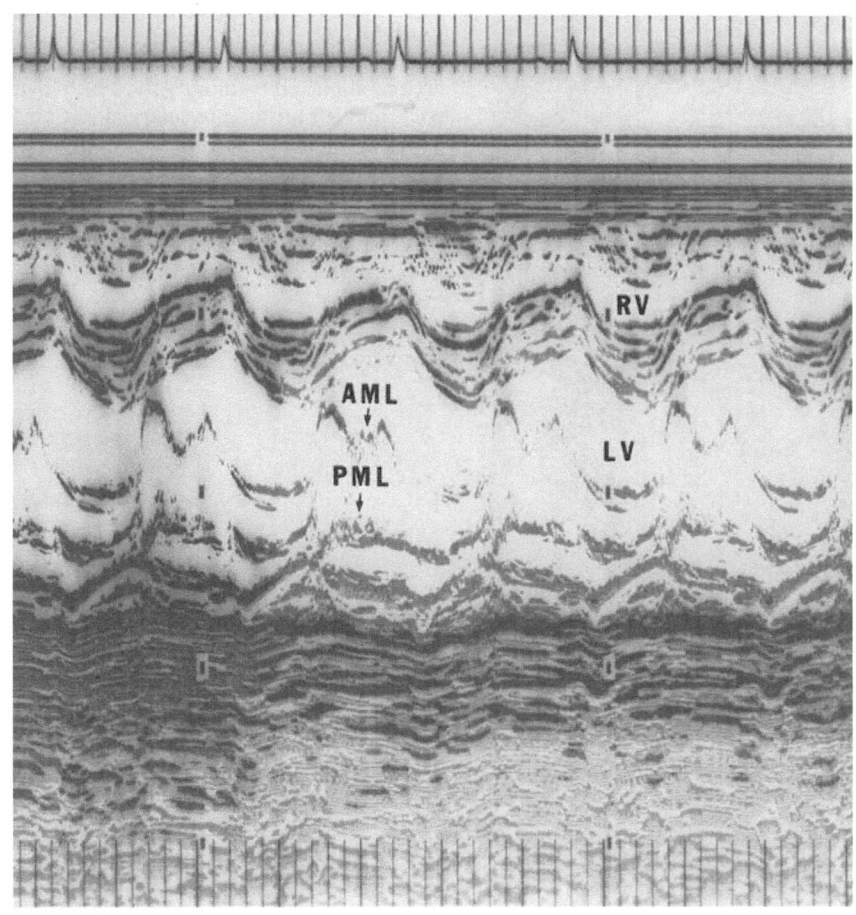

B

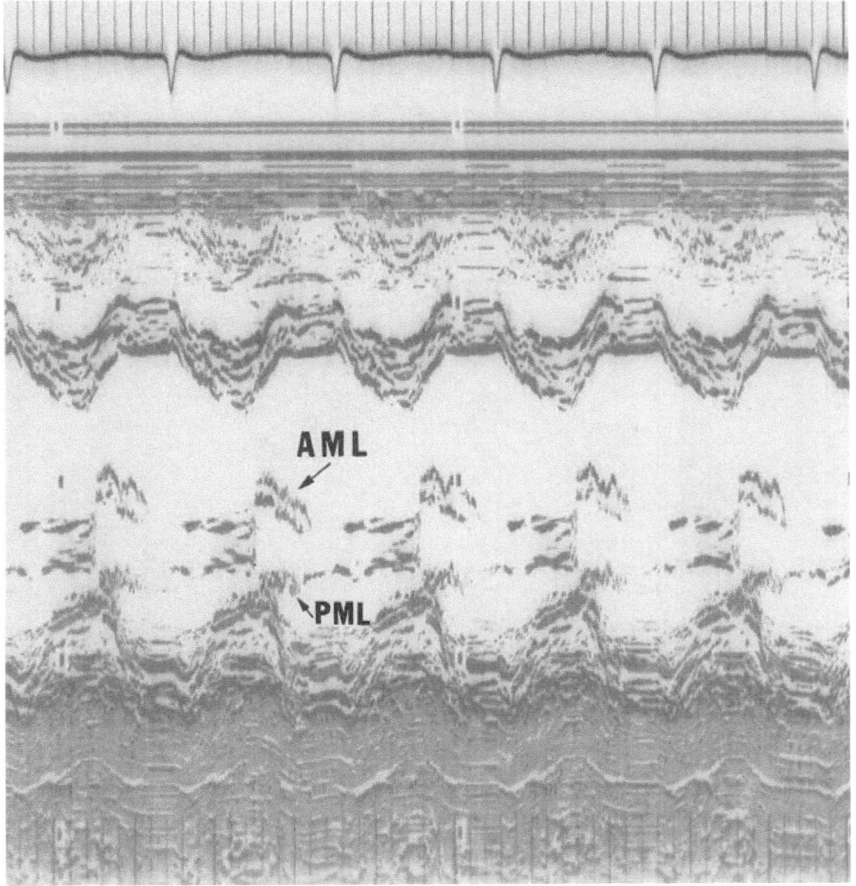

C

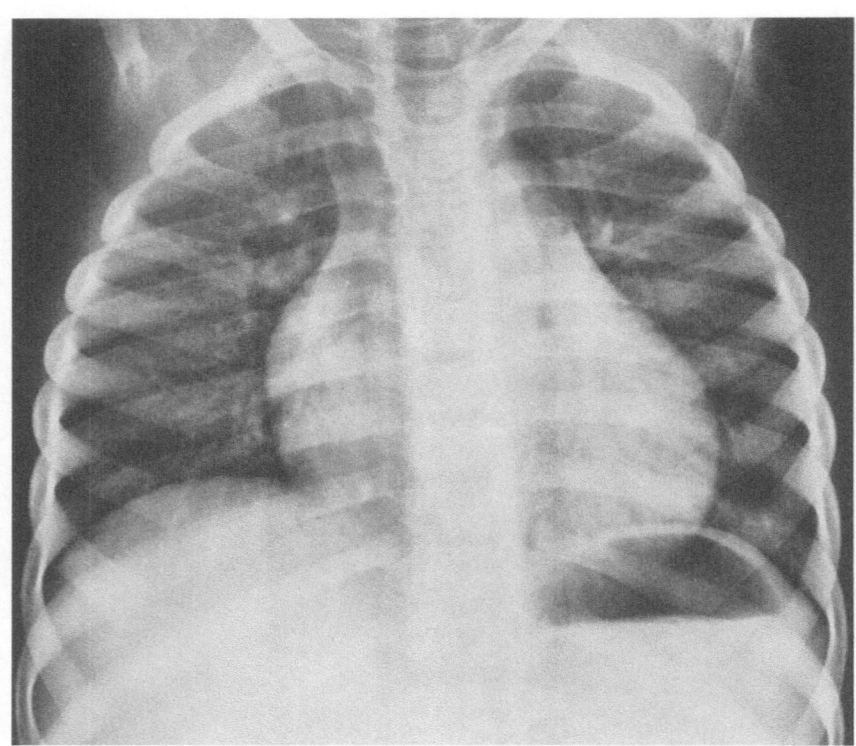

A

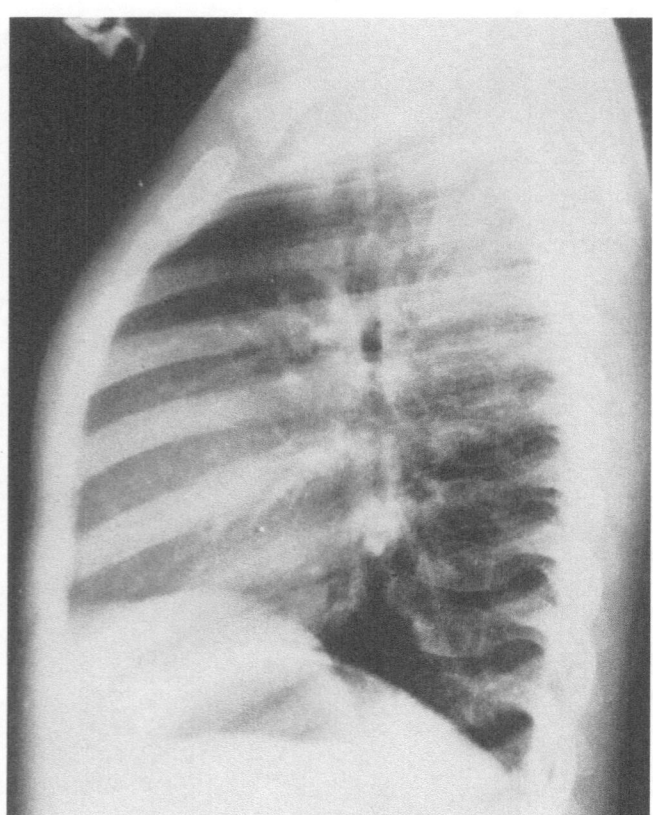

B

Fig. 7–55. *Patent ductus arteriosus in a 4-year-old boy.* The frontal and lateral chest roentgenograms demonstrate pulmonary overcirculation and cardiomegaly. The left ventricle and left atrium are enlarged, the aortic arch is prominent, and the main pulmonary artery is dilated. (Same patient as Fig. 7–58.)

Fig. 7–56. *Calcified aneurysm of a patent ductus arteriosus in a 44-year-old woman.*

A The frontal plain chest roentgenogram shows pulmonary overcirculation and cardiomegaly, with left ventricular enlargement. The ascending aorta is prominent. The aneurysmal ductus arteriosus projects over the aortic arch and proximal descending aorta. In contrast to calcification of the aortic arch, which occurs mainly in the upper wall, calcification of the ductus arteriosus occurs chiefly along the inferior border.

B An LAO view of the aortogram in the same patient demonstrates the aneurysmal patent ductus arteriosus and the large left-to-right shunt into the main pulmonary artery.

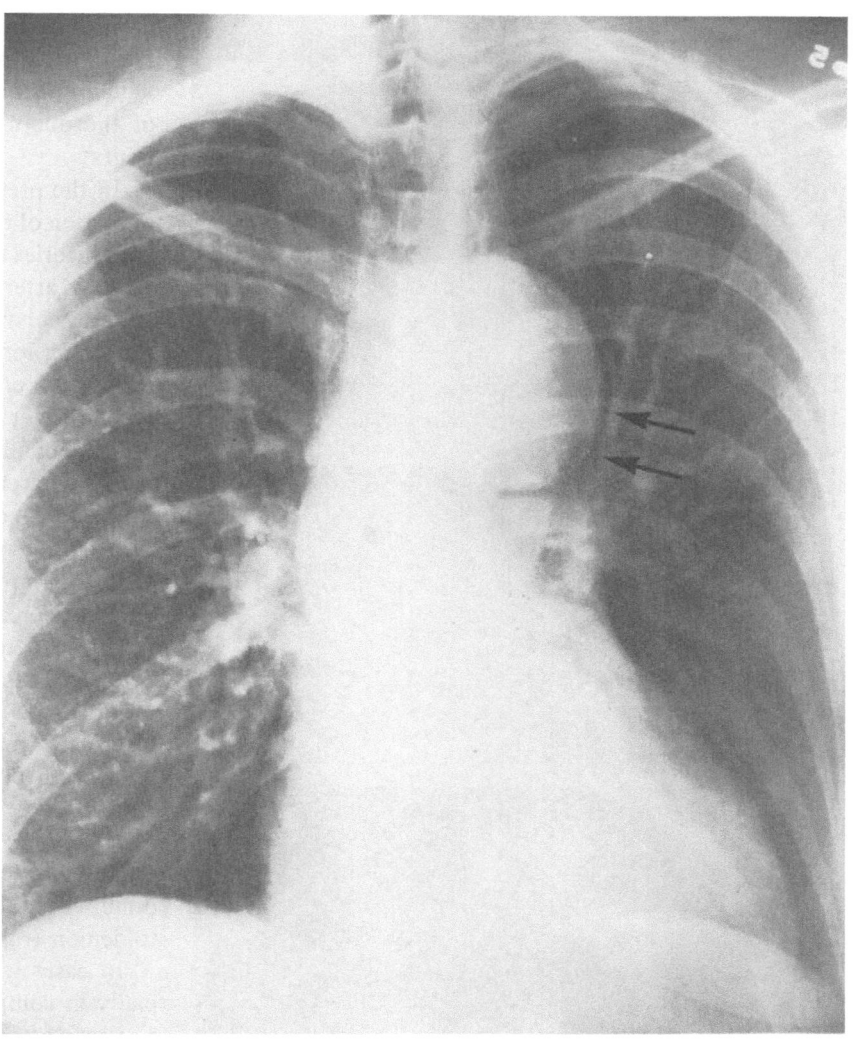

A

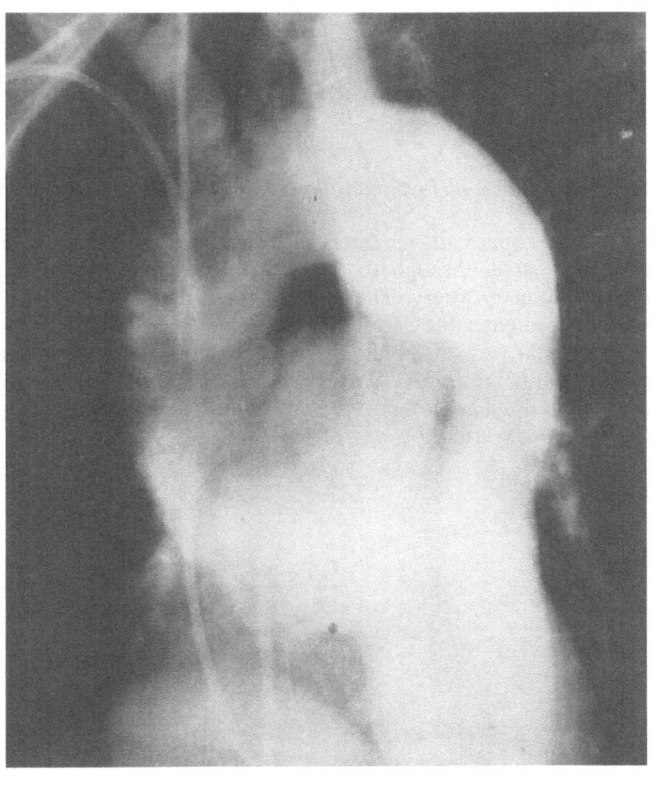

B

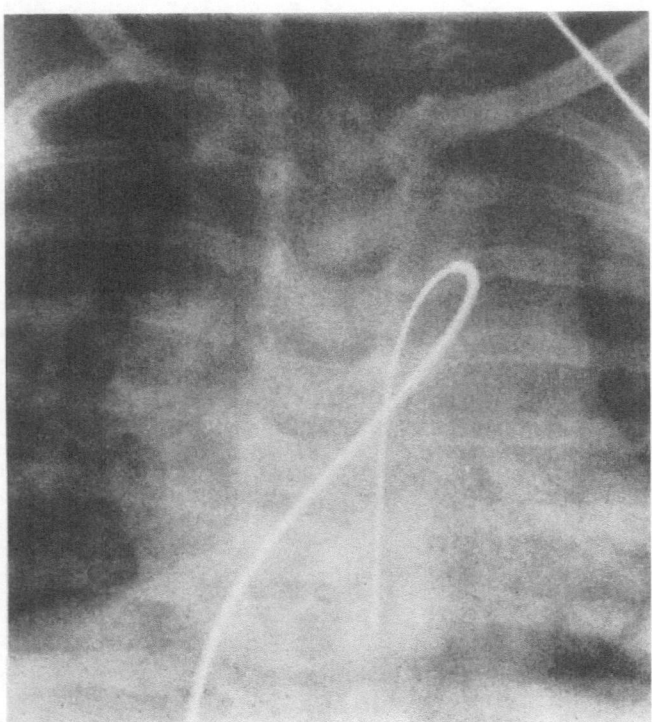

A

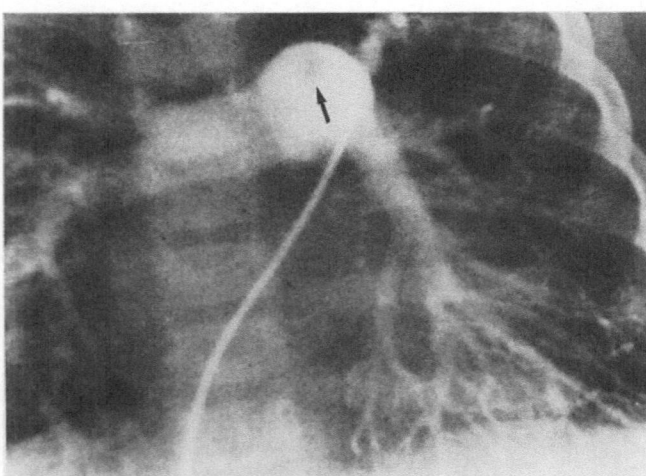

B

Fig. 7-57. *Treble-clef configuration of the catheter in patent ductus arteriosus.*

A The venous catheter enters the heart from the inferior vena cava and passes through the right atrium, right ventricle and main pulmonary artery. The catheter then traverses the ductus arteriosus to enter the descending aorta.

B Frontal view of a pulmonary angiogram in a child with a patent ductus arteriosus. A negative jet (*arrow*) in the dome of the main pulmonary artery represents unopacified blood entering the pulmonary artery by way of the ductus.

are complicated by rupture, embolism or infection. Ductal aneurysm should be differentiated from a "ductus bump," which is a normal variant caused by transient dilatation of the ductus arteriosus in the postnatal period (24–48 hours).

In the presence of PDA with Eisenmenger physiology, dilatation of the pulmonary trunk and right and left pulmonary arteries occurs with constriction of the interlobar pulmonary arteries (pruned-tree appearance). Other features include enlargement of the RV, a normal-sized or small ascending aorta, and calcification of the pulmonary arteries. Rarely hypertrophic osteoarthropathy may develop with Eisenmenger syndrome.

Hemodynamics The catheter easily traverses the ductus, forming a treble-clef configuration on AP fluoroscopy (Fig. 7-57A). In patients with left-to-right shunt via PDA, cardiac catheterization will demonstrate an oxygen step-up in the main pulmonary artery. The size of the ductal shunt cannot be accurately calculated because of sampling error due to inadequate mixing (or streaming) in the pulmonary arteries. Pulmonary artery pressures may or may not be elevated.

Contrast Studies (Fig. 7-58) In children with isolated PDA with classic continuous (machinery) murmurs and no sign of associated defect and in premature infants with characteristic clinical and echocardiographic findings, the ductus is often closed surgically without angiography. If doubt exists about the diagnosis, angiography is necessary to demonstrate the ductus and to define associated defects.

In cases with other defects in addition to PDA, especially in complex cases and in those in which pulmonary resistance is increased, the ductal shunt may be bidirectional or right to left. Clinical findings and even oxygen saturation may not be reliable to determine presence or absence of associated PDA in those cases. It may be necessary to inject contrast material on the right side if a left-to-right ductal shunt is not present on the aortogram. In cases of VSD the ventricular level shunt often obscures the ductus on the left ventriculogram. A separate aortogram is necessary in these cases to exclude an associated PDA.

Treatment In premature infants, ductal closure may be promoted by improvement in oxygenation, correction of acidosis and fluid restriction. If these methods fail, or if the left-to-right shunt is contributing to respiratory decompensation, pharmacological closure may be attempted with prostaglandin inhibitors such as aspirin and indomethacin. If the ductus remains open or reopens thereafter, or if prostagandin inhibitors are contraindicated, surgical closure can be performed fairly safely in even the smallest premature infants.

In term babies, prostaglandin inhibition is generally unsuccessful, and spontaneous closure is unlikely after a few months of age. Surgical closure is performed if the left-to-right shunt produces symptoms or if it complicates other defects such as a large VSD.

In older children, PDA is surgically closed to prevent

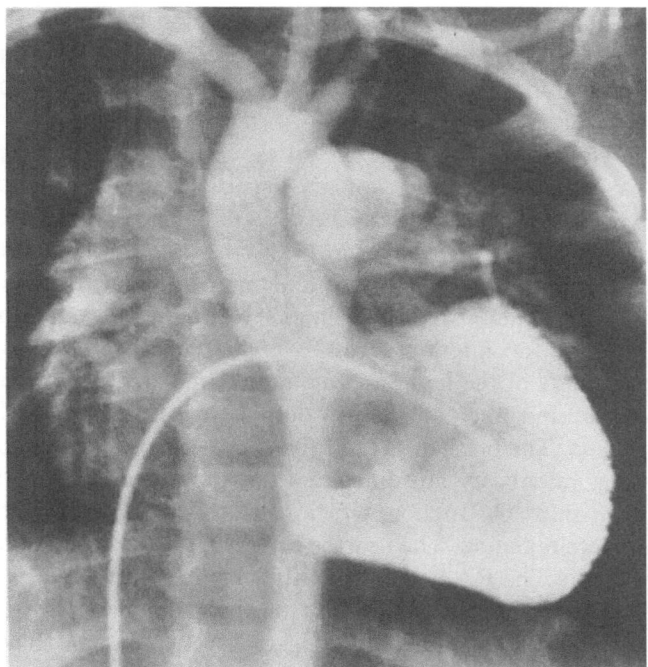

A

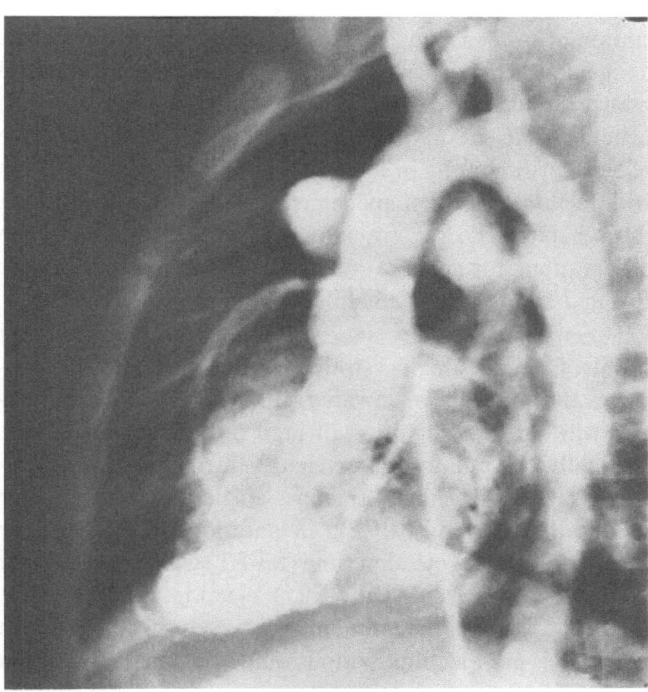

B

Fig. 7–58. *Patent ductus arteriosus in a 4-year-old boy (patient in Fig. 7–55).* **A** and **B** are frontal and lateral views of the left ventriculogram. The catheter was passed from the inferior vena cava into the right atrium and then through the foramen ovale and left atrium into the left ventricle. The ductus arteriosus connects the ductus diverticulum to the left pulmonary artery near the bifurcation of the main pulmonary artery.

progressive pulmonary hypertension if the shunt is large and to prevent bacterial endocarditis even if the shunt is small. The risk in closing a PDA during childhood is very low. In adults, on the other hand, the ductus may be calcified or aneurysmal so that surgical repair represents a significant risk. Under these circumstances a small asymptomatic ductus in an adult may be observed without surgery.

A recent innovation for closure of the ductus arteriosus consists of insertion of a plug using a combined venous and arterial catheter technique. This method might be especially useful in cases in which other forms of closure are inappropriate because of a patient's clinical condition. Closure of a ductus by any technique is contraindicated in patients with Eisenmenger physiology, because acute right heart obstruction and acute or chronic right heart failure generally will supervene.

Persistence of the Fetal Circulation (PFC Syndrome)
This syndrome of persistence of the fetal circulation (PFC) occurs in infants born at term or near term. It is characterized by tachypnea and cyanosis associated with abnormal postnatal persistence of pulmonary hypertension and a right-to-left shunt through the foramen ovale or the ductus arteriosus or both. Some affected infants die from progressive systemic hypoxia; others survive with complete resolution of the pulmonary hypertension.
Clinical Features The clinical presentation includes RV decompensation, cyanosis and pulmonary undercirculation on chest roentgenography. A murmur of tricuspid insufficiency may be present.

In addition to RV failure and a right-to-left shunt, LV failure may also complicate the course. An important predisposing factor in this syndrome is chronic fetal distress, which may cause hypertrophy of the pulmonary arteriolar musculature. Gestational diabetes may be an example of this. Perinatal asphyxia, aspiration, hyperviscosity, hypocalcemia, hypoglycemia and acidosis also contribute. The differential diagnosis of respiratory distress and cyanosis in newborn infants at term includes pulmonary disease (e.g., meconium aspiration, congenital diaphragmatic hernia, airway obstruction), disturbance of the central nervous system, hematological disorders (e.g., methemoglobinemia), congenital heart disease, hyaline membrane disease and PFC syndrome without an anatomic heart defect. The most important of these entities to exclude are congenital heart defects, some of which may be palliated temporarily by prostaglandins, but which require immediate referral to a cardiac center for definitive diagnosis and treatment.

An important differential feature that may distinguish cyanosis due to lung disease from that due to a heart defect is the response to correction of metabolic disturbances and to the administration of oxygen. In the PFC syndrome the pulmonary resistance is often reduced by these measures so that oxygenation occurs. In the absence of response to oxygen a vasodilator such as tolazoline (Priscoline) may be administered to reduce pulmonary vascular resistance. These therapeutic measures are carried out in rapid sequence in many nurseries. Failure to raise arterial concentration of oxygen is evidence for the presence of a cyanotic congenital heart defect, although severe PFC may respond poorly or have a delayed response. Echocardiography is usually sufficient to identify cyanotic heart defects. Use of echocardiography in nurseries outside of cardiac centers will facilitate early management of PFC by identifying those babies who require subspecialty referral. Follow-up observations for signs of pulmonary hypertension and for RV and LV failure are helpful.

Echocardiography The *signs of pulmonary hypertension* follow: Comparison of systolic time intervals of the pulmonary valve and the aortic valve on M-mode echocardiography will aid in recognition of high pulmonary resistance. Normally the pulmonary or right ventricular pre-ejection period (RPEP) is shorter than the aortic or left ventricular pre-ejection period (LPEP). In addition, the pulmonary (right ventricular) ejection time (RVET) is normally longer than the aortic (left ventricular) ejection time (LVET). As the pressures in the pulmonary artery approach systemic levels the pre-ejection periods and ventricular ejection times of the two ventricles become equal—that is, the RPEP becomes longer and the RVET becomes shorter (Fig. 7–59A-B). The ratio of RPEP/RVET to LPEP/LVET tends to exaggerate these changes and is used by Hirschfeld et al. in their studies to correlate systolic time intervals with pulmonary artery pressure. Persistence of abnormal pulmonary systolic time intervals in spite of treatment in infants with PFC is a poor prognostic sign. Other signs of high pulmonary resistance are absence of the pulmonary "a kick" and mid systolic closure of the pulmonary valve.

Signs of myocardial failure include RV failure, indicated by an increase in the RV diameter 7–59C. On 2-D echocardiography the ventricular septum bulges into the LV, and the atrial septum bulges into the LA. LV failure, if present, produces dilatation of the LV along with a decreased shortening fraction and ejection rate (velocity of circumferential fiber shortening) and enlargement of the LA.

Location of right-to-left shunt may be determined by injection of small amounts of saline, green dye, or the baby's own blood through a venous catheter. With PFC the contrast agent should appear first in the RA and then immediately proceed to the LA, indicating an atrial level right-to-left shunt. Shunts at the atrial level also occur with cyanotic heart defects (e.g., total anomalous pulmonary venous drainage, Ebstein anomaly of the tricuspid valve). A shunt at the ventricular level or an isolated great vessel level shunt should not occur with PFC. The presence of either should suggest another diagnosis. During injection of contrast material, tricuspid insufficiency secondary to RV failure might also be recognized by its negative washout effect.

Establishing the absence of a cyanotic congenital heart defect: The presence of all valves and chambers, with normal spatial relations and intact septa, is usually enough evidence of an anatomically normal heart. Total anomalous pulmonary venous return (TAPVR), which produces echocardiographic findings similar to those of PFC, may be difficult to distinguish from PFC. Demonstration of the openings of the pulmonary veins into the LA by 2-D echocardiography excludes TAPVR (see also description of TAPVR).

Radiological (Plain Film) Features The pulmonary vascular pattern reflects precapillary hypertension (high pulmonary vascular resistance). The main pulmonary artery may reach huge proportions, projecting over the apex of the left hemithorax (Fig. 7–60) and may simulate a thymic density. The proximal pulmonary arteries are dilated, whereas the interlobar vessels are attenuated. Thus the periphery of the lungs appears undercirculated. A curious feature in some patients is a dotted appearance of vessels on end. The mechanism and the appearance of the pulmonary vascularity are different from those occurring with right-sided obstruction, which causes a typical pattern of undercirculation. The heart is enlarged, on occasion markedly so. The RA and RV are the chambers involved.

Except for the appearance of the pulmonary vessels, these plain film findings may suggest severe pulmonic stenosis, pulmonary atresia with intact ventricular septum and tricuspid insufficiency, or Ebstein anomaly. Hypoplastic left heart syndrome and total anomalous pulmonary venous drainage may be difficult to distinguish because the same heart chambers are enlarged in both entities (RA, RV, main pulmonary artery); however, pulmonary venous hypertension (postcapillary hypertension) is generally present with hypoplastic LV rather than precapillary hypertension. D-transposition may be excluded because of differences in the patterns of pulmonary circulation. If a baby with a congenital heart defect also has PFC syndrome, distinction on plain chest films may be impossible.

Hemodynamics At catheterization severe pulmonary hypertension is found with right-to-left shunting via the foramen ovale and ductus arteriosus. The amount of right-to-left shunting depends on the severity of the increase in pulmonary resistance and the level of the systemic pressure.

Contrast Studies Pulmonary angiography demonstrates a large pulmonary trunk and a right-to-left ductal shunt. The proximal pulmonary arteries taper abruptly, while the interlobar vessels are attenuated and may be tortuous. The peripheral vessels appear sparse. The ductus arteriosus is usually huge, often with the same dimensions as the descending aorta. Aortography or left ventriculography shows dilution of the contrast medium in the descending aorta during ventricular systole because of the right-to-left shunt through the ductus (Fig. 7–61). On cine aortography the descending aorta fills intermittently. No congenital heart defect is identified.

Treatment Relief of pulmonary arteriolar spasm is essential to treatment. Oxygen is administered by headbox, by nasal prongs or by endotracheal intubation, with constant positive airway pressure. Vasodilators such as tolazoline (Priscoline) are administered as bolus injections or as intravenous infusions. In addition, abnormalities of sodium, potassium, glucose, calcium and pH must be corrected,

Fig. 7–59. *M-mode echocardiograms in a one-day-old infant with persistent fetal circulation.*

A Aortic valve for systolic time intervals (*LPEP* = 65 msec, *LVET* = 180 msec); **B** pulmonic valve for systolic time intervals (RPEP = 65 msec, RVET = 210 msec, RPEP/RVET = .31); **C** right and left ventricular cavities; **D** Tricuspid valve.

The purpose of the echocardiogram is: 1) to exclude the diagnosis of cyanotic congenital heart defects, 2) to evaluate severity of pulmonary hypertension, and 3) to evaluate left ventricular function.

In this patient the aortic valve is posterior and toward the right and the pulmonic valve superior and leftward. Thus, normal orientation of the great arteries excludes dextrotransposition of the great arteries. The systolic time intervals of the left ventricle are normal. The right ventricle has a long RPEP/RVET (normal 0.16 to 0.30) indicating elevation of the pulmonary resistance. Flattening of the atrial kick ("*a*") on the pulmonic valve tracing (**B**) also indicates elevation of the pulmonary resistance. (*Continued*)

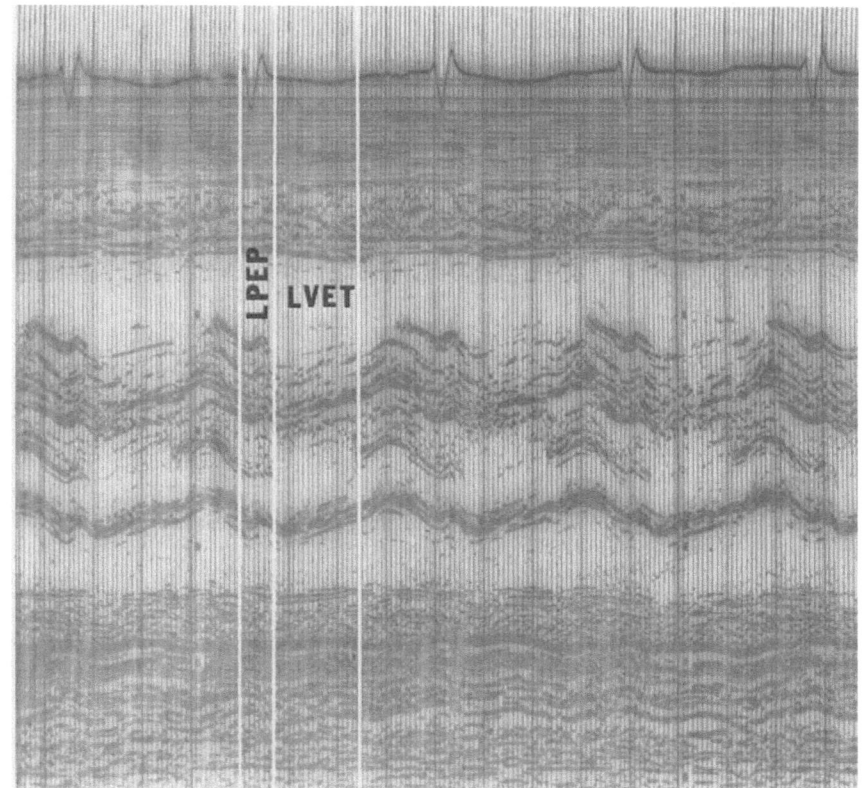

A

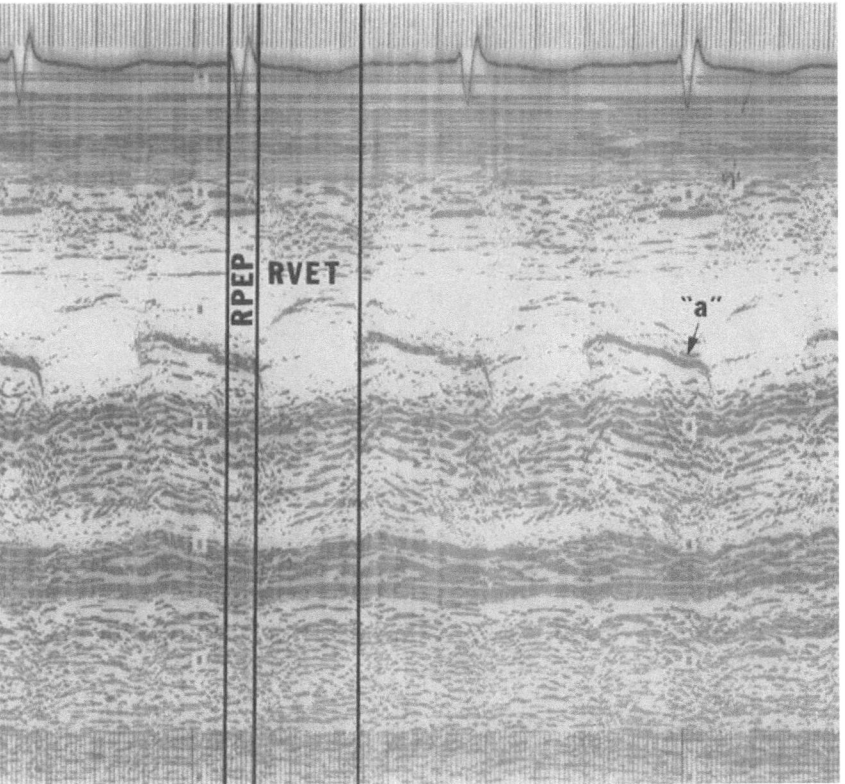

B

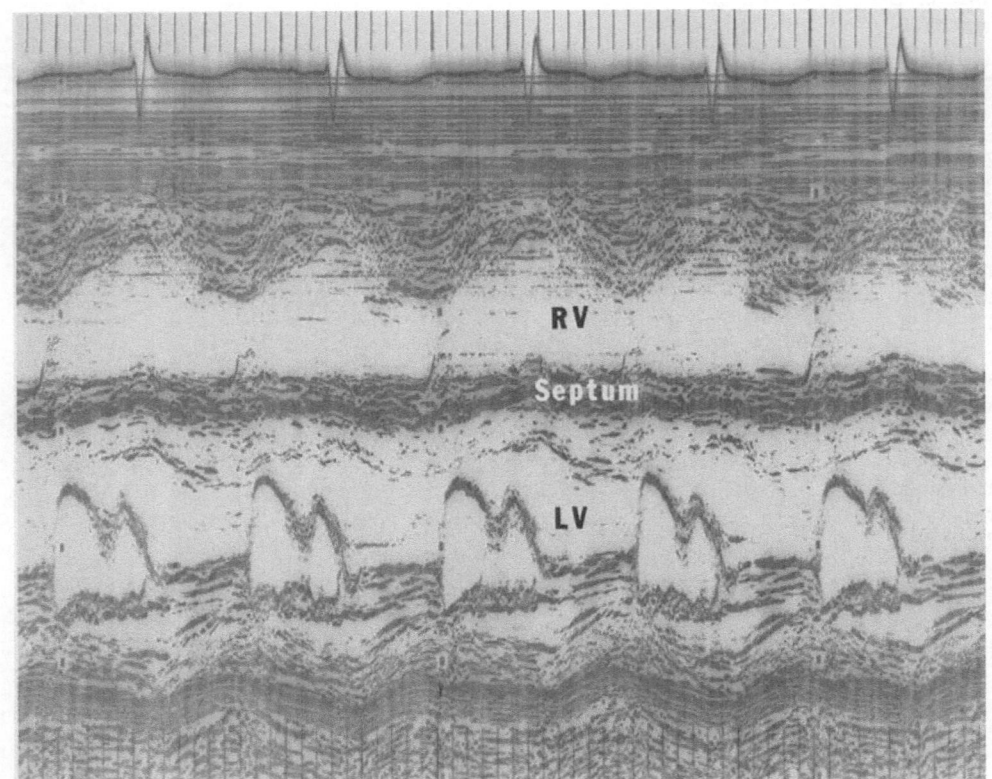

C

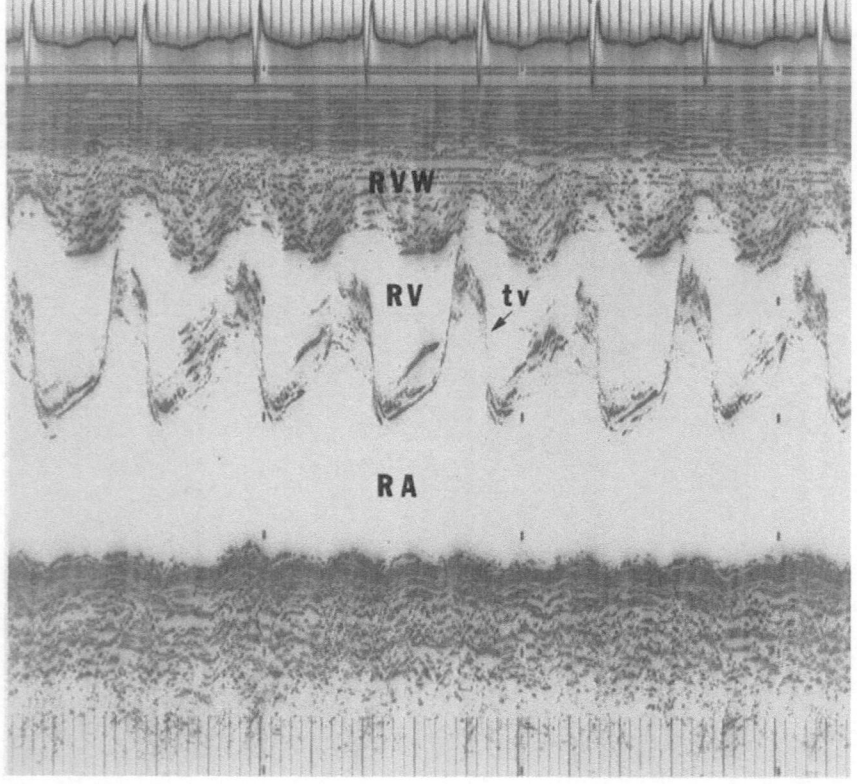

D

Fig. 7–59 (*Cont.*). In **C** the right ventricular cavity (*RV*) is slightly dilated, and the right ventricular free wall (*RVW*) is hyperkinetic. Left ventricular (*LV*) contractions are normal. The ventricular septum is thickened, suggesting some intrauterine stress. In **D** presence of the tricuspid valve (*tv*) excludes the diagnosis of tricuspid atresia. A 2-dimensional study (not shown) confirms normal cardiac anatomy and dilatation of the right ventricle. Contrast echocardiography demonstrated a right-to-left shunt at the atrial level. *RA* = right atrium.

Fig. 7–60. *Persistent fetal circulation in a 1-day-old baby.* The chest roentgenogram demonstrates marked undercirculation with moderate cardiomegaly. The main pulmonary artery is markedly enlarged, almost reaching the left thoracic apex. The right atrium is also enlarged. The rounding of the cardiac apex in this case is due to right ventricular hypertrophy and dilatation.

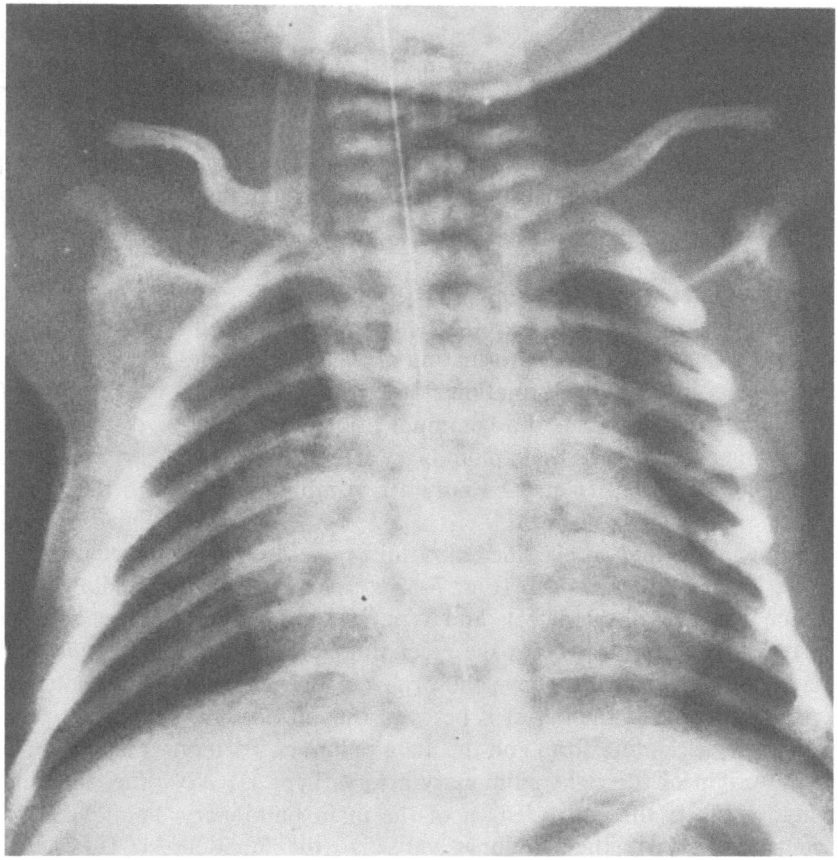

Fig. 7–61. *Persistent fetal circulation in the patient in Fig. 7–60.* A lateral view of the left ventriculogram reveals a normal-sized left ventricle that is retrodisplaced by a markedly enlarged right ventricle. The wide sweep of the right coronary artery confirms right ventricular dilatation. The ascending aorta and brachiocephalic vessels are densely opacified, while the descending aorta beyond the ductus is only faintly opacified because of dilution resulting from the right-to-left shunt through the ductus arteriosus. Mitral insufficiency may have been induced by the catheter. Pulmonary pressure was at systemic levels. Right-to-left shunts at the atrial and ductal levels were observed. No anatomical cardiac defect was noted. Incidentally, note the presence of four brachiocephalic vessels, the third being the left vertebral artery, which originates directly from the aorta rather than from the subclavian artery.

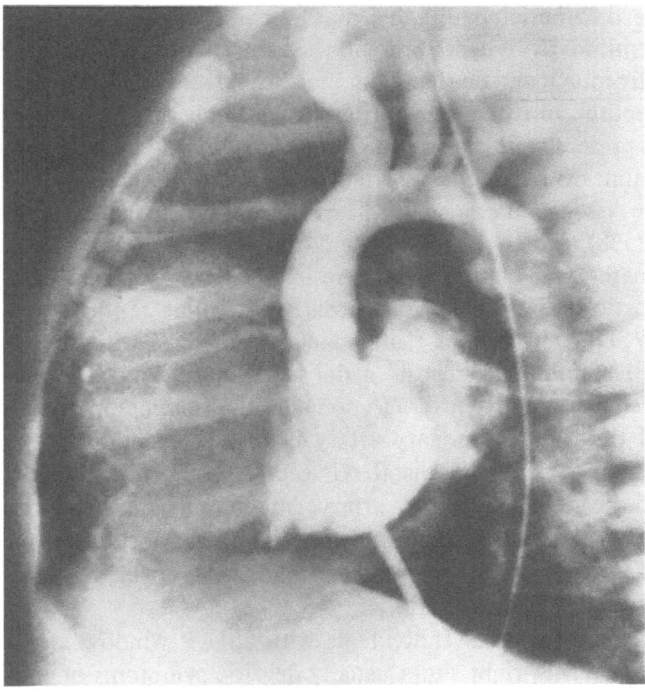

while the body temperature and degree of hydration are maintained.

Cardiac inotropes such as dopamine are administered if ventricular dysfunction is a significant factor. During resolution, pulmonary resistance decreases and the right-to-left shunt resolves. The ductus arteriosus may remain patent for a short time, causing a large left-to-right shunt and congestive heart failure.

Aorticopulmonary Window

Aorticopulmonary septal defect or fenestration (AP window) is a relatively rare malformation of the great arteries that results from faulty formation of the truncoconal septum. The defect consists of a communication between the ascending aorta and the main pulmonary artery. The defect is usually large, but it may be only a few millimeters in size.

AP window may be classified into three types according to its location (Mori et al.) (Fig. 7–62): type I, proximal defect; type II, distal defect; and type III, total defect. In type I the defect involves the ascending aorta and the main pulmonary artery above the origin of the coronary arteries. In type II the defect is between the left posterior wall of the ascending aorta and the main pulmonary artery at the origin of the right pulmonary artery. Type III AP window affects the entire length of the main pulmonary artery from above the semilunar valves to the junction of the right pulmonary artery.

An AP window of type III and truncus arteriosus must be differentiated. In AP window two distinct anatomical semilunar valves are present, the ventricular septum is usually intact, and neither great vessel overrides the ventricular septum. In truncus arteriosus only a single semilunar valve is present, with a ventricular septal defect, and the common trunk overrides the ventricular septum.

Associated congenital heart defects are not uncommon (25%). These include patent ductus arteriosus (PDA), coarctation of the aorta, atresia of the aortic arch, right aortic arch, subaortic stenosis, ventricular septal defect (VSD), tetralogy of Fallot, bicuspid or fenestrated aortic valve, pulmonic stenosis, atrial septal defect, mitral insufficiency, coronary arterial anomalies and anomalous origin of the right pulmonary artery from the ascending aorta. The association of distal AP septal defect, aortic origin of the right pulmonary artery, intact ventricular septum, PDA and interruption or coarctation of the aortic isthmus has been reported sporadically and may represent a new syndrome (Berry et al.).

Clinical Features Individuals with an AP window and a large left-to-right shunt usually develop symptoms of congestive heart failure in the neonatal period or early in infancy. The pulses are bounding, reminiscent of PDA. The

murmur is heard loudest anteriorly at the base of the heart. In the neonate and even in older children with high pulmonary resistance the murmur may be systolic rather than continuous. The electrocardiographic findings are similar to those occurring in patients with a large PDA. In the presence of pulmonary hypertension the clinical features of AP window mimic those of PDA or VSD with pulmonary hypertension. A greater tendency for bidirectional shunting exists, however, with an AP window.

Echocardiography Recent reports indicate that 2-D echocardiography (short axis view at the level of the great vessels) can image a break in the AP septum in instances of AP window (Fig. 7–63). Echocardiographic demonstration of two semilunar valves excludes the diagnosis of truncus arteriosus. Other echocardiographic features are similar to those observed with PDA and VSD (enlarged LA, dilated hyperkinetic LV, and signs of pulmonary arterial hypertension).

Radiological (Plain Film) Features Roentgenograms of the chest reflect the size of the left-to-right shunt. The pulmonary vasculature may be normal if the defect is small or markedly overcirculated if the defect is large. With large defects, pulmonary venous hypertension is an associated feature (Fig. 7–64A). The LV and LA are enlarged, and the pulmonary arteries are dilated. The ascending aorta may be dilated, but may not be discernible on plain films of the chest.

Hemodynamics In patients with AP window, manipulation of the catheter into the aorta from the main pulmonary artery is difficult. If the catheter crosses the AP window it passes directly up into the ascending aorta. This feature is in contrast to the ease with which a catheter can be passed into the descending aorta from the pulmonary artery in a downward direction through a PDA (Fig. 7–57). The hemodynamics are virtually indistinguishable from those encountered in a patient with a large PDA. A bidirectional shunt is more likely with AP window than with PDA.

Contrast Studies Retrograde biplane aortography is the most useful technique to accurately delineate the size and type of AP window and to distinguish it from PDA. However, the high risk of the arterial approach in sick infants often forces a venous approach. Therefore one should be familiar with the findings on pulmonary arteriography and ventriculography. Two semilunar valves must be identified to exclude truncus arteriosus. If the semilunar valves cannot be demonstrated on aortography, then ventriculography may be necessary. Fig. 7–64 illustrates the findings on pulmonary arteriography, left ventriculography and aortography.

Treatment Closure with a transaortic patch during total cardiopulmonary bypass constitutes the preferred surgical method for repair of AP window.

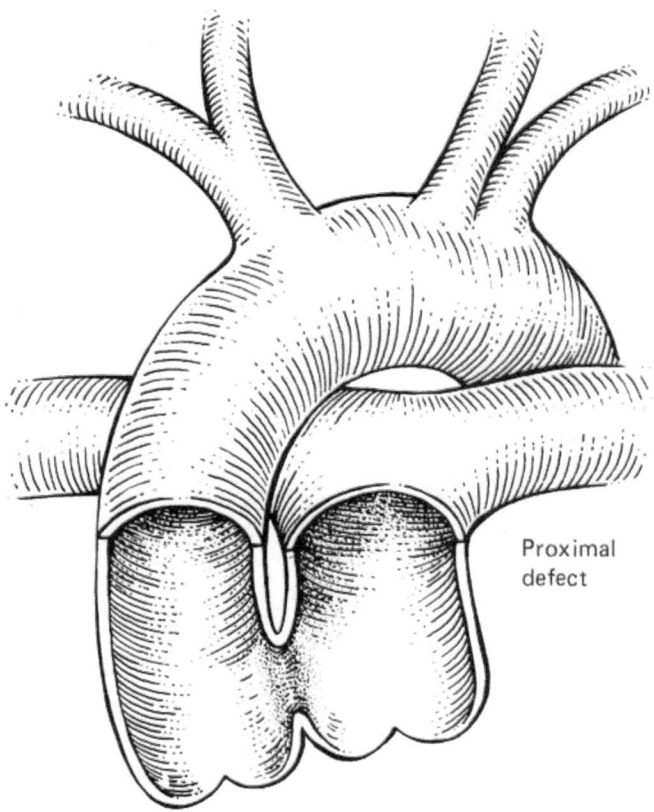

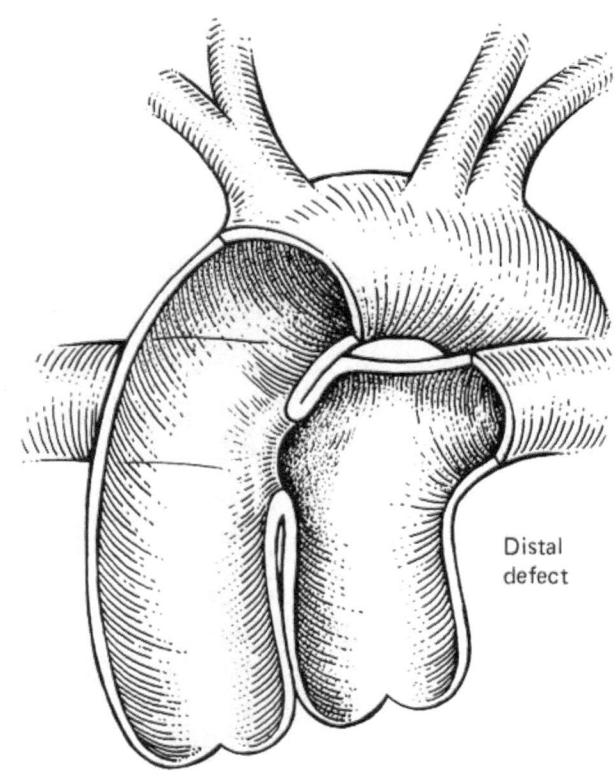

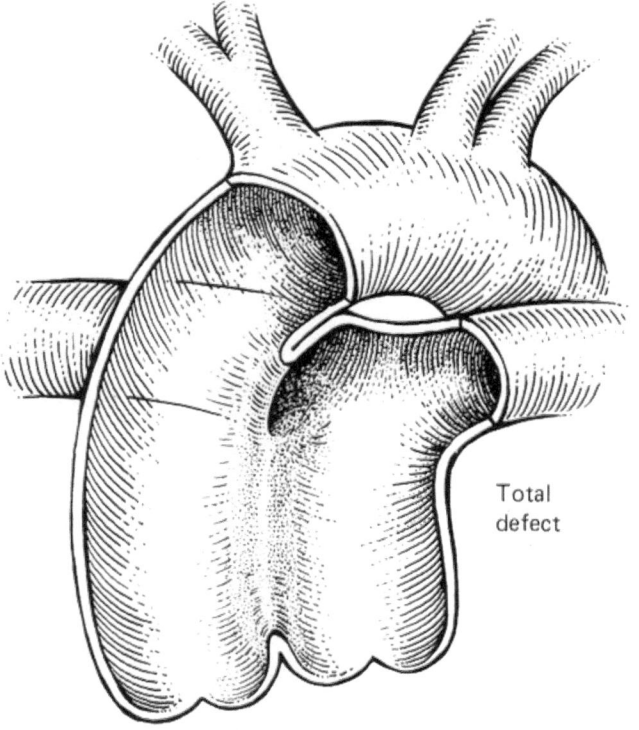

Fig. 7–62. *Types of aorticopulmonary window.* Type I is a proximal defect in the aorticopulmonary septum; type II is a distal defect; and type III consists of total absence of the aorticopulmonary septum from the semilunar valves to the origin of the right pulmonary artery.

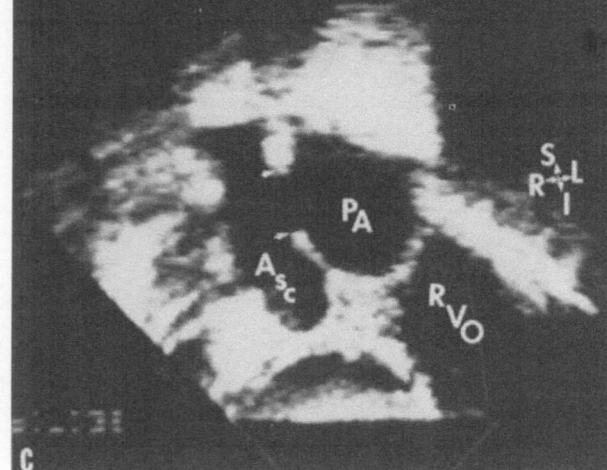

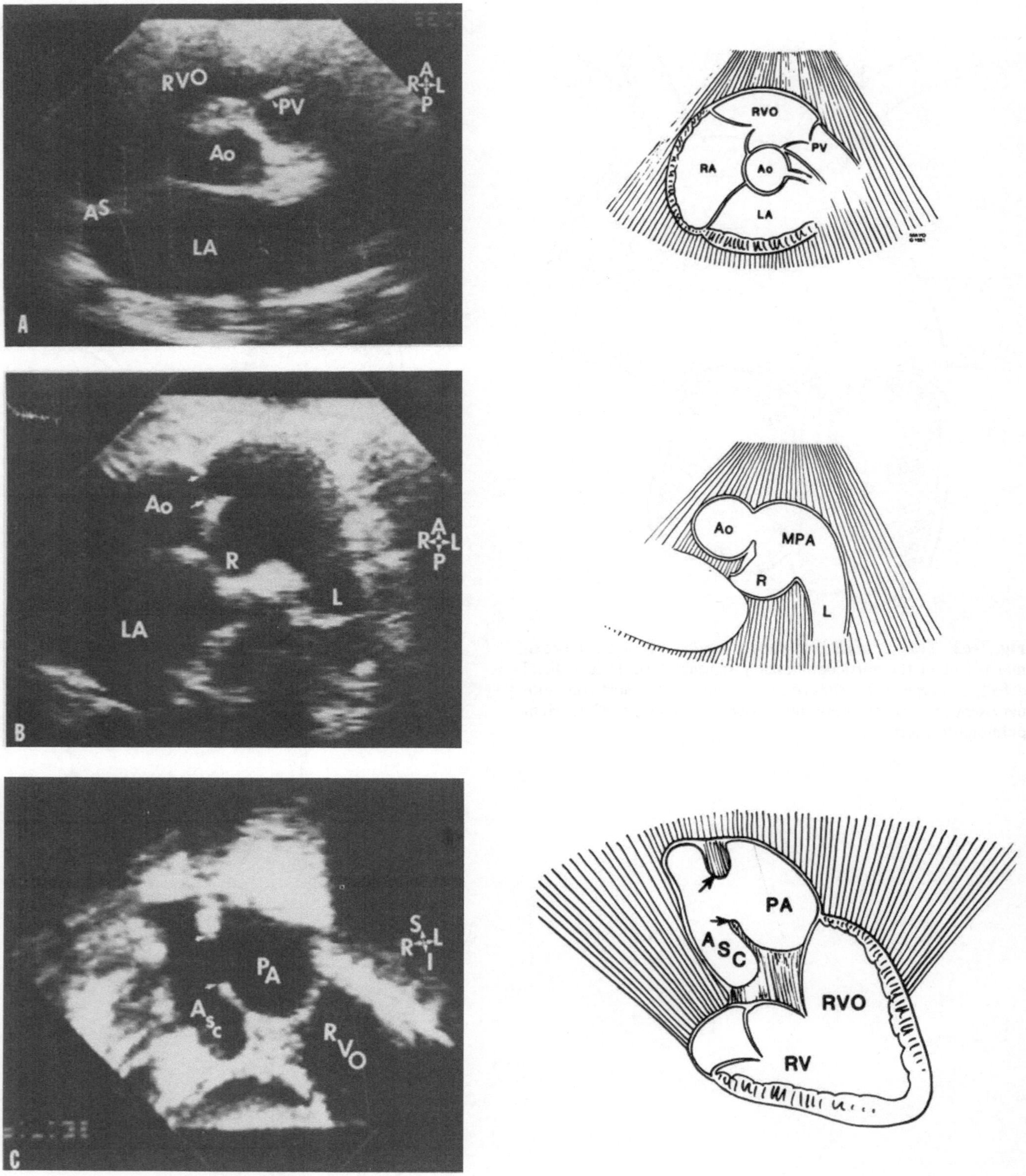

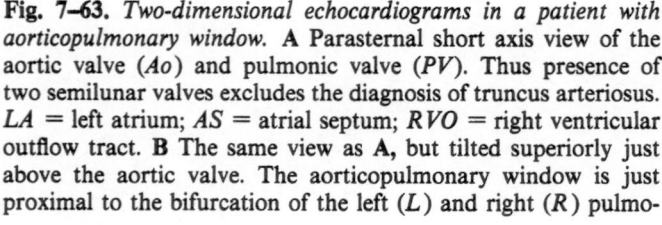

Fig. 7–63. *Two-dimensional echocardiograms in a patient with aorticopulmonary window.* **A** A Parasternal short axis view of the aortic valve (*Ao*) and pulmonic valve (*PV*). Thus presence of two semilunar valves excludes the diagnosis of truncus arteriosus. *LA* = left atrium; *AS* = atrial septum; *RVO* = right ventricular outflow tract. **B** The same view as **A,** but tilted superiorly just above the aortic valve. The aorticopulmonary window is just proximal to the bifurcation of the left (*L*) and right (*R*) pulmo- nary arteries. **C** A subxiphoid view showing the ascending aorta (*Asc*) and the main pulmonary artery (*PA*). Again the large aorti- copulmonary window is evident (*arrows*). Reprinted with permis- sion from Rice MJ, Seward JB, Hagler DJ, Mair DD, Tajik AJ (1982) Visualization of aortopulmonary window by two-di- mensional echocardiography. Mayo Clin Proc 57:482–487. (Cour- tesy of Mary J. Rice, M.D.)

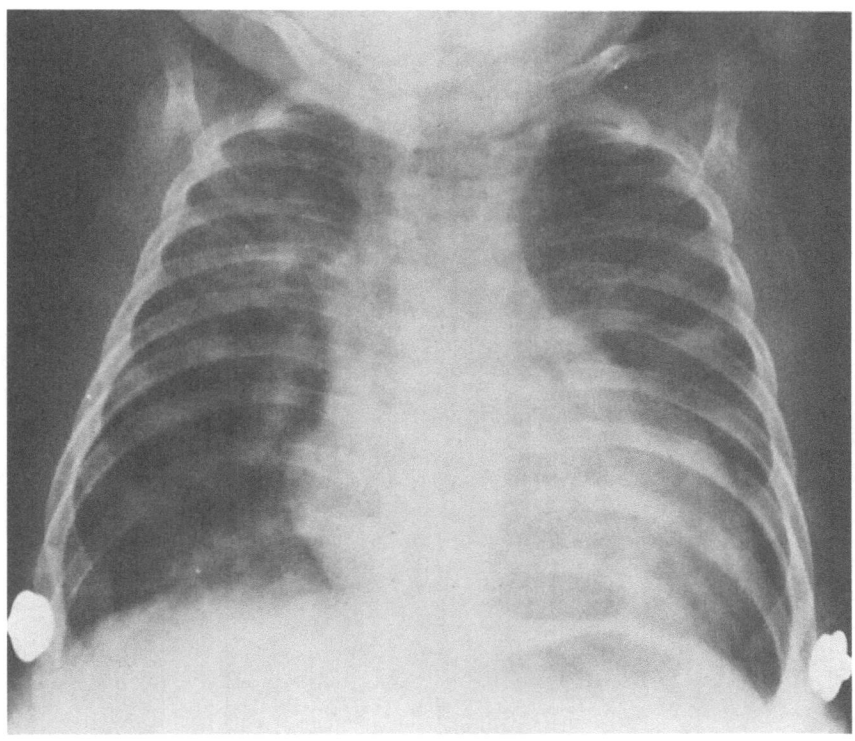

A

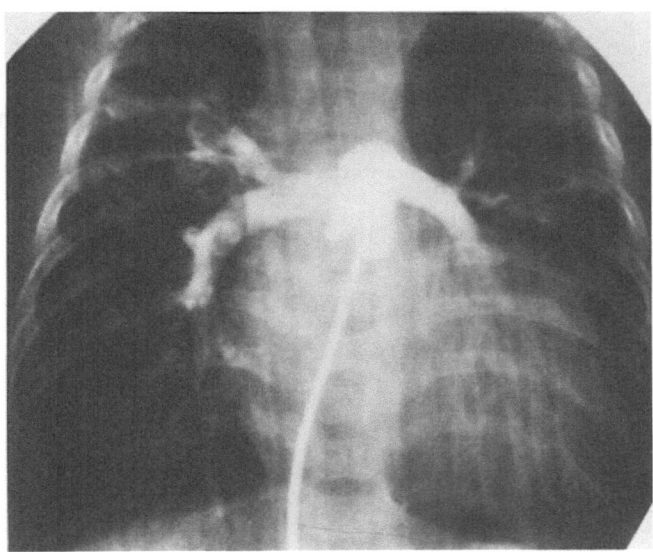

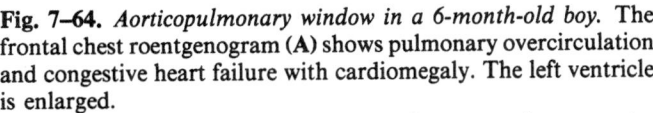

B

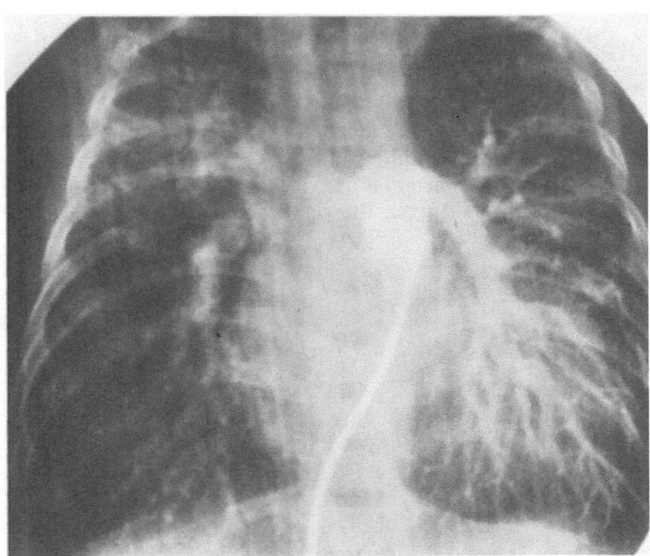

C

Fig. 7–64. *Aorticopulmonary window in a 6-month-old boy.* The frontal chest roentgenogram (**A**) shows pulmonary overcirculation and congestive heart failure with cardiomegaly. The left ventricle is enlarged.

Angiographic findings in type II (distal) aorticopulmonary window. On injection in the main pulmonary artery (**B** and **C**) there is intermittent dilution of contrast material in the right pulmonary artery, while the left pulmonary artery remains opacified throughout the injection. This finding of intermittent de-opacification of the right pulmonary artery by unopacified blood from the aorta indicates presence of an aorticopulmonary window rather than a patent ductus arteriosus. A ductus arteriosus differs from aorticopulmonary window in that it connects the left pulmonary artery near its origin or the main pulmonary artery at its bifurca-

tion. Therefore, a patent ductus arteriosus would not selectively deopacify the right pulmonary artery. Compare these pictures with the pulmonary angiogram from a patient with patent ductus arteriosus (Fig. 7–57B), in which unopacified blood enters the main pulmonary artery from above.

On left ventriculography (**D**) the right pulmonary artery fills at the same time as the ascending aorta but before the aortic arch and descending aorta. Again, this feature contrasts with the findings in patent ductus arteriosus in which the pulmonary trunk and both branches of the pulmonary artery are opacified at the same time as the descending aorta (Fig. 7–58B). The aorta arises normally from the left ventricle. A ventricular septal defect is not present, and the aorta does not override the ventricular septum.

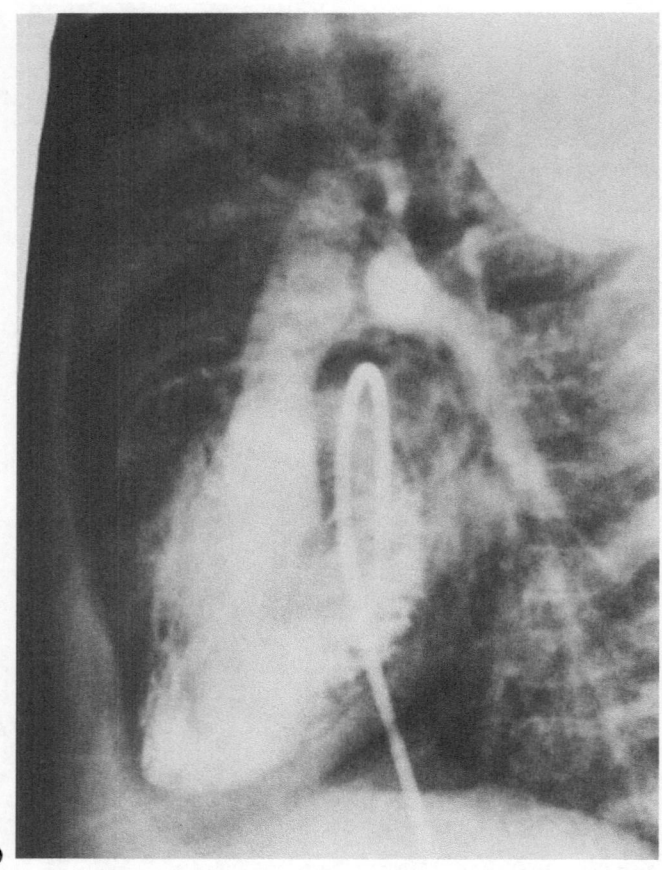

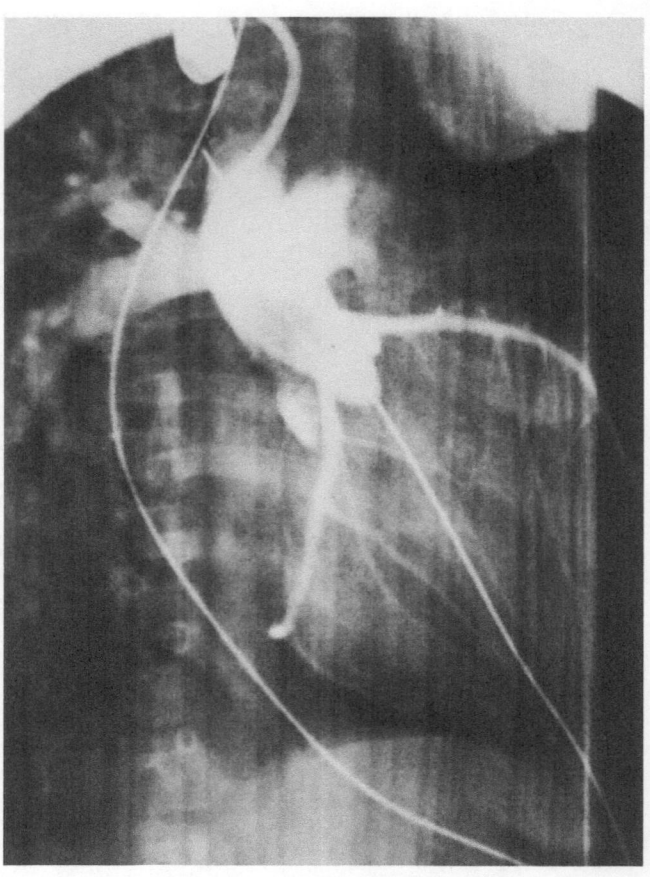

D

E

On aortography (E) the ascending aorta and both pulmonary arteries are opacified simultaneously. Note that the distal segment of the left pulmonary artery is not visualized, because it is perfused by unopacified blood from the right ventricle. The aortic valve is clearly identified. The aorta is not broad based, and the coronary arteries arise normally from the aortic root thus excluding truncus arteriosus. See also truncus arteriosus (Figs. 7–112 to 7–115).

Bibliography

Atrial Septal Defect

Bedford DE (1960) The anatomical types of atrial septal defect. Their incidence and clinical diagnosis. Am J Cardiol 6:568–574

Cohn LH, Morrow AG, Braunwald E (1967) Operative treatment of atrial septal defects: Clinical and hemodynamic assessments in 175 patients. Br Heart J 29:725–734

Diamond MA, Dillon JC, Haine CL, Chang S, Feigenbaum H (1971) Echocardiographic features of atrial septal defect. Circulation 43:129–135

Ferrell RL, Jones B, Lucas RV Jr (1966) Simultaneous occurrence of the Holt-Oram and the Duane syndromes. J Pediatr 69:630–634

Gorlin RJ, Cervenka J, Anderson RC, Sank JJ, Bevis WD (1970) Robin's syndrome. Am J Dis Child 119:176–178

Hagan AD, Francis GS, Sahn DJ, Karliner JS, Friedman WE, O'Rourke RA (1974) Ultrasound evaluation of systolic anterior septal motion in patients with and without right ventricular volume overload. Circulation 50:248–254

Harley HRS (1958) The sinus venosus type of interatrial septal defect. Thorax 13:12–27

Harris LC, Osborne WP (1966) Congenital absence or hypoplasia of the radius with ventricular septal defect: Ventriculoradial dysplasia. J Pediatr 68:265–272

Holt M, Oram S (1960) Familial heart disease with skeletal malformations. Br Heart J 22:236–242

Hunt CE, Lucas RV Jr (1973) Symptomatic atrial septal defect in infancy. Circulation 47:1042–1048

Hynes KM, Frye RL, Brandenburg RO, McGoon DC, Titus JL, Guiliani ER (1974) Atrial septal defect (secundum) associated with mitral regurgitation. Am J Cardiol 34:333–338

James LS, Burnard ED, Rowe RD (1961) Abnormal shunting through the foramen ovale after birth (abstr). Am J Dis Child 102:550

Kato K (1924) Congenital absence of the radius with review of the literature and report of three cases. J Bone Joint Surg 6:589–626

Keith A (1903) The anatomy of valvular mechanism around the venous orifices of the right and left auricles with some observations on the morphology of the heart. J Anat 37:2

Kyger ER, Frazier OH, Cooley DA, Gillette PC, Reul GJ Jr, Sandiford FM, Wukasch DC (1978) Sinus venosus atrial septal defect: Early and late results following closure in 109 patients. Ann Thorac Surg 25:44–50

Levin AR, Spach MS, Boineau JP, Canent RV Jr, Capp MP, Jewett PH (1968) Atrial pressure-flow dynamics in atrial septal defects (secundum type). Circulation 37:476–488

Lieppe W, Scallion R, Behar VS, Kisslo JA (1977) Two-dimensional echocardiographic finding in atrial septal defect. Circulation 56:447–456

Nadas AS, Fyler DC (1972) Pediatric cardiology, (3rd edn). Saunders, Philadelphia, pp 317–348

Nasser FN, Tajik AJ, Seward JB, Hagler DJ (1981) Diagnosis of sinus venosus atrial septal defect by two-dimensional echocardiography. Mayo Clin Proc 56:568–572

Phillips SJ, Okies JE, Henken D, Sunderland CO, Starr A (1975) Complex of secundum atrial septal defect and congestive heart failure in infants. J Thorac Cardiovasc Surg 70:696–700

Pocock WA, Barlow JB (1971) An association between the billowing posterior mitral leaflet syndrome and congenital heart disease, particularly atrial septal defect. Am Heart J 81:720–722

Rastelli GC, Rahimtoola SH, Ongley PA, McGoon DC (1968) Common atrium: Anatomy, hemodynamics, and surgery. J Thorac Cardiovasc Surg 55:834–841

Sanz G, Nadal-Ginard B, Mata LA, Buentello L (1973) The upper limb-cardiovascular syndrome (Holt-Oram Syndrome). A survey and a report of four cases. Clin Pediatr 12:687–691

Tandon R, Edwards JE (1974) Atrial septal defect in infancy. Common association with other anomalies. Circulation 49:1005–1010

Ticzon AR, Damato AN, Caracta AR, Russo G, Foster JR, Lau SH (1976) Interventricular septal motion during preexcitation and normal conduction in Wolff-Parkinson-White syndrome. Am J Cardiol 37:840–847

Titus JL, Rastelli GC (1976) Anatomic features of persistent common atrioventricular canal. In: Feldt RH (ed) Atrioventricular canal defects. Saunders, Philadelphia, pp 13–35

Vazquez-Perez J, Frontera-Izquierdo P (1979) Anomalous drainage of the right superior vena cava into the left atrium as an isolated anomaly. Rare case report. Am Heart J 97:89–91

Young D (1973) Later results of closure of secundum atrial septal defect in children. Am J Cardiol 31:14–22

Persistence of the Left Superior Vena Cava

Raghib G, Ruttenberg HD, Anderson RC, Amplatz K, Adams P, Edwards JE (1965) Termination of the left superior vena cava in left atrium, atrial septal defect, and absence of coronary sinus. A developmental complex. Circulation 31:906–918

Tuchman H, Brown JF, Huston JH, Weinstein AB, Rowe GG, Crumptom CW (1956) Superior vena cava draining into left atrium. Another cause for left ventricular hypertrophy with cyanotic congenital heart disease. Am J Med 21:481–484

Endocardial Cushion Defects

Aziz KU, Paul MH, Muster AJ, Idriss FS (1979) Positional abnormalities of atrioventricular valves in transposition of the great arteries including double outlet right ventricle, atrioventricular valve straddling and malattachment. Am J Cardiol 44:1135–1145

Baron MG, Wolf BS, Steinfeld L, Van Mierop LHS (1964) Endocardial cushion defects. Specific diagnosis by angiocardiography. Am J Cardiol 13:162–175

Bass JL, Bessinger FB Jr, Lawrence C (1978) Echocardiographic differentiation of partial and complete atrioventricular canal. Circulation 57:1144–1150

Bierman FZ, Williams RG (1979) Subxiphoid two-dimensional imaging of the interatrial septum in infants and neonates with congenital heart disease. Circulation 60:80–90

Eshaghpour E, Turnoff HB, Kingsley B, Kawai N, Linhart JW (1975) Echocardiography in endocardial cushion defects: A preoperative and postoperative study. Chest 68:172–177

Espino-Vela J, Murad-Netto S, Rubio-Alverez R (1960) Differential diagnosis between persistent atrioventricular canal and the combination of atrial and ventricular septal defects. Am J Cardiol 6:589–597

Hagler DJ, Tajik AJ, Seward JB, Mair DD, Ritter DG (1979) Real-time wide-angle sector echocardiography: Atrioventricular canal defects. Circulation 59:140–150

Lang LW, Sahn DJ, Allen HD, Goldberg SJ (1979) Subxiphoid

cross-sectional echocardiography in infants and children with congenital heart disease. Circulation 59:513–524

Macartney FJ, Rees PG, Daly K, Piccoli GP, Taylor JFN, DeLeval MR, Stark J, Anderson RH (1979) Angiocardiographic appearances of atrioventricular defects with particular reference to distinction of ostium primum atrial septal defect from common atrioventricular orifice. Br Heart J 42:640–656

Neufeld HN, Titus JL, Dushane JW, Burchell HB, Edwards JE (1961) Isolated ventricular septal defect of the persistent common atrioventricular canal type. Circulation 23:685–695

Rastelli GC, Kirklin JW, Kincaid OW (1967) Angiocardiography of persistent common atrioventricular canal. Mayo Clin Proc 42:200–209

Rastelli GC, Rahimtoola SH, Ongley PA, McGoon DC (1968) Common atrium: Anatomy, hemodynamics, and surgery. J Thorac Cardiovasc Surg 55:834–841

Titus JL, Rastelli GC (1976) Anatomic features of persistent common atrioventricular canal. In: Atrioventricular canal defects Feldt RH (ed) WB Saunders Co., Phila, London, Toronto pp 13–35

Williams RG, Rudd M (1974) Echocardiographic features of endocardial cushion defects. Circulation 49:418–422

Partial Anomalous Pulmonary Venous Return

Dalith F, Neufeld H (1960) Radiological diagnosis of anomalous pulmonary venous connection: A tomographic study. Radiology 74:1–18

Dotter CT, Hardisty NM, Steinberg I (1949) Anomalous right pulmonary vein entering the inferior vena cava: Report of two cases diagnosed during life by angiography and cardiac catheterization. Am J Med Sci 218:31–36

Morrow AG, Awe WC, Aygen MM (1962) Total unilateral anomalous pulmonary venous connection with intact atrial septum. Diagnostic features and a method of surgical correction. Am J Cardiol 9:933–937

Snellen HA, Albers FH (1952) The clinical diagnosis of anomalous pulmonary venous drainage. Circulation 6:801–816

Snellen HA, Dekker A (1963) Anomalous pulmonary venous drainage in relation to left superior vena cava and coronary sinus. Am Heart J 66:184–196

Scimitar Syndrome

Halasz NA, Halloran KH, Liebow AA (1956) Bronchial and arterial anomalies with drainage of the right lung into the inferior vena cava. Circulation 14:826–846

Jue KL, Amplatz K, Adams P Jr, Anderson RC (1966) Anomalies of great vessels associated with lung hypoplasia. Am J Dis Child 111:35–44

Kittle CF, Crockett JE (1962) Vena cava bronchochovascular syndrome—a triad of anomalies involving the right lung: Anomalous pulmonary vein, abnormal bronchi and systemic pulmonary arteries. Ann Surg 156:222–233

Mascarenhas E, Javier RP, Samet P (1973) Partial anomalous pulmonary venous connection and drainage. Am J Cardiol 31:512–518

Neill CA, Ferencz C, Sabinston DC, Sheldon H (1960) The familial occurrence of hypoplastic right lung with systemic arterial supply and venous drainage "scimitar syndrome." Bull Johns Hopkins Hosp 107:1–21

Roehm JOF, Jr., Jue KL, Amplatz K (1966) Radiographic features of the scimitar syndrome. Radiology 86:856–859

Pulmonary Sequestration

Boyd GL (1953) Intralobar pulmonary sequestration. Dis Chest 24:162–172

Gerle RD, Jaretzki A, Ashley CA, Berne AS (1968) Congenital bronchopulmonary-foregut malformation. Pulmonary sequestration communicating with the gastrointestinal tract. N Engl J Med 278:1413–1419

Heithoff KB, Sane SM, Williams HJ, Jarvis CJ, Carter J, Kane P, Brennom W (1976) Bronchopulmonary-foregut malformations. A unifying etiological concept. Am J Roentgenol 126:46–55

Price DM (1946) Lower accessory pulmonary artery with intralobar sequestration of lung: A report of seven cases. J Pathol Bacteriol 58:457–467

Savic B, Birtel FJ, Tholen W, Funke HD, Knoche R (1979) Lung sequestration: Report of seven cases and review of 540 published cases. Thorax 34:96–101

Total Anomalous Pulmonary Venous Return

Behrendt DM, Aberdeen E, Waterson DJ, Bonham-Carter RE (1972) Total anomalous pulmonary drainage in infants. Circulation 46:347–356

Burroughs JI, Edwards JE (1960) Total anomalous pulmonary venous connection. Am Heart J 59:913–931

Darling RC, Rothney WB, Craig JM (1957) Total pulmonary venous drainage into the right side of the heart. Report of 17 autopsied cases not associated with other major cardiovascular anomalies. Lab Invest 6:44–64

Elliott LP, Edwards JE (1962) The problem of pulmonary venous obstruction in total anomalous pulmonary venous connection to the left innominate vein (editorial). Circulation 25:913–915

Everhart FJ, Korns ME, Amplatz K, Edwards JE (1967) Intrapulmonary segment in anomalous pulmonary venous connection. Resemblance to scimitar syndrome. Circulation 35:1163–1169

Gatham GE, Nadas AS (1970) Total anomalous pulmonary venous connection: Clinical and physiologic observations of 75 pediatric patients. Circulation 42:143–154

Hastreiter AR, Paul MH, Molthan ME, Miller RA (1962) Total anomalous pulmonary venous connection with severe pulmonary venous obstruction. A clinical entity. Circulation 25:916–928

Kauffman SL, Ores CN, Andersen DH (1962) Two cases of total anomalous pulmonary venous return of the supracardiac type with stenosis simulating infradiaphragmatic drainage. Circulation 25:376–382

Lester RG, Mauck HP, Grubb WL (1966) Anomalous pulmonary venous return to the right side of the heart. Semin Roentgenol 1:102–119

Lucas RV Jr, Anderson RC, Amplatz K, Adams P Jr, Edwards JE (1963) Congenital causes of pulmonary venous obstruction. Pediatr Clin North Am 10:781–837

Mortera C, Tynan M, Goodwin AW, Hunter S (1977) Infradiaphragmatic total anomalous pulmonary venous connection to portal vein. Diagnostic implications of echocardiography. Br Heart J 39:685–687

Paquet M, Gutgesell M (1975) Echocardiographic features of total anomalous pulmonary venous connection. Circulation 51:599–605

Rabinowitz JG, Liu L, Lindner A (1969) Asplenia associated with infradiaphragmatic total anomalous pulmonary venous return and esophageal varices. Radiology 93:350–352

Sahn DJ, Allen HD, Lange LW, Goldberg SJ (1979) Cross-sectioned echocardiographic diagnosis of the sites of total anomalous pulmonary venous drainage. Circulation 60:1317–1325

Snider AR, Ports TA, Silverman NH (1979) Venous anomalies of the coronary sinus: Detection by M-mode, two-dimensional and contrast echocardiography. Circulation 60:721–727

Turley K, Tucker WY, Ullyot DJ, Ebert PA (1980) Total anomalous pulmonary venous connection in infancy: Influence of age and type of lesion. Am J Cardiol 45:92–97

Rupture of Sinus of Valsalva into a Cardiac Chamber

Cooperberg P, Mercer EN, Mulder DS, Winsberg F (1974) Rupture of a sinus Valsalva aneurysm. Report of a case diagnosed preoperatively by echocardiography. Radiology 113:171–172

Davidsen HG, Petersen O, Thompsen G (1958) Roentgenologic findings in 5 cases of congenital aneurysm of the aortic sinuses (sinuses of Valsalva). Acta Radiol 49:205–217

Edwards JE, Burchell HB (1956) Specimen exhibiting the essential lesion in aneurysm of the aortic sinus. May Clin Proc 31:407–412

Edwards JE, Burchell HB (1957) The pathological anatomy of deficiencies between the aortic root and the heart, including aortic sinus aneurysms. Thorax 12:125–139

Fishbein MC, Obma R, Roberts WC (1975) Unruptured sinus of Valsalva aneurysm. Am J Cardiol 35:918–922

Goetz AA, Graham WH (1956) Aneurysm of the sinus of Valsalva associated with coarctation. Radiology 67:416–418

Haraoka S, Ueda M, Saito D, Ogino Y, Yoshida H, Kusuhara S (1978) Echocardiographic findings of a case of sinus of Valsalva aneurysm ruptured into left ventricle: Abnormal echoes in the left ventricular outflow tract. J Cardiogr 8:293–301

Herson RN, Symons M (1946) Ruptured congenital aneurysm of the posterior sinus of Valsalva. Br Heart J 8:125–129

Lillehei CW, Stanley P, Varco RL (1957) Surgical treatment of ruptured aneurysms of the sinus of Valsalva. Ann Surg 146:459–472

Matsumoto M, Matsuo H, Beppu S, Yoshioka Y, Kawashima Y, Nimura Y, Abe H (1976) Echocardiographic diagnosis of ruptured aneurysm of sinus of Valsalva. Report of two cases. Circulation 53:382–389

Meyer J, Wukasch DC, Hallman GL, Cooley DA (1975) Aneurysm and fistula of the sinus of Valsalva. Clinical considerations and surgical treatment in 45 patients. Ann Thorac Surg 19:170–179

Nimura Y, Abe H (1976) Echocardiographic diagnosis of ruptured aneurysm of sinus of Valsalva. Report of two cases. Circulation 53:382–389

Nishimura K, Hibi N, Kato T, Fukui Y, Arakawa T, Tatematsu H, Miwa A, Tada H, Kambe T (1976) High speed ultrasonocardiotomography: Echographic manifestation of right sinus of Valsalva aneurysm ruptured into right ventricle. J Cardiogr 6:149–159

Rothbaum DA, Dillon JC, Chang S, Feigenbaum H (1974) Echocardiographic manifestation of right sinus of Valsalva aneurysm. Circulation 49:768–771

Sakakibara S, Konno S (1962) Congenital aneurysm of the sinus of Valsalva anatomy and classification. Am Heart J 63:405–424

Sakakibara S, Konno S (1968) Congenital aneurysm of the sinus of Valsalva associated with ventricular septal defect. Anatomical aspects. Am Heart J 75:595–603

Sawyers JL, Adams JE, Scott HW Jr (1957) Surgical treatment for aneurysms of the aortic sinuses with aorticoatrial fistula. Experimental and clinical study. Surgery 41:26–42

Shapiro JH, Jacobson HG, Rubenstein BM, Poppel MH, Schwedel JB (1963) Calcification in sinus of Valsalva aneurysm. In: Calcifications of the heart. Thomas, Springfield, Ill, pp 18–25

Steinberg I, Finby N (1957) Roentgen manifestations of unperforated aortic sinus aneurysms. Report of three new cases. Am J Roentgenol 77:263–273

Left Ventricular–Right Atrial Communication

Baron MG, Wolf BS, Grishman A, Van Mierop LHS (1964) Aneurysm of the membranous septum. Am J Roentgenol 91:1303–1313

Braunwald E, Morrow AG (1960) Left ventriculo-right atrial communication. Diagnosis by clinical, hemodynamic and angiographic methods. Am J Med 28:913–920

Elliott LP, Gedgaudas E, Levy MJ, Edwards JE (1965) The roentgenologic findings in left ventricular-right atrial communication. Am J Roentgenol 93:304–314

Gerbode F, Hultgren H, Melrose D, Osborn J (1958) Syndrome of left ventricular-right atrial shunt. Successful surgical repair of defect in five cases, with observation of bradycardia on closure. Ann Surg 148:433–446

Kramer RA, Abrams HL (1962) Radiologic aspects of operable heart disease. VII. Left ventricular-right atrial shunts. Radiology 78:171–179

Laurichesse J, Ferrane J, Renais J, Scebat L, Lenegre J (1964) Communication entre le ventricule gauche et l'oreillette droite. Arch Mal Coeur 57:703–724

Mills P, McLaurin L, Smith C, Murray G, Craige E (1977) Echocardiographic findings in left ventricular to right atrial shunts. Br Heart J 39:594–597

Nordenstrom B, Ovenfors CO (1960) Septal defect between the left ventricle and the right atrium diagnosed by cardioangiography. Acta Radiol 54:393–396

Perry EL, Burchell HB, Edwards JE (1949) Congenital communication between the left ventricle and the right atrium: Co-existing ventricular septal defect and dobule tricuspid orifice. Proc Staff Meet Mayo Clin 24:198–206

Russell E, Spindola-Franco H, Eisenberg R (1978) Left ventricular-right atrial communication with aneurysm of the membranous interventricular septum. Br J Radiol 51:463–466

Sakakibara S, Konno S (1963) Left ventricular-right atrial communication. Ann Surg 158:93–99

Congenital Coronary Arteriovenous Fistulas

Agusti R, Liebman J, Ankeney J, Macleod CA, Linton DS, Wiltsie R (1967) Congenital right coronary artery to left atrium fistula. Am J Cardiol 19:428–433

Berman DA, Alexander CS, Adicoff A, Sako Y (1965) Coronary arteriovenous fistula. Report of an unusual case simulating atrial septal defect. Am J Cardiol 15:853–855

Bjork VO, Bjork L (1965) Coronary artery fistula. J Thorac Cardiovasc Surg 49:921–930

Colbeck JC, Shaw JM (1954) Coronary aneurysm with arteriovenous fistula. Am Heart J 48:270–274

Eguchi S, Nitta H, Asano K, Tanaka M, Hoshino K (1970) Congenital fistula of the right coronary artery to the left ventricle. Am Heart J 80:242–246

Gobel FL, Anderson CF, Baltaxe HA, Amplatz K, Wang Y (1970) Shunts between the coronary and pulmonary arteries with normal origin of the coronary arteries. Am J Cardiol 25:655–665

Habermann JH, Howard ML, Johnson ES (1963) Rupture of the coronary sinus with hemopericardium. A rare complication of coronary arteriovenous fistula. Circulation 28:1143–1144

Jaffe RB, Glancy DL, Epstein SE, Brown BG, Morrow AG (1973) Coronary arterial-right heart fistulae. Long-term observations in seven patients. Circulation 47:133–143

Lee SH, Fisher B, Fisher ER, Little A (1962) Arteriovenous fistula and bacterial endocarditis. Surgery 52:463–467

Lowe JE, Oldham HN, Jr, Sabinston DC Jr (1981) Surgical management of congenital coronary fistulas. Ann Surg 194:373–380

Newcombe CP, Whitaker W, Keates PG (1964) Coronary arteriovenous fistulae. Thorax 19:16–21

Ogden JA (1971) Surgical correction of congenital coronary defects. II. Coronary artery-cardiac chamber fistulas. Conn Med 35:168–172

Ogden JA, Stansel HC Jr (1972) Coronary arterial fistulas terminating in the coronary venous system. J Thorac Cardiovasc Surg 63:172–182

Rodgers DM, Wolf NM, Barrett MJ, Zuckerman GL, Meister SG (1982) Two-dimensional echocardiographic features of coronary arteriovenous fistula. Am Heart J 104:872–874

Sloman G, Macphee A, Fairley K (1965) An unusual coronary arteriocameral fistula. Am J Cardiol 15:856–861

Isolated Ventricular Septal Defect

Alpert BS, Cook DH, Varghese PJ, Rowe RD (1979) Spontaneous closure of small ventricular septal defects: Ten year follow-up. Pediatrics 63:204–206

Barash BA, Freedman L, Opitz JM (1970) Anatomic studies in the 18–trisomy syndrome. Birth Defects 6 (4):3–15

Baron MG, Wolf BS, Steinfeld L, Gordon AJ (1963) Left ventricular angiocardiogram in the study of ventricular septal defect. Radiology 81:223–235

Blank CE (1960) Apert's syndrome (a type of acrocephalosyndactyly); observations on British series of 39 cases. Ann Hum Genet 24:151–164

Breg WR, Steele MW, Miller OJ, Warburton D, deCapoa A, Allderdice PW (1970) The cri du chat syndrome in adolescents and adults: Clinical finding in 13 older patients with partial deletion of the short arm of chromosome no. 5(5p-). J Pediatr 77:782–791

Capelli H, Andrade JL, Somerville J (1983) Classification of the site of ventricular septal defect by 2-dimensional echocardiography Am J Cardiol 51:1474–1480

Engel MA (1972) Ventricular septal defect: Status report from the 70's. Cardiovasc Clin 4:282–304

Freedom RM, Culham JAG, Rowe RD (1977) Angiography of subaortic obstruction in infancy. Am J Roentgenol 129:813–824

Friedman WF, Mehrizi A, Pusch AL (1964) Multiple muscular ventricular septal defects. Circulation 32:35–42

Gasul BM, Dillon RF, Vrla V, Hait G (1957) Ventricular septal defects. Their natural transformation into those with infundibular stenosis or into the cyanotic or noncyanotic type of tetralogy of Fallot. JAMA 164:847–853

Gibson DA, Uchida IA, Lewis AJ (1963) A review of the 18–trisomy syndrome. Med Biol 13:80–88

Goor DA, Lillehei CW, Rees R, Edwards JE (1970) Isolated ventricular septal defect. Development basis for various types

and presentation of classification. Chest 58:468–482

Greenwood RD, Sommer A, Rosenthal A, Craenen J, Nadas A (1977) Cardiovascular abnormalities in the Beckwith-Wiedemann syndrome. Am J Dis Child 131:293–294

Heath D, Edwards JE (1958) The pathology of hypertensive pulmonary vascular disease: A description of six grades of structural changes in the pulmonary arteries with special reference to congenital cardiac septal defects. Circulation 18:533–547

Jain V, Subramanian S, Lambert EC (1969) Concomitant development of infundibular pulmonary stenosis and spontaneous closure of ventricular septal defect. An unusual variant in the natural history of ventricular septal defect. Am J Cardiol 24:247–254

King DL, Steeg CN, Ellis K (1973) Visualization of ventricular septal defects by cardiac ultrasonography. Circulation 48:1215–1220

Kirklin JW, Appelbaum A, Bargeron LM Jr (1976) Primary repair versus banding for ventricular septal defects in infants. In: Langford Kidd BS, Rowe RD (eds). The child with congenital heart disease after surgery. Futura Publishing Co., Mount Kisco, NY, pp 3–9

Kirklin JW, Harshbarger HG, Donald DE, Edwards JE (1957) Surgical correction of ventricular septal defect: Anatomic and technical considerations. J Thorac Cardiovasc Surg 33:45–59

Lincoln C, Jamieson S, Joseph M, Shinebourne E, Anderson RH (1977) Transatrial repair of ventricular septal defects with reference to their anatomic classification. J Thorac Cardiovasc Surg 74:183–190

Maron BJ, Ferrans VJ, White RI Jr (1973) Unusual evolution of acquired infundibular stenosis in patients with ventricular septal defect. Clinical and morphologic observations. Circulation 48:1092–1103

Moncada R, Bicoff JP, Arcilla RA, Agustsson MH, Lendrum BL, Gasul BM (1963) Retrograde left ventricular angiocardiography in ventricular septal defects. Am J Cardiol 11:436–446

Riggs T, Mehta S, Hirschfeld S, Borkat G, Liebman J (1979) Ventricular septal defect in infancy. A combined vectocardiographic and echocardiographic study. Circulation 59:385–394

Santamaria H, Soto B, Ceballos R, Bargeron LM Jr, Coghlan HC, Kirklin JW (1983) Angiographic differentiation of types of ventricular septal defects. Am J Roentgenol 141:273–281

Soto B, Becker AE, Moulaert AJ, Lie JT, Anderson RH (1980) Classification of ventricular septal defects. Br Heart J 43:332–343

Spranger JW, Opitz JM, Bidder U (1971) Heterogeneity of chondrodysplasia punctata. Humangenetik 11:190–212

Stevenson JG, Kawabori I, Dooley TK, Guntheroth WG (1978) Diagnosis of ventricular septal defect by pulsed doppler echocardiography-sensitivity, specificity, limitations. Circulation 58:322–326

Subramanian S (1976) Ventricular septal defect: Problems of repair in infancy. In: Langford Kidd BS, Rowe RD (eds) The child with congenital heart disease after surgery. Futura Publishing Co., Mount Kisco, NY, pp 11–24

Valdes-Cruz LM, Pieroni DR, Roland JM, Shematek JP (1977) Recognition of residual postoperative shunts by contrast echocardiographic techniques. Circulation 55:148–152

Watson H, McArthur P, Somerville J, Ross D (1969) Spontaneous evolution of ventricular septal defect into isolated pulmonic stenosis. Lancet 2:1225–1228

Ventricular Septal Defect with Aortic Insufficiency

Aziz KV, Cole RB, Paul MH (1979) Echocardiographic features of supracristal ventricular septal defect with prolapsed aortic valve leaflet. Am J Cardiol 43:854–859

Girod DA, Raghib G, Adams P Jr, Anderson RC, Wang Y, Edwards JE (1966) Cardiac malformations associated with ventricular septal defect. Am J Cardiol 17:73–82

Karpawich PP, Duff DF, Mullins CE, Cooley DA, McNamara DG (1981) Ventricular septal defect with associated aortic valve insufficiency. Progression of insufficiency and operative results in young children. J Thorac Cardiovasc Surg 82:182–189

Mardelli TJ, Morganroth J, Naito M, Chen CC (1980) Cross-sectional echocardiographic detection of aortic valve prolapse. Am Heart J 100:295–301

Nadas AS, Thilenius OG, LaForge CG, Hauck AJ (1964) Ventricular septal defect with aortic regurgitation. Medical and pathological aspects. Circulation 29:862–873

Pugliese LP, Eufrate S (1980) Interventricular septal defect with aortic insufficiency—surgical considerations. Thorac Cardiovasc Surg 28:173–176

Sakakabara S, Konno S (1962) Congenital aneurysm of the sinus of Valsalva; anatomy and classification. Am Heart J 63:405–424

Somerville J, Brando A, Ross DN (1970) Aortic regurgitation with ventricular septal defect. Surgical management and clinical features. Circulation 41:317–330

Tatsuno K, Konno S, Ando M, Sakakibara S (1973) Pathogenetic mechanisms of prolapsing aortic valve and aortic regurgitation associated with ventricular septal defect. Anatomical, angiographic, and surgical considerations. Circulation 48:1028–1037

Taussig HB, Seaman SJH (1940) Severe aortic insufficiency in association with a congenital malformation of the heart of Eisenmenger type. Johns Hopkins Med J 66:156–165

Van Praagh R, McNamara JJ (1968) Anatomic types of ventricular septal defect with aortic insufficiency: Diagnostic and surgical considerations. Am Heart J 75:604–619

Patent Ductus Arteriosus

Abrams HL (1958) Persistence of fetal ductus function after birth. The ductus arteriosus as an avenue of escape. Circulation 18:206–226

Alzamora V, Rotta A, Battilana G, Abugattas R, Rubio C, Bouroncle J, Zapata C, Santa-Maria E, Binder T, Subiria R, Paredes D, Pando B, Graham GG (1953) On the possible influence of great altitudes on the determination of certain cardiovascular anomalies. Preliminary report. Pediatrics 12:259–262

Berdon WE, Baker DH, James LS (1965) The ductus bump. A transient physiologic mass in chest. Roentgenograms of newborn infants. Am J Roentgenol 95:91–98

Binet JF, Conso JF, Losay J, Narcy PH, Raynaud EJ, Beaufils FR, Dor C, Bruniaux J (1978) Ductus arteriosis sling: Report of a newly recognized anomaly and its surgical correction. Thorax 33:72–75

Bloom KR, Rodrigues L, Swan EM (1977) Echocardiographic evaluation of left-to-right shunt in ventricular septal defect and persistent ductus arteriosus. Br Heart J 39:260–265

Campbell M (1961) Place of maternal rubella in the aetiology of congenital heart disease. Br Med J 1:691–696

Castellanos A, Hernandez FA (1967) Size of ascending aorta in congenital cardiac lesions and other heart diseases. Acta Radiol 6:49–64

Clyman RI, Mauray F, Roman C, Rudolph AM, Heymann MA (1980) Circulating prostaglandin E_2 concentrations and patent ductus arteriosus in fetal and neonatal lambs. J Pediatr 97:455–461

Coggin CJ, Parker KR, Keith JD (1970) Natural history of isolated patent ductus arteriosus and the effect of surgical correction: Twenty years' experience at the Hospital for Sick Children, Toronto. Can Med Assoc J 102:718–720

Currarino G, Jackson JH Jr (1970) Calcification of the ductus arteriosus and ligamentum botalli. Radiology 94:139–142

Falcone MW, Perloff JK, Roberts WC (1972) Aneurysms of the non-patent ductus arteriosus. Am J Cardiol 29:422–426

Friedman WF, Hirschklau MJ, Printz MP, Pitlick PT, Kirkpatrick SE (1976) Pharmacologic closure of patent ductus arteriosus in the premature infant. N Engl J Med 295:526–529

Gittenberger-DeGroot AC, Van Ertbruggen I, Moulaert AJMG, Harinck E (1980) The ductus arteriosus in the preterm infant: Histologic and clinical observations. J Pediatr 96:88–93

Hallman GL, Rosenberg HS (1964) Bilateral patent ductus arteriosus: Case report. Angiology 15:140–144

Heiner DC, Nadas AS (1958) Patent ductus arteriosus in association with pulmonic stenosis. A report of 6 cases with additional noncardiac congenital anomalies. Circulation 17:232–242

Heitz F, Fouron JC, van Doesburg NH, Bard H, Teasdale F, Chessex P, Davignon A (1984) Value of systolic time intervals in the diagnosis of large patent ductus arteriosus in fluid-restricted and mechanically ventilated preterm infants. Pediatrics 74:1069–1074

Higgins CB, Rausch J, Friedman WF, Hirschklau MJ, Kirkpatrick SE, Goergen TG, Reinke RT (1977) Patent ductus arteriosus in preterm infants with idiopathic respiratory distress syndrome. Radiographic and echocardiographic evaluation. Radiology 124:189–196

Johnson GL, Breart GL, Gewitz MH, Brenner JI, Lang P, Dooley KJ, Ellison RC (1983) Echocardiographic characteristics of premature infants with patent ductus arteriosus. Pediatrics 72:864–871

Kirks DR, McCook TA, Serwer GA, Oldham HN Jr (1980) Aneurysm of the ductus arteriosus in the neonate. A J R 134:573–576

Pochaczevsky R, Dunst ME (1972) Coexistent pulmonary artery and aortic arch calcification. Its significance and association with patent ductus arteriosus. Am J Roentgenol 116:141–145

Porstmann W, Wierny L, Warnke H, Gerstberger G, Romaniuk PA (1971) Catheter closure of patent ductus arteriosus; 62 cases treated without thoracotomy. Radiol Clin North Am 9:203–218

Rudolph AM (1970) The changes in the circulation after birth. Their importance in congenital heart disease. Circulation 41:343–359

Sahn DJ, Vaucher Y, Williams DE, Allen HD, Goldberg SJ, Friedman WF (1976) Echocardiographic detection of large left to right shunts and cardiomyopathies in infants and children. Am J Cardiol 38:73–79

Sato K, Fujino M, Kozuka T, Naito Y, Kitamura S, Nakano S, Ohyama C, Kawashima Y (1975) Transfemoral plug closure of patent ductus arteriosus. Experience in 61 consecutive cases treated without thoracotomy. Circulation 51:337–341

Steinberg I (1963) Left-sided patent ductus arteriosus and right-sided aortic arch. Angiocardiographic findings in three cases. Circulation 28:1138

Steinberg I (1964) Roentgenography of patent ductus arteriosus. Am J Cardiol 13:698–707

Tutassaura H, Goldman B, Moes CAF Mustard WT (1969) Spontaneous aneurysm of the ductus arteriosus in childhood. J Thorac Cardiovasc Surg 57:180–184

Whitley JE, Rudhe U, Herzenberg H (1963) Decreased left lung vascularity in congenital left to right shunts. Acta Radiol 1:1125–1131

Williams B, Toong Ling JI, Leight L, McGaff CJ (1963) Patent ductus arteriosus and osteoarthropathy. Arch Intern Med 111:346–350

PFC Syndrome

Bauer CR, Tsipuras D, Fletcher BD (1974) Syndrome of persistent pulmonary vascular obstruction of the newborn: Roentgen findings. Am J Roentgenol 120:285–290

Burnell RH, Joseph MC, Lees MH (1972) Progressive pulmonary hypertension in newborn infants. Am J Dis Child 123:167–170

Gersony WM (1973) Persistence of the fetal circulation: A commentary. J Pediatr 82:1103–1106

Gersony WM, Duc GV, Sinclair JC (1969) "PFC" syndrome (Persistence of the fetal circulation). Circulation 40:III–87

Hirschfeld S, Meyer R, Schwartz DC, Korfhagen J, Kaplan S (1975) The echocardiographic assessment of pulmonary artery pressure and pulmonary vascular resistance. Circulation 52:642–650

Levin DL, Cates L, Newfeld EA, Muster AJ, Paul MH (1975) Persistence of the fetal cardiopulmonary circulatory pathway: Survival of an infant after a prolonged course. Pediatrics 56:58–63

Naeye RL, Shochat SJ, Whitman V, Maisels MJ (1976) Unsuspected pulmonary vascular abnormalities associated with diaphragmatic hernia. Pediatrics 58:902–906

Riggs T, Hirschfeld S, Fanaroff A, Liebman J, Fletcher B, Meyer R (1977) Persistence of fetal circulation syndrome: An echocardiographic study. J Pediatr 91:626–631

Siassi B, Goldberg SJ, Emmanouilides GC, Higashino SM, Lewis E (1971) Persistent pulmonary vascular obstruction in newborn infants. J Pediatr 78:610–615

Aortopulmonary Window

Agius PV, Rushworth A, Connolly N (1970) Anomalous origin of left coronary artery from pulmonary artery associated with an aortopulmonary septal defect. Br Heart J 32:708–710

Bellon EM, Borkat G, Whitman V, Perrin EV (1974) Unusual catheter course in aortic arch atresia associated with aortopulmonary window. Br J Radiol 47:144–146

Berry TE, Bharati S, Muster AJ, Idriss FS, Santucci B, Lev M, Paul MH (1982) Distal aortopulmonary septal defect, aortic origin of the right pulmonary artery, intact ventricular septum, patent ductus arteriosus and hypoplasia of the aortic isthmus: A newly recognized syndrome. Am J Cardiol 49:108–116

Coleman EN, Barclay RS, Reid JM, Stevenson JG (1967) Congenital aortopulmonary fistula combined with persistent ductus arteriosus. Br Heart J 29:571–576

Deverall PB, Lincoln JCR, Aberdeen E, Bonham-Carter RE, Waterston DJ (1969) Aortopulmonary window. J Thorac Cardiovasc Surg 57:479–486

Donaldson RM, Ballester M, Richards AF (1982) Diagnosis of aorticopulmonary window by two-dimensional echocardiography. Cathet Cardiovasc Diagn 8:185–189

Fisher EA, DuBrow IW, Eckner FAO, Hastreiter AR (1974) Aorticopulmonary septal defect and interrupted aortic arch: A diagnostic challenge. Am J Cardiol 34:356–359

Gula G, Chew C, Radley-Smith R, Yacouls M (1978) Anomalous origin of the right pulmonary artery from the ascending aorta associated with aortopulmonary window. Thorax 33:265–269

Hurwitz RA, Ruttenberg HD, Fonkalsrud E (1967) Aortopulmonary window, ventricular septal defect and mesoversion. Am J Cardiol 20:566–570

Ito K, Kohguchi N, Ohkawa Y, Akasaka T, Ohara H, Takarada M, Aoki H, Ogata M, Nishibatake M, Fukatsu O, Matsushima K (1977) Total one-stage repair of interrupted aortic arch associated with aortic septal defect and patent ductus arteriosus. J Thorac Cardiovasc Surg 74:913–917

Johansson L, Michaelsson M, Westerholm CJ, Aberg T (1978) Aortopulmonary window: A new operative approach. Ann Thorac Surg 25:564–567

Meisner H, Schmidt-Habelmann P, Sebering F, Klinner W (1968) Surgical correction of aorto-pulmonary septal defects. Dis Chest 58:750–758

Mori K, Ando M, Takao A, Ishikawa S, Imai Y (1978) Distal type of aortopulmonary window. Report of 4 cases. Br Heart J 40:681–689

Neufeld HN, Lester RG, Adams P, Anderson RC, Lillehei CW, Edwards JE (1962) Aorticopulmonary septal defect. Am J Cardiol 9:12–25

Parker BM, Burford TH, Carlsson EC, Buchner EF (1963) The diagnosis of aortico-pulmonary septal defect. Am Heart J 65:534–541

Rice MJ, Seward JB, Hagler DJ, Mair DD, Tajik AJ (1982) Visualization of aortopulmonary window by two-dimensional echocardiography. Mayo Clin Proc 57:482–487

Richardson JV, Doty DB, Rossi NP, Ehrenhaft JL (1979) The spectrum of anomalies of aortopulmonary septation. J Thorac Cardiovasc Surg 78:21–27

Rosenquist GC, Taylor JFN, Stark J (1974) Aortopulmonary fenestration and aortic atresia. Report of an infant with ventricular septal defect, persistent ductus arteriosus, and interrupted aortic arch. Br Heart J 36:1146–1148

Wright JS, Freeman R, Johnston JB (1968) Aortopulmonary fenestration. J Thorac Cardiovasc Surg 55:280–283

Chapter 7, Section 2
Admixture Lesions

An admixture lesion is one in which systemic venous blood and pulmonary venous blood are mixed, because all the blood flows through a single chamber (see Venous Admixture in the introduction to this chapter). Central to recognition on plain films is the presence of pulmonary overcirculation in a patient with cyanosis. The most common defects that produce this combination of features are dextrotransposition of the great vessels (D-TGA), atrioventricularis communis (A-V communis), single ventricle, some forms of double-outlet right ventricle, truncus arteriosus and total anomalous pulmonary venous return (Table 7–4). Although uncomplicated levotransposition of the great vessels (L-TGA) is not an admixture lesion, it is included here because it is a form of transposition of the great vessels. Total anomalous pulmonary venous drainage, a classic admixture lesion, has been described with partial anomalous pulmonary venous drainage (an atrial level left-to-right shunt) because they share embryological features. A-V communis, an admixture lesion that does not always result in cyanosis, has been included with ostium primum atrial septal defect, since both are forms of endocardial cushion defect. Tricuspid atresia with transposition of the great vessels is classified with other forms of tricuspid atresia in the section entitled "Right Heart Obstruction."

Transposition of the Great Arteries

Transposition of the great arteries is defined as discordance of the ventriculoarterial connections, that is, the aorta originates from the morphological (anatomical) right ventricle and the pulmonary artery from the morphological left ventricle. Normally in situs solitus (Fig. 7–65A) the aortic valve is posterior, inferior and right sided, while the pulmonary artery is anterior, superior and left sided. The aorta arises from the left ventricle and is in fibrous continuity with the mitral valve. (This normal anatomical relationship is called aortic-mitral fibrous continuity.) The pulmonary artery arises from the right ventricle and is separated from the tricuspid valve by conal musculature (crista supraventricularis). Thus the pulmonary valve in normal hearts has no fibrous continuity with the tricuspid valve. In hearts with abnormal relationships of the great arteries the conal musculature is called conus, and its position relative to the great arteries (subaortic or subpulmonic) is important to the description of these complex defects. Transposition of the great arteries is characterized by a reversal of the normal ventriculoarterial connections.

In the typical forms of transposition of the great vessels

Table 7–4. Admixture Lesions
(Increased Pulmonary Blood Flow with Cyanosis)

D-TGA with or without VSD
A-V communis (Atrioventricular canal)
Total anomalous pulmonary venous return (supradiaphragmatic)
Tricuspid atresia with transposition of the great vessels
Truncus arteriosus communis without pulmonic stenosis
Single ventricle without pulmonic stenosis
Double-outlet right ventricle with subpulmonary VSD (Taussig Bing)
Criss-cross heart

the aorta arises above the morphological right ventricle and is separated from the tricuspid valve by the conus. Thus the aorta has no fibrous continuity to the atrioventricular valve (aortic-tricuspid discontinuity). On the other hand, the pulmonary artery arises above the morphological left ventricle, and in the absence of conus the pulmonary valve is in fibrous continuity with the mitral valve (pulmonary-mitral fibrous continuity). Depending on the location of the aorta (left or right sided), transposition of the great arteries in situs solitus may be divided into two principal groups: dextrotransposition of the great arteries (D-TGA) (Fig. 7–65B) and levotransposition of the great arteries (L-TGA) (Fig. 7–65D). Some rarely encountered variants of transposition do not conform strictly to these patterns. These include criss-cross heart (see p. 425) and atypical dextrotransposition of the great arteries (Fig. 7–65C). Also described in this section is an entity known as ventricular inversion without transposition of the great arteries (isolated ventricular inversion) (Fig. 7–65E). The great vessels are usually transposed in patients with single ventricle. This entity is discussed separately. The descriptions in this section assume the presence of situs solitus unless specified otherwise. Situs solitus refers to the fact that the anatomical right atrium is on the right side and the left atrium is on the left.

The loop rule of Van Praagh is often used to aid in predicting the locations of the ventricles and the great arteries in transposition complexes. The loop rule states that the great vessel orientation (D or L) is usually the same as the ventricular loop (D or L). Thus, in individuals with right-sided aortic valve (normal and D-TGA), the ventricles are in D-loop (the right ventricle is on the right). On the other hand, in individuals with left-sided aortic valve (situs inversus and L-TGA), the anatomical right ventricle should be on the left (L-loop).

Fig. 7–65. *The normal heart and four types of transposition of the great vessels.* **A** represents a normal heart in situs solitus, a term that indicates that the right atrium is on the right side and the left atrium is on the left side. In the normal heart, concordance exists among the atria, the ventricles and the great arteries, indicating that the right and left atria are connected to the right and left ventricle respectively, and that the aorta arises from the morphological left ventricle and the pulmonary artery arises from the right ventricle. The aortic valve and the mitral valve are in fibrous continuity (aortic-mitral fibrous continuity). The pulmonary valve is separated from the tricuspid valve by the crista supraventricularis* (pulmonary-tricuspid discontinuity).

B represents dextrotransposition of the great vessels (D-TGA) in situs solitus. Atrioventricular concordance is present; however, the connections of the great arteries are reversed (ventriculoarterial discordance). This means that the aorta arises from the right ventricle and the pulmonary artery from the left ventricle. Conal muscle (conus)* is present within the right ventricle, separating the aorta from the tricuspid valve (aortic-tricuspid discontinuity). Conus is absent from the left ventricle, and pulmonary-mitral fibrous continuity exists.

C represents a rare form of dextrotransposition of the great vessels (D-TGA) called atypical D-TGA. The connections are the same as in **B,** and the patients are cyanotic; however, conus within the left ventricle separates the pulmonary valve from the mitral valve (pulmonary-mitral discontinuity). The pulmonary valve is elevated and displaced anteriorly by the subpulmonic conus, producing an almost normal external appearance of the heart. The pulmonary artery arises anterior, superior and to the left of the aorta. Conus is not present within the right ventricle, and therefore fibrous continuity exists between the aortic and tricuspid valves.

D represents levotransposition of the great vessels (L-TGA) in situs solitus—It is called corrected transposition because the connections do not result in cyanosis. Atrioventricular discordance (A-V discordance) as well as ventriculoarterial discordance (V-A discordance) exist. A-V discordance indicates that the ventricles are inverted with the morphological left ventricle being connected to the right atrium, while the right ventricle is connected to the left atrium. V-A discordance indicates that the aorta arises from the morphological right ventricle, while the pulmonary artery arises from the left ventricle. Pulmonary-mitral fibrous continuity exists unless a bilateral conus is present. The conus within the right ventricle separates the aortic valve from the tricuspid valve and elevates the aortic valve, displacing it anteriorly. Thus the aortic valve is superior, anterior and to the left of the pulmonary valve.

E represents another rare form called isolated ventricular inversion. Atrioventricular discordance exists with ventriculoarterial concordance. In other words, the left ventricle is connected to the right atrium and the right ventricle to the left atrium, while the aorta arises above the morphological left ventricle and the pulmonary artery above the right ventricle. The conus within the morphological right ventricle separates the pulmonary valve from the tricuspid valve, elevates it and displaces it anteriorly. Again the external appearance of the heart is almost normal (the pulmonary valve is superior, anterior and to the left); however, the pulmonary and systemic circulations are in parallel as in D-TGA, resulting in cyanosis.

RA = right atrium; *LA* = left atrium; *RV* = right ventricle; *LV* = left ventricle; *Ao* = aortic valve; *PA* = pulmonary valve.

* Conal muscle or conal musculature represents the muscle of the conus septum. In normal hearts the crista supraventricularis is the part of the conus septum that separates the pulmonary valve from the tricuspid valve. In complex congenital heart defects (e.g., transpositions), muscle separating a semilunar valve from an atrioventricular valve is called conus. Some authors have used the word *conus* to refer to the infundibulum or outflow tract of the right ventricle. In this text, *conus* refers to the muscle itself, rather than to the lumen of the right ventricular outflow tract. In these diagrams the conus is represented by a kidney-shaped structure partly surrounding one of the semilunar valves. This shape bears no relationship to the anatomical or angiographic appearance of the conus.

Dextrotransposition of the Great Arteries

In this type of transposition the aortic valve is anterior and right sided. D-loop, atrioventricular concordance and ventriculoarterial discordance are present. D-loop indicates that the morphological right ventricle (RV) is right sided. Atrioventricular concordance signifies that the RV is connected to the right atrium (RA) and the left ventricle (LV) to the left atrium (LA). Ventriculoarterial discordance indicates that the aorta arises above the RV and the pulmonary artery originates above the LV. Interposition of the subaortic conus (conal musculature) results in fibrous discontinuity between the aortic valve and the tricuspid valve. Pulmonary–mitral valve fibrous continuity is present because conus is not present within the LV. The aortic valve is anterior, superior and to the right while the pulmonary valve is posterior, inferior and to the left. The transposed aorta gives rise to the coronary ostia. The right coronary artery (RCA) usually originates from the posterior cusp and the left coronary artery (LCA) from the anterior cusp. The left circumflex artery may branch off from the RCA. Rarely the origin of the RCA may be anterior and that of the LCA posterior. Other unusual coronary artery patterns have been described, including single coronary artery and absence of the left circumflex artery.

Defects frequently found in association with D-TGA include ostium secundum atrial septal defect (ASD), dilated foramen ovale, ventricular septal defect (VSD) and patent ductus arteriosus (PDA). Rarely a LV-RA communication is associated. A PDA is present in at least 50% of newborns with D-TGA, but the ductus tends to close within the first weeks of life. Obstruction to the LV outflow (pulmonic stenosis) is not uncommon (approximately 40%), usually resulting from membranous or fibromuscular subpulmonary stenosis. Other causes of pulmonic obstruction include pulmonary valvar stenosis (unicuspid valve), anomalous attachment of the mitral valve (anterior leaflet) to the ventricular septum at the LV outlet (with or without parachute deformity), accessory mitral or pulmonary valve tissue, or both, and protrusion of the septal leaflet of the tricuspid valve through a VSD. On occasion an aneurysm of the membranous septum may bulge into the LV outflow tract. Less commonly, the obstruction to pulmonary blood flow is due to interposition of a muscular segment (LV conus) between the pulmonary and mitral valves (atypical D-TGA). Other complicating malformations include stenosis or atresia of the tricuspid or mitral valve, atrioventricular canal and coarctation of the aorta.

Pathophysiology During fetal life, oxygenated blood enters

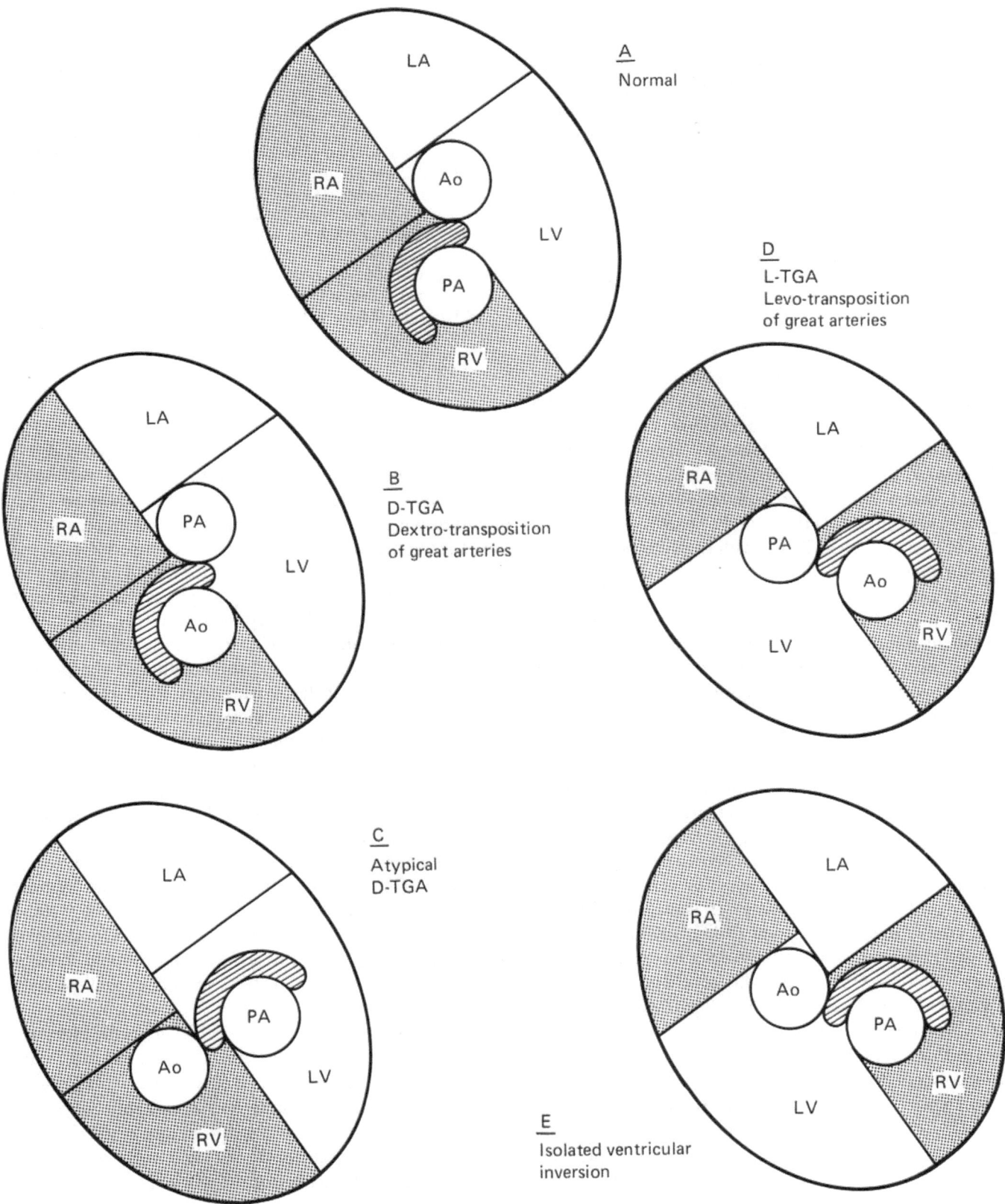

the circulation via the inferior vena cava; part of it crosses the foramen ovale. Thus both circulations receive oxygenated blood. Growth of the fetus is normal. Shortly after birth of an infant with D-TGA the fetal communications tend to close, and the aorta receives systemic venous blood exclusively while the pulmonary artery receives the pulmonary venous blood. Thus the two circulations are in parallel, and a communication is needed for interchange between them. Of the possible communications, an ASD is preferable, because it allows free mixing between the two circulations. Pulmonary venous hypertension is less severe in babies with ASD than in individuals with competent foramen ovale. In infants with intact ventricular septum the ASD results in higher oxygen saturation (due to mixing between the systemic venous and pulmonary venous blood), without a marked increase in pulmonary blood flow or pulmonary pressure. In infants with D-TGA and VSD, in whom the principal clinical feature is heart failure, the presence of an associated ASD results in lower left atrial pressure and a decrease in the severity of heart failure.

Clinical Features Male predominance is reported, in an approximate ratio of 3:1. A family history of diabetes is frequently encountered. Babies with transposition are often large for their gestational age.

Infants with an intact ventricular septum or with a small VSD are markedly cyanotic from birth (the foramen ovale and ductus arteriosus tend to close rapidly). Cyanosis, tachypnea, and hepatomegaly (indicating hypoxia and heart failure) appear within days. Acidosis signals a rapid downhill course.

In the presence of a VSD the predominant clinical feature is congestive heart failure, with mild or minimal cyanosis. This group of infants and those with a large PDA have the worst prognosis if surgical therapy is not instituted promptly. Infants surviving with a large VSD or PDA and pulmonary hypertension are likely to develop irreversible changes due to pulmonary hypertension (Eisenmenger physiology) by the age of 2 years. In some, these changes begin even within the first year of life. Infants with VSD and mild to moderate pulmonic stenosis have the best prognosis without surgery. D-TGA with severe pulmonic stenosis and VSD produces a picture resembling tetralogy of Fallot. The predominant features are early and severe cyanosis with decreased pulmonary blood flow.

Echocardiography The characteristic feature of D-TGA is the anterior, superior, right-sided position of the aortic valve (Fig. 7-66A). If the anterior great vessel is found on the right by M-mode in a cyanotic baby with situs solitus, D-TGA is strongly suspected. The pulmonary valve is to the left, posterior and inferior (Fig. 7-66B). Fibrous continuity between the pulmonary valve and the mitral valve is observed in uncomplicated D-TGA (Fig. 7-67).

In an infant whose aortic valve is directly anterior to the pulmonary valve, comparison of the systolic time intervals of the two valves can distinguish the aortic valve from the pulmonary valve (Fig. 7-66). The valve that shows a longer pre-ejection period and shorter ventricular ejection

Fig. 7-66. *Dextrotransposition of the great vessels* (D-TGA). M-mode echocardiograms through (A) the aortic valve (Ao.V) and (B) the pulmonary valve (PV). The time lines are 10 msec apart. The operator has indicated that the anterior semilunar valve (A) is toward the right and superior, while the posterior semilunar valve (B) is toward the left and inferior. The right ventricular preejection period (RPEP) is 70 msec, and the right ventricular ejection time (RVET) is 150 msec. The left ventricular preejection period (LPEP) is 55 msec and the left ventricular ejection time (LVET) is 180 msec. The RPEP is longer than the LPEP, and the RVET is shorter than the LVET. These are the reverse of normal, indicating that the aortic valve arises from the right ventricle while the pulmonic valve arises from the left ventricle. These systolic time intervals along with the relative positions of the semilunar valves represent strong evidence for D-TGA.

RA = right atrium; RVOT = right ventricular outflow tract; LA = left atrium.

time is the aortic valve. On 2-D echocardiography a rightward anterior vessel and a leftward posterior vessel are identified on the short axis at the base of the heart (Fig. 7-68). If the transducer is rotated 90 degrees the ascending aorta is imaged in the long axis as it arcs superiorly, giving off the brachiocephalic vessels (Fig. 7-69). The main pulmonary artery curves posteriorly as it arises from the heart and gives off the pulmonary branches (Fig. 7-69). As reported by Bierman and Williams, the subxiphoid transverse view shows a dramatic presentation of the pulmonary artery and branches arising from the LV, almost as they appear on left ventriculography in the RAO view (Fig. 7-70A). The subxiphoid transverse view shows the aorta arising from the RV (Fig. 7-70C). The aorta may be followed to the transverse arch. If a VSD is present the defect may be visualized by 2-D echocardiography on long-axis and four-chamber views.

Subpulmonic stenosis is suggested by a narrow LV outflow tract (Fig. 7-71A), marked flutter or mid systolic closure of the pulmonary valve and on occasion by systolic anterior motion of the mitral valve (Fig. 7-72). Doppler echocardiography from the apex window should demonstrate the site of stenosis (valvar, subvalvar) and estimate its severity.

During follow-up prior to surgical repair, serial measurements of pulmonary systolic time intervals can aid in detecting changes in pulmonary vascular resistance. Hirshfeld et al. have reported the normal values and anticipated values in infants with D-TGA and low pulmonary resistance. Progressive prolongation of the left ventricular pre-ejection period (LPEP), shortening of the left ventricular ejection time (LVET) or increase in LPEP/LVET suggests increasing pulmonary vascular resistance. After balloon atrial septostomy or surgical septectomy, defects in the atrial septum are imaged best in the subxiphoid view (Fig. 7-73). After surgical repairs at the atrial level the baffles can be recognized within the atrial cavity (see Fig. 7-85D-I). Caval obstruction is indicated by dilatation of the superior vena cava (SVC) or inferior vena cava (IVC) or by delayed ap-

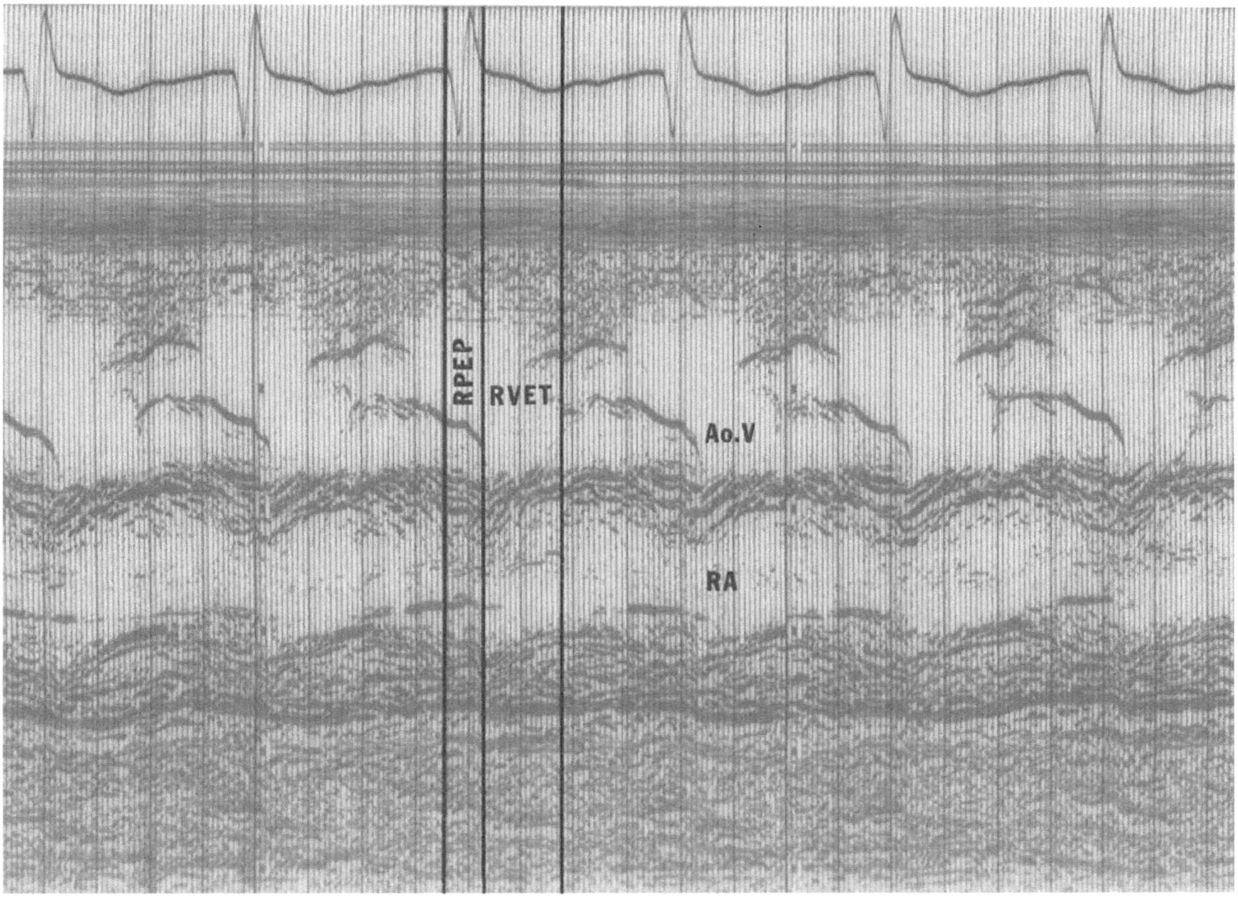

A

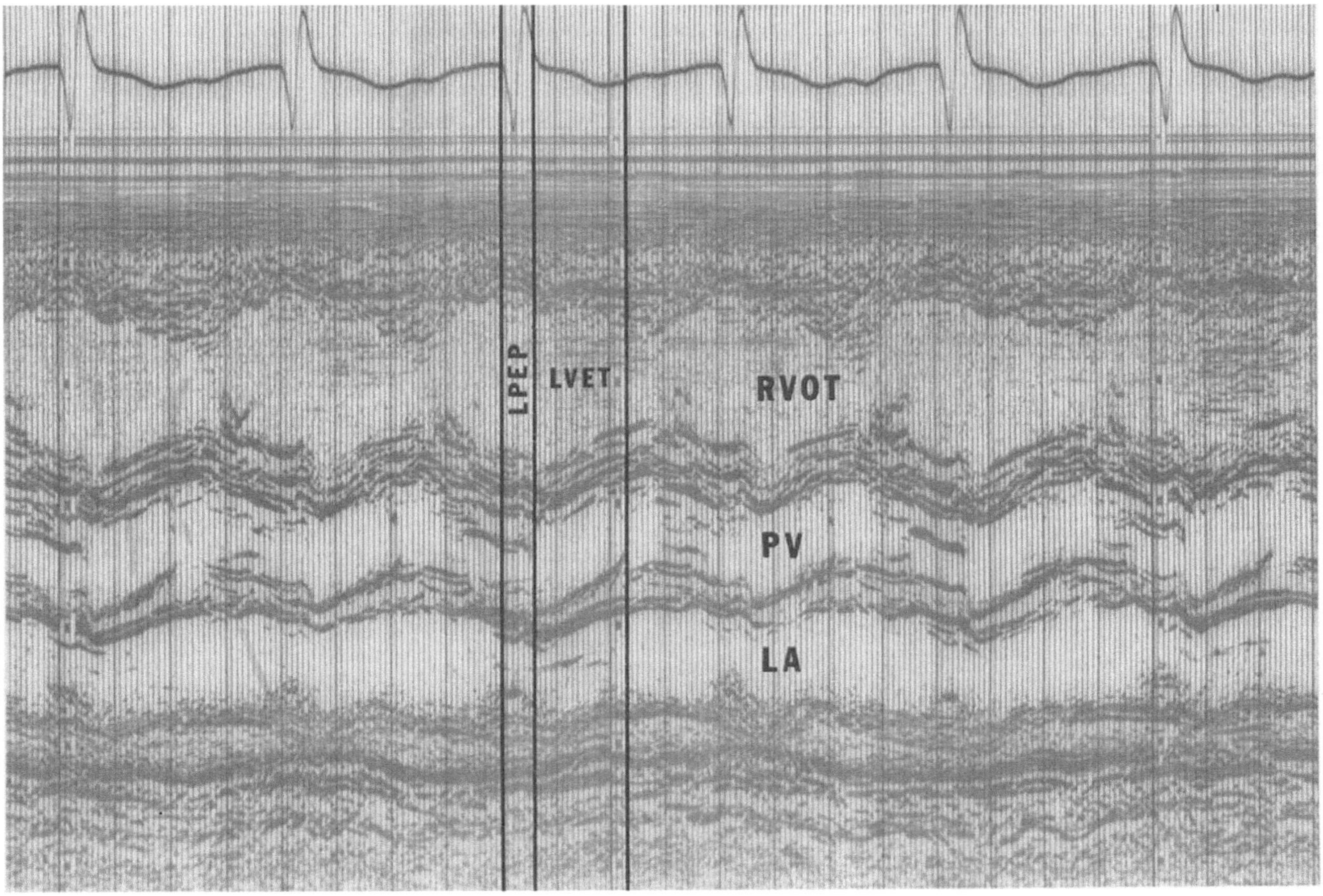

B

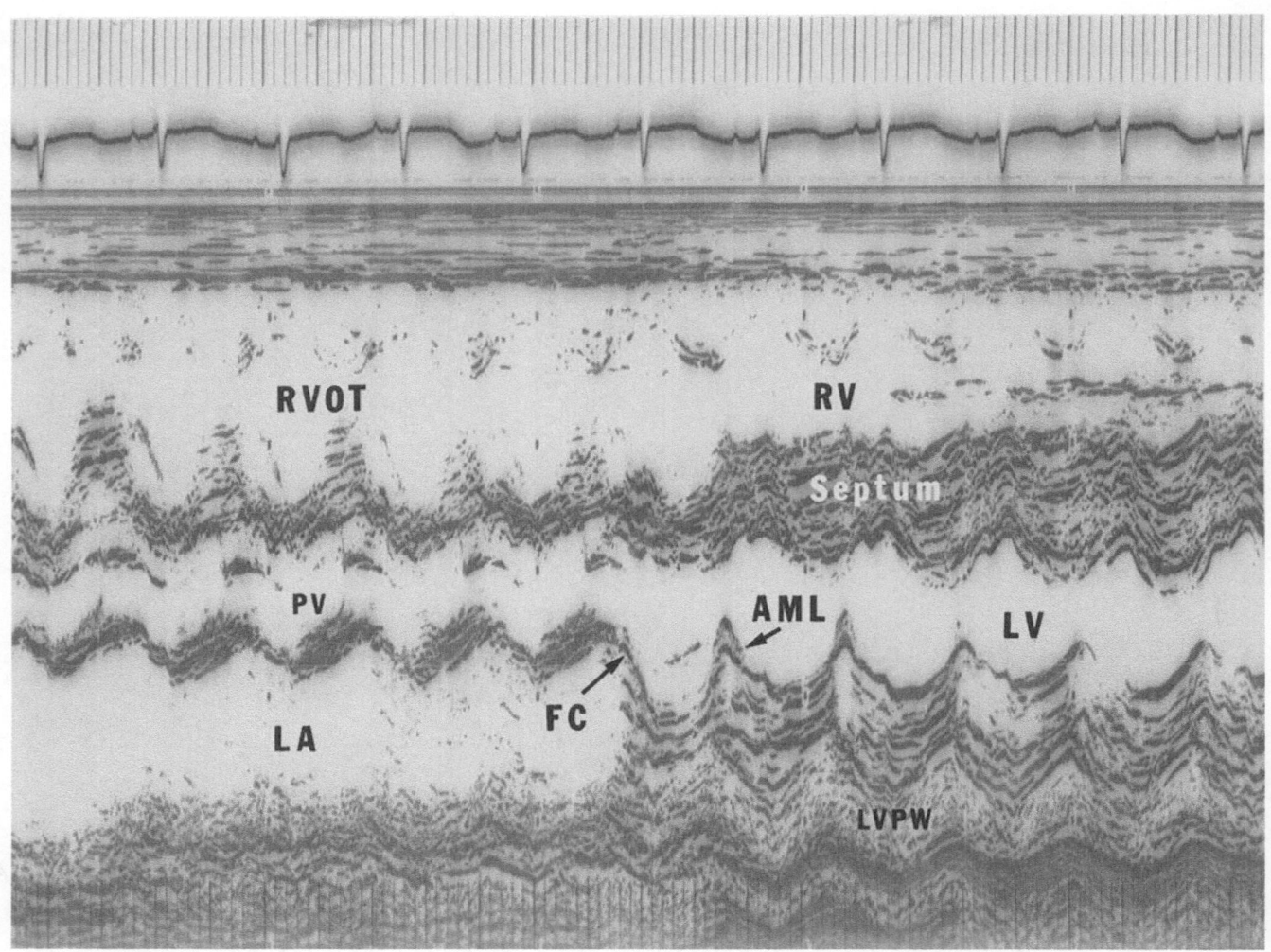

Fig. 7–67. *Pulmonary-mitral fibrous continuity in dextrotransposition of the great arteries* (D-TGA). An arc scan from the pulmonary valve (*PV*) through the left ventricular outflow tract into the left ventricle (*LV*) indicates that the pulmonary valve is in fibrous continuity (*FC*) with the anterior leaflet of the mitral valve (*AML*). This arc scan looks exactly like an arc scan through the left ventricular outflow tract in a normal baby. The diagnosis of D-TGA is made by determining that this semilunar valve is posterior (further from the transducer) and to the left, while the other semilunar valve (the aortic valve) is identified anterior (closer to the transducer) and toward the right. Systolic time intervals are confirmatory (see Fig. 7–66).

LA = left atrium; *LVPW* = posterior wall of the left ventricle; *RV* = right ventricle; *RVOT* = right ventricular outflow tract.

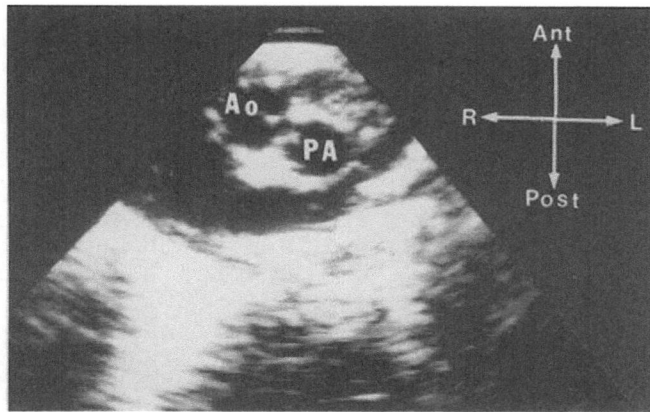
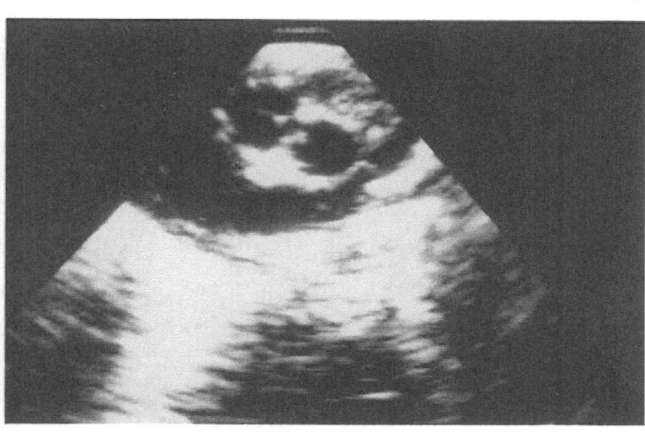

Fig. 7–68 *Parasternal short axis view of a two-dimensional echocardiogram in an infant with D-TGA.* **A** *with labels;* **B** *without labels. The anterior great vessel is on the right* (*Ao*) *and the posterior great vessel is on the left* (*PA*). *This great vessel orientation is consistent with dextrotransposition of the great vessels.*

The space behind the great vessels represents the atria. No echoes of atrial septum are present, a finding that may be due to technique rather than due to absence of the atrial septum. *Ao* = aorta; *PA* = pulmonary artery.

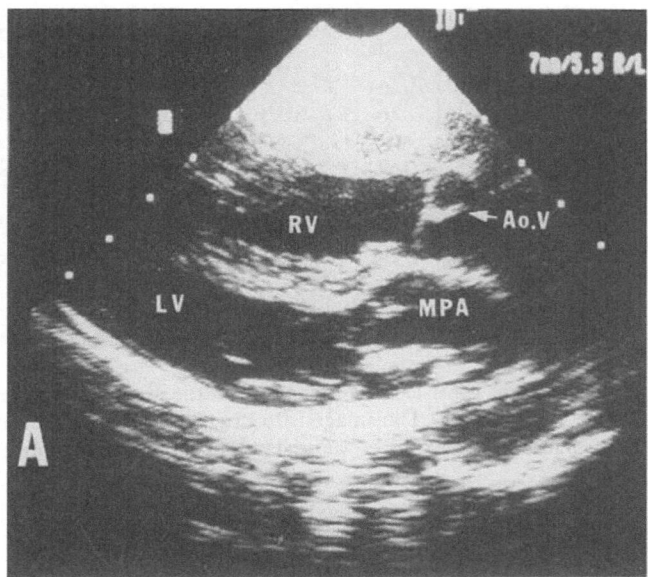
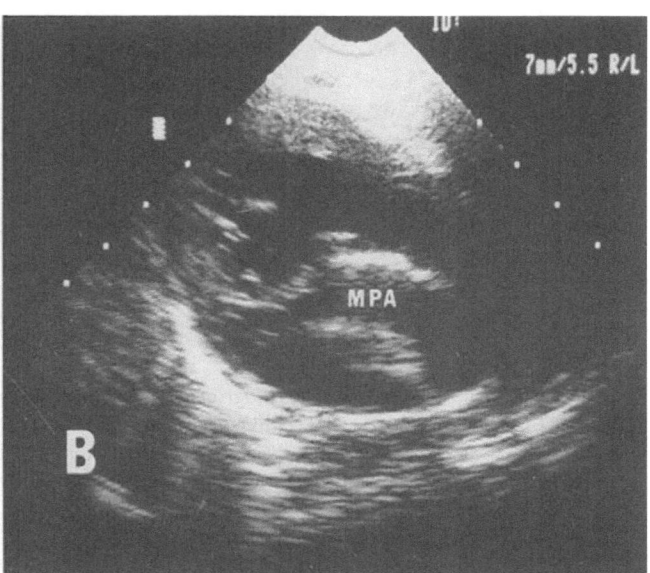

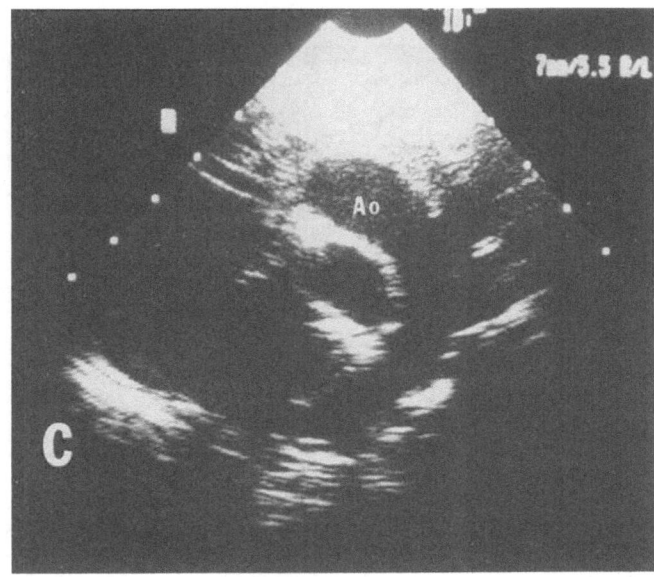

Fig. 7–69. *The characteristic appearance of the great arteries in the long axis view in a patient with D-TGA. In* **A** *the main pulmonary artery* (*MPA*) *arises above the left ventricle* (*LV*) *and curves immediately posteriorly to give off the pulmonary branches. The aortic valve* (*Ao.V*) *is also identified above the right ventricle* (*RV*) *and is anterior and superior to the pulmonary valve. In* **B** *the curvature of the MPA is outlined more completely than in* **A.** *In* **C** *the aorta* (*Ao.*) *forms a broad arch as it curves posteriorly.*

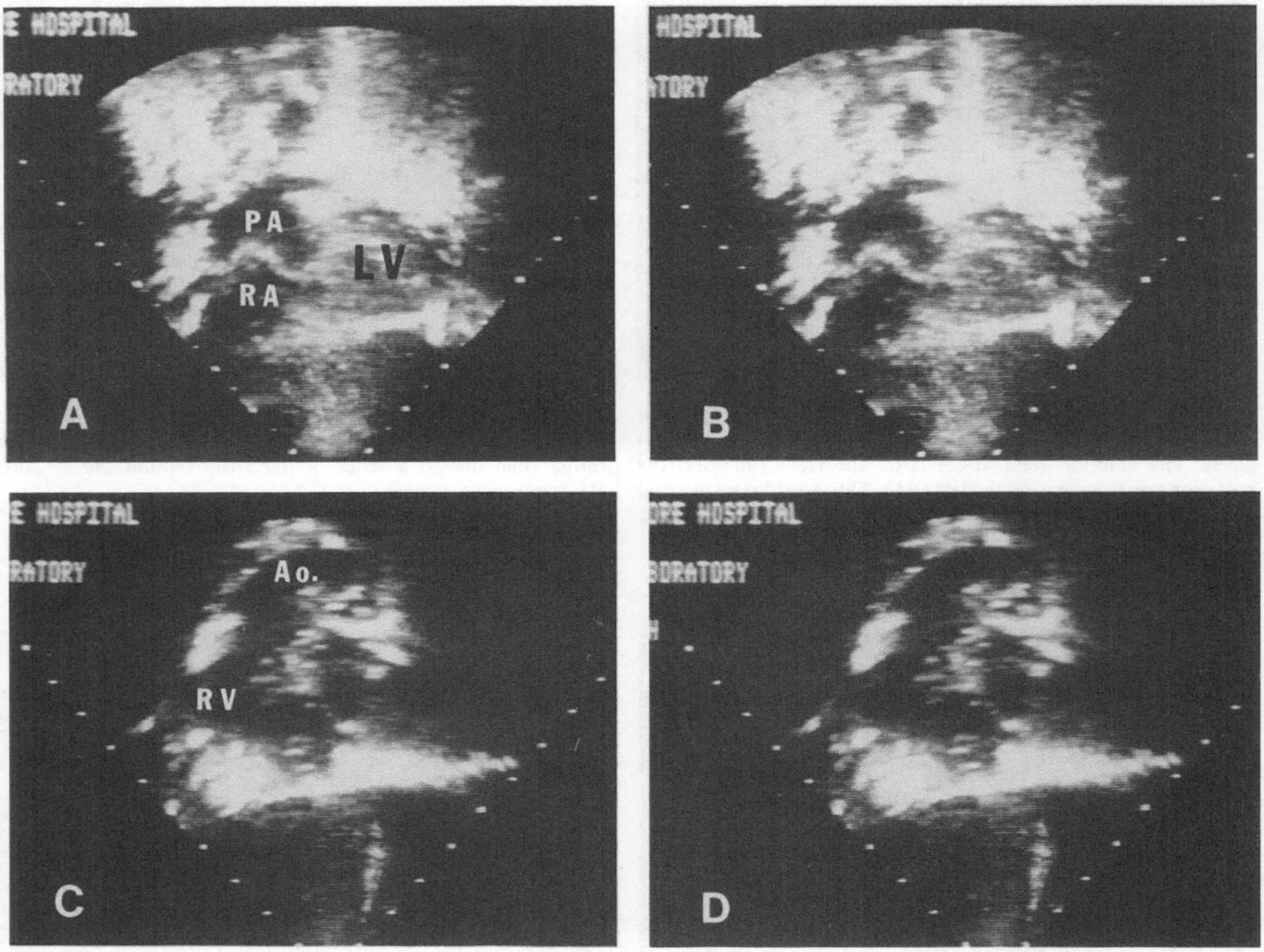

Fig. 7–70. *Two-dimensional echocardiogram (subxiphoid transverse view) in D-TGA.* In **A** and **B** the pulmonary artery (*PA*), identified because of its two branches, arises from the left ventricle (*LV*). In **C** and **D** the transducer is angled anteriorly to demonstrate the right ventricle (*RV*) from which the aorta (*Ao.*) arises. *RA* = right atrium. The images are oriented so that the heart is upright as if the subject were standing facing the examiner.

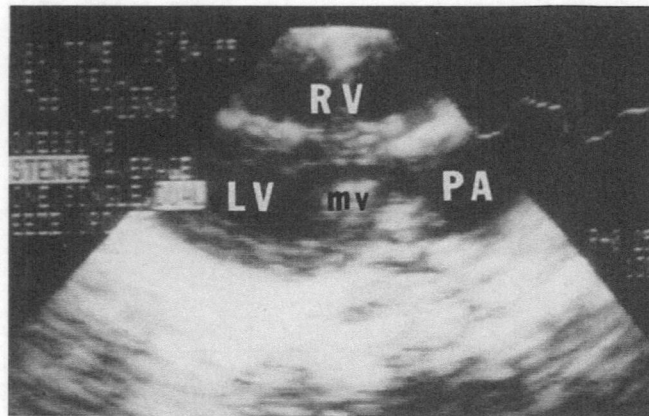
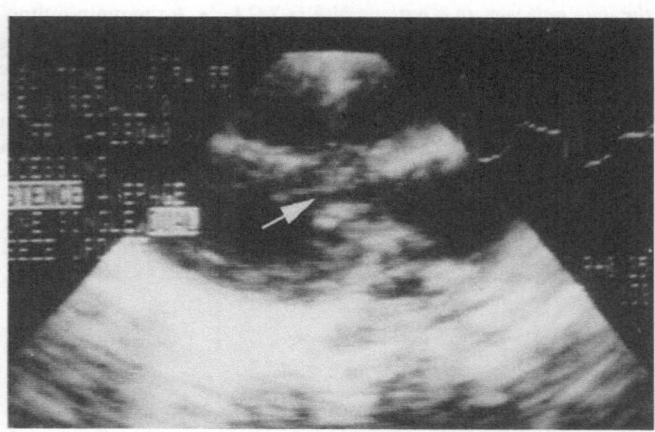

Fig. 7–71. *Left ventricular outflow tract obstruction in D-TGA.* A parasternal long axis view of the left ventricle (*LV*) shows narrowing of the left ventricular outflow tract (*arrow*) because of fibrous tissue attached to the septum and to the anterior leaflet of the mitral valve (*mv*). The left atrium is not identified behind the pulmonary artery. *RV* = right ventricle; *PA* = main pulmonary artery.

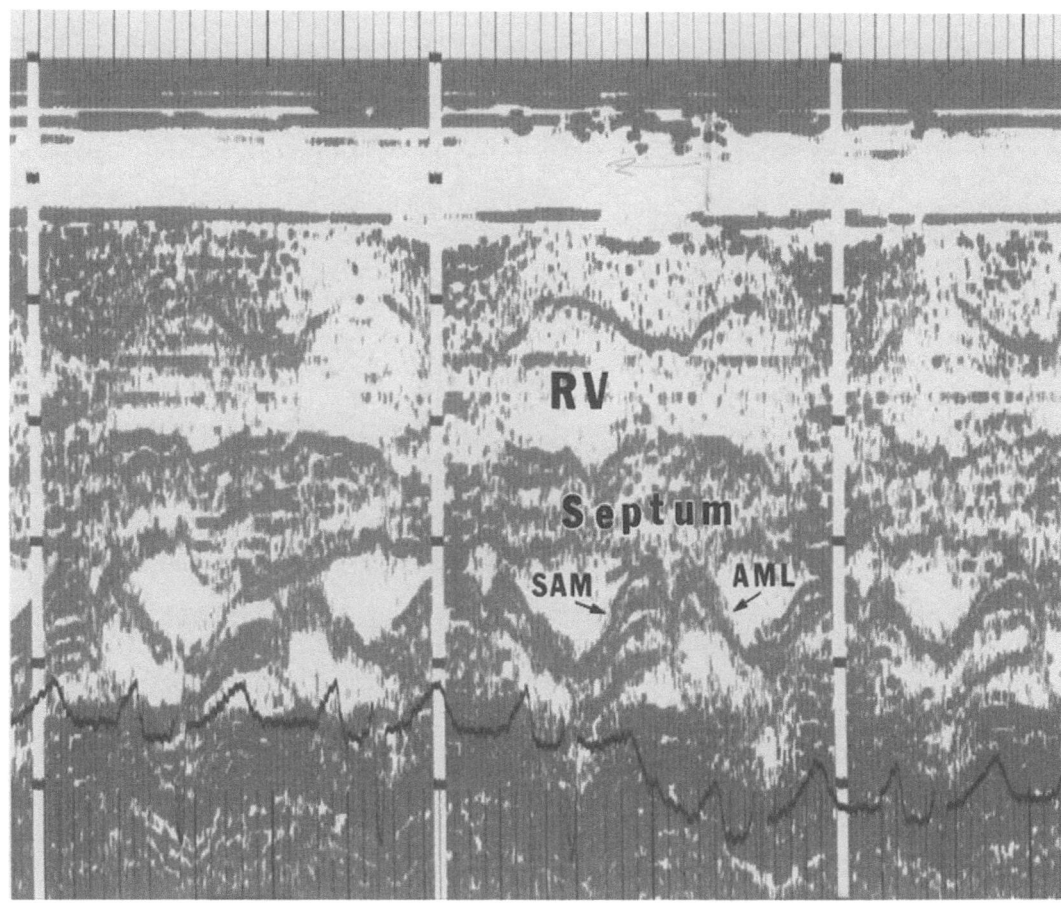

A

Fig. 7–72. A *Left ventricular outflow tract obstruction in D-TGA.* This M-mode echocardiogram shows systolic anterior motion (*SAM*) of the anterior leaflet of the mitral valve similar to that occurring with hypertrophic obstructive cardiomyopathy (HOCM). The normal diastolic opening motion of the anterior mitral leaflet (*AML*) occurs immediately after the SAM. In this instance, septal thickening is due to right ventricular hypertrophy rather than left ventricular hypertrophy. The pathological features of the obstruction are different from those of HOCM. With D-TGA a fibrous subpulmonic membrane or tunnel narrows the left ventricular outflow tract, whereas with HOCM the massively hypertrophied septum bulges into the left ventricular outflow tract. (*Continued*)

pearance or absence of contrast material in the systemic venous atrium after peripheral injection during ultrasonography. Doppler echocardiography is helpful in identifying presence or absence of flow in the SVC if that vessel is occluded or high velocity in the SVC or IVC if either is partly obstructed (see Fig. 7–85G).

Radiological (Plain Film) Features The radiological appearance in D-TGA shows a wide variation in the size of the heart and in the appearance of the pulmonary vasculature. The typical plain film findings of D-TGA occur in individuals with no pulmonary stenosis and relatively low pulmonary vascular resistance. The heart may be normal in size at birth, but it usually enlarges by the age of 2 months. An egg-shaped heart with a narrow vascular pedicle and pulmonary overcirculation is often considered classic for D-TGA (Fig. 7–74). The pulmonary artery segment is absent, because the pulmonary artery is situated more toward the midline, behind the aorta. The vascular pedicle in the LAO or lateral projections is wider than normal. The aortic arch is nearly always left sided. A right aortic arch suggests associated pulmonic stenosis. If the ascending aorta can be identified in instances of D-TGA, its curve is convex toward the right, similar to normal. If the ascending aorta curves toward the left side, L-TGA

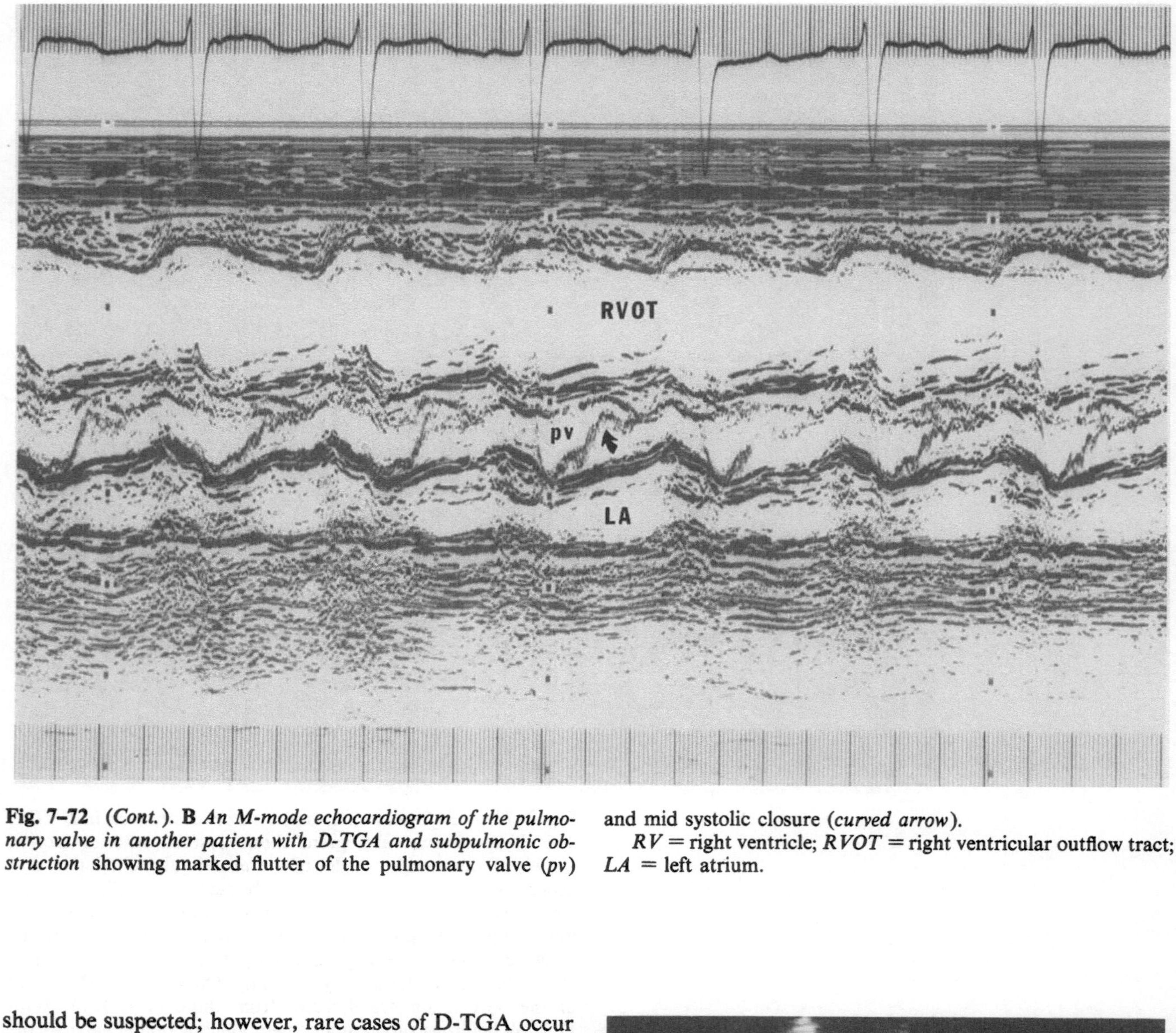

RVOT

pv

LA

B

Fig. 7–72 (Cont.). **B** *An M-mode echocardiogram of the pulmonary valve in another patient with D-TGA and subpulmonic obstruction* showing marked flutter of the pulmonary valve (pv) and mid systolic closure (*curved arrow*).

RV = right ventricle; $RVOT$ = right ventricular outflow tract; LA = left atrium.

should be suspected; however, rare cases of D-TGA occur with the aorta curving toward the left (Fig. 7–75). A markedly narrowed vascular pedicle is observed if the aorta ascends at the midline with no rightward or leftward curvature. A midline ascending aorta is occasionally present in normal infants.

The appearance of the pulmonary vasculature depends primarily on the pulmonary vascular resistance. Thus normal vasculature or the pattern of undercirculation is often present in the newborn (Fig. 7–76). Either set of findings will progress to overcirculation as resistance falls. In infants with pulmonic stenosis, pulmonary undercirculation will persist (Fig. 7–77). In many instances the configuration of the heart is nonspecific (Fig. 7–78); nevertheless the features of cardiomegaly and pulmonary overcirculation in a cyanotic baby should lead to suspicion of the presence of D-TGA. High left atrial and pulmonary venous pressures in infants with heart failure result in superimposition of the radiological pattern of pulmonary venous hypertension. This occurs especially in infants with large PDA or VSD. Signs of increased pulmonary vascular resistance

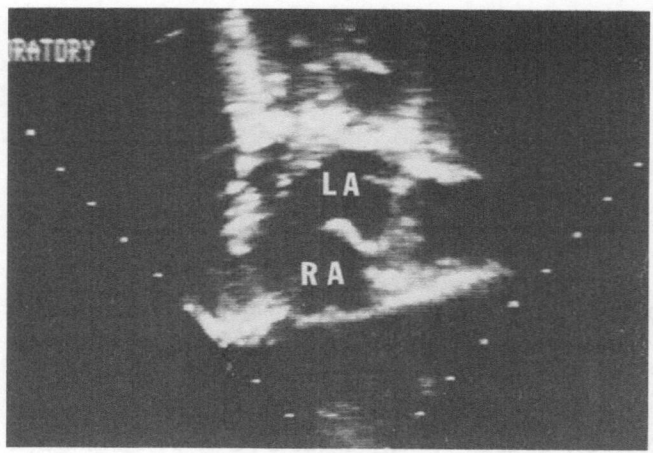

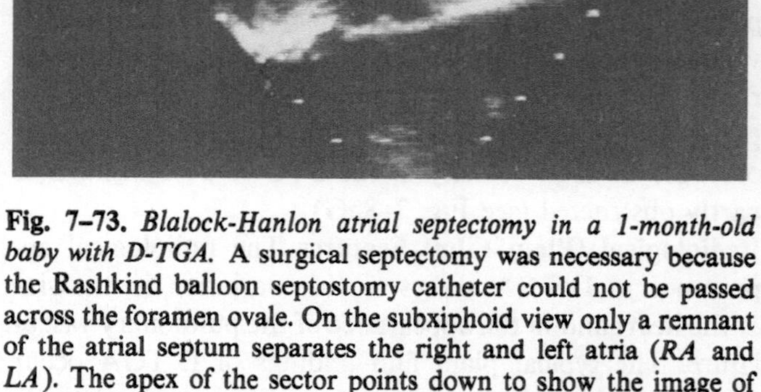

Fig. 7–73. *Blalock-Hanlon atrial septectomy in a 1-month-old baby with D-TGA.* A surgical septectomy was necessary because the Rashkind balloon septostomy catheter could not be passed across the foramen ovale. On the subxiphoid view only a remnant of the atrial septum separates the right and left atria (*RA* and *LA*). The apex of the sector points down to show the image of the heart upright, as if the baby were standing opposite the observer. (Same patient as in Fig. 7–70.)

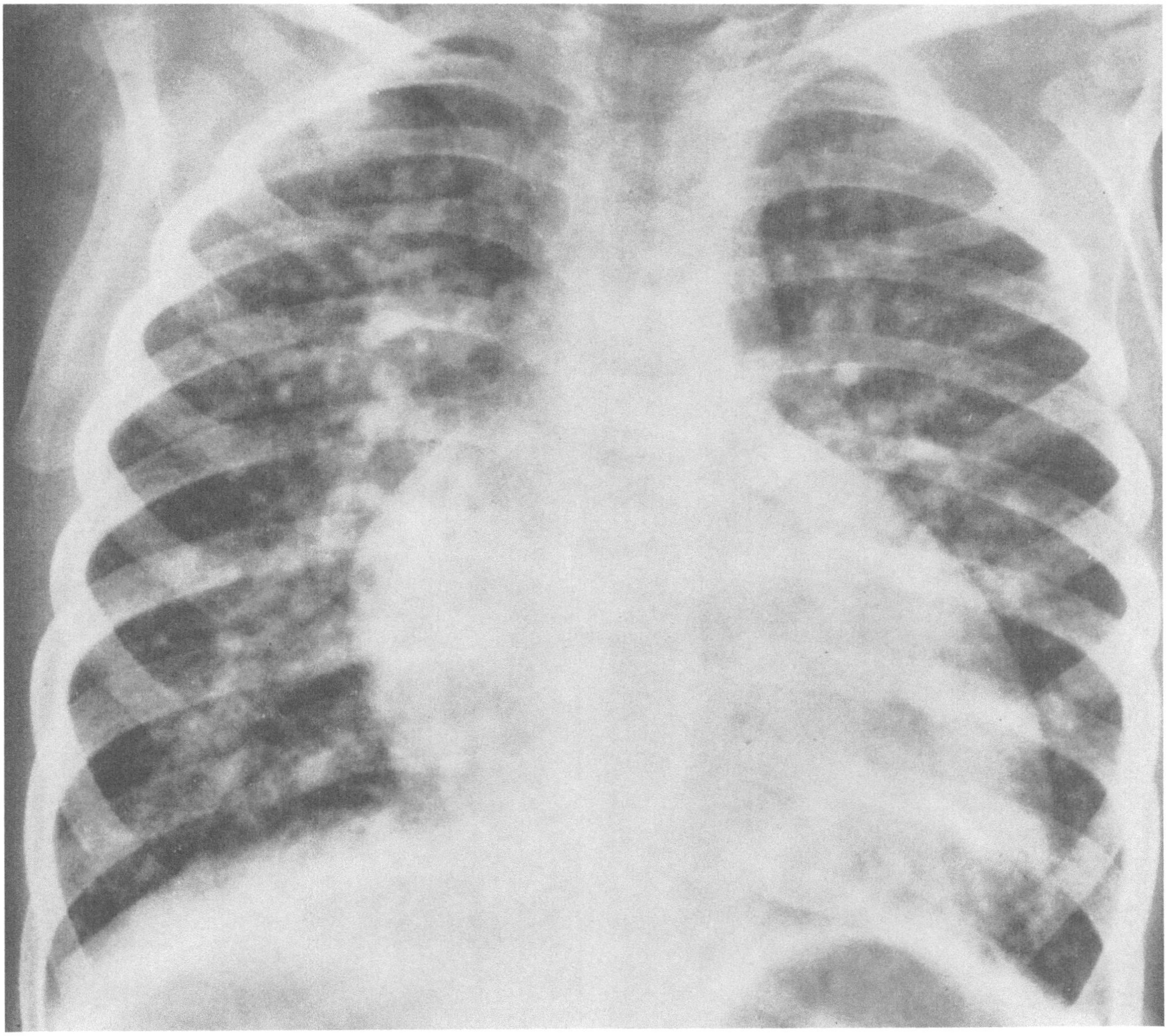

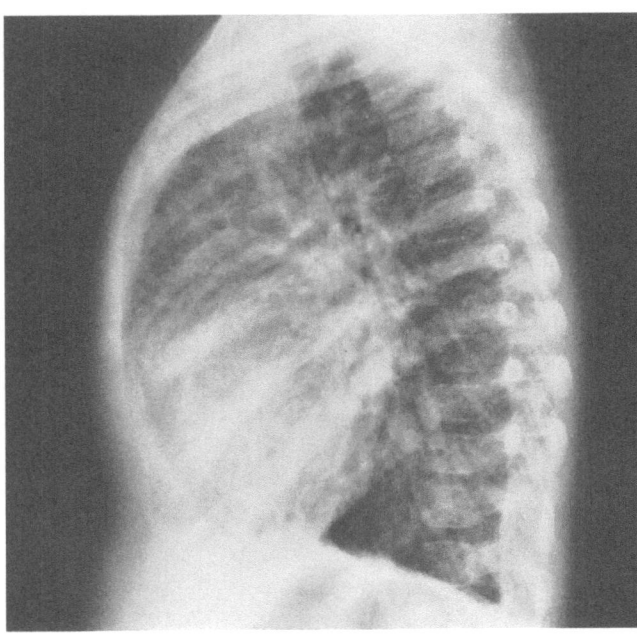

A

B

Fig. 7–74. *The characteristic plain film findings of D-TGA* consist of pulmonary overcirculation, an egg-shaped heart and a narrow vascular pedicle. Such radiological features occur only in patients without pulmonic stenosis and without increase in pulmonary vascular resistance. These roentgenograms of the chest are from a 1½-year-old boy with D-TGA, without pulmonic stenosis and with normal pulmonary vascular resistance. A balloon septostomy had been performed in the newborn period.

On the PA film (**A**) pulmonary overcirculation is present. The heart is enlarged, predominantly right ventricular and right atrial in configuration, producing an egg-shaped contour. The vascular pedicle is narrow because the pulmonary artery is behind the aorta rather than lateral to it. The lateral film (**B**) shows pulmonary overcirculation and right ventricular enlargement.

Although this particular cardiac configuration is considered classic, many cases of D-TGA show a nonspecific cardiac contour. The presence of cardiomegaly and pulmonary overcirculation in a cyanotic infant must suggest dextrotransposition.

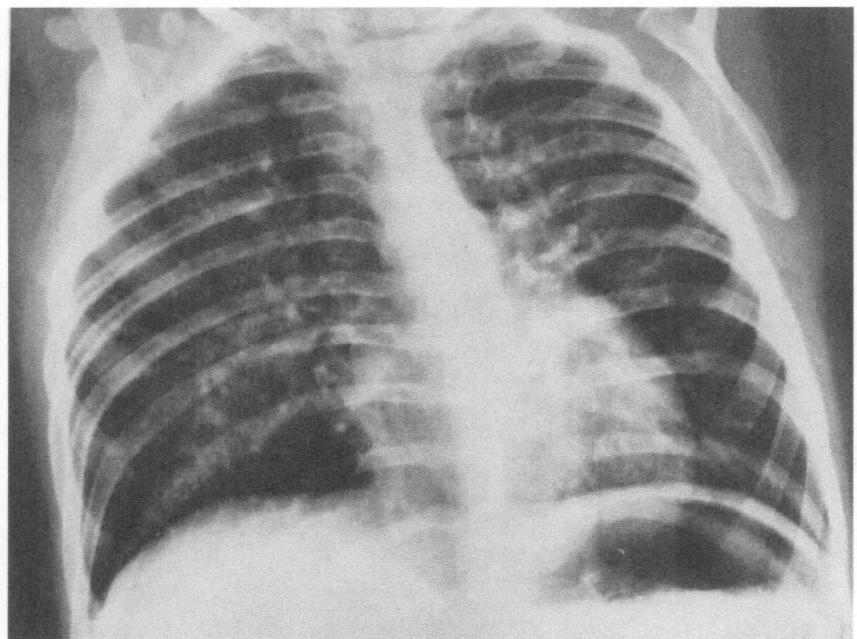

A

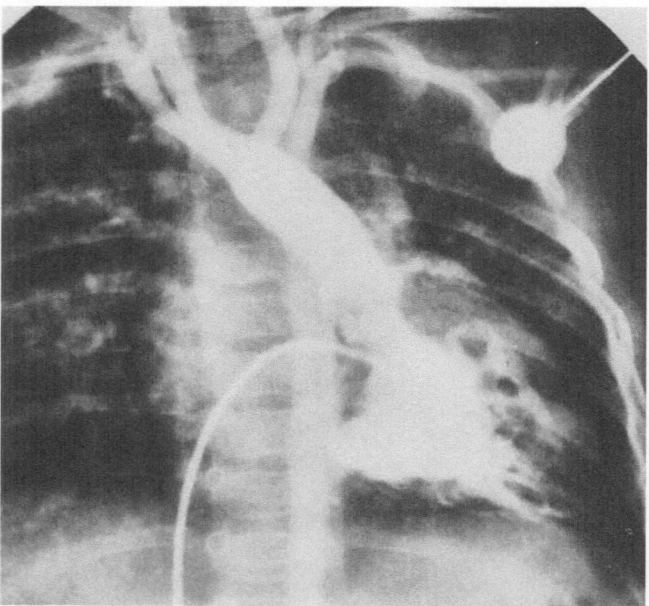

B

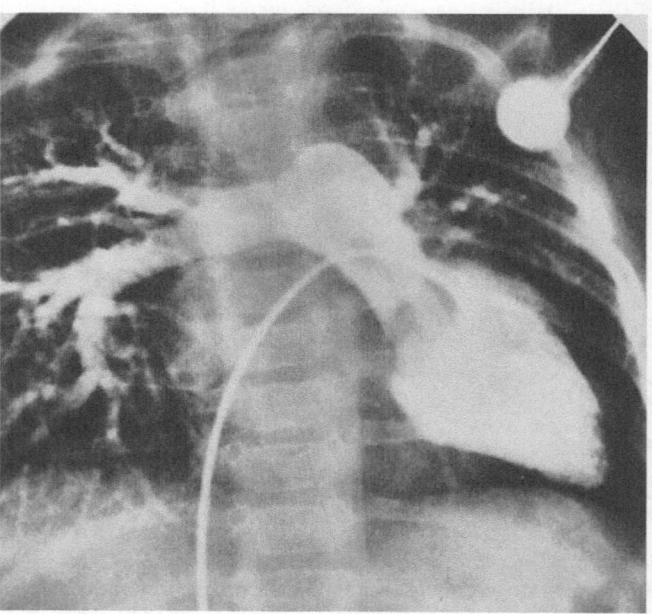

C

Fig. 7–75. *D-TGA with leftward convexity of the ascending aorta.*
A Frontal plain roentgenogram of the chest; B right ventriculogram; C left ventriculogram.

In A the vascular pedicle is markedly narrowed, and the convexity of the ascending aorta is slightly toward the left. In *B*
the configuration of the aorta is confirmed. D-TGA is the most
tenable diagnosis because the aorta arises from the right ventricle
and the pulmonary artery arises from the left ventricle (C).

Usually the ascending aorta in D-TGA is convex toward the
right; on occasion the convexity is toward the front so that the
aorta ascends in the midline with no rightward or leftward curvature. Only rarely in D-TGA is the aorta observed to be convex
toward the left; thus, when the aorta curves toward the left,
the diagnoses to be considered are levotransposition of the great
arteries, single ventricle with levotransposition (levomalposition)
of the great arteries, and, rarely, criss-cross heart rather than
D-TGA.

Fig. 7-76. *D-TGA with patent ductus arteriosus and high pulmonary resistance in a newborn baby.* The lungs have the appearance of undercirculation and the heart is not enlarged. This is a frequent radiographic feature in a neonate with D-TGA.

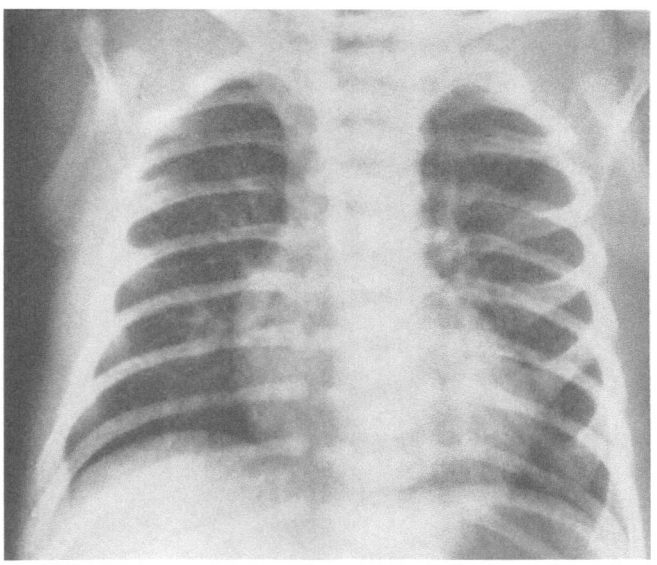

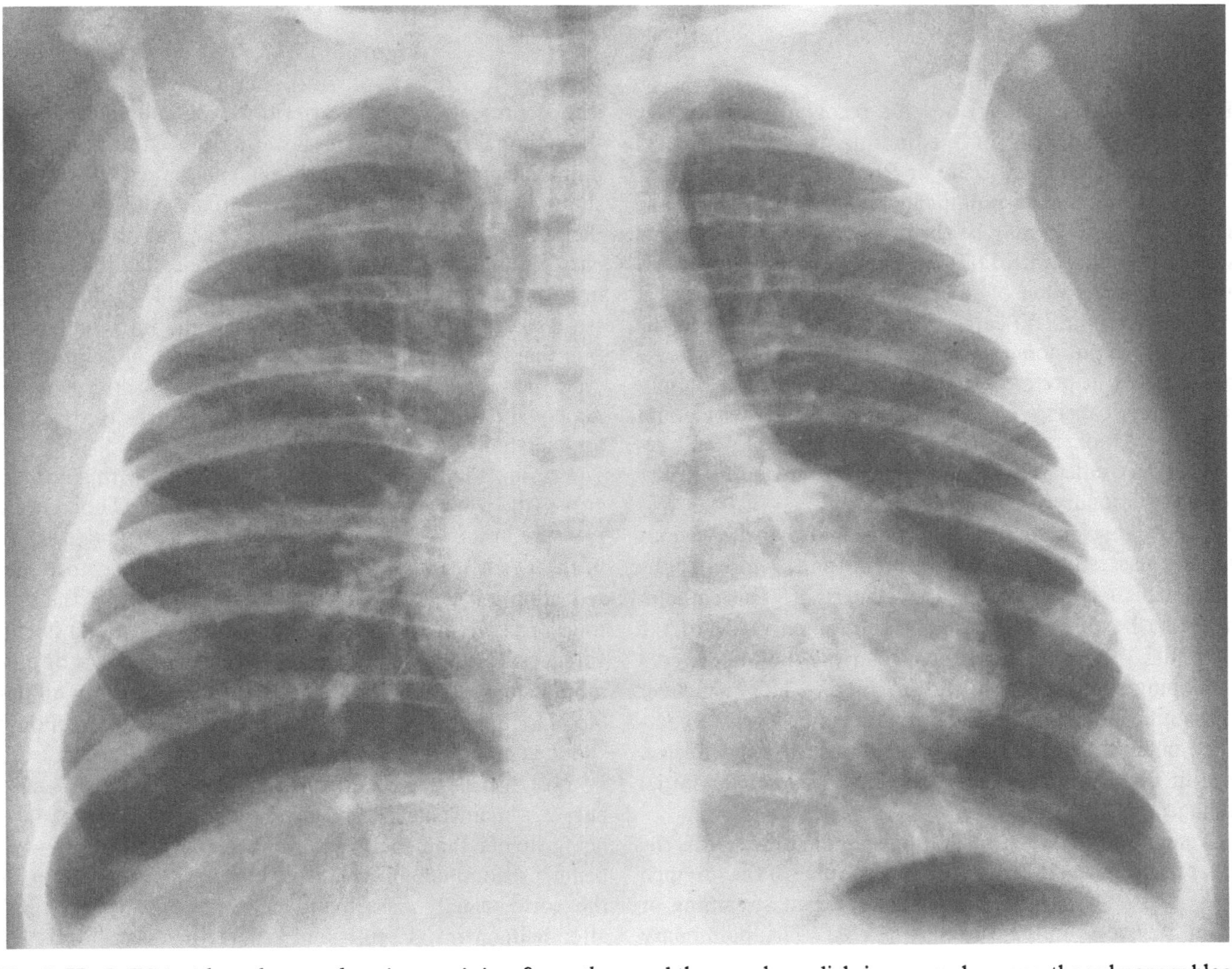

Fig. 7-77. *D-TGA with moderate pulmonic stenosis in a 9-month-old girl.* The heart has the shape of an egg lying on its side, and the vascular pedicle is narrow; however, the pulmonary blood flow is normal.

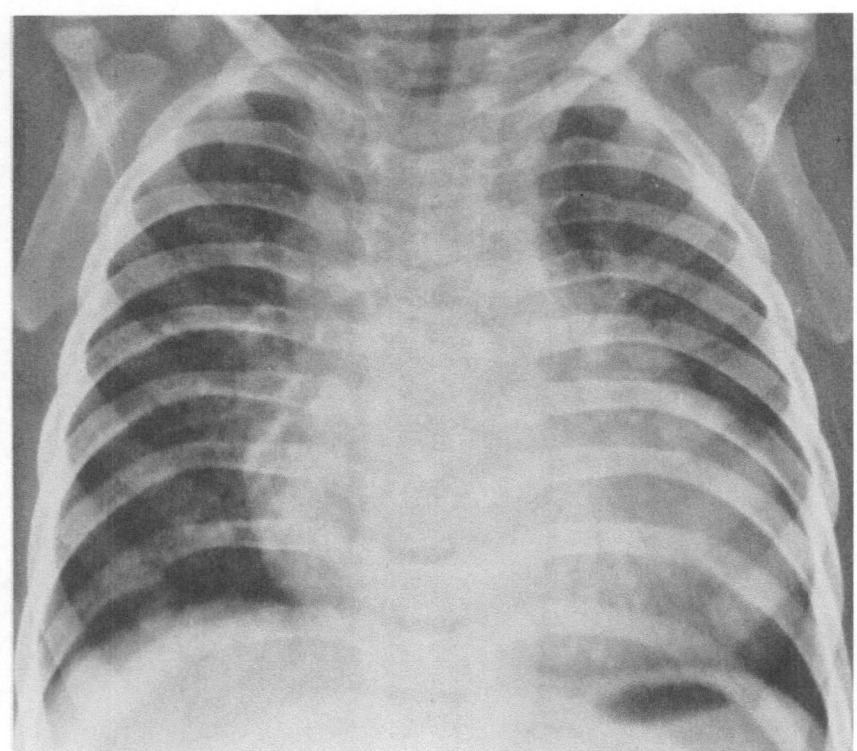

Fig. 7–78. *D-TGA in a 1-year-old boy with minimal subpulmonic stenosis.* Pulmonary overcirculation is present as is biventricular enlargement. The vascular pedicle is not narrow. Thus the cardiac configuration is not characteristic. Nevertheless, D-TGA is a likely diagnosis because of pulmonary overcirculation in the presence of severe cyanosis. Other admixture lesions should also be considered (e.g., truncus arteriosus, single ventricle, double-outlet right ventricle).

(Eisenmenger physiology) may be recognized during the second or third year of life in infants with untreated D-TGA and significant VSD or PDA.

The distribution of pulmonary blood flow between the right and left lungs may be asymmetrical in D-TGA. This is because infants with D-TGA often have an exaggerated rightward inclination of the main pulmonary artery as it emerges from the LV, causing an acute angle between the main and left pulmonary arteries. This anatomical arrangement results in preferential perfusion of the right pulmonary artery, causing overcirculation on the right side and undercirculation on the left. Angiocardiography and radionuclide studies have documented an unequal distribution of pulmonary blood flow.

Hemodynamics In a newborn with D-TGA the venous catheter passes from the RA through the RV to enter the aorta, which is anterior and on the right. The catheter may also be directed through the foramen ovale to the LA and LV. The main pulmonary artery may be entered by looping the catheter in the LA or LV. This maneuver has significant risk in a newborn, and is not always undertaken in this age group because the pressures and oxygen data in the pulmonary artery are not essential for initial management.

A step-up in oxygen saturation may be detected in the RA, reflecting an ASD or incompetent valve of the foramen ovale. A step-up in the RV might represent streaming or might reflect shunting through a VSD. The pulmonary veins are generally fully saturated while the LA is usually mildly desaturated, indicative of bidirectional atrial shunt-

ing. If present, a ductus arteriosus generally shunts into the pulmonary artery, thus lowering the saturation of the pulmonary artery. The sum of the anatomical left-to-right shunts (e.g., into the pulmonary circuit) and the sum of the anatomical right-to-left shunts (e.g., out of the pulmonary circuit) are equal, and together are called the bidirectional shunt, or the effective pulmonary blood flow ($\dot{Q}ep$, see also section on hemodynamics in the introduction to this chapter). The $\dot{Q}ep$ indicates the volume of desaturated systemic venous blood entering the lungs to be oxygenated. An equal amount of oxygenated blood returns to the body for metabolism.

Pressures in the RA are generally normal with a normal curve (the a wave is larger than the v wave). The systolic pressure in the RV is equal to aortic pressure. The pressure in the LA is usually elevated prior to balloon septostomy, reflecting left ventricular failure. In the newborn the systolic pressure in the LV (the pulmonary ventricle) is elevated, reflecting high pulmonary vascular resistance or pulmonic stenosis or both. Balloon atrial septostomy allows blood to flow freely between the two atria. The bidirectional shunt at the atrial level increases, and the mean pressure in the LA becomes equal to that in the RA. The pressure curves remain characteristic for each atrium, the a wave being higher than the v wave in the RA, and the v wave being predominant in the LA. The oxygen saturation in the aorta usually rises to no more than 70 (pO$_2$ = 35) after balloon atrial septostomy; nevertheless, acidosis resolves and the baby remains comfortable. If oxygen saturation fails to rise and acidosis persists after an adequate balloon atrial septostomy, increase of pulmonary resistance may be the cause, and an infusion of prostaglandin E_1 may result in improvement.

In older infants and children with D-TGA, pulmonary blood flow, pulmonary blood pressure and pulmonary vascular resistance must be determined, and the presence and severity of left ventricular outflow tract obstruction (pulmonic stenosis) must be determined in preparation for definitive surgery.

Patients with elevation of LV pressure secondary to VSD or pulmonary artery band (but not those with severe valvar pulmonic stenosis) may be candidates for an anatomical correction (arterial switch, Jatene). Those with low pressure in the LV are not candidates, as the LV cannot take over systemic pressure, and are generally referred for interatrial baffle repair (Mustard, Senning). Individuals with severe subpulmonic LV outflow tract obstruction may require a prosthetic conduit to reestablish connection between the ventricle and the pulmonary artery. High pulmonary vascular resistance (Eisenmenger physiology) may occur within the first year of life in infants with D-TGA with or without VSD. This complication is a contraindication for repair of VSD or PDA. Occasionally a palliative Mustard procedure may be of benefit in patients with D-TGA and Eisenmenger syndrome.

Contrast Studies Biplane selective angiocardiography establishes the diagnosis of D-TGA by demonstrating the position of the ventricles, the conus and the origins of the great vessels. Figure 7–79 shows normal right and left

ventriculograms to compare with those occurring with D-TGA.

The first injection, in an infant with D-TGA, should be made in the LV (Fig. 7–80). On recirculation, the LA and LV reopacify so that the degree of bidirectional shunting at the atrial level (if present) can be estimated. A VSD is diagnosed by right ventriculography (Fig. 7–81). Coarctation of the aorta can be diagnosed by either a right ventriculogram or an aortogram. Subpulmonic stenosis, either fibrous or fibromuscular, is a fairly frequently associated defect and should be carefully sought. A compound axial view with cranial tilt is very helpful in assessing these lesions (Figs. 7–81, 7–82).

Treatment In 1966 Rashkind and Miller introduced a nonsurgical method for atrial septostomy, demonstrating its effectiveness as a palliative measure in transposition of the great arteries, total anomalous pulmonary venous return, tricuspid atresia and in some cases of mitral atresia.

Atrial septostomy is performed as part of the diagnostic cardiac catheterization. A 6.5 F balloon septostomy catheter is advanced to the RA and across the foramen ovale into the LA. The position of the catheter is confirmed by advancing its tip into a pulmonary vein during biplane fluoroscopy.

The balloon is inflated in the LA with dilute contrast medium to a diameter of 1.0–1.5 cm. (Fig. 7–83); then, under fluoroscopic control, it is withdrawn across the atrial septum with an abrupt, short tug. The pullback motion

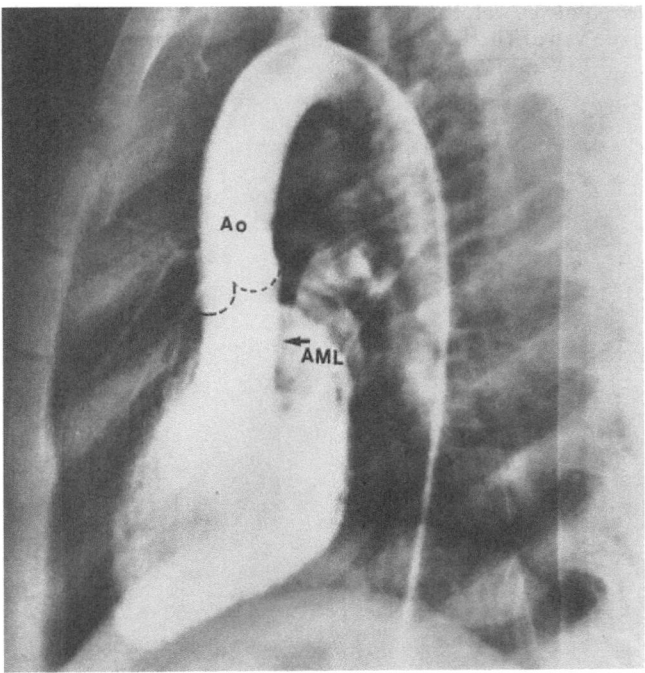

A

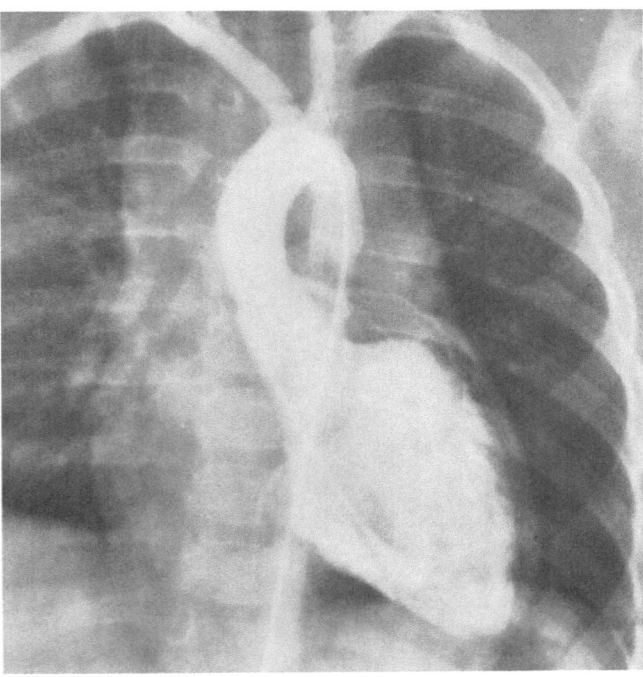

B

Fig. 7–79. A and **B** *Aortic-mitral fibrous continuity in the normal left ventricle.* **A** Lateral view, and **B** frontal view of left ventriculogram. The left ventricle is recognized by its characteristic shape and by its lack of coarse trabeculations. It has no conus muscle, and therefore the aortic valve (*dashed line*) is in fibrous continuity with the anterior leaflet of the mitral valve (*AML*). Fibrous continuity is best demonstrated on the lateral view during diastole. The aortic valve is posterior and inferior to the pulmonary valve. On the frontal view (**B**) the aortic valve arises to the right of the pulmonary valve. (*Continued*)

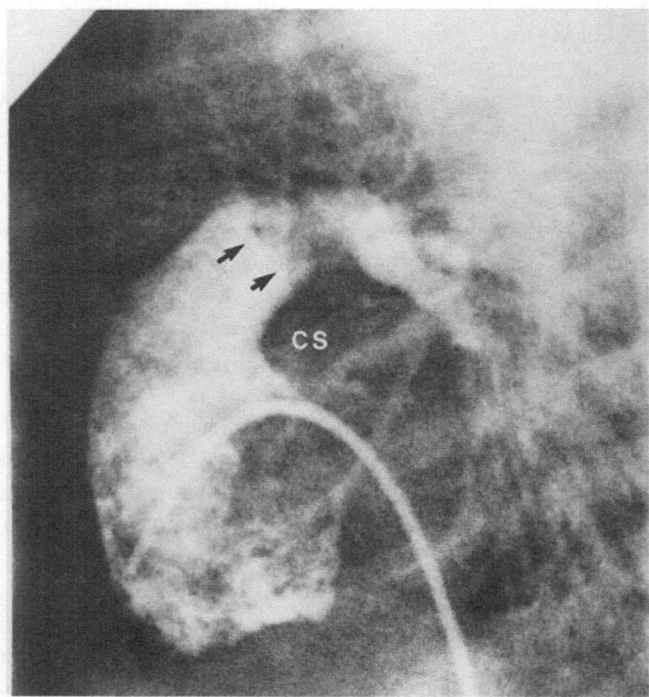

C

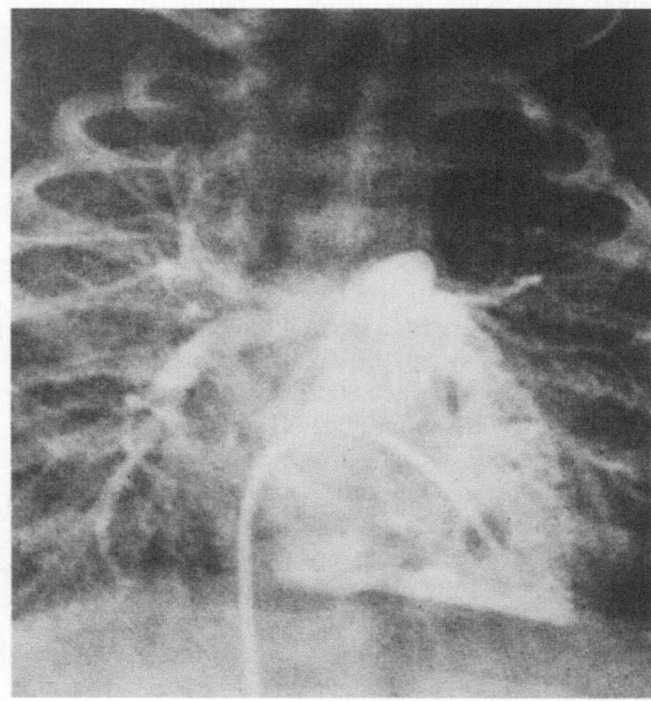

D

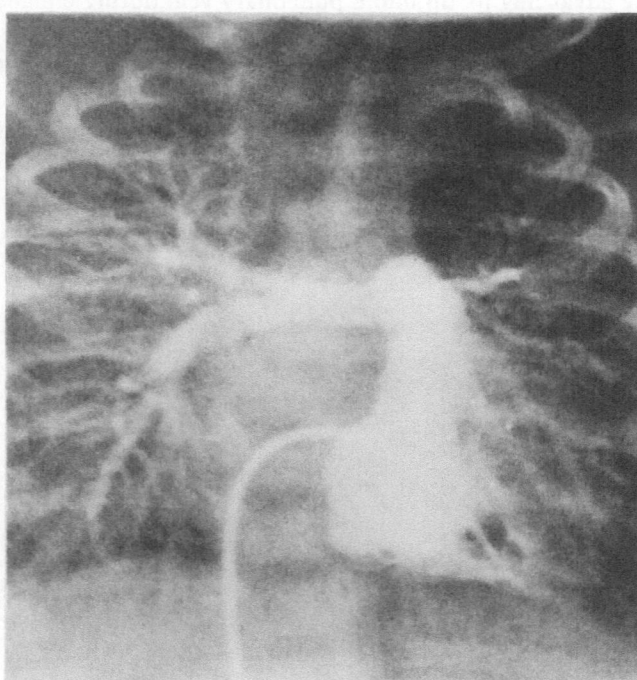

Fig. 7–79 (*Cont.*). *Crista supraventricularis separating the pulmonary valve from the tricuspid valve in the normal right ventricle* (*pulmonary-tricuspid discontinuity*) *from a different patient.* **C** lateral view; **D** and **E** frontal view of a right ventriculogram during diastole and systole. The right ventricle is recognized by its characteristic shape and coarse trabeculations and by the presence of the crista supraventricularis (*CS*), which separates the pulmonic valve (*arrows*) from the tricuspid valve. The CS is recognized here on the lateral film during diastole when the tricuspid valve is open. On the frontal film the right ventricular outflow tract crosses anterior to the left ventricular outflow tract so that the pulmonic valve is anterior, superior, and to the left of the aortic valve. The CS is better outlined during systole (**E**).

E

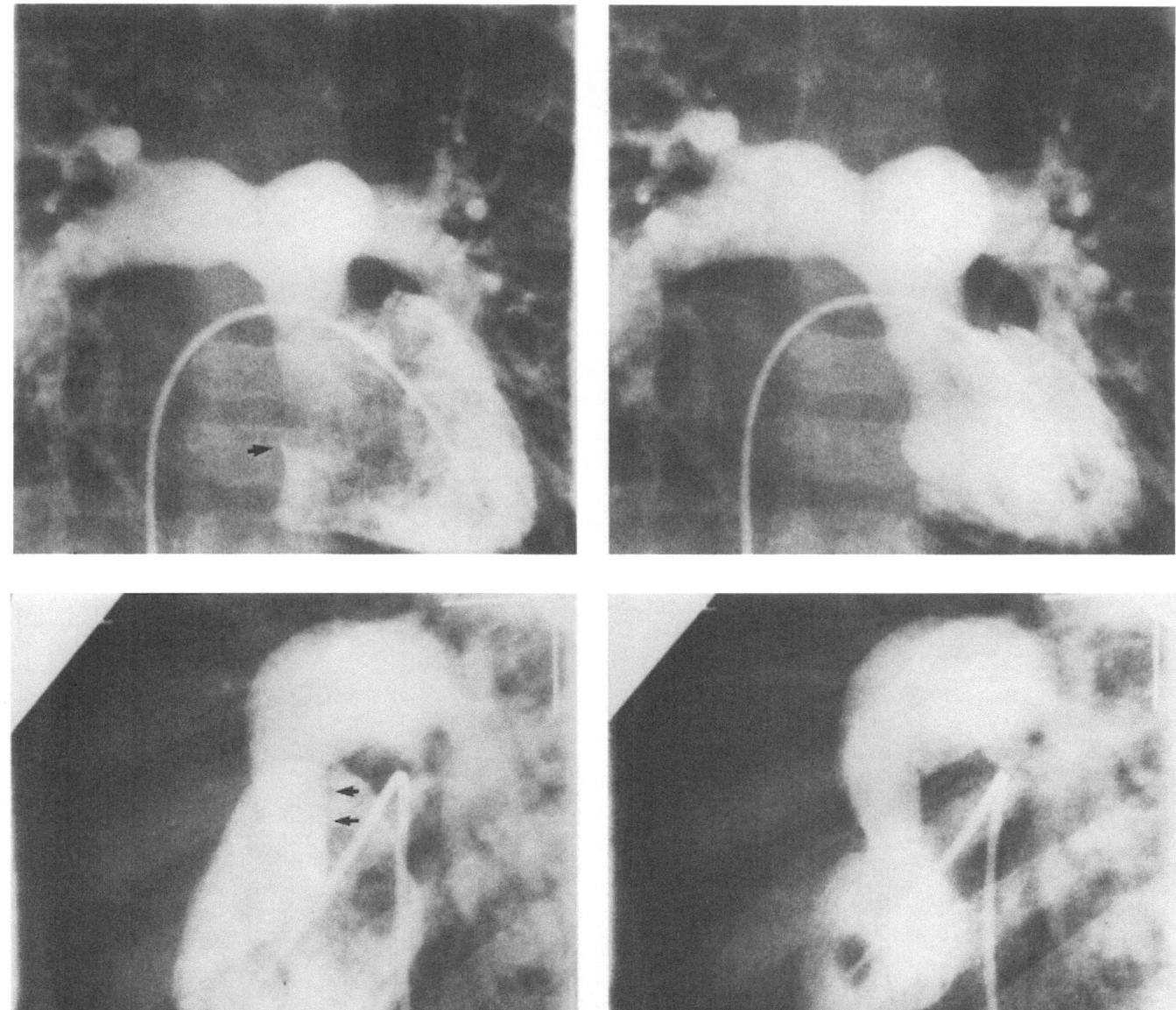

Fig. 7–80. *Angiographic findings in D-TGA.* The first injection in a baby suspected of having D-TGA is a left ventriculogram. **A** and **B** Frontal views of the left ventricle; **C** and **D** lateral views of the left ventricle.

The anatomical left ventricle is identified because it is ellipsoid and because its trabeculations are not coarse. Note: this left ventricle is not a typical ellipsoid because it has a type III configuration of the mitral valve, high fulcrum (*arrow*) without notching of the fornix. [See also Fig. 4–36 for morphology of the normal left ventricle.] In D-TGA the pulmonary artery arises from the left ventricle. Mitral-pulmonary fibrous continuity is recognized best on the lateral film during diastole (**C**, *arrows*). The pulmonary valve is posterior, inferior and toward the left relative to the aortic valve. (*Continued*)

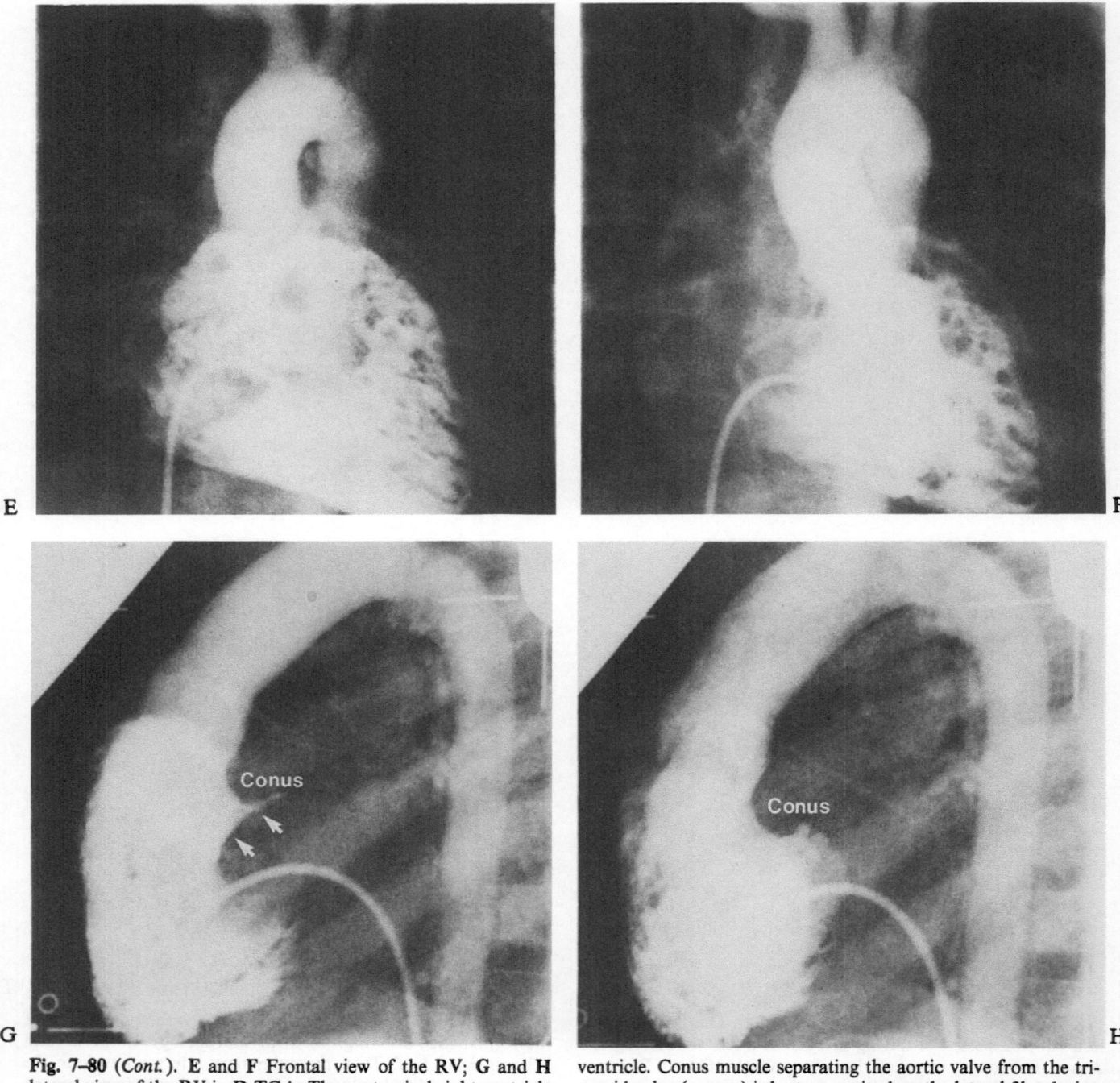

E

F

G

H

Fig. 7–80 (*Cont.*). E and F Frontal view of the RV; G and H lateral view of the RV in D-TGA. The anatomical right ventricle is identified because it is characteristically triangular and because its trabeculations are coarse. The aorta arises above the right ventricle. Conus muscle separating the aortic valve from the tricuspid valve (*arrows*) is best recognized on the lateral film during diastole (G). The aortic valve is anterior, superior and toward the right.

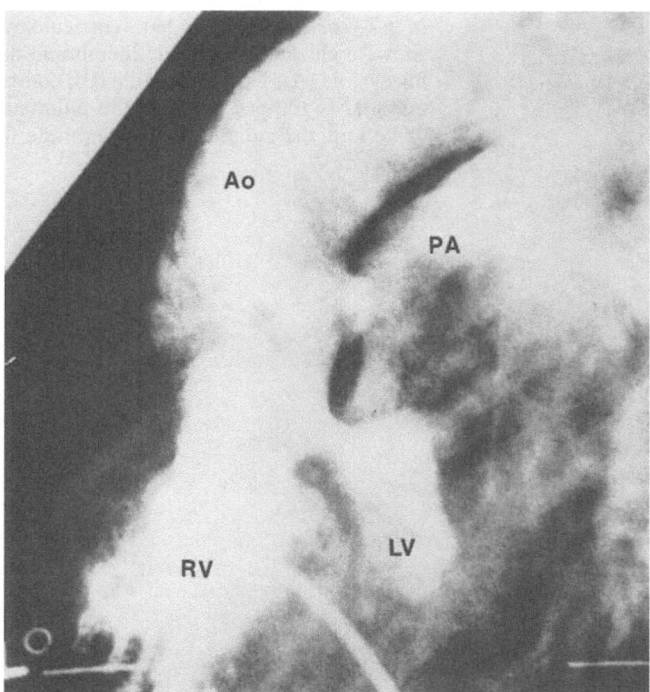

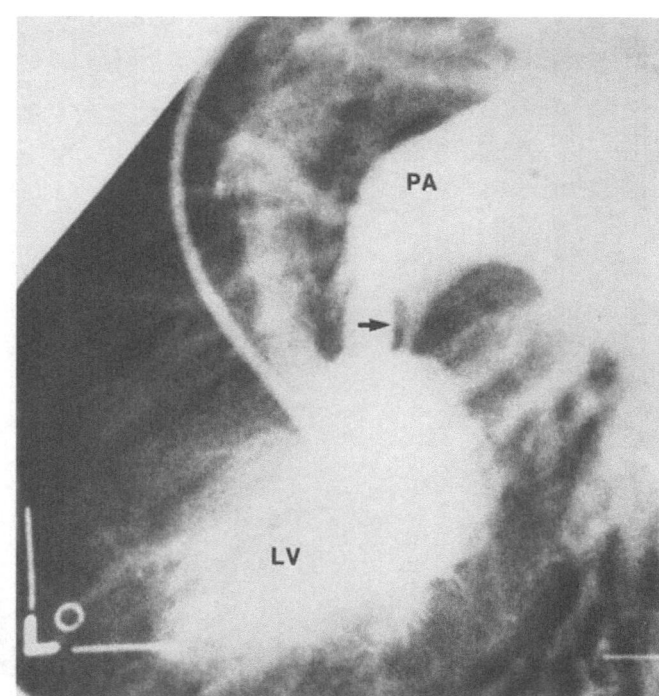

A   B

Fig. 7–81. *D-TGA with ventricular septal defect, valvar pulmonic stenosis and subvalvar pulmonic stenosis.* The lateral view of the right ventriculogram (**A**) shows the shunt from the right ventricle (*RV*) into the left ventricle (*LV*) through a subaortic ventricular septal defect. The lateral view of the left ventriculogram (**B**) shows a thickened, domed pulmonic valve (*arrow*). In **C,** the compound LAO view of the left ventriculogram with cranial tilt (hepatoclavicular view), a thick subpulmonic membrane is demonstrated (*arrow*). Note that an arterial approach was used for left ventriculography. The catheter was passed from the aorta into the RV and then through the subaortic VSD into the LV. *PA* = pulmonary artery. *PV* = pulmonic valve; *Ao* = aorta; *PA* = pulmonary artery; *RV* = right ventricle; *LV* = left ventricle.

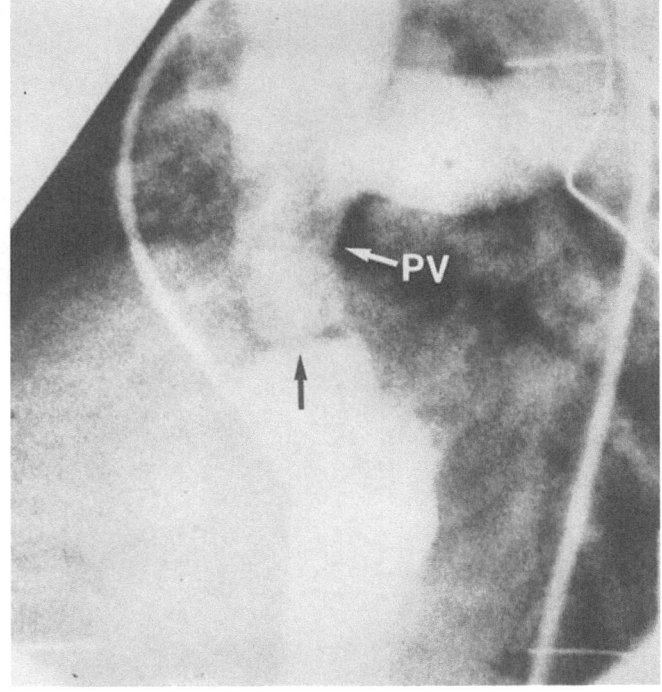

C

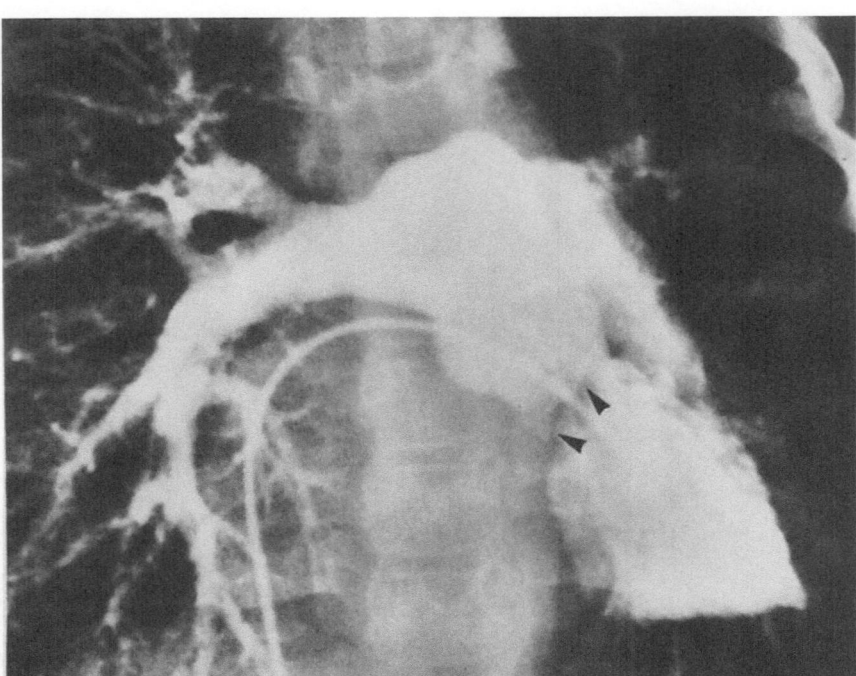

A

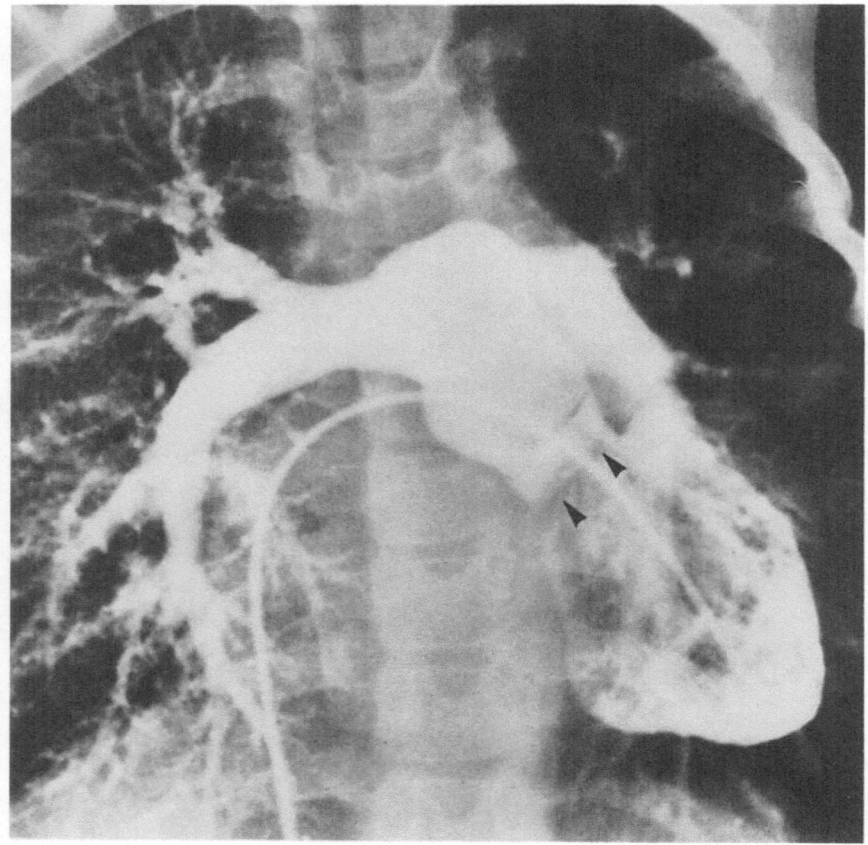

B

Fig. 7–82. *D-TGA and subpulmonic stenosis in a 7-year-old boy.* The left ventriculogram shows a thick subpulmonic membrane during systole (**A**). During diastole (**B**), contrast material is trapped between the pulmonary valve and the subpulmonic membrane (*arrowheads*).

Fig. 7–83. *Balloon atrial septostomy (Rashkind procedure) in D-TGA.* The position of the catheter is verified by advancing it into a pulmonary vein during fluoroscopic observation and then withdrawing it to the left atrium. The balloon is then inflated with dilute contrast material and withdrawn across the atrial septum with a sharp tug that brings it to the inferior vena cava. A tearing sensation may be felt by the operator.

Signs of a successful atrial septostomy are: (1) equalization of the right and left atrial pressures; (2) bidirectional atrial level shunting by oxygen saturation data; (3) improved mixing across the atrial septum on repeat left ventricular angiography; (4) improved arterial oxygen saturation. The procedure may be repeated several times to achieve these results.

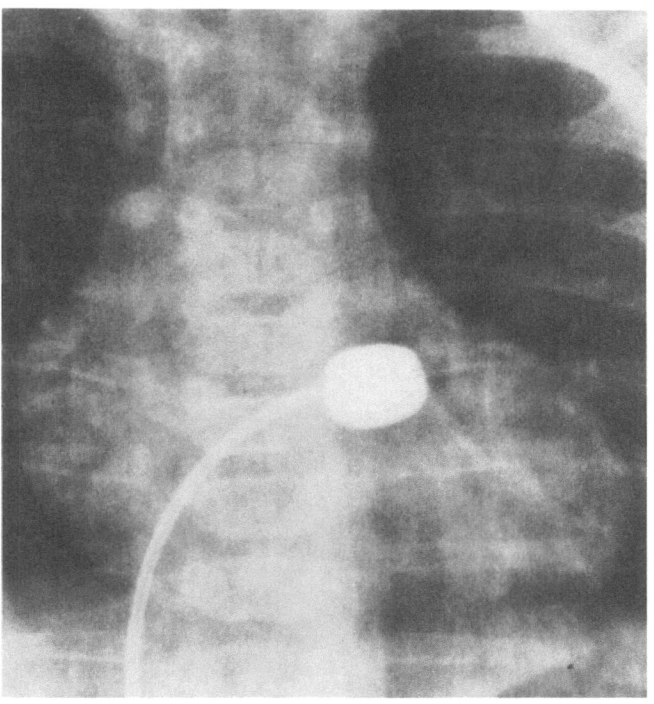

should carry the balloon from the LA to the right atrial–inferior vena cava junction in a single movement. If the procedure is performed properly the operator feels a snap as the flap of the foramen ovale is torn. The procedure is repeated several times. A satisfactory balloon septostomy is indicated by the following: no further resistance is met on pullback, the presence of bidirectional shunting across the atrial septum by O_2 saturation data, satisfactory oxygen saturation in the aorta (75%–85%) and disappearance of the LA-RA pressure gradient. The venous return phase of a postseptostomy left ventriculogram is also helpful in corroborating adequate mixing at the atrial level.

Complications of balloon septostomy include those inherent in the performance of cardiac catheterization in addition to occasional injury to the inferior vena cava, damage to atrioventricular valves (resulting from inadequate confirmation of catheter position) and balloon rubber embolization (rupture of balloon). In some infants, mixing remains inadequate after balloon atrial septostomy. Usually mixing is inadequate because high pulmonary resistance limits pulmonary blood flow. Prostaglandin E_1 may be required to maintain arterial oxygen saturations at acceptable levels until pulmonary resistance decreases.

Atrial septostomy is a short-term palliative method in that the initial high saturation levels obtained may not be maintained beyond 2–3 months. Total correction or further palliative surgery is then necessary.

Palliative surgical procedures for transposition include creation of an atrial defect to allow atrial mixing (Blalock-Hanlon, Sterling-Edwards, inflow occlusion) and proce-

dures to decrease or increase pulmonary blood flow (e.g., pulmonary artery banding, shunt operations).

"Complete" repair requires rechanneling of the pulmonary and systemic circulations at the atrial, ventricular or great artery level. The Mustard (Fig. 7–84, 7–85, 7–86), Senning (Fig. 7–87) and Schumacher procedures redirect the venous streams at the atrial level by means of baffles (Mustard) or infoldings of atrial tissue (Senning, Schumacher), so that pulmonary venous blood returns to the RV and is pumped to the systemic circulation. The anatomical RA, which previously carried systemic venous blood now becomes the physiological LA (or pulmonary venous atrium), and carries pulmonary venous blood; the opposite occurs for the new systemic venous atrium. After the Mustard procedure the coronary sinus is sometimes left to drain with the pulmonary venous blood into the RV, causing mild systemic desaturation.

The Rastelli procedure is used for D-TGA with large VSD and severe pulmonic stenosis. A large intraventricular baffle is used to direct blood from the LV through the VSD and out through the aorta. The pulmonary artery is tied off proximally. A valved conduit is sewn to the ventriculotomy incision in the RV and anastomosed distally to the main pulmonary artery. As a result, the LV pumps into the aorta and the RV supplies the lungs.

The Jatene procedure consists of transection and reimplantation of the ascending aorta and main pulmonary artery so that the aorta arises from the LV and the pulmonary artery from the RV. The coronary arteries are also reimplanted with a cuff of aortic tissue into the root of the

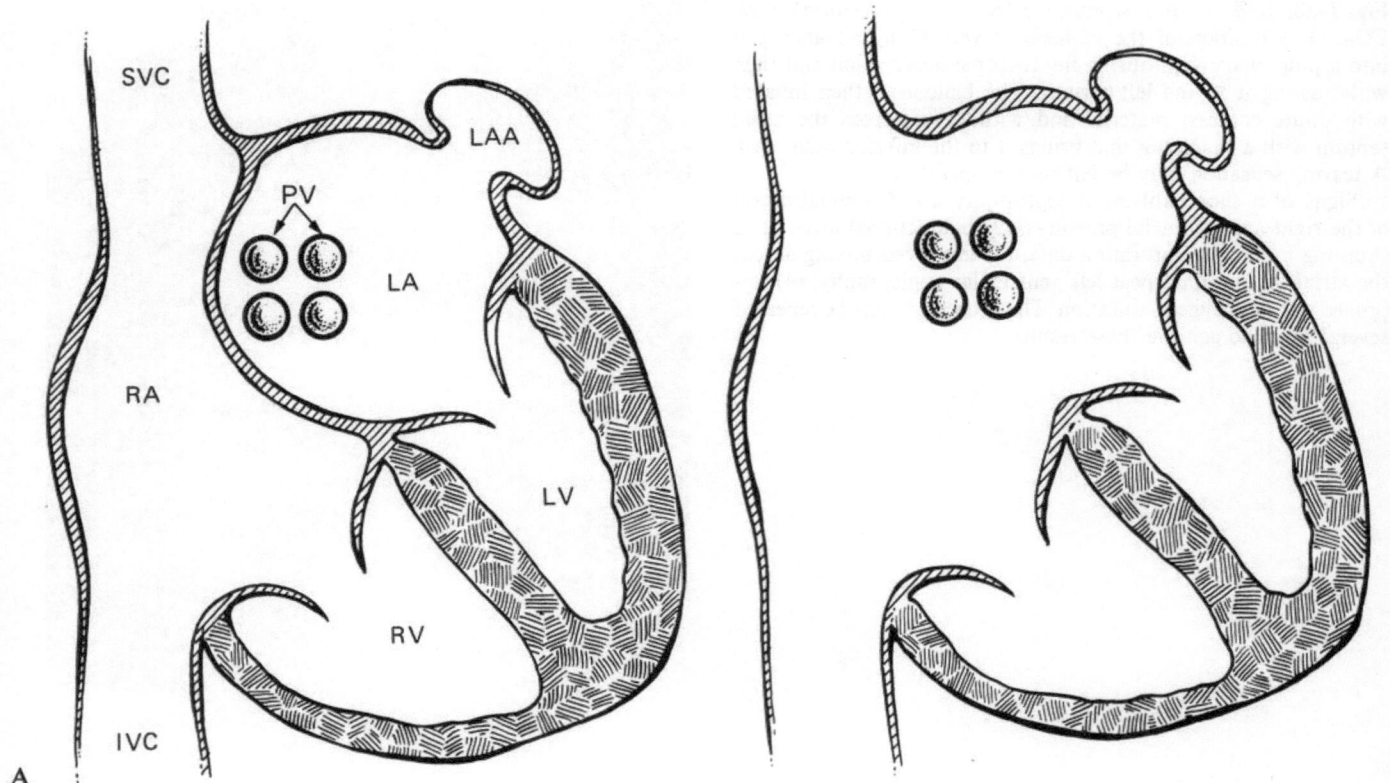

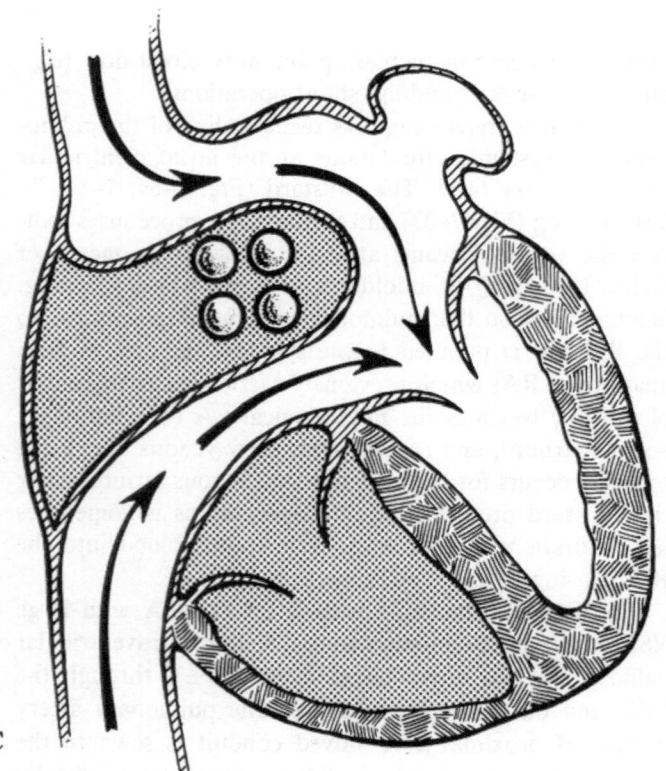

Fig. 7–84. *The Mustard procedure for repair of D-TGA.* The Mustard procedure reroutes the venous streams in the atria by replacing the atrial septum with a baffle that diverts blood from the superior vena cava (*SVC*) and inferior vena cava (*IVC*) so that it can enter the left ventricle. Pulmonary venous blood flows into the right ventricle.

In **A** the positions of the SVC, IVC and pulmonary veins (*PV*), are shown relative to the positions of the atrial septum and ventricles. In **B** the atrial septum has been removed. In **C** the baffle has been sewn in such a way that it partially surrounds the SVC and IVC. The baffle curves medially, surrounding the pulmonary veins and directing their flow to the right ventricle while flow from the SVC and IVC is directed toward the left ventricle. The flow of systemic venous blood is indicated by the *arrows*. The pulmonary venous blood passes on the right side of the baffle to enter the right ventricle. The newly created physiological left atrium, which carries pulmonary venous blood, might be called the pulmonary venous atrium, and the new physiological right atrium might be called the systemic venous atrium.

Note that the left atrial appendage (*LAA*) and most of the anatomical left atrium now form part of the systemic venous atrium. Similarly, the openings of the pulmonary veins and most of the anatomical right atrium are now part of the pulmonary venous atrium.

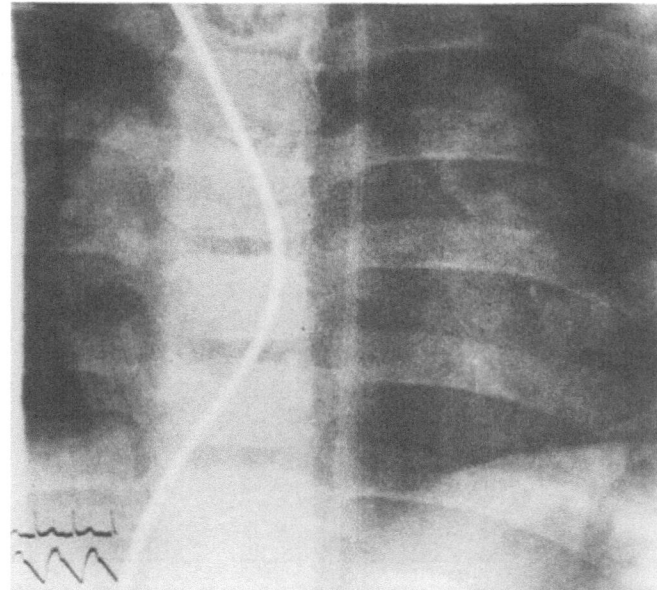

A

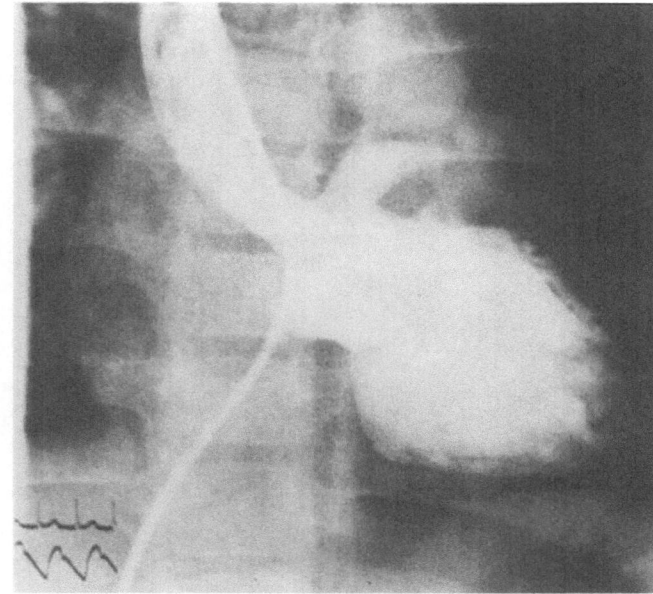

B

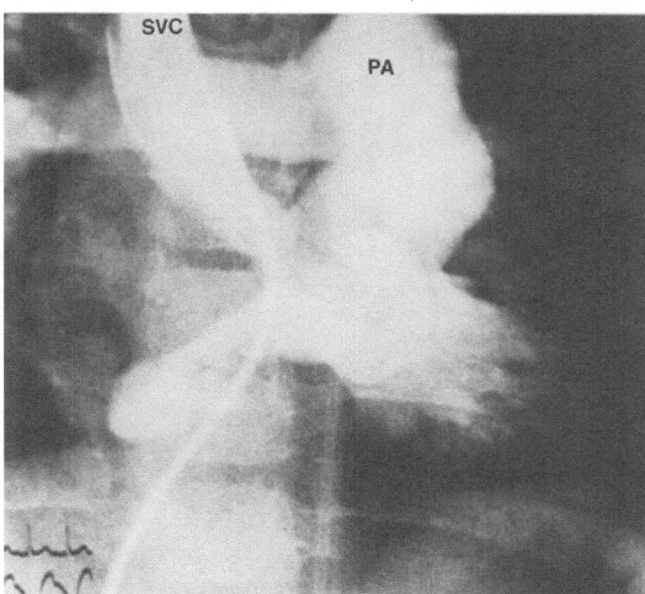

C

Fig. 7–85. *Mustard procedure (interatrial baffle) for dextrotransposition of the great vessels: angiographic and echocardiographic findings.* **A, B,** and **C** are frames from a frontal view of an injection of contrast medium into the superior vena cava (SVC). **A** demonstrates the position of a catheter entering the inferior vena cava (IVC) and passing through the systemic venous atrium to reach the SVC. The catheter curves medially within the atrium following the curve of the interatrial baffle. **B** is a frame from the injection showing contrast medium filling the upper limb of the baffle, the systemic venous atrium and the left ventricle. The left atrial appendage is part of the systemic venous atrium. **C** is a later frame from the same injection showing filling of the upper and lower limbs of the interatrial baffle. The left ventricle gives origin to the pulmonary artery. No obstruction to systemic venous flow is identified.

D, D′, E–I are two-dimensional echocardiograms of a different patient who had a Mustard procedure for D-TGA. **D** and **D′** represent a frame from a parasternal long axis view of the left ventricle (*LV*). The pulmonary artery (*PA*) arises above the LV. The systemic venous atrium (*sva*) is a small chamber behind the mitral valve. A corner of the pulmonary venous atrium (*pva*) is superior to the sva. The aorta (*Ao.*) travels behind the heart near the pva. (*Continued*)

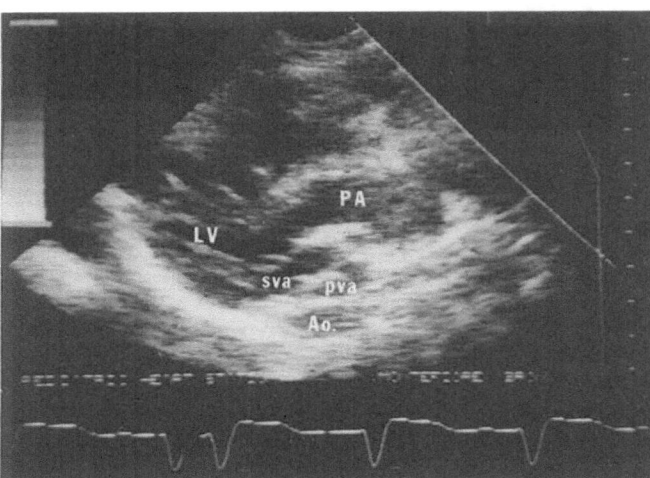

D

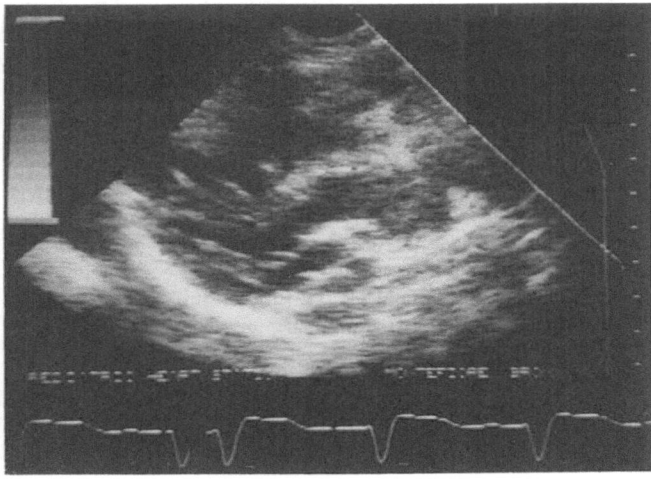

D′

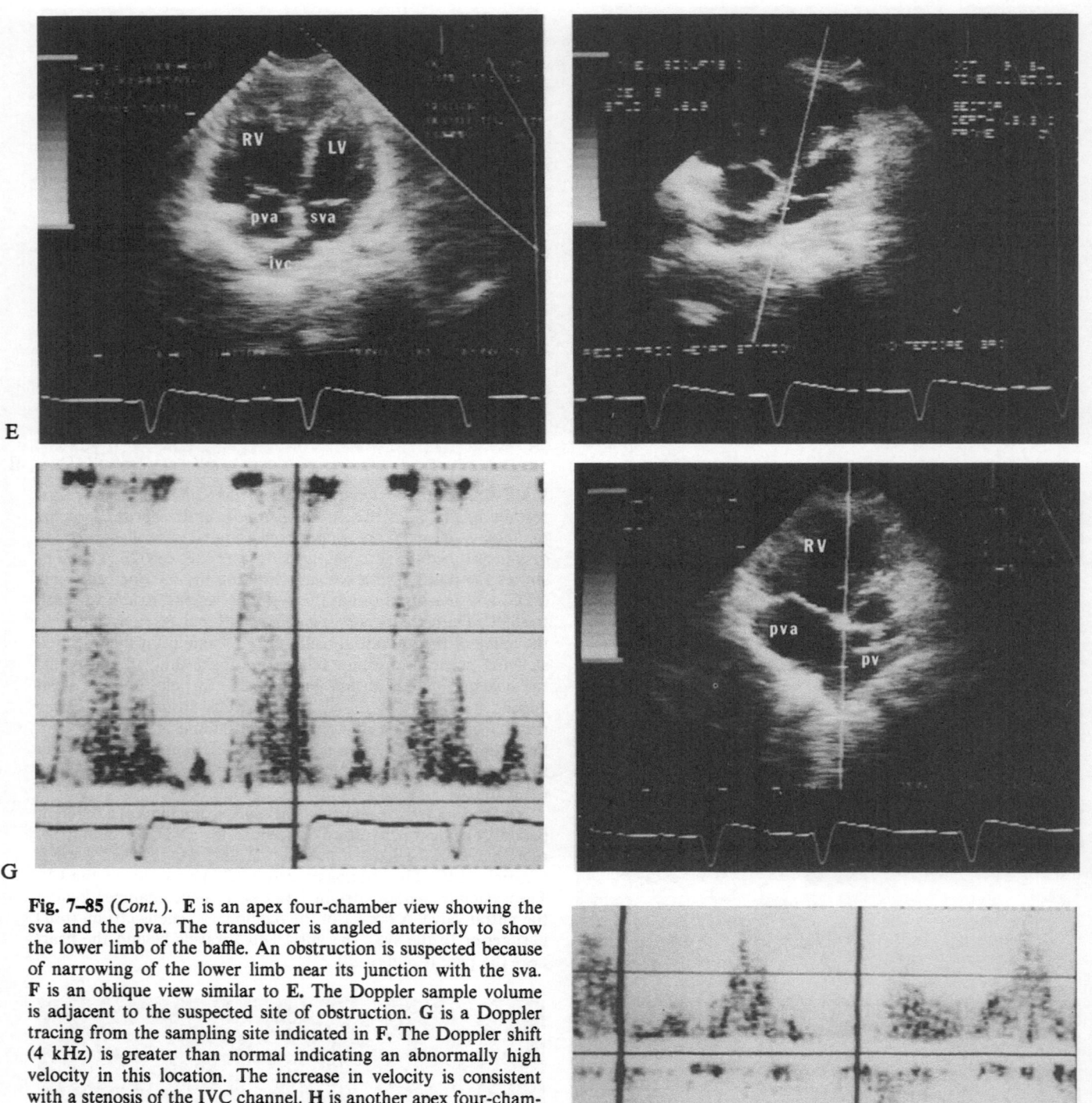

Fig. 7–85 (*Cont.*). **E** is an apex four-chamber view showing the sva and the pva. The transducer is angled anteriorly to show the lower limb of the baffle. An obstruction is suspected because of narrowing of the lower limb near its junction with the sva. **F** is an oblique view similar to **E**. The Doppler sample volume is adjacent to the suspected site of obstruction. **G** is a Doppler tracing from the sampling site indicated in **F**. The Doppler shift (4 kHz) is greater than normal indicating an abnormally high velocity in this location. The increase in velocity is consistent with a stenosis of the IVC channel. **H** is another apex four-chamber view angulated more posteriorly than in **E** to show the pulmonary venous channel. This channel is not obstructed, and the pulmonary veins (*pv*) are normal. The Doppler sample volume is adjacent to the entrance of the pulmonary veins into the pva. **I** is a Doppler tracing from the sampling site indicated in **H**. The Doppler shift is normal (1 kHz) indicating normal velocity of flow thus excluding obstruction.

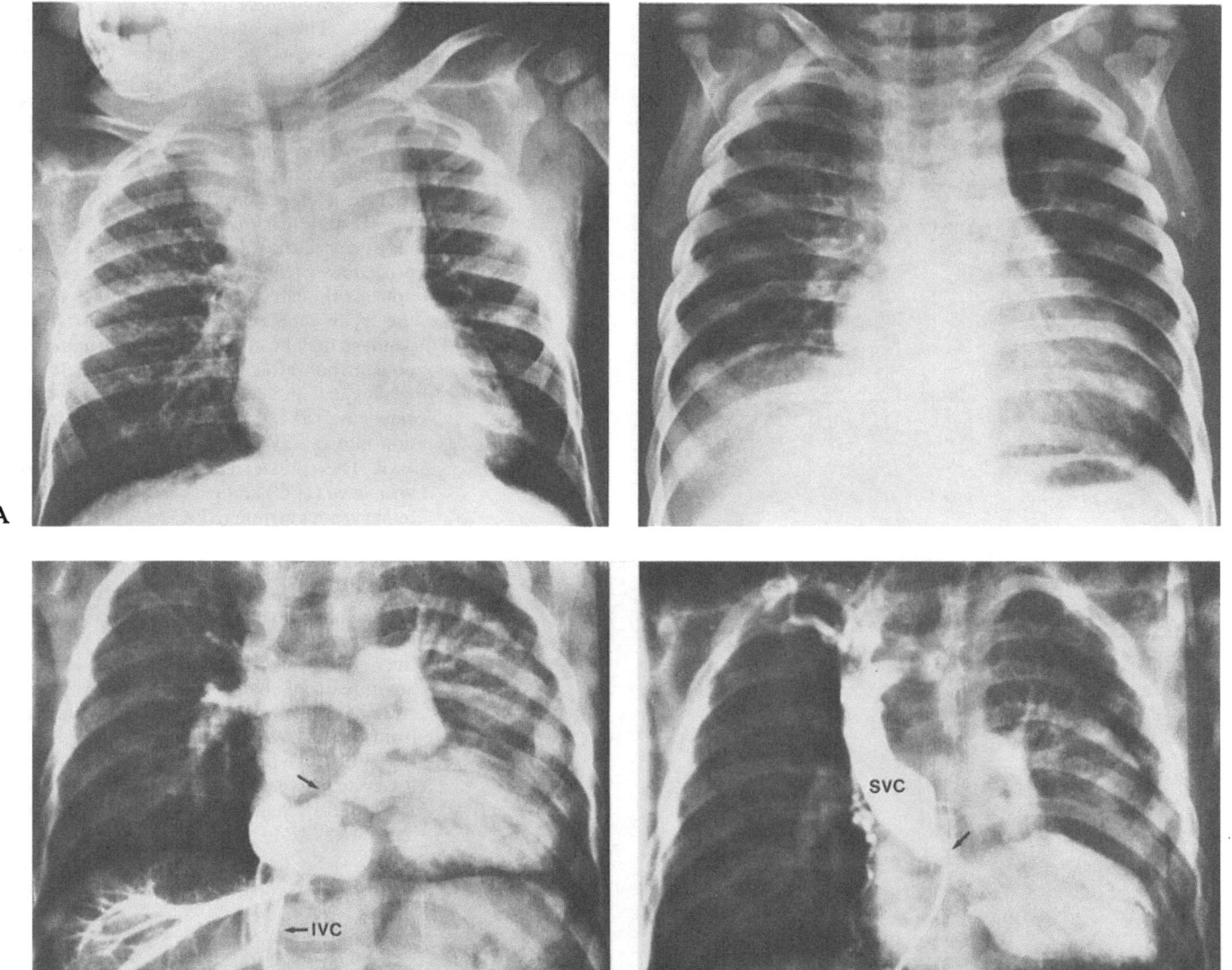

Fig. 7–86. *Venous obstruction after the Mustard repair for D-TGA.* **A** Frontal plain film of the chest in a 2-year-old boy with severe venous obstruction; **B** frontal plain film in a different patient in whom findings are less severe; **C** frontal view of injection of contrast medium into the inferior vena cava; **D** injection of contrast medium into the superior vena cava.

A demonstrates mild cardiomegaly with right ventricular enlargement. Marked widening of the mediastinum represents distention of the superior vena cava and the left innominate, the azygos and the hemiazygos veins. Pleural fluid is present around the apices. This distribution of the pleural fluid is probably a result of the film's being obtained with the baby supine. On angiography (**C** and **D**), severe obstruction of the superior and inferior venae cavae was noted. **B** The superior mediastinum is widened because of dilatation of the veins. Minimal fluid is present in the pleura and in the minor fissure. The right hemidiaphragm is elevated, suggesting subpulmonic effusion. These findings are not as obvious as in **A**; however, in a child after the Mustard procedure for D-TGA, they should lead to strong suspicion of venous obstruction. **C** After injection of contrast medium into the inferior vena cava (*IVC*), obstruction (*arrow*) is present in the lower limb of the baffle. The saccular structure is part of the anatomical right atrial chamber included within the baffle along-with the IVC. **D** After injection of contrast medium into the superior vena cava (*SVC*), obstruction (*arrow*) is seen in the upper limb of the interatrial baffle.

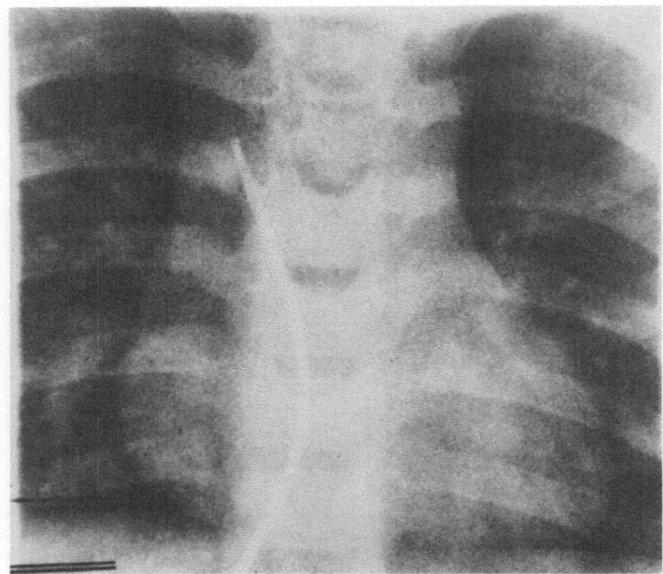

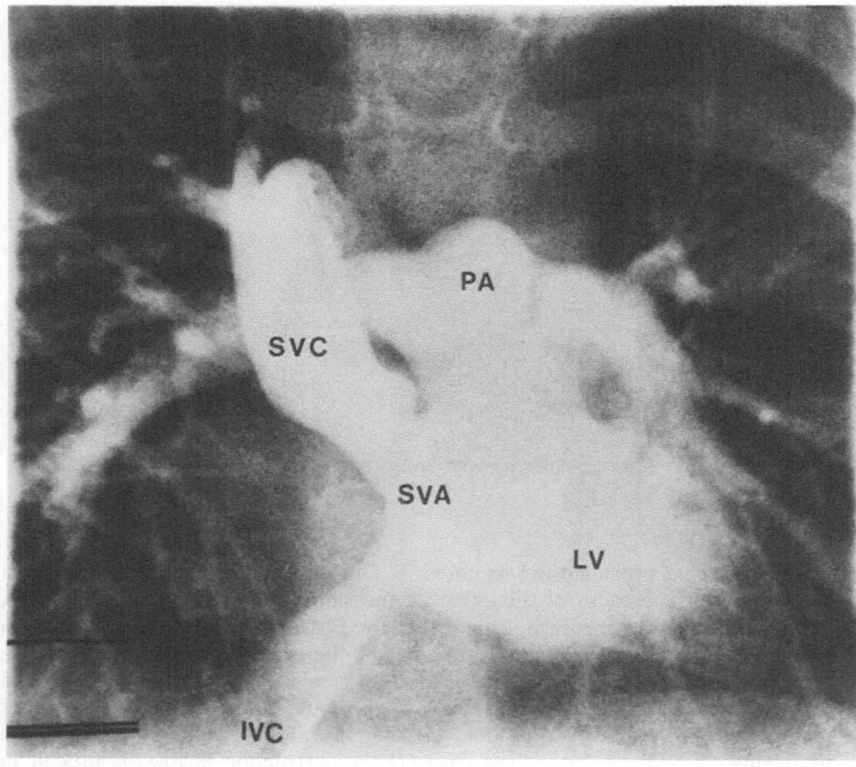

Fig. 7–87. *Senning procedure for repair of D-TGA.* This procedure uses infoldings of native atrial tissue to redirect the venous streams. The left atrial appendage is often invaginated and used to replace tissue missing because of the balloon septostomy. The angiographic appearance is similar to that of the Mustard procedure (Fig. 7–85), except that the left atrial appendage is outlined after the Mustard procedure but not after the Senning procedure (Note: a modified Senning procedure performed in some centers does not use the left atrial appendage as part of the repair, and therefore the left atrial appendage may be attached to the systemic venous atrium after the Senning repair.). **A** a venous catheter with its tip in the superior vena cava (*SVC*); **B** frontal view of an injection into the SVC.

A The catheter enters from the inferior vena cava (*IVC*) and passes through the systemic venous atrium (*SVA*) to enter the superior vena cava (*SVC*). The catheter curves in the atrium because it is deviated by the wall separating the systemic from the pulmonary venous atrium. This catheter position is characteristic for either the Mustard or the Senning procedure. In patients without an interatrial baffle the catheter passes straight up just within the right heart border from the IVC through the right atrium into the SVC. **B** An injection in the SVC opacifies the systemic venous atrium, the IVC (by reflux), the left ventricle (*LV*) and the pulmonary artery (*PA*).

new aorta. The pulmonary artery may be directed either to the right or to the left of the ascending aorta. In some instances the pulmonary artery is lengthened by means of a short tubular prosthesis.

The arterial "switch" procedure was introduced fairly recently. The early mortality was high. As criteria are developed to identify patients who can benefit from it, and as appropriate age for elective repair is determined, the results are becoming more acceptable. The procedure is considered applicable during the newborn period while the LV remains at systemic pressure because of high pulmonary resistance, and later in infancy in patients with persistent elevation of LV pressure due to VSD or pulmonary artery band. The arterial switch is generally not performed in the presence of pulmonic stenosis.

All the surgical procedures just described improve oxygen supply to the tissues. The atrial procedures can be performed in many centers with low risk during the first year of life. Definitive repair should be performed electively by 12 to 18 months of life to prevent the complications of long-term cyanosis (e.g., stroke, brain abscess) and pulmonary overcirculation (pulmonary vascular obstructive disease).

The most common complication of the atrial operations is arrhythmia. Other difficulties include shunts in either direction across the atrial septum, obstruction to pulmonary venous return, and obstruction to the superior or inferior vena cava (Fig. 7–86). Obstruction to the superior vena cava may cause hydrocephalus. Obstruction of the inferior vena cava may cause ascites and may prevent the catheter from entering the heart. In addition, the tricuspid valve may become insufficient, either acutely at the time of surgery or later during long-term follow-up. After the Mustard and Senning procedures the RV remains the systemic ventricle. Numerous reports indicate that RV volume is larger than normal, that the ejection fraction of the RV is reduced, and that response to stress (e.g., methoxamine challenge) is blunted.

After the arterial switch procedure, acute coronary artery obstruction has occurred because of compression by the pulmonary artery. Supravalvar pulmonic stenosis has occurred in patients who have received tubular prostheses to extend the main pulmonary artery. In contrast to the inter-atrial procedures, the LV becomes the systemic ventricle after the switch (Jatene procedure). Early reports indicate that the function of the LV is normal after the arterial switch. These findings support efforts to recommend this procedure for patients who can tolerate it.

Levotransposition of the Great Arteries

Levotransposition (L-TGA) is also called corrected transposition and represents atrioventricular and ventriculoarterial discordance. The incidence of L-TGA is less than 1.0% of all cases of congenital heart defects. The male-female ratio is approximately 2:1. Uncomplicated L-TGA is not an admixture lesion. It is included here because its embryology is similar to that of other transpositions.

In this type of transposition, ventricular inversion is present (L-loop in situs solitus). In other words, the morphological RV is left sided, and the morphological LV is right sided. The aorta emerges from the left-sided morphological RV above the conus (subaortic conus). This entity thus conforms to the loop rule of Van Praagh. The pulmonary artery arises from the right-sided morphological LV. A subpulmonic conus is seldom present. The aortic valve is anterior, superior and to the left of the pulmonary valve. The atrioventricular (A-V) valves (mitral and tricuspid) follow their respective ventricles, resulting in mitral-pulmonary fibrous continuity. The subaortic conus prevents tricuspid–aortic valve fibrous continuity. A-V discordance occurs because the atria are in situs solitus (morphological RA on the right side of the LA), and the ventricles are inverted. The double discordance (atrioventricular and ventriculoarterial) corrects the physiological abnormality. Thus, systemic venous blood reaches the lungs to be oxygenated, and the oxygenated blood returns to the body. In this way, associated defects with L-TGA have the same effect on the circulation as they would in a normal heart (e.g., VSD results in a left-to-right shunt; VSD plus pulmonic stenosis in L-TGA would result in symptoms and hemodynamics similar to those of tetralogy of Fallot). In uncomplicated cases the pulmonary veins and the venae cavae (systemic veins) drain into their respective atria.

The coronary arteries are inverted (Fig. 7–88). Thus the anterior coronary artery arises from the anterior sinus of Valsalva and the posterior coronary from the posterior sinus. The noncoronary sinus is anterior and to the left. The anterior coronary artery is similar to a left main coronary artery. It gives off an anterior descending and a right-sided circumflex artery which supply branches to the anatomical LV. The posterior coronary artery runs in the left A-V groove to the crux of the heart. Then, as with a normal right coronary artery, it gives off a posterior descending coronary artery and a crux artery. The posterior coronary artery thus supplies the posterior aspect of the anatomical RV, the basal ventricular septum and the diaphragmatic wall of the anatomical LV. This pattern represents a fairly standard example of coronary artery distribution. Many variations exist, just as in normal hearts (see also Fig. 7–102E).

The conduction system is abnormal because of malalignment between the atrial and ventricular septa. The A-V node is anteriorly placed in the atrial septum, and the proximal bundle of His penetrates the ventricular septum anterior to the membranous septum or anterior to the VSD, if one is present, rather than posteriorly as in the normal individual. The bundle branches are inverted as are the ventricles. The abnormal position of the proximal bundle of His may account for some occurrences of heart block in patients with L-TGA. At the time of cardiac surgery, mapping of the bundle of His may be necessary to avoid complete heart block. The Wolff-Parkinson-White syndrome and supraventricular tachycardias also occur more frequently in L-TGA than in normal hearts.

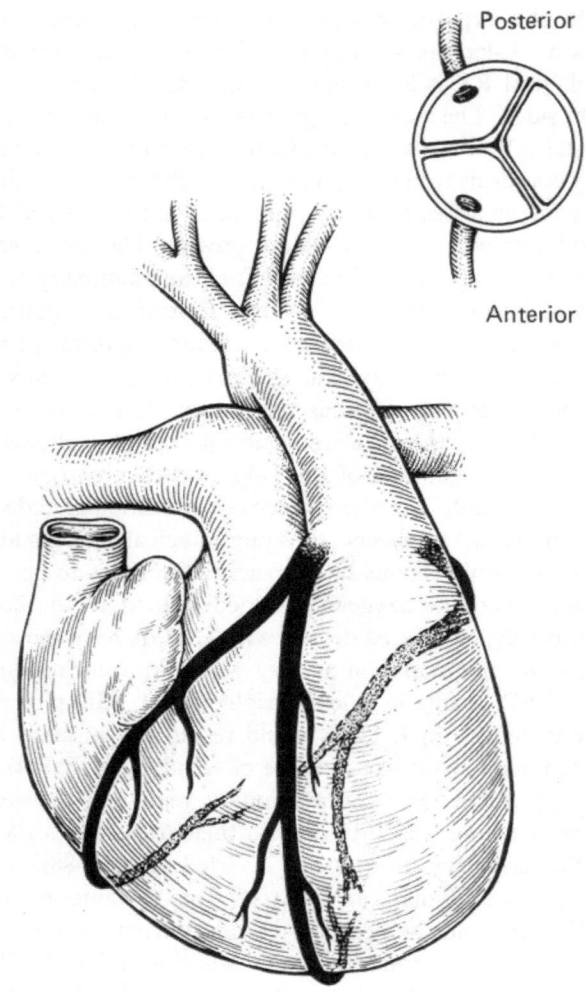

Posterior

Anterior

Fig. 7–88. *Coronary arteries in levotransposition of the great vessels (L-TGA).* This diagram of the external view of the heart demonstrates a typical pattern of the coronary arteries in relation to the inverted ventricles. The anterior coronary artery (ACA) arises from the anterior (right) coronary cusp, descending in the anterior interventricular sulcus. The ACA gives off an anterior descending branch similar to a left anterior descending coronary artery, and a right-sided circumflex artery that courses in the right atrioventricular groove. These vessels supply the anatomical left ventricle. The posterior coronary artery (PCA) arises from the posterior (left) cusp, coursing in the left atrioventricular goove to the crux of the heart, where it divides into a posterior descending (PD) coronary artery and a crux artery (CA). The PCA supplies the posterolateral and diaphragmatic walls of the anatomical right ventricle. The PD artery supplies the basal interventricular septum, while the CA supplies the diaphragmatic surface of the anatomical left ventricle. See also Fig. 7–102E.

Associated intracardiac defects are very common. The most frequent are VSD and pulmonic stenosis. A VSD is present in approximately 75% of patients with L-TGA. The VSD usually occurs in the membranous septum. The membranous septum in these patients is larger than in normal individuals because of malalignment between the interatrial and interventricular septa.

Pulmonary stenosis may be valvar or subvalvar. Subvalvar stenosis is usually membranous or fibromuscular. Subvalvar stenosis may also be due to accessory mitral tissue or rarely to a parachute deformity of the right A-V valve, aneurysm of the membranous septum or deformity of the muscular septum. Ebstein malformation of the tricuspid valve (left A-V valve) may be present. The association of L-TGA and single ventricle is discussed later in this section in Single Ventricle.

In summary, although the systemic and pulmonary circuits are in series in L-TGA, and, physiologically speaking, the circulation is normal, the hearts in this entity rarely, if ever, function normally.

Clinical Features The clinical features and the age at presentation are determined by presence or absence of associated defects. Complete heart block may occur in a fetus with L-TGA and the diagnosis made, on occasion, during fetal echocardiography as part of the evaluation for persistent fetal bradycardia. Infants may have congestive heart failure secondary to a large VSD, or cyanosis due to VSD and pulmonic stenosis.

L-TGA may be detected in older children and adults during evaluation for murmurs or arrhythmias. The characteristic auscultatory finding in L-TGA, without significant intracardiac defects, is a loud aortic second sound caused by the anteriorly placed aorta. Murmurs and the cardiac impulse vary with the intracardiac defects and overload patterns. The electrocardiogram may show abnormally directed initial (septal) forces because of the inversion of the ventricular septum. As a result a Q wave is produced in the right precordium (V_1, V_2) with absence of the septal Q wave in V_5 and V_6. Patterns of hypertrophy reflect the cardiac overload. Prolongation of the PR interval is common, as is complete heart block, Wolff-Parkinson-White syndrome and supraventricular tachycardia.

Echocardiography On M-mode the positions of the great vessels suggest a normal pattern. The anterior great vessel is superior and toward the left (Fig. 7–89A) and the posterior great vessel is inferior and toward the right (Fig. 7–89B). Systolic time intervals differentiate the aortic valve (left, anterior, superior) from the pulmonic valve (right, posterior, inferior) in most cases. The aortic valve has a longer pre-ejection period and a shorter ventricular ejection time than does the pulmonary artery. An arc scan from the pulmonic valve to the mitral valve (right A-V valve) demonstrates pulmonary-mitral continuity (Fig. 7–90). An arc scan from the aortic valve to the tricuspid valve (left A-V valve indicates a marked break in continuity corresponding to the conus (Fig. 7–91). These images are difficult or impossible to obtain in some patients. The major diffi-

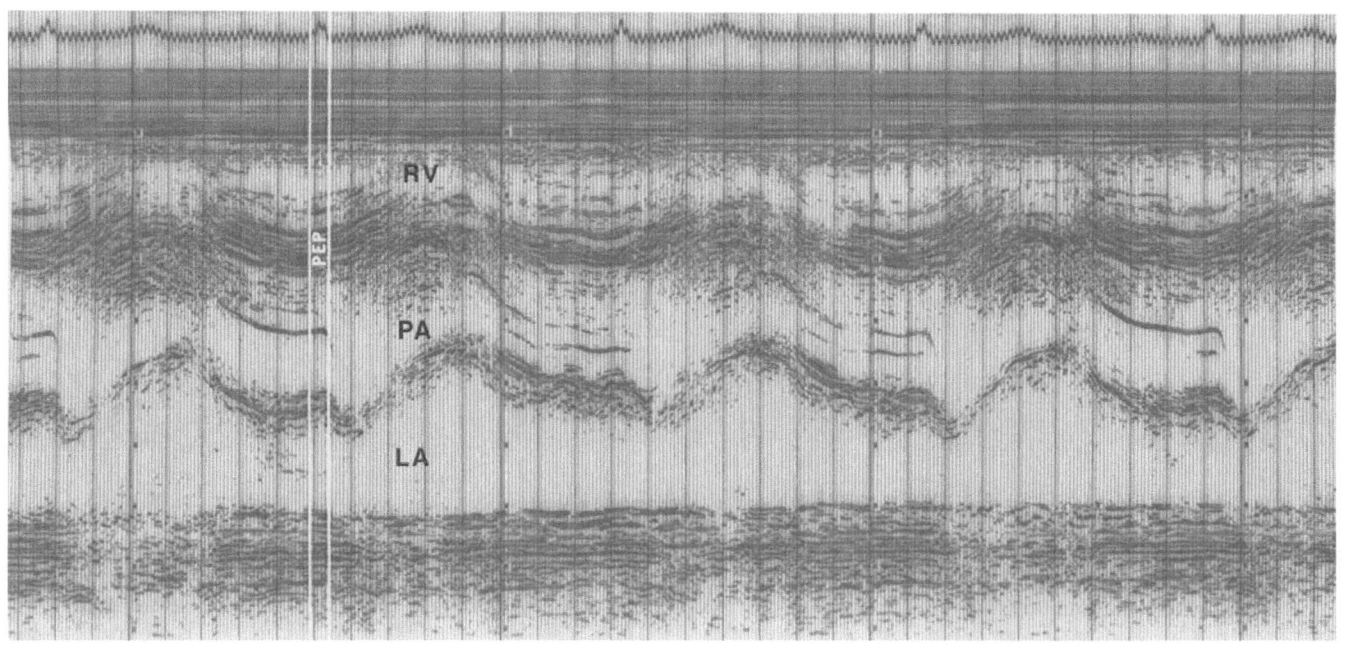

A

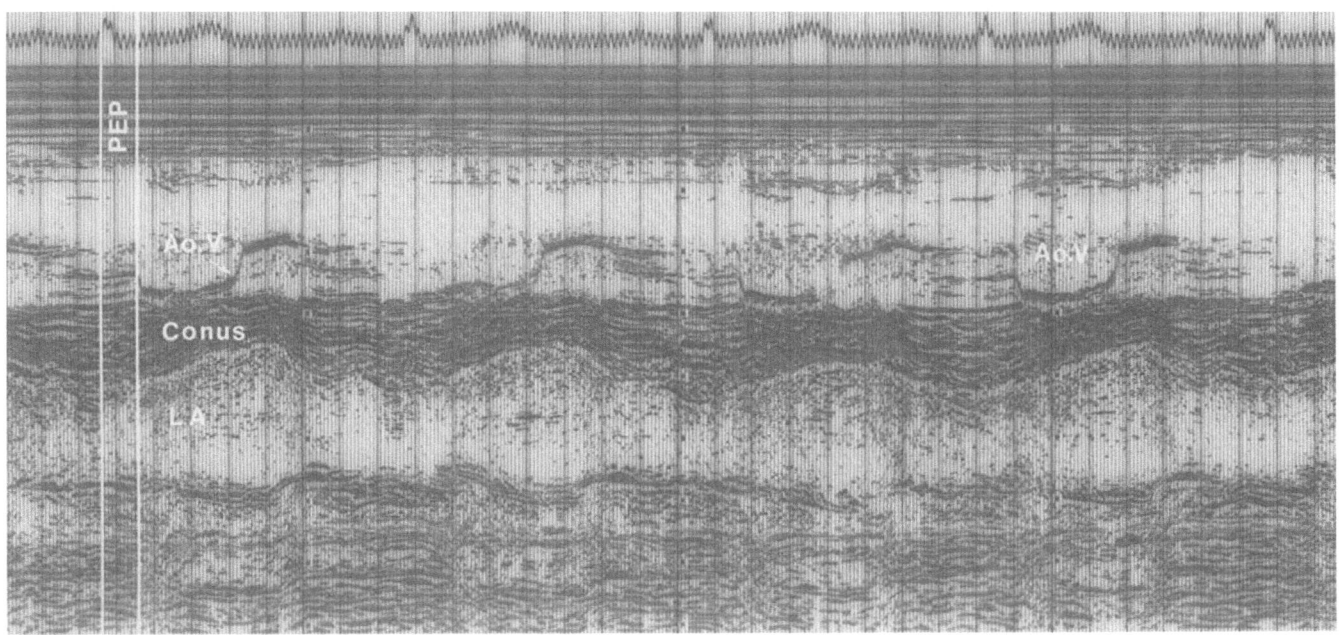

B

Fig. 7–89. *M-mode echocardiogram of the semilunar valves in L-TGA.* **A** Pulmonic valve; **B** aortic valve. The time lines are 10 msec apart. **A** The posterior semilunar valve was identified while the transducer was positioned in the fourth left intercostal space and directed slightly toward the right. **B** The anterior semilunar valve was demonstrated by changing the angle of the transducer superiorly and toward the left. This relationship of the great vessels is consistent with normal position or with L-TGA. The pre-ejection period *(PEP)* of the posterior semilunar valve is 40 msec while the PEP of the anterior valve is 80 msec. As a result, the anterior valve is likely to be the aortic valve and the orientation of the great vessels indicative of L-TGA. Although two-dimensional echocardiography has largely supplanted this method of distinguishing the aortic from the pulmonic valve, M-mode echocardiography remains useful in determining systolic time intervals for assessment of pulmonary resistance.

Ao.V = aortic valve; *LA* = left atrium; *RV* = right ventricle; *PA* = pulmonary artery.

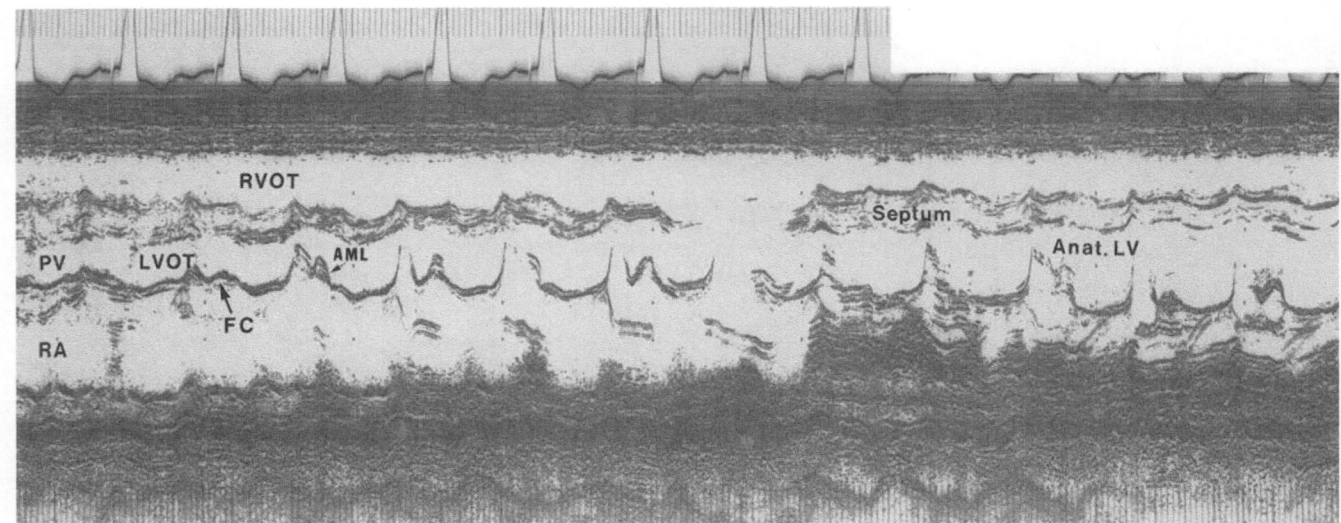

Fig. 7–90. *M-mode echocardiogram in a 4-year-old boy with L-TGA and complete heart block* (note pacemaker artifact on the ECG). An arc scan from the pulmonic valve (*PV*) to the mitral valve (right atrioventricular valve, *AML*) demonstrates pulmonary-mitral fibrous continuity (*FC*). This image is obtained by first angling the transducer from the left sternal border toward the right to demonstrate the pulmonic valve. The transducer is then directed inferiorly and farther toward the right to encounter the mitral valve within the right-sided ventricle (anatomic left ventricle, *Anat. LV*). Often the mitral valve is so far to the right of the sternum that this arc scan is impossible to achieve in L-TGA. The dropout of echoes in the septum is an artifact and does not represent a ventricular septal defect.

RA = right atrium; *RVOT* = right ventricular outflow tract; *LVOT* = left ventricular outflow tract.

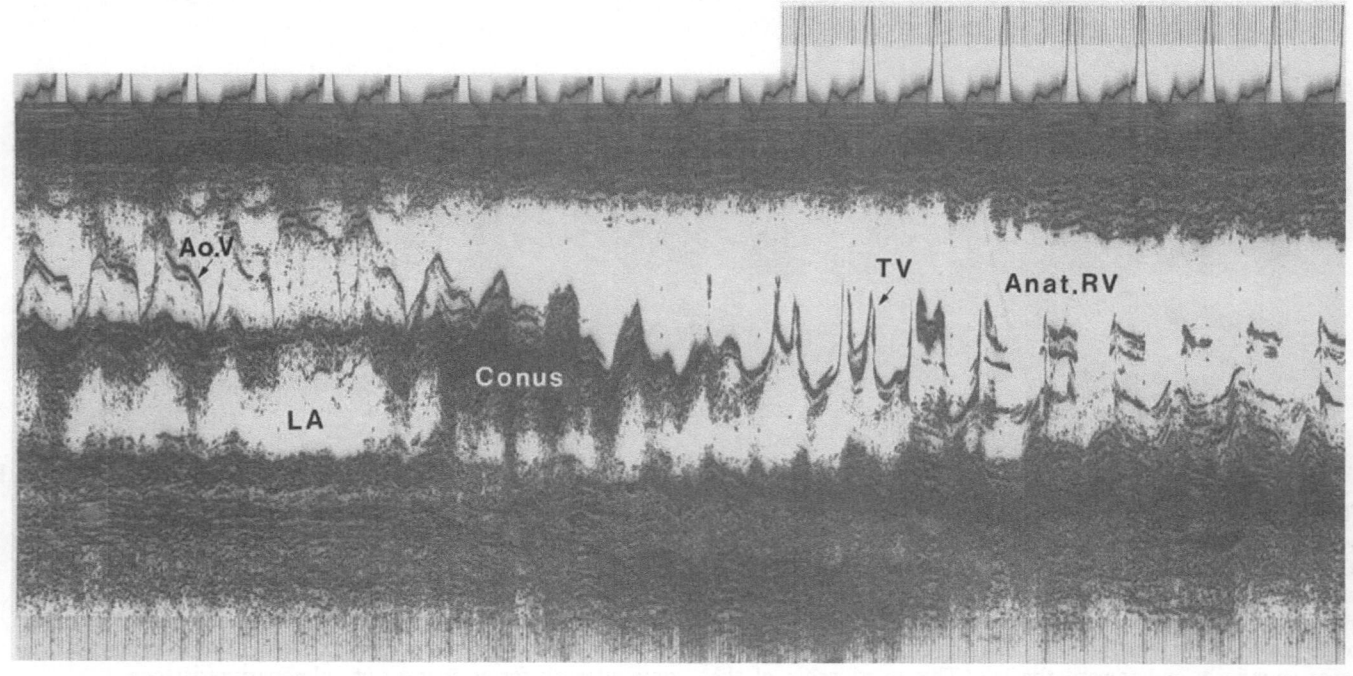

Fig. 7–91. *M-mode arc scan from the aortic to the tricuspid valve (left-sided atrioventricular valve) in a 4-year-old boy with L-TGA* (patient in Fig. 7–90) reveals a marked break in continuity corresponding to interposition of the conus muscle. To obtain this image the transducer is placed along the left sternal border and is first directed far to the left and superiorly to identify the aortic valve (*Ao.V*). It is then scanned inferiorly and leftward to encounter the tricuspid valve (*TV*) within the left-sided ventricle (anatomic right ventricle, *Anat. RV*). *LA* = left atrium.

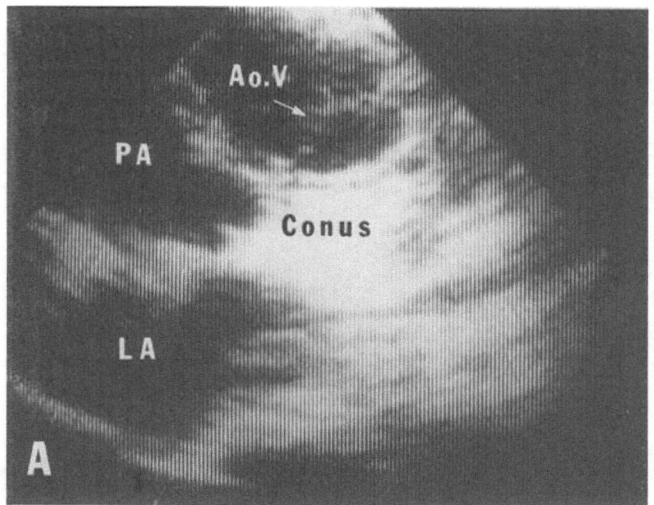

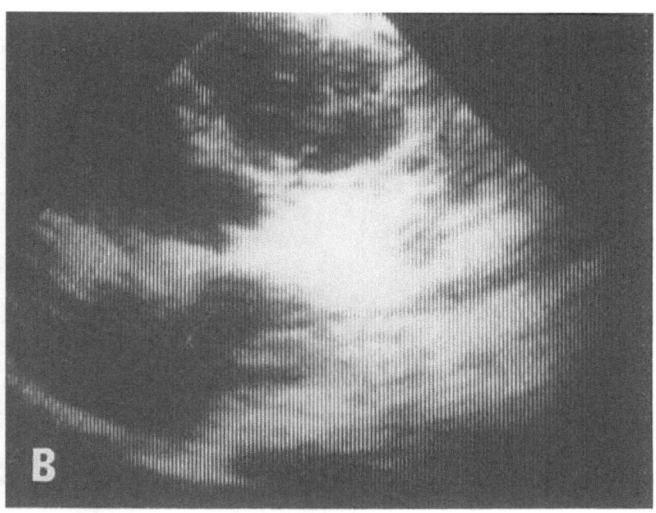

Fig. 7–92. *Two-dimensional echocardiograms in L-TGA.* **A** with labels; **B** without labels. The short axis view at the level of the great vessels demonstrates the anterior semilunar valve (*Ao.V*) to the left and the posterior semilunar valve (*PA*) to the right. This image differs from normal in that two circles are present and occurs because the two great arteries ascend in parallel. With normally related great arteries the right ventricular outflow tract wraps around the aortic valve anteriorly, so that the image produced is that of a "circle and sausage" (see Fig. 2–20). LA = left atrium

culty in imaging L-TGA by M-Mode occurs because the ventricular septum lies in a sagittal plane, parallel to the sound beam. Thus the ventricular septum reflects poorly and is difficult to image. Dropout of echoes may lead to suspicion of a large VSD or even a single ventricle, in spite of the presence of an intact septum. If the septum is not recognized, an arc scan might be obtained from the pulmonic valve across the septum to the left A-V valve. This might be mistakenly interpreted as aortic-mitral fibrous continuity. In instances of L-TGA with VSD the pulmonic and tricuspid valves may actually be continuous across the VSD, increasing the opportunity for error. Thus, while M-mode may define the great vessel orientation, it is not always helpful in evaluating the intracardiac relationships.

On 2-D echocardiography the positions of the great vessels are defined by a short axis view at the level of the great vessels (Fig. 7–92). A long axis view of the left-sided vessel will show the superior sweep of an ascending aorta (Fig. 7–93). Serial cross sections of the right-sided vessel will reveal the bifurcation and the main pulmonary branches (see Fig. 7–126), identifying that vessel as pulmonary. Long axis views of the RV may demonstrate the conus (Fig. 7–94). Long axis views of the LV (Fig. 7–95) may demonstrate subpulmonic obstruction or valvar pulmonic stenosis. Apical and subxiphoid four-chamber views (Figs. 7–96 and 7–97) may aid in identifying complex intracardiac relationships such as mitral-pulmonary fibrous continuity, and VSD. Of note on the four-chamber view is that the left A-V valve (tricuspid) is attached to the septum closer to the apex than is the right A-V valve (mitral)

(Fig. 7–96). This pattern is the reverse of normal. In addition, the moderator band is in the left-sided ventricle (anatomical RV) rather than in the right-sided ventricle (Figs. 7–96 and 7–97). As each image is recorded in these complex cases the position of the transducer must be clearly indicated so that the images can be used later to reconstruct the anatomy.

Radiological (Plain Film) Features Because of the abnormal position of the great arteries, the image of a normal vascular pedicle (formed by the triad of the ascending aorta on the right, aortic arch and main pulmonary artery on the left) is not observed. Instead the vascular pedicle tends to be narrow (Fig. 7–98). The ascending aorta and the outflow tract of the left-sided morphological RV produce a slightly convex upper left heart border (Fig. 7–98), a straight left heart border (Fig. 7–99) or a shoulder-like configuration of the left heart border (Fig. 7–100). The main pulmonary artery is not border forming. Instead, the main and left pulmonary arteries may produce a density within the cardiac silhouette (Fig. 7–99), causing an impression on the left side of the esophagus below the level of the aortic indentation. On occasion the right pulmonary artery is tilted upward, producing a steep downward slope of its branches as they turn to supply the lower lobe of the right lung. This anatomical arrangement of the right pulmonary artery and its branches produces a characteristic waterfall appearance on the frontal plain roentgenograms (Fig. 7–98). A prominent pulmonary artery may displace the superior vena cava to the right, producing a density along the right upper heart border (Figs. 7–99, 7–100), which may be mistaken for the ascending aorta.

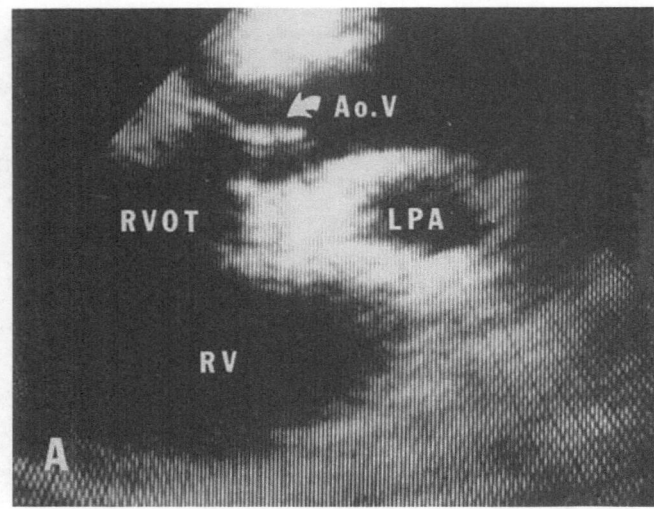

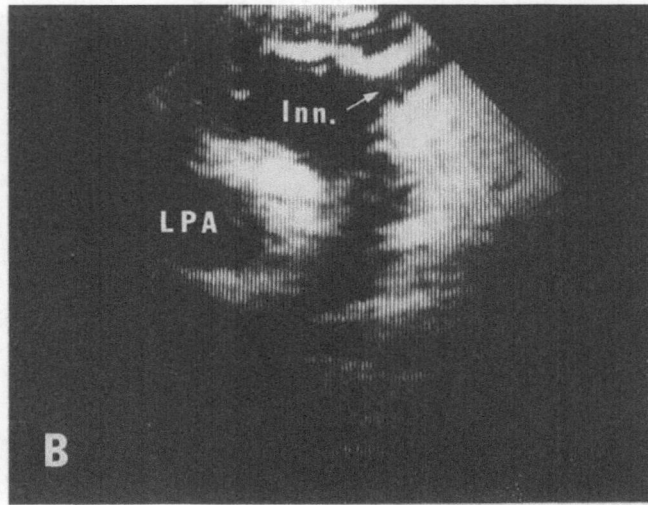

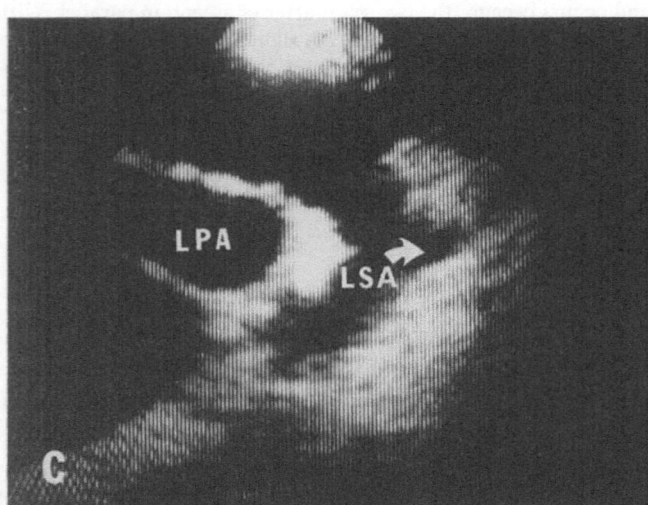

Fig. 7–93. *Long axis of the aorta in L-TGA.* These two-dimensional echocardiograms are obtained from the second left intercostal space or the suprasternal notch. **A** represents the aortic valve (*Ao. V*), which is anterior (near the chest wall) as it arises from the right ventricular outflow tract (*RVOT*). *RV* = right ventricle. **B** represents the ascending aorta and the innominate artery (*Inn.*). **C** delineates the aortic arch, left subclavian (*LSA*) artery and descending aorta. The left pulmonary artery (*LPA*) is behind and below the aortic arch in all views. See Fig. 7–126 for a long axis view of the main pulmonary artery (*MPA*) in levotransposition. The *MPA* curves immediately posteriorly to form the pulmonary branches.

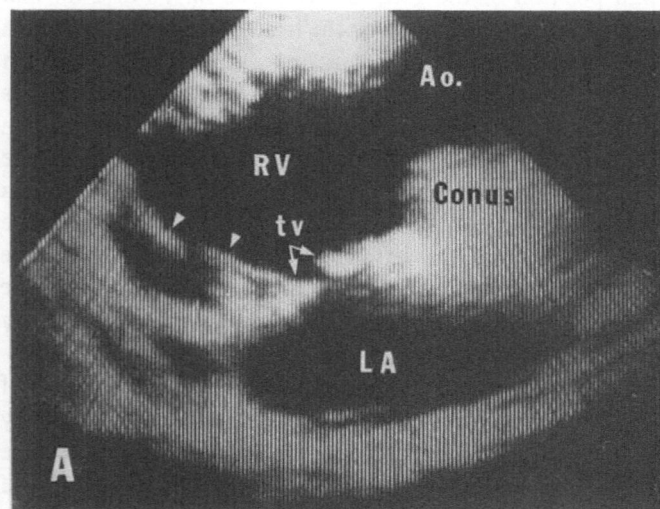

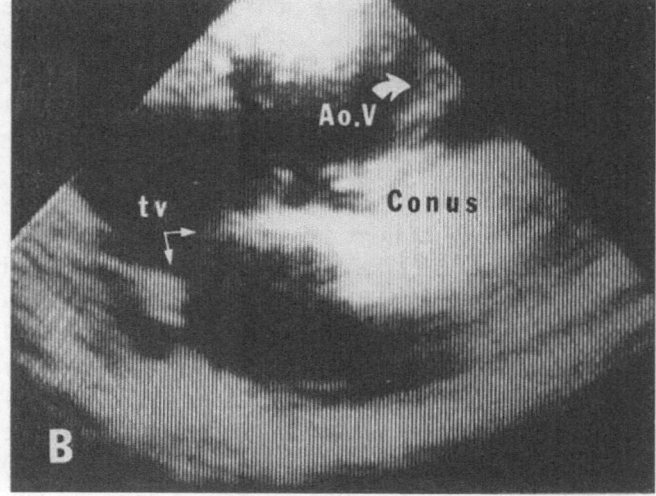

Fig. 7–94. *Two-dimensional echocardiogram in L-TGA.* **A** systole; **B** diastole. This parasternal long axis view identifies the anatomic right ventricle (*RV*).

A The right ventricle is recognized during systole because of the conus muscle that separates the semilunar valve from the atrioventricular valve (*tv*). The atrioventricular valve follows the ventricle; therefore this valve is a tricuspid valve. This tricuspid valve is thickened. Clinically and on ventriculography, tricuspid insufficiency was present. *LA* = left atrium; *Ao.* = ascending aorta; *arrowheads* = chordae tendineae of tricuspid valve. **B** The tricuspid valve is open and the aortic valve (*Ao. V*) is closed during diastole. The outflow tract of the right ventricle is best appreciated in **A**.

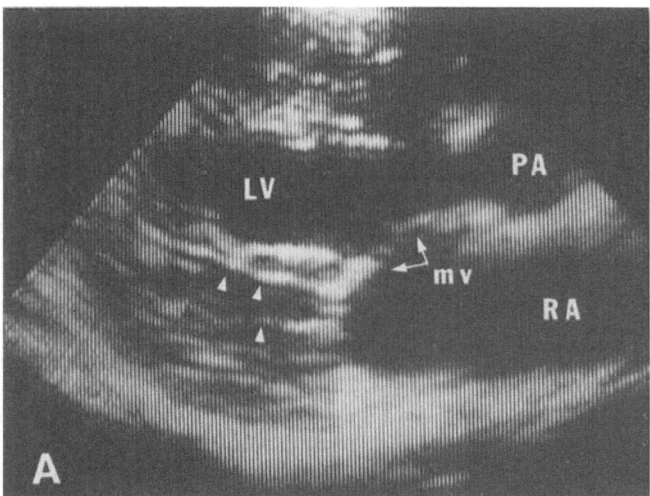

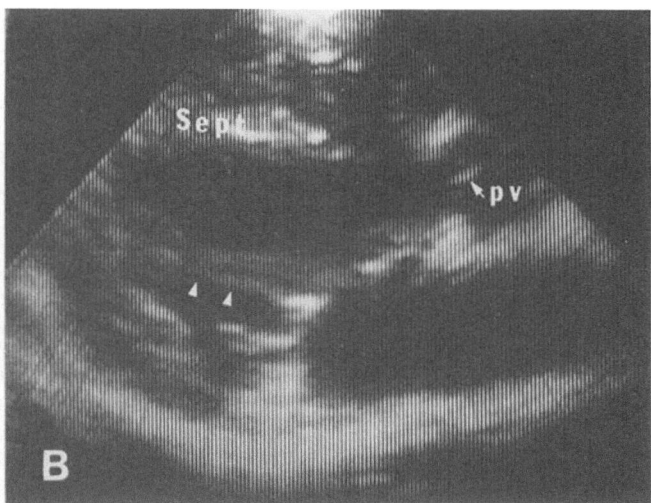

Fig. 7–95. *Parasternal long axis view of the anatomic left ventricle in L-TGA.* **A** Late systole; **B** early diastole. This view is obtained by angling the transducer far toward the right from the left sternal border. This angle is used to demonstrate the tricuspid valve and right ventricular apex in normal persons.

A During late systole the mitral valve (*mv*) is closed, and the pulmonary valve is open. **B** During early diastole the pulmonary valve (*pv*) is closed and the mitral valve remains closed.

Pulmonary-mitral fibrous continuity is demonstrated in both **A** and **B**. The shape of the ventricle is that of a normal left ventricle. This view is very difficult to obtain, especially in patients with mesocardia or dextrocardia.

LV = anatomical left ventricle; *PA* = pulmonary artery; *RA* = right atrium; *arrowheads* = chordae tendineae; *Sept* = interventricular septum.

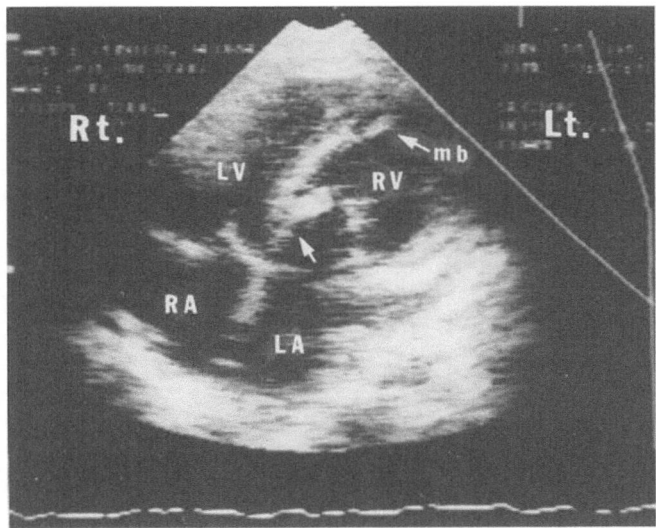

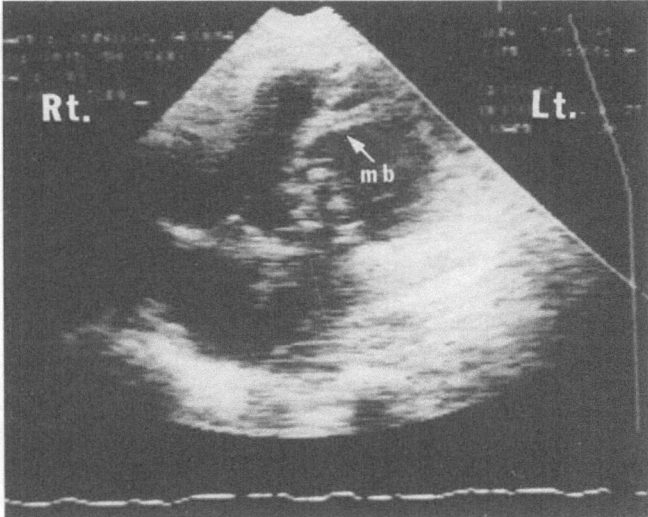

Fig. 7–96. *Apex 4-chamber view of a two-dimensional echocardiogram in a 36-year-old man with L-TGA and with a ventricular septal defect and pulmonic stenosis.* The patient's right side (*Rt.*) and left side (*Lt.*) are indicated. The insertion of the left-sided atrioventricular valve (A-V valve, *arrow*) is slightly distal to the insertion of the right sided A-V valve. Thus, the left-sided A-V valve is likely to be the anatomic tricuspid valve. *LV* = anatomic left ventricle; *RV* = anatomic right ventricle; *RA* = right atrium; *LA* = left atrium; *mb* = moderator band.

Fig. 7–97. *Same patient as in Fig. 7–96.* The moderator band (*mb*) is present in the left-sided ventricle; thus, the left-sided ventricle represents the anatomic right ventricle. Features in Figs. 7–96 and 7–97 indicate ventricular inversion.

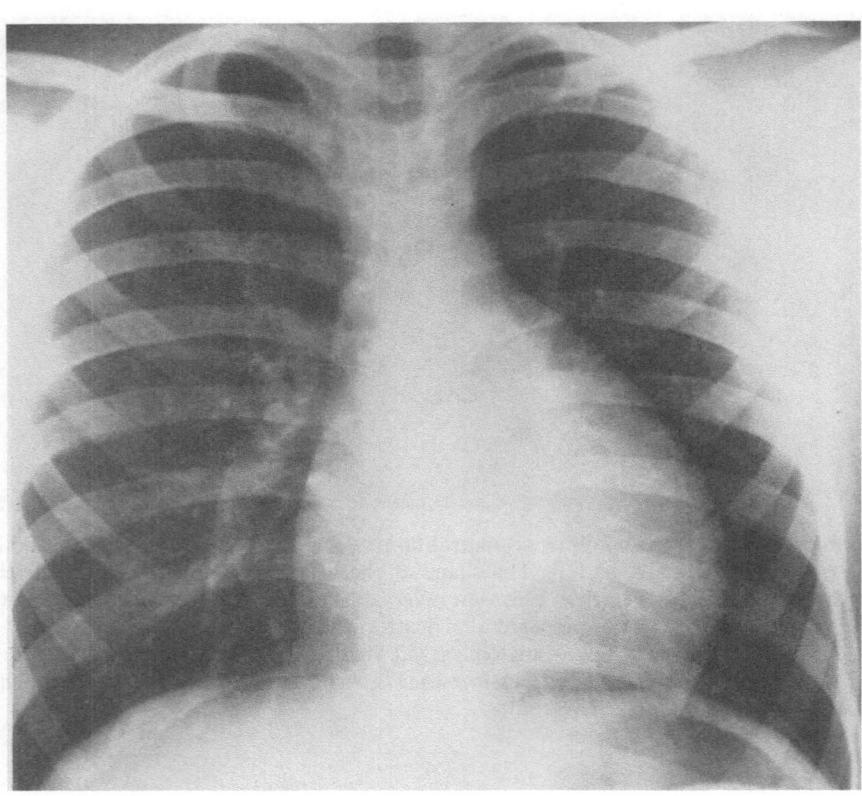

A

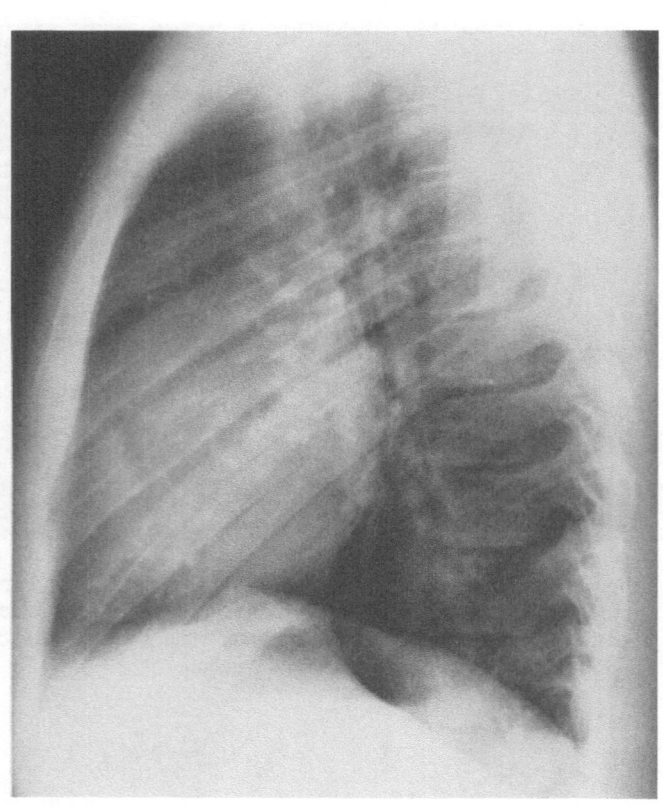

B

Fig. 7–98. *The characteristic convex left heart border in L-TGA.* **A** In this 11-year-old boy with L-TGA, ventricular septal defect and subpulmonic stenosis, mild cardiomegaly is shown on the frontal projection. Convexity of the left heart border is produced by the right ventricular outflow tract and ascending aorta. This convexity of the left heart border may occasionally be difficult to distinguish from a thymus.

B Failure to identify the thymus on the lateral projection should lead to the correct diagnosis.

In this patient a radiolucent line, representing the epicardial fat, outlines the myocardium separating it from the pericardium. (The presence of this line excludes the thymus.) The main pulmonary artery is medial to the ascending aorta. The right pulmonary artery illustrates the characteristic waterfall appearance. Pulmonary overcirculation is absent because pulmonic stenosis limits pulmonary blood flow. (Same patient as in Fig. 7–101, 7–102, 7–104).

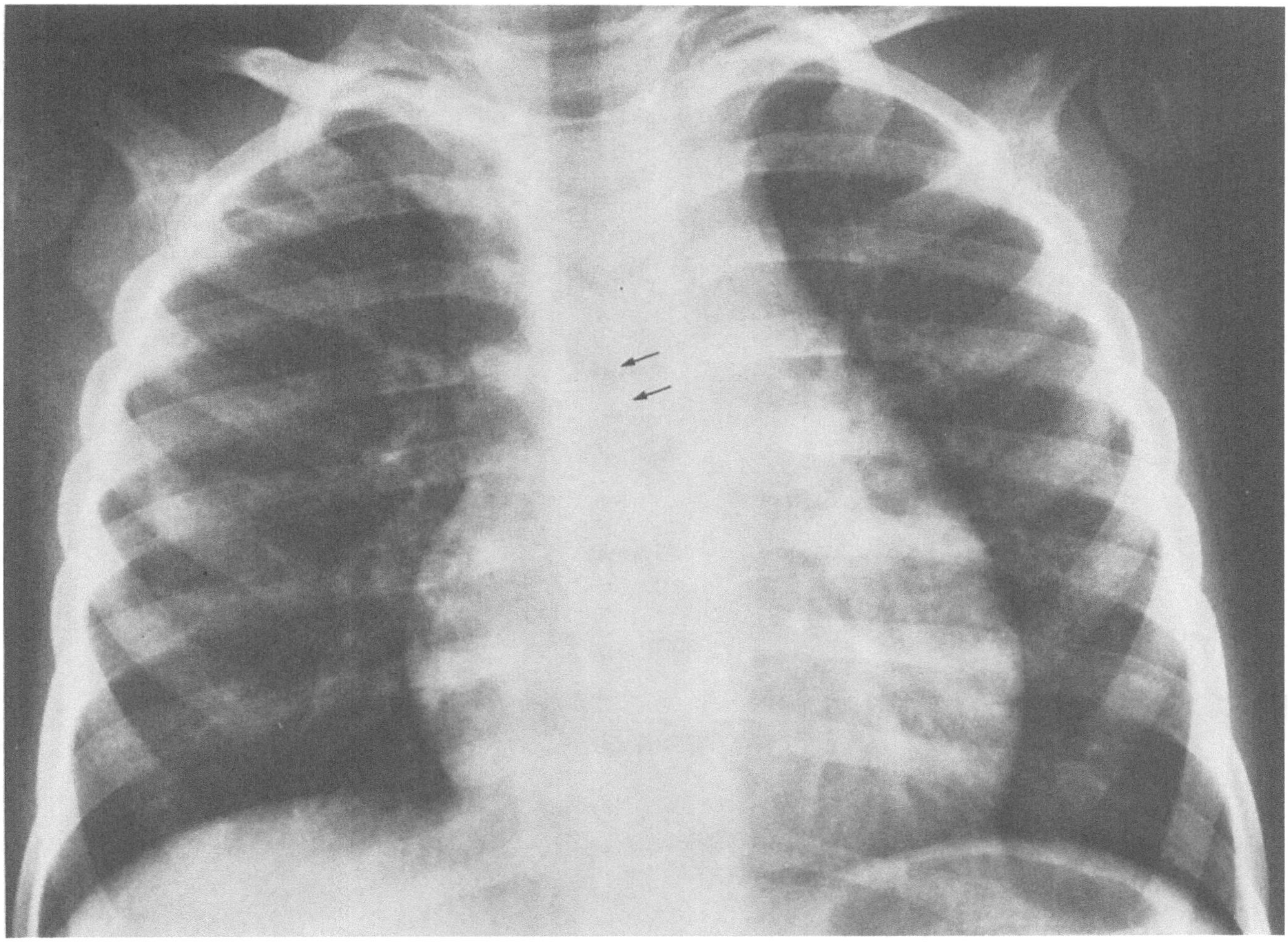

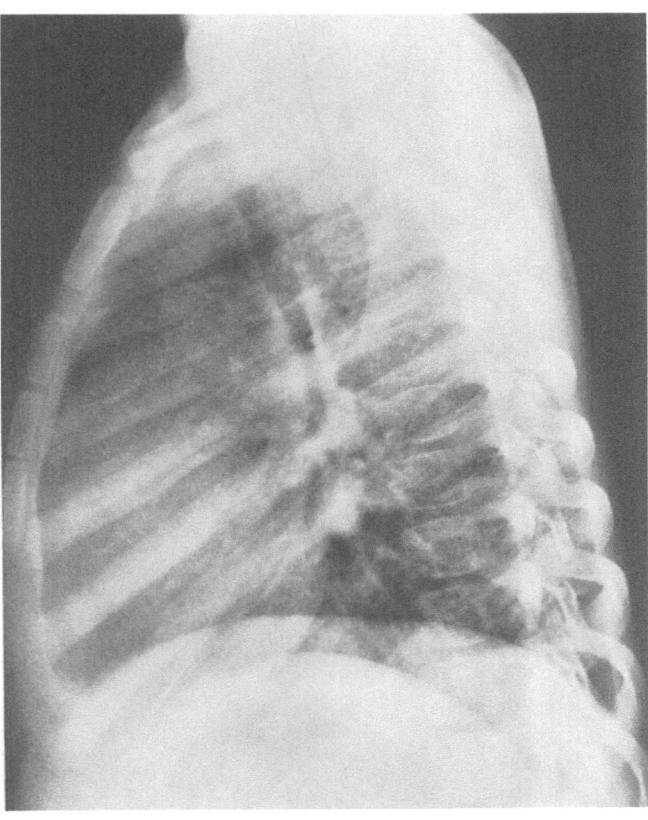

A

Fig. 7–99. *Roentgenogram of the chest in a 3-year-old girl with L-TGA and pulmonic stenosis.* The left heart border is straight rather than convex. In this patient, straightening of the left heart border is due to the abnormal position of the aorta as it arises from the outflow tract of the right ventricle and should not be mistaken for enlargement of the left atrium. Other causes of straightening of the left heart border include (1) idiopathic dilatation of the left atrial appendage; (2) thymus (normal or abnormal); (3) dilatation of the right ventricular outflow tract; (4) aneurysm of the outflow tract of the right ventricle; (5) pericardial defect; (6) pericardial cyst and (7) L-TGA. Absence of a corresponding density on the lateral view is usually helpful in excluding thymus, pericardial cyst and left atrial enlargement. In this patient the main feature other than straightening of the left heart border is the medial location of the main pulmonary artery (*arrows*). The left pulmonary artery is also visualized through the density of the heart.

B

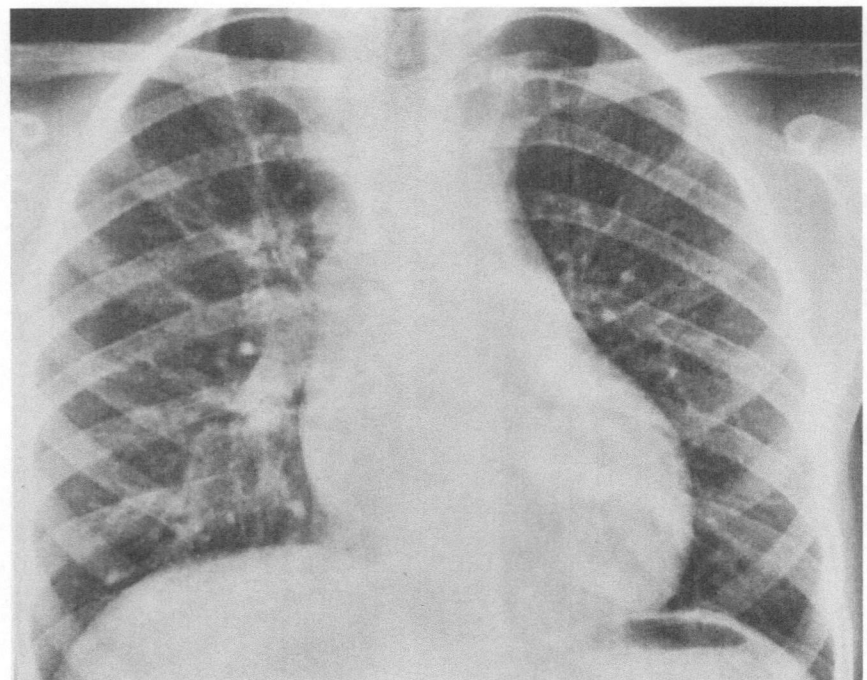

A

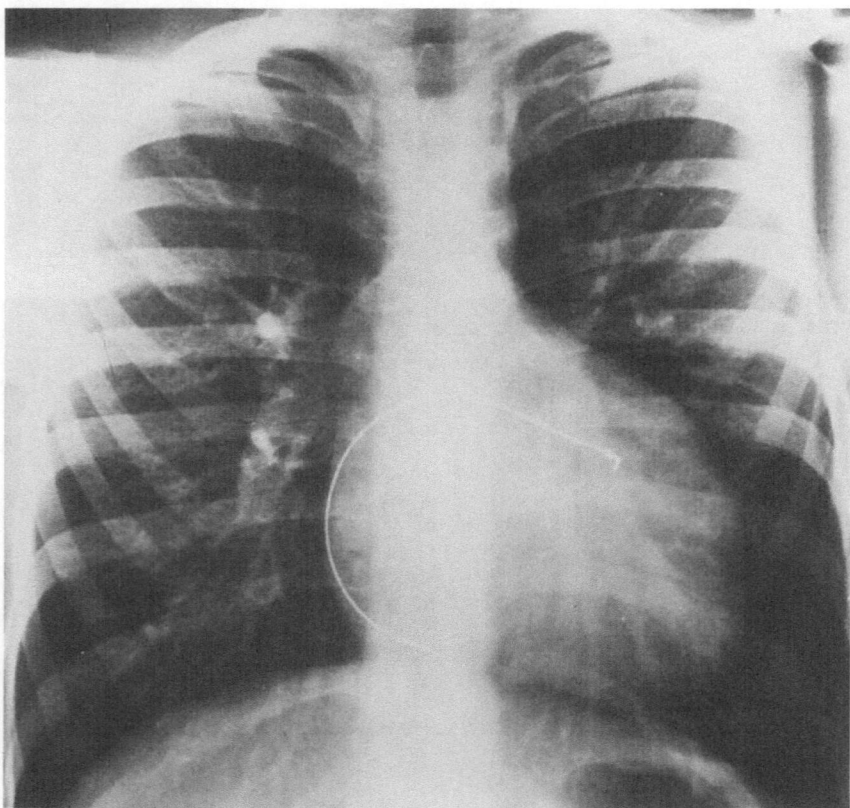

B

Fig. 7–100. *Shoulder-like configuration ("bump") of the left heart border in a 7-year-old girl with L-TGA and in an 8-year-old boy with L-TGA with complete heart block after repair of a ventricular septal defect.* **A** In the girl this bump is formed by the outflow tract of the right ventricle (see angiogram, Fig. 7–103). **B** In the boy the bump is observed to be more prominent and somewhat higher, representing the junction between the right ventricular outflow tract and the aortic valve.

Poststenotic dilatation of the main pulmonary artery may result in a prominent convexity of the upper right heart border. Because the ventricular septum has a somewhat horizontal orientation, it may be represented by a notch (septal notch) in the left heart border on the frontal projection. The notch is at the apex if the RV is well developed, but is difficult to recognize in this location. If the RV is rudimentary as in patients with single ventricle, then the septal notch is higher in location and easier to identify.

The pulmonary vasculature is variable, but because of the frequent presence of large VSDs, overcirculation is often noted. The pulmonary vascularity may be normal or decreased (pulmonary undercirculation) in the presence of pulmonic stenosis.

Hemodynamics Pressures and oxygen contents in the cardiac chambers are normal, and the systemic circulation is fully saturated in patients without septal defects or pulmonic stenosis; however, most patients have defects such as ASD, VSD and pulmonic stenosis. In such instances the hemodynamics will reflect the associated defects. Intra-

cardiac electrophysiological studies may be indicated in individuals with heart block or other arrhythmias.

Contrast Studies Of the various catheter positions, the one characteristic of L-TGA is that of a retrograde catheter in the ascending aorta (Fig. 7–101A and B). Instead of looping medially and posteriorly in the transverse arch as it does in normal individuals (Fig. 7–101C and D), the catheter curves laterally toward the left heart border. Of course, the lateral view will show the catheter to lie anteriorly (Fig. 7–101B). The venous catheter may have an apparently normal passage to the right-sided ventricle (Fig. 7–101A and B). The pulmonary artery will be entered posteriorly and somewhat medially. Injection into the anatomical RV (systemic ventricle) will demonstrate the abnormal position of the aorta and inversion of the ventricles (Fig. 7–102). Injection into the anatomical RV will also delineate the distribution of the coronary arteries (Fig. 7–102E) and will demonstrate such associated defects as VSD, tricuspid insufficiency (or Ebstein malformation of the tricuspid valve) and coarctation of the aorta if present. Injection

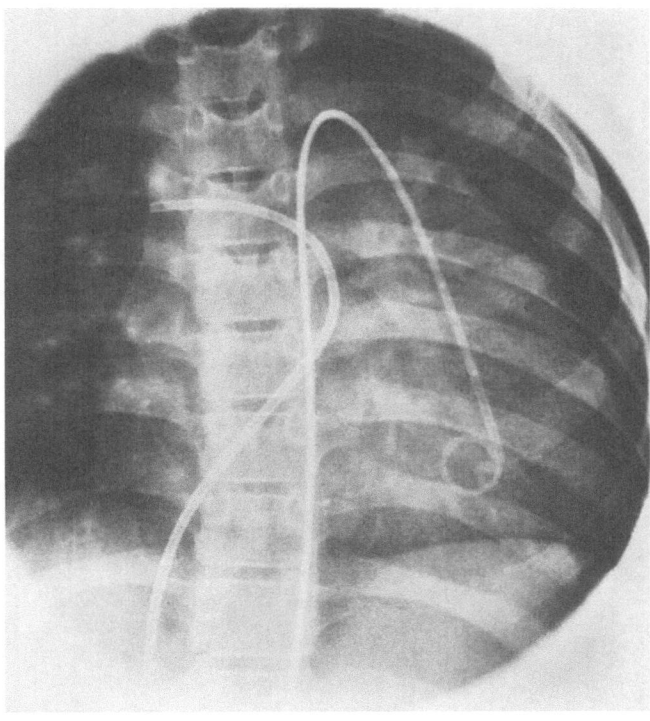

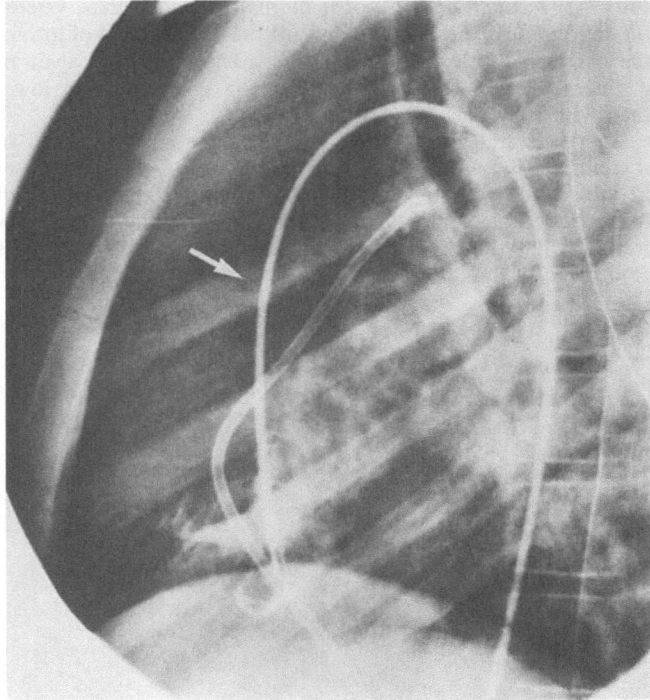

A   B

Fig. 7–101. *The position of a retrograde aortic catheter in L-TGA.* (Same patient as in Fig. 7–98, 7–102, 7–104.) **A** Frontal view of a catheter in the anatomic right ventricle in L-TGA. **B** Lateral view of the catheter in L-TGA. **C** and **D** are from a patient with normally related great vessels (patient in Fig. 7–79A and B) for comparison. **C** Frontal view of a catheter in the left ventricle; **D** Lateral view.

A The retrograde arterial catheter (pigtail catheter) ascends in the thoracic aorta to the left of the spine. In the aortic arch it curves toward the left to enter the ascending aorta and anatomical right ventricle. As the heart contracts the catheter may rotate, so that on the frontal view the descending portion of the catheter may intermittently cross its ascending portion, high up in the ascending aorta.

B The aortic catheter (*arrow*) curves anteriorly to enter the

aortic arch. The catheter tip is in the anatomical right ventricle. If this catheter were in the apex of the heart it would appear more anteriorly near the chest wall (the lateral view of the retrograde catheter is not helpful in diagnosing L-TGA, without the frontal view).

A second catheter, the venous catheter, follows a course that is indistinguishable from normal on the frontal view (**A**) as it enters the right atrium and passes through the anatomic left ventricle and main pulmonary artery to reach the right pulmonary artery.

In the lateral view (**B**) the venous catheter enters the pulmonary artery posterior to the position of the aortic catheter. This abnormal position of the catheters mandates the diagnosis of transposition of the great arteries, and suggests L-TGA. (*Continued*)

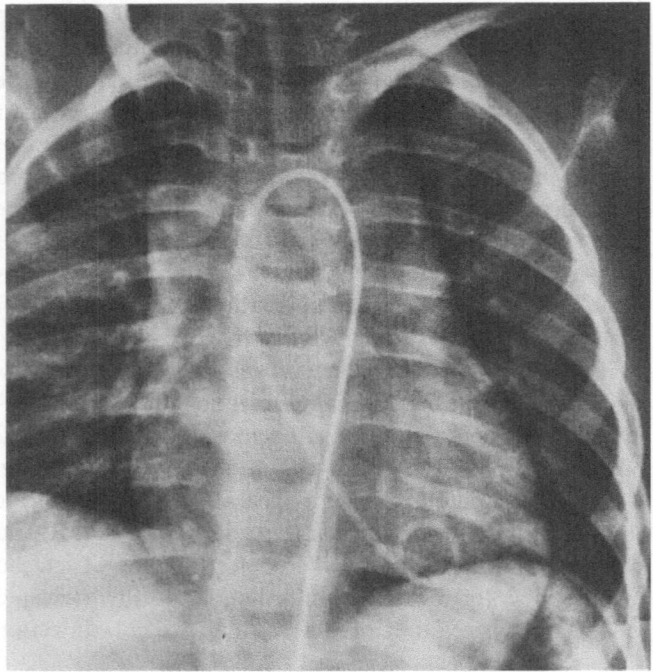

C

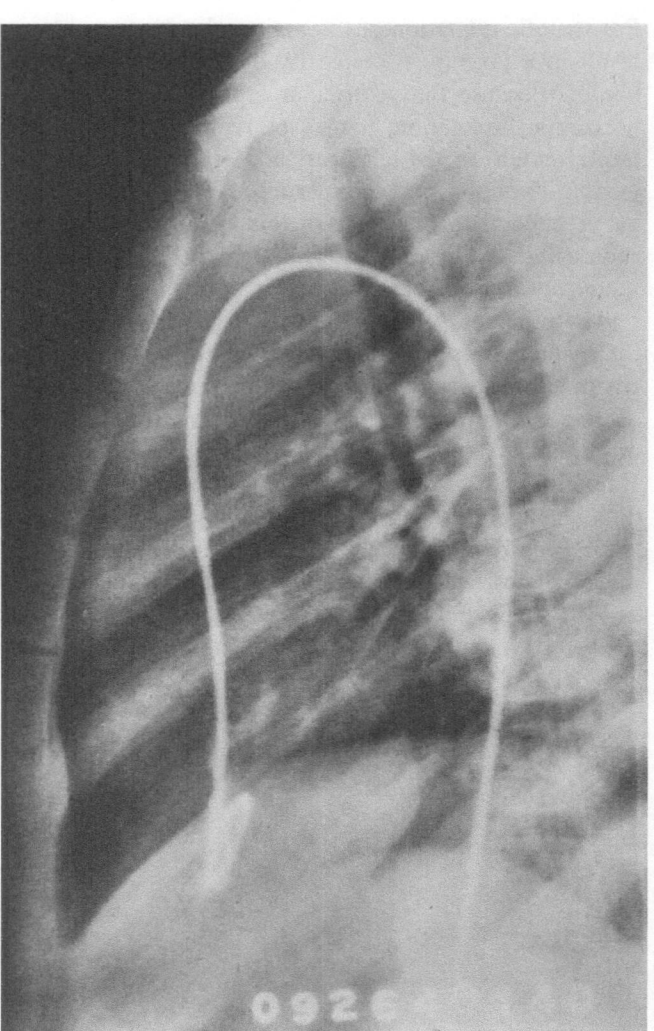

Fig. 7–101 (*Cont.*). In **C**, with normally related great vessels, the retrograde catheter curves toward the right instead of toward the left as it reaches the aortic arch, passing laterally again as it enters the left ventricle. The crossing point is much lower than with L-TGA.

In the lateral view (**D**) the course of the aortic catheter in this normal person appears similar to that of the aortic catheter in the patient with L-TGA. Thus, the characteristic course of the aortic catheter in L-TGA is recognized in the frontal projection, while the characteristic course of the venous catheter is recognized in the lateral view.

D

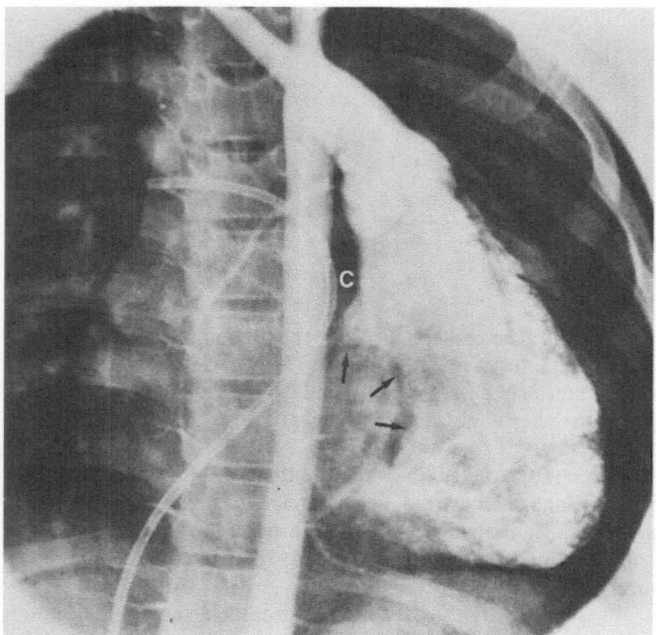

A

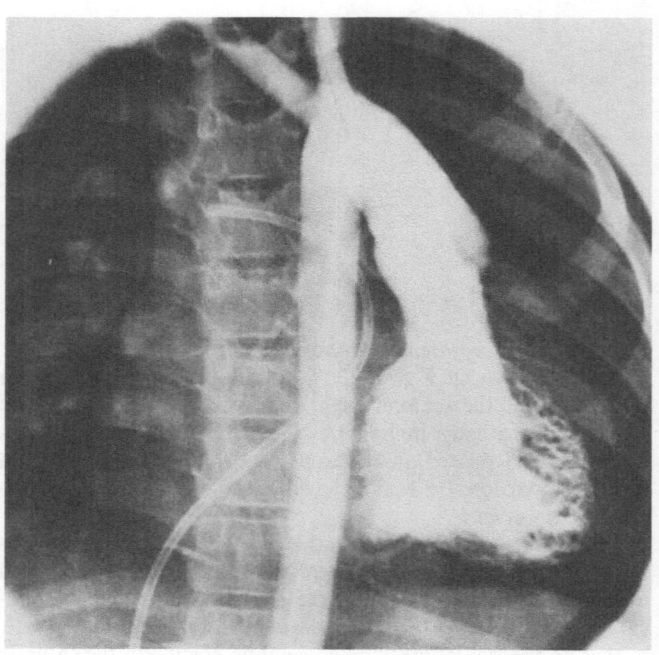

B

Fig. 7–102. *Injection into the anatomic right ventricle in L-TGA* (Patient in Figs. 7–98, 7–101, 7–104). In the frontal view (**A**) during diastole and (**B**) systole the right ventricular outflow tract and the ascending aorta account for the convexity of the left heart border. The shape of the ventricle and its trabeculations identify the chamber as a right ventricle (*RV*); (*Continued*)

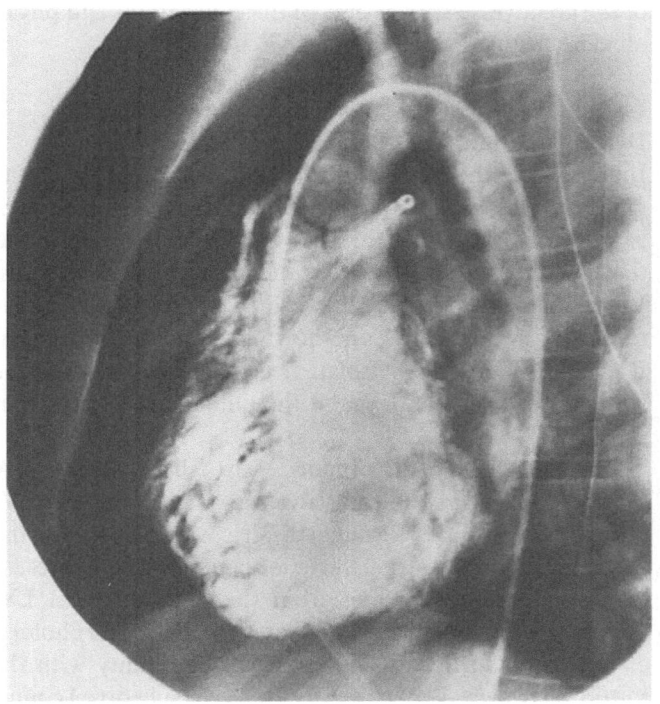

C

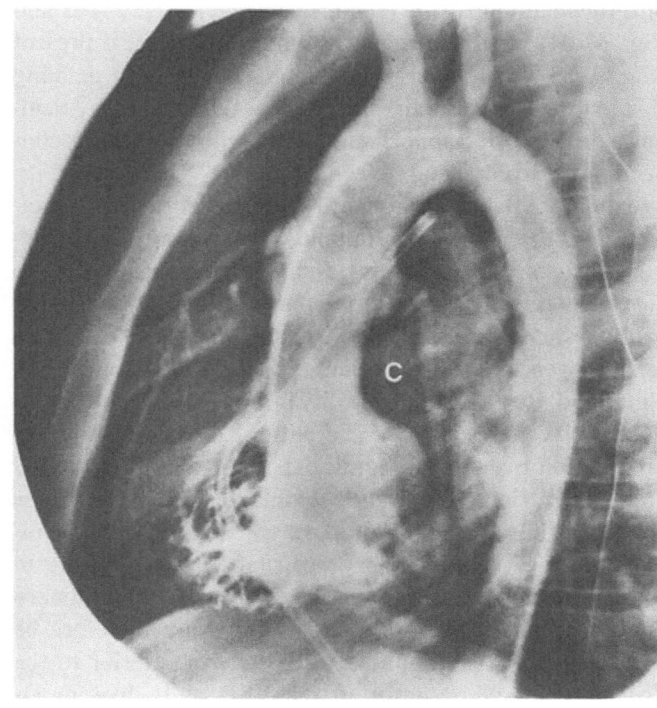

D

Fig. 7-102 (*Cont.*) The atrioventricular valve is tricuspid because it is associated with a right ventricle. In normal ventricles and in ventricular inversion the atrioventricular valves follow their respective ventricles. The conus (*c*) separates the tricuspid valve (*arrows*) from the aortic valve. The aorta arises along the left heart border, ascends obliquely and superiorly and then descends on the left side of the spine. The convexity of the ascending aorta toward the left is characteristic of L-TGA. In almost all instances of L-TGA, the ventricular loop is "L," which means that the anatomical right ventricle is on the left (this is known as the loop rule).

On the lateral projection (**C**) during diastole the typical appearance of the anatomical right ventricle is demonstrated and in (**D**) during systole the subaortic conus becomes evident. In **E** (lateral view late in the series to show the coronary arteries) the courses of the coronary arteries are outlined. The anterior (right) coronary artery (*ACA*) divides into an anterior descending coronary artery (*AD*), which runs in the anterior interventricular sulcus, and a right-sided circumflex (*RCX*), which runs in the right atrioventricular groove. The posterior (left) coronary artery (*PCA*) runs in the left atrioventricular groove to the crux of the heart, where it divides into a posterior descending coronary artery (*PD*) and a crux artery (see also Fig. 7-88.)

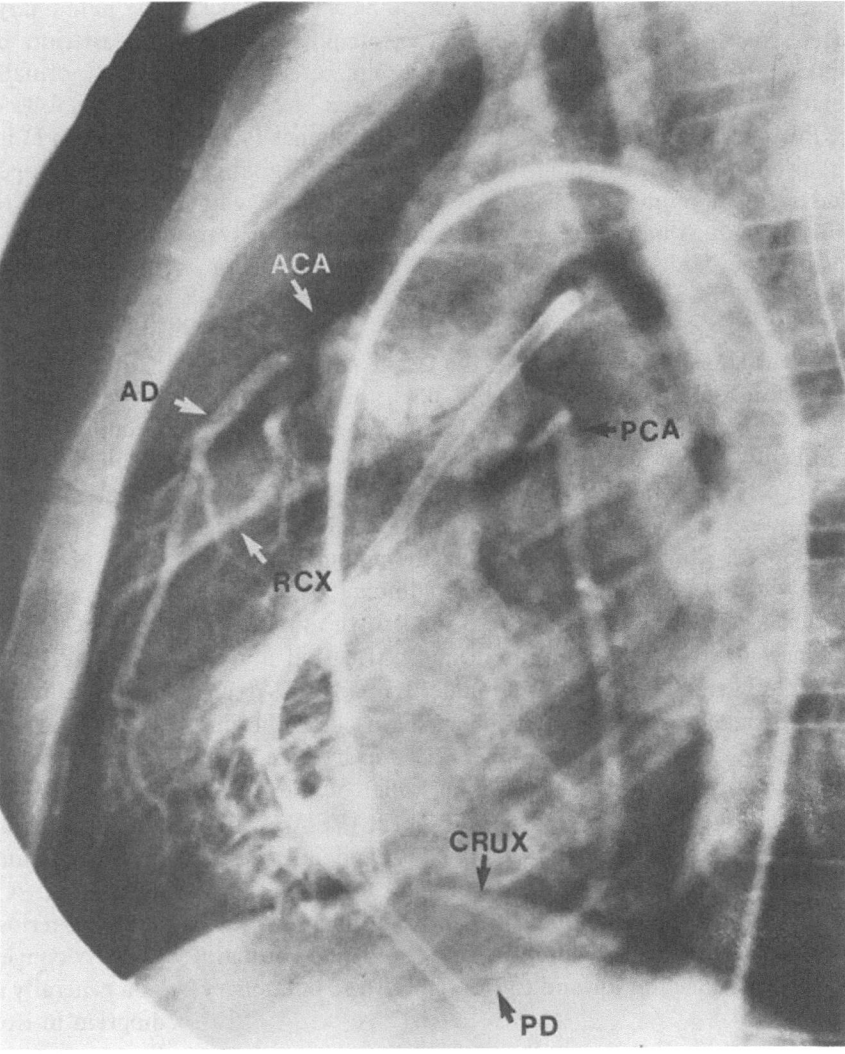

E

into the anatomical LV (venous ventricle) (Fig. 7–103 and Fig. 7–104) will delineate subpulmonic stenosis, if present (Fig. 7–104). The lateral view is most helpful in defining this lesion. The recirculation phase of this study may demonstrate associated abnormalities of pulmonary venous connection or atrial septal defect.

Treatment Medical treatment is determined by the associated defect (e.g., VSD, pulmonic or subpulmonic obstruction, tricuspid regurgitation). Infants requiring surgery are generally referred for palliation (e.g., pulmonary artery band, systemic-to-pulmonary shunt) rather than definitive repair. Even when intracardiac repair is delayed until mid childhood, the reported mortality is high and the postoperative results are only fair. The pattern of coronary artery distribution over the anatomical LV leaves only a limited area for ventriculotomy. The proximal bundle of His passes anterior to the pulmonary outflow tract, so that the definitive repair of subpulmonary obstruction often results in complete heart block. Reconstruction of the pulmonary outflow tract by the use of a conduit may therefore be necessary. The distal bundle of His passes anterior to the VSD, instead of posterior to the VSD as it does in D-loop. Intraoperative electrophysiological mapping of the bundle of His reduces the incidence of complete heart block after repair of VSD in L-TGA. Tricuspid regurgitation is difficult to repair, and prosthetic valve replacements are relatively poorly tolerated in growing children.

Postoperative complications include arrhythmias (some requiring pacemaker implantation), tricuspid regurgitation and residual pulmonic stenosis. Residua associated with valved conduits include obstruction and pulmonary valvar insufficiency. Infective endocarditis may also occur postoperatively.

Atypical Dextrotransposition of the Great Arteries

In this uncommon disorder (Fig. 7–65C) the external appearance of the heart is normal even though the connections and hemodynamics are those of (D-TGA). As with typical D-TGA the pulmonary trunk arises from the LV, and the aorta arises from the RV. Unlike D-TGA the conus has developed within the LV, separating the pulmonary valve from the mitral valve, raising the pulmonary valve and displacing it anteriorly and toward the left. In most cases, absence of a RV conus results in aortic-tricuspid fibrous continuity. In a few instances an underdeveloped RV (subaortic) conus is present, preventing aortic-tricuspid fibrous continuity. The posterior cusp of the aortic valve is in fibrous continuity with the anterior leaflet of the mitral valve through the ventricular septal defect (VSD), which is subaortic when viewed from the RV and infracristal when viewed from the LV. The coronary arteries usually have normal distribution, but they may be transposed (i.e., the anterior descending artery arises from the left coronary artery but runs anterior and to the right of the pulmonary trunk).

It is important to recognize that the conus muscle can lie within the LV, resulting in normal spatial relationships

of the great vessels, even though the connections and physiological features are those of D-TGA.

Isolated Ventricular Inversion (Atrioventricular Discordance and Ventriculoarterial Concordance)

Inversion of the ventricles without transposition of the great arteries (isolated ventricular inversion, Fig. 7–65E) is a rare malformation that has been reported both in patients with situs solitus and patients with situs inversus. Ventricular inversion in situs solitus means that the anatomical LV is situated on the right and the anatomical RV on the left. With isolated ventricular inversion the aorta arises from the LV and the pulmonary artery from the RV.

Atrioventricular discordance exists because the RA empties through the mitral valve into the anatomical LV, and the LA empties through the tricuspid valve into the anatomical RV. Ventriculoarterial concordance is present because the aorta emerges from the morphological LV, and the pulmonary artery originates from the morphological RV. The aortic valve is in fibrous continuity with the mitral valve because of absence of the LV (subaortic) conus. The RV (subpulmonic) conus is well developed, separating the pulmonary from the tricuspid valve. The aortic valve is posterior, inferior and to the right of the pulmonary valve (normally related great arteries). Thus this disorder does not follow the loop rule, which states that if the ventricles are in D-loop (RV to the right) the great vessels should be in dextroposition (normal position or D-TGA). In this abnormality the ventricles are in L-loop, and the great vessels are in "normal" position (aorta to the right and posterior). The right coronary ostium is anterior, giving rise to the left anterior descending and right circumflex arteries to supply the LV; the left coronary ostium is posterior, supplying the left-sided, posterior, morphological RV through right ventricular branches; thus the coronary distribution is inverted, as are the ventricles.

Clinical Features Although the great arteries are normally oriented with a normal relationship to the ventricles and atrioventricular (A-V) valves, the physiological features are those of (D-TGA) because both the aorta and cavae are to the right of the cardiac septa, and therefore both carry deoxygenated blood. Thus, as with D-TGA, associated defects (ASD, VSD, PDA) are needed for survival.

The clinical presentation of isolated ventricular inversion is like that of typical D-TGA. The babies are observed to be cyanotic and acidotic soon after birth, with death ensuing if inadequate intracardiac communication exists. An atrial septal defect may allow survival for a few months or years if enough oxygenated blood crosses to the systemic circulation. A large ventricular septal defect or a patent ductus arteriosus should facilitate oxygenation, but unfortunately congestive heart failure and pulmonary hypertension generally supervene (see also D-TGA). The electrocardiogram in isolated ventricular inversion reveals a normal P wave axis, consistent with situs solitus and a QRS complex suggestive of ventricular inversion.

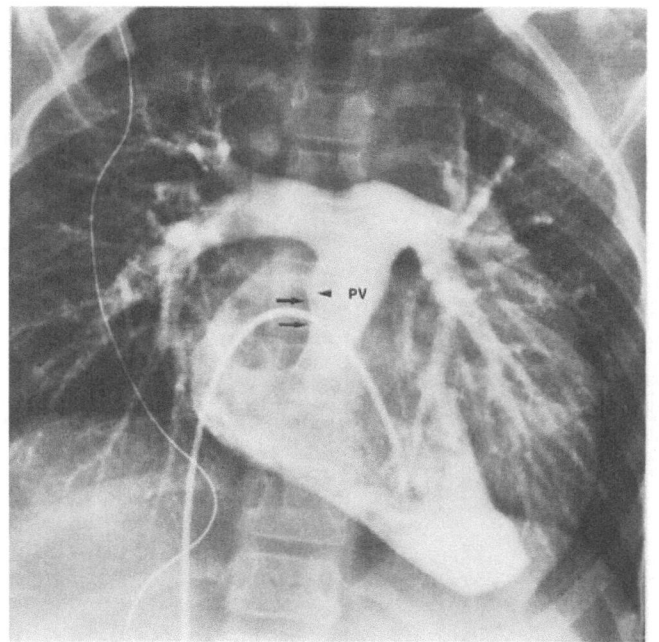

A

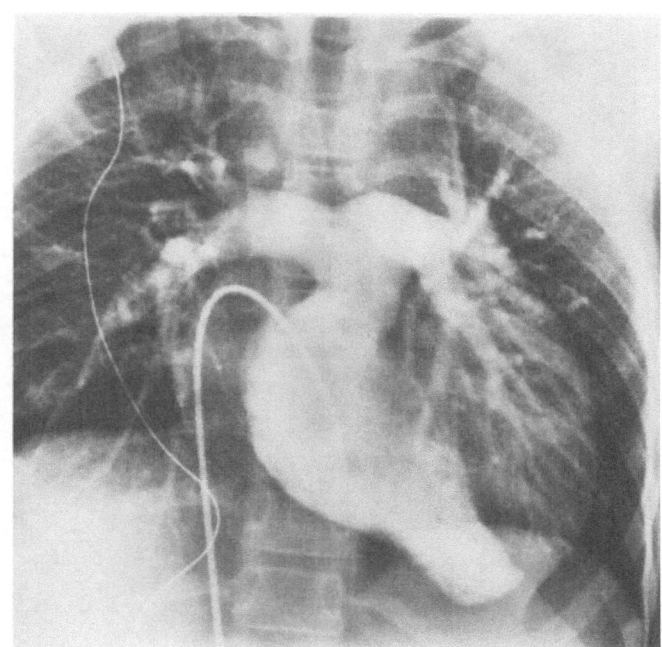

B

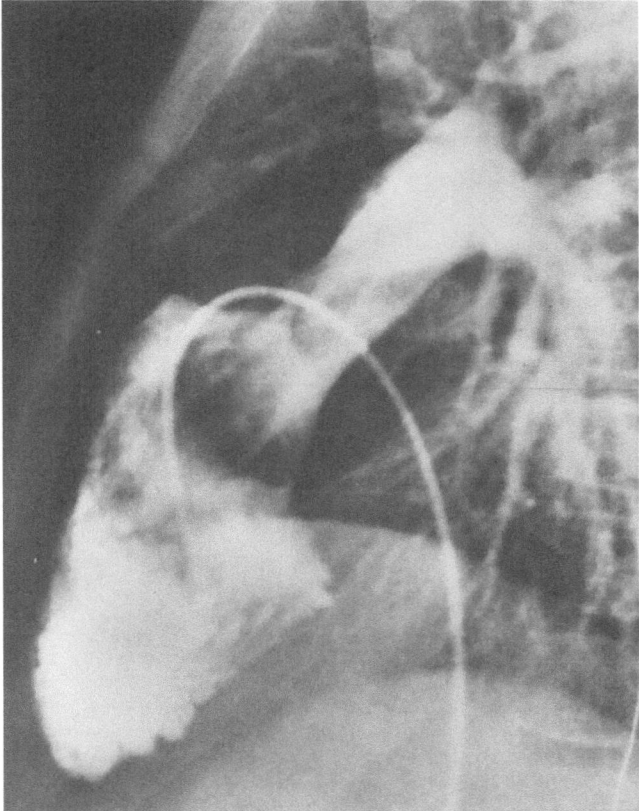

C

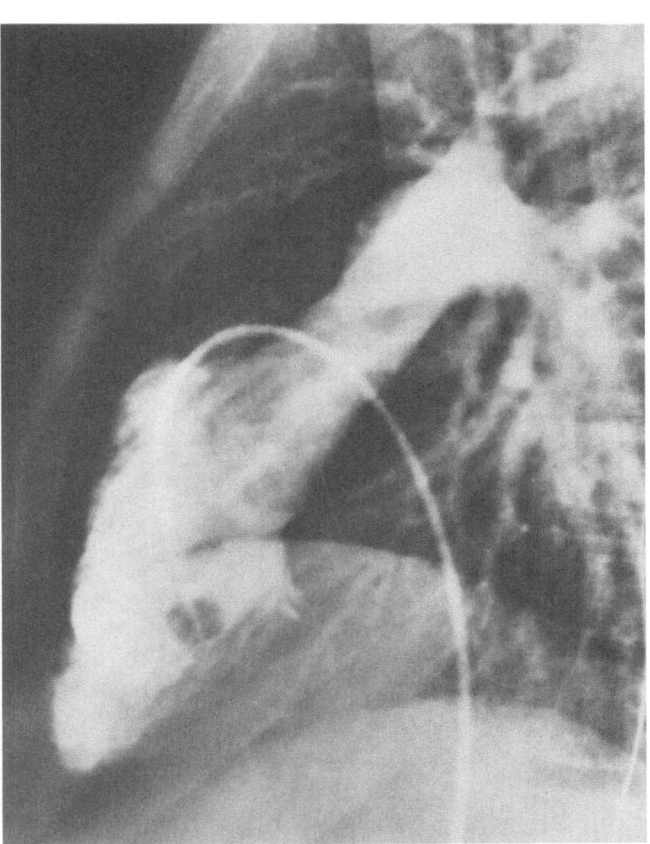

D

Fig. 7-103. *The anatomic left ventricle in L-TGA.* **A** Frontal view, diastole; **B** frontal view, systole; **C** lateral view, diastole; **D** lateral view, systole.

A and **B** The characteristic shape and lack of coarse trabeculations identify this ventricle as a left ventricle. Again the atrioventricular valve (*arrows*) follows the ventricle, and therefore in this instance is a mitral valve. Conus is not identified during diastole or during systole, ensuring that pulmonary-mitral fibrous continuity is present (*arrowhead*). The pulmonary valve (*PV*) is in the middle of the cardiac silhouette, to the right of and inferior to the aortic valve.

C The mitral valve opens normally. Note that this ventricle has a type III mitral valve apparatus, indicating a high fulcrum, without notching of the fornix (see Fig. 4-36 for a description of the types of mitral valve). The pulmonary valve is inferior and posterior to the aortic valve. Again conus is not evident during diastole or systole.

The course of the venous catheter is from inferior vena cava to the right atrium through the mitral valve into the anatomical left ventricle. (Same patient as Fig. 7-100A.)

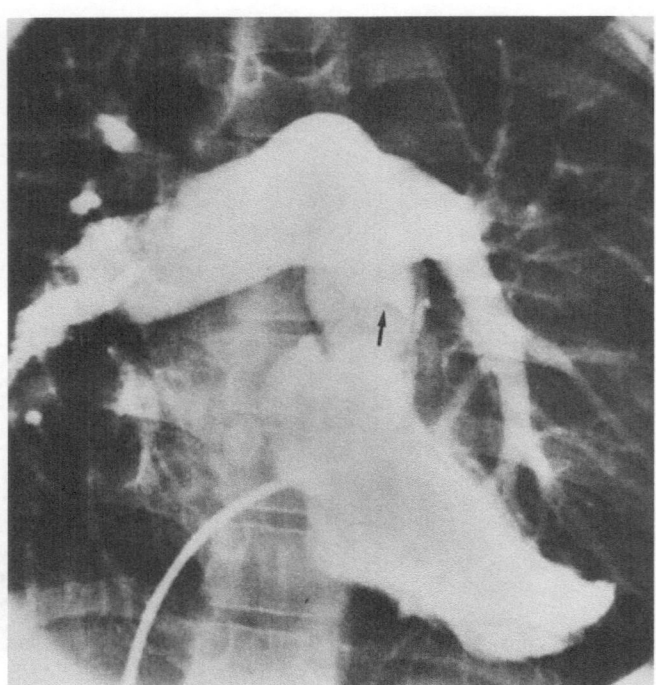

A

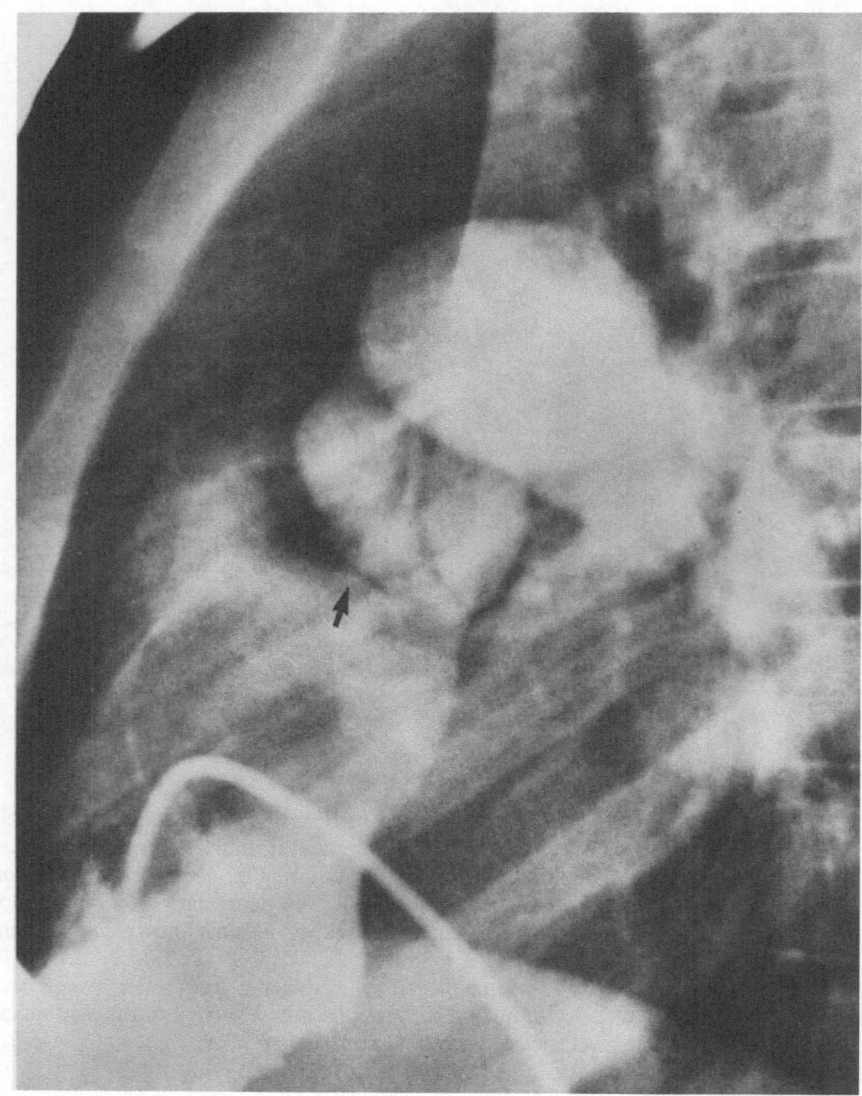

B

Fig. 7–104. *Subvalvar pulmonic stenosis in an 11-year-old boy with L-TGA.* (Same patient as in Figs. 7–98, 7–101A and B and 7–102). **A** Frontal view, systole, and **B** lateral view, diastole, of a left ventricular angiogram. **A** The typical findings of levotransposition of the great arteries are noted. The pulmonary valve is thickened and domed during systole (arrow). **B** A lucent line (*arrow*), representing a subpulmonic membrane, is noted.

Echocardiography The aortic valve is to the right and posterior, with the pulmonary valve situated toward the left, anterior and superior. This arrangement is consistent with normally related great arteries. Arc scans from the great arteries to the ventricles may provide an indication of the ventriculoarterial connections. Although the authors have no experience with echocardiography in this malformation, it is anticipated that 2-D echocardiography would be superior in the imaging of the ventricular septum, conus and connections of the great arteries.

Radiological (Plain Film) Features On plain films the heart is usually enlarged with a normal vascular pedicle that is consistent with normally related great arteries. The apex of the heart is usually to the left, but it may be midline or to the right. Pulmonary overcirculation occurs in the absence of obstruction to pulmonary flow. The plain film and electrocardiographic findings of situs solitus without transposition of the great arteries in a patient with cyanosis should strongly suggest the diagnosis of isolated ventricular inversion.

Contrast Studies Angiocardiography is definitive in establishing the diagnosis by demonstration of the position and relationship of the great vessels to the ventricles and the A-V valves. The presence or absence of associated malformations (e.g., tricuspid atresia) is also established.

Treatment Balloon atrial septostomy is indicated; however, in the presence of premature closure of the foramen ovale, this procedure is impracticable, and surgical septectomy is mandated. If a large ventricular septal defect is present a pulmonary band may be necessary. Corrective procedures, such as the Mustard or Senning operation, should be successful.

Criss-Cross Heart

Criss-cross heart (Fig. 7–105) is another rare malformation in which the external appearance of the heart is not consistent with the internal connections. In this abnormality, rotation of the ventricles occurs after establishment of atrioventricular and ventriculoarterial connections, moving

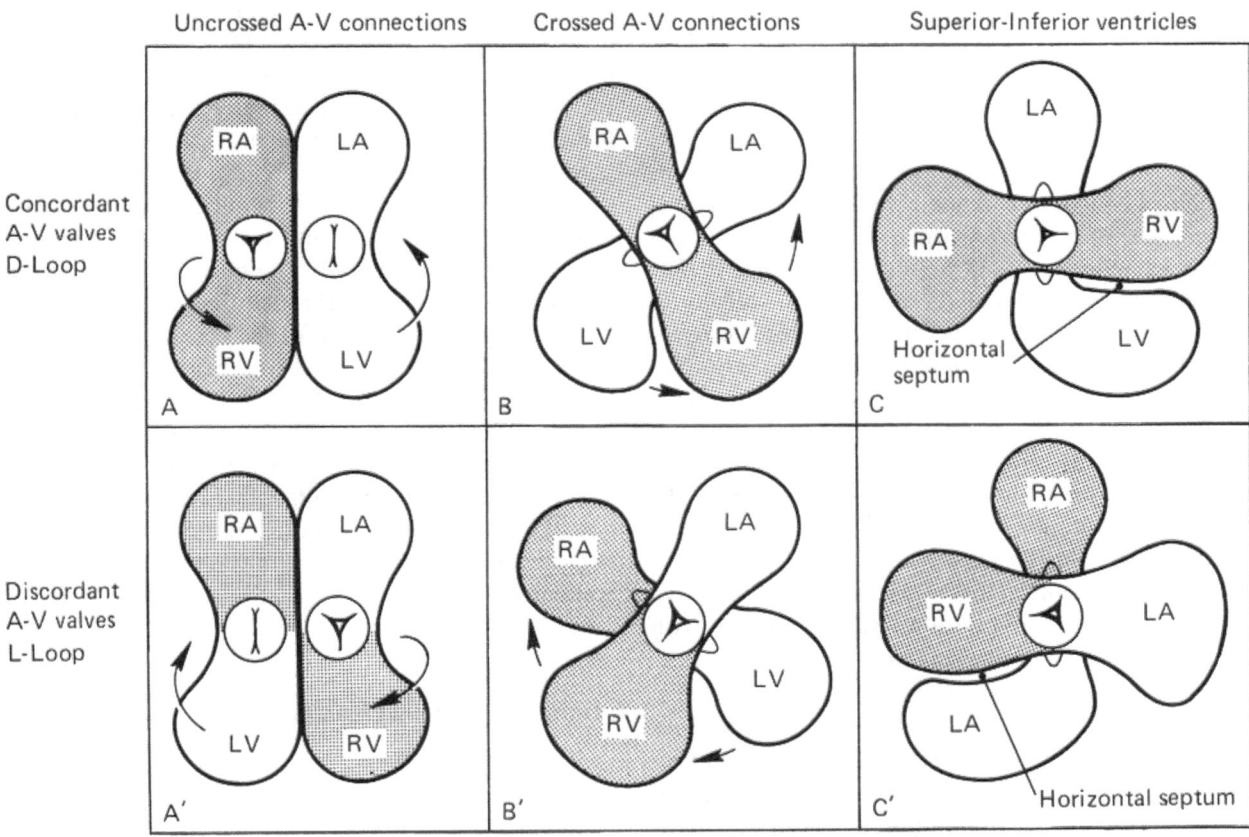

Fig. 7–105. *Criss-cross heart.* **A** and **A′** Normal (uncrossed) atrioventricular connections. **A** represents concordant atrioventricular connections (RA → RV; LA → LV) and **A′** represents discordant atrioventricular connections (RA → LV; LA → RV) in situs solitus. The curved arrows indicate the direction in which the ventricles will rotate. The first rotation (**B** and **B′**) brings the right ventricle to the side opposite its original position, but leaves its connections intact. **C** and **C′** The second rotation creates a horizontal septum while raising the right ventricle above the left ventricle (superior-inferior ventricles). These rotations are used only to delineate the anatomical features and do not serve to explain the pathogenesis of criss-cross heart. Some authors consider the horizontal septum to result from failure of descent of the right ventricular outflow tract rather than superior rotation of the septum later in development.

RA = right atrium; *RV* = right ventricle; *LA* = left atrium; *LV* = left ventricle. Modified from Attie F, Munoz-Castellanos L, Ovseyevitz J, Flores-Delgado I, Testelli MR, Buendia A, Kuri J, Molina B (1980) Crossed atrioventricular connections. Am Heart J 99:163–172

both ventricles and their atrioventricular (A-V) valves to the side opposite their original positions. A horizontal septum, present in many instances, results in superior-inferior ("upstairs-downstairs") ventricles (Fig. 7–105 C and C'). The tricuspid valve and the RV are superior to the mitral valve and LV. Crossed A-V connections have occurred in situs solitus as well as in situs inversus, and the connections have been concordant as well as discordant. Thus the ventricles no longer occupy their original positions but maintain their connections. The result is crossed A-V connections, each ventricle being on the side opposite the atrium to which it is connected.

Clinical Features Criss-cross heart is most frequently encountered with transposition of the great arteries. Because the aorta arises from the shifted RV it is also on the side opposite where it is expected. Thus a criss-cross heart with the connections of D-TGA will give the external appearance of L-TGA, since the RV and aorta are shifted to the left. A criss-cross heart with connections of L-TGA will have an external appearance reminiscent of D-TGA, inasmuch as the RV and aorta are shifted to the right.

Ventricular septal defect (VSD), pulmonic stenosis and "straddling" of an A-V valve are frequently associated with criss-cross heart. In addition to transposition of the great arteries, double-outlet right ventricle has been reported.

Echocardiography On M-mode echocardiography the aortic valve is anterior and superior and may be toward the right or the left. The tricuspid valve is superior to the mitral valve. M-mode arc scans reveal discontinuity between the aortic and tricuspid valve and may or may not show tenuous pulmonary-mitral fibrous continuity. The connections are unusual, and the operator is unlikely to delineate them on arc scans. In contradistinction, 2-D echocardiography may be most helpful in assessing these complex anomalies and in identifying associated intracardiac defects. In cases with superior-inferior ventricles the unusual positions of the transducer required to image the structures are a prominent feature. The long axis of the LV is obtained by rotating the transducer counterclockwise from its usual position. This is because the ventricular septum is nearly horizontal (Fig. 7–106). In this view are demonstrated the elongated outflow tract of the LV with tenuous pulmonary-mitral fibrous continuity. The ventricular septal defect is also identified in this view.

The short axis view at the level of the great arteries shows the aortic valve to be anterior, with the right ventricular outflow tract (RVOT) crossing anterior to the LV so that the aorta is on the side opposite the RV. This is in contradistinction to the findings with regular D-TGA or L-TGA in which the RVOT does not cross anteriorly. The two semilunar valves instead form two juxtaposed circles with the aortic valve anterior and to the right in D-TGA and anterior and to the left in L-TGA. (See also Fig. 7–68 for D-TGA and Fig. 7–92 for L-TGA.)

In the four-chamber views (apex or subxiphoid) the abnormal horizontal position of the ventricular septum is again noted, and straddling of an A-V valve is demonstrated, if present. Thus, in the authors' experience, the 2-D echocardiographic features of criss-cross heart are the elongated LV outflow tract, the apparent crossing of the RV outflow tract in front of the LV outflow tract and the abnormal position of the ventricular septum.

Radiological (Plain Film) Features On roentgenograms of the chest the size of the heart and the pulmonary circulation reflect the connections and intracardiac defects. The most common occurrence is in situs solitus with D-TGA. The RV and aortic valve are shifted to the left, and the ascending aorta has a leftward convexity; as a result the left heart border may have a convexity or shoulder configuration, similar to L-TGA (Fig. 7–107; also compare with Fig. 7–98). In cases with a horizontal septum a septal notch may be recognized high along the left heart border, similar to that occurring with single ventricle with a left-sided outflow tract. If the connections are those of L-TGA in situs solitus, but the RV is shifted to the right and the aorta is convex toward the right, then the cardiac silhouette will be reminiscent of D-TGA, while the connections are those of L-TGA.

Contrast Studies Angiocardiography is diagnostic, demonstrating both the connections and the positions of the cardiac chambers and great vessels (Fig. 7–108). As an example, in a patient with D-TGA and crossed A-V connections the RA injection shows continuity between the RA and RV. The tricuspid valve is high, so the contrast medium travels vertically within the RA before it crosses through the tricuspid valve. The RV is superior and on the left, being bounded inferiorly by the horizontal septum (Fig. 7–108A and B). Because of the horizontal position of the ventricular septum, flow through the VSD will be vertical. The aorta arises from the RV, and because of the abnormal position of the RV the aorta is on the left, and its convexity is toward the left, as in L-TGA. Injection into the LA demonstrates connection between the LA and LV. If the mitral valve straddles the ventricular septum both ventricles will opacify, creating difficulty in defining this connection. The LV is inferior, and its outflow tract is elongated and stenotic, yet pulmonary-mitral fibrous continuity is maintained.

Truncus Arteriosus Communis

Truncus arteriosus (TA) (Fig. 7–109) is an uncommon cardiovascular anomaly (1%–4%) in which a single arterial trunk originates from a single semilunar valve at the base of the heart. This single arterial trunk gives rise directly to the systemic, coronary and pulmonary arteries. No infundibulum (RV outflow tract) is present in TA. This definition excludes other congenital heart anomalies in which atresia of either semilunar valve results in one great vessel receiving the entire cardiac output. Thus, aortic atresia and truncus solitarius pulmonalis are excluded. Pulmonary atresia and ventricular septal defect (pseudotruncus; for-

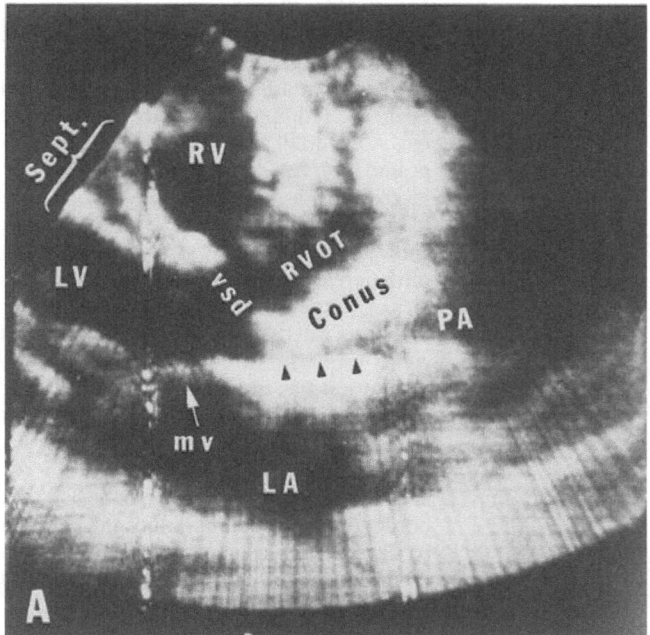
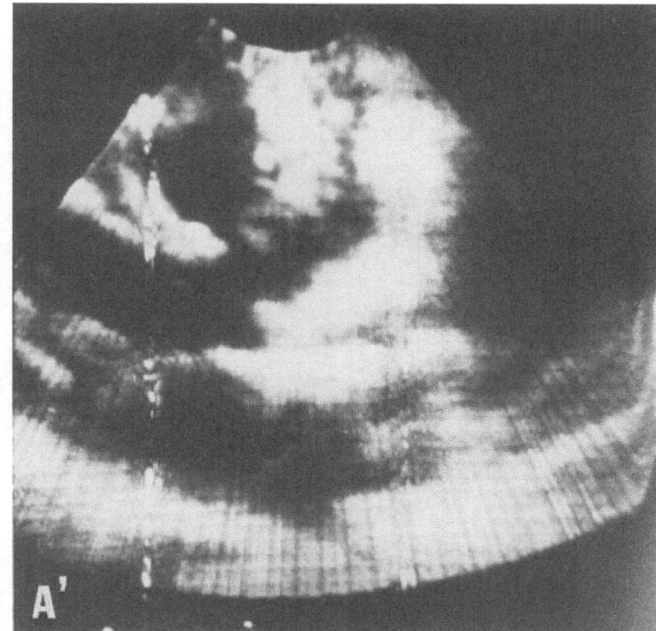

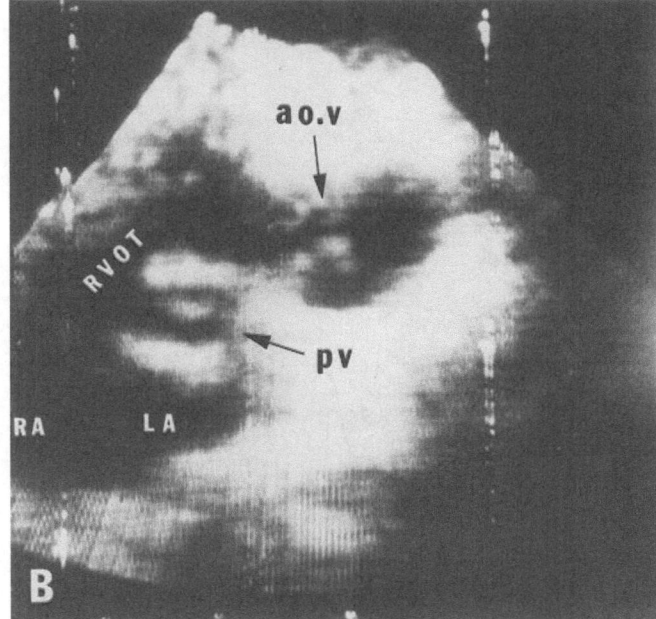

Fig. 7–106. *Two-dimensional echocardiograms in criss-cross heart in situ solitus with connections of D-TGA and superior-inferior ventricles (horizontal septum).* (A) Long axis view of the left ventricle (with labels); A′ without labels. The transducer is rotated counterclockwise from the angle ordinarily used in obtaining this view. Even though the left ventricular outflow tract (*arrowheads*) is elongated, pulmonary-mitral fibrous continuity is maintained. The septum (*Sept.*) points toward the sternum. The ventricular septal defect (*vsd*) is identified.

B is a short axis view at the level of the great vessels. The anterior valve is larger than the posterior valve. Since this patient has marked pulmonary undercirculation the smaller valve is assumed to be the pulmonary valve (pulmonic stenosis). The great vessels are therefore in the position of L-TGA (aorta anterior and left); however, the right ventricular outflow tract (*RVOT*) is observed to cross in front of the pulmonary valve and can be followed to the tricuspid valve, demonstrating the connection between the right atrium and right ventricle. Thus the connections of D-TGA are demonstrated by two-dimensional echocardiography, even though the relationship of the great vessels is that of L-TGA.

RV = right ventricle; *LV* = left ventricle; *Sept.* = septum; *vsd* = ventricular septal defect; *PA* = pulmonary artery; *mv* = mitral valve; *LA* = left atrium; *RA* = right atrium; *pv* = pulmonary valve; *ao.v* = aortic valve. (Same patient as in Figs. 7–107B and 108.)

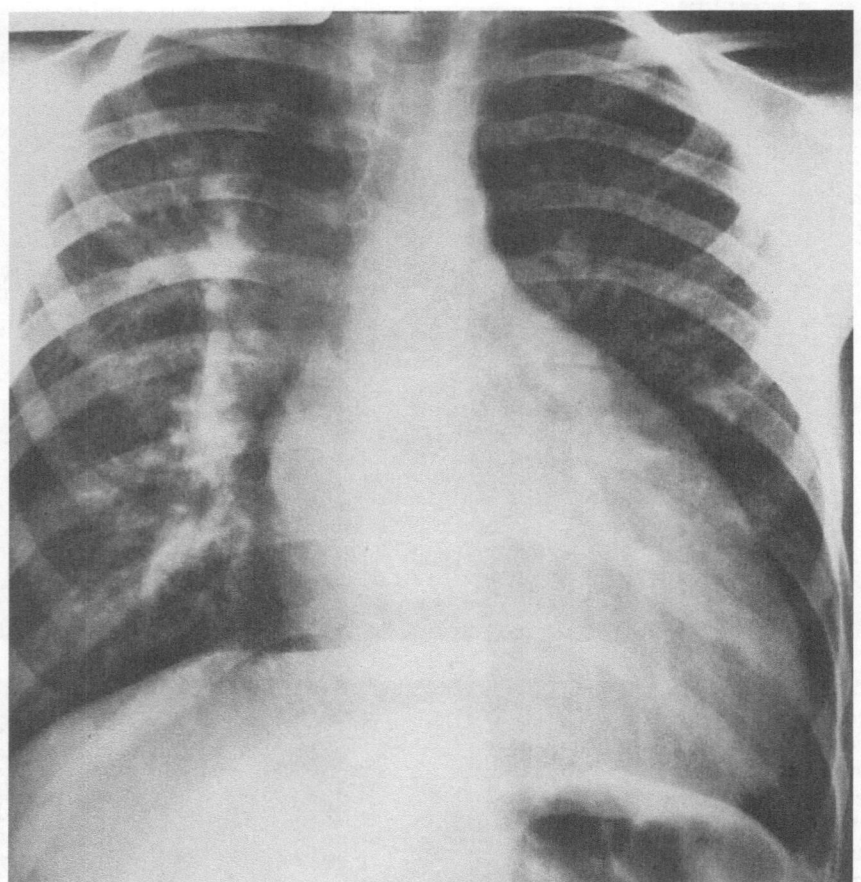

A

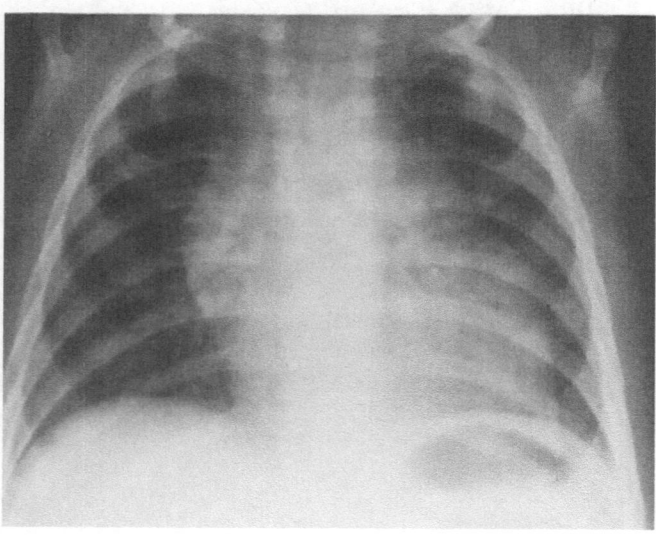

B

Fig. 7–107. *Plain films in two patients with criss-cross heart.* Both patients have situs solitus and connections of D-TGA.

A is from a 6-year-old boy with minimal cyanosis. Pulmonary overcirculation is present. A waterfall appearance of the right-sided pulmonary vessels is noted. The heart is enlarged with a shoulder configuration of the left heart border. Cardiac catheterization showed criss-cross heart with transposition of the great arteries, superior-inferior ventricles, a large ventricular septal defect and moderate valvular pulmonary stenosis. The right ventricle is connected to the right atrium but has been shifted toward the left. The aorta arises from the right ventricle and is convex toward the left. The outflow tract of the right ventricle and the ascending aorta account for the convexity of the left heart border. The roentgenogram of the chest may be interpreted as consistent with L-TGA with ventricular septal defect; however, crisscross heart should also be considered.

B is from a 4-month-old cyanotic boy. Associated findings at cardiac catheterization were ventricular septal defect, severe pulmonic stenosis and straddling mitral valve. Pulmonary undercirculation is present, and the heart is mildly enlarged. A shoulder configuration of the left heart border is identified. (Same patient as Figs. 7–106 and 108.)

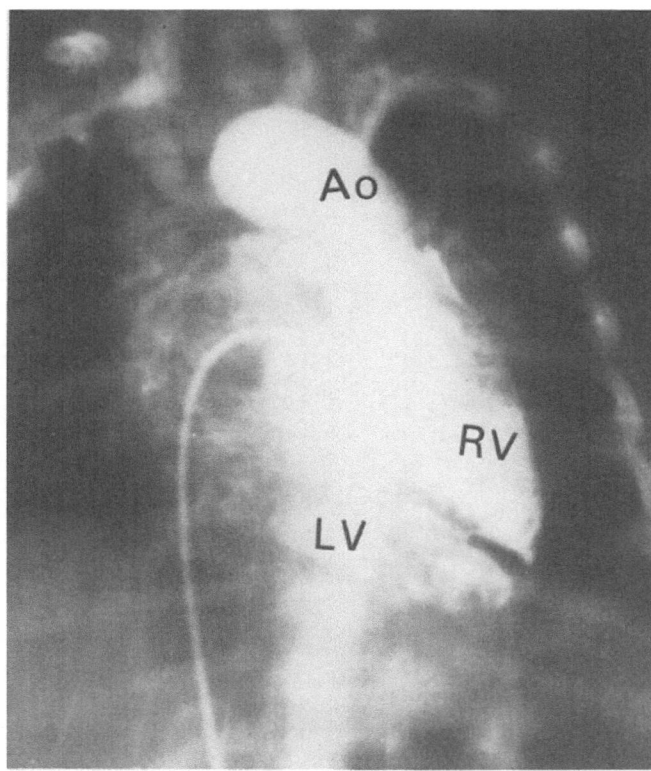

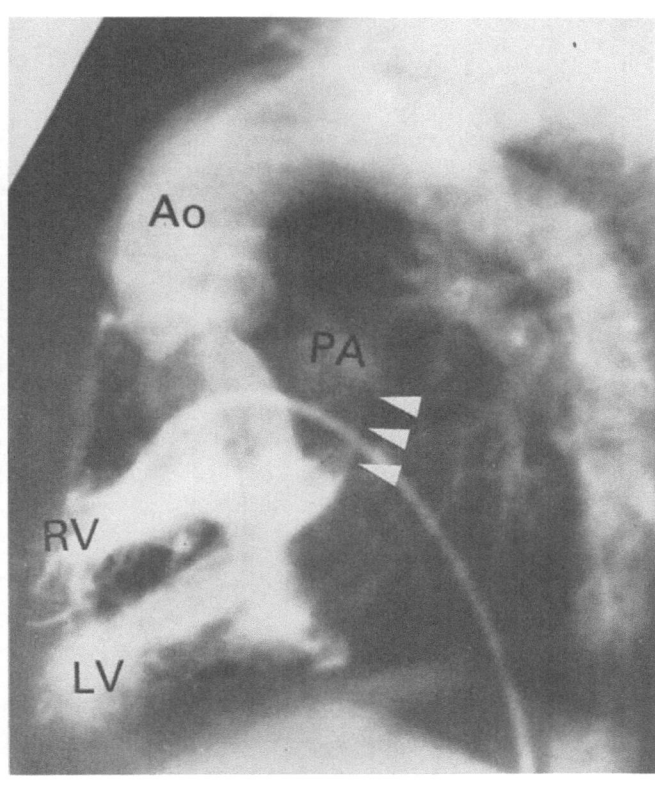

A   B

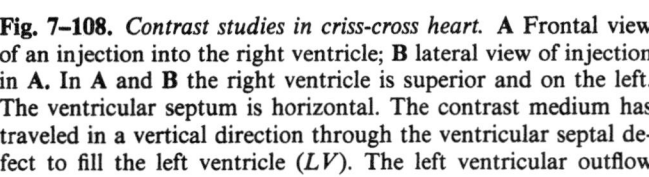

Fig. 7-108. *Contrast studies in criss-cross heart.* **A** Frontal view of an injection into the right ventricle; **B** lateral view of injection in **A**. In **A** and **B** the right ventricle is superior and on the left. The ventricular septum is horizontal. The contrast medium has traveled in a vertical direction through the ventricular septal defect to fill the left ventricle (*LV*). The left ventricular outflow tract (*arrowheads*) is stenotic because of elongation. No subpulmonic diaphragm or ectopic muscle is present. The anterior mitral leaflet is stretched; however, pulmonary-mitral fibrous continuity is maintained. The pulmonary artery (*PA*) arises from the left ventricle. (Same patient as in Figs. 7-106 and 107B.)

merly known as Collett and Edwards truncus type IV) is currently classified within the spectrum of tetralogy of Fallot rather than as TA, because in almost every such instance careful angiographic or pathological studies show a main pulmonary artery and central pulmonary vessels, either patent or represented by cordlike structures. The following features distinguish pulmonary atresia from TA. (1) In pulmonary atresia there usually is an infundibulum (RV outflow tract), whereas no infundibulum is present in TA; and (2) the lungs are perfused by systemic vessels from the descending aorta in pulmonary atresia, while at least one pulmonary artery arises from the truncus in TA.

In the great majority of patients with TA the truncus overrides the ventricular septum with mitral–truncal valve fibrous continuity and tricuspid–truncal valve discontinuity. The discontinuity is caused by the interposition of muscle (the ventriculoinfundibular fold). In a few patients, because of poor development or absence of the ventriculoinfundibular fold, fibrous continuity between the mitral and tricuspid valves and continuity between the tricuspid and truncal valves (mitral-tricuspid-semilunar valve continuity) occur. Rarely, discontinuity exists between the truncal valve and both the mitral and the tricuspid valves. In other rare examples the truncal valve arises solely from either the RV or LV.

TA is almost invariably associated with a ventricular septal defect (VSD). In rare instances, dysplastic tissue arises from the crest of the ventricular septum and attaches to the commissures of the truncal valve, so that no VSD is present (TA communis with intact ventricular septum). For the most part, the truncal valve is tricuspid (60%–70%), but it may be quadricuspid or bicuspid. Five- and even six-leaflet truncal valves have also been reported. The truncal leaflets are often thickened, polypoid and myxomatous, and truncal stenosis or incompetence (prolapsing leaflets) may be observed. The origin of the coronary arteries is extremely variable, often preventing identification of the semilunar leaflets by the coronary distribution. A right aortic arch is present in approximately 25% of cases. Interruption of the aortic arch has been reported sporadically in association with TA and with aorticopulmonary septal defects (AP window). Classification of TA is based on the presence or absence of the main pulmonary artery and the site of origin of the pulmonary branches from the common trunk (Fig. 7-109). In type I truncus, the most common type, the main pulmonary artery is a branch of the common trunk. The pulmonary trunk is short and gives origin to the right and left pulmonary arteries. In type II the right and left pulmonary arteries arise separately but close to each other from the posterior wall of the truncus. In type III the pulmonary arteries arise separately from the lateral aspect of the truncus. In some instances

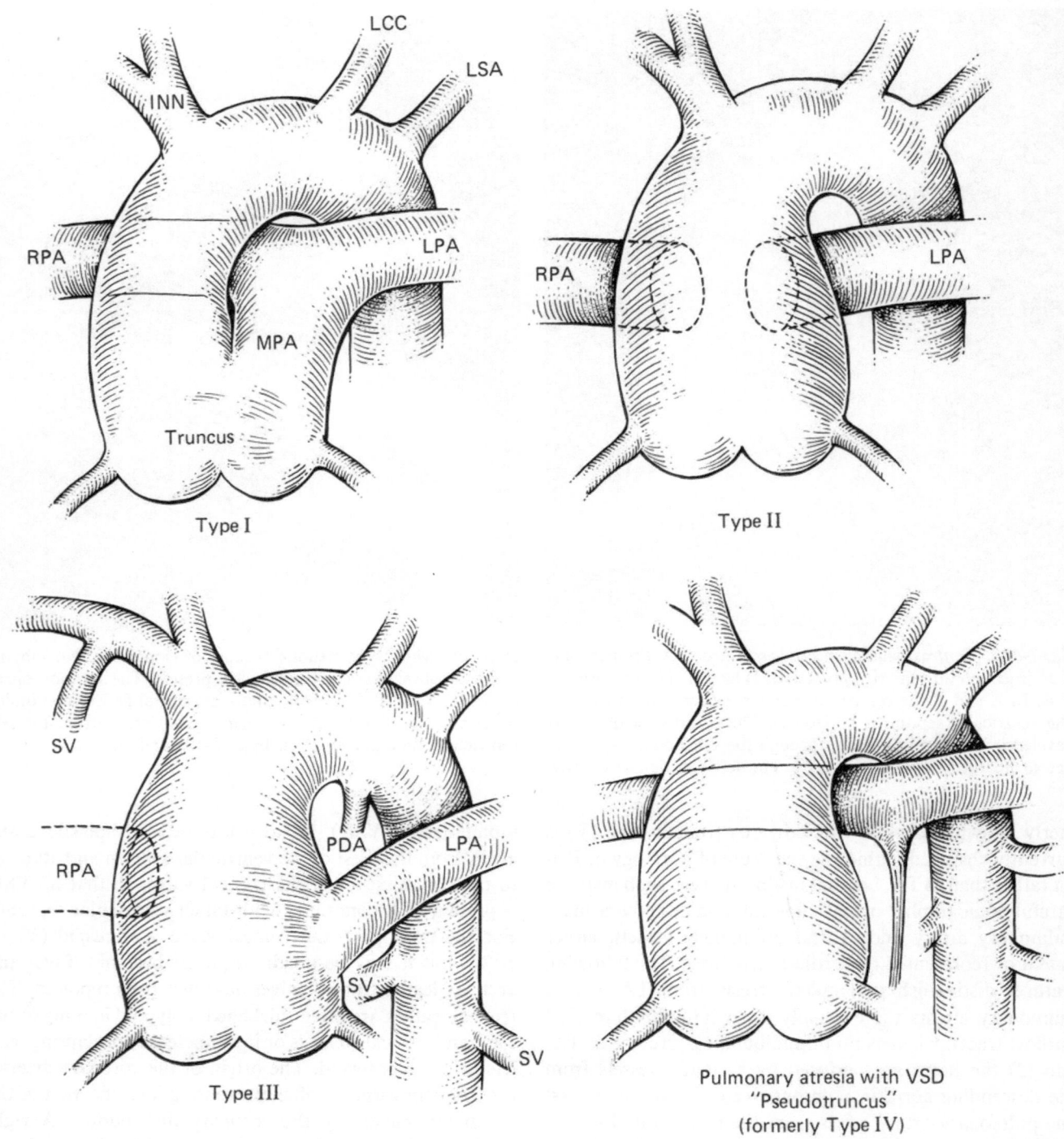

Fig. 7-109. *The types of truncus arteriosus.* These are defined by the location of the origins of the pulmonary arteries. In **type I** a main pulmonary artery arises from the main trunk, giving off the left and right pulmonary arteries. In **type II** the pulmonary arteries arise separately from the back of the truncus. In **type III** (mixed type), one of the lungs is perfused by a true pulmonary artery arising from the ascending portion of the main trunk; the other lung is perfused by a systemic vessel that may originate from the arch of the aorta, from the descending aorta, from a peripheral vessel such as the innominate or even from a patent ductus arteriosus. (Any vessel arising from the undersurface of the aortic arch is considered a ductus arteriosus). The classification by Collet and Edwards included as type III examples in which both pulmonary arteries originated from the lateral aspect of the main trunk.

The original classification of Collet and Edwards also included **type IV** in which the lungs are perfused exclusively by systemic vessels from the descending aorta. Careful angiographic and pathological examination in this last group of patients has revealed remnants of a main pulmonary artery and proximal pulmonary vessels in almost every instance. Therefore Sotomora and Edwards and others have categorized these cases as examples of ventricular septal defect with pulmonary atresia (pseudotruncus) rather than truncus arteriosus. The distinction is important because treatment is different. The pulmonary arteries in pseudotruncus can be used for shunt procedures, and even for complete repair.

INN = innominate artery; *LCC* = left common carotid artery; *LSA* = left subclavian artery; *RPA* = right pulmonary artery; *LPA* = left pulmonary artery; *MPA* = main pulmonary artery; *SV* = systemic vessel; *PDA* = patent ductus arteriosus.

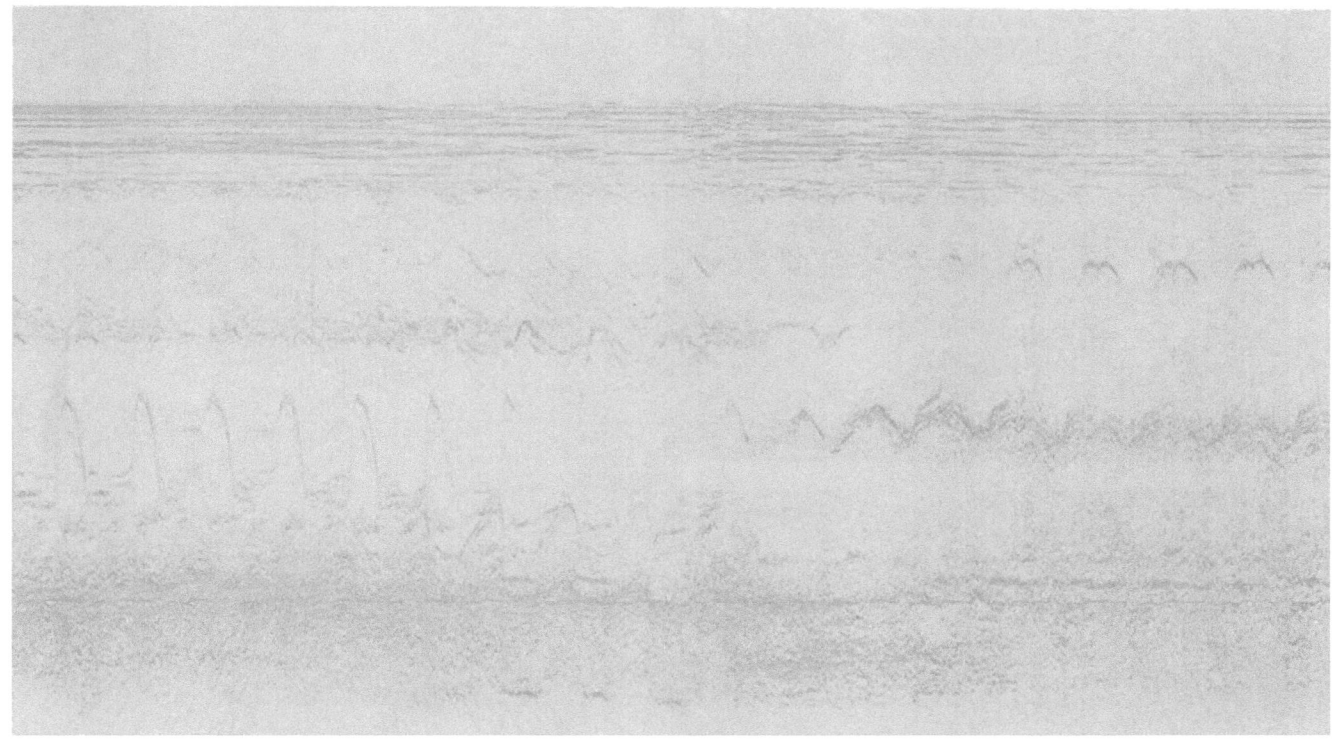

Fig. 7–110. *M-mode echocardiogram in a 29-year-old woman with truncus arteriosus.* The arc scan from the left ventricle to the truncus arteriosus demonstrates overriding of the truncus above the ventricular septum. A pulmonary valve could not be identified. Overriding of the aorta also occurs with tetralogy of Fallot. Fail-

ure to identify a pulmonary valve on M-mode does not exclude severe tetralogy of Fallot or pulmonary atresia. Thus the M-mode echocardiogram for severe tetralogy of Fallot and for truncus arteriosus may be indistinguishable.

one pulmonary artery may be absent; in such individuals systemic vessels supply the lung not perfused by the truncus. All types of TA may be complicated by pulmonic stenosis. It should be stressed that the pathological aspects and classification of TA discussed here apply to hearts in situs solitus with atrioventricular (A-V) concordance. Truncus arteriosus may also occur in situs inversus or situs ambiguus, with or without A-V concordance.

Clinical Features The clinical features are variable and depend on the size of the pulmonary arteries and the degree of pulmonary vascular resistance. In patients with large pulmonary arteries without significant pulmonary stenosis and without increased pulmonary resistance, heart failure and retardation of growth are the presenting manifestations. Cyanosis may not be apparent. Frequently a thrill, a systolic ejection murmur, a single loud second heart sound, a low-pitched mid diastolic rumble, cardiomegaly and bounding pulses are present. The electrocardiogram often demonstrates biventricular hypertrophy and a rightward axis. Patients with unrestrictive flow to the lungs may go on to develop the physiological changes of the Eisenmenger syndrome. Patients with pulmonic stenosis or increased pulmonary resistance have cyanosis.

Echocardiography The M-mode echocardiographic features of TA include a large truncal root that overrides the interventricular septum, mitral valve–truncal valve fibrous continuity, and an enlarged RV (Fig. 7–110). Differentiation from tetralogy of Fallot may be difficult. Detec-

tion of a pulmonary valve excludes truncus. Two-dimensional echocardiography (Fig. 7–111) shows a large overriding great vessel in both TA and pseudotruncus. High parasternal short axis and subxiphoid views may demonstrate the origin of the pulmonary arteries from the common trunk (Fig. 7–111). Diastolic fluttering of the anterior leaflet of the mitral valve and LV surface of the interventricular septum may be observed in the presence of insufficiency of the truncal valve.

Radiological (Plain Film) Features Pulmonary overcirculation is usually present (Fig. 7–112). In patients with associated pulmonic stenosis, pulmonary undercirculation may be observed. Cardiomegaly is frequent, usually with RV predominance, characterized by rounding and uplifting of the cardiac apex (Fig. 7–113). The pulmonary artery segment varies from a pronounced concavity to a bulge; not infrequently the junction of the vascular pedicle and the base of the heart may present as a sharp angulation, instead of a rounded concavity (Fig. 7–113). On occasion a bump or shelf configuration of the left heart border occurs (Fig. 7–114), representing the fornix of the LV (the anterobasal segment), which is border forming in TA (Fig. 7–113B). Normally this segment is obscured by the outflow tract of the RV and by the main pulmonary artery. This configuration may be indistinguishable from the shoulder configuration noted in levotransposition of the great arteries, single ventricle with left-sided outlet chamber, and criss-cross heart. Rarely in type I, two prominences may be observed

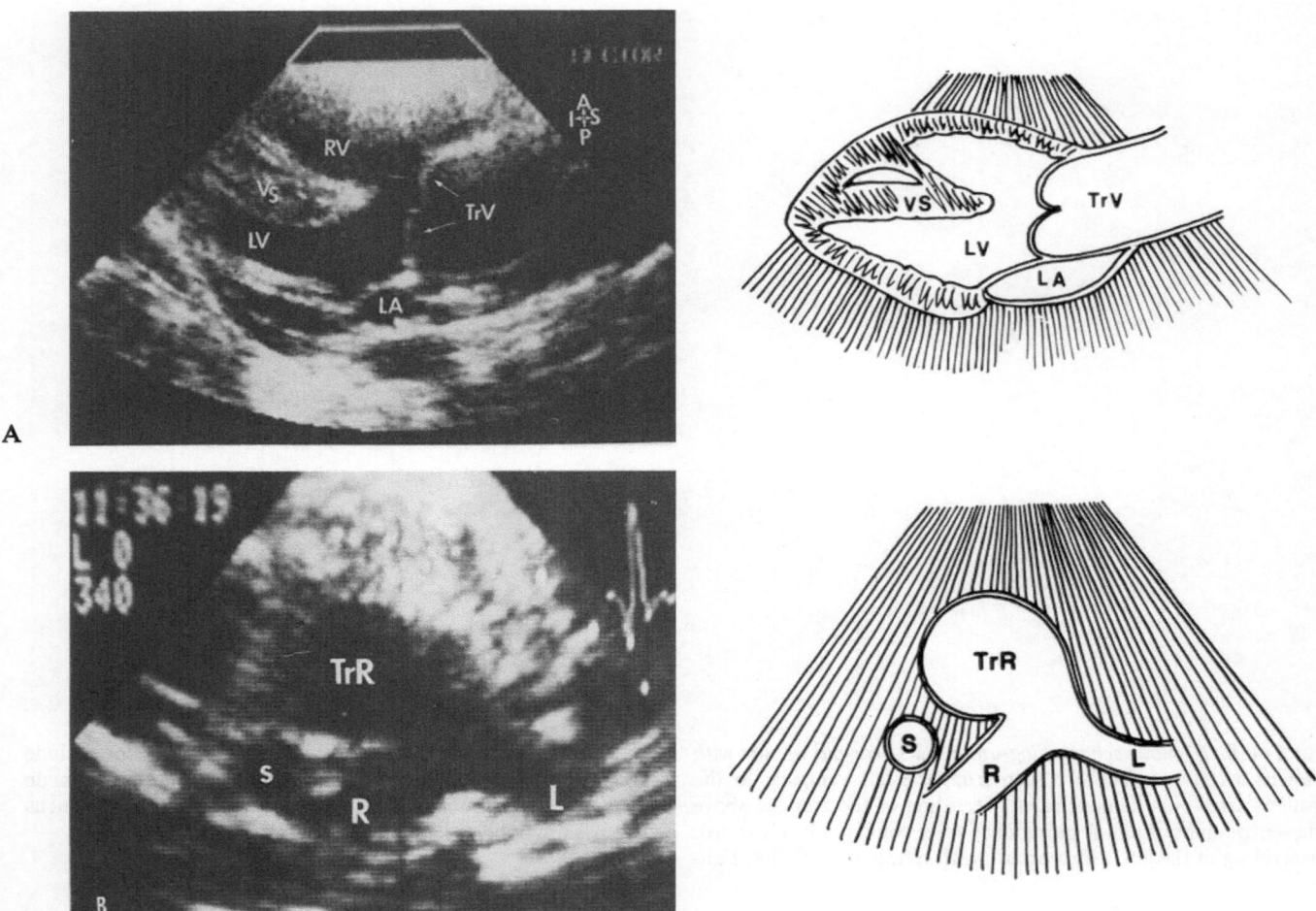

Fig. 7–111. *Two-dimensional echocardiography in truncus arteriosus.* **A** Parasternal long-axis view showing overriding of the truncal valve (*TrV*) above the ventricular septum (*VS*). Fibrous continuity is maintained between the truncal valve and the mitral valve. *RV* = right ventricle; *LA* = left atrium; *LV* = left ventricle. **B** High parasternal short-axis view of the truncal root (*TrR*) just above the valve demonstrates origin of the pulmonary arteries from the posterolateral surface. *R* = right pulmonary artery; *L* = left pulmonary artery; *s* = superior vena cava. Careful scanning in patients with truncus arteriosis fails to demonstrate a right ventricular outflow tract or pulmonic valve anterior to the truncal valve. Reprinted with permission from Rice MJ, Seward JB, Hagler DJ, Mair DD, Tajik AJ (1982) Definitive diagnosis of truncus arteriosis by two-dimensional echocardiography. Mayo Clin Proc 57:476–481.

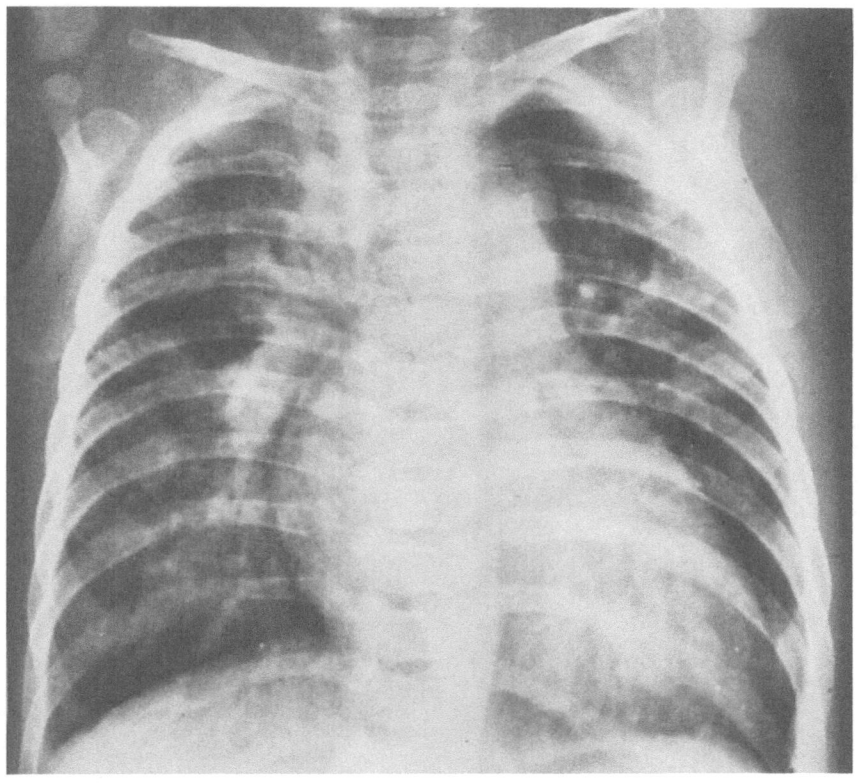

A

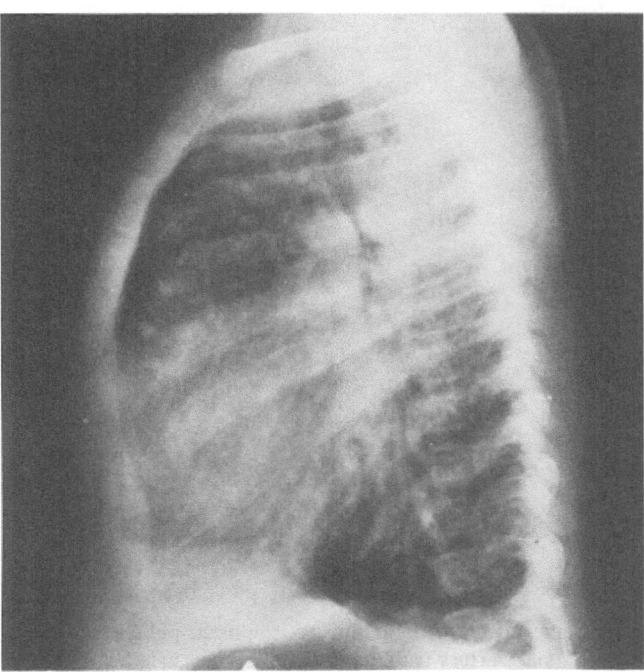

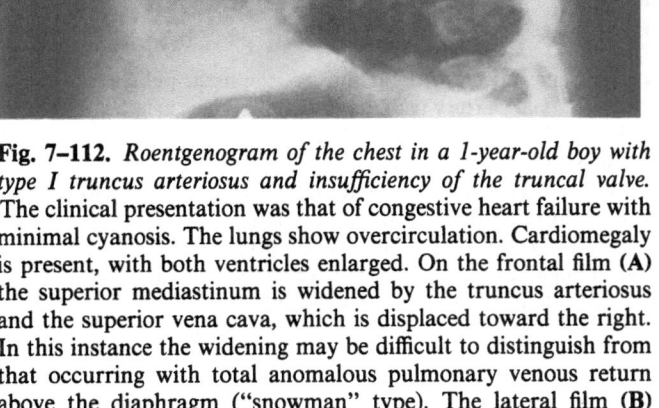

B

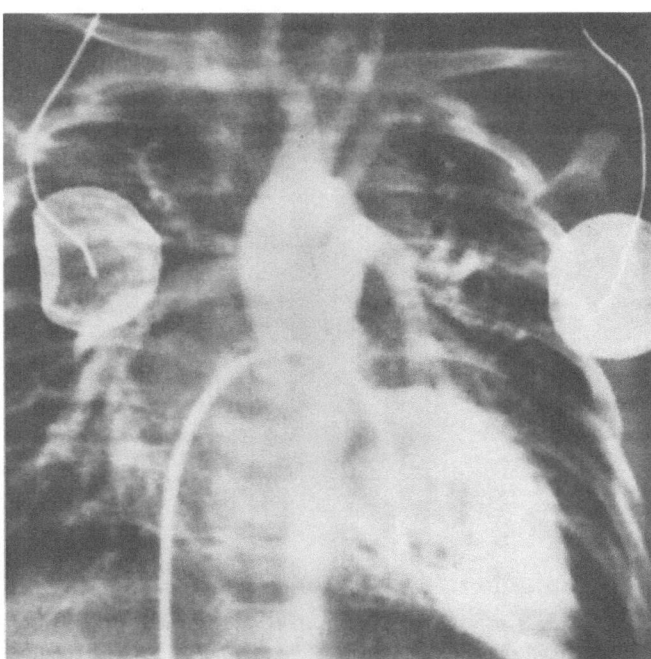

C

Fig. 7–112. *Roentgenogram of the chest in a 1-year-old boy with type I truncus arteriosus and insufficiency of the truncal valve.* The clinical presentation was that of congestive heart failure with minimal cyanosis. The lungs show overcirculation. Cardiomegaly is present, with both ventricles enlarged. On the frontal film (**A**) the superior mediastinum is widened by the truncus arteriosus and the superior vena cava, which is displaced toward the right. In this instance the widening may be difficult to distinguish from that occurring with total anomalous pulmonary venous return above the diaphragm ("snowman" type). The lateral film (**B**) fails to identify a mass density along the trachea anteriorly, excluding total anomalous pulmonary venous return (compare with Fig. 7–27B). The bump on the left side of the vascular pedicle (upper segment of the left heart border) is caused by the high position of the left pulmonary artery. The frontal view of the left ventriculogram (**C**) confirms the position of the left pulmonary artery. This is a type I truncus arteriosus. The main pulmonary artery arises just above the truncal valve, giving origin to the pulmonary artery branches. As noted on the plain films the aortic arch is left-sided.

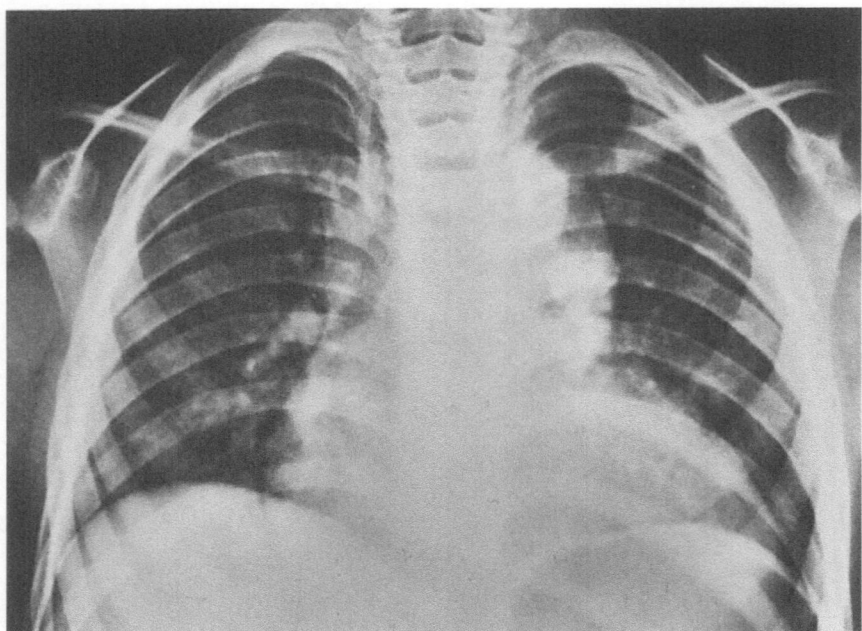

A

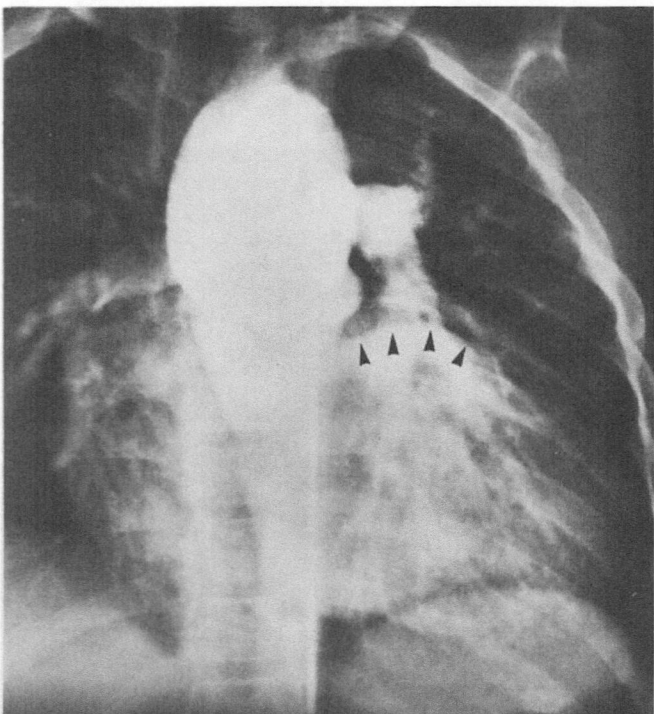

B

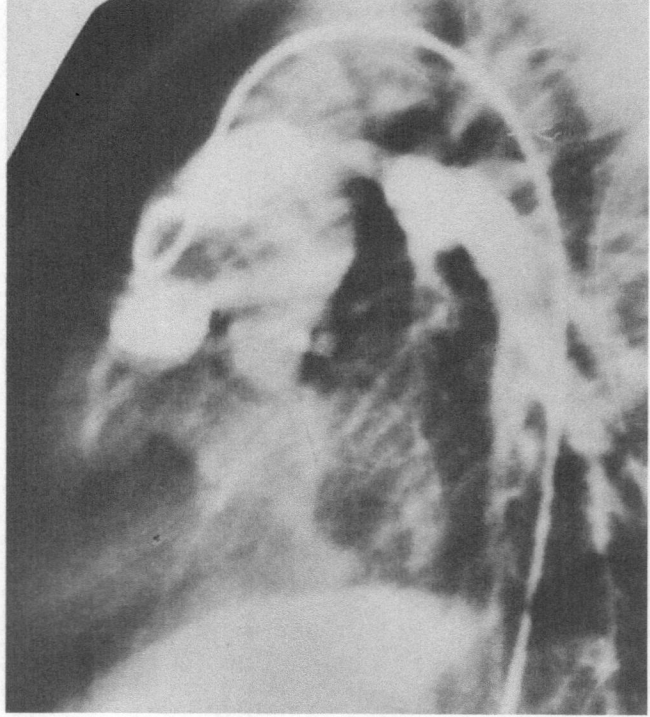

C

Fig. 7–113. *The vascular pedicle in truncus arteriosus.* **A** represents a frontal projection in this 4-year-old child with truncus arteriosus type I after main pulmonary artery banding. The mediastinum is widened; the cardiac apex is elevated. The junction of the vascular pedicle and the base of the heart forms a sharp angulation rather than a rounded concavity. The density lateral to the aortic arch and descending aorta is caused by the left pulmonary artery as it descends. (Note: poor inspiration partly obscures the apex.)

The frontal view of an injection into the truncus (**B**) demonstrates the position of the left pulmonary artery. The lateral view of the same injection (**C**) delineates the main pulmonary artery, the pulmonary artery band and the pulmonary arteries. The truncal valve has four cusps. The left ventricle is opacified as a result of the severe truncal insufficiency. On the frontal view the fornix of the left ventricle (the anterobasal segment) (*arrowheads*) is border forming because the infundibulum and main pulmonary artery are not present. The fornix forms the lower limb of the sharp angulation between the base of the heart and the vascular pedicle. It also causes the shelf configuration of the left heart border in Fig. 7–114A from a different patient.

in the region of the pulmonary trunk (Zamora et al.); the lower prominence is caused by the main pulmonary artery and the upper prominence by the left pulmonary artery. The left pulmonary artery forms the second density lateral to the vascular pedicle noted in Fig. 7–112. The truncus is usually very large, and a right arch is often found (approximately 25%). The aortic arch tends to occupy a higher position than is normal, and the ascending portion may form a marked convexity to the right.

Hemodynamics Admixture of systemic and pulmonary venous blood occurs because the common trunk overrides the ventricles, and both ventricles pump into it. Thus an oxygen "step-up" may be present in the RV or in the TA. The LA and LV may be fully saturated, while the truncus has less saturation. Oxygen saturation in the pulmonary artery is the same as in the truncus. Oxygen saturation of systemic blood will depend on the size of the pulmonary vessels and on the degree of pulmonary vascular resistance. The systolic pressures in the truncus, pulmonary arteries and in both ventricles are at systemic levels. In the presence of pulmonic stenosis the pressure in the pulmonary artery is lower than that in the truncus.

Contrast Studies Angiocardiography defines the type of TA and associated cardiovascular malformations (e.g., interruption of aortic arch). The truncus gives rise directly to systemic, coronary and pulmonary arteries (Fig. 7–115). The RV lacks an infundibulum. The presence or absence of pulmonic stenosis and truncal insufficiency can be determined. On occasion a proximal AP window may present difficulties in differentiation. Identification of two semilunar (aortic and pulmonary) valves and a RV infundibulum establishes the diagnosis of AP window. It may be difficult to distinguish TA and associated aortic arch interruption from distal AP window with aortic arch interruption. Again the presence of two semilunar valves indicates an AP window. A VSD is almost invariably present in TA, but rare in AP window.

Pulmonary atresia with VSD (pseudotruncus) should be distinguished from TA with severe pulmonic stenosis. A pulmonary artery arising from the truncus is characteristic of TA, whereas in pseudotruncus both lungs are perfused by systemic vessels from the aortic arch, the descending aorta or the peripheral vessels. Another feature that distinguishes pulmonary atresia from TA is the presence of an infundibulum (RV outflow tract) in pulmonary atresia, whereas no infundibulum is present with TA. In patients with pulmonary atresia and atresia of the RV infundibulum, differentiation from TA by ventriculography may be difficult. If pulmonary atresia with VSD is suspected, careful examination of the angiograms and probably additional injections are necessary to demonstrate the main pulmonary artery and the peripheral pulmonary vessels (See also section, Tetralogy of Fallot).

Treatment Complete correction of TA consists of closure of the VSD, leaving the truncus arising from the LV. The pulmonary arteries are detached from the truncus and attached to the RV, using a valved conduit (Fig. 7–116).

This procedure is now available for children under 1 year of age without obstructive pulmonary vascular disease. Primary complete repair in infancy appears to have lower overall mortality than banding of the pulmonary artery followed later by complete repair.

Postoperative Findings After complete repair using homograft reconstruction of the RV outflow tract, calcification of the graft may be noted on plain films (Fig. 7–117) or by fluoroscopy. On angiography, stenosis at any level of the graft may be observed. Persistent VSD may also be demonstrated. Right bundle-branch block secondary to the right ventriculotomy is a common finding.

Single Ventricle

This malformation is a complex congenital heart disorder, characterized by a single or common ventricular chamber that receives the atrial flow by way of two atrioventricular (A-V) valves or through a single A-V valve in individuals with A-V communis. In those with two A-V valves, both may be patent or one may be atretic. The ventricular output may exit directly into the great vessels or it may exit partly or completely through a rudimentary outflow chamber.

Four types of single ventricle may be identified by angiocardiography and pathological studies. When the trabecular pattern of the main chamber is reminiscent of a LV, the chamber is called a single ventricle of the LV type (or single LV). This pattern represents the most common variety of single ventricle. When the shape and trabecular pattern resemble a RV, it is known as single RV (single ventricle of the RV type). If the main chamber resembles neither a LV nor a RV, an undifferentiated single ventricle is present (rare form). A fourth type of single ventricle is known as an undivided ventricle or common ventricle. Characteristics resembling both ventricles are present, but the ventricular septum is absent. The undivided ventricle may, in fact, be an extreme manifestation of a ventricular septal defect rather than a true single ventricle.

The morphology of the A-V valves in single ventricle is often impossible to determine. Therefore in this text they are designated right-sided or left-sided A-V valves rather than tricuspid or mitral valves. The A-V valves have five ways to connect with the single ventricle: (1) two patent A-V valves connecting with the single ventricle (double-inlet left ventricle, double-inlet right ventricle), (2) right A-V valve atresia, (3) left A-V valve atresia, (4) common A-V valve (A-V communis; this is most common with asplenia), (5) straddling of the left or right A-V valve into the rudimentary chamber.

Conus muscle is interposed between the A-V valves and semilunar valves except in rare cases in which the conus is attenuated. Thus, semilunar to A-V valve fibrous continuity is rare in single ventricle. It is important to understand that the diagnosis of semilunar to A-V valve fibrous continuity or discontinuity by echocardiography or angiography may be inaccurate. The fibrous tissue between the valves

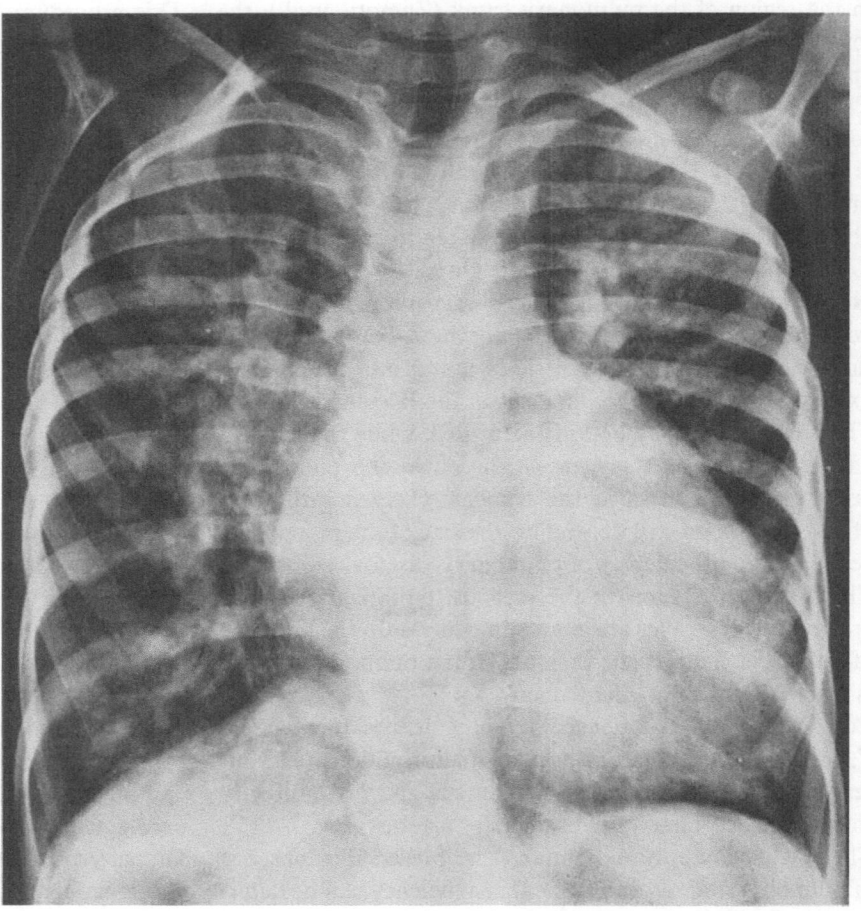

A

Fig. 7–114. *Shelf configuration of the left heart border in truncus arteriosus.* A and B are roentgenograms of the chest in a 2-year-old girl with type II truncus arteriosus. C and D are frontal and lateral views of an injection of contrast medium into the truncus arteriosus. Pulmonary overcirculation is present. Both ventricles and the left atrium are enlarged. The aortic arch is left-sided. On the frontal film (A) the main pulmonary artery is not identified, while on the lateral film the left pulmonary artery is not visualized in its normal location because of its unusual course (see angiogram frame D). This configuration of a sharp angulation or "shelf" below the pulmonary artery segment represents the fornix of the left ventricle. (Compare with aortogram in Fig. 113B from a different patient which confirms the position of the fornix of the left ventricle).

On the aortogram (C and D) the pulmonary arteries arise from the posterior wall of the truncus just above the semilunar sinuses, while on the lateral view the separate origins of each pulmonary artery account for the findings noted on the lateral film of the chest. The left pulmonary artery descends directly inferiorly and does not arch posteriorly as it does normally. Nevertheless, a normal relationship of the left pulmonary artery to the hyparterial bronchus is maintained. Truncal insufficiency is not identified. An incidental finding is the left circumflex artery arising from the right coronary artery.

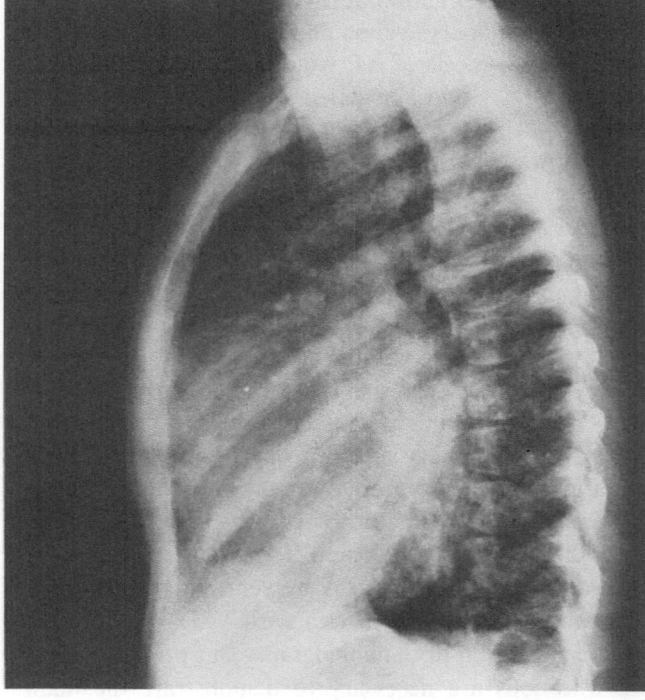

B

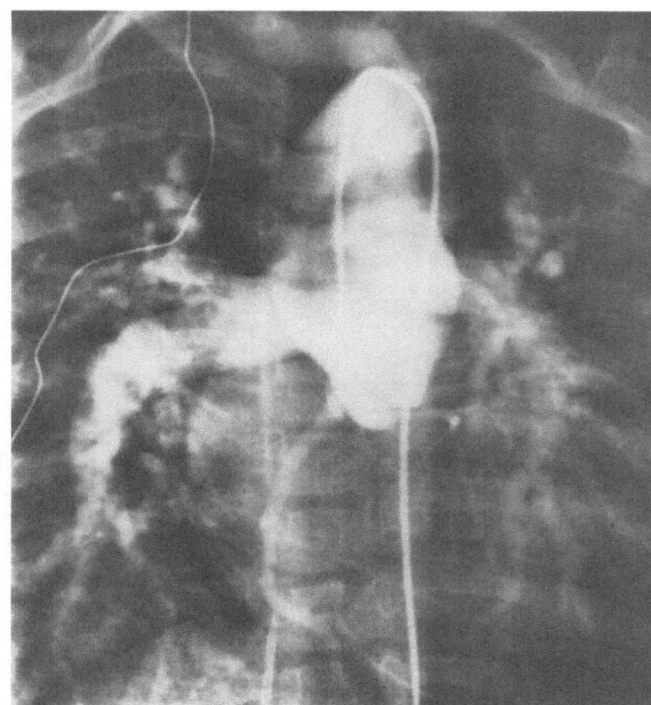

C

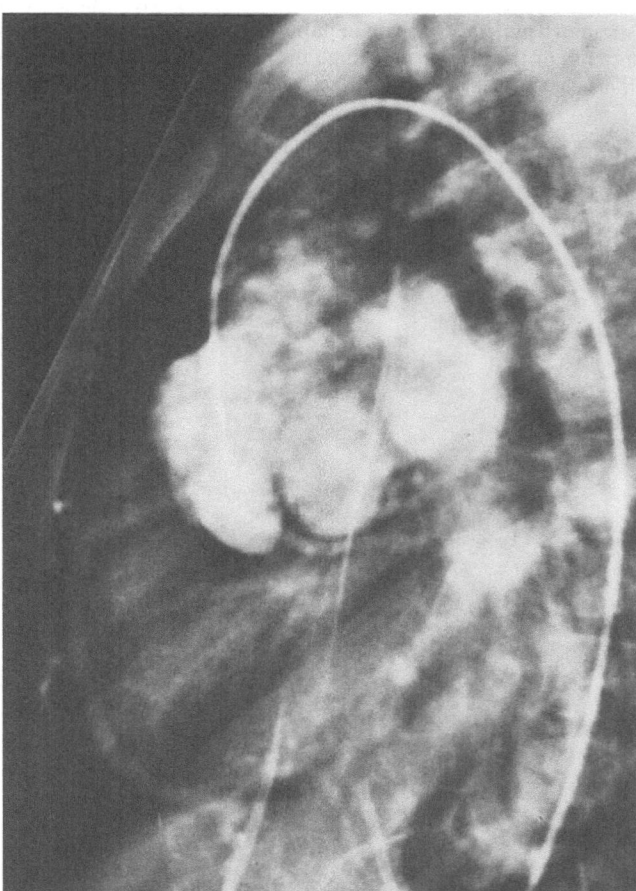

D

can elongate so that continuity may extend over a fairly long distance. On the other hand, a narrow band of conus tissue that cannot be identified by echocardiography or angiography may interrupt fibrous continuity even though the valves are close together. In the authors' experience with angiography in single ventricle, the typical appearance of fibrous continuity between the semilunar and A-V valves does not occur. If typical findings of semilunar to A-V valve fibrous continuity are present, one should consider diagnoses other than single ventricle.

In both LV and RV types of single ventricle a rudimentary outlet chamber usually receives part or all of the ventricular flow. In the single ventricle of the LV type the outlet chamber is considered to represent a RV chamber without an inlet portion. In the RV type the rudimentary chamber suggests a LV that has no atrioventricular connection (Shinebourne). In the authors' experience, single ventricle of the RV type often has no outlet chamber although conus muscle surrounds the origins of both great vessels.

The opening between the main chamber and the rudimentary outlet chamber is called a bulboventricular foramen. Some authors also refer to this opening as a ventricular septal defect (VSD). The opening is usually very large, but may be restrictive at birth or may become restrictive later in life, causing subaortic or subpulmonic stenosis. Conus muscle within the outlet chamber may also produce stenosis.

The rudimentary outlet chamber associated with the LV type of single ventricle is identified at the base of the heart on the right side ("normally related" infundibular chamber) or on the left side ("inverted" infundibular chamber). This chamber may give rise to both great arteries, one great artery or, on occasion, no great artery. Most commonly a single vessel, usually the aorta, arises from the outlet chamber. The other great artery arises from the main chamber. Even when both great vessels originate from the outlet chamber the aorta tends to arise anteriorly. Thus in single ventricle the great arteries are virtually always transposed. If the outlet chamber is on the right, the aorta will be in the position of D-TGA and will often be convex toward the right. If the outlet chamber is on the left, the aorta will be in a position reminiscent of L-TGA and will often be convex toward the left. These relationships of the great vessels can be called D-TGA and L-TGA respectively or D-malposition and L-malposition. Single ventricle with D-TGA and straddling of the right-sided A-V valve into the rudimentary chamber bears the eponym Lambert heart. The rare configuration of single ventricle with the pulmonary artery arising from the outlet chamber (normally related great vessels) is designated Holmes heart. If no great vessel arises from the rudimentary chamber, the chamber has the appelation ventricular pouch. Ventricular pouches occur on the right or left at the base of the heart or even at the diaphragmatic surface. As with rudimentary outlet chambers, the ventricular pouch may receive a straddling A-V valve.

Pulmonic stenosis frequently complicates single ventri-

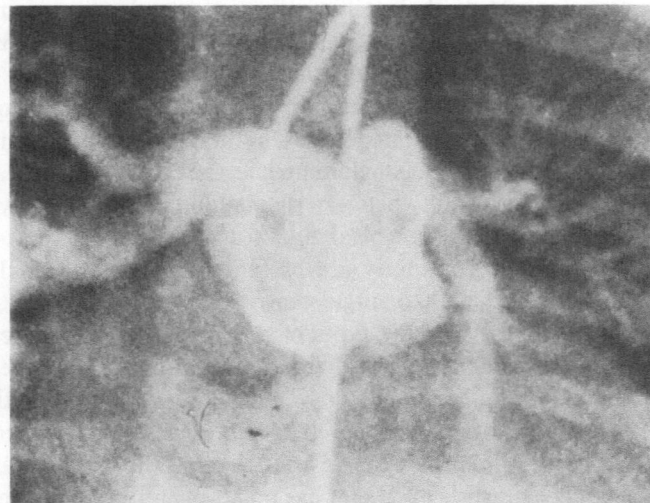

A

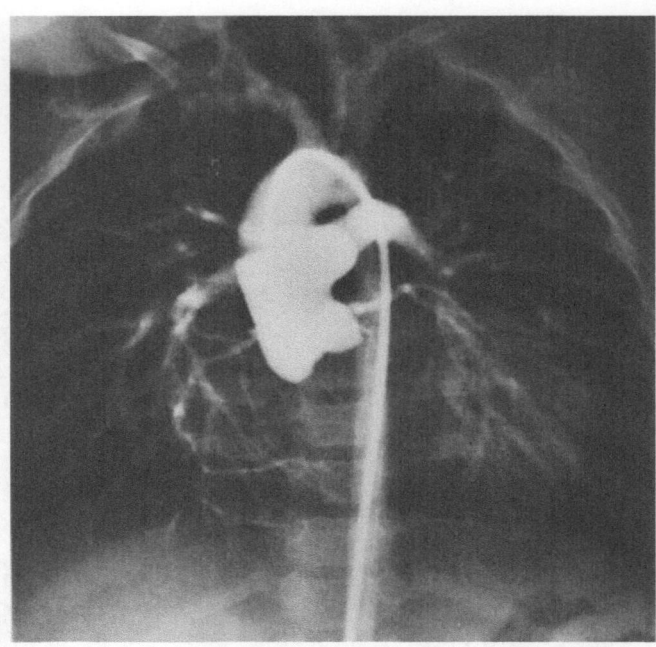

B

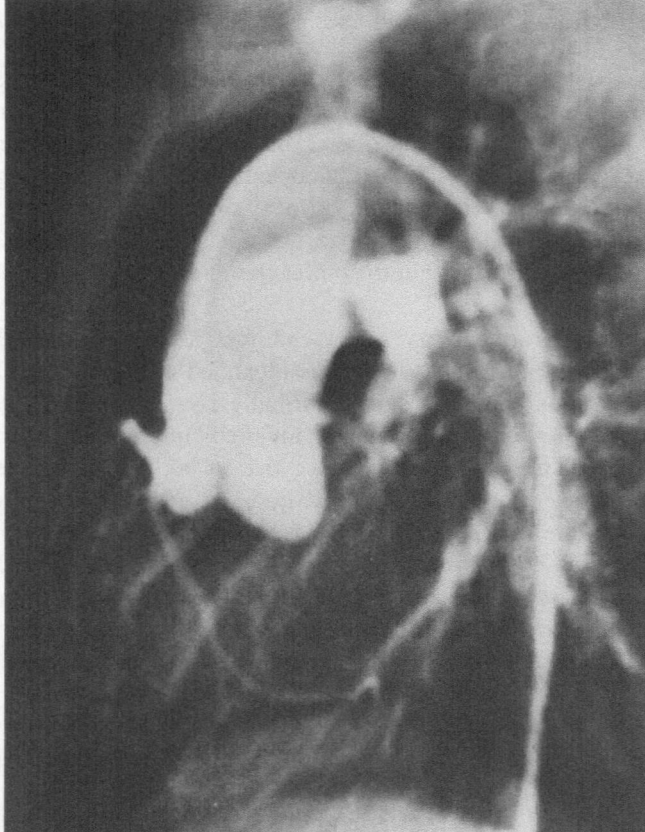

C

Fig. 7–115. *Two types of origin of the main pulmonary artery in type I truncus arteriosus.* **A** is the frontal view of an aortogram. In this patient the main pulmonary artery arises just above the truncal valve. **B** and **C** are frontal and lateral views of an aortogram in a patient whose main pulmonary artery arises as a distinct branch of the main trunk some distance above the truncal valve. The coronary arteries and systemic vessels are well delineated.

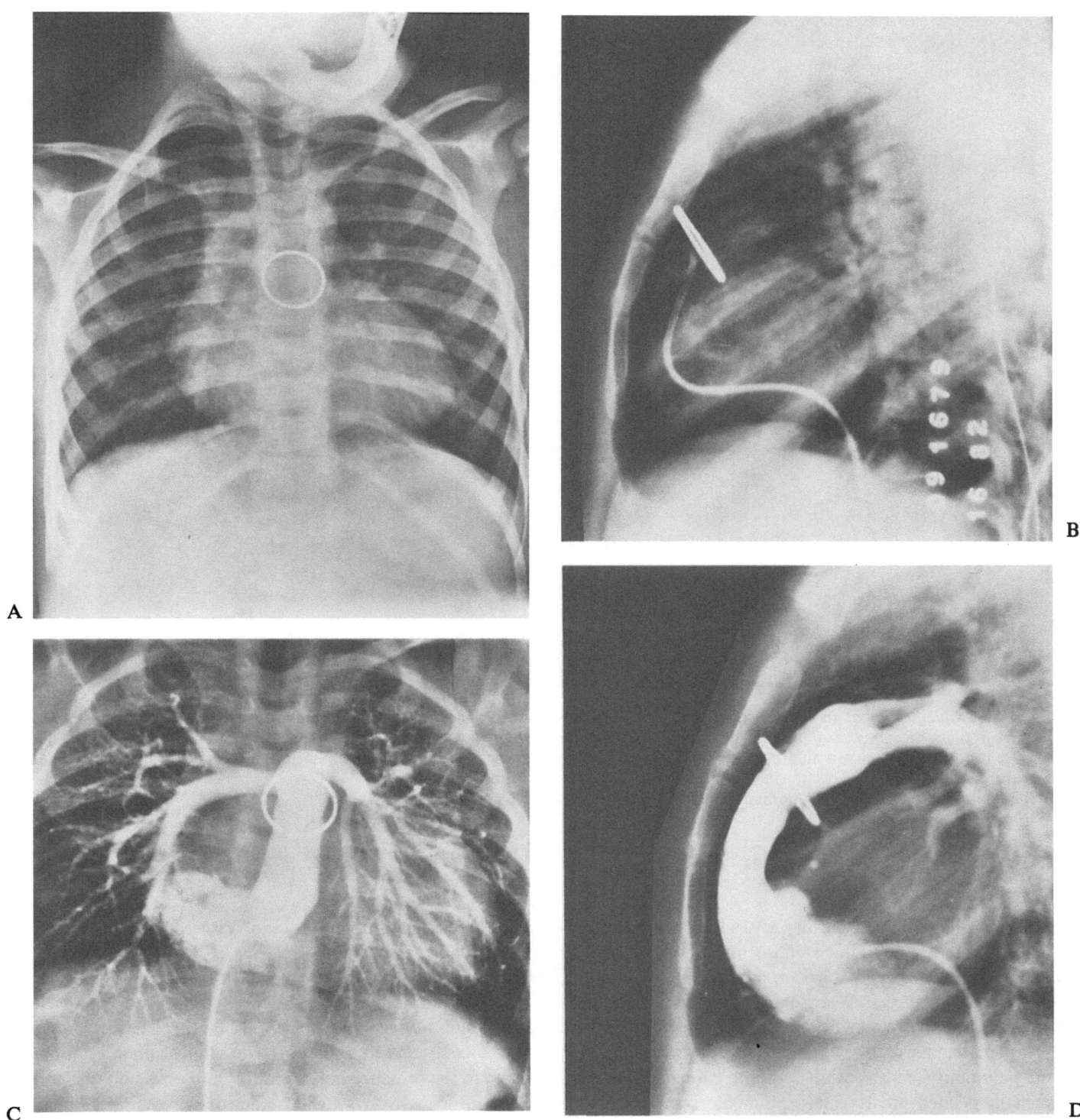

Fig. 7–116. *A valved conduit in a 2-year-old girl following repair of type I truncus arteriosus at age 7 months.* The frontal roentgenogram of the chest (**A**) and a lateral film with a catheter in the conduit (**B**) demonstrate the position of the porcine heterograft valve that is part of the conduit opacified in the frontal and lateral angiograms (**C** and **D**). Stenosis is not identified at any site.

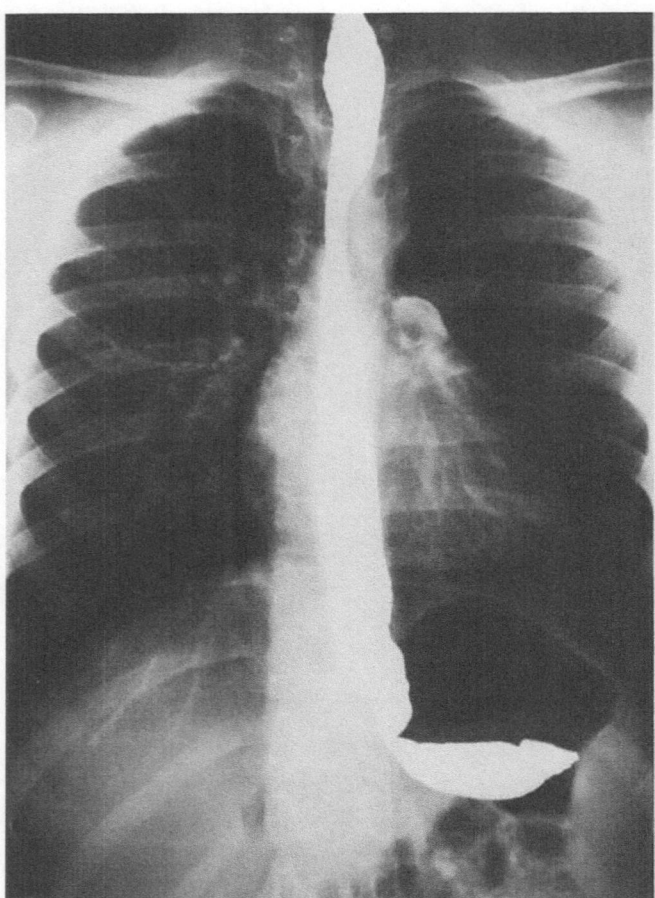

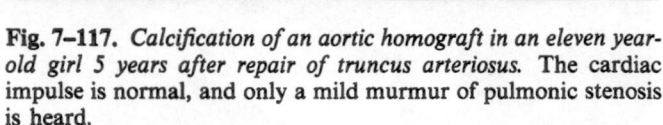

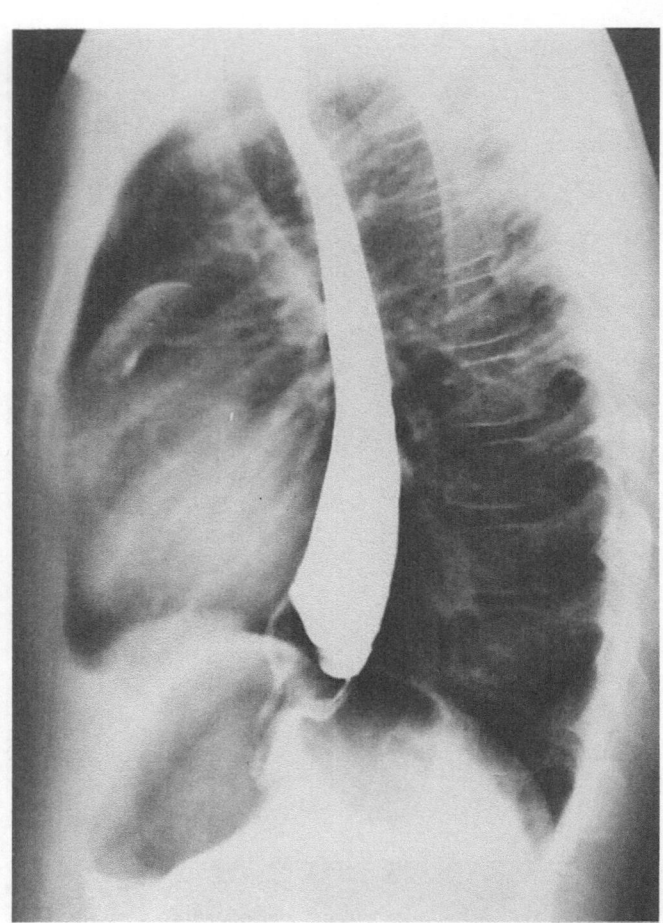

A   B

Fig. 7–117. *Calcification of an aortic homograft in an eleven year-old girl 5 years after repair of truncus arteriosus.* The cardiac impulse is normal, and only a mild murmur of pulmonic stenosis is heard.

The pulmonary circulation is normal. The aortic arch is left-sided. The heart is mildly enlarged with an elevated apex and slight convexity of the left heart border. Calcium outlines the aortic homograft that connects the right ventricle to the main pulmonary artery.

cle. When the pulmonary artery arises from the main ventricular chamber, pulmonic stenosis may be valvar or may be caused by a fibrous diaphragm or fibromuscular tunnel. When both great vessels arise from the outlet chamber the pulmonary valve may be deformed by the high pressure aorta, so that its cross section assumes a crescent shape and pulmonic stenosis results. In the rare instance with normally related great vessels, pulmonic stenosis may be caused by obstruction at the bulboventricular foramen or within the infundibular chamber. Subaortic stenosis may be caused by the same mechanisms (valvar stenosis, narrow subaortic conus, restrictive bulboventricular foramen). In cases without an outlet chamber, valvar stenosis or a fibromuscular membrane may involve either or both outflow tracts. Coarctation of the aorta, patent ductus arteriosus and interruption of the aortic arch may also be associated. Noncardiac defects (e.g., hydroureter, imperforate anus), may be encountered, particularly in infants who do not survive the neonatal period. Single ventricle is one of the malformations occurring with the asplenia syndrome (see also the section, Abnormalities of Visceroatrial Situs, later in this chapter).

Clinical Features All individuals with single ventricle have venous admixture because they have only one ventricle into which all venous blood flows. Nevertheless, cyanosis may or may not be apparent. The clinical manifestations relate to the presence or absence of pulmonic stenosis, aortic stenosis and A-V valve insufficiency or stenosis. Babies born with single ventricle and severe pulmonic stenosis will have cyanosis, whereas those infants with wide-open pulmonary circulation will develop congestive heart failure, secondary to pulmonary overcirculation. Between these extremes, individuals with single ventricle and moderate pulmonic stenosis may remain mildly cyanotic, but compensation may be maintained through childhood and even into early adult life.

A-V valve insufficiency with single ventricle will contribute to heart failure. Left-sided A-V valve stenosis or atresia with a small foramen ovale will produce pulmonary venous congestion like that occurring with hypoplastic left-heart

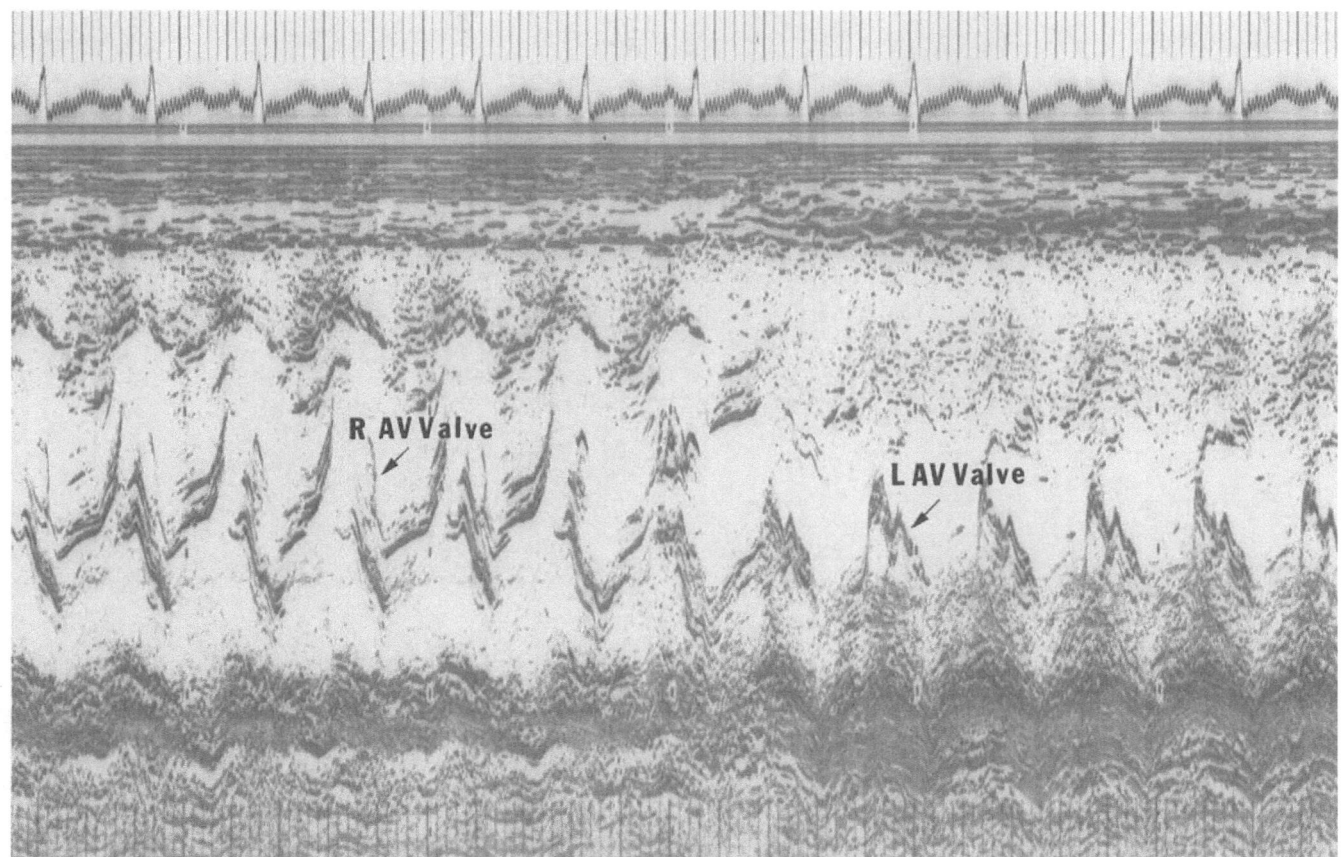

Fig. 7–118. *M-mode echocardiogram in single ventricle.* The transducer is placed at the left of the sternum and is angled from right to left to obtain this tracing. Two atrioventricular valves are present within a single ventricular chamber. The right atrioventricular valve (*R AV valve*) is slightly anterior (closer to the transducer) and has a larger excursion than does the left atrioventricular valve (*L AV valve*). If these two valves were at the same distance from the transducer and had the same excursion they could not be distinguished by M-mode as separate valves. If the presence of two A-V valves cannot be established then the possibility of atrioventricularis communis (atrioventricular canal) or atresia of one A-V valve exists.

syndrome. Atresia of the right A-V valve will force systemic venous drainage to cross the foramen ovale from right to left, to enter the ventricle, and the physiological changes will mimic tricuspid atresia. Subaortic stenosis may be asymptomatic, but it may produce valvular cardiomyopathy and the gradual onset of congestive heart failure.

The physical findings are varied, depending on the associated intracardiac defects. Semilunar valve stenosis or stenosis of the bulboventricular foramen or A-V valve insufficiency may result in systolic murmurs and thrills. Heaves and gallops accompany cardiac overload secondary to the foregoing or to an increase in pulmonary blood flow. The anteriorly placed aorta produces a loud second sound in most instances. A separate pulmonic component of the second sound is not often heard. Thus the physical examination is noncontributory except for the assessment of the presence and severity of cyanosis and congestive heart failure. The electrocardiogram usually shows sinus rhythm, although prolonged PR interval, second-degree heart block or complete heart block may be present. The P wave axis

provides a clue to abnormalities of visceroatrial situs. Atrial hypertrophy may indicate right or left atrial overload, secondary to factors already described. The QRS axis is variable and may point toward the left and superiorly. Absence of progression from RV to LV QRS complexes across the precordium, as well as absence of septal Q waves in all precordial leads, suggests the diagnosis of single ventricle.

Echocardiography On M-mode, single ventricle is suspected when two A-V valves are imaged within a single ventricular chamber (Fig. 7–118). Absence of the ventricular septum as demonstrated by M-mode may be misleading, however, because a septum that lies parallel to the plane of the echo beam may not be visible. This potentially misleading feature occurs especially in L-TGA with VSD. On the other hand, large papillary muscles may be mistaken for ventricular septum when no septum is present (Fig. 7–119A). If the A-V valves are equidistant from the transducer, it may be difficult to determine by M-mode whether one or two A-V valves are present. If only one A-V valve is present, tricuspid atresia, single ventricle with left or

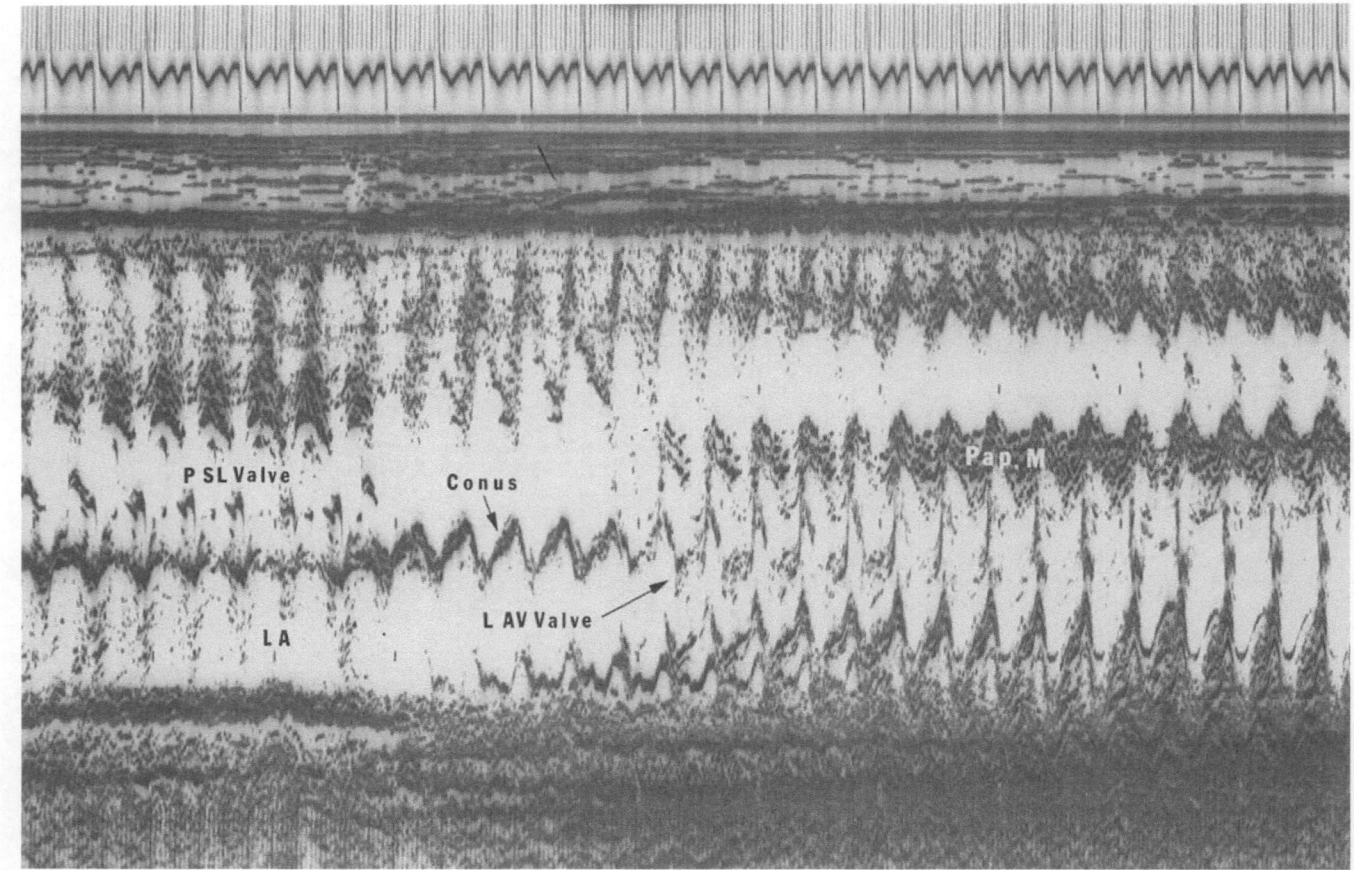

A

Fig. 7–119. *Relationship of the semilunar to the atrioventricular valves in a newborn with single ventricle showing conus muscle interposed between both semilunar valves and their respective atrioventricular valves.*

A is an arc scan from the posterior semilunar valve (*P SL Valve*) to the left atrioventricular valve (*L AV Valve*). Between the posterior wall of the root of the great vessel and the anterior leaflet of the L AV valve a long segment of fairly thick tissue is encountered, representing conus muscle. Further toward the apex a large papillary muscle (*Pap. M*) was interpreted as ventricular septum. The angiogram (Fig. 7–131) showed a single ventricle with conus muscle below each semilunar valve and with no remnant of a ventricular septum.

B is an arc scan from the right atrioventricular valve (*Rt AV Valve*) to the anterior semilunar valve (*Ant SL Valve*). Again conus is interposed between the root of this great vessel and the atrioventricular valve. The Ant SL Valve is on the right and superior, suggesting dextrotransposition of the great arteries. C is an arc scan from the left (posterior) semilunar valve to the right atrioventricular valve (*Rt AV Valve*). No intervening ventricular septum is encountered. The atrioventricular valve is anterior, apparently attached near the middle or the front of the posterior semilunar valve (*Post SL Valve*).

LA = left atrium; *RA* = right atrium. Same patient as in Figs. 7–120 and 7–131.

right A-V valve atresia, or atrioventricularis communis (A-V communis) must be included in the differential diagnosis. The connections between the semilunar valves and A-V valves rarely appear as typical fibrous continuity; almost always muscle is interposed (Fig. 7–119A and B). The right A-V valve may appear to be attached near the anterior wall of the posterior great vessel (Fig. 7–119C). The orientation of the great vessels is determined by identifying the position and angle of the transducer as the semilunar valves are demonstrated. If the pulmonary resistance is less than the systemic resistance, the systolic time intervals should allow one to differentiate the aortic valve from the pulmonic valve (Fig. 7–120A and B). Marked flutter

of the pulmonary valve may indicate subpulmonic stenosis (diaphragm or fibrous tunnel). Flutter or mid systolic closure of the aortic valve (if it arises from the outlet chamber) may indicate obstruction of the bulboventricular foramen (VSD).

Thus, M-mode echocardiography provides a useful screening technique, but leaves much to be desired as a method for diagnosing single ventricle.

Two-dimensional echocardiography, on the other hand, often provides definitive diagnoses and even permits a degree of subclassification, especially if a variety of echo windows and transducer angles are used. The apex and subxiphoid four-chamber views (Fig. 7–121) are most effective

Rt AV Valve
Ant SL Valve
Conus
RA
LA

B

Post SL Valve
Conus
Rt AV Valve
RA

C

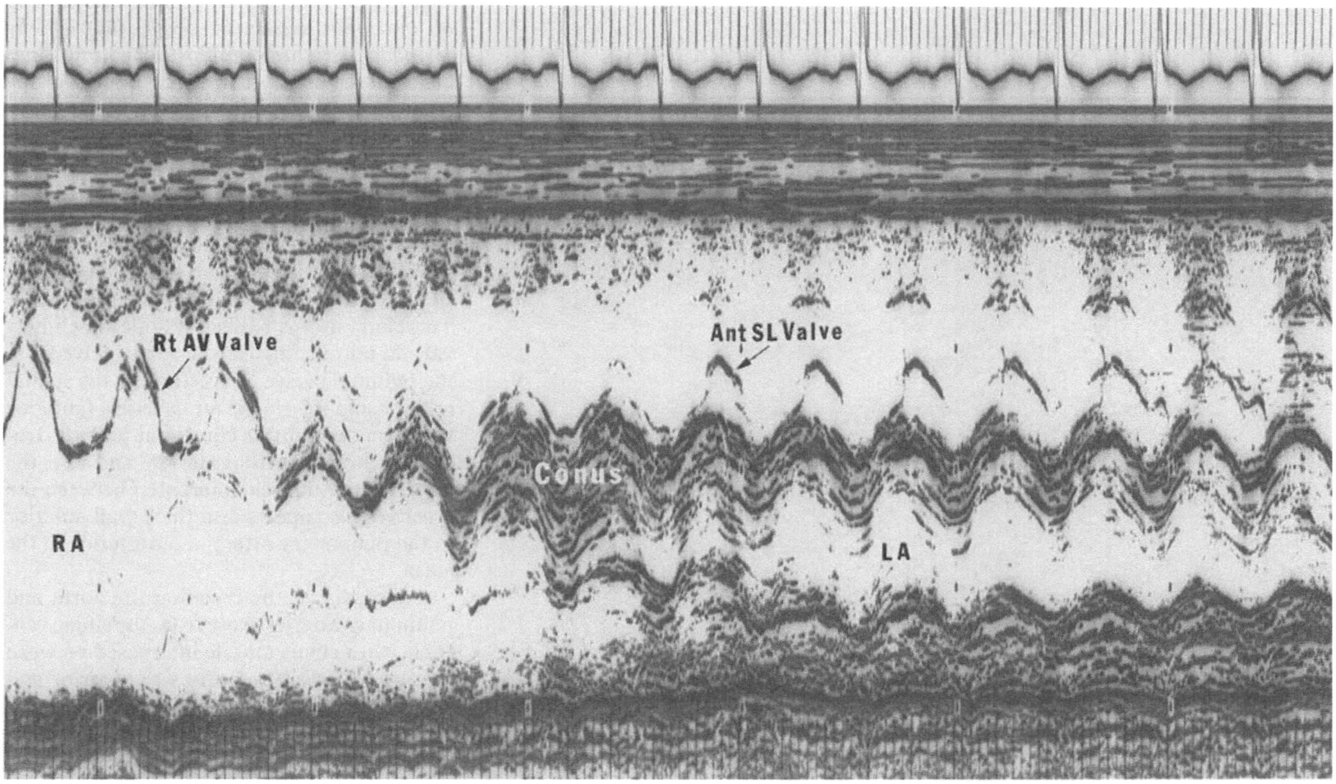

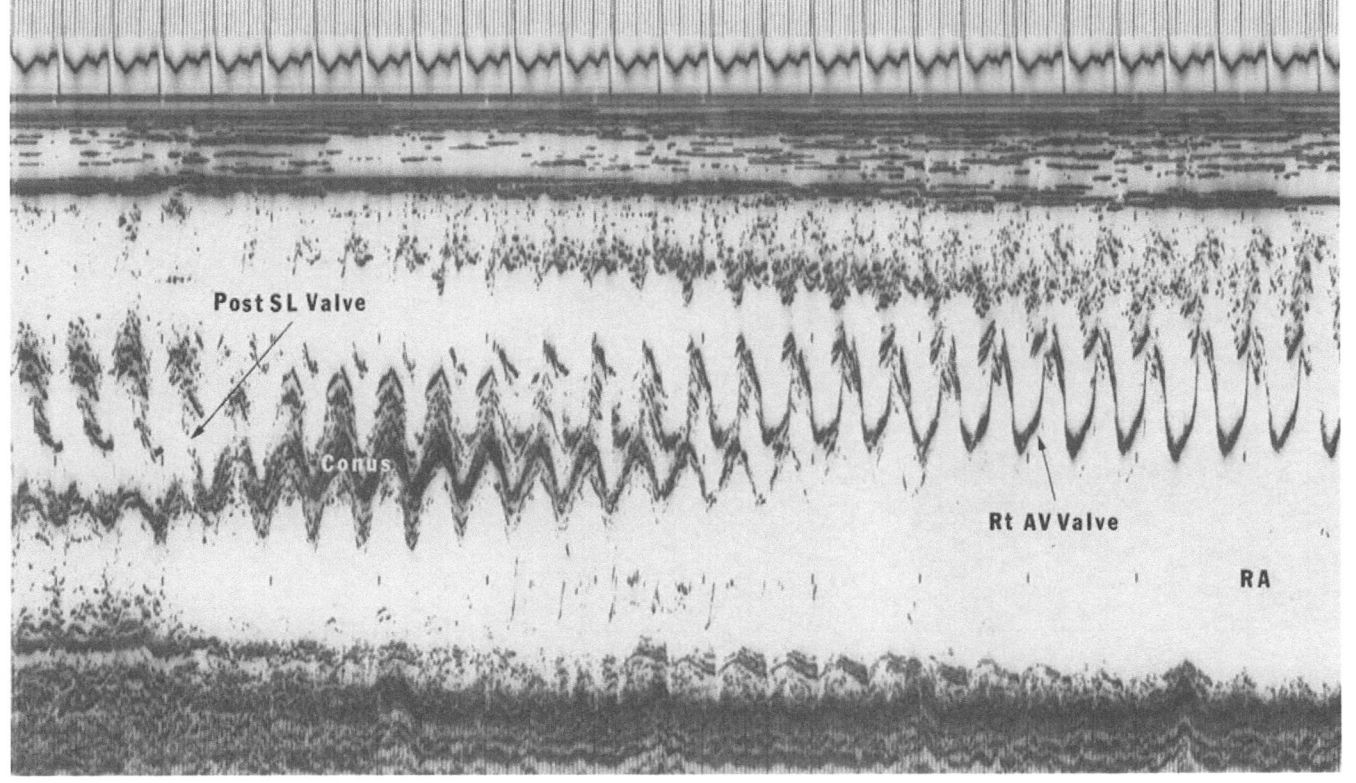

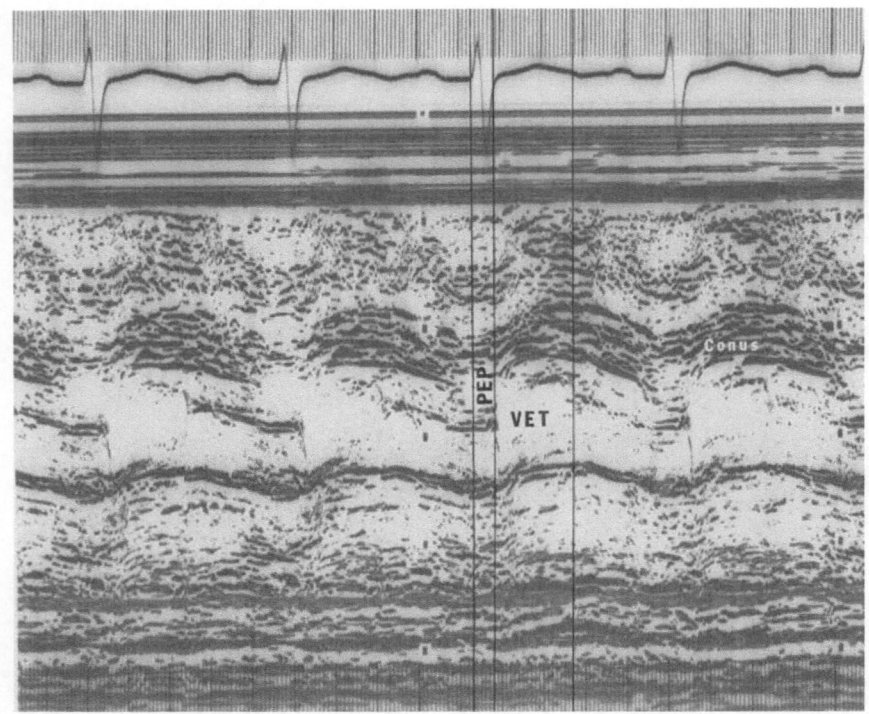

A

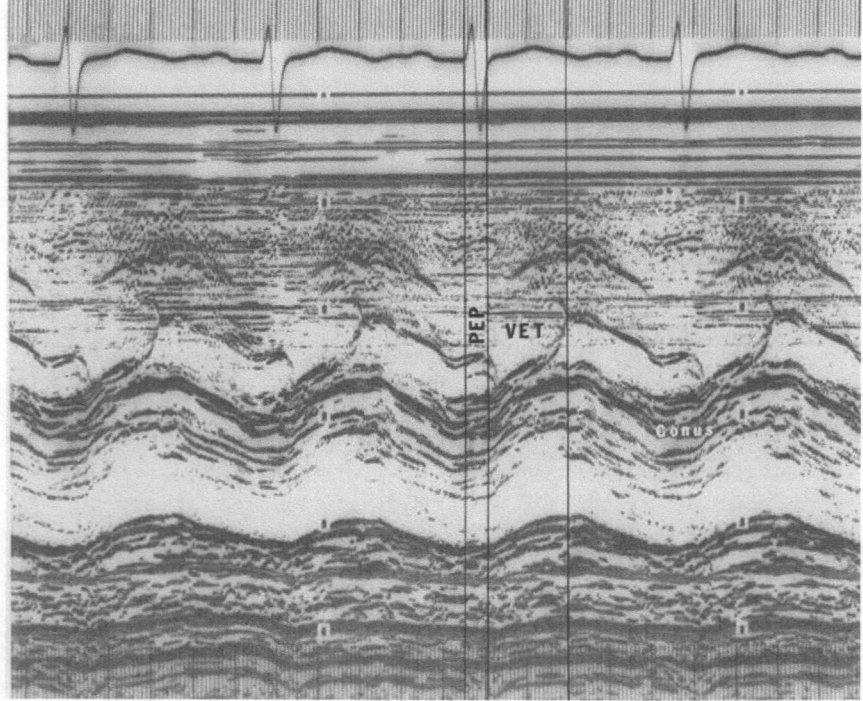

B

Fig. 7–120. *Determination of the relationship of the great vessels in single ventricle by M-mode echocardiography.* The time lines are 10 msec apart. **A** M-mode tracing of the posterior, inferior, left-sided semilunar valve; **B** M-mode tracing of the anterior, superior, right-sided semilunar valve. The operator has recorded the position of the hand-held M-mode transducer while each tracing was being recorded. In addition, the pre-ejection period (*PEP*) of each valve is 55 msec, and the ejection times (*VET*) are 195 msec. Therefore, in this patient systolic time intervals do not distinguish the aortic valve from the pulmonic valve. Nevertheless, the spatial relationship of the great arteries (anterior vessel on the right) is consistent with dextro-transposition (aorta anterior and on the right). Conus muscle interposed between the great vessels appears as a thick wall anterior to the pulmonary artery and posterior to the aorta.

At cardiac catheterization the aorta and pulmonary arteries arose from the single ventricle, with conus muscle interposed between the two vessels. The aorta was anterior and on the right. The pulmonary and systemic pressures and resistances were equal. (Patient in Figs. 7–119 and 7–131).

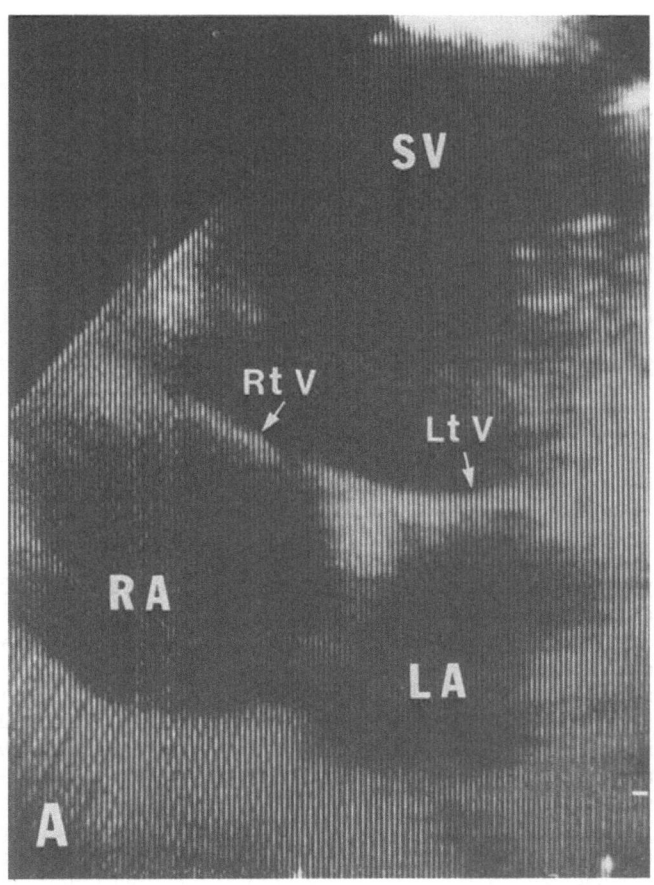

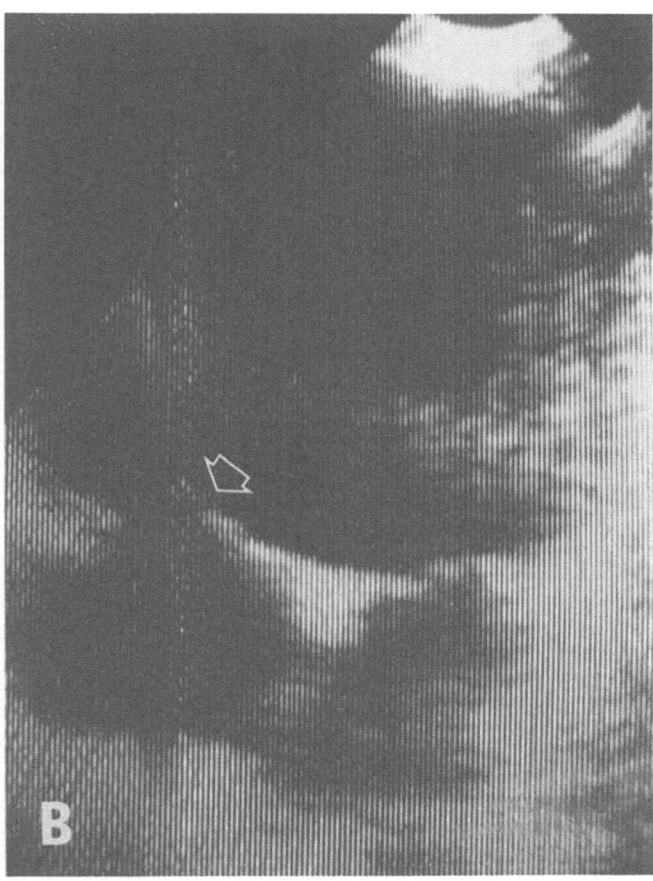

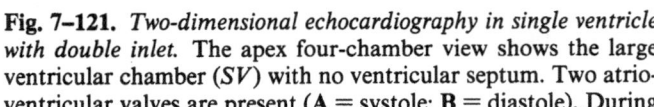

Fig. 7–121. *Two-dimensional echocardiography in single ventricle with double inlet.* The apex four-chamber view shows the large ventricular chamber (*SV*) with no ventricular septum. Two atrioventricular valves are present (**A** = systole; **B** = diastole). During diastole their attachment to the atrial septum is demonstrated. (The open arrow points to the open right A-V valve.) *Lt V* = left atrioventricular valve; *Rt V* = right atrioventricular valve; *LA* = left atrium. *RA* = right atrium.

in the study of single ventricle. A single ventricular cavity is demonstrated with no intervening ventricular septum (care must be exercised to differentiate large papillary muscles from ventricular septum). The A-V valves are demonstrated along with the atrial septum. Atretic or imperforate A-V valves can be recognized by a bar of bright echoes or by a moving diaphragm between the affected atrium and the ventricle. A-V communis appears as a single large A-V valve that extends across the single chamber, with the atrial septum posterior to the chamber (Fig. 7–122).

A blind ventricular pouch or a posterior rudimentary chamber may also be identified near the crux of the heart, using the apex views. A parasternal short axis view near the apex also allows visualization of the single ventricular chamber. Rotation and angulation slightly higher may demonstrate the bulboventricular foramen (VSD) as well as the rudimentary outlet chamber (Fig. 7–123). Careful search in this plane may show entry of one or more papillary muscles into the rudimentary chamber, confirming the diagnosis of straddling A-V valves. The long axis view at the base of the heart demonstrates conus interposed between the semilunar and A-V valves (Fig. 7–124). The short axis view at the base of the heart (Fig. 7–125), together with high parasternal long axis views and suprasternal views (Fig. 7–126), will differentiate the great vessels and indicate their orientation.

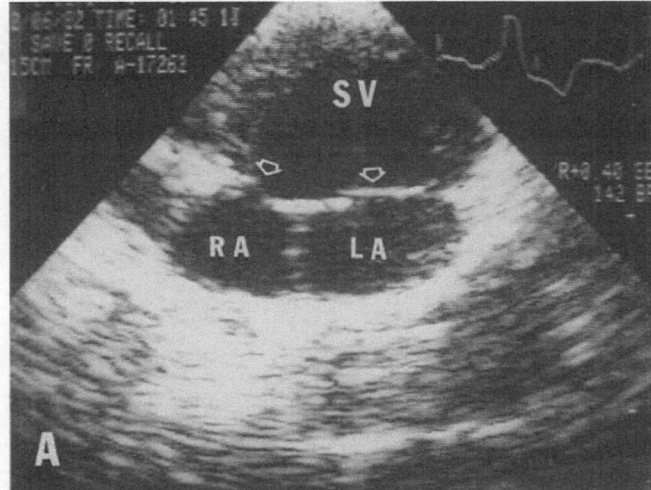

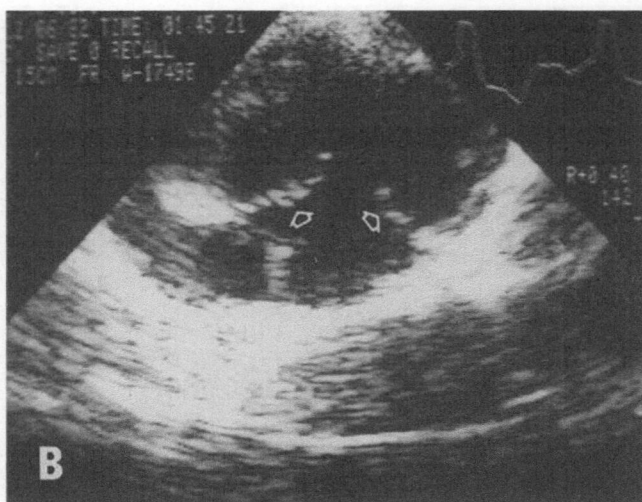

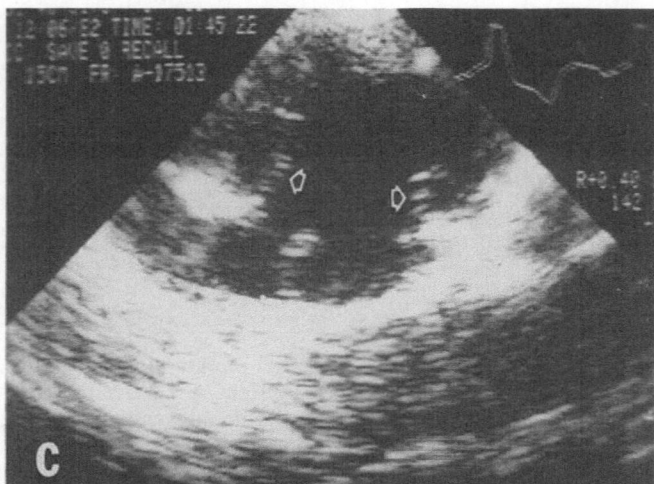

Fig. 7–122. *Two-dimensional echocardiogram in single ventricle with atrioventricular canal (A-V communis).* This 9-year-old with asplenia and levocardia had a pulmonary artery banding procedure as an infant. As in Fig. 7–121 the apex four-chamber view delineates the single ventricular chamber (*SV*). The *open arrows* in each frame indicate the leaflets of the common atrioventricular valve. During systole (**A**) while the atrioventricular valve is closed it appears the same as in Fig. 7–121. During early diastole (**B**) and later during diastole (**C**); however, no attachments are demonstrated between the atrioventricular valve and the atrial septum. The opening of the atrioventricular valve stretches across the entire width of the ventricle. The tip of the atrial septum appears bulbous, reminiscent of the appearance of the atrial septum in A-V communis without single ventricle.

RA = right atrium; *LA* = left atrium.

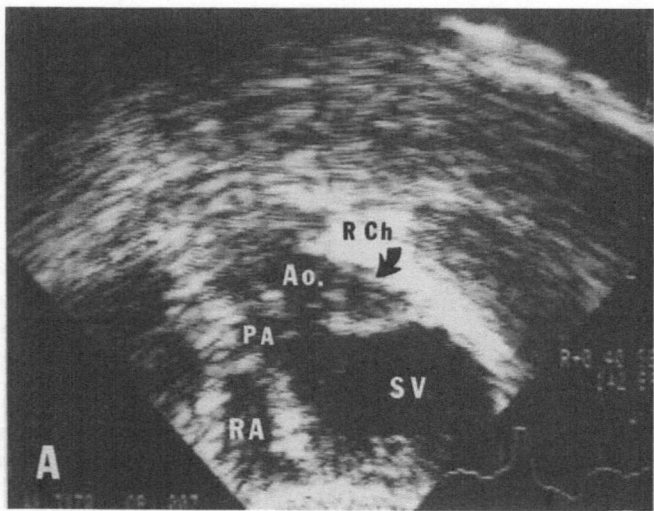

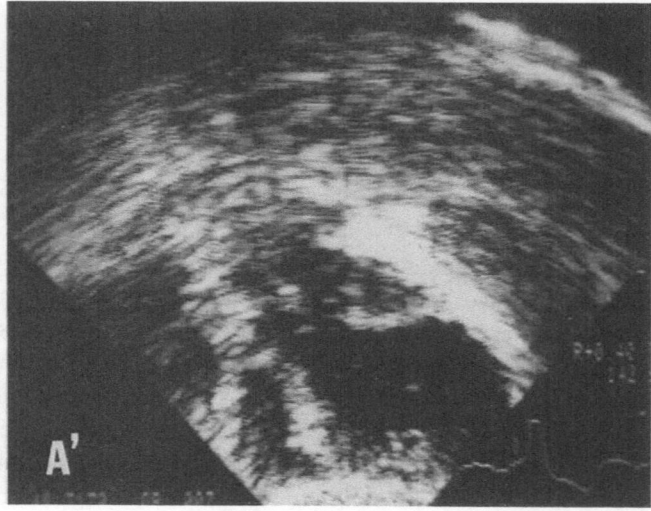

Fig. 7–123. *Subxiphoid oblique view of the patient in Fig. 7–122 to show the position of the rudimentary chamber and the great arteries.* **A** with labels; **A′** without labels. The sector is electronically inverted so that the orientation of the heart is similar to that observed on angiography. The ventricle (*SV*) has the shape of a left ventricle. The rudimentary chamber (*R Ch, curved arrow*) is at the base of the heart and on the left. The two great arteries arise side by side. The left-sided semilunar valve (the aortic valve, *Ao.*) arises from the rudimentary chamber, while the pulmonary artery (*PA*) arises from the main chamber. *RA* = right atrium.

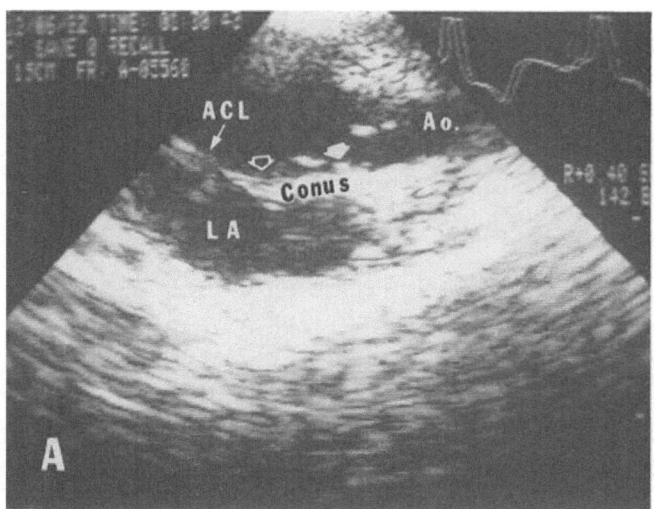
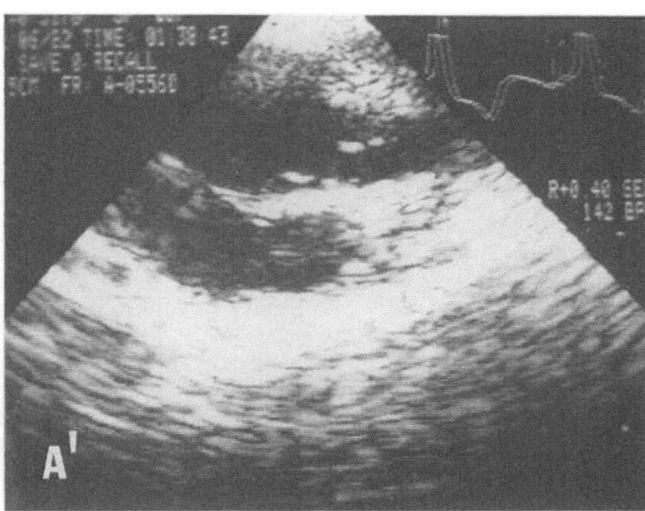

Fig. 7–124. *Semilunar to atrioventricular valve connection in single ventricle.* (Patient in Fig. 7–122 and 7–123). **A** with labels; **A'** without labels. This parasternal long axis view of the aortic valve (*Ao.*) and the anterior leaflet of the common atrioventricular valve (*ACL*) during diastole shows conus muscle interposed between the aortic and atrioventricular valves. This image is differ-ent from that occurring with aortic-mitral fibrous continuity because the fulcrum of the atrioventricular valve (*open arrow*) is separated from the root of the aorta (*closed arrow*) by thick, highly reflective tissue, representing conus muscle. *LA* = left atrium.

Fig. 7–125. *Great vessel relationships in single ventricle.* (Patient in Fig. 7–122 to 7–124). This short axis view of the great vessels demonstrates that the aorta (*Ao.*) and pulmonary artery (*PA*) are side by side. On angling superiorly the right-sided great vessel narrows to become indistinct (at the site of the pulmonary artery band), while the left-sided great vessel continues upward to form the arch of the aorta (not shown).

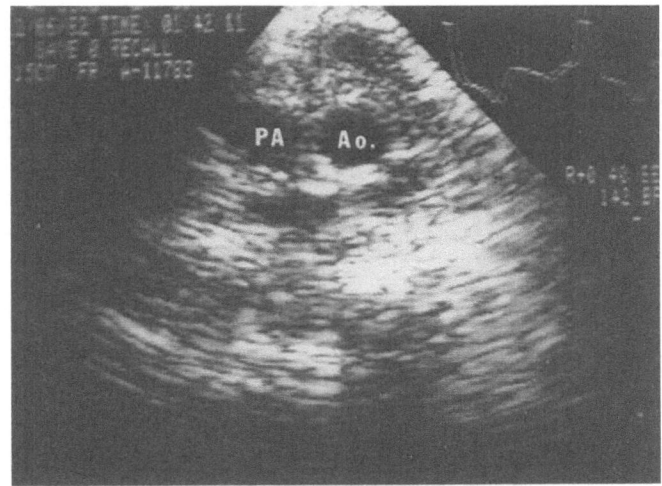

Radiological (Plain Film) Features Overcirculation of the pulmonary vasculature is usually present, but a normal pattern or even undercirculation may be noted, depending on the presence or absence of pulmonic stenosis or increased pulmonary resistance. The heart may be normal in size or enlarged. If pulmonary blood flow is increased the heart may be grossly enlarged. The apex of the heart may be on the left, in the middle or on the right (levocardia, mesocardia or dextrocardia). The normal triad of densities formed by the ascending aorta, the aortic arch and descending aorta, and the pulmonary artery is not present. Instead, in cases with right-sided outlet chamber, the vascular pedicle may be narrow because the aortic arch curves anteriorly or slightly toward the right within the cardiac silhouette, while the pulmonary artery arises directly behind the aorta. The cardiac contour with a right-sided outlet chamber and pulmonic stenosis may resemble that of tetralogy of Fallot (coeur en Sabot). In patients without pulmonic stenosis the cardiac contour resembles D-TGA (egg-shaped heart) (Fig. 7–127).

Radiological features most characteristic of single ventricle occur in patients with a left-sided outlet chamber (Fig. 7–128). In such cases the aorta forms the left upper heart border as it curves anteriorly and toward the left, or it may curve directly anteriorly so that a narrow vascular pedicle is observed (Fig. 7–129). On occasion a right aortic arch is present (Fig. 7–130). The aortic valve and rudimentary chamber form a bulge or shoulder configuration along

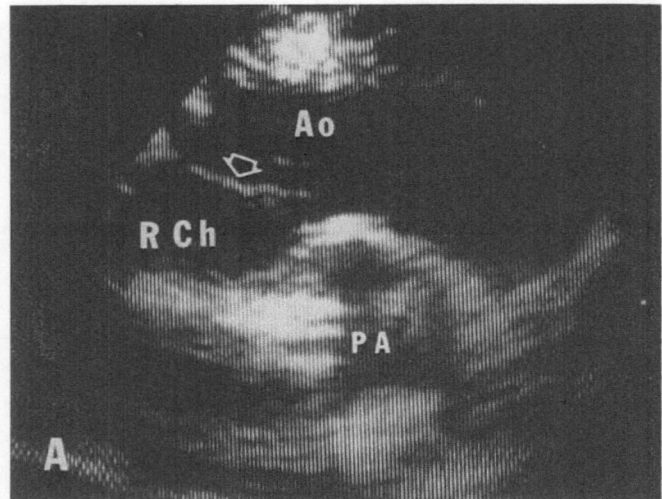

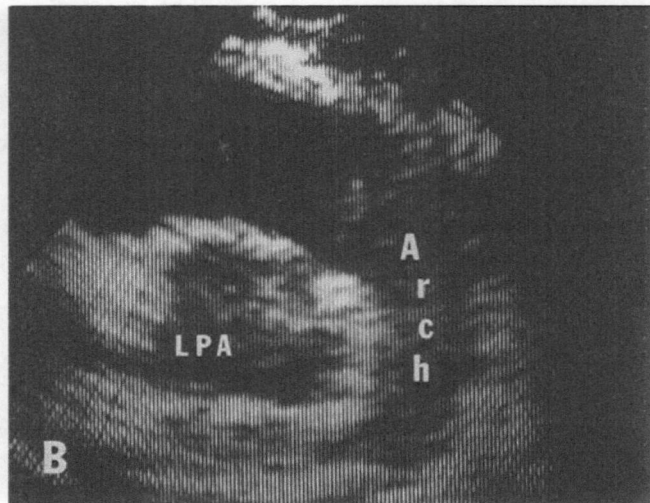

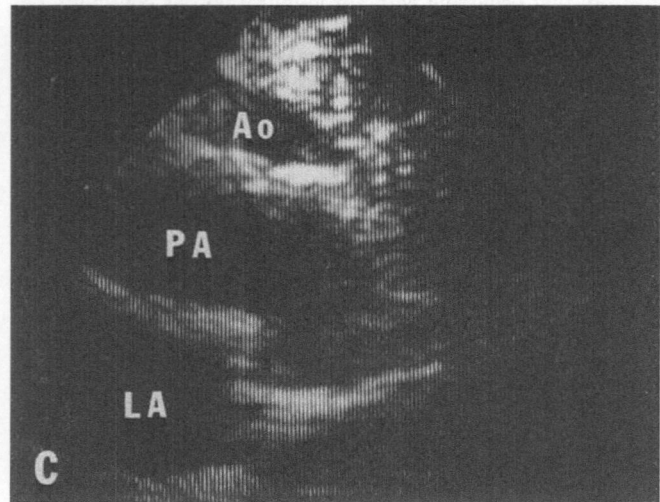

Fig. 7–126. *The great vessels in single ventricle with left-sided rudimentary outflow tract.* (Patient in Fig. 7–121). In **A** and **B** the anterior, left-sided great vessel (*Ao*) arises from the rudimentary chamber (*R Ch*), ascending to form the aortic arch. The *open arrow* indicates the aortic valve. The main and left pulmonary arteries (*PA,LPA*) are below the aortic arch. In **C** the posterior, right-sided great vessel (*PA*) arises from the main ventricular chamber, curving posteriorly to give origin to the pulmonary artery branches. *Ao* = aorta; *LA* = left atrium.

the left upper heart border, similar to that occurring with L-TGA (Figs. 7–128 to 7–130). The groove separating the rudimentary chamber from the main ventricular chamber is designated the septal notch (arrow in Figs. 7–128 to 7–130). This notch occurs high along the left heart border in cases of single ventricle, whereas it occurs near the apex, if at all, in cases of L-TGA. The main pulmonary artery arises posteriorly and medially in most instances of single ventricle, often indenting the left side of the esophagus at or below the carina. This feature is apparent especially when the pulmonary artery is dilated. The cascade or waterfall appearance of the right pulmonary artery and its branches occurring with L-TGA may also be noted in cases of single ventricle with a left-sided aorta. Thus the cardiac configuration in single ventricle may not be diagnostic or may have an appearance suggesting D-TGA, L-TGA or, on occasion, tetralogy of Fallot. The presence of the shoulder configuration of the left heart border with a septal notch high along the left heart border should indicate a diagnosis of single ventricle with left-sided outlet chamber (a high septal notch is also present in rare cases of crisscross heart).

Hemodynamics The physiological changes vary with the associated anomalies. In an individual with uncomplicated single ventricle, mixing at the ventricular level is indicated by a large oxygen step-up between the RA and the main ventricular chamber. The aortic and pulmonic O_2 saturation is usually the same as that in the ventricular chamber. Only a few cases have been reported with streaming from the left A-V valve into the rudimentary chamber, so that the aorta is fully saturated at the time of cardiac catheterization. Streaming occurs especially with straddling A-V valves. In the absence of pulmonic stenosis, pressure in the lungs is systemic, and pulmonary blood flow is determined by pulmonary vascular resistance. Pulmonary stenosis decreases pulmonary blood flow and pressure. In the

Fig. 7–127. *Pulmonary overcirculation and pulmonary venous hypertension with single ventricle.* This 7-week-old baby had severe congestive heart failure but no clinical cyanosis. The heart is enlarged, its contour being reminiscent of D-TGA, because the vascular pedicle is narrow and the heart is egg shaped. Cardiac catheterization demonstrated a single ventricle of the right ventricular type, with atresia of the left atrioventricular valve and a restrictive atrial septal defect. The aortic valve was on the right and the pulmonary valve on the left. The ascending aorta was hypoplastic. Coarctation of the aorta and a patent ductus arteriosus were also present.

When the aortic valve is on the right in single ventricle, the cardiac contour may be that of D-TGA, or it is nonspecific in configuration.

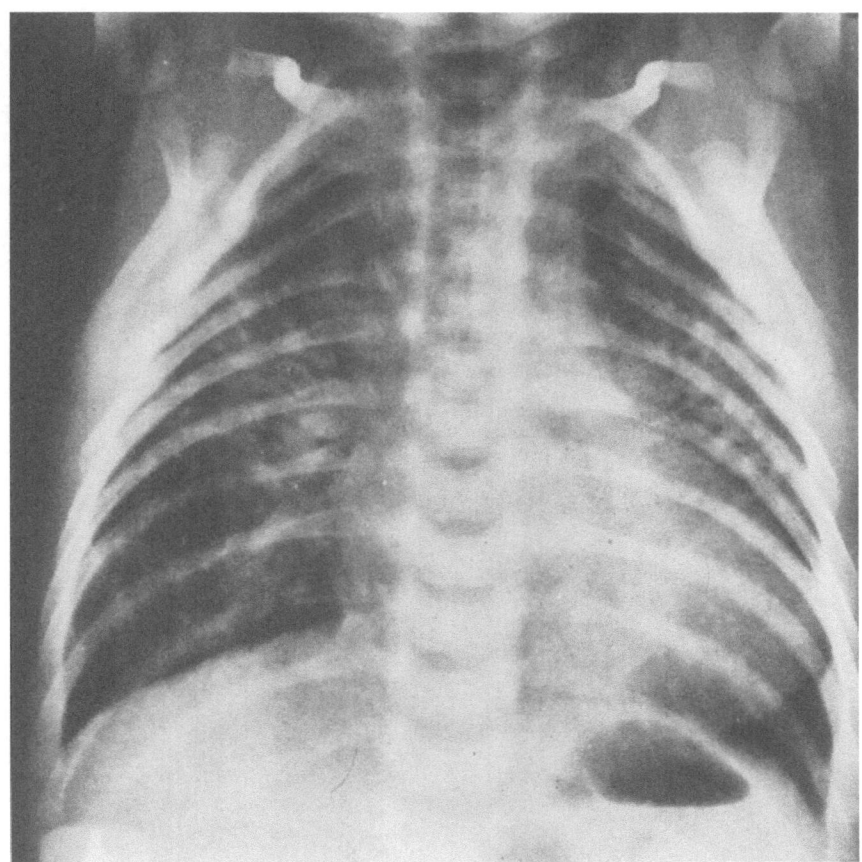

presence of severe pulmonic stenosis or atresia, pulmonary blood flow is markedly reduced and O_2 saturations are low.

The ventricular, aortic and pulmonic pressures are identical, unless pulmonic or aortic stenosis is present. Stenosis of the bulboventricular foramen may produce a pressure difference between the main ventricular chamber and the rudimentary chamber, affecting either the pulmonary or systemic circulation, depending on which great vessel arises from the outlet chamber. Pressures in the atria reflect pulmonary venous return or A-V valve function or both. A markedly increased pulmonary blood flow, stenosis of the left atrioventricular valve and insufficiency of the left atrioventricular valve all cause elevation of the LA pressure. The RA pressure will be elevated, with right A-V valve obstruction and a restrictive foramen ovale.

Contrast Studies Biplane frontal and lateral techniques are supplemented by axial views as necessary. If single ventricle

is suspected clinically, by chest roentgenography or by echocardiography then the initial injection of contrast material is in the main ventricular chamber. The type of single ventricle is determined by the trabecular pattern during ventricular systole. Course trabeculations indicate a RV type (Fig. 7–131), whereas fine trabeculations are characteristic of a LV type (Fig. 7–128C and D). In some instances the pattern is not sufficiently specific for characterization. Also ascertained from the initial injection are the number, patency, insufficiency or atresia of the A-V valves; the presence and location of pouches or rudimentary outlet chambers; and unusual ventriculoarterial connections such as those present in Holmes heart (Fig. 7–132). Stenosis of the bulboventricular foramen is recognized if present. Injection of contrast medium in the atria may be necessary to determine the presence or absence of the A-V valves and the atrial septum (Fig. 7–133). Injection of contrast material into the great arteries and systemic veins may

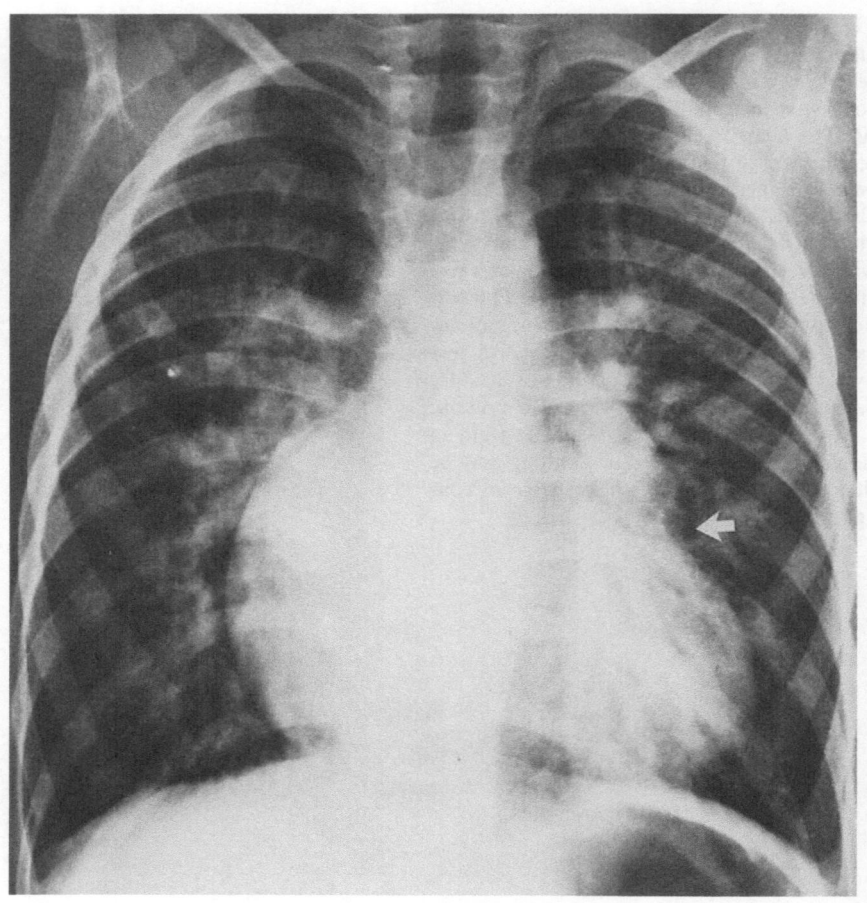

A

Fig. 7–128. *Radiological features characteristic of single ventricle of the left ventricular type with a left-sided rudimentary chamber.* **A** and **B** Frontal and lateral roentgenograms of the chest; **C** and **D** frontal and lateral angiograms. **A** and **B** Pulmonary overcirculation is present. The heart is enlarged, and both atria are dilated. The bump on the left heart border is formed by the rudimentary outlet chamber and the ascending aorta. The septal notch (*arrow*) indicates the groove formed by the septum between the main chamber and the outlet chamber. The frontal angiogram (**C**) demonstrates the position of the outlet chamber and the curve

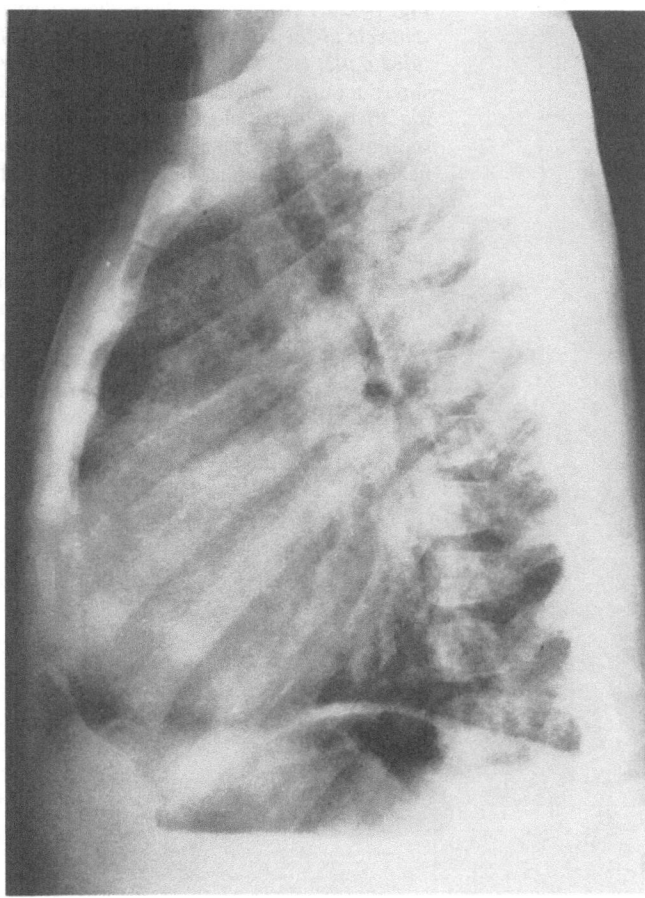

B

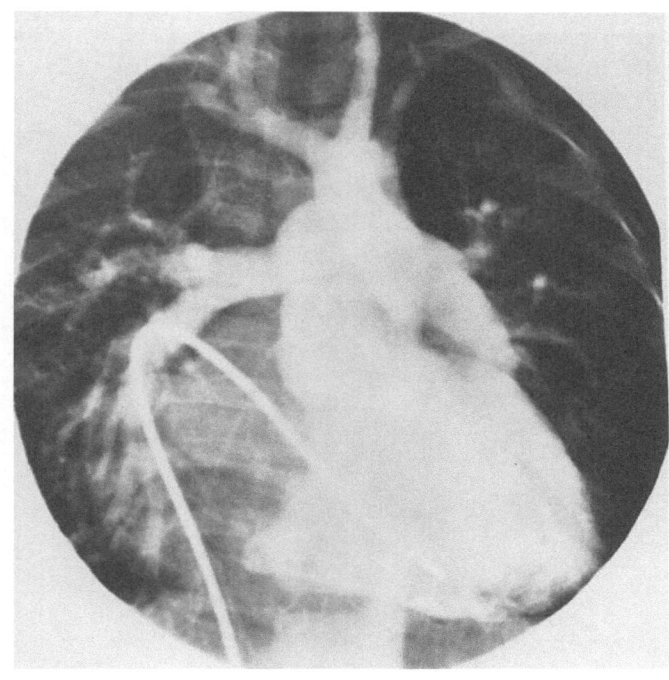

C

of the ascending aorta on the left. The position of the septum separating the outlet chamber from the main chamber corresponds to the septal notch on the PA roentgenogram of the chest. **D** The lateral angiogram shows the great vessels to be superimposed (side by side). A pulmonary artery band is noted (*arrow*). When the aortic valve is on the left in single ventricle the cardiac contour may be that of L-TGA. The high septal notch makes single ventricle more likely; however, criss-cross heart with horizontal septum should also be considered. Same patient as in Fig. 7–133.

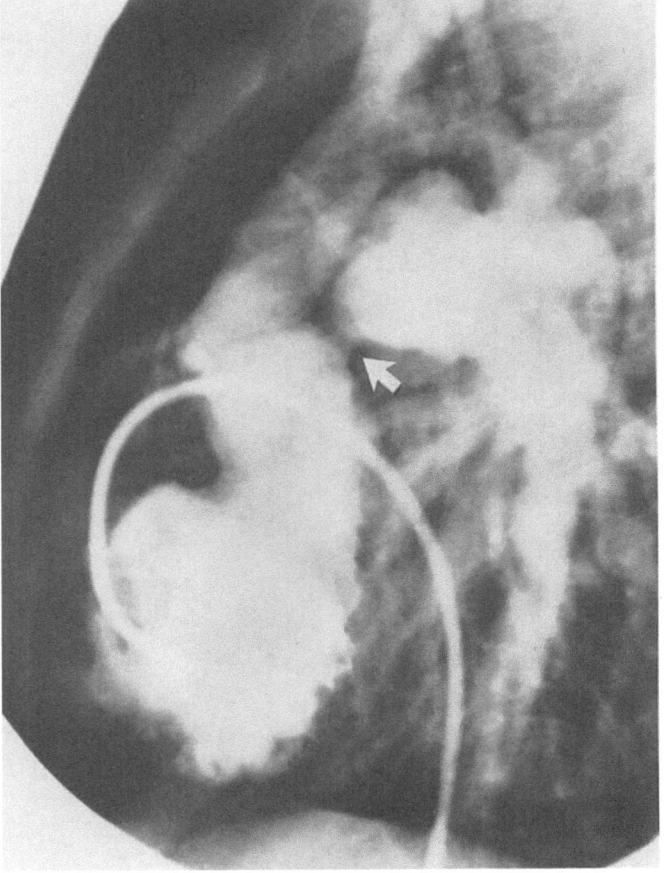

D

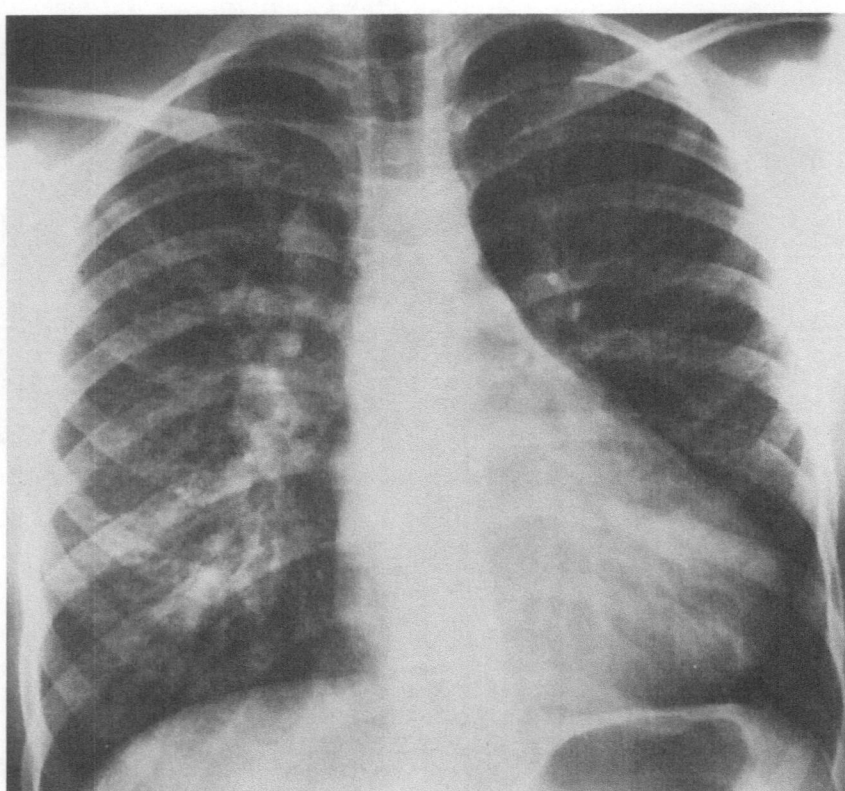

A

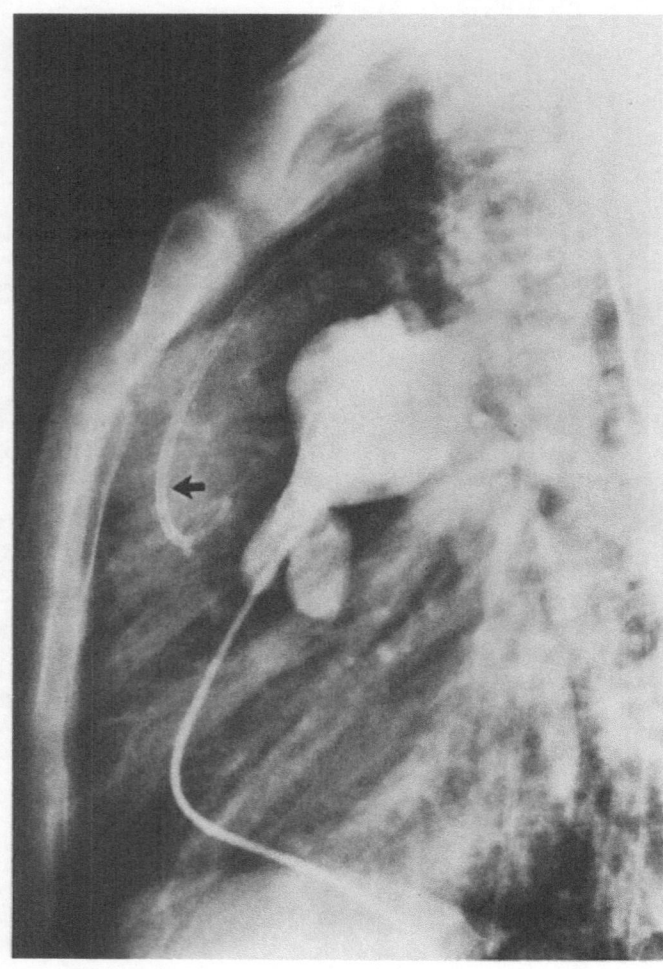

B

Fig. 7–129. *Narrow vascular pedicle in single ventricle of the left ventricular type with left-sided outlet chamber.* The PA chest film **(A)** shows a bump and septal notch corresponding to the outlet chamber and ventricular septum. The vascular pedicle is relatively narrow because the aorta curves toward the right and anteriorly. On the lateral film **(B)** of a pulmonary artery angiogram the mediastinum is noted to be widened by the ascending aorta, which curves anteriorly in front of the pulmonary artery. The *arrow* indicates a catheter in the ascending aorta. Injection of contrast medium through the second catheter into the pulmonary artery demonstrates a pulmonary artery band.

Fig. 7-130. *Right-sided aortic arch with single ventricle of the left ventricular type and left-sided outlet chamber.* Pulmonary overcirculation and an enlarged heart are present. The characteristic bump and septal notch (*arrow*) are evident along the left heart border (as demonstrated in Fig. 7-128). In this patient the aortic arch and proximal two-thirds of the descending aorta are on the right side (right aortic arch).

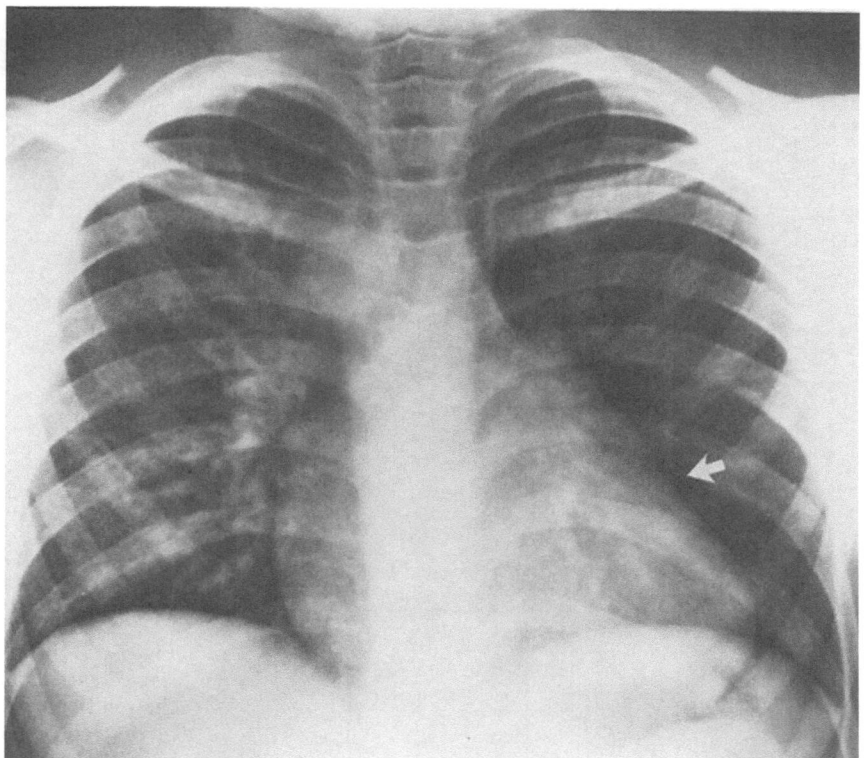

be necessary to identify associated anomalies such as patent ductus arteriosus, coarctation of the aorta and anomalous venous connections.

Treatment Initial palliation includes systemic-to-pulmonary artery shunts for infants with inadequate pulmonary blood flow and pulmonary artery banding for those infants with congestive heart failure secondary to excessive pulmonary blood flow. It is important that associated patent ductus arteriosus or coarctation of the aorta be repaired if either abnormality is contributing to symptoms.

Complete repair by an intracardiac septation procedure is possible in patients with two A-V valves. Electrophysiological mapping is essential to avoid suturing through the conducting system. A previously placed pulmonary artery band or shunt must be taken down and pulmonic stenosis, if present, relieved at the same time. If the pulmonary outflow tract is narrow, a procedure utilizing a conduit (Rastelli) is necessary. If the subaortic outflow tract is on

the right side, septation will leave the aorta attached to the systemic venous ventricle. Thus, in addition to an intracardiac septation procedure, the creation of an interatrial baffle (Mustard procedure) will be necessary. The mortality reported for these types of repairs is high, especially if a palliative procedure had been performed previously. At the present time the Fontan procedure (connection from the RA directly to the pulmonary artery) is preferred over septation procedures for individuals with single ventricle whose pulmonary vascular resistance is low. The Fontan procedure may also benefit those with only one A-V valve.

Postoperative findings include residual ventricular level shunts in either direction, residual pulmonic stenosis and obstruction of the superior or inferior limb of a Mustard baffle. The various arrhythmias, which include atrial and ventricular ectopic rhythms as well as first-, second- and third-degree heart block, are frequently encountered, either immediately postoperatively or as late sequelae.

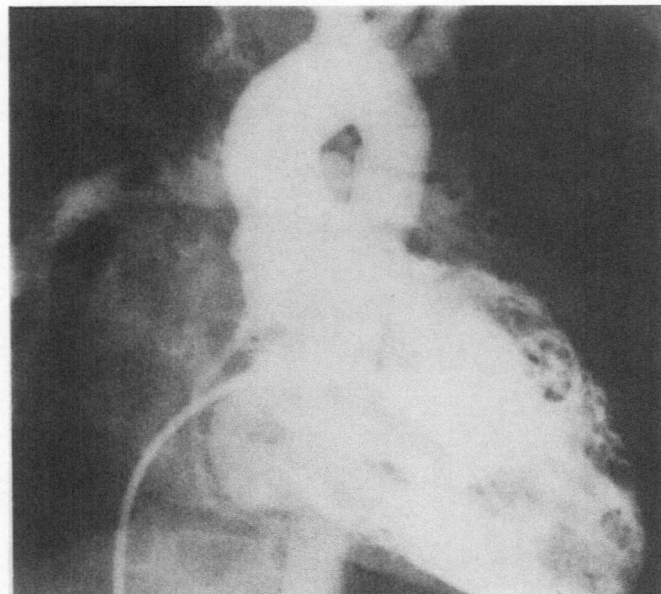

A

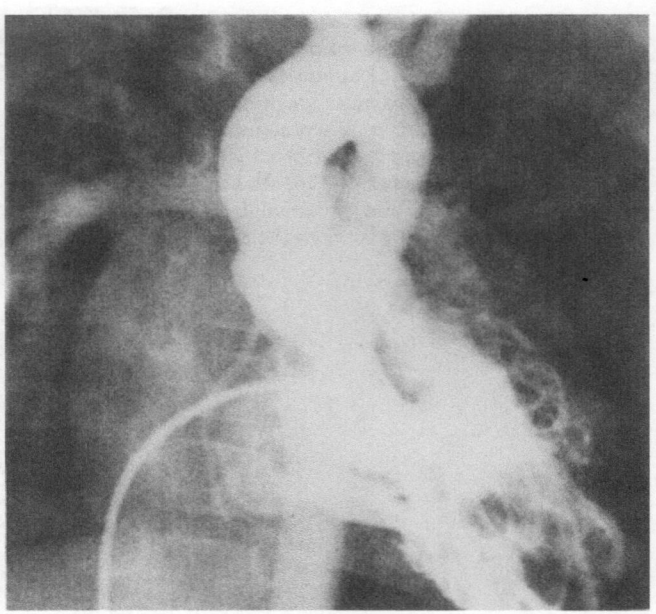

B

Fig. 7–131. *Characteristic angiographic findings in a patient with single ventricle of the right ventricular type.* **A** Frontal view of the ventriculogram in diastole; **B** same, in systole; **C** lateral view of the ventriculogram in diastole; **D** same, in systole; **E** LAO view of a second ventriculogram with cranial angulation (four-chamber view). The aorta is anterior and to the right of the pulmonary valve. In all views the coarse trabeculations are characteristic of a right ventricle. Two patent atrioventricular valves are noted in the ventricular chamber on viewing the ciné film. Conus muscle separating the semilunar valves from the atrioventricular valves is best demonstrated on the axial view (**E**). No outlet chamber is present. A ventricular pouch along the posterolateral wall inferiorly is noted on the lateral view (**C** and **D**). No connections are demonstrated between this pouch and the atrioventricular valves. A pulmonary artery band is also demonstrated in the lateral and axial views. Same patient as in Figs. 7–119 and 7–120.

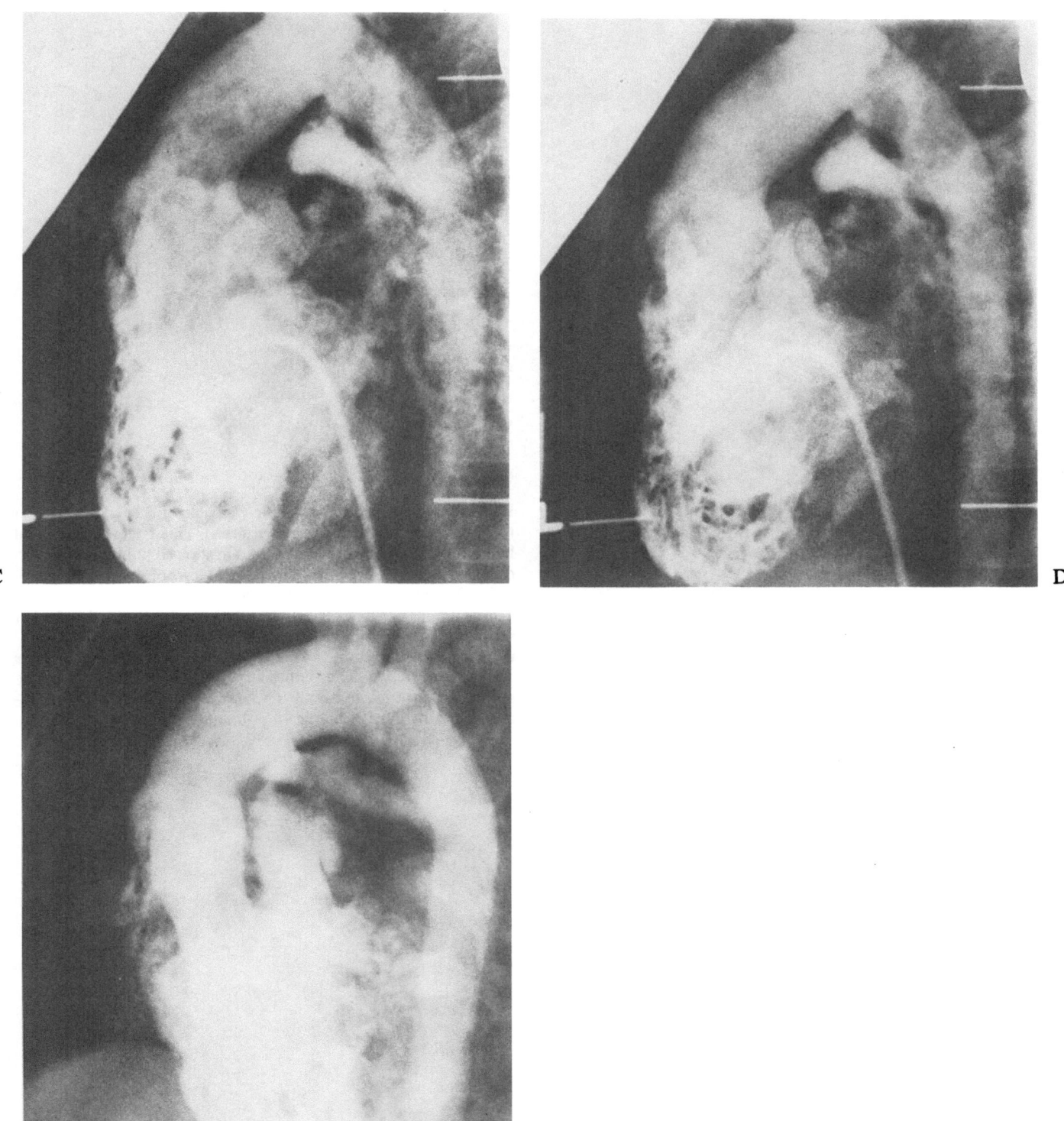

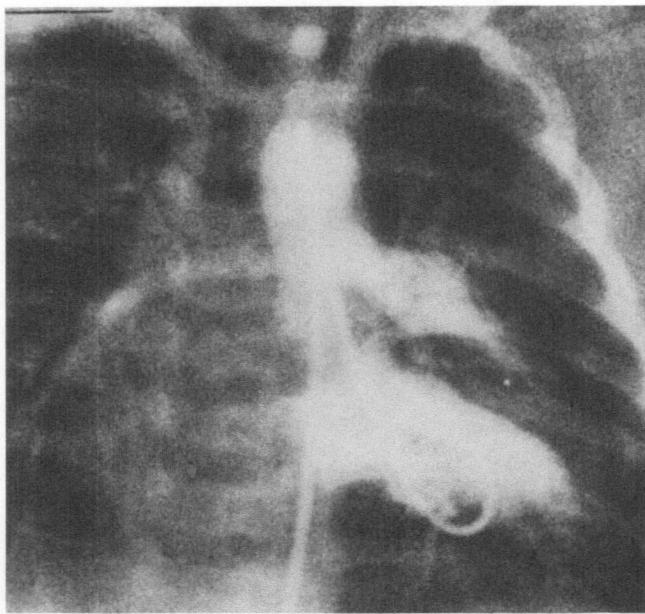

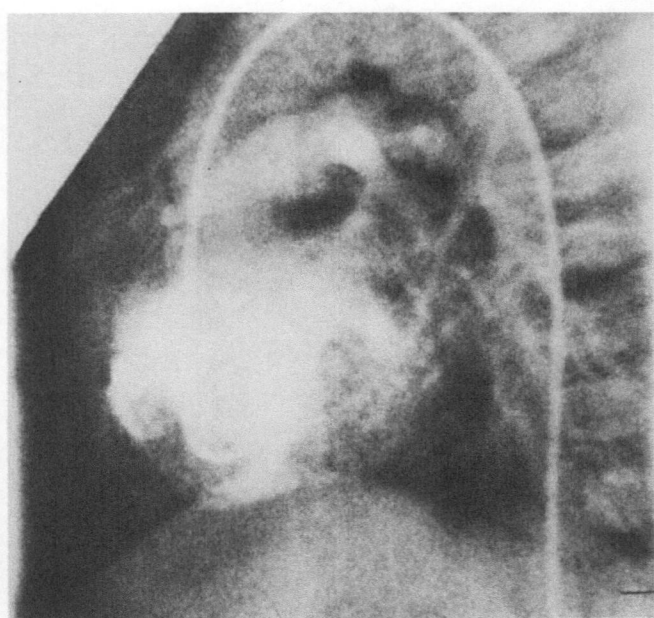

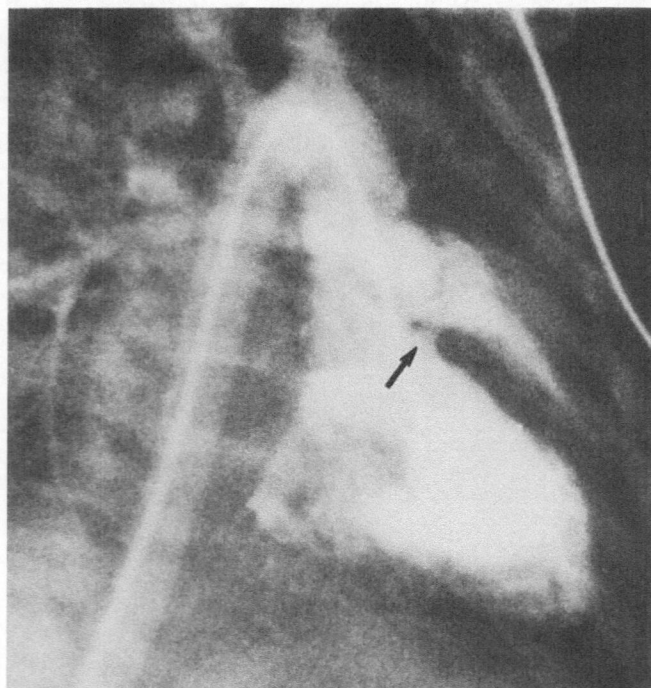

Fig. 7–132. *Holmes Heart* (single ventricle of the left ventricular type with normally related great arteries). This 1-month-old infant had cyanosis. The chest roentgenogram showed pulmonary under-circulation. **A** and **B** Frontal and lateral views of a ventriculogram; **C** RAO view of a second ventriculogram with cranial angulation. The main chamber has fine trabeculations characteristic of a left ventricle. The pulmonary artery arises from the left-sided rudimentary outlet chamber. The bulboventricular foramen (*arrow* in **C**) is restrictive. The pulmonary valve is thickened, and the pulmonary arteries are small. The restrictive bulboventricular foramen results in obstruction to pulmonary blood flow.

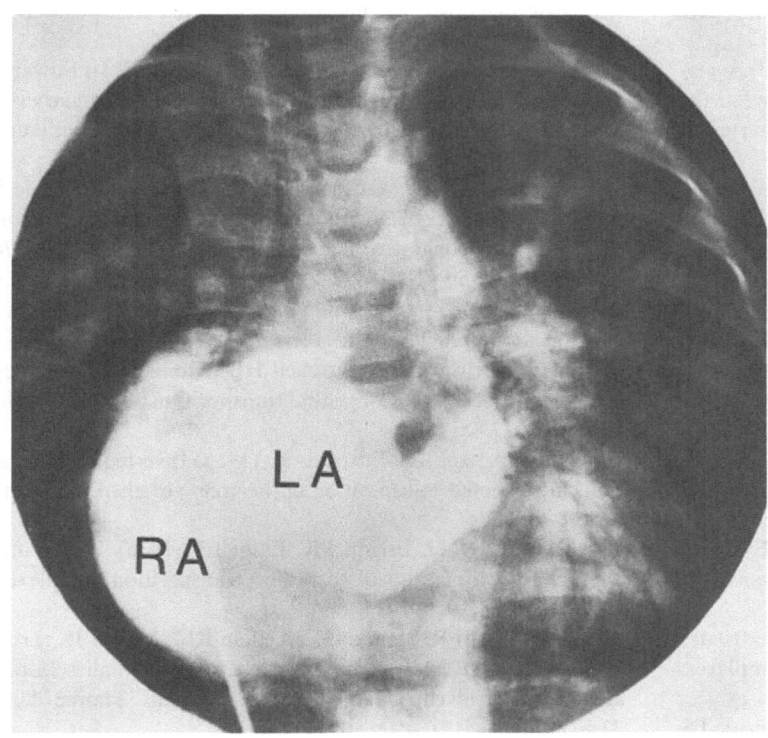
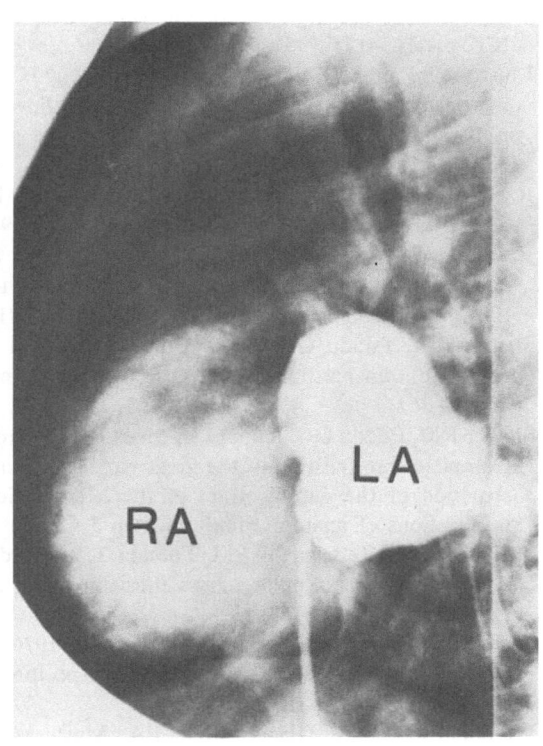

A   B

Fig. 7–133. *Atresia of the left atrioventricular valve in single ventricle* (Patient in Fig. 7–128). **A** Frontal view; **B** lateral view of an injection into the left atrium (*LA*) demonstrate no exit from that chamber except through a restrictive foramen ovale. The right atrium (*RA*) is enlarged.

Bibliography

Dextrotransposition of the Great Arteries

Bierman FZ, Williams RB (1979) Prospective diagnosis of d-Transposition of the great arteries in neonates by subxiphoid, two-dimensional echocardiography. Circulation 60:1496–1502

de la Cruz MV, Arteaga M, Espino-Vela J, Quero-Jimenez, M, Anderson RH, Diaz GF (1981) Complete transposition of the great arteries: Types and morphogenesis of ventriculoarterial discordance. Am Heart J 102:271–281

Duncan WJ, Freedom RM, Rowe RD, Olley PM, Williams WG, Trusler GA (1981) Echocardiographic features before and after the Jatene procedure (anatomical correction) for transposition of the great vessels. Am Heart J 102:227–232

Elliot LP, Carey LS, Adams P Jr, Edwards JE (1963) Left ventricular-right atrial communication in complete transposition of the great vessels. Am Heart J 66:29–35

Elliot LP, Neufeld HN, Anderson RC, Adams P Jr, Edwards JE (1963) Complete transposition of the great vessels. I. An anatomic study of 60 cases. Circulation 27:1105–1117

Foster JR, Damato AN, Kline LE, Akhtar M, Ruskin J (1976) Congenitally corrected transposition of the great vessels: Localization of the site of complete atrioventricular block using His bundle electrograms. Am J Cardiol 38:383–387

Fox LS, Kirklin JW, Pacifico AD, Waldo AL, Bargeron LM (1976) Intracardiac repair of cardiac malformations with atrioventricular discordance. Circulation 54:123–127

Graham TP Jr, Atwood GF, Boucek RJ Jr, Boerth RC, Bender HW Jr (1975) Abnormalities of right ventricular function following Mustard's operation for transposition of the great arteries. Circulation 52:678–684

Hirschfeld SS, Meyer RA, Kaplan S (1975) Measurement of right and left ventricular systolic time intervals by echocardiography. Circulation 51:304–309

Jatene AD, Fontes VF, Sauza LCB, Paulista PP, Neto CA, Sousa JEMR (1982) Anatomic correction of transposition of the great arteries. J Thorac Cardiovasc Surg 83:20–26

Jarmakani JMM, Canent RV Jr (1974) Preoperative and postoperative right ventricular function in children with transposition of the great vessels. Circulation 50:II39–II45.

Lange PE, Onnasch DG, Stephan E, Wessel A, Radley-Smith R, Yacoub MH, Regensburger D, Bernhard A, Heintzen PH (1981) Two-stage anatomic correction of complete transposition of the great arteries: Ventricular volumes and muscle mass. Herz 6:336–343

Mahony L, Turley K, Ebert P, Heymann MA (1982) Long-term results after atrial repair of transposition of the great arteries in early infancy. Circulation 66:253–258

Muster AJ, Paul MH, Van Grondelle A, Conway JJ (1976) Abnormal distribution of the pulmonary blood flow between the two lungs in transposition of the great arteries. In: Langford Kidd BS, Rowe RD (eds) The child with congenital heart disease after surgery. Futura Publishing Co., Mount Kisco, NY, pp. 165–178

Muster AJ, Paul MH, Van Grondelle A, Conway JJ (1976) Asymmetric distribution of the pulmonary blood flow between the right and left lungs in d-transposition of the great arteries. Am J Cardiol 38:352–361

Rashkind WJ (1971) Atrioseptostomy by balloon catheter in congenital heart disease. Radiol Clin North Am 9:193–202

Rashkind WJ, Miller WW (1966) Creation of an atrial septal defect without thoracotomy. A palliative approach to complete transposition of the great arteries. JAMA 196:991–992

Shaher RM, Puddu GC (1966) Coronary arterial anatomy in complete transposition of the great vessels. Am J Cardiol 17:355–361

Shaher RM, Puddu GC, Khoury G, Moes F, Mustard WT (1967) Complete transposition of the great vessels with anatomic obstruction of the outflow tract of the left ventricle. Surgical implications of anatomic findings. Am J Cardiol 19:658–670

Shrivatstava S, Tadavarthy SM, Fukuda T, Edwards JE (1976) Anatomic causes of pulmonary stenosis in complete transposition. Circulation 54:154–159

Tonkin IL, Kelley MJ, Bream PR, Elliot LP (1976) The frontal chest film as a method of suspecting transposition complexes. Circulation 53:1016–1025

Waldman JD, Paul MH, Newfeld EA, Muster AJ, Idriss FS (1977) Transposition of the great arteries with intact ventricular septum and patent ductus arteriosus. Am J Cardiol 39:232–238

Yacoub M, Bernhard A, Lange P, Radley-Smith R, Keck E, Stephan E, Heintzen P (1980) Clinical and hemodynamic results of the two-stage anatomic correction of simple transposition of the great arteries. Circulation: I190–I196

Levotransposition of the Great Arteries

Allwork SP, Bentall HH, Becker AE, Cameron H, Gerlis LM, Wilkinson JL, Anderson RH (1976) Congenitally corrected transposition of the great arteries: Morphologic study of 32 cases. Am J Cardiol 38:910–923

Cardell BS (1956) Corrected transposition of the great vessels. Br Heart J 18:186–192

Carey LS, Ruttenberg HD (1964) Roentgenographic features of congenital corrected transposition of the great vessels. Am J Roentgenol 92:623–651

Dekker A, Mehrizi A, Vengsarker AS (1965) Corrected transposition of the great vessels with Ebstein malformation of the left atrioventricular valve: An embryologic analysis and two case reports. Circulation 31:119–126

de la Cruz MV, Arteaga M, Espino-Vela J, Quero-Jimenez M, Anderson RH, Diaz GF (1981) Complete transposition of the great arteries: Types and morphogenesis of ventriculoarterial discordance. Am Heart J 102:271–281

Ellis K, Morgan BC, Blumenthal S, Anderson DH (1962) Congenital corrected transposition of the great vessels. Radiology 79:35–50

Hagler DJ, Tajik AJ, Seward JB, Edwards WD, Mair DD, Ritter DG (1981) Atrioventricular and ventriculoarterial discordance (corrected transposition of the great arteries). Wide-angle two-dimensional echocardiographic assessment of ventricular morphology. Mayo Clin Proc 56:591–600

King DL, Steeg CN, Ellis K (1973) Demonstration of transposition of the great arteries by cardiac ultrasonography. Radiology 107:181–186

Lester RG, Anderson RC, Amplatz K, Adams P (1960) Roent-

genologic diagnosis of congenitally corrected transposition of the great vessels. Am J Roentgenol 83:985–997

Levy MJ, Lillehei CW, Elliot LP, Carey LS, Adams P Jr, Edwards JE (1963) Accessory valvular tissue causing subpulmonary stenosis in corrected transposition of great vessels. Circulation 27:494–502

Nagle JP, Cheitlin MD, McCarty RJ (1971) Corrected transposition of the great vessels without associated anomalies: Report of a case with congestive failure at age 45. Chest 60:367–370

Okamura K, Konno S (1973) Two types of ventricular septal defect in corrected transposition of the great arteries: Reference to surgical approaches. Am Heart J 85:483–490

Schiebler GL, Edwards JE, Burchell HB, DuShane JW, Ongley PA, Wood EH (1961) Congenital transposition of great vessels. Pediatrics 27:851–888

Todd DB, Anderson RC, Edwards JE (1965) Inverted malformations in corrected transposition of the great vessels. Circulation 32:298–300

Tonkin IL, Kelly MJ, Bream PR, Elliot LP (1976) The frontal chest film as a method of suspected transposition complexes. Circulation 53:1016–1025

Williams WG, Suri R, Shindo G, Freedom RM, Morch JE, Trusler GA (1981) Repair of major intracardiac anomalies associated with atrioventricular discordance. Ann Thorac Surg 31:527–531

Atypical Dextrotransposition of the Great Arteries

Marin-Garcia J, Edwards JE (1980) Atypical d-transposition of the great arteries: Anterior pulmonary trunk. Am J Cardiol 46:507–510

Van Praagh R, Perez-Trevino C, Lopez-Cuellar M, Baker FW, Zuberbuhler JR, Quero M, Perez VM, Moreno F, Van Praagh S (1971) Transposition of the great arteries with posterior aorta, anterior pulmonary artery, subpulmonary conus and fibrous continuity between aortic and atrioventricular valves. Am J Cardiol 28:621–631

Wilkinson JL, Arnold R, Anderson RH, Acerete F (1975) 'Posterior' transposition reconsidered. Br Heart J 37:757–766

Isolated Ventricular Inversion

de la Cruz MV, Espino-Vela J, Attie F, Munoz CL (1967) An embryologic theory for ventricular inversions and their classification. Am Heart J 73:777–793

Espino-Vela J, de la Cruz MV, Munoz-Castellanos L, Plaza L, Attie F (1970) Ventricular inversion without transposition of the great vessels in situs inversus. Br Heart J 32:292–303

Quero-Jimenez M, Raposo-Sonnenfeld IR (1975) Isolated ventricular inversion with situs solitus. Br Heart J 37:293–304

Van Praagh R, Van Praagh S (1966) Isolated ventricular inversion. A consideration of the morphogenesis, definition and diagnosis of nontransposed and transposed great arteries. Am J Cardiol 17:395–406

Criss-Cross Heart

Anderson RH, Shinebourne EA, Gerlis LM (1974) Criss-cross atrioventricular relationships producing paradoxical atrioventricular concordance or discordance. Their significance to nomenclature of congenital heart disease. Circulation 50:176–180

Attie F, Munoz-Castellanos L, Jacobo Ovseyevitz J, Flores-Delgado I, Testelli MR, Buendia A, Kuri J, Molina B (1980) Crossed atrioventricular connections. Am Heart J 99:163–172

de la Cruz MV, Berrazueta JR, Arteaga M, Attie F, Soni J (1976)

Rules for diagnosis of arterioventricular discordances and spatial identification of ventricles. Crossed great arteries and transposition of the great arteries. Br Heart J 38:341–354

Guthaner D, Higgins CB, Silverman JF, Hayden WG, Wexler L (1976) An unusual form of the transposition complex. Uncorrected levo-transposition with horizontal ventricular septum: Report of two cases. Circulation 53:190–195

Truncus Arteriosus Communis

Allwork SP, Bentall RHC (1973) Case Report. Truncus solitarius pulmonalis. Br Heart J 35:977–980

Assad-Morell JL, Seward JB, Tajik AJ, Hagler DJ, Giuliani ER, Ritter DG (1976) Echo-phonocardiographic and contrast studies in conditions associated with systemic arterial trunk overriding the ventricular septum. Truncus arteriosus, tetralogy of Fallot, and pulmonary atresia with ventricular septal defect. Circulation 53:663–673

Becker AE, Becker MJ, Edwards JE (1971) Pathology of the semilunar valve in persistent truncus arteriosus. J Thorac Cardiovasc Surg 62:16–26

Bharati S, McAllister HA Jr, Rosenquist GC, Miller RA, Tatooles CJ, Lev M (1974) The surgical anatomy of truncus arteriosus communis. J Thorac Cardiovasc Surg 67:501–510

Calder L, Van Praagh R, Van Praagh S, Sears WP, Corwin R, Levy A, Keith JD, Paul MH (1976) Truncus arteriosus communis. Clinical angiocardiographic and pathologic findings in 100 patients. Am Heart J 92:23–38

Carr I, Bharati S, Kusnoor VS, Lev M (1979) Truncus arteriosus communis with intact ventricular septum. Br Heart J 42:97–102

Chung KJ, Alexson CG, Manning JA, Gramiak R (1973) Echocardiography in truncus arteriosus. The value of pulmonic valve detection. Circulation 48:281–286

Collett RW, Edwards JE (1949) Persistent truncus arteriosus: A classification according to anatomic types. Surg Clin North Am 29:1245–1270

Crupi G, Macartney FJ, Anderson RH (1977) Persistent truncus arteriosus. A study of 66 autopsy cases with special reference to definition and morphogenesis. Am J Cardiol 40:569–578

Davis GD, Fulton RE, Ritter DG, Mair DD, McGoon DC (1978) Congenital pulmonary atresia with ventricular septal defect: Angiographic and surgical correlates. Radiology 128:133–144

Edwards JE (1976) Persistent truncus arteriosus: A comment (editorial) Am Heart J 92:1–2

French JW, Silverman NH, Martin RP, Schiller NB, Popp RL (1976) Examination of operative patients with conotruncal abnormalities using an ultrasonic wide angle scanner (abstr). Circulation 54:II–46

Goldberg MJ, McGregor M (1958) Persistent truncus arteriosus: Report of a case with atypical radiologic features. Am Heart J 55:360–365

Goor DA, Lillehei CW (1975) Congenital malformation of the heart. Embryology, anatomy, and operative considerations. Grune & Stratton, New York, pp 154–168

Hagler DJ, Tajik AJ, Seward JB, Mair DD, Ritter DG (1980) Wide-angle two-dimensional echocardiographic profiles of conotruncal abnormalities. Mayo Clin Proc 55:73–82

Henry WL, Maron BJ, Griffith MS, Epstein SE (1975) Differential diagnosis of abnormalities of the great arteries by real-time two-dimensional echocardiography. Circulation 51:281

Lev M, Saphir O (1942) Truncus arteriosus communis persistens. J Pediatr 20:74–88

Mair DD, Ritter DG, Danielson GK, Wallace RB, McGoon

DC (1977) Truncus arteriosus with unilateral absence of a pulmonary artery. Criteria for operability and surgical results. Circulation 55:641–647

Marin-Garcia J, Tonkin ILD (1982) Two-dimensional echocardiographic evaluation of persistent truncus arteriosus. Am J Cardiol 50:1376–1379

McCue CM, Lester RG, Bosher L Jr, Mauck HP Jr (1964) Persistent truncus arteriosus. A clinical correlation with the pathologic anatomy. Dis Chest 46:507–523

McFaul RC, Mair DD, Feldt RH, Ritter DG, McGoon DC (1976) Truncus arteriosus and previous pulmonary arterial banding: Clinical and hemodynamic assessment. Am J Cardiol 38:626–632

Moes CAF, Freedom RM (1980) Aortic arch interruption with truncus arteriosus or aorticopulmonary septal defect. Am J Roentgenol 135:1011–1016

Nadal-Ginnard B, Malpartida F, Espino-Vela J (1972) Inversion ventricular con tronco comun. Arch Inst Cardiol Mex 42:181–192

Poirier RA, Berman MA, Stansel HC Jr (1975) Current status of the surgical treatment of truncus arteriosus. J Thorac Cardiovasc Surg 69:169–182

Rice MJ, Seward JB, Hagler DJ, Mair DD, Tajik AJ (1982) Definitive diagnosis of truncus arteriosus by two-dimensional echocardiography. Mayo Clin Proc 57:476–481

Riggs TW, Paul MH, Pajcic S (1982) Two dimensional echocardiographic prospective diagnosis of common truncus arteriosus in infants. Am J Cardiol 50:1380–1384

Shrivastava S, Edwards JE (1977) Coronary arterial origin in persistent truncus arteriosus. Circulation 55:551–554

Sotomora RF, Edwards JE (1978) Anatomic identification of so-called absent pulmonary artery. Circulation 57:624–633

Stark J, Gandhi D, de Leval M, Macartney F, Taylor JFN (1978) Surgical treatment of persistent truncus arteriosus in the first year of life. Br Heart J 40:1280–1287

Taussig HB (1947) Clinical and pathological findings in cases of truncus arteriosus in infancy. Am J Med 2:26

Thiene G, Bortolotti B, Gallucci V, Terribile V, Pellegrino PA (1976) Anatomical study of truncus arteriosus communis with embryological and surgical considerations. Br Heart J 38:1109–1123

Tingelstad JB, Robertson LW (1976) Fluttering of the interventricular septum. The result of truncal insufficiency. Chest 69:119–120

Van Mierop LHS, Patterson DF, Schnarr WR (1978) Pathogenesis of persistent truncus arteriosus in light of observations made in a dog embryo with the anomaly. Am J Cardiol 41:755–762

Van Praagh R (1976) Classification of truncus arteriosus communis (TAC) (editorial) Am Heart J 92:129–132

Van Praagh R, Van Praagh S (1965) The anatomy of common aorticopulmonary trunk (truncus arteriosus communis) and its embryologic implications. A study of 57 necropsy cases. Am J Cardiol 16:406–426

Victorica BE, Krovetz LJ, Elliott LP, Van Mierop LHS, Bartley TD, Gessner IH, Schiebler GL (1969) Persistent truncus arteriosus in infancy. A study of 14 cases. Am Heart J 77:13–25

Zamora C, Jain SC, Munoz-Castellanos L, Testelli M (1980) Truncus arteriosus communis, an unusual anatomical variant of type I. Cathet Cardiovasc Diagn 6:81–87

Single Ventricle

Anderson RH, Becker AE, Wilkinson JL (1975) Proceedings:

Morphogenesis and nomenclature of univentricular hearts. Br Heart J 37:781–782

Anderson RH, Becker AE, Wilkinson JL, Gerlis LM (1976) Morphogenesis of univentricular hearts. Br Heart J 38:558–572

Anderson RH, Wilkinson JL, Gerlis LM, Smith A, Becker AE (1977) Atresia of the right atrioventricular orifice. Br Heart J 39:414–428

Anselmi G, Armas SM, de la Cruz MV, de Pisani F, Blanco P (1968) Diagnosis and classification of single ventricle. Am J Cardiol 21:813–829

Becker AE, Wilkinson JL, Anderson RH (1980) Atrioventricular conduction tissues: A guide in understanding the morphogenesis of the univentricular heart. In: Van Praagh R and Takao A (eds) Etiology and morphogenesis of congenital heart disease. Futura Publishing Co., Mount Kisco, New York, pp 489–514

Bharati S, Lev M (1975) The course of the conduction system in single ventricle with inverted (L−) loop and inverted (L−) transposition. Circulation 51:723–730

Carey LS, Ruttenberg HD (1964) Roentgenographic features of common ventricle with inversion of the infundibulum. Corrected transposition with rudimentary left ventricle. Am J Roentgenol 92:652–668

Chesler E, Joffe HS, Vecht R, Beck W, Schrire V (1970) Ultrasound cardiography in single ventricle and the hypoplastic left and right heart syndromes. Circulation 42:123–129

de la Cruz MV, Miller BL (1968) Double-inlet left ventricle. Two pathological specimens with comments on the embryology and on its relation to single ventricle. Circulation 37:249–260

Edie RN, Malm JR (1976) Surgical repair of single ventricle. In: Langford Kidd BS, Rowe RD (eds.) The child with congenital heart disease after surgery. Futura Publishing Co., Mount Kisco, New York, pp 35–54

Elliott LP (1978) An angiocardiographic and plain film approach to complex congenital heart disease: Classification and simplified nomenclature. Curr Probl Cardiol 3(3):1–64

Elliott LP, Anderson RC, Edwards JE (1964) The common cardiac ventricle with transposition of the great vessels. Br Heart J 26:289–301

Elliott LP, Gedgaudas E (1964) The roentgenologic findings in common ventricle with transposition of the great vessels. Radiology 82:850–865

Feldt RH, Mair DD, Danielson GK, Wallace RB, McGoon DC (1981) Current status of the septation procedure for univentricular heart. J Thorac Cardiovasc Surg 82:93–97

Jacoub MH, Radley-Smith R (1976) Use of a valved conduit from right atrium to pulmonary artery for "correction" of single ventricle. Circulation 54:63–70

Kozuka T, Sato K, Fujino M, Kawashima Y, Nosaki T (1973) Roentgenographic diagnosis of single ventricle. Analysis of 42 cases. Am J Roentgenol 119:512–523

Lambert EC (1951) Single ventricle with a rudimentary outlet chamber. Case report. Bull Johns Hopkins Hosp 88:231–238

Liberthson RR, Paul MH, Muster AJ, Arcilla RA, Eckner FAO, Lev M (1971) Straddling and displaced atrioventricular orifices and valves with primitive ventricles. Circulation 43:213–226

Macartney FJ, Partridge JB, Scott O, Deverall PB (1976) Common or single ventricle. An angiographic and hemodynamic study of 42 patients. Circulation 53:543–554

Marin-Garcia J, Tandon R, Moller JH, Edwards JE (1974) Common (single) ventricle with normally related great vessels. Circulation 49:565–573

Marin-Garcia J, Tandon R, Moller JH, Edwards JE (1974) Single ventricle with transposition. Circulation 49:994–1004

Morgan AD, Krovetz LJ, Bartley TD, Green JR Jr, Shanklin DR, Wheat MW Jr, Schiebler GL (1966) Clinical features of single ventricle with congenitally corrected transposition. Am J Cardiol 17:379–388

Mortera C, Hunter S, Terry G, Tynan M (1977) Echocardiography of primitive ventricle. Br Heart J 39:847–855

Muñoz-Castellanos L, de la Cruz MV, Cieslinski A (1973) Double inlet right ventricle: Two pathological specimens; with comments on embryology. Br Heart J 35:292–297

Quero M (1970) Atresia of the left atrioventricular orifice associated with a Holmes heart. Circulation 39:739–744

Quero M (1972) Coexistence of single ventricle with atresia of one atrioventricular orifice. Circulation 46:794–798

Quero Jiménez M, Pérez Martínez VM, Maitre Azćarete MJ, Merino Batres G, Moreno Granados F (1973) Exaggerated displacement of the atrioventricular canal towards the bulbus cordis (rightward displacement of the mitral valve). Br Heart J 35:65–74

Sahn DJ, Harder JR, Freedom RM, Duncan WJ, Rowe RD, Allen HD, Valdez-Cruz L, Goldberg SJ (1982) Cross-sectional echocardiographic diagnosis and subclassification of univentricular hearts: Imaging studies of atrioventricular valves, septal structures and rudimentary outflow chambers. Circulation 66:1070–1077

Seward JB, Tajik AJ, Hagler DJ, Guiliani ER, Gau GT, Ritter DG (1977) Echocardiogram in common (single) ventricle: Angiographic-anatomic correlation. Am J Cardiol 39:217–225

Shinebourne EA, Lau K, Calcaterra G, Anderson RH (1980) Univentricular heart of right ventricular type: clinical, angiographic and electrocardiographic features. Am J Cardiol 46:439–445

Shinebourne EA, Macartney FJ, Anderson RH (1976) Sequential chamber localization: The logical approach to diagnosis in congenital heart disease. Br Heart J 38:327–340

Somerville J, Becu L, Ross D (1974) Common ventricle with acquired subaortic obstruction. Am J Cardiol 34:206–214

Soto B, Bertranou EG, Bream PR, Souza A Jr, Bargeron LM Jr (1979) Angiographic study of univentricular heart of right ventricular type. Circulation 60:1325–1334

Tynan MJ, Becker AE, Macartney FJ, Quero-Jimenez M, Shinebourne EA, Anderson RH (1979) Nomenclature and classification of congenital heart disease. Br Heart J 41:544–553

Van Praagh R, Ongley PA, Swan HJC (1964) Anatomic types of single or common ventricle in man. Morphologic and geometric aspects of 60 necropsied cases. Am J Cardiol 13:367–386

Van Praagh R, Van Praagh S, Vlad P, Keith JD (1965) Diagnosis of the anatomic types of single or common ventricle. Am J Cardiol 15:345–366

Chapter 7, Section 3
Right Heart Obstruction

Obstructive abnormalities of the right side of the heart occur at all levels, from the pulmonary arteries (e.g., primary pulmonary hypertension) to the right atrium and systemic veins (e.g., tumor of the right atrium, superior vena cava syndrome). In the classification developed by the authors of this work (Table 7–5), simple defects are those that cause obstruction at a single level of the right heart, but do not include a septal defect. Valvar pulmonic stenosis with intact ventricular septum is an example of a simple defect.

Complex defects consist of combinations of obstruction of the right side of the heart and one or more septal defects. Ventricular septal defect with pulmonic stenosis and a single ventricle with pulmonic stenosis constitute examples of complex defects. Tricuspid atresia is also a complex defect, because it includes a right-to-left shunt at the atrial level, and because a ventricular septal defect is almost always associated.

In this chapter most of the simple lesions are included, and in addition, tricuspid atresia, tetralogy of Fallot and variants of tetralogy of Fallot. Idiopathic dilatation of the main pulmonary artery is included because its appearance on chest roentgenograms is similar to that of valvar pulmonic stenosis. Uhl anomaly is described with other cardiomyopathies. Tumors of the heart are dealt with in a separate chapter. Many of the complex lesions such as A-V communis and pulmonic stenosis, or single ventricle and pulmonic stenosis, are included in other sections because pulmonic stenosis is a part of the complex rather than being the primary lesion.

Primary (Idiopathic) Pulmonary Hypertension

The clinical diagnosis of primary pulmonary hypertension (PPH) is made by exclusion after all known causes of pulmonary hypertension have been excluded. PPH is a rare disorder occurring in both children and adults. In adults PPH is more common in women, but in children no sex predilection has been established.

This clinical entity represents the end stage of a vasoconstrictive process that causes chronically increased pulmonary resistance. PPH is usually progressive and leads to premature death. At autopsy the pulmonary arteries show atherosclerotic plaque, medial hypertrophy, intimal fibrosis and plexiform aneurysms, which are the same changes occurring with pulmonary hypertension from definitive causes. On pathological studies PPH is distinct from recurrent or chronic pulmonary thromboembolism and from pulmonary venoocclusive disease.

Table 7–5. Right Heart Obstruction
(*Normal to Decreased Pulmonary Blood Flow, with or without Cyanosis*)

1. Simple
   Primary (idiopathic) pulmonary hypertension
   Peripheral pulmonic stenosis (PPS)
      Diffuse
      Localized (multiple or single)
      Supravalvar
   Unilateral agenesis of a pulmonary artery
   Valvar pulmonic stenosis (PS) including dysplastic pulmonary valve
   Subvalvar pulmonic stenosis
      Stenosis of the os infundibuli (subpulmonic membrane)
      Hypertrophic cardiomyopathy (including asymmetrical septal hypertrophy)
      Anomalous muscle bundle (two-chambered RV)
      Accessory tricuspid valve tissue
   Tricuspid stenosis (rare)
   Ebstein anomaly with or without PS
   Cor triatriatum dexter
   Uhl anomaly
   Heart tumors
2. Complex
   Tetralogy of Fallot and variants
      (Pseudotruncus, absence of pulmonary valve, absence of left pulmonary artery, left hemitruncus)
   Ventricular septal defect and PS
   PS and Atrial septal defect (trilogy of Fallot)
   PS and Aortic stenosis (e.g., fetal hydantoin syndrome)
   PS (or atresia) with:
      D-TGA
      A-V communis (atrioventricular canal)
      Single ventricle
      L-TGA and VSD
      Truncus arteriosus
      Double-outlet right ventricle (DORV)
      Criss-cross Heart
   Pulmonary atresia with intact ventricular septum with or without tricuspid insufficiency
   Tricuspid atresia (TA)
      Tricuspid atresia with D-TGA

The *clinical features* are manifestations of pulmonary hypertension and limited cardiac output. Cyanosis may be secondary to a right-to-left shunt either in the lungs or through a patent foramen ovale. Symptoms of fatigue, dyspnea and pain in the chest are common, while syncope and pulmonary hemorrhage may occur, connoting a grave prognosis.

On physical examination a right ventricular heave and a loud pulmonary second sound are characteristic. A pulmonary ejection click, a right-sided S_4 and a diastolic murmur of pulmonary regurgitation may also be encountered.

461

With right ventricular failure the murmur of tricuspid regurgitation may be audible, and the neck veins may be distended with increased a and v waves. Late in the course of the disorder, hepatomegaly and ascites are present.

Electrocardiograms show signs of hypertrophy of the right ventricle (RV) and the right atrium (RA).

M-mode echocardiography shows evidence of pulmonary hypertension (e.g., absence of "atrial kick" on the pulmonary valve tracing, long right ventricular pre-ejection period, short right ventricular ejection time, mid systolic closure of the pulmonary valve) (Fig. 7–134A). The RV is dilated, and the ventricular septum does not move (flat), or moves paradoxically during ventricular systole (Fig. 7–134C). The E-to-F slope of the mitral valve is reduced. This finding does not indicate mitral stenosis, but may be secondary to slow filling of the left ventricle (LV). The posterior leaflet of the mitral valve moves normally (Fig. 7–134C). *On 2-D echocardiography* the ventricular septum bulges into the LV during systole. Echocardiography excludes mitral stenosis, which may be a causative factor in pulmonary hypertension.

On *roentgenograms of the chest* (Figs. 7–135A and B), the heart is usually enlarged with predominance of the RV and RA. The most striking feature is dilatation of the central pulmonary arteries and abrupt tapering of their interlobar branches (precapillary pulmonary hypertension, the pruned-tree appearance). Although this pattern is easy to recognize in adults it may not be readily apparent on PA chest films in children because the dilated central pulmonary vessels may be mistaken for hilar adenopathy. The lateral projection is helpful in children because the left pulmonary artery is clearly outlined in this view, excluding a tumor or lymphadenopathy. At the same time, abrupt tapering of the interlobar branches is clearly defined. Evidence of postcapillary pulmonary hypertension (pulmonary venous hypertension) on roentgenograms of the chest should suggest other causes of pulmonary hypertension (e.g., mitral stenosis, pulmonary venoocclusive disease). Nuclear scanning for pulmonary perfusion may differentiate PPH from gross thromboembolic disease, but not from chronic microembolism.

Cardiac catheterization, and especially pulmonary angiography, has a high risk in patients with PPH, on occasion precipitating an acute increase in pulmonary resistance with RV failure. If performed, cardiac catheterization provides definitive evidence of pulmonary hypertension and increased pulmonary resistance, excluding congenital heart defects such as ventricular septal defect (VSD) and patent ductus arteriosus (PDA) with reactive pulmonary vascularity in which surgery may lead to a fall in pulmonary pressure. The angiograms may demonstrate thromboemboli, leading to consideration of the use of anticoagulants. Therapy for PPH generally is ineffective. Vasodilators such as oxygen, diazoxide, hydralazine, tolazoline, isoproterenol and prostacyclin have all been reported to lower pulmonary resistance in patients with PPH, but reversal of the underlying process does not occur.

Pulmonic Stenosis

Obstruction to the RV may be at the valvar, subvalvar (infundibular, subinfundibular) or supravalvar level. Valvar pulmonic stenosis is the most common of the three and occurs as an isolated anomaly or in association with other congenital heart defects and with systemic disorders.

Valvar Pulmonic Stenosis
Isolated Pulmonic Stenosis Isolated pulmonary stenosis (PS) is a common congenital lesion, accounting for approximately 6% of all congenital heart defects. Abnormalities of the pulmonic valve can be grouped as follows: typical valvar pulmonic stenosis (commissural PS), bicuspid pulmonary valve, quad ricuspid pulmonary valve, dysplastic pulmonary valve and pulmonary valve atresia. The typical form of pulmonic stenosis occurs with a normally formed tricuspid pulmonary valve. Thickening of the free edges of the valve and fusion of the commissures result in limitation of the systolic excursion of the leaflets (doming). The severity of reduction of the valvar area depends on the degree of thickening and fusion. Hypertrophy of the RV and poststenotic dilatation of the pulmonary trunk are commonly observed.

A dysplastic pulmonary valve is composed of three distinct but thickened and rigid leaflets with little or no commissural fusion. Such valves are usually stenotic, although a few have been reported to be regurgitant, with little or no stenosis. The pulmonary anulus is usually hypoplastic, with the hypoplasia extending into the most proximal pulmonary trunk. The cusps are filled with masses of embryonic connective tissue (abnormal spongiosa). Angiographically the valve is markedly thickened and limited in motion. Failure of reconstitution of the semilunar sinuses in diastole is noted. Poststenotic dilatation generally is lacking.
Other, Uncommon, Types of Isolated Congenital Pulmonic Stenosis. A bicuspid pulmonary valve may be found as an isolated anomaly, but is usually observed with tetralogy of Fallot. In tetralogy of Fallot with a bicuspid pulmonary valve the anulus and the main pulmonary artery tend to be hypoplastic. PS is usually mild in isolated bicuspid pulmonary valve, but in tetralogy of Fallot it tends to be severe. Angiographically a bicuspid pulmonary valve is reminiscent of an open clam shell or Pac Man (see Fig. 7–161).

Quadricuspid semilunar valves are highly unusual. The pulmonary valve is affected more often (93%) than the aortic valve and more commonly in males (65%). A quadricuspid pulmonic valve tends to function normally. If function is abnormal, then regurgitation is more common than stenosis. Association with other congenital heart defects is rare, but it has been reported in combination with atrial septal defect (ASD) (primum and secundum), VSD, and PDA. Endocarditis occurs infrequently. A quadricuspid aortic valve, on the other hand, is less common, has equal sex distribution and functions abnormally (insufficiency is more common than stenosis). In the cases reported, insuffi-

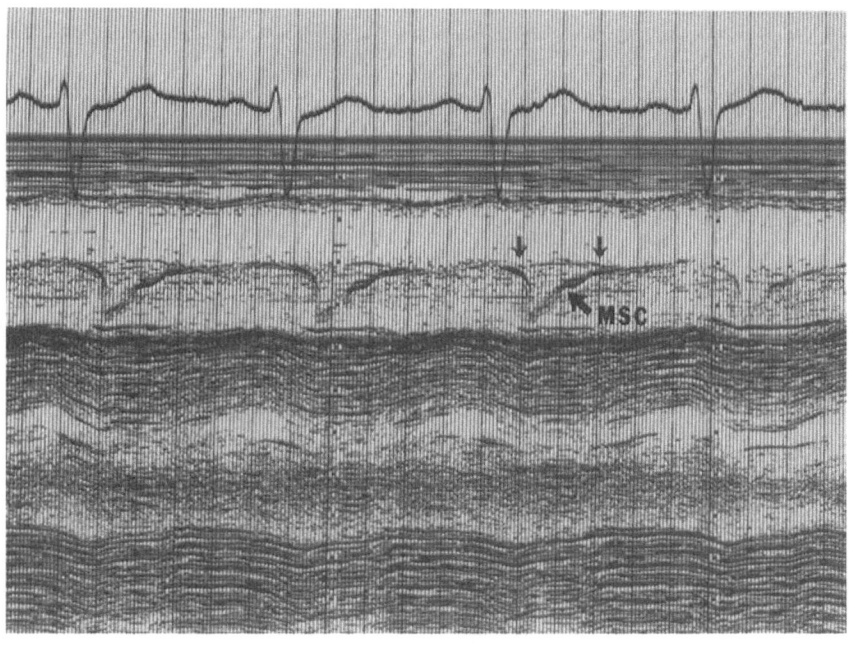

A

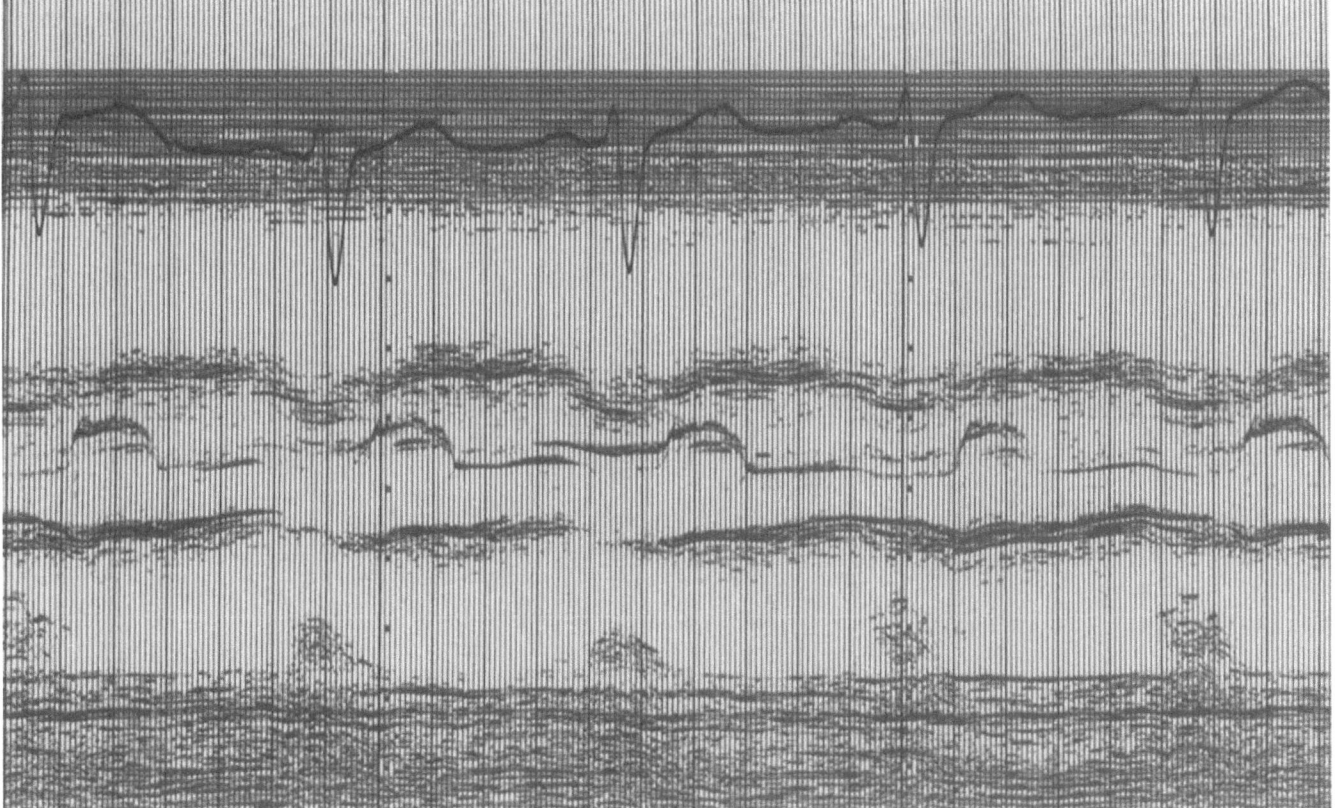

B

Fig. 7–134. *M-mode echocardiogram in a 6-year-old boy with primary pulmonary hypertension.* **A** pulmonic valve; **B** aortic valve; **C** right and left ventricle with mitral valve and tricuspid valve: **D** tricuspid valve. The time lines are 10 msec apart. In **A** the opening and closing motion of the pulmonary valve is indicated by *small arrows.* The tracing shows signs of severe pulmonary hypertension (e.g., flat diastolic slope, absence of "atrial kick," long right ventricular pre-ejection period [120 msec], short right ventricular ejection time [180 msec] and a notch indicating mid-systolic closure [*MSC*] of the pulmonary valve). The aortic valve tracing (**B**) shows an abnormally long pre-ejection period (110 msec) and a short left ventricular ejection time (170 msec), indi-cating elevation of the systemic vascular resistance or left ven-tricular failure. In **C** the left ventricle contracts poorly, but has a normal diameter while the right ventricle (*RV*) is markedly dilated. The ventricular septum moves abnormally (paradoxically) during ventricular systole. Part of the tricuspid valve (*TV*) is within the RV anterior to the septum. The E-to-F slope of the mitral valve is reduced; however, the valve is not thickened, and the posterior leaflet moves posteriorly during ventricular systole. *MV* = mitral valve. In **D** the tricuspid valve (*TV*) is displaced toward the left (medially) because of the enlargement of the right atrium and right ventricle. It is therefore imaged more easily than usual.

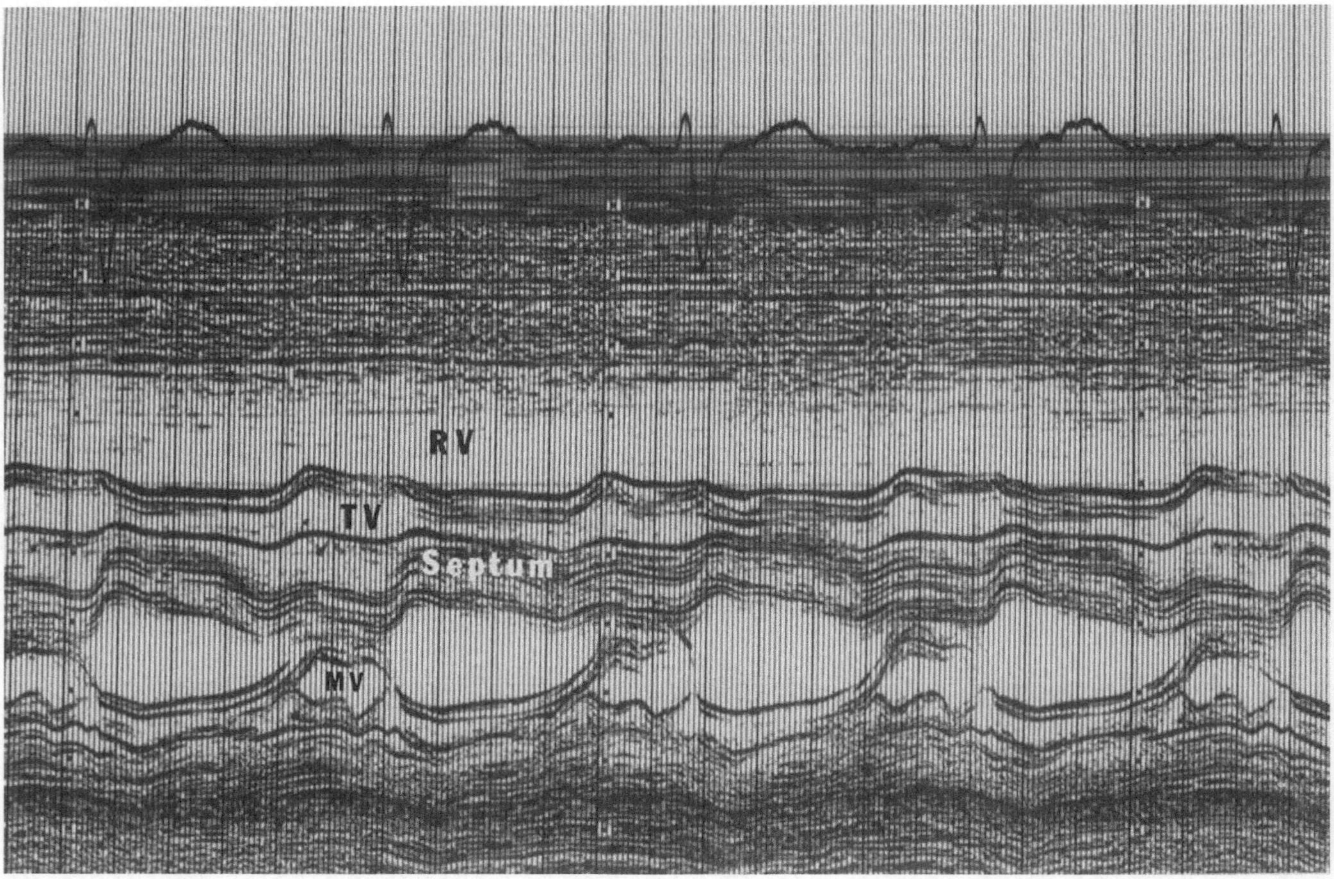

C

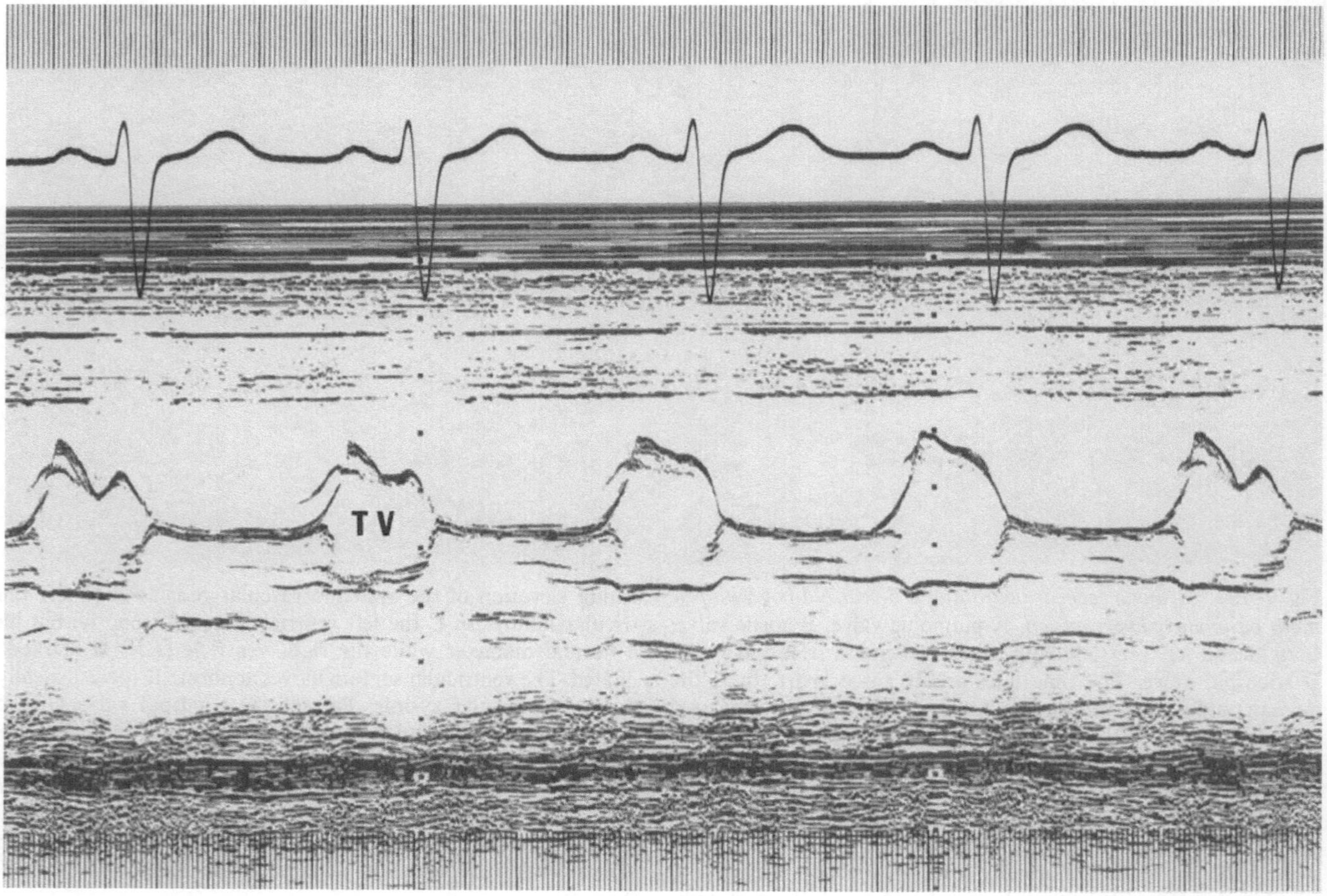

D

Fig. 7–135. *Roentgenogram of the chest in a 6-year-old boy with primary pulmonary hypertension and clinical signs of right heart failure.* The heart is enlarged. The retrosternal clear space is obliterated by the dilated right ventricle and right atrium. On the frontal view **(A)** the pulmonary trunk and the right main pulmonary artery are dilated. The right pulmonary artery is rounded, simulating hilar adenopathy. The interlobar vessels taper abruptly (the pruned-tree appearance), resulting in a paucity of vessels to the lungs. **B** is a cone down view of the right hemithorax showing the dilated right pulmonary artery. On the lateral film **(C)** the dilated left pulmonary artery with abrupt tapering of the interlobar vessels is conclusive evidence for precapillary pulmonary hypertension.

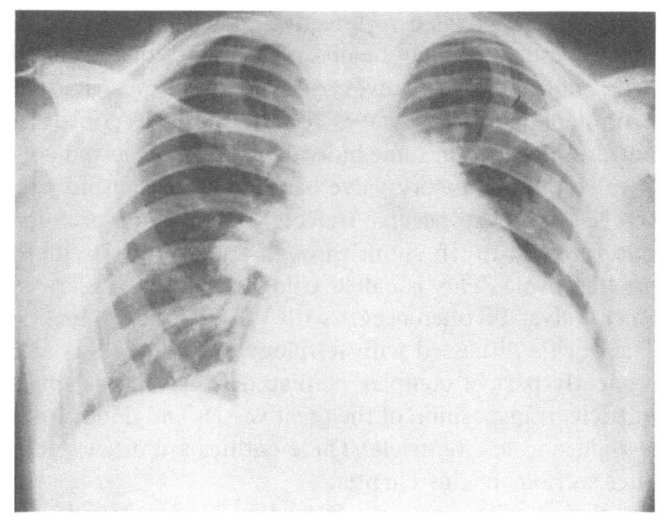

A

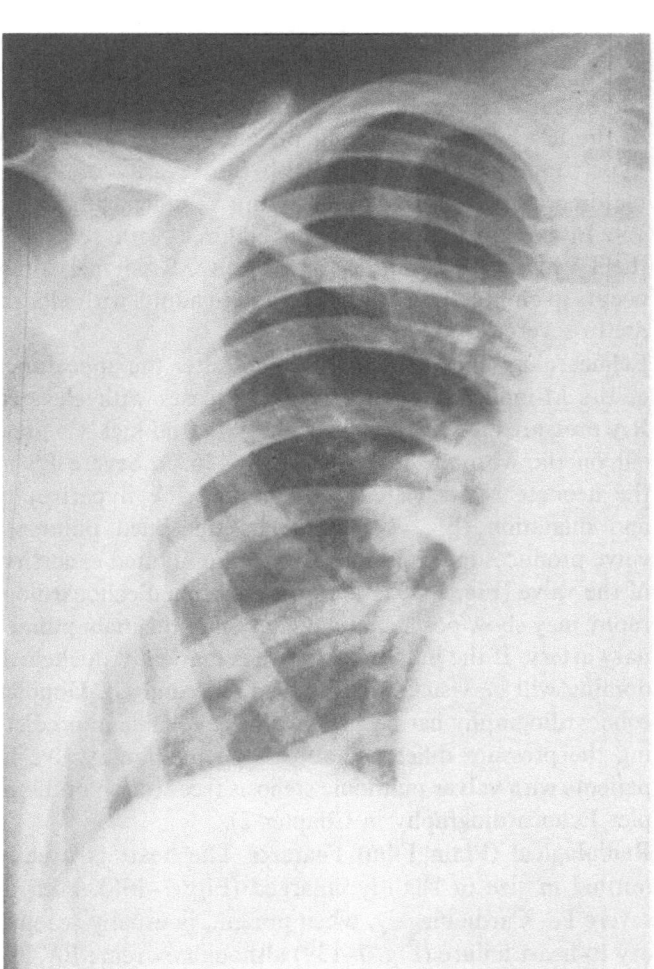

B

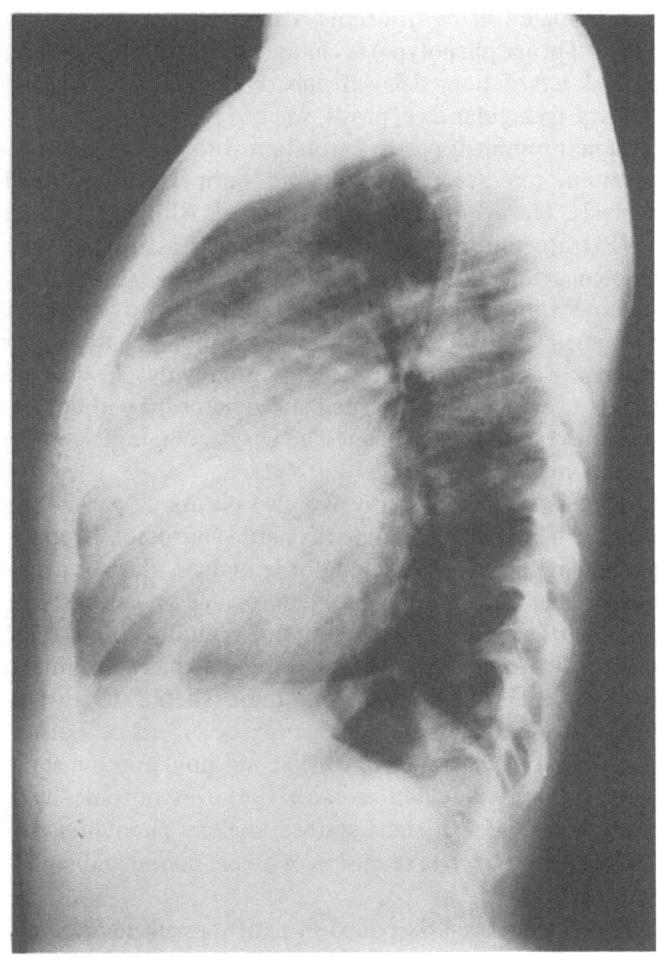

C

ciency was not related to infective endocarditis. Multiple small fenestrations may be observed in both quadricuspid aortic and pulmonary valves. Association of quadricuspid aortic and pulmonary valves has not been described; in contrast, however, in some individuals with a bicuspid aortic valve the pulmonary valve has also been bicuspid.

Associated Cardiovascular Defects Severe PS on occasion causes a right-to-left shunt through an ASD or stretched foramen ovale. This is called trilogy of Fallot (described later). Valvar PS often occurs with VSD. This combination of defects is discussed with tetralogy of Fallot. PS is also frequently part of complex cardiac defects such as single ventricle, transposition of the great vessels and double-outlet right and left ventricle. These entities are discussed in other sections of this chapter.

Association with Systemic Disorders Noonan syndrome (also called male Turner syndrome or pseudo-Turner syndrome, male Ullrich syndrome, Turner phenotype, and XX or XY Turner phenotype) is characterized by short stature, mental retardation, delayed puberty, hypertelorism, low-set ears, triangular face, ptosis, webbed neck, dental malocclusion, prominent pectus carinatum with distal pectus excavatum, undescended testes and normal chromosomal analysis. The syndrome may be familial. Although PS and a VSD are the most common anomalies associated with Noonan syndrome, other heart malformations (e.g., supravalvar PS, pulmonary branch stenosis, ASD, dysplasia of the aortic valve and hypertrophic cardiomyopathy) may be present. The pulmonary valve is usually dysplastic, consisting of thickened, shortened and rigid cusps without significant commissural fusion. The cusps contain prominent fibrous masses.

Dysplastic pulmonary valve also occurs as part of the multiple lentigines syndrome (leopard syndrome). Leopard is a mnemonic of Gorlin et al. for lentigines, electrocardiographic conduction disturbances, ocular hypertelorism, pulmonary stenosis, abnormalities of genitalia, retardation of growth and deafness (sensorineural). It has a dominant mode of inheritance. This syndrome should be distinguished from a similar clinical entity described by Forney et al. (Forney syndrome), in which congenital mitral insufficiency is present. Children with Forney syndrome have conductive deafness, short stature, skeletal anomalies (fusion of cervical vertebrae, fusion of carpal bones) and multiple "freckles."

PS has also been described in patients with neurofibromatosis, Laurence-Moon-Biedl syndrome, trisomy 18 and trisomy 13–15. PS is rare in trisomy 21. Even though maternal rubella is frequently associated with patent ductus arteriosus and pulmonary branch stenosis, pulmonary valvar stenosis may also be present.

Carcinoid syndrome causes an acquired form of tricuspid and pulmonary valve deformity, resulting in tricuspid insufficiency and pulmonic stenosis. Holt et al. described a typical hourglass appearance of the pulmonary valve in the carcinoid syndrome.

Clinical Features Children with PS are generally asymptomatic. A few children and adults with severe PS have fatigue on exertion. Cyanosis with severe (critical) PS is caused by shunting through a patent foramen ovale or ASD (trilogy of Fallot). Infants with critical PS may show signs of heart failure.

On physical examination in individuals with mild PS the findings are an early systolic ejection click at the second left intercostal space and a systolic ejection murmur in the same location. With moderate to severe stenosis a RV heave is present, and a thrill palpated at the left upper sternal border may extend up into the suprasternal notch. On auscultation, with moderate to severe PS, the systolic ejection click occurs earlier than with mild PS, and the murmur is louder and longer, on occasion continuing beyond the aortic component of the second sound. With severe PS the pulmonary second sound (P_2) is delayed and may be faint or inaudible. In adults with RV decompensation a fourth sound may be heard. On electrocardiography the extent of the right axis deviation and the magnitude of the R wave over the right precordium (V_3R, V_1) (RV hypertrophy) correlate well with the severity of PS. In children, upright T waves in V_3R and V_1 indicate moderate PS. In normal children and in children with severe PS the T waves in V_3R and V_1 are negative. RA hypertrophy occurs in children with severe PS and in adults with moderate to severe PS.

Echocardiography Mild PS does not alter the appearance of the M-mode echogram. In severe cases with elevated RA pressure an increased pulmonary "atrial kick" is present on the M-mode tracing (Fig. 7–136A). Severe PS in the neonate is associated with marked RV hypertrophy and dilatation (Fig. 7–137A). The thickened pulmonic valve produces multiple echoes, showing limited excursion of the valve (Fig. 7–137B). Two-dimensional echocardiography may show poststenotic dilatation of the main pulmonary artery. If the pulmonary valve is markedly thickened, doming will be visualized (Fig. 7–136 B and C). Doppler echocardiography has been shown to be reliable in predicting the pressure difference across the pulmonic valve in patients with valvar pulmonic stenosis (see section on Doppler Echocardiography in Chapter 2).

Radiological (Plain Film) Features The heart is usually normal in size or slightly enlarged (Fig. 7–138), even in severe PS. Cardiomegaly, when present, is usually secondary to heart failure (Fig. 7–139) although extreme RV hypertrophy may be a factor (Fig. 7–140).

The pulmonary vascularity is normal or decreased, nevertheless, the pulmonary blood flow measured at catheterization is normal except in severe cases of PS.

Poststenotic dilatation of the pulmonary trunk and left pulmonary artery is often observed on plain roentgenograms (Fig. 7–138). In addition, the left lung is preferentially perfused, rather than the right as with normal persons (Fig. 7–138). The inequality in the pulmonary vasculature between the two lungs is confirmed by radionuclide lung

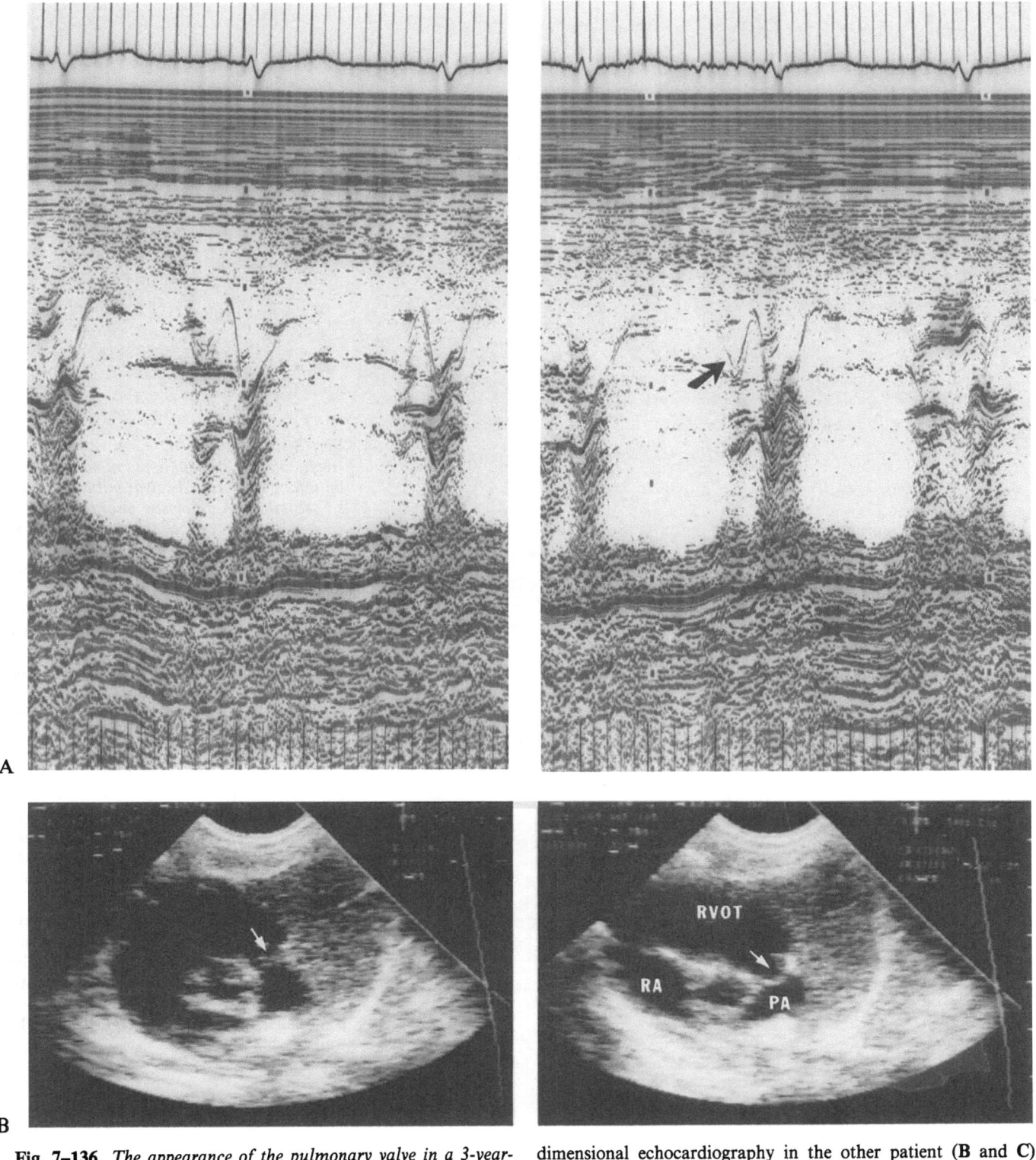

Fig. 7–136. *The appearance of the pulmonary valve in a 3-year-old boy with severe valvar pulmonic stenosis due to typical (commissural) valvar pulmonic stenosis.* A M-mode; B and C two-dimensional echocardiograms in a one month old infant with valvar pulmonic stenosis. On the M-mode (A) a prominent atrial kick (*arrow*) precedes the opening of the pulmonic valve. On two-dimensional echocardiography in the other patient (B and C) the parasternal short axis view at the level of the great vessels during diastole (B) shows the thickened pulmonic valve (*arrow*) extending straight across the anulus. During systole (C) doming of the pulmonic valve occurs (*arrow*), the valve becoming convex toward the pulmonary artery. *RVOT* = right ventricular outflow tract; *RA* = right atrium; *PA* = pulmonary artery.

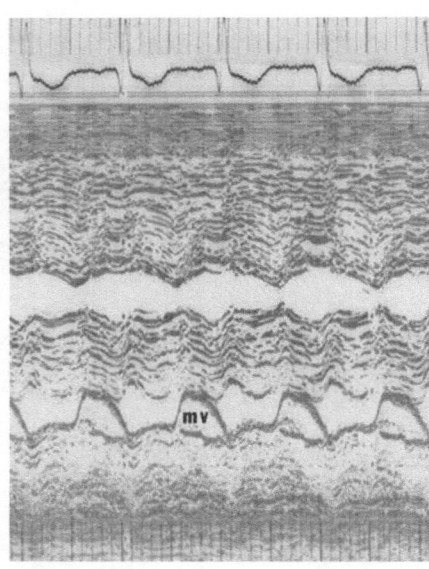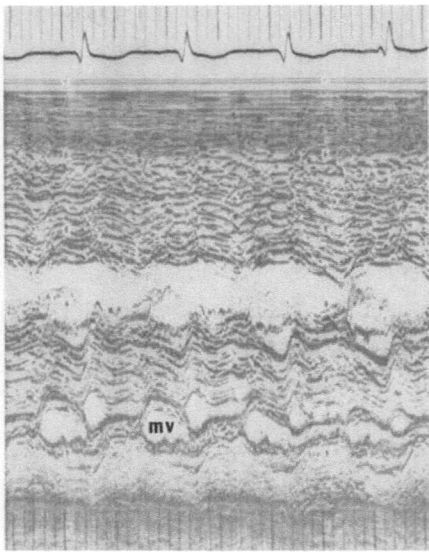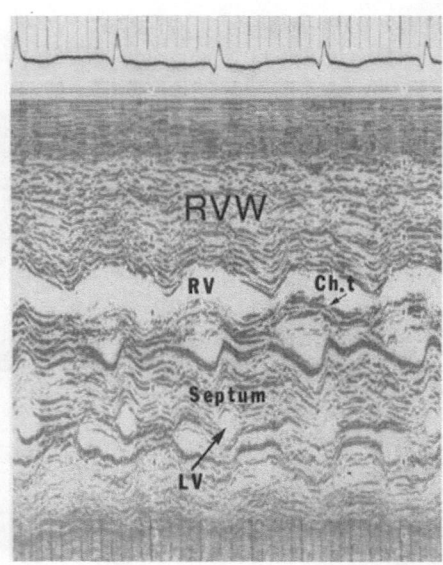

A

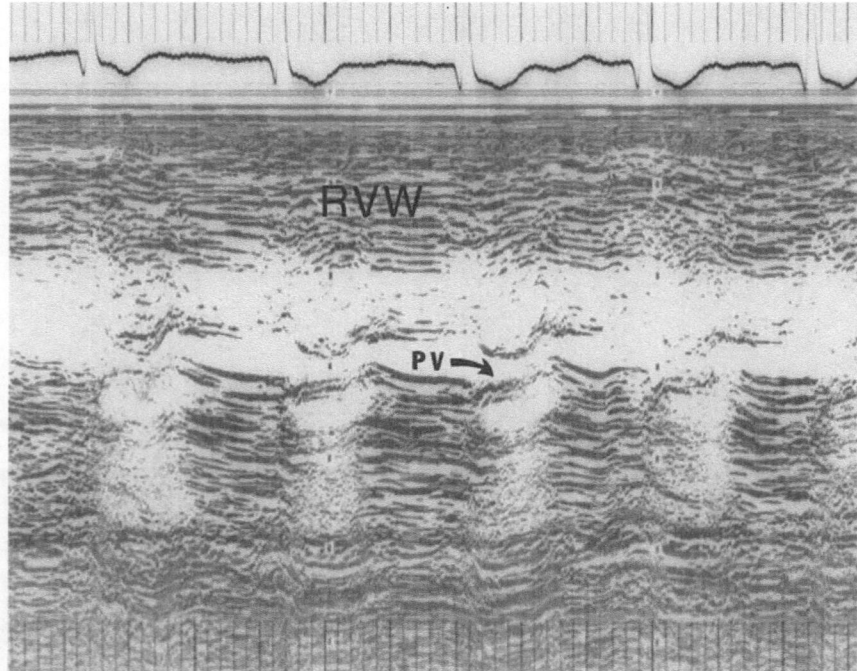

B

Fig. 7–137. *Marked right ventricular hypertrophy and an immobile pulmonary valve in an infant with critical valvar pulmonic stenosis secondary to dysplastic pulmonary valve.*

A is a composite of three sections of an M-mode echocardiogram. The transducer was angled through an arc from the level of the mitral valve (*mv*) to the level of the cavity of the left ventricle (*LV*). The free wall of the right ventricle (*RVW*) and the ventricular septum are massively thickened. The right ventricular cavity (*RV*) is of normal diameter, and the chordae tendineae of the tricuspid valve (*Ch.t*) are imaged within it. The diameter of the left ventricular cavity is very small, however, this finding may be partly due to the position of the transducer. On angiography the left ventricle was normal in size, but was markedly retrodisplaced. The left ventricular free wall is thickened, and the E-to-F slope of the mitral valve is decreased, both suggesting abnormal function of the left ventricle.

B is an M-mode echocardiogram through the pulmonary valve (*PV*). The valve vibrates during ventricular systole, but its excursion is very limited. The atrial kick is not accentuated in this patient, even though pulmonic stenosis is severe. *RVW* = right ventricular wall.

Fig. 7–138. *Poststenotic dilatation of the pulmonary trunk and preferential flow to the left lung in a 13-year-old boy with moderate valvar pulmonic stenosis.* The vessels of the left lung, and especially those of the left upper lobe, are dilated in comparison to those on the right. Although preferential flow to the left lung may on occasion be observed in normal individuals, it is a sign of valvar pulmonic stenosis. The size of the heart is normal on the frontal view (**A**) but the lateral film (**B**) shows obliteration of the retrosternal clear space by the dilated right ventricular outflow tract and main pulmonary trunk. Although poststenotic dilatation of the pulmonary trunk is characteristic of valvar pulmonic stenosis, it may be absent in some patients with pulmonic stenosis. If dilatation is present, its extent does not correlate with the severity of the stenosis.

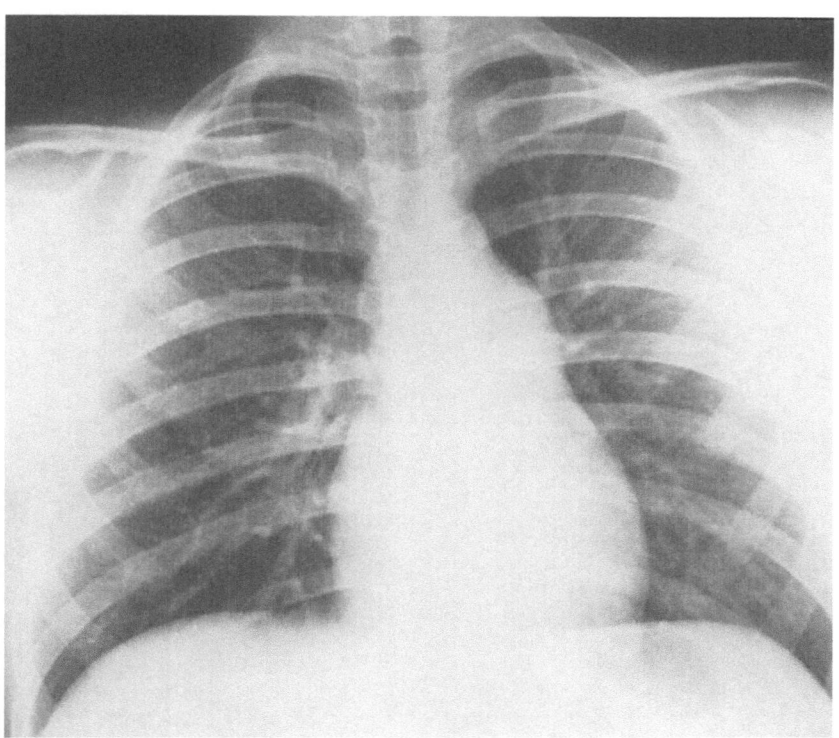

A

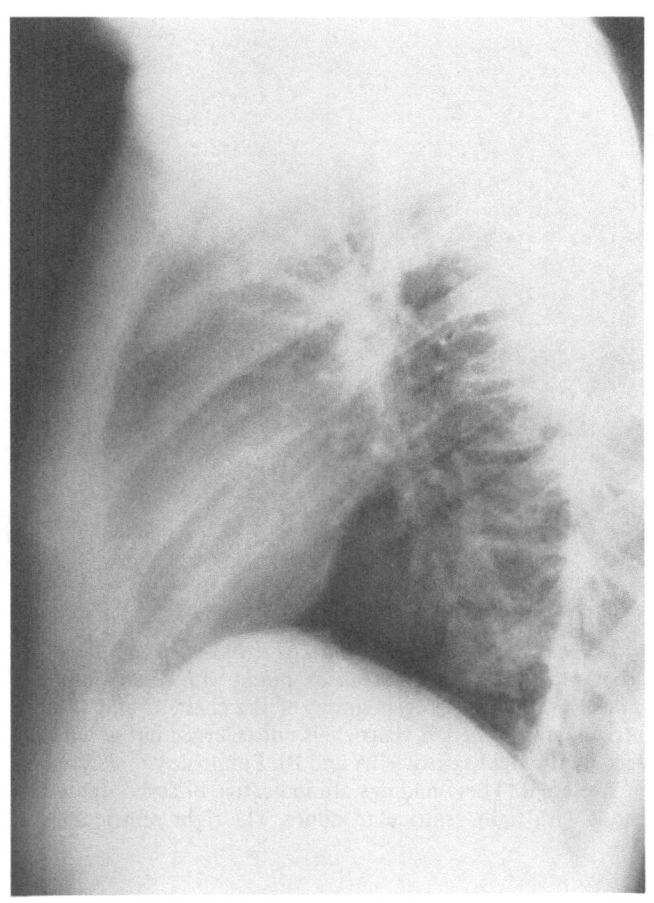

B

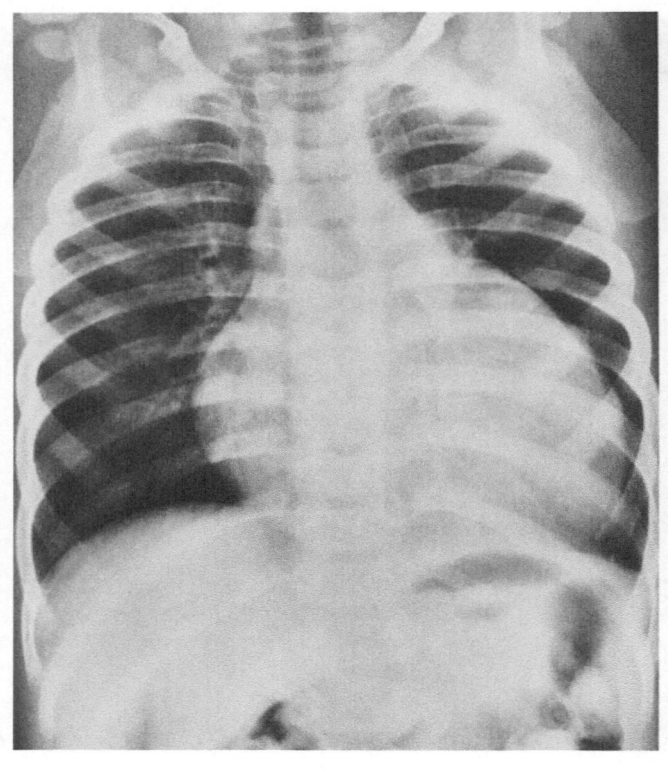

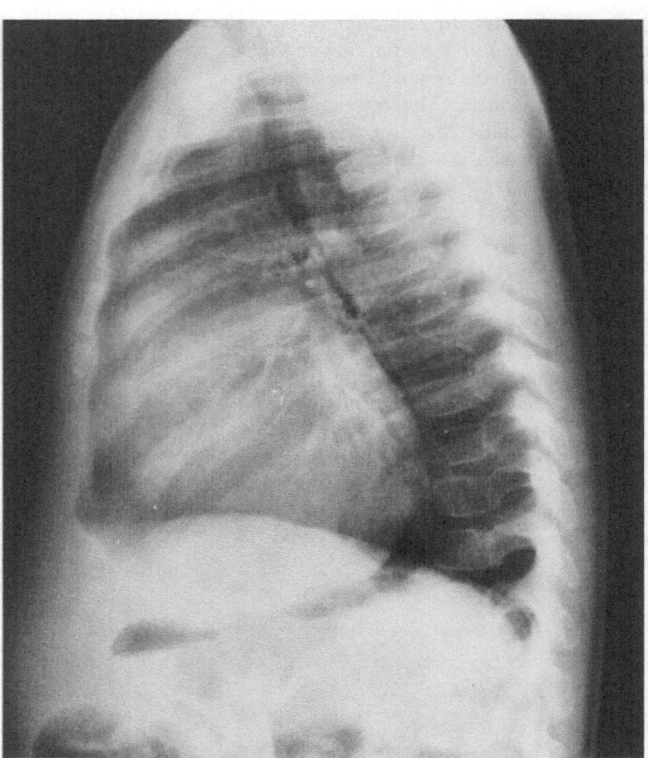

A

B

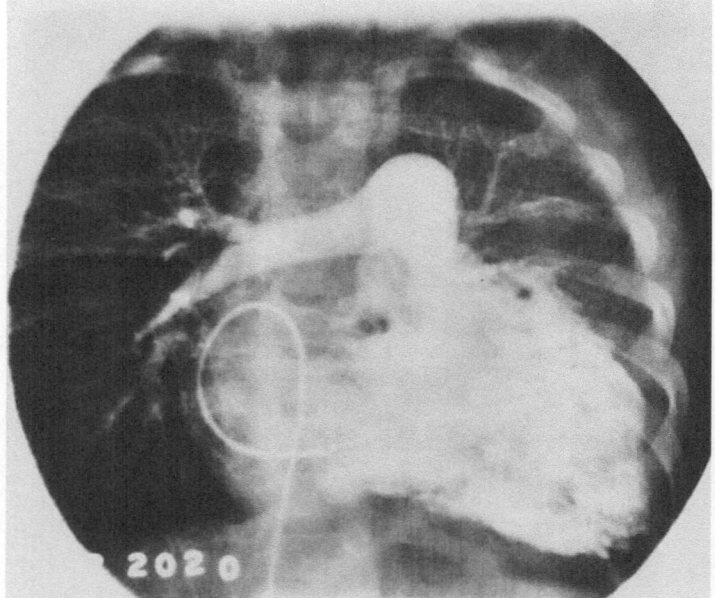

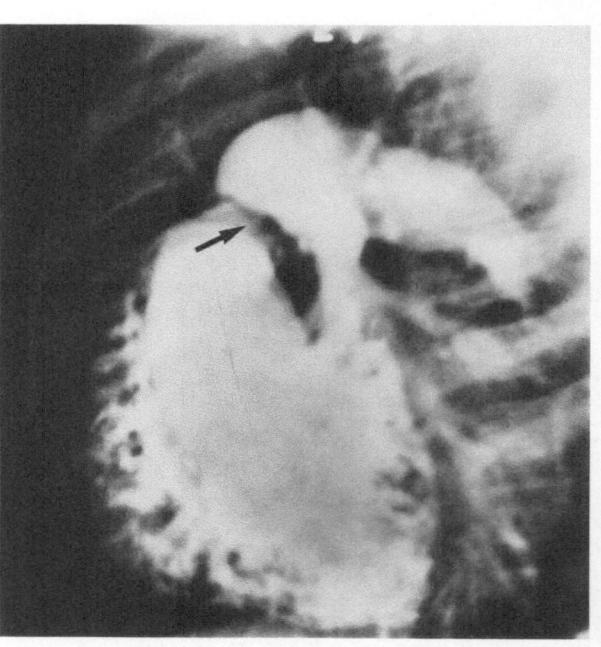

C

D

Fig. 7–139. *Cardiomegaly with marked right ventricular and moderate right atrial enlargement in an infant with severe pulmonic stenosis.* **A** and **B** Roentgenograms of the chest; **C** and **D** right ventriculogram. The left ventricle is not enlarged but is retrodisplaced by the right ventricle (**A** and **B**). Pulmonary undercirculation is present. These findings are indicative of severe pulmonic stenosis with right ventricular failure. The right ventriculogram in the frontal (**C**) and lateral (**D**) projections confirms marked dilatation of the right ventricle, along with a thickened immobile pulmonary valve (*arrow*). The size of the right ventricle changed very little from diastole to systole, indicating right ventricular dysfunction. The dilated right ventricle forms the left heart border giving it a convex appearance.

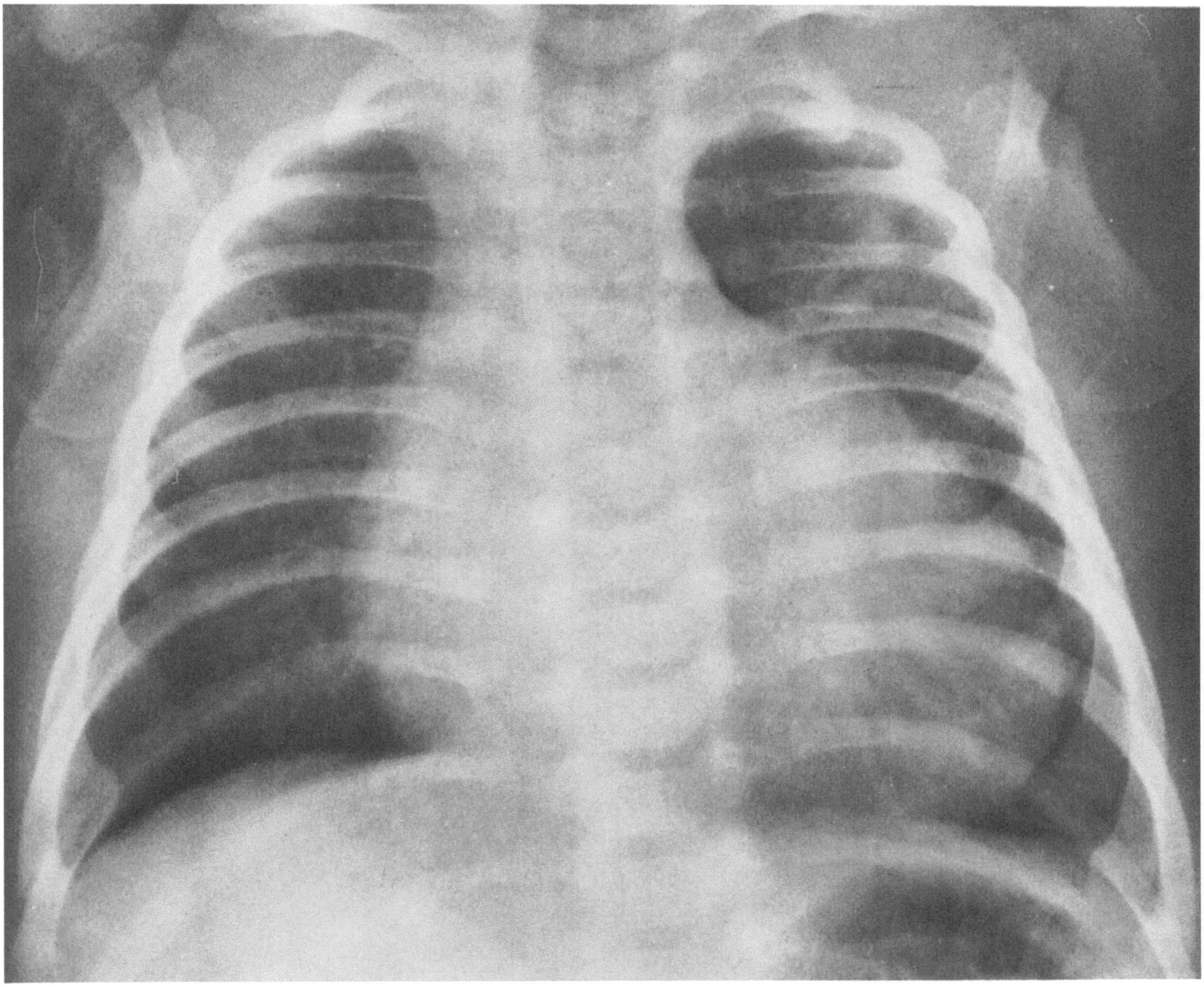

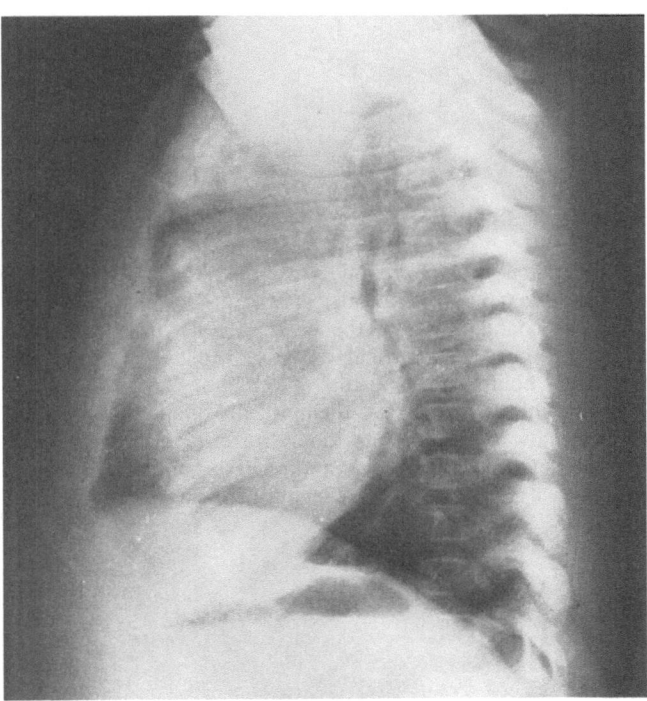

A

B

Fig. 7–140. *Marked cardiomegaly and pulmonary undercirculation in a 5-month-old boy with critical pulmonic stenosis due to a dysplastic pulmonary valve.* **A** and **B** Frontal and lateral chest films; **C** to **F** frames from the right ventriculogram. Generalized cardiomegaly is secondary to extreme right ventricular hypertrophy. The cardiac apex is rounded and uplifted.

On the lateral film, retrodisplacement of the left ventricle and left atrium by the hypertrophied right ventricle might be mistaken for left atrial and left ventricular enlargement. The normal size of the left atrium on the frontal film and the absence of pulmonary venous hypertension aid in differentiating these findings from those of left ventricular enlargement. Obliteration of the retrosternal clear space also suggests that the right ventricle and not the left ventricle is responsible for the cardiomegaly. The features on the plain films in other infants with critical valvar pulmonic stenosis may be impossible to distinguish from left ventricular enlargement. (*Continued*)

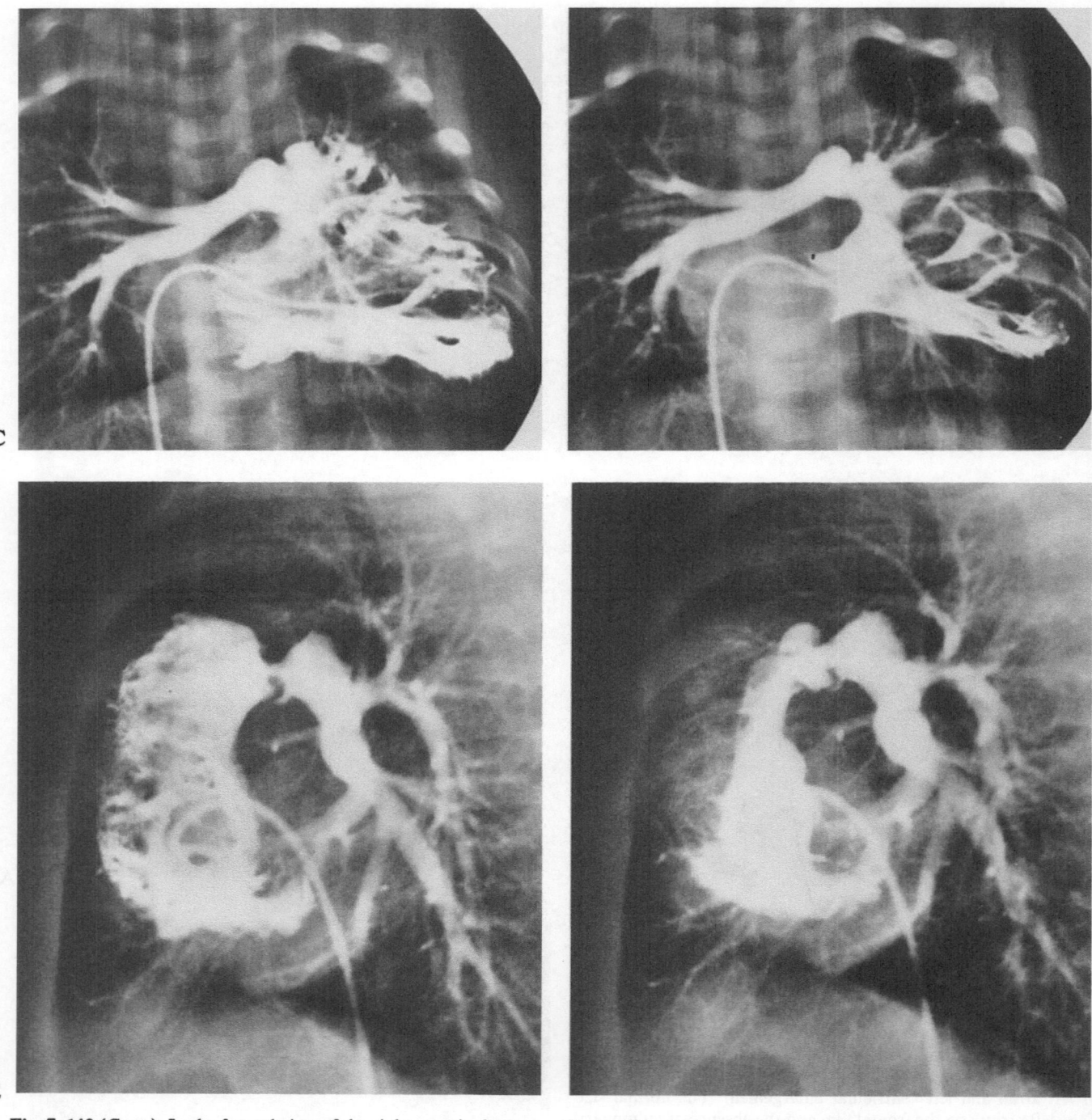

C

D

E

F

Fig. 7–140 (*Cont.*) In the frontal view of the right ventriculogram during diastole (C) the right ventricle is border forming, accounting for the configuration of the heart. Massive trabeculations impinge on the right ventricular cavity, which during systole (D) is nearly obliterated, with the trabeculations becoming more prominent. On the lateral view the markedly dilatated right ventricular outflow tract obliterates the retrosternal clear space (E). Hyperkinetic contractions and marked trabeculations are also noted in this view. Marked thickening of the right ventricular free wall and the enlarged papillary muscles are noted during systole (F). The left ventricle is displaced posteriorly. The leaflets of the pulmonic valve are replaced by small nubbins of tissue that do not move. The sinuses of Valsalva are outlined during ventricular systole. The pulmonary anulus is small. Poststenotic dilatation of the main pulmonary trunk is not identified. The appearance of the pulmonic valve and absence of poststenotic dilatation are characteristic of a dysplastic pulmonary valve.

imaging and by pulmonary angiography. In extreme examples, normal perfusion of the right lung accompanies hyperperfusion (overcirculation) of the left lung. Calcification of the pulmonary valve is rare. A sustained rise in the RV systolic pressure secondary to severe PS, previous pulmonary valvotomy and bacterial endocarditis have been mentioned as possible predisposing factors for calcium deposition in the pulmonary valve.

Hemodynamics In pulmonic stenosis with intact ventricular septum the RV pressure is increased. Mean pressure and pulse pressure in the main pulmonary arteries and branches are low. Withdrawal of a catheter from the main pulmonary artery across the pulmonic valve reveals a sharp rise in the pressure as the catheter tip is drawn into the RV (Fig. 7–141). In mild to moderate PS, normal cardiac output is maintained. In severe cases, decreased cardiac output with increased tissue oxygen extraction occurs. (Clinically the low venous O_2 saturation causes peripheral cyanosis.) With cardiac decompensation or tricuspid insufficiency, elevated RA pressure sometimes results in a right-to-left shunt across the foramen ovale and systemic desaturation. Clinically this is manifested as central cyanosis.

Contrast Studies Right ventriculography demonstrates doming and thickening of the pulmonary valve during systole (Fig. 7–142A, B and C). Reconstitution (visualization) of the semilunar sinuses during diastole usually indicates commissural PS. Absence of motion of the leaflets during systole and failure to see the pulmonic sinuses of Valsalva in diastole suggests unicuspid PS or dysplastic pulmonary valve.

Presence, degree and type of infundibular PS must be determined. Two types of infundibular stenosis may be distinguished—dynamic and fixed. In dynamic infundibular stenosis (Fig. 7–143) the crista supraventricularis is hypertrophied. The outflow tract of the RV (infundibulum) opens during diastole and constricts during systole. This usually resolves after valvotomy; however, infundibulectomy may be required in severe cases at the time of valvotomy. Fixed infundibular stenosis is characterized by diffuse narrowing of the infundibulum with virtually no change during systole and diastole. The narrowing is due to severe muscle hypertrophy and scarring. Infundibular resection, outflow patch or both will be necessary for relief of obstruction caused by fixed infundibular stenosis.

Hypertrophy of the RV correlates with the severity of the PS. Underdevelopment of the RV and hypoplasia of the tricuspid valve have been described in association with critical PS during infancy.

Treatment The long-term prognosis of mild valvar PS is good, although prophylaxis against infective endocarditis is recommended (i.e., antibiotics prior to dental or surgical procedures). The severity of the stenosis generally remains unchanged over time, although progression has been reported in a few cases. Relief of stenosis is recommended if the pressure difference across the valve is greater than 70 mm of Hg (moderate to severe PS) with a normal cardiac output. Surgery is urgent in infants with critical PS and heart failure.

Repair consists of incision of the valve along the commissures, if commissures can be identified. If no commissures are delineated the valve is divided into three sections. The incisions are carried to the base of the leaflet. The resultant regurgitation of the pulmonic valve seems to be tolerated well. After repair of severe PS the infundibulum may contract in such a way as to obstruct the RV outflow tract (dynamic infundibular stenosis), sometimes resulting in a mild to moderate pressure difference between the RV and the pulmonary outflow tract. If cardiac output is maintained after discontinuation of cardiac bypass this narrowing may be left alone as it regresses spontaneously in time. If the gradient is severe, infundibular resection or an outflow patch may be necessary.

Stenosis due to dysplastic pulmonary valve is relieved by excising the nubbins of tissue that represent the valvar leaflets. If the anulus is small an outflow patch is necessary to assure adequate relief of the stenosis.

Recently balloon valvuloplasty has been successful in relieving PS (Fig. 7–142D and E). This technique has been used in adults and children with typical valvar pulmonic stenosis (commisural fusion). It would not be expected to succeed in patients with dysplastic pulmonary valve.

Idiopathic Dilatation of the Pulmonary Artery

Idiopathic dilatation of the pulmonary artery is a benign congenital malformation that does not affect cardiac function in any appreciable degree. The etiology is unknown in most cases. Espino-Vela found cystic medial necrosis in some patients, suggesting a forme fruste of Marfan syndrome. Affected individuals are asymptomatic.

A pulmonic systolic murmur is usually present, while an ejection click is sometimes heard. The electrocardiogram is normal. The plain chest roentgenogram reveals various degrees of dilatation of the pulmonary artery in the presence of a normal-sized heart. At catheterization, pressures and oxygen saturations are found to be normal. A small pressure gradient across the pulmonic valve may be encountered in the presence of normal RV pressure. It is believed by some observers that this pressure gradient may be due to deceleration of blood flow in the dilated pulmonary artery, rather than to true obstruction of the pulmonary valve. Angiocardiography shows dilatation of the pulmonary trunk without evidence of associated heart defects.

The appearance of the dilated main pulmonary artery on chest films may be mistaken for a hilar mass or for poststenotic dilatation occurring with valvar pulmonic stenosis. Clinical correlation will assist in differentiation. Dilatation of the main pulmonary artery also occurs with Marfan syndrome, Larsen syndrome and Ehlers-Danlos syndrome. One report (Teitelbaum and Altman) describes dilatation of the interlobar pulmonary branches reminiscent of an arteriovenous fistula on chest roentgenograms.

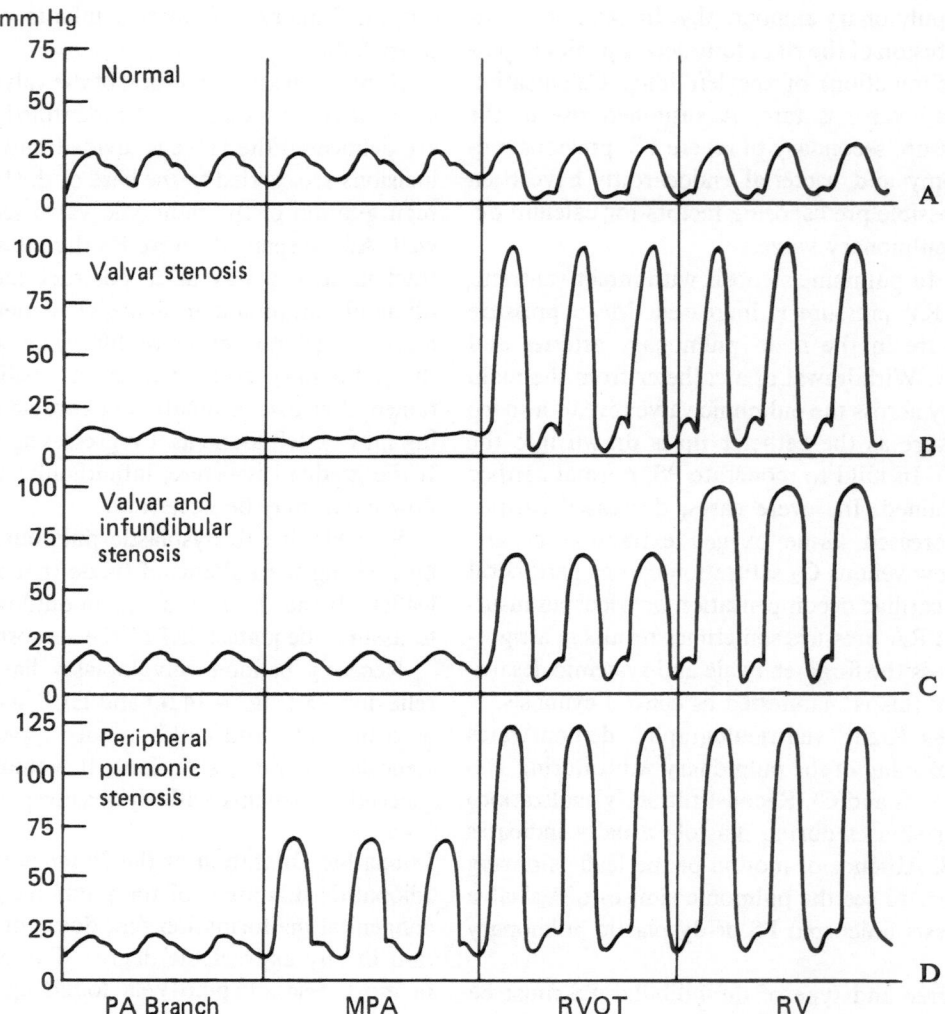

Fig. 7–141. *Comparison of pressure tracings in various types of pulmonic stenosis.* These tracings are recorded as an end-hole catheter is withdrawn from the pulmonary artery to the right ventricle. **A** is a normal curve. The pulmonary artery pressure is recognized by a dicrotic notch and by a descending pressure curve during diastole. In contrast, the pressure in the right ventricle rises during diastole and an "atrial kick" occurs just before the onset of systole. **B** represents a tracing during withdrawal in a patient with valvar pulmonic stenosis. The pressure in the pulmonary artery is damped. The decrease in pressure just above the pulmonary valve is caused by a Venturi effect. The pressure tracing from the right ventricle has a large atrial kick and elevated systolic pressure with a sharp angulation at its peak. **C** shows a characteristic tracing occurring with a combination of valvar and infundibular stenosis. A tracing similar to this can be obtained in patients with tetralogy of Fallot who have this combination of lesions. The pulmonary artery tracing is damped, but the descent of the pressure during diastole is recognized. As the catheter is withdrawn to the infundibular chamber the systolic pressure is higher and the pressure rises during diastole. This part of the tracing is therefore recognized as a ventricular tracing (the infundibular or "third" chamber). The body of the right ventricle

has a higher pressure. Note that the top of this pressure curve is rounded rather than peaked, unlike valvar pulmonic stenosis.

In **D**, a tracing from a patient with valvar pulmonic stenosis and peripheral pulmonic stenosis, two areas of stenosis are present as well. The first pressure change occurs between a pulmonary branch and the main pulmonary artery. Both of the distal pressures descend during diastole and are therefore recognized as being from the pulmonary artery. The highest pressure, from the ventricle, is recognized as such because the tracing shows a rise in pressure during diastole.

Note that these are idealized drawings. If the holes at the tip of the catheter are spaced widely apart the withdrawal curve may simulate combined stenosis when only one stenotic lesion is present. Arrhythmias occur frequently during withdrawal, so that such tracings cannot always be used to determine the level or levels of stenosis. (Modified from Plauth WH, et al: In Hurst JW et al (eds); The Heart, 5th ed. New York, McGraw-Hill, 1982, p. 749.)

PA branch = a branch of the pulmonary artery; *MPA* = main pulmonary artery; *RVOT* = outflow tract of the right ventricle; *RV* = body of the right ventricle.

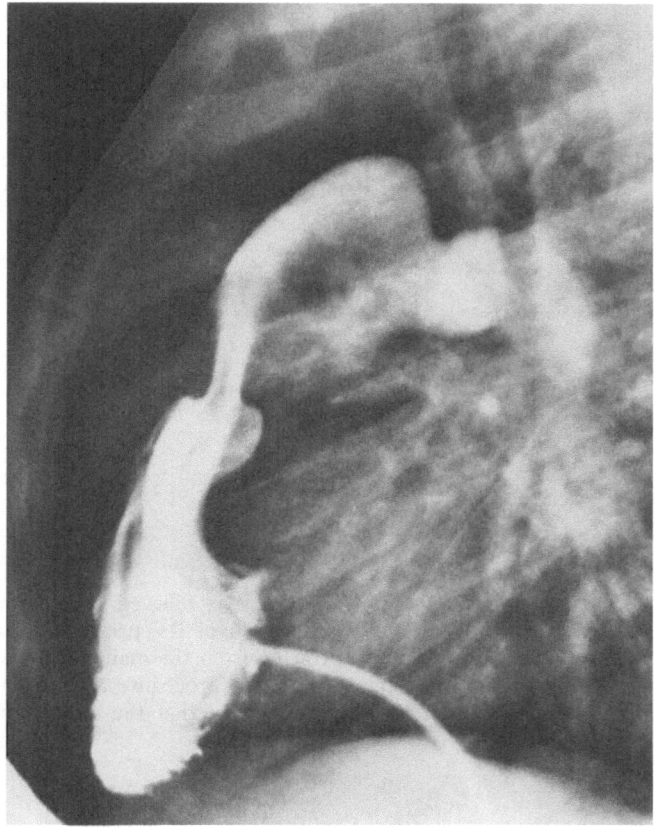

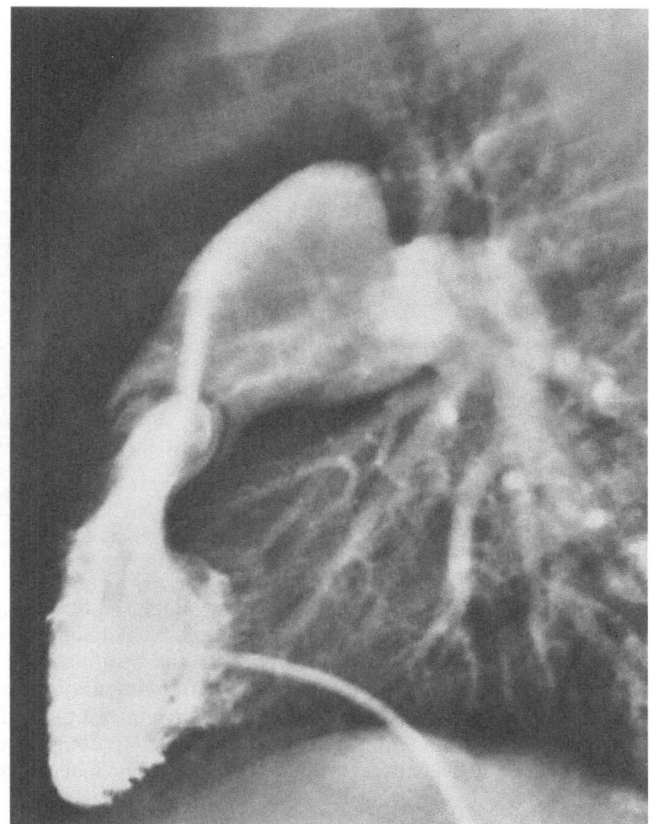

A

B

Fig. 7–142. *The appearance of the pulmonary valve in typical valvar pulmonary stenosis in a 1-year-old girl.* The right ventriculogram shows a distinct jet through the pulmonary valve during systole **(A).** Later during the injection **(B)** systolic doming of the pulmonary valve is demonstrated along with the jet. During diastole **(C)** the sinuses of Valsalva reconstitute as the pulmonary valve closes.

Marked poststenotic dilatation of the pulmonary trunk and left pulmonary artery is present on all three frames. The jet, systolic doming of the valve, reconstitution during diastole and poststenotic dilatation of the pulmonary trunk are characteristic angiographic features of typical valvar pulmonic stenosis (commissural fusion). *(Continued)*

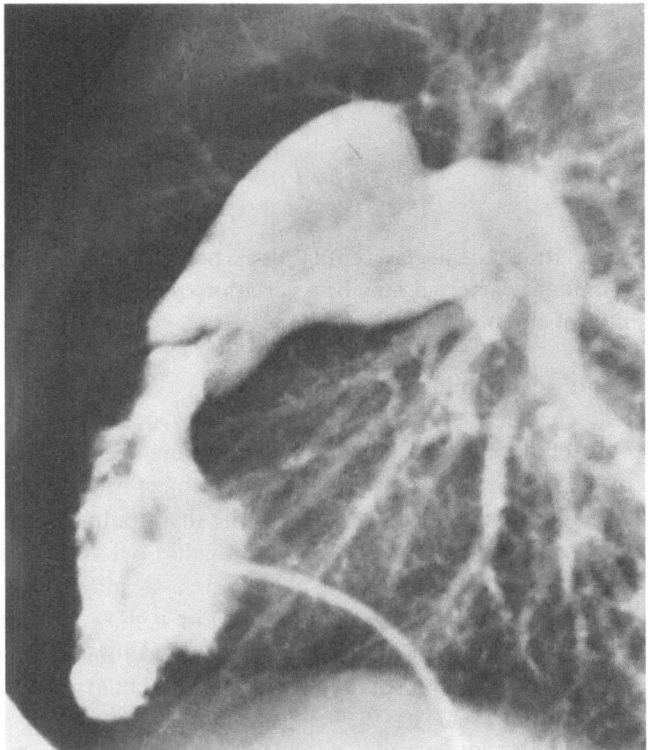

C

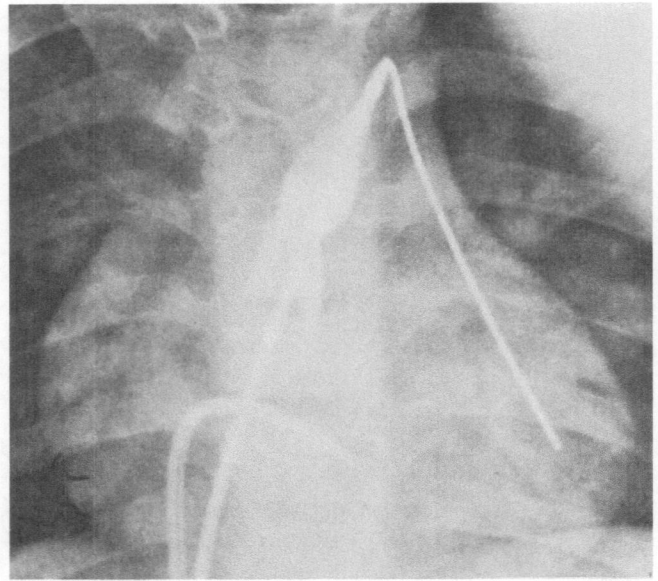

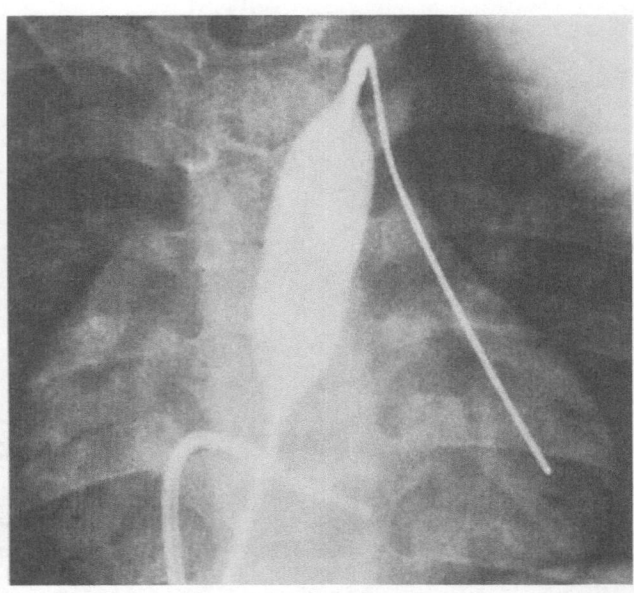

D

E

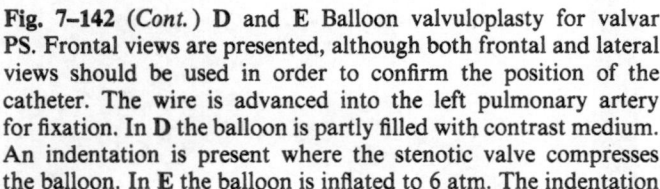

Fig. 7–142 (*Cont.*) **D** and **E** Balloon valvuloplasty for valvar PS. Frontal views are presented, although both frontal and lateral views should be used in order to confirm the position of the catheter. The wire is advanced into the left pulmonary artery for fixation. In **D** the balloon is partly filled with contrast medium. An indentation is present where the stenotic valve compresses the balloon. In **E** the balloon is inflated to 6 atm. The indentation disappears indicating that the stenosis is relieved. The second catheter in the RV is for measurement of RV pressure during the procedure. A withdrawal tracing from the main pulmonary artery to the RV is obtained after the procedure as well as a right ventriculogram in order to confirm that the stenosis has been relieved.

Even though this last entity does not involve the main pulmonary artery it may be a variation of idiopathic dilatation of the pulmonary artery.

Supravalvar Pulmonic Stenosis

The stenosis may affect the pulmonary artery above the valve and either or both of its main branches. Narrowing of the pulmonary arteries may involve one or more arteries. A single stenosis usually involves the main pulmonary artery or its proximal right or left branches, while multiple stenoses are usually peripheral. The stenosis may be a discrete area of narrowing (coarctation) or it may be diffuse (long segment or the entire artery, so called tubular hypoplasia). Poststenotic dilatation of the pulmonary arteries is usually present.

Peripheral pulmonic stenosis (PPS) is frequently encountered as part of the rubella embryopathy. Other heart defects commonly associated with congenital rubella are patent ductus arteriosus, pulmonic valve stenosis and atrial septal defect. Stenosis of other vessels may also be part of the rubella embryopathy (e.g., aorta, coronary, cerebral, mesenteric, renal arteries) together with cataracts, microphthalmia, deafness, thrombocytopenia, hepatitis and blood dyscrasias. In the absence of rubella infection, supravalvar PS or peripheral PS may be associated with ventricular and atrial septal defects, tetralogy of Fallot and supravalvular aortic stenosis (Williams syndrome).

Clinical Features A systolic murmur in an unusual location and distribution over the lung may suggest PPS. Rarely a continuous murmur may be present, simulating patent ductus arteriosus. The pulmonary second sound may be accentuated because of high pressure in the main pulmonary artery proximal to the stenosis. Electrocardiography shows RV hypertrophy in severe cases; however, the findings may be altered by the associated lesions. Other signs of fetal rubella infection should be sought in infants and children with PPS.

Echocardiography On 2-D echocardiography, stenosis of the main pulmonary artery is imaged in the long axis view, and branch PS is best demonstrated from the suprasternal notch or subxiphoid position. The pulmonary branches are perpendicular to the Doppler beam; and therefore prediction of the level of stenosis or the severity of stenosis in PPS is difficult by Doppler.

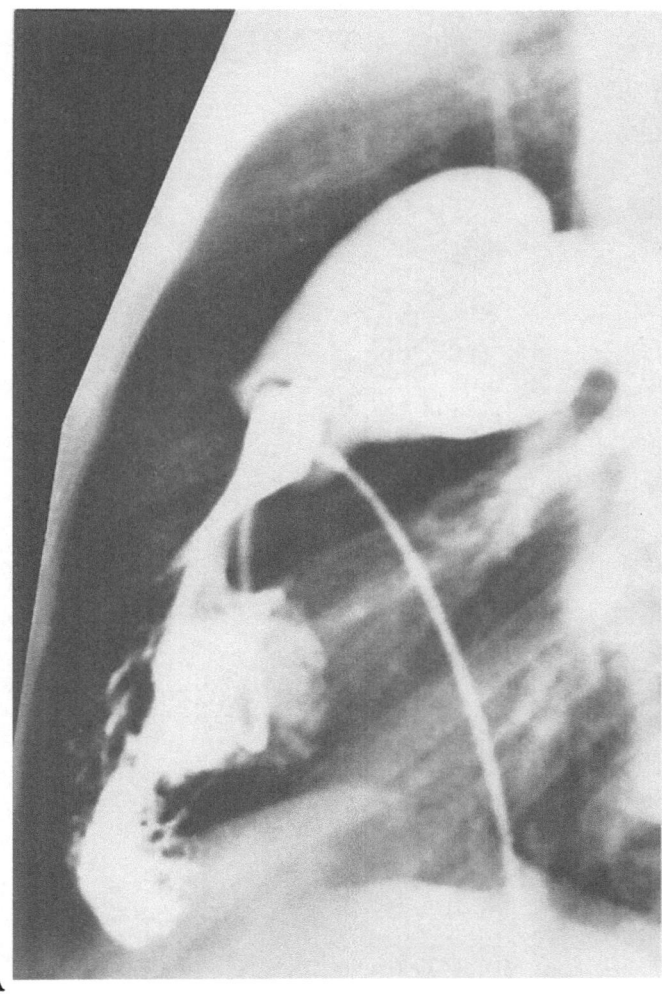

A

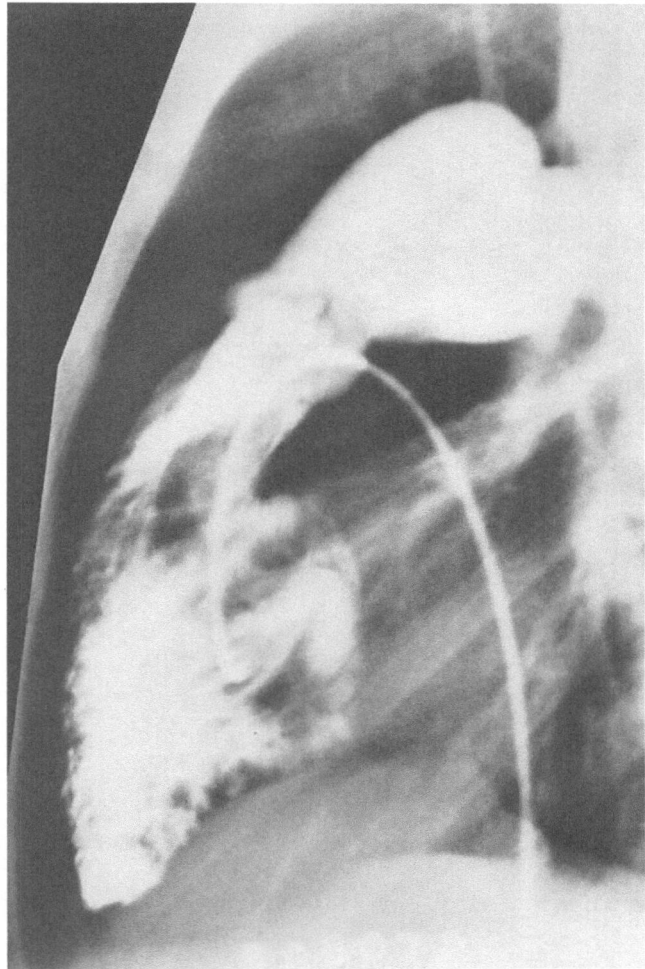

B

Fig. 7–143. *Dynamic infundibular pulmonic stenosis in severe valvar pulmonic stenosis.* The infundibulum constricts during systole **(A)** but distends during diastole **(B).** The right ventricle is hypertrophied. Systolic doming of the pulmonary valve and poststenotic dilatation of the pulmonary trunk are noted. Dynamic infundibular stenosis should be differentiated from fixed infundibular stenosis, which usually occurs in tetralogy of Fallot. In fixed stenosis the infundibulum remains narrow during diastole.

Radiological (Plain Film) Features The chest roentgenogram is usually not diagnostic for supravalvar PS. However, in patients with multiple peripheral branch stenoses and marked poststenotic dilatation a nodular or fusiform vascular pattern or "sausagization" of the pulmonary arteries may be observed (Fig. 7–144). In some cases, marked poststenotic dilatation of the pulmonary arteries has been mistaken for a pattern of pulmonary overcirculation or even a mass density. Severe unilateral pulmonary branch stenosis results in unilateral pulmonary undercirculation with contralateral overcirculation (see Fig. 1–15). The RV may be enlarged in moderate to severe cases.

Hemodynamics At catheterization the diagnosis of supravalvar PS may be suggested by an abrupt increase in pressure during withdrawal of the catheter from a peripheral pulmonary artery to the main pulmonary artery (Fig. 7–141). Hypertension proximal to the stenosis is present, except in patients with associated valvar PS. If the stenoses are beyond the reach of the catheter or if the catheter fails to pass an area of stenosis the diagnosis of primary pulmonary hypertension may be entertained erroneously. **Contrast Studies** Selective injections in the RV or pulmonary artery are diagnostic (Figs. 7–144 to 7–146). The type, number and location of the stenoses can be assessed accurately. Special angulated views may be required. An aortogram should be obtained in patients with peripheral PS to exclude PDA and supravalvular aortic stenosis.

Treatment An isolated coarctation of the main pulmonary artery might be patched if the stenosis is severe. Discrete narrowing of the branches might also benefit from a reconstructive procedure. Diffuse or multiple stenoses do not lend themselves to repair. Balloon angioplasty has been recommended even though it may not always be successful.

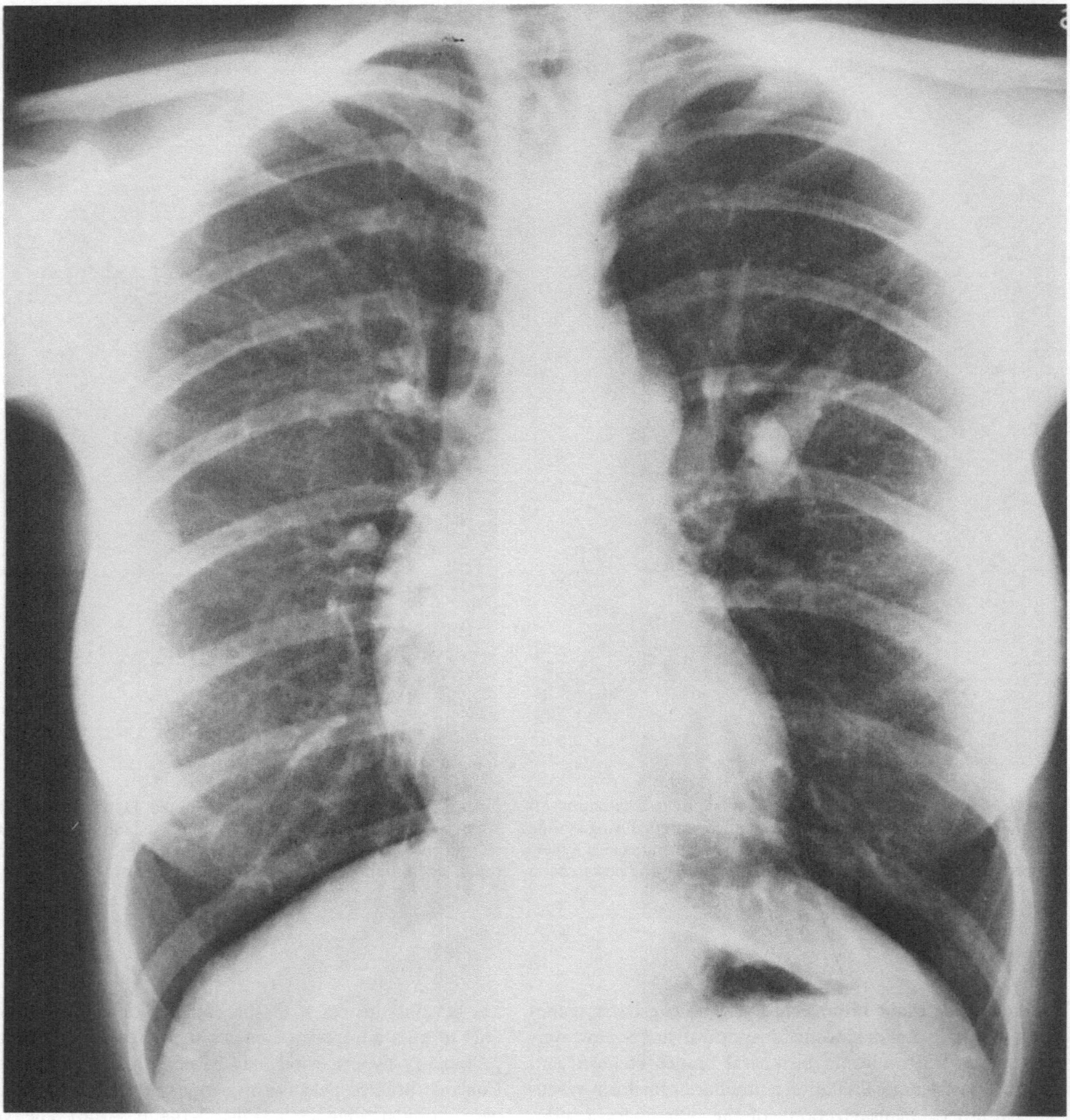

A

Fig. 7–144. *Multiple peripheral pulmonic stenoses causing fusiform dilatation ("sausagization") of the pulmonary artery branches in a 19-year-old girl with mental retardation.* **A** The main pulmonary artery is dilated. The size of the heart is normal. The pulmonary angiogram **(B)** delineates the multiple stenoses of the pulmonary branches with poststenotic dilatation.

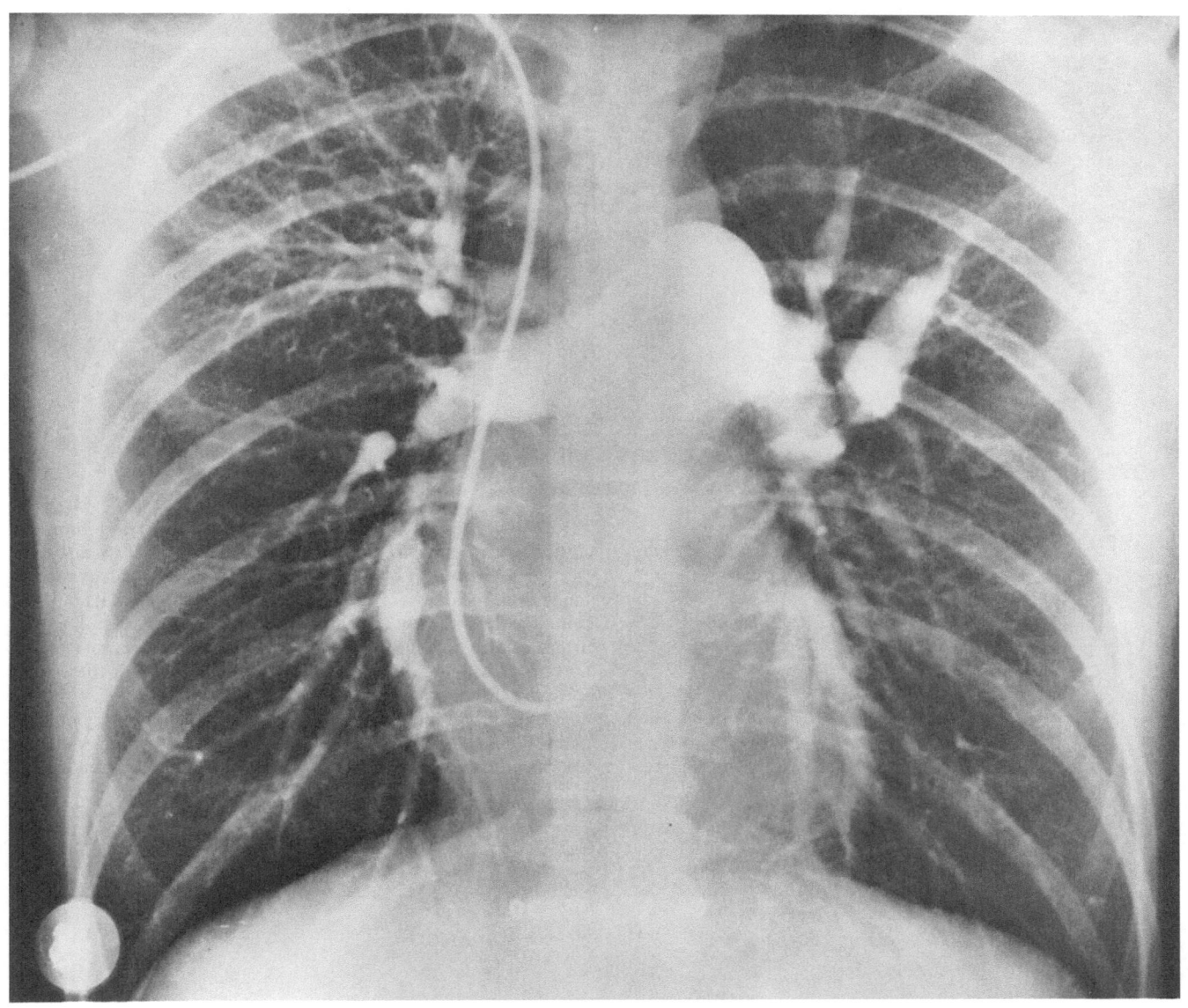

B

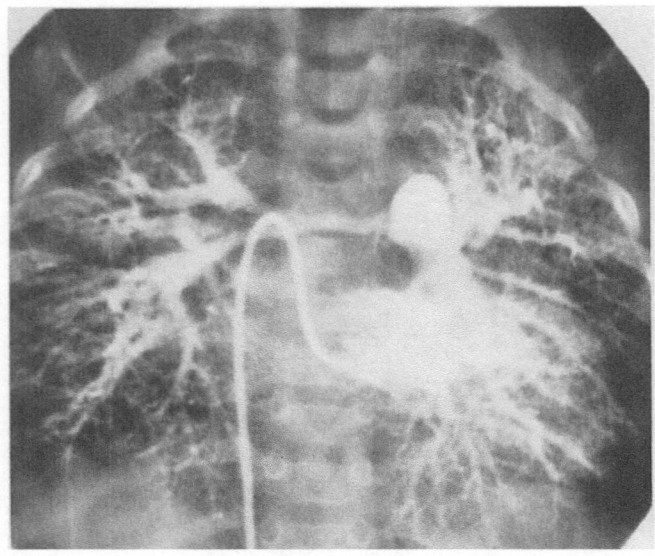

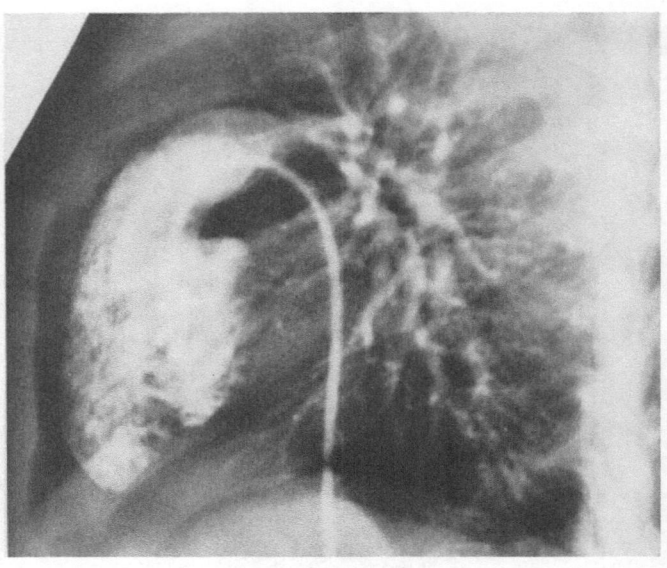

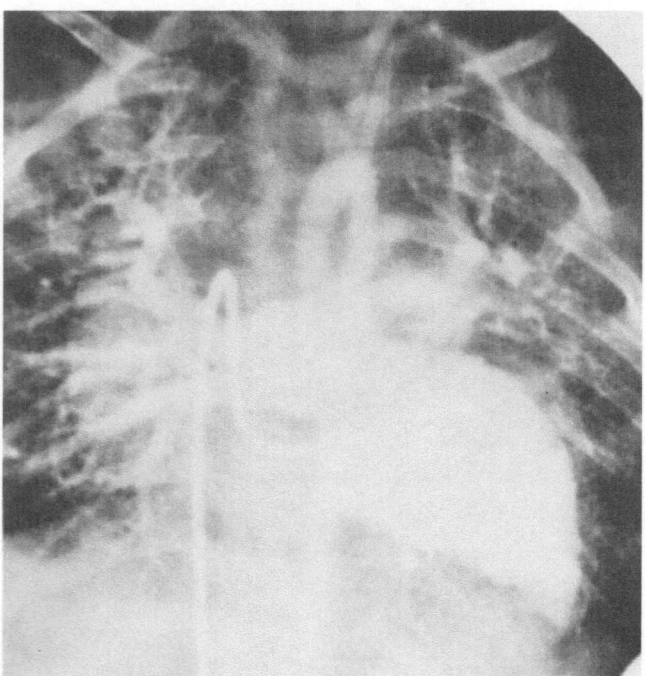

Fig. 7–145. *Diffuse narrowing of the pulmonary artery branches in a 10-month-old girl without signs of rubella embryopathy.* In the frontal view (**A**) of the right ventriculogram, narrowing extends from the origin of the right pulmonary artery to its bifurcation. The lateral view (**B**) shows that the distal main pulmonary artery is also involved. In the levophase (**C**) the lumen of the aorta is also markedly narrowed in comparison with the size of the left ventricle.

At autopsy 6 months later the walls of the pulmonary arteries and of the aorta were thickened and irregular. A younger sibling also has the clinical findings of peripheral pulmonic stenosis.

Fig. 7–146. *Stenosis of the right pulmonary artery in a 17-year-old girl who also has moderate valvar pulmonic stenosis.* Preferential perfusion of the left lung is present.

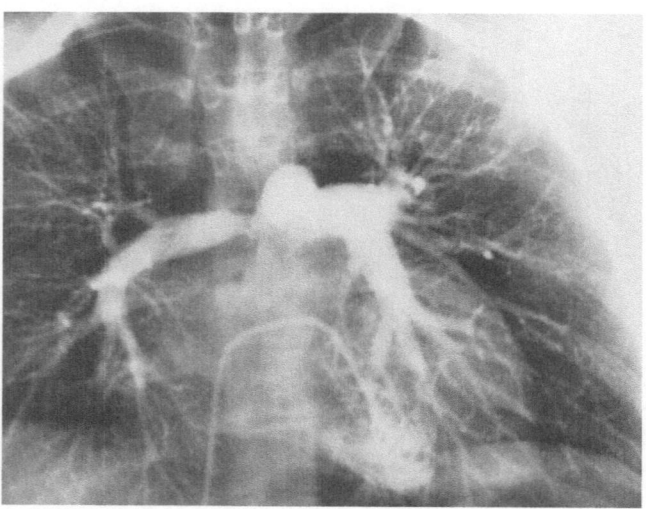

Subvalvar Pulmonic Stenosis

Discussed in the following are anomalous muscle bundle (two-chambered right ventricle), stenosis of the os infundibuli (discrete subpulmonic stenosis), hypertrophic cardiomyopathy (including asymmetrical septal hypertrophy) and accessory tricuspid valve tissue. Fixed infundibular stenosis is part of tetralogy of Fallot, while dynamic infundibular stenosis occurs with valvar pulmonic stenosis. Neoplasms of the right heart are described in Chapter 8.

Anomalous Muscle Bundle (Two-Chambered Right Ventricle or Double Chambered Right Ventricle)

Subinfundibular obstruction of the RV by anomalous muscle bundle (AMB) is an unusual form of obstruction of the RV outflow tract. The RV is divided into a proximal high-pressure chamber and a distal low-pressure chamber. The obstruction is caused by an AMB or multiple muscle bundles of either abnormal or normal bulbar muscle. AMB may occur either just below the crista supraventricularis or in the proximal portion of the body of the RV. On occasion multiple AMBs are present. Ventricular septal defect is the most frequently associated malformation. Coexisting pulmonic valve stenosis, pulmonary atresia and persistent ductus arteriosus have also been described. AMB may also occur as an isolated anomaly.

The *clinical features* may be reminiscent of PS, VSD or tetralogy of Fallot. Approximately half the patients with AMB are asymptomatic. The others have varying degrees of exercise intolerance, increased number of respiratory infections in infancy or growth failure. Cyanosis may occur with a high degree of obstruction due to AMB in association with VSD. On auscultation a loud harsh pansystolic murmur or systolic ejection murmur is heard. A palpable thrill is often associated. The absence of a systolic ejection click, and the location of the murmur along the mid to lower left sternal border rather than in the second left intercostal space should lead one to consider subvalvar pulmonic stenosis rather than valvar pulmonic stenosis in a patient with signs of RV obstruction. The electrocardiogram most often shows right ventricular hypertrophy; although combined hypertrophy may be present in patients with a large VSD. A few patients with AMB have normal electrocardiograms.

M-mode echocardiography may be used to evaluate the relationship of the aorta to the septum in cases with findings similar to tetralogy of Fallot. Absence of overriding of the aortic valve above the septum would merit consideration of other forms of obstruction of the right ventricular outflow tract. Two-dimensional echocardiography may identify the AMB (Goldberg et al). Doppler echocardiography identifies disturbance of flow and a high velocity jet within the right ventricle which must be distinguished from that associated with VSD.

The *radiological findings* are not specific for this entity and relate to the associated defects. The heart and pulmonary vascularity may be normal (Fig. 7–147A). However, the findings of ventricular septal defect with left-to-right shunt or those of tetralogy of Fallot (either pink or blue) may be observed.

At catheterization a systolic pressure gradient is present within the RV. The obstruction usually lies below the infundibulum. Serial cardiac catheterizations in some patients have demonstrated absence of or minimal intraventricular pressure gradient initially with subsequent progression in obstruction. A hemodynamically obstructive AMB should be differentiated from discrete or diaphragmatic infundibular stenosis (stricture), diverticulum of the RV and Ebstein malformation.

The AMB is better demonstrated in the frontal and right anterior oblique projections. One or more radiolucent bands cross the ventricular cavity below the infundibulum. On occasion, AMB may occur in the outflow tract of the RV (Fig. 7–147B and C). These unusual cases may be difficult to differentiate from tetralogy of Fallot. The associated ventricular septal defect is usually below the AMB, but it may be above it.

Stenosis of the Infundibular Ostium (os infundibuli)

Infundibular ostial stenosis (discrete subpulmonary stenosis) is caused by a fibromuscular ring between the conus (infundibulum) and the body of the RV. The resulting narrowing of the RV lumen is located just above the papillary muscle of the conus (muscle of Lancisi). The infundibular chamber (between the obstruction and the pulmonary valve) is normal in size or larger than normal and is devoid of trabeculations. The RV proximal to the stenosis is hypertrophied. The pulmonary valve is usually normal, but it may be stenosed. Infundibular ostial stenoses are rigid, fixed stenotic rings that require excision to relieve the obstruction. This anomaly is observed on occasion in tetralogy of Fallot.

Asymmetrical Septal Hypertrophy

Asymmetrical septal hypertrophy (ASH) usually involves the LV wall and septum, but in some severe cases obstruction to the RV outflow tract may occur (Bernheim syndrome). Biplane biventricular simultaneous injection in the RAO-LAO or frontal-lateral projections precisely delineate this anomaly (see Hypertrophic Cardiomyopathy in Chapter 6).

Accessory Tricuspid Valve Tissue

Accessory tricuspid valve tissue is an uncommon cause of RV outflow tract obstruction. The anomalous tricuspid tissue may occur as a free-floating leaflet (parachute-like sac) or a mass of tissue attached by chordae tendineae to rudimentary papillary muscles arising usually from the septal papillary muscle. The abnormal tissue obstructs the RV outflow tract during systole and floats back into the RV sinus during diastole, mimicking a pedunculated tumor on angiography. The anomalous tricuspid tissue does not form or contribute to the function of the tricuspid valve. Accessory valvular tissue has been noted in the subaortic

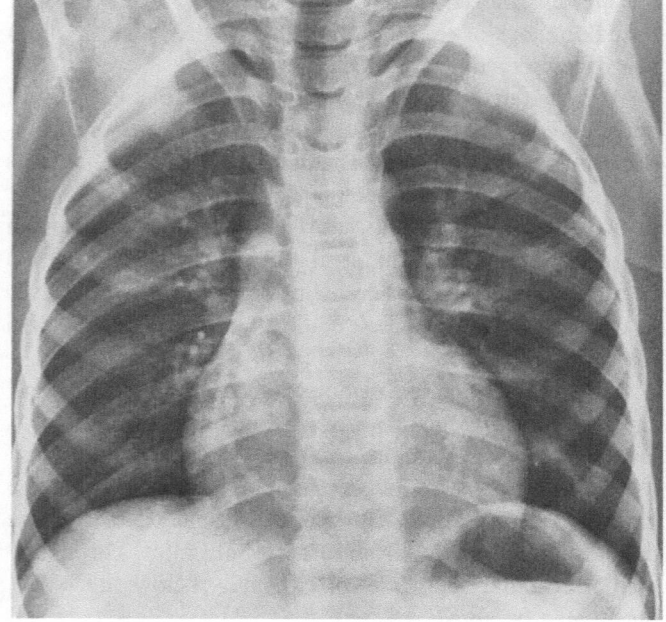

A

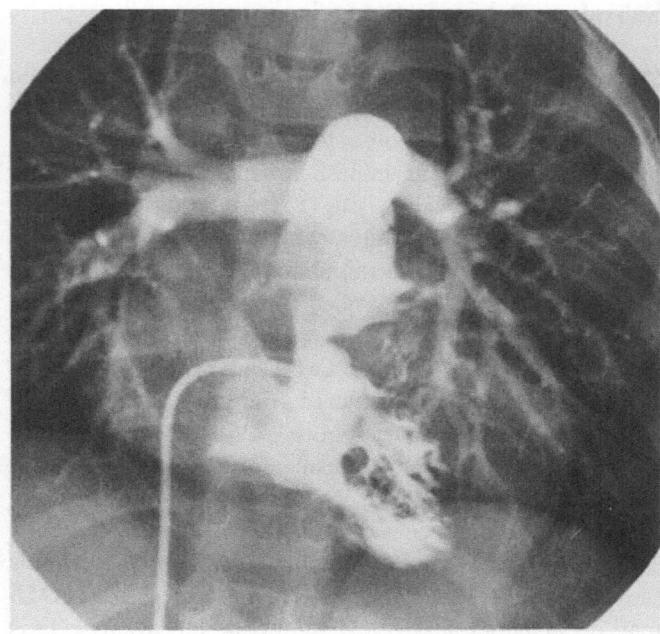

B

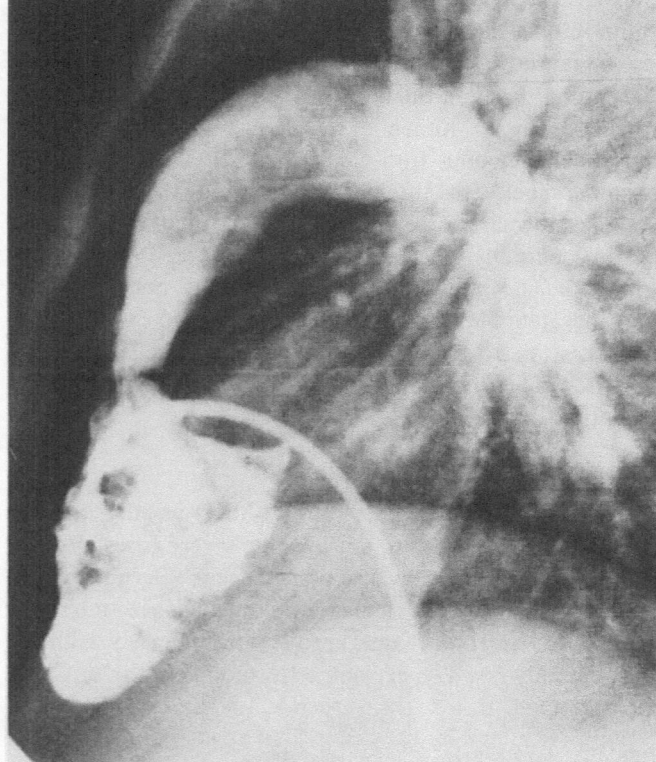

C

Fig. 7–147. *Anomalous muscle bundle (two-chambered right ventricle).* **A** Frontal chest roentgenogram; **B** and **C** frontal and lateral frames of a right ventriculogram. On the plain film the heart is not enlarged, and the pulmonary vasculature is normal. The right ventriculogram shows an anomalous muscle bundle at the level of the ostium of the right ventricular outflow tract, which divides the right ventricle into two compartments. The compartment proximal to the anomalous muscle bundle has high pressure and is hypertrophied. The outflow portion has lower pressure and is dilated. On left ventriculography (not illustrated) a small infracristal ventricular septal defect and an aneurysm of the membranous septum were demonstrated.

and subpulmonic regions and in association with levo-transposition of the great arteries.

Stenosis of the Tricuspid Valve

Tricuspid stenosis (TS) is rarely encountered as an isolated congenital defect. Hypoplasia of the tricuspid valve may be part of other congenital heart defects (e.g., Uhl anomaly, severe pulmonary stenosis with hypoplastic RV, pulmonary

atresia). In adults, TS occurs on occasion with mitral stenosis as part of chronic rheumatic heart disease. In addition to hypoplasia of the anulus, TS may be due to accessory tricuspid valve tissue or secondary to tissue derived from a venous valve (cor triatriatum dexter). Schlesinger et al. described tricuspid stenosis due to commissural fusion of a bicuspid atrioventricular valve in the RV. Their impression was that of a congenital deformity rather than a rheumatic process.

The differential diagnosis of TS includes other deformities of the tricuspid valve (e.g., Ebstein anomaly, tumors of the right side of the heart).

Clinical features in isolated TS consist of fatigue and peripheral cyanosis (venous hypoxia) due to limited cardiac output, venous engorgement, hepatomegaly and peripheral edema. A diastolic rumble may be present which varies with respiration. The electrocardiogram and chest films show right atrial enlargement. The M-mode echocardiogram demonstrates thickening and abnormal motion of the tricuspid valve similar to that occurring with mitral stenosis. The 2-D echocardiogram may indicate the small size of the anulus. Tumors and vegetations of the right heart are excluded by echocardiography.

Cardiac catheterization shows a diastolic gradient across the tricuspid valve. The angiogram demonstrates thickening, doming and limitation of motion of the tricuspid valve in patients with commissural fusion. Hypoplasia, accessory tricuspid valve tissue, Ebstein anomaly with small or imperforate orifice, cor triatriatum dexter and right atrial tumors are also delineated.

Ebstein Anomaly of the Tricuspid Valve

Ebstein anomaly consists of displacement of the tricuspid valve into the RV, resulting in "atrialization" of part of the RV. Hemodynamic effects include tricuspid insufficiency, a large RA, and often, a right-to-left atrial shunt through a stretched foramen ovale or secundum ASD. Displacement or malattachment of the tricuspid valve varies from a mild form with minimal or no symptoms to a severe form incompatible with life. The posterior leaflet is usually the most severely deformed and malattached, while the medial (septal) leaflet is often deformed and attached to the interventricular septum. The anterior leaflet is the least affected and may be the only functioning part of the valve. Distal to the displaced leaflets the RV is formed by a small portion of the apical sinus and the outflow tract. The infundibulum (outflow tract) is usually thick and may be obstructed. The RV proximal to the displaced leaflets (atrialized portion) and RA form a single large cavity with thin walls. Thinning of the RV wall resembles that occurring in Uhl anomaly (parchment RV) but to a lesser degree. In levotransposition of the great vessels the tricuspid valve is on the left. Therefore the rare occurrence of Ebstein anomaly with levotransposition produces clinical and hemodynamic manifestations resembling mitral insufficiency. "Ebstein malformation" of the mitral valve with normally related great arteries is extremely rare. The mitral leaflets are dysplastic, and the anterior leaflet is displaced into the LV to the level of the posteromedial papillary muscle. Mitral-aortic fibrous continuity is maintained.

Associated defects are unusual. They include left-to-right shunts (patent ductus arteriosus, ventricular septal defect, endocardial cushion defect), mitral valve abnormalities (mitral valve prolapse, supravalvular mitral ring, dysplasia of the mitral leaflets), tricuspid abnormalities (mus-

cular tricuspid leaflets with partial Uhl anomaly, rarely tricuspid stenosis, imperforate tricuspid valve) and coarctation of aorta. Ebstein anomaly has also been reported in association with other forms of obstruction to the right heart. The case reported by Huhta et al. showed pulmonary atresia with a double-chambered RV. Gerlis and Anderson described a patient with Ebstein anomaly, cor triatriatum dexter, imperforate tricuspid valve and pulmonary atresia.

Clinical Features The clinical picture is variable as a result of the wide spectrum of abnormalities and the presence or absence of associated malformations.

In the neonatal period, because of the high pulmonary resistance, infants may develop severe tricuspid insufficiency and a right-to-left shunt at the atrial level with heart failure and pronounced cyanosis. A decrease in the pulmonary resistance in these infants results in improvement of symptoms. In older patients the symptoms are closely related to the degree of tricuspid insufficiency, right-to-left shunting and RV performance. Cyanosis and dyspnea are usually present and peripheral edema may be present. Many patients show dysrhythmias. On auscultation the first and second heart sounds are widely split, with prominent third and fourth sounds. Tricuspid insufficiency murmurs in systole, as well as diastolic flow rumbles, are common.

The electrocardiogram may show a Wolff-Parkinson-White (WPW) syndrome, which is almost always type B. In the absence of WPW pre-excitation syndrome, the PR interval is often prolonged, the QRS complex is of low voltage, with an indeterminate axis and complete right bundle-branch block. RA enlargement is common, with strikingly enlarged P waves. Supraventricular tachycardias are common.

Echocardiography M-mode echocardiography shows a large RV, paradoxical ventricular septal motion (RV volume overload), increased excursion of the tricuspid valve and abnormally delayed closing of the tricuspid valve as compared to mitral closure. The tricuspid E-F slope is decreased. The tricuspid valve echoes are displaced toward the left (Fig. 7–148). Two-dimensional echocardiography, using an apical four-chamber view, demonstrates the displacement of the tricuspid leaflets toward the apex of the RV and delineates the atrialized portion of the RV (Fig. 7–149). (Normally the tricuspid valve is attached less than 1 cm closer to the apex than is the mitral.)

In the cyanotic neonate it is essential to demonstrate a patent pulmonary valve in addition to features of Ebstein anomaly. Management of pulmonary atresia with tricuspid insufficiency differs markedly from Ebstein anomaly without pulmonic stenosis.

Radiological (Plain Film) Features The pulmonary vasculature may be normal but is usually decreased. Pulmonary overcirculation is rare. If present, it indicates an associated left-to-right shunt, often due to a VSD or PDA. The configuration of the heart may be normal or may show mild enlargement of the RA (Fig. 7–150) or gross cardiomegaly with a huge RA⁻ and RV. The typical appearance (Fig.

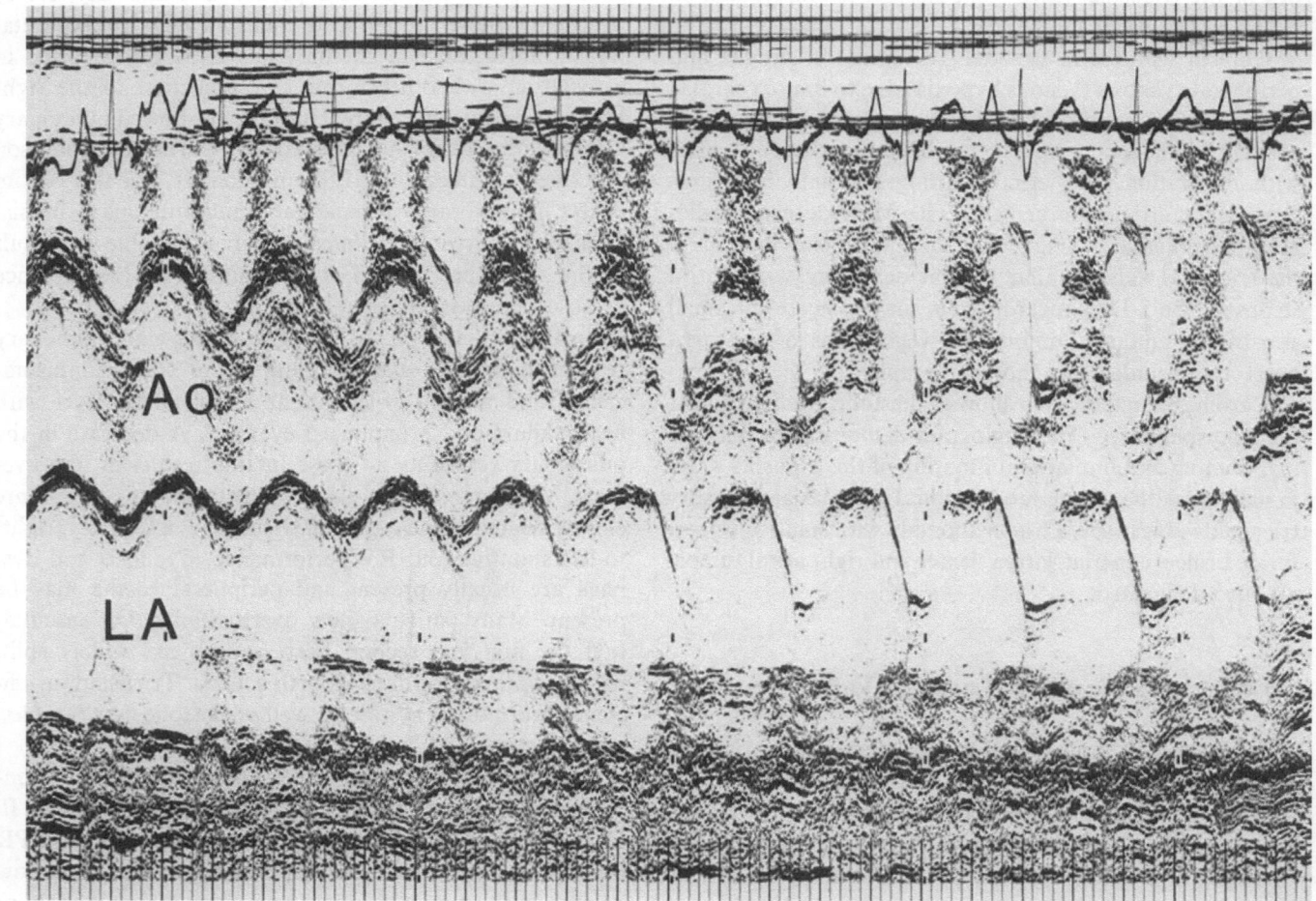

A

Fig. 7–148. *M-mode echocardiography in a 2-year-old boy with Ebstein anomaly.* **A** *is an arc scan from the aortic root* (*Ao.*) *to the ventricles.* (Note that this arc scan is continuous across pages 484 and 485.) The right ventricle (*RV*) is enlarged, and the septum moves paradoxically (anteriorly during ventricular systole). The tricuspid valve (*TV*) is demonstrated throughout the entire length of the right ventricle, even as the transducer is directed toward the apex. This feature indicates displacement of the tricuspid valve toward the apex of the right ventricle. **B** is a tracing of the mitral (*MV*) and tricuspid valves (*TV*). The tricuspid valve closes 0.04 msec later than the mitral valve. In this infant the closure of the tricuspid valve is not delayed; delayed closure of the tricuspid valve ($>$0.06 sec) is reported in adults with Ebstein anomaly. *LV* = left ventricle; *LA* = left atrium; *AML* = anterior mitral leaflet.

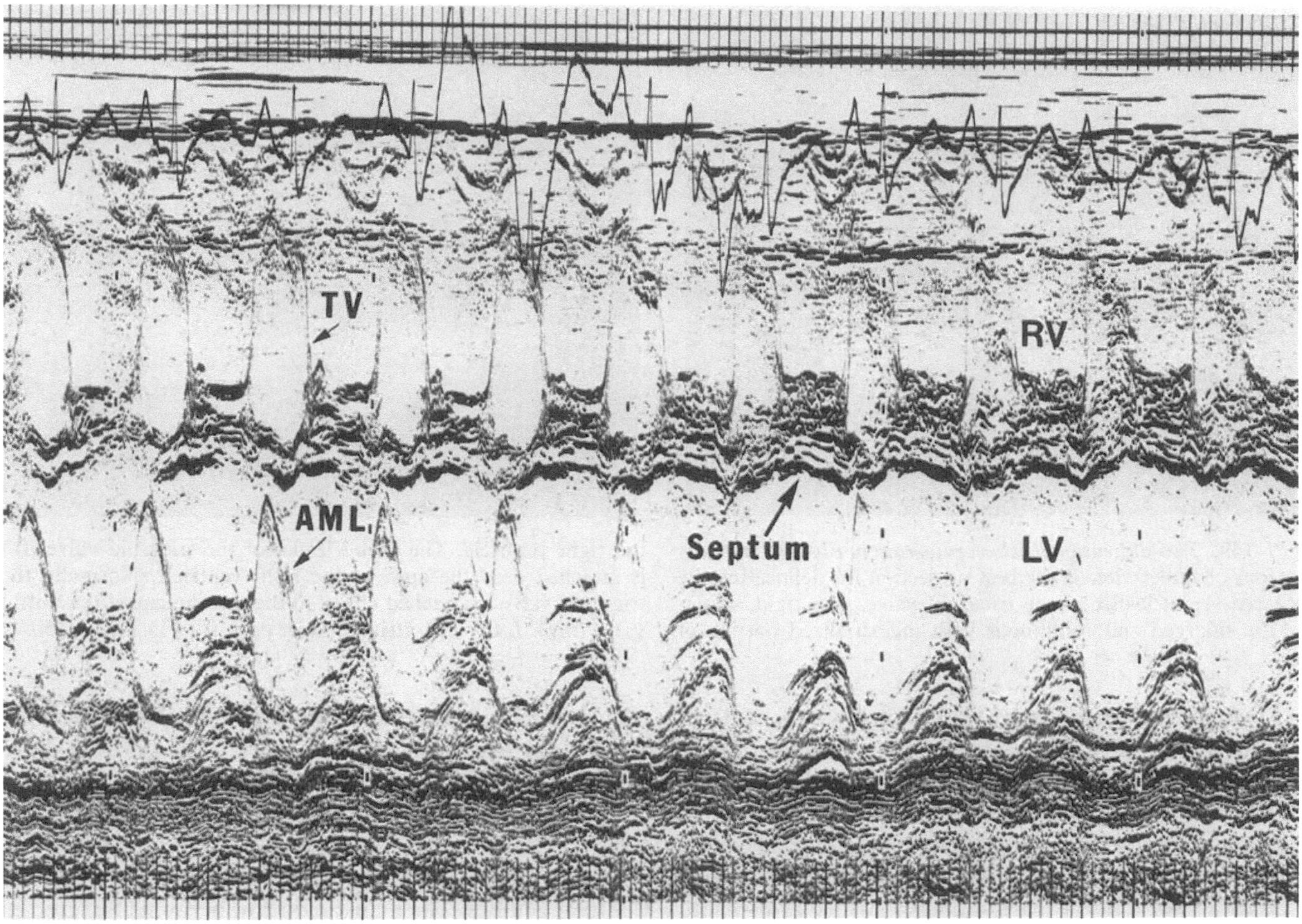

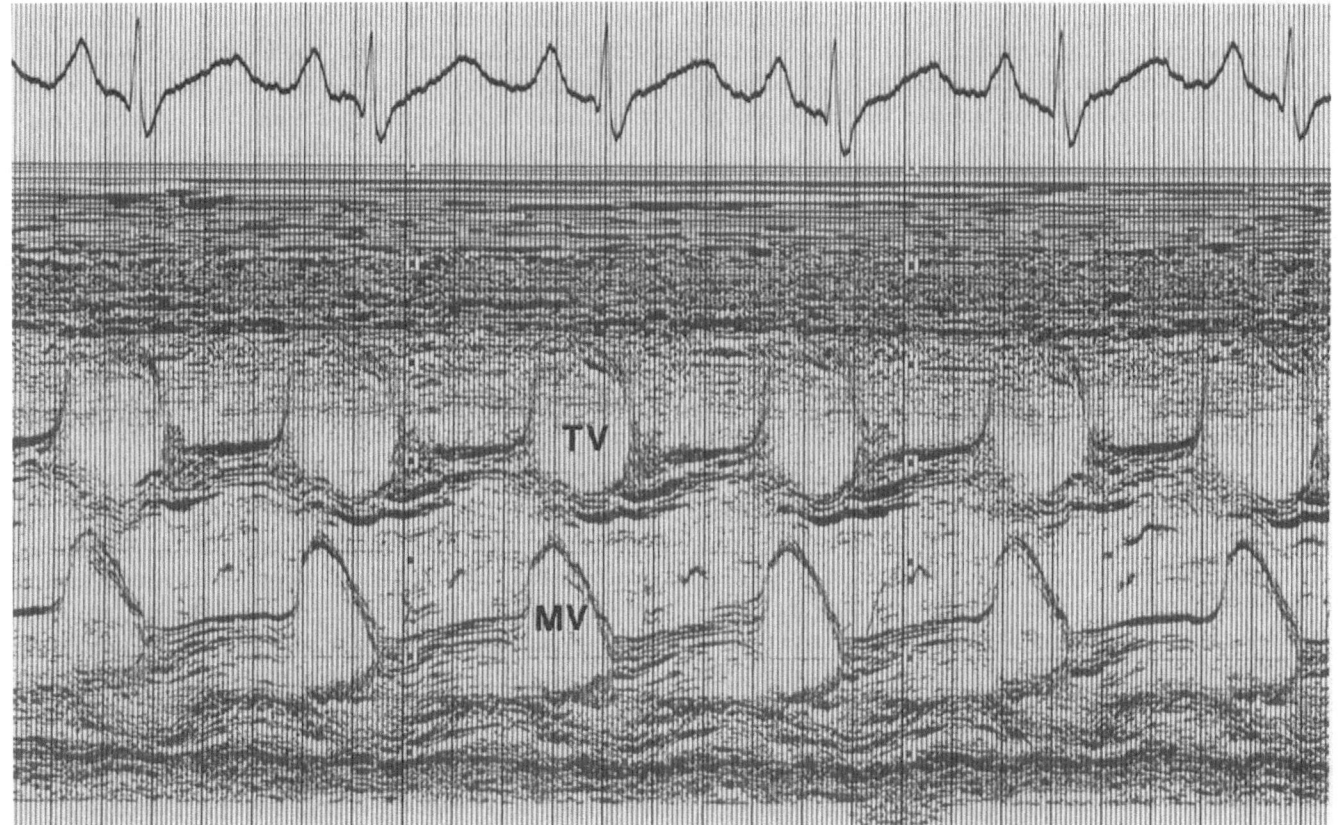

A

B

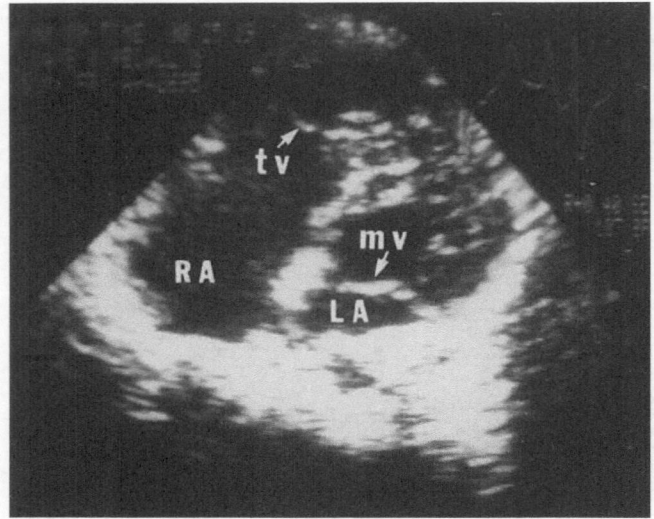

A

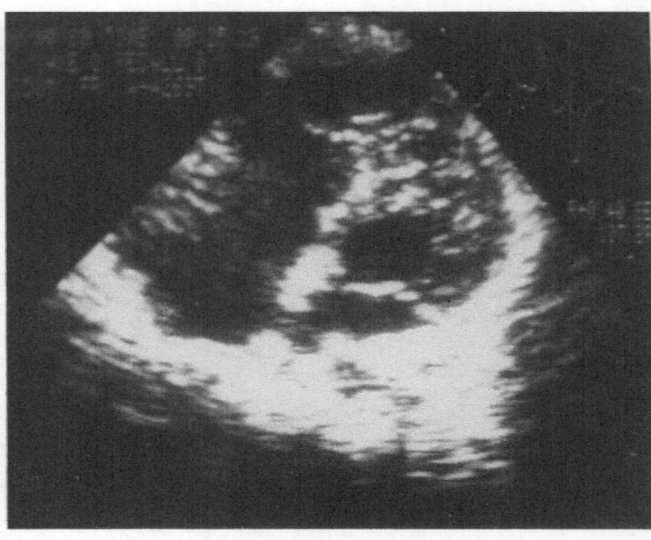

B

Fig. 7–149. *Two-dimensional echocardiogram in Ebstein anomaly.* The four-chamber view is the best projection for delineating the displaced septal leaflet of the tricuspid valve. The right atrium (*RA*) is enlarged and continuous with the atrialized portion of the right ventricle. The septal leaflet of the tricuspid valve (*tv*) is attached near the apex of the right ventricle. Normally the tricuspid valve is attached closer to the attachment of the mitral valve (*mv*). *LA* = left atrium. Same patient as in Fig. 7–150.

7–151) is that of a large heart with a narrow waist (inconspicuous main pulmonary artery and small aortic arch). The RA may reach huge proportions, especially in neonates (see Fig. 1–6). The left heart border shows a wide convexity, with its maximum curvature in the region corresponding to the atrioventricular junction. This characteristic convexity is cast by the outflow tract of the RV, which is displaced by the combination of the large RA and the atrialized RV. The convexity of the left heart border caused by the RV outflow tract in conjunction with the lengthening and increased convexity of the right heart border produced by the dilated RA accounts for the characteristic boxlike or globular heart configuration observed in Ebstein anomaly. The LA and LV are not enlarged.

In the neonatal period, infants with pulmonary atresia with an intact interventricular septum and tricuspid insufficiency and those with tricuspid atresia and a restrictive interatrial communication may have plain film findings similar to those occurring with Ebstein anomaly (see Fig. 7–175).

Hemodynamics At catheterization the pressures in the pulmonary artery and functioning RV are usually normal; however, the RV end-diastolic pressure may be elevated. The RA pressure is elevated and shows a prominent V wave with a steep Y descent. The RA pressure may be normal in a very large and compliant RA. Determinations of oxygen saturation often show a right-to-left shunt at the atrial level, with systemic arterial desaturation.

A characteristic finding in Ebstein anomaly at catheterization is the pattern of the intracardiac electrocardiogram obtained simultaneously with pressure tracings during withdrawal of a catheter from the RV through the atrialized portion of the RV and into the RA (Fig. 7–152).

Recordings in the functioning RV cavity reveal a ven-

tricular electrocardiogram along with a RV pressure curve. Recordings from the atrialized portion of the RV show persistence of the ventricular electrocardiogram, whereas the pressure contour changes to that characteristic of a RA. When the true RA is entered, the electrocardiogram as well as the pressure tracing are those of the RA.

Contrast Studies The main angiocardiographic features in Ebstein anomaly in the frontal view are those of tricuspid insufficiency and a notch in the diaphragmatic wall caused by the displacement of the posterior leaflet. In fact, two notches are present, the first notch representing the site of the tricuspid anulus situated between the large RA and the RV and the second notch defining the displaced posterior leaflet of the tricuspid valve. The area between the two notches is the atrialized portion of the RV (Figs. 7–150D, 7–151C). On occasion the RA, the atrialized portion of the RV and the functioning distal RV result in a trilobed appearance on the frontal view. In extreme cases the huge RA forms the entire anterior and posterior outlines of the cardiac silhouette on the lateral view (Fig. 7–151D). Cine studies demonstrate that the atrialized portion of the RV and the functioning RV contract in synchrony.

Treatment Several surgical techniques (prosthetic replacement of the tricuspid valve, plication and anuloplasty, and combinations thereof) have been used with variable results. Danielson et al. have adopted a combination of plication of the free wall of the atrialized portion of the RV, posterior tricuspid anuloplasty and RA reduction. This procedure has resulted in satisfactory early and late results in most patients. In patients with refractory disturbances of the rhythm secondary to the WPW syndrome, intraoperative electrophysiological mapping and surgical division of accessory Kent bundle pathways have been performed.

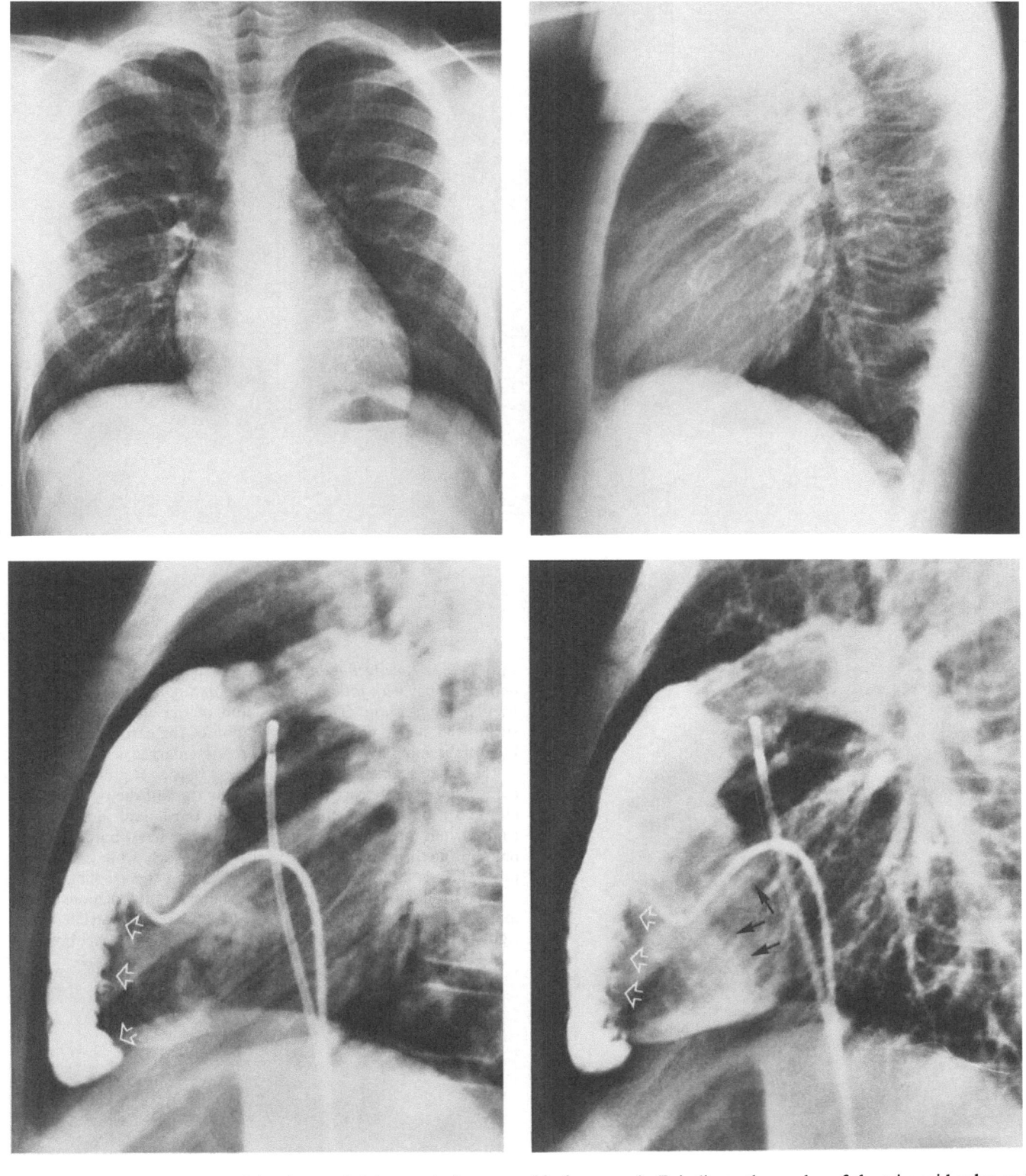

Fig. 7–150. *Roentgenograms of the chest and right ventriculogram in a 10-year-old asymptomatic boy with Ebstein anomaly.* The frontal film of the chest (**A**) shows right atrial enlargement and slight straightening of the left heart border. In the lateral view (**B**) the retrosternal clear space is obliterated. The lateral view of the right ventriculogram reveals dense filling of the outflow tract of the right ventricle (**C**) and subsequent opacification of the atrialized portion of this chamber (**D**). The *open arrows* in C indicate the displaced septal leaflet of the tricuspid valve. The *black arrows* in **D** indicate the anulus of the tricuspid valve and the *open arrows* the displaced attachment of the septal leaflet of the tricuspid valve. These two anatomical structures are the landmarks that delimit the atrialized portion of the right ventricle. Note the electrode catheter used to record simultaneous pressure and intracardiac electrograms during withdrawal of the catheter from the outflow tract of the right ventricle through the atrialized portion of the right ventricle and into the right atrium (see text) (Same patient as in Fig. 7–149).

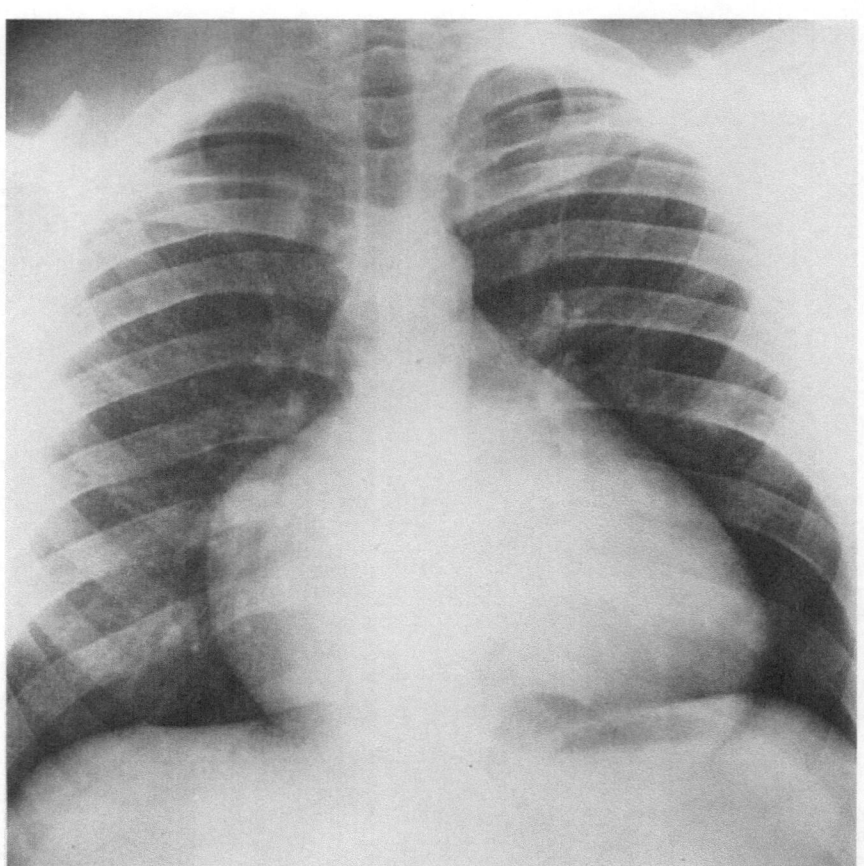

A

Fig. 7–151. *Roentgenogram of the chest and angiogram in an adolescent boy with fatigue on exertion and paroxysmal supraventricular tachycardia.* The frontal film of the chest (**A**) demonstrates the classic boxlike configuration of the cardiac silhouette in Ebstein anomaly. The heart is grossly enlarged with squaring of the lower segment of the right heart border (right atrium), a convex left heart border (dilated outflow tract of the right ventricle) and a narrow vascular pedicle. On the lateral film (**B**) the right atrium forms the anterior and posterior heart borders, thus obliterating the retrosternal clear space anteriorly while extending posteriorly behind the inferior vena cava and the esophagus.

The frontal view of the right ventriculogram (**C**) demonstrates marked dilatation of the right atrium and right ventricle. The right ventricle accounts for the convexity of the left heart border.

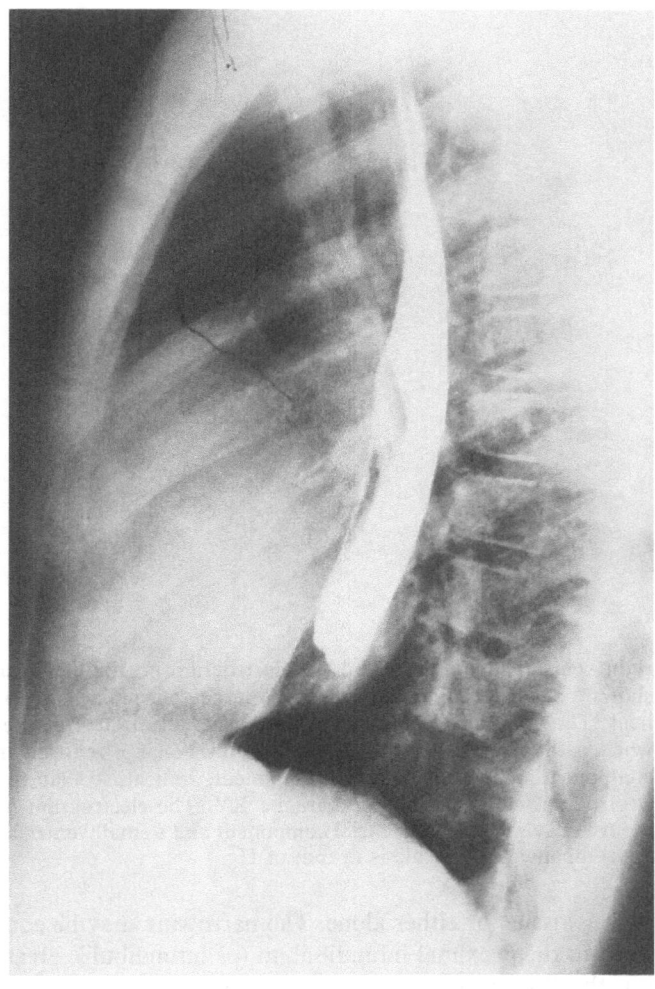

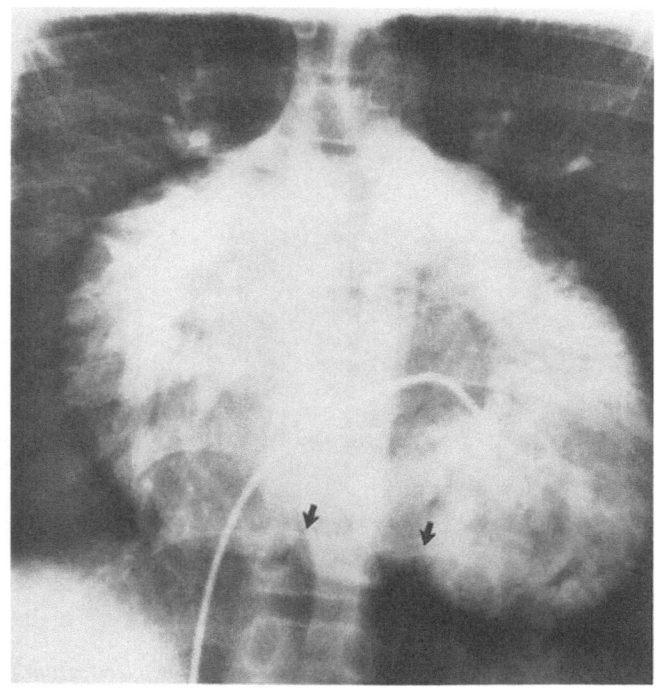

C

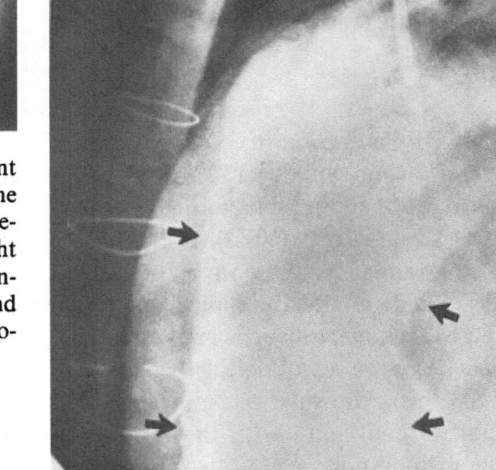

D

B

The two notches on the diaphragmatic surface (*arrows*) represent the normal tricuspid anulus and the displaced attachment of the septal and posterior leaflets of the tricuspid valve. The area between the notches represents the atrialized portion of the right ventricle. The lateral view of the right ventriculogram (**D**) demonstrates a huge right atrium that forms both the anterior and posterior borders of the heart. The right ventricle (*arrows*) projects within the right atrium.

RV   Atr. RV   RA

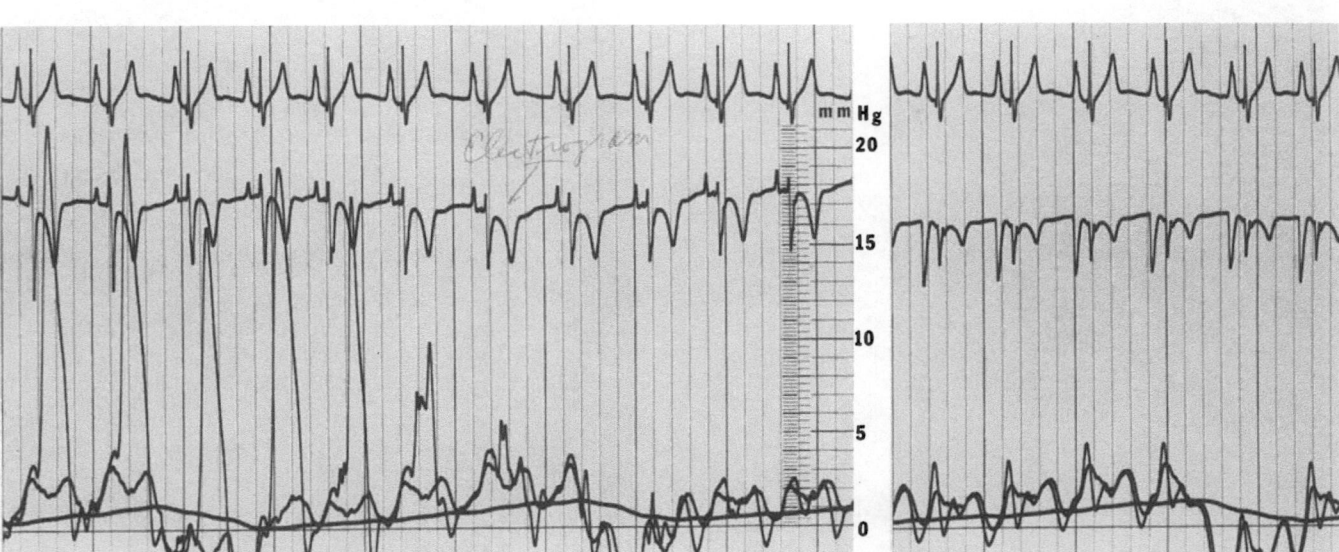

Fig. 7–152. *Pressure tracings and an intracardiac electrogram in a 10 year old boy with Ebstein anomaly.* The recording on the left of the scale is during withdrawal of an electrode catheter from the right ventricle (*RV*) through the displaced tricuspid valve into the atrialized portion of the right ventricle (*Atr.RV*). The tracing on the right of the scale was recorded while the catheter was in the true right atrium (*RA*) proximal to the anulus of the tricuspid valve. The pressure tracing in the RV is a typical right ventricular pressure, and the electrogram in that chamber shows a small atrial component and a large ventricular component. The pressure tracing in the Atr.RV is an atrial pressure, whereas the electrogram in the Atr.RV shows a large ventricular component and a small atrial component, indicating that the electrogram comes from the anatomic RV. The electrogram in the true RA shows a large atrial component and a small ventricular component. The scale is in mm of Hg.

Tetralogy of Fallot

Tetralogy of Fallot (TOF) is the most common form of cyanotic heart disease beyond infancy (30%). The four basic features of this malformation are pulmonary stenosis or atresia, ventricular septal defect (VSD), overriding of the aorta and right ventricular hypertrophy. The pulmonary stenosis and the VSD determine the clinical and radiological findings. The VSD is large, subaortic and infracristal in location. Two basic types of septal defects occur: With the usual form of VSD the aortic valve has a biventricular origin and shows fibrous continuity with the mitral and tricuspid valves. The membranous septum is rudimentary (flap). Thus the posteroinferior border of the defect is formed by valvular and membranous tissue. The bundle of His runs in the muscular septum along its junction with the membranous flap. In the second type (relatively infrequent) the defect is encircled by a muscular rim, the proximal conus septum (right posterior division of the septal band) preventing aorticotricuspid fibrous continuity. In this group the membranous septum is well formed and is situated below the proximal conus septum. The conduction system is away from the edge of the defect. Lev and Eckner believe this second type of VSD represents a perforation of the crista supraventricularis. Intermediate variations between type I and II VSDs may be encountered.

The pulmonary stenosis is usually infundibular, although valvular stenosis may also be present. Infundibular stenosis is usually due to a combination of muscular and fibrous tissue, or either alone. The narrowing may be confined to the proximal infundibulum (os infundibuli), creating the "third" or infundibular chamber from the unaffected outflow tract of the RV. In other instances the stenosis involves the entire outflow tract of the RV so that the infundibulum is narrow. These two varieties account for the majority of cases. In both, the infundibulum is normal in length or even elongated. In the second variety the pulmonary valve and pulmonary artery are also narrow. A third variety occurs in which the infundibulum is hypoplastic. In these patients the infundibulum is short and narrow, and the VSD appears to be more anterior and closer to the pulmonary valve. The pulmonary ring and the main pulmonary artery are narrow.

Stenosis of the pulmonic valve may be mild, moderate or severe. Atresia of the valve is present in 20% of patients with TOF. The pulmonary valve may be bicuspid in up to 50% of patients, unicuspid in 10% and absent in 3%. In all forms of TOF the size of the main pulmonary artery corresponds to the severity of the pulmonic stenosis. If the degree of pulmonic stenosis is not severe, the main pulmonary artery may be normal or, rarely, large. Poststenotic dilatation is uncommon, but may occur with tight stenosis of the pulmonic valve.

TOF with pulmonary atresia is also called pseudotruncus arteriosus. In this entity the only outlet from the heart is an enlarged aorta. The infundibulum of the RV ends blindly at the site of the pulmonary valve, but is attached by a ligament to the main pulmonary artery, which extends downward from the pulmonary artery branches. These branches, incidentally, are usually patent. Perfusion to the lungs is by way of the ductus arteriosus or systemic collateral vessels from the descending aorta, subclavian arteries and intercostal arteries, or it may be via both. TOF with pulmonary atresia was previously designated type IV truncus arteriosus, particularly when the infundibulum and the main pulmonary artery were atretic. The entity is now excluded from the group of cases with truncus arteriosus because almost all such patients have a fibrous remnant of the infundibulum and pulmonary artery and in most instances the pulmonary branches are patent. Demonstration of the pulmonary arteries is mandatory in patients with pseudotruncus, because these arteries determine the surgical approach and the prognosis.

The most common cardiac defect associated with TOF is a right aortic arch (25%), usually with mirror-image branching but occasionally with an aberrant left subclavian artery. Other associated defects include patent ductus arteriosus, atrial septal defect (pentalogy of Fallot), coronary artery anomalies (e.g., origin of the left anterior descending artery from the right coronary artery in approximately 9%, and coronary arteriovenous fistula), anomalous systemic or pulmonary veins, pulmonary artery branch stenosis, intraarteriolar thrombi, absence of the pulmonary valve (TOF with pulmonary regurgitation syndrome), absence of the left pulmonary artery, ectopic origin of the left pulmonary artery from the ascending aorta (TOF with left hemitruncus), congenital pericardial defect and, very rarely, supravalvar mitral stenosis.

Clinical Features Presentation and clinical course are determined by the severity of the pulmonic stenosis. Infants with pulmonary atresia (pseudotruncus) depend upon a patent ductus arteriosus or large systemic collaterals for pulmonary blood flow. They become severely cyanotic and acidotic simultaneously with the initial closure of the ductus arteriosus. On the other hand, rare patients with so-called pink TOF do not exhibit cyanosis during infancy or childhood. The degree of cyanosis in the usual case of TOF is intermediate between these extremes.

Infants with TOF and mild pulmonic stenosis at birth may even show signs of a large left-to-right shunt during the newborn period. Toward the end of the first year of life a bidirectional shunt develops, and thereafter a right-to-left shunt. The clinical course in these is indistinguishable from that of infants with large VSD who exhibit heart failure initially, but then become cyanotic with increasing pulmonary vascular resistance (Eisenmenger syndrome). Many infants with TOF are asymptomatic initially, but gradually cyanosis, clubbing and rising hemoglobin and hematocrit levels develop as pulmonary blood flow becomes inadequate. At first, cyanosis may occur only during crying. When the baby begins to stand and walk, dyspnea and cyanosis may develop on exertion. Some toddlers with TOF squat during mild exertion. It is thought that this posture reduces systemic venous return from the lower body and redirects blood from the legs into the pulmonary circulation

and into the brain. Cyanotic "spells" may occur in patients with TOF when oxygen supply is critically low. These spells are typically described as progressive tachypnea, tachycardia, emotional irritability and anxiety followed by diaphoresis and on occasion by a seizure or loss of consciousness. During the somnolent period after the spell, color returns and heart rate and breathing rate return to normal. Anoxic spells, dyspnea, cyanosis on mild exertion or rising hematocrit levels indicate mandatory surgical intervention.

The physical findings include a loud murmur in infancy with a single second sound and a right ventricular heave. The murmur may become softer as pulmonary flow decreases. The electrocardiogram shows normal dominance of the RV at birth but, because of persistent RV hypertension, fails to show regression of RV forces as the baby grows. Right ventricular hypertrophy may thus be diagnosed later during the first year of life.

The long-term natural history of TOF includes progressive cyanosis and acidosis with intolerance to effort. Paradoxical emboli lead to stroke and brain abscess. Infective endocarditis is relatively frequent. During the second and third decade of life, RV failure and arrhythmias occur as fibrous tissue replaces the chronically hypoxic muscle. In patients not having operation death may be due to severe cyanosis, stroke, infection or arrhythmia.

Echocardiography (Fig. 7–153) The characteristic finding on ultrasound study of children with TOF is overriding of the aortic valve above the ventricular septum. This abnormality is readily imaged on M-mode by an arc scan from the aortic valve to the LV (Fig. 7–153A) or by a long axis two-dimensional view (Fig. 7–153B). Overriding of the aorta is also demonstrated in truncus arteriosus. Identification of a pulmonic valve separate from the aortic valve allows these two groups of defects to be differentiated. The presence of aortic-mitral fibrous continuity separates TOF with severe overriding of the aorta from double-outlet RV except in rare cases of double-outlet RV in which the fibrous connection is elongated.

Two-dimensional sector scans also allow measurement of the main pulmonary artery and pulmonary artery branches. This permits planning for shunting procedures in infancy, and for surgical correction later.

Radiological (Plain Film) Features The classic features of TOF include a normal or nearly normal heart size with a rounded and uplifted cardiac apex and a concave pulmonary artery segment (coeur en sabot, boot-shaped heart). The aorta is prominent and the pulmonary vascularity is decreased (pulmonary undercirculation) (Fig. 7–154).

A right aortic arch is present in approximately 25% of cases of TOF (Figs. 7–154B to 7–157). The right-sided aortic arch widens the superior mediastinum on the right and produces a characteristic indentation on the right side of the trachea near its bifurcation. The barium-filled esophagus also displays an indentation on the right side. In TOF the right aortic arch usually shows mirror-image branching of the brachiocephalic vessels and does not cause

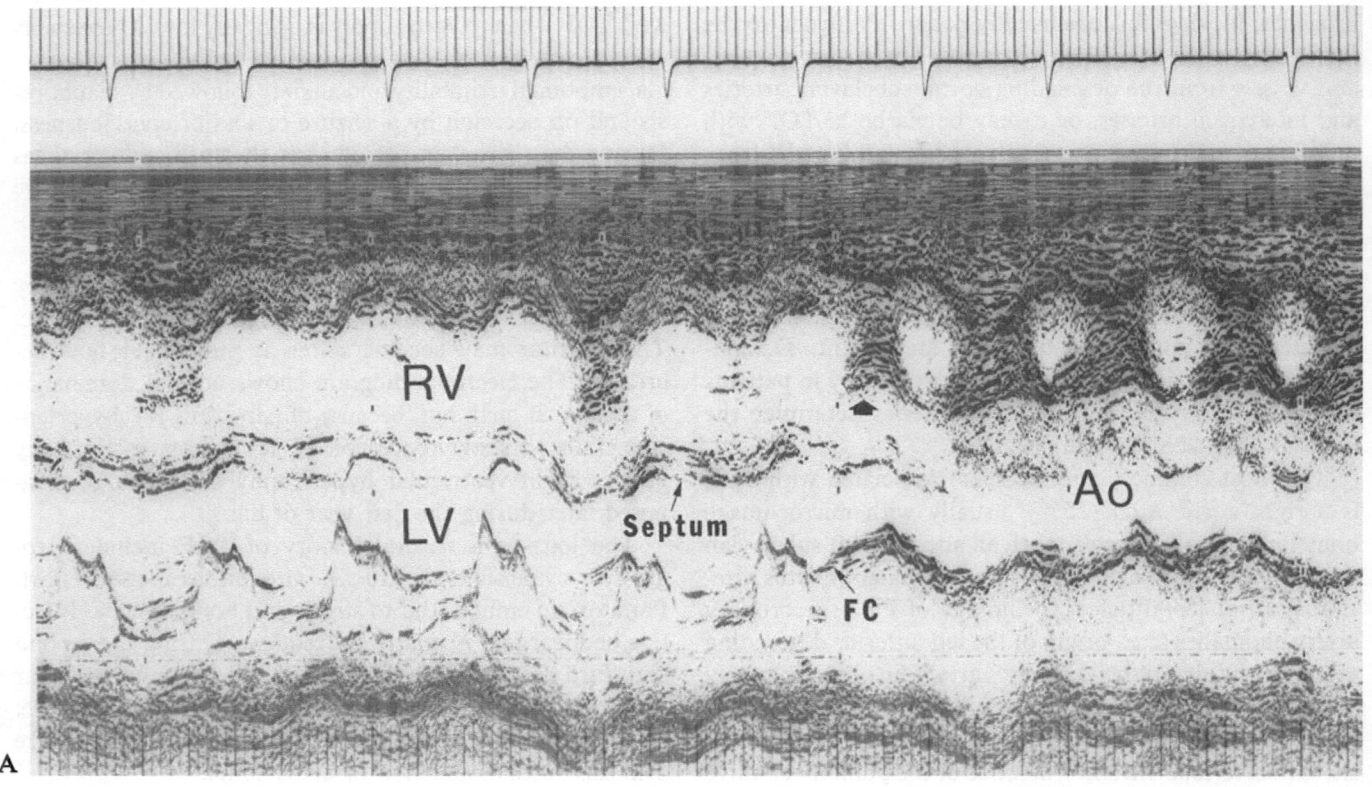

A

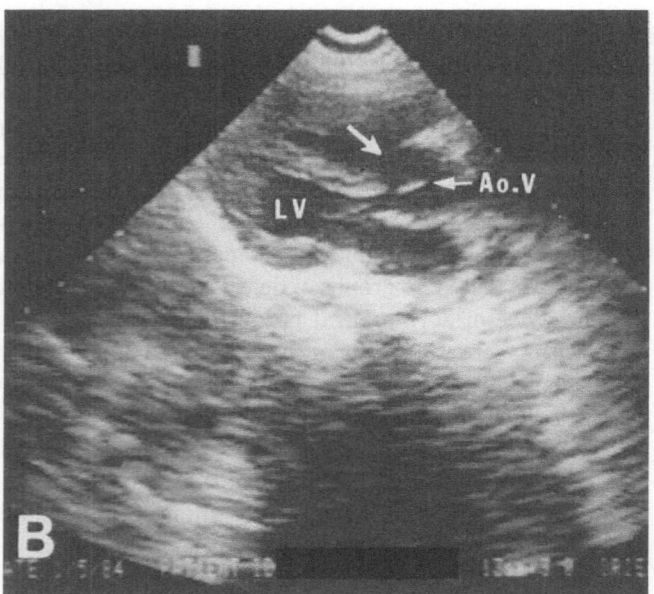

B

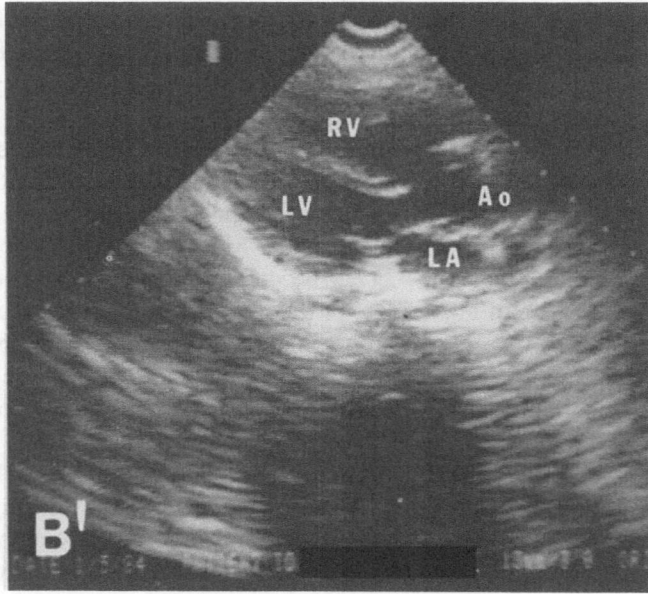

B'

Fig. 7–153. *Echocardiography in tetralogy of Fallot.* **A** is an M-mode arc scan showing overriding of the aorta in a 2-year-old girl with severe tetralogy of Fallot. The aorta (*Ao*) is larger than normal. The anterior wall of the aortic root (*broad arrow*) and the top of the ventricular septum are not continuous. Instead, the top of the ventricular septum appears in the middle of the aortic root, indicating overriding of the aorta. The space between the septum and the anterior wall of the aortic root corresponds to the ventricular septal defect. The aortic valve and the mitral valve are in fibrous continuity (*FC*). Aortic-to-mitral valve fibrous continuity excludes double-outlet right ventricle. Overriding of the aorta also occurs with truncus arteriosus. If a separate pulmonary valve is demonstrated, truncus is exluded. Minimal diastolic flutter of the mitral valve is noted, although the aortogram showed no aortic regurgitation. The mechanism of this flutter may be the right-to-left shunt during diastole impinging upon the anterior leaflet of the mitral valve. *RV* = right ventricle; *LV* = left ventricle.

B and **B'** represent a long axis sector scan of the ventricles in a different patient during diastole and systole. Aortic override is again demonstrated along with aortic-to-mitral valve fibrous continuity. The ventricular septum appears in the middle of the aortic root. The ventricular septal defect is indicated by an *arrow*. *RV* = right ventricle; *LV* = left ventricle; *Ao.V* = aortic valve; *Ao* = aortic root.

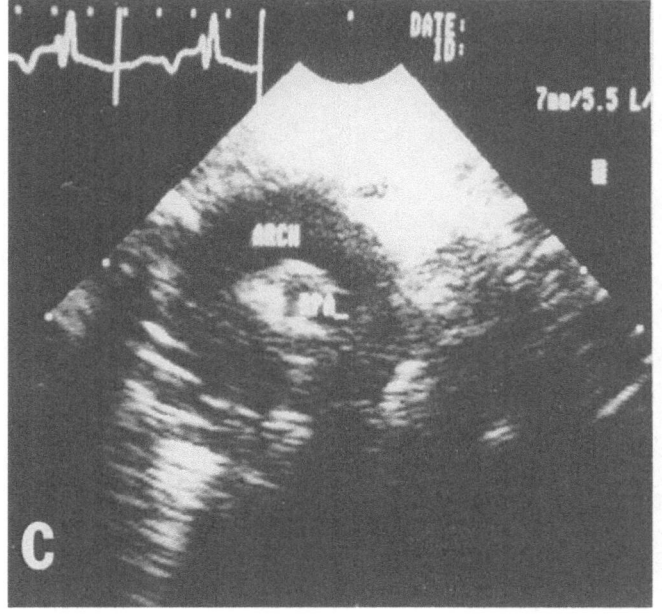
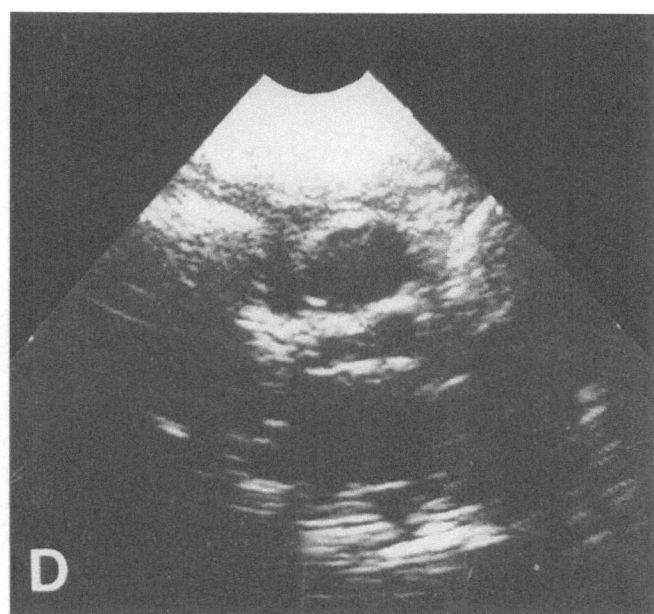
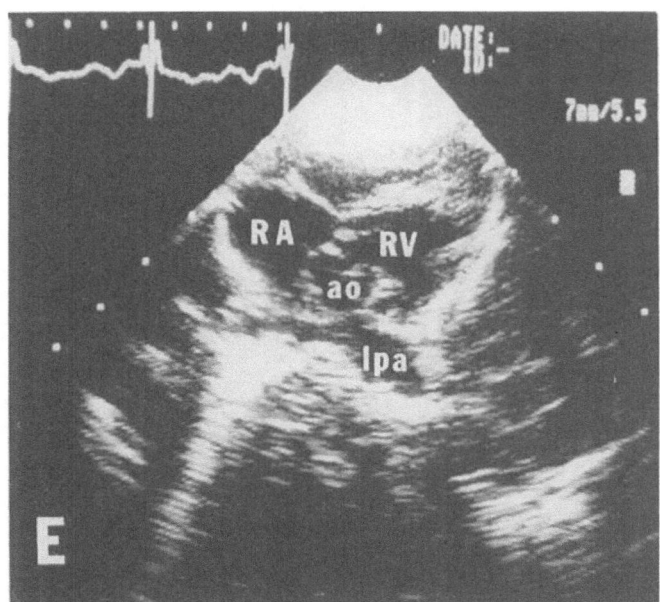
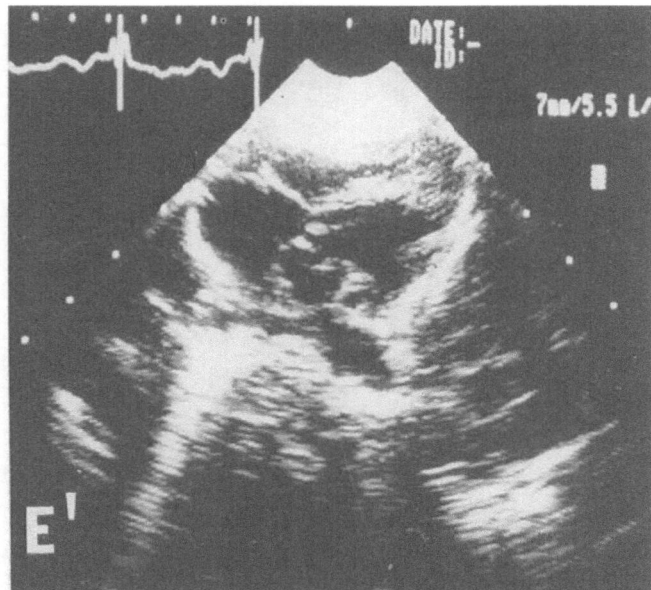

C and **D** are views from the suprasternal notch, parallel (**C**) and perpendicular (**D**) to the arch of the aorta (*arch*). In **C** the aortic arch surrounds the right pulmonary artery, which passes under it. In **D** the aortic arch appears as a circle with the right pulmonary artery cut along its length. From these two views the right pulmonary artery is measured; its size is important when a palliative shunting procedure is planned. RPA = right pulmonary artery.

E and **E′** represent a subxiphoid oblique view of the ventricles and great arteries in a neonate with tetralogy of Fallot. The apex of the right ventricle is at the top of the illustration (closest to the transducer). The transducer is angled through the aortic valve, but posterior to the arch of the aorta. At this angle the pulmonary arteries are demonstrated behind the aortic root. Again the position and size of the pulmonary branches are important surgical considerations. This view is also very helpful in demonstrating infundibular narrowing if present. *RA* = right atrium; *RV* = right ventricle; *ao* = aorta; *lpa* = left pulmonary artery. (*Continued*)

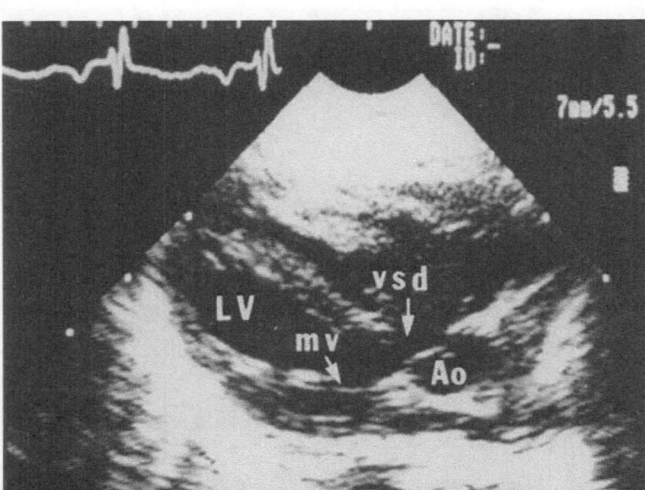

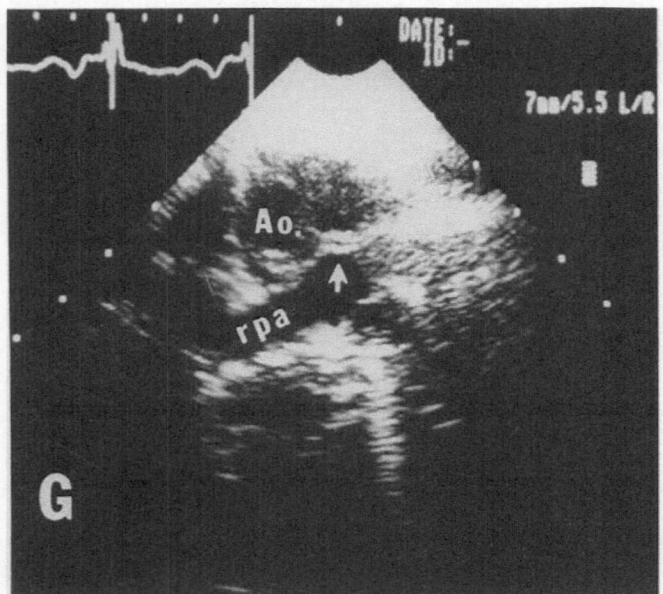

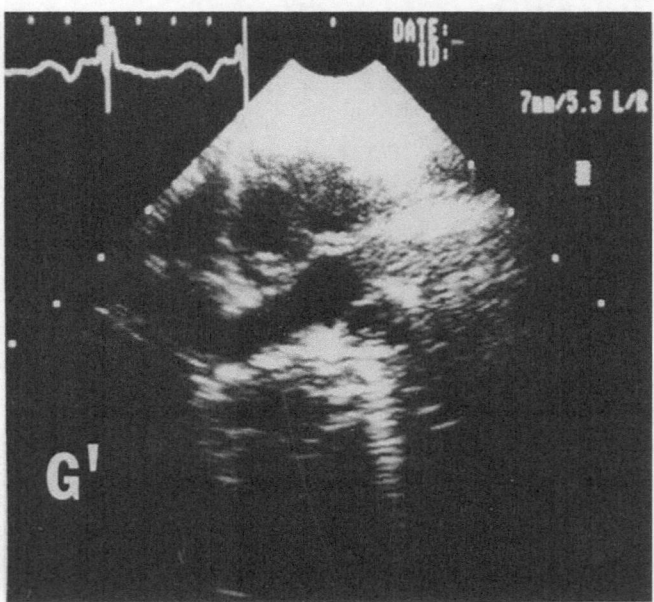

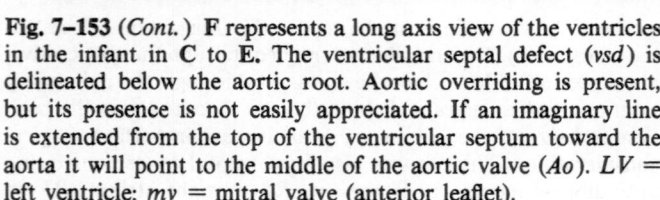

Fig. 7–153 (*Cont.*) **F** represents a long axis view of the ventricles in the infant in **C** to **E**. The ventricular septal defect (*vsd*) is delineated below the aortic root. Aortic overriding is present, but its presence is not easily appreciated. If an imaginary line is extended from the top of the ventricular septum toward the aorta it will point to the middle of the aortic valve (*Ao*). *LV* = left ventricle; *mv* = mitral valve (anterior leaflet).

G and **G'** represent a short axis view at the level of the great arteries in the same patient. The pulmonic valve (*arrow*) is thickened and does not open during systole. These findings indicate atresia or critical pulmonic stenosis. Nevertheless, the valve moves posteriorly during ventricular systole so that its motion on M-mode is similar to that of a patent pulmonic valve. *Ao.* = aorta; *rpa* = right pulmonary artery.

Fig. 7–154. *Tetralogy of Fallot with a left aortic arch* (**A**) *and tetralogy of Fallot with a right aortic arch* (**B**). **A** In this roentgenogram of the chest in a patient with tetralogy of Fallot the heart is of normal size. The apex is uplifted and rounded secondary to hypertrophy of the right ventricle. The pulmonary artery segment is concave. Pulmonary undercirculation is present. The arch of the aorta is left sided. **B** is a roentgenogram of the chest in a 2-year-old boy with pseudotruncus. The heart is enlarged with rounding and uplifting of the apex and concavity of the main pulmonary artery segment (boot-shaped heart). The aortic arch is on the right, indenting the trachea.

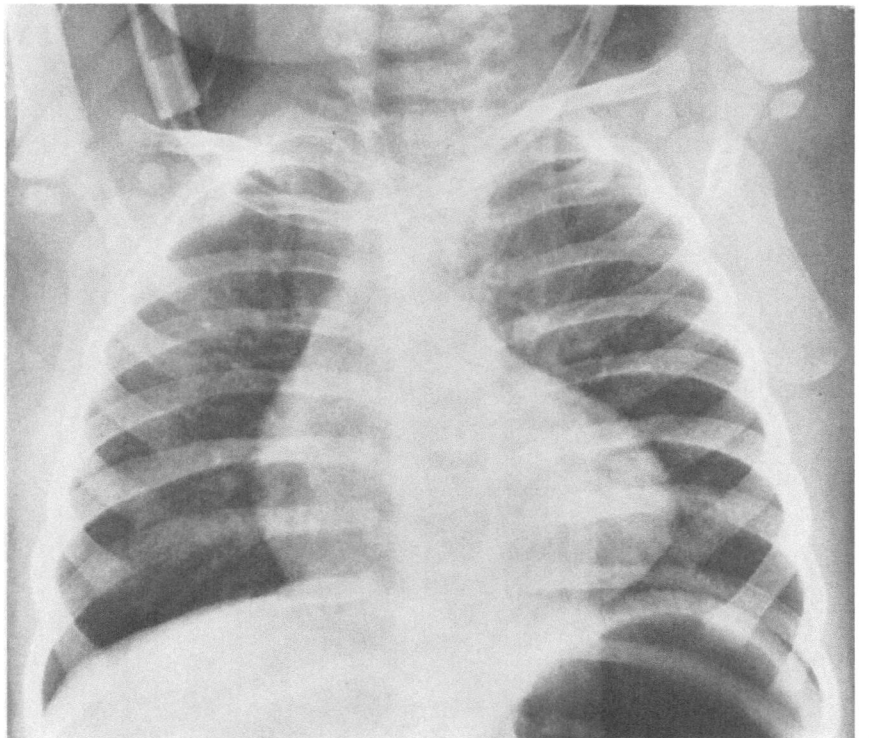

A

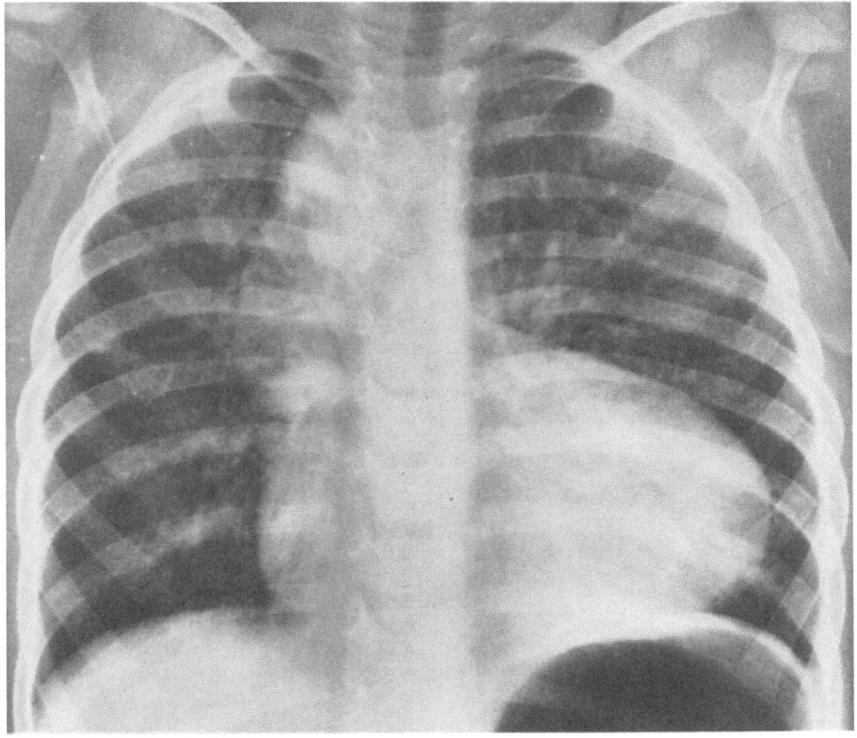

B

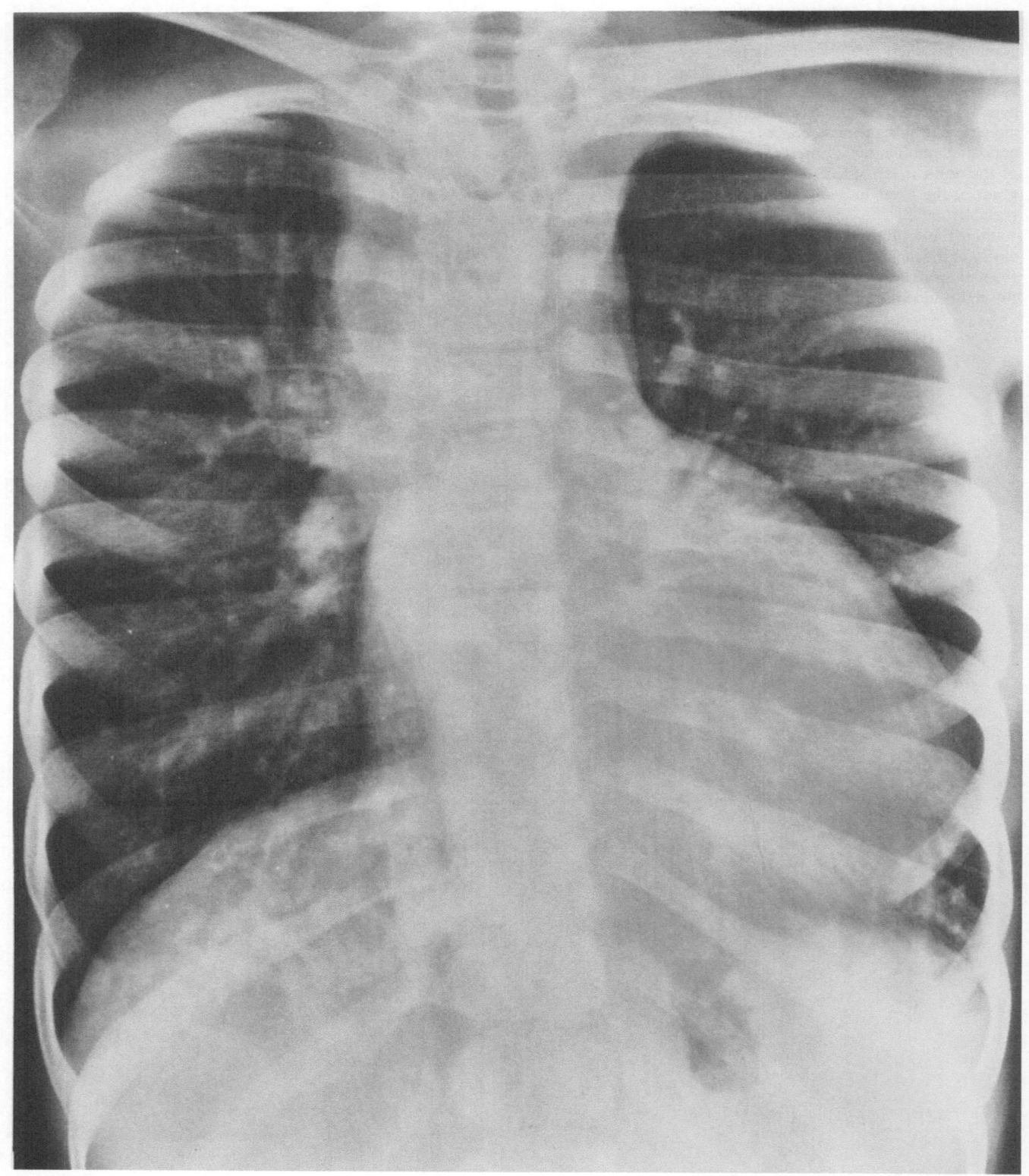

A

Fig. 7–155. *Variegated appearance of the pulmonary vasculature in pulmonary atresia (pseudotruncus), with systemic collateral circulation to the lung.* **A** Frontal film of the chest; **B** frame from the frontal view of a right ventriculogram; **C** a later frame from the right ventriculogram in B; **D** subtraction film from an angiogram illustrating the origin of the systemic collateral vessels from the descending thoracic aorta. **A** The right upper and middle lobes show overcirculation. The left upper lobe also shows dilatation of the pulmonary arteries. The right lower lobe has a small

area of overcirculation adjacent to the cardiophrenic angle. The remainder of the lungs shows undercirculation. The heart is enlarged with a right-sided aortic arch.

The right ventriculogram (**B**) demonstrates a hypoplastic pulmonary outflow tract with atresia of the pulmonary valve. The right ventricle fills the aorta through the ventricular septal defect (right-to-left shunt). **C** systemic collateral vessels from the descending thoracic and abdominal aorta (celiac axis) supply the lungs. The vessels to the right upper lobe and lower lobes are

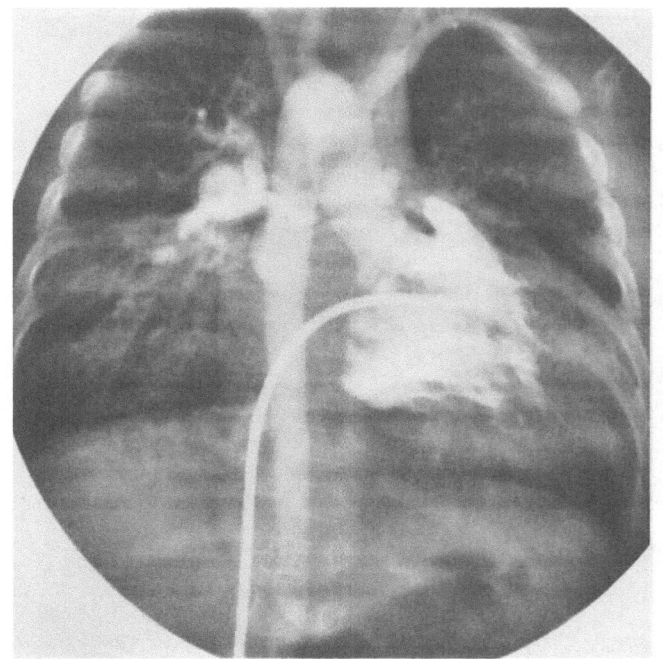

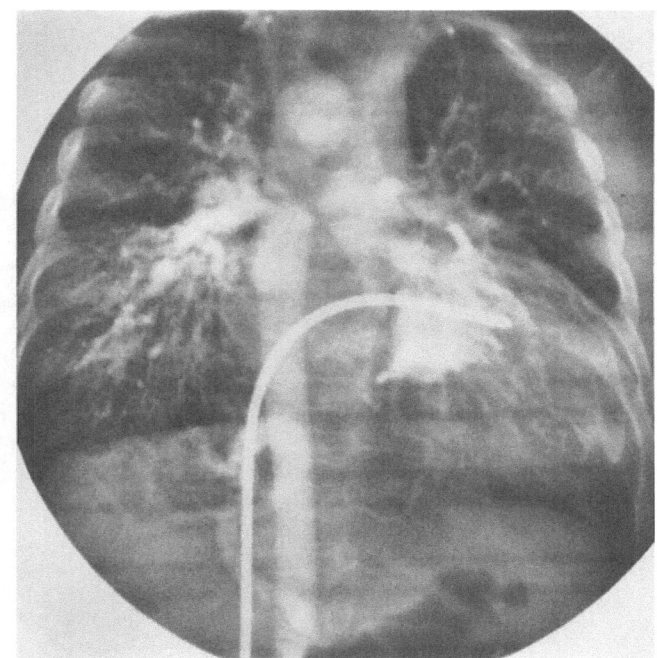

B

C

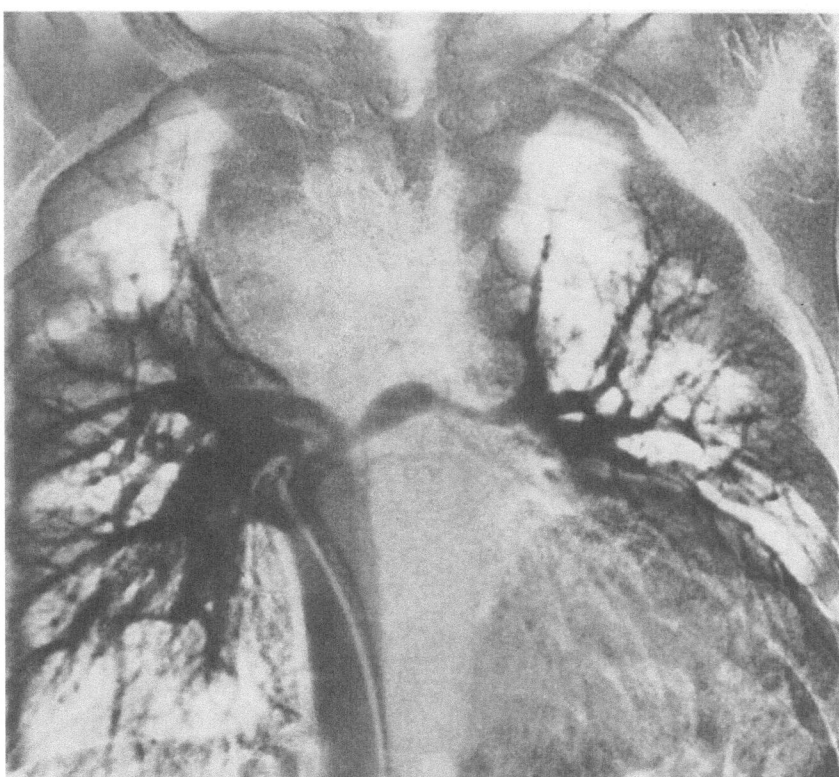

D

not stenotic, and pulmonary overcirculation is present in those areas. The subtraction film **(D)** shows stenosis of the left pulmonary artery, while the peripheral vessels to the left upper lobe show poststenotic dilatation.

Note the right aortic arch with mirror-image branching **(B).** The innominate artery is on the left, and the right carotid and right subclavian arteries arise as the second and third branches on the right.

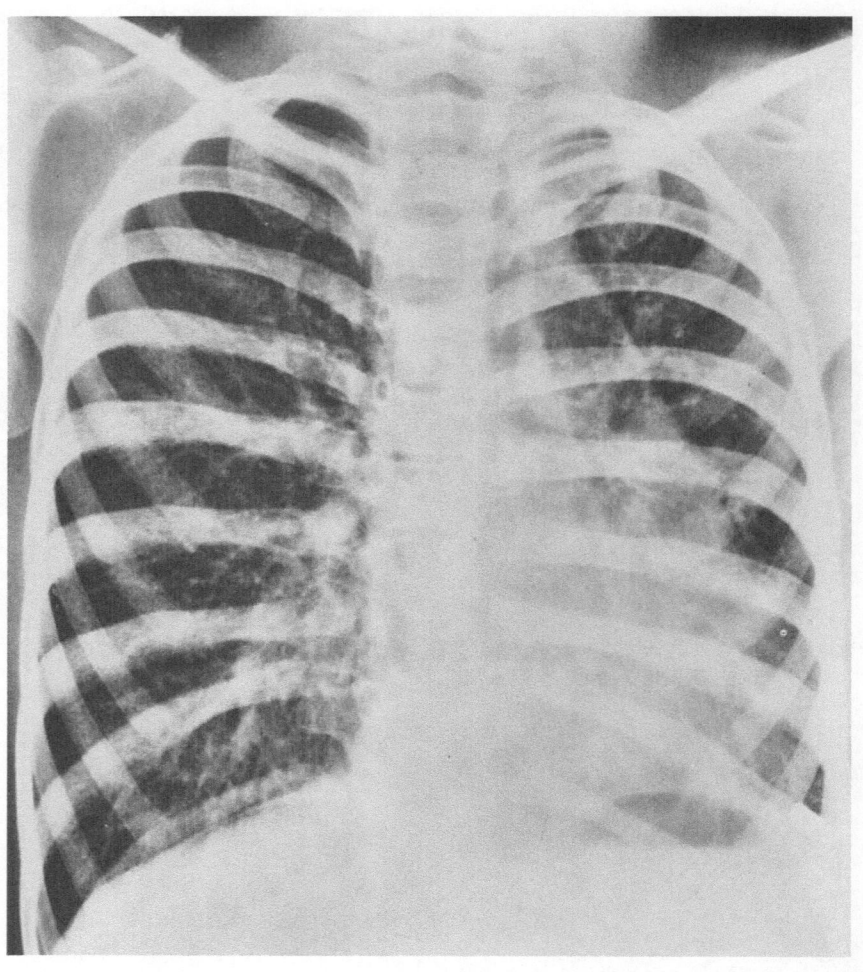

A

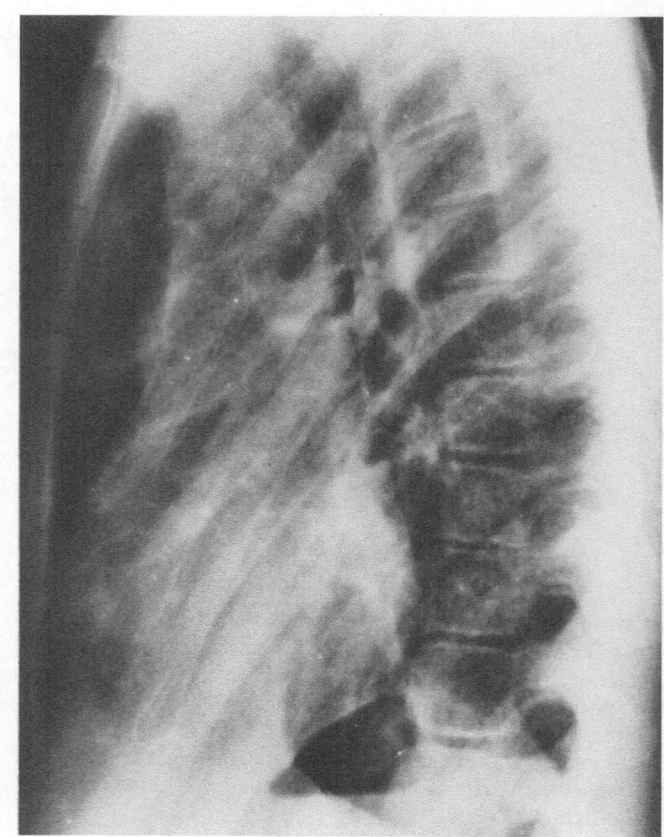

B

Fig. 7–156. *Hypoplasia of the left lung due to absence of the left pulmonary artery in a 7-year-old girl with tetralogy of Fallot.* On the frontal projection (**A**) the mediastinum is shifted to the left because of loss of volume of the left lung. No distinct left pulmonary artery is identified. Pulmonary undercirculation is present on the left. The trachea is indented on the right by a right-sided aortic arch. On the lateral view (**B**) the density normally formed by the left pulmonary artery is absent. Because of a clinical history of cyanosis, tetralogy of Fallot and absence of the left pulmonary artery may be suspected rather than unilateral pulmonary fibrosis secondary to an inflammatory process (unilateral hyperlucent lung, Swyer-James syndrome). The right ventriculogram (**C**) demonstrates a hypertrophied right ventricle

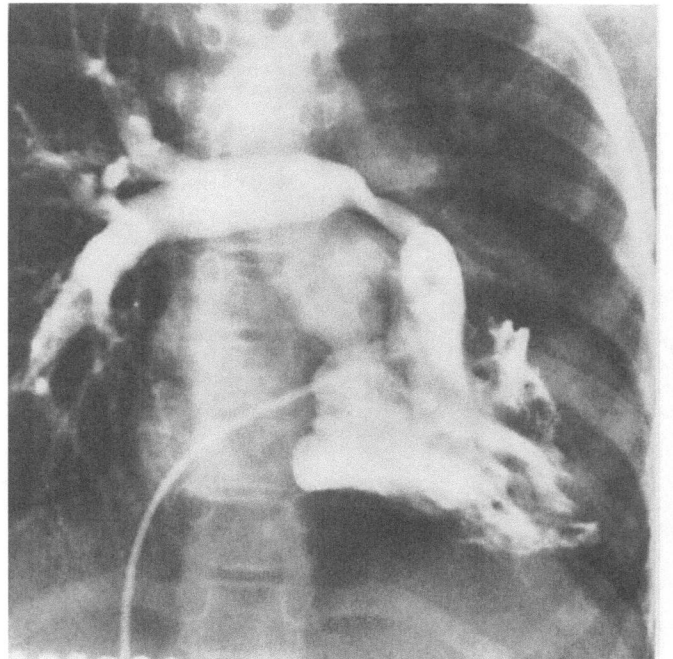

C

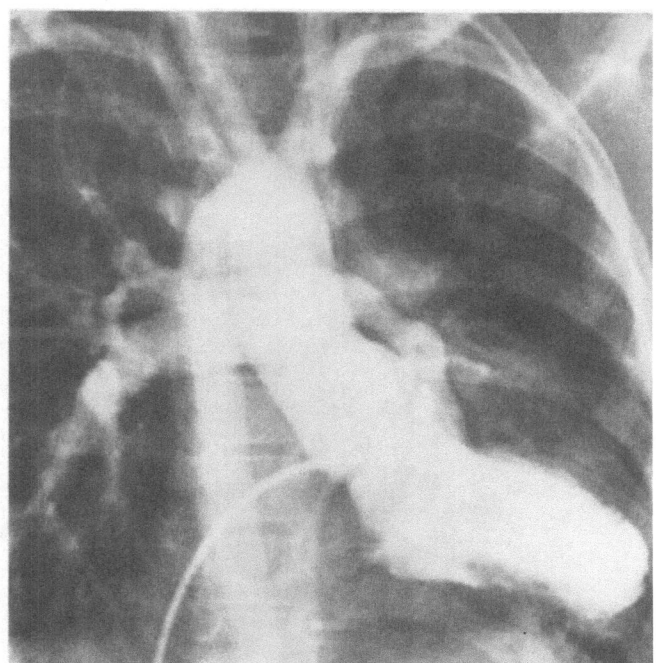

D

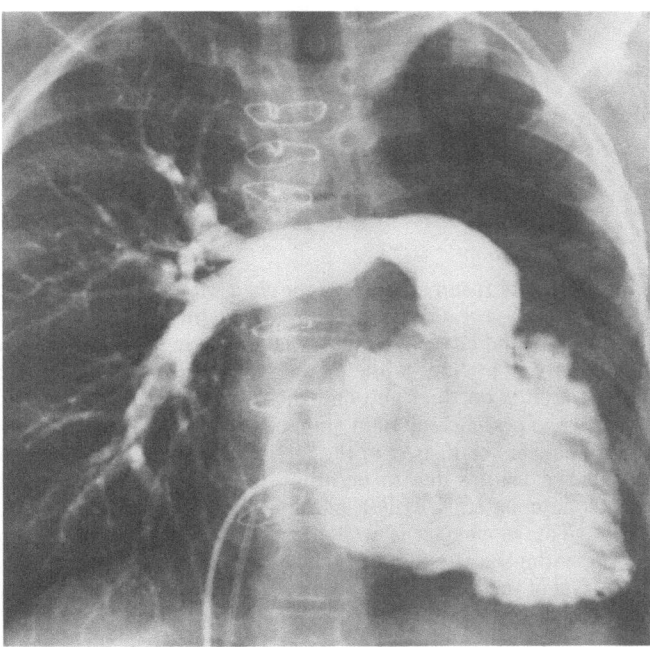

E

with a right-to-left shunt at the ventricular level that fills the aorta faintly. The pulmonary valve is hypoplastic and stenosed. The main pulmonary artery is also hypoplastic. The left pulmonary artery is absent. The left ventriculogram (**D**) shows the right-sided aortic arch with mirror-image branching. The infundibulum and pulmonary artery fill by way of the ventricular septal defect (the shunt is bidirectional). At surgery the ventricular septal defect was repaired, and the outflow tract of the right ventricle and the main pulmonary artery were widened by a pericardial patch. The postoperative right ventriculogram (**E**) delineates the wide infundibulum and main pulmonary artery. No right-to-left shunt is evident.

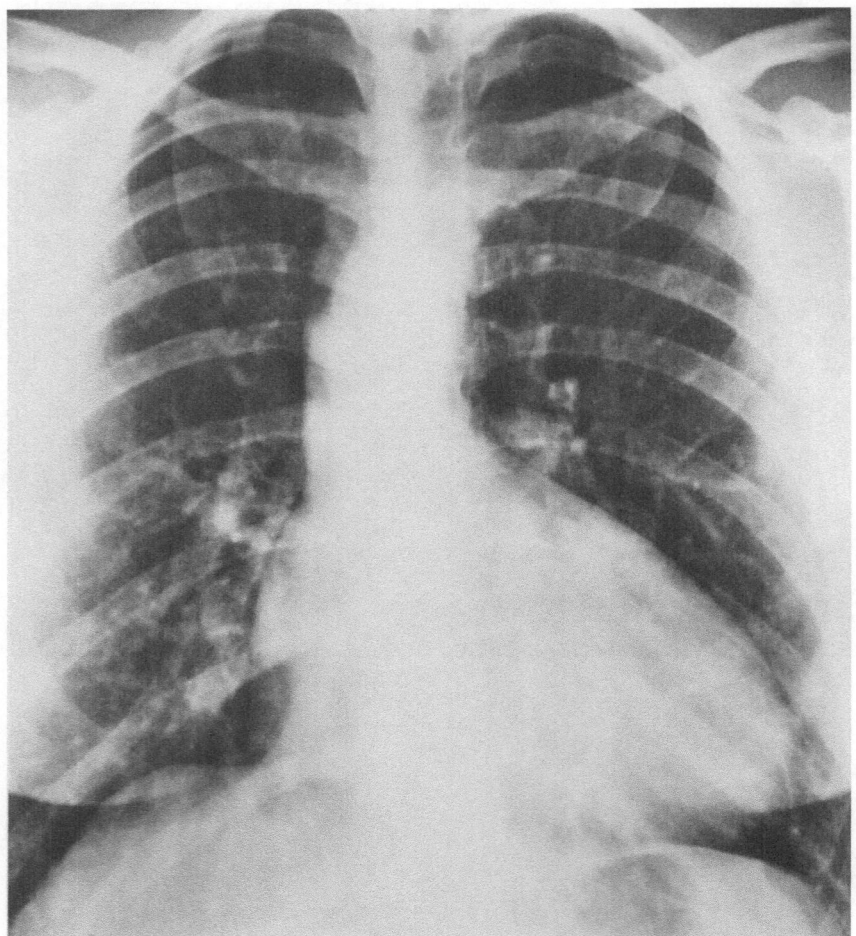

A

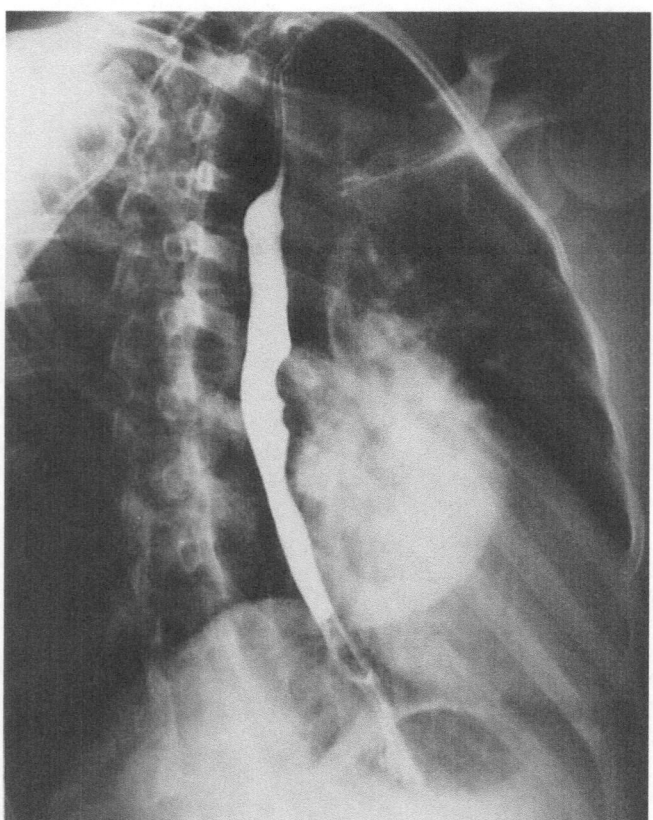

B

Fig. 7–157. *A roentgenogram of the chest with a barium esophagogram in a 25-year-old woman with severe tetralogy of Fallot (pseudotruncus)* and large systemic vessels supplying the lungs. **A** Cardiomegaly is present, with the apex uplifted and rounded. The aortic arch is on the right, and the main pulmonary segment is concave. The left and right pulmonary arteries have relatively small calibers compared to the interlobar vessels, which are distended, a feature due to perfusion of the interlobar vessels by systemic collaterals. **B** is a barium esophagogram in the RAO view. The esophagus is well filled, and multiple indentations, representing large systemic collaterals, are present anteriorly at the level of the hilus. This finding was confirmed by aortography.

Fig. 7–158. *Pulmonary overcirculation secondary to a Waterston anastomosis (ascending aorta to right pulmonary artery) in tetralogy of Fallot.* The heart is larger than in the preoperative film in this patient (Fig. 7–154A), and the pulmonary blood flow is increased. Pulmonary overcirculation is most marked on the right. The Blalock-Taussig anastomosis (subclavian to pulmonary artery) and the polytetrafluoroethylene (Gore-Tex) tubular prosthesis are preferred in some centers because excessive pulmonary blood flow occurs less frequently with these two operative procedures.

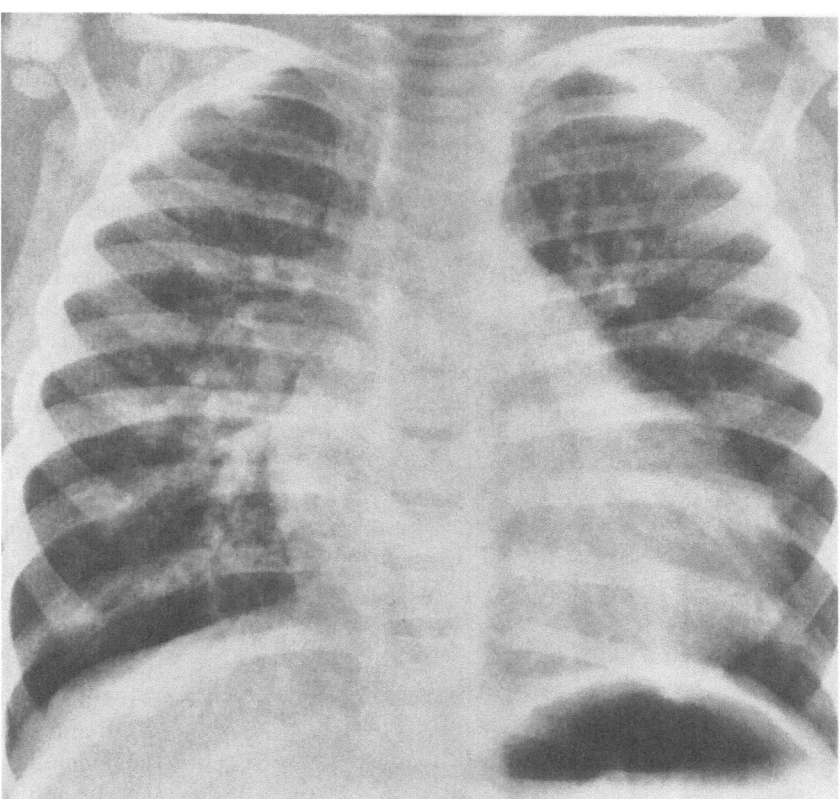

an indentation on the barium esophagogram posteriorly (Fig. 7–157). A right aortic arch with an aberrant left subclavian artery, which usually occurs as an isolated defect, indents the esophagus, thus allowing differentiation between the two most common varieties of right aortic arch. Indentations secondary to large bronchial collaterals in pseudotruncus are usually multiple; they indent the esophagus anteriorly and at a lower level, usually in the area of the hilus (Fig. 7–157B). These various indentations should not be confused with an aberrant left subclavian artery or with mediastinal lymph nodes.

Variations of the classic features of TOF depend on the severity of the pulmonic stenosis and the presence of associated malformations. The heart may be normal in size or enlarged. The pulmonary artery segment may be concave, may be normal, or may even bulge because of poststenotic dilatation of the pulmonary trunk or dilatation of the infundibulum. The aorta is usually large, and the pulmonary vasculature may be normal, decreased or even increased (noncyanotic tetralogy of Fallot or "pink" tetralogy). The authors have observed patients with a variegated pulmonary vascular pattern—that is, areas of overcirculation interspersed with areas of undercirculation (Fig. 7–155). This pattern occurs in patients with TOF and pulmonary atresia (pseudotruncus) with systemic collateral vessels to the lungs. The collateral vessels without stenosis result in pulmonary overcirculation, whereas collateral vessels with stenosis cause diminished vascularity. Absence of a pulmonary artery will result in ipsilateral hypoplasia of the lung (Fig. 7–156). An ectopic pulmonary artery arising from the aorta will be accompanied by severe overcirculation (see Fig. 7–223 in section on hemitruncus).

Aorta-to-pulmonary artery shunt procedures performed for palliation of TOF may result in unilateral or bilateral pulmonary overcirculation (Fig. 7–158). Aneurysmal dilatation of the right or left pulmonary artery (or both) occurs with TOF and absence of the pulmonary valve (see Fig. 7–164; also see discussion of hemitruncus).

Hemodynamics The pressures in the RV and LV are usually equal, whereas low pressure is encountered in the pulmonary artery. On withdrawal of the catheter from the main pulmonary artery through the infundibulum into the RV a pressure gradient is recorded. On occasion an additional gradient is observed at the pulmonary valve (Fig. 7–141). The severity of the resistance across the RV outflow tract and pulmonary valve determines the degree of right-to-left shunting. In mild cases the shunt may be left-to-right with high O_2 saturation in the RV. In moderately severe cases a bidirectional shunt is demonstrated. The usual finding, however, is of predominantly or solely right-to-left shunting (absence of or minimal oxygen "step-up" in the RV). Even though the shunt is through the VSD, the extent of desaturation (severity of right-to-left shunting) is best determined in the aorta and peripheral arteries, rather than in the LV. The oxygen saturation of the LA is normal, while the LV saturation is usually intermediate between that of the LA and aorta. LA desaturation may indicate tricuspid insufficiency or RV failure, resulting in

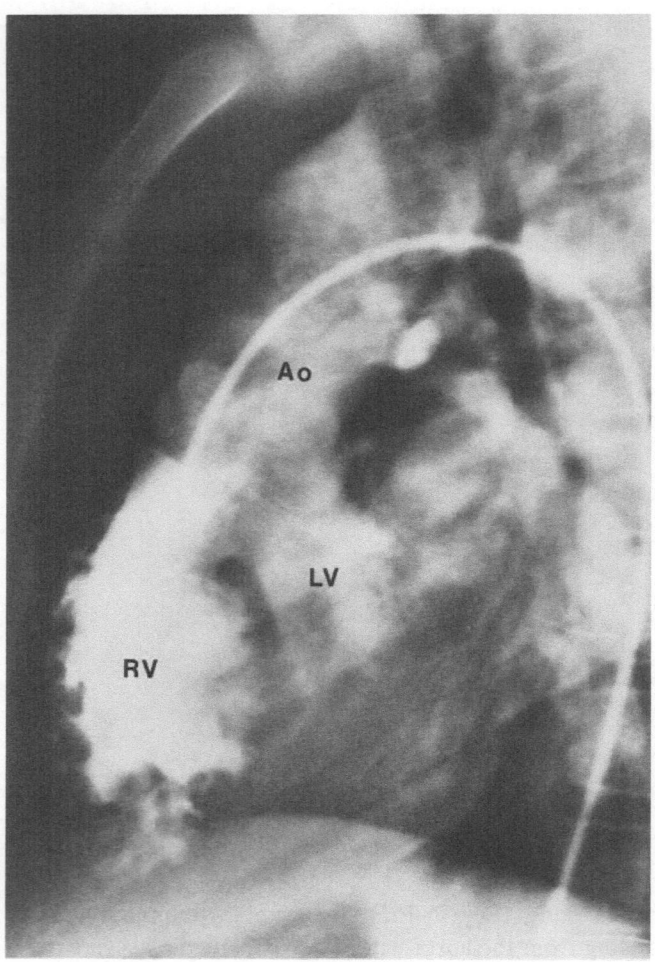

Fig. 7–159. *Right ventricular angiogram (lateral projection) in a 5-year-old girl with tetralogy of Fallot.* The VSD shunts from right to left, and the aortic valve overrides the ventricular septum. RV = right ventricle; LV = left ventricle; Ao = aorta. Note that the catheter enters the right ventricle through the aortic valve.

a right-to-left atrial shunt. In the presence of a palliative systemic-to-pulmonary shunt an oxygen step-up may be sensed in the pulmonary artery. If the shunt is large, pulmonary pressure may be elevated.

Contrast Studies The typical angiographic features of TOF are overriding of the aorta above the ventricular septum and a VSD with a right-to-left shunt (Fig. 7–159), best demonstrated by right ventriculography in the lateral view. The right ventriculogram is also useful for demonstration of the site of obstruction (stenosis or atresia). The frontal view is particularly helpful in assessment of infundibular stenosis (Fig. 7–160A). Obstruction of the os infundibuli results in a third chamber, representing the infundibulum, which intrinsically is relatively unaffected (Fig. 7–160B and C). The presence and degree of stenosis or atresia of the pulmonary valve are also assessed. A bicuspid pulmonary valve is frequently demonstrated (Fig. 7–161). Its appearance has been noted to resemble a bivalve clam, but the authors believe the appearance is more like "Pac Man" with the mouth open. With atresia of the pulmonary valve the outflow tract of the RV ends blindly (Fig. 7–155B).

The left ventriculogram demonstrates fibrous continuity between the aortic valve and the mitral valve, excluding double-outlet right ventricle. The coronary arteries, ductus arteriosus, palliative shunt procedures, and systemic collateral vessels are also evaluated through a left ventriculogram or aortogram. Assessment of coronary artery anatomy may require a selective injection. Palliative shunts are imaged to determine their size and to ascertain the presence of damage to the pulmonary arteries associated with the shunt (e.g., kinking and occlusion). In individuals with pulmonary atresia, injection into the shunt or into a systemic collateral vessel may be the only way to assess the sizes and origins of the pulmonary arteries (Figs. 7–155B to D, 7–162). In such studies the main pulmonary artery tapers to form the shape of a bird's beak pointing toward the RV outflow tract; the distance between the artery and the RV outflow tract is important in planning surgery.

Associated defects that may be delineated on angiography are absence of the left pulmonary artery, left hemitruncus, absence of the pulmonary valve and A-V communis (see appropriate section for descriptions of these entities). **Treatment** Emergency treatment of newborn infants with TOF and severe cyanosis (pulmonary atresia, pseudotruncus) includes maintenance of patency of the ductus arteriosus by infusion of prostglandin E_1 until surgery can be performed. Cyanotic spells are treated with oxygen, sodium bicarbonate, and morphine. Once cyanotic spells are manifest surgical treatment becomes urgent as brain damage and death may result from further spells. Propranolol is occasionally used to control spells if surgery must be delayed.

Two surgical approaches are available for TOF: palliative and complete repair. Palliative procedures include "shunt" operations to augment pulmonary blood flow (systemic artery-to-pulmonary artery anastomosis; e.g., subclavian artery to pulmonary artery [Blalock-Taussig], aorta to left pulmonary artery [Potts], ascending aorta to right pulmonary artery [Waterston, Cooley], prosthetic tubular grafts—a Gore-Tex graft [polytetrafluoroethylene]). The Brock operation is another palliative procedure, consisting of pulmonary valvulotomy for the relief of pulmonic stenosis. A similar approach to palliation involves a pulmonary outflow patch without repair of VSD. Definitive repair of TOF includes closure of the VSD and relief of the pulmonic stenosis by means of cardiopulmonary bypass or total circulatory arrest (deep hypothermia). A RV outflow tract patch is usually interposed by means of a vertical ventriculotomy. If necessary, the ventriculotomy is extended across the pulmonary valve ring to the bifurcation of the pulmonary artery. Babies are normally considered for definitive repair by the age of 2 years. Contraindications to primary repair of TOF during infancy include atresia of the infundibulum or pulmonary trunk, severely hypoplastic pulmonary arteries and anomalous origin of the left anterior descending artery from the right coronary artery. Coexistence of an A-V communis also greatly increases the risk of total repair in infancy. Palliative procedures are often recommended

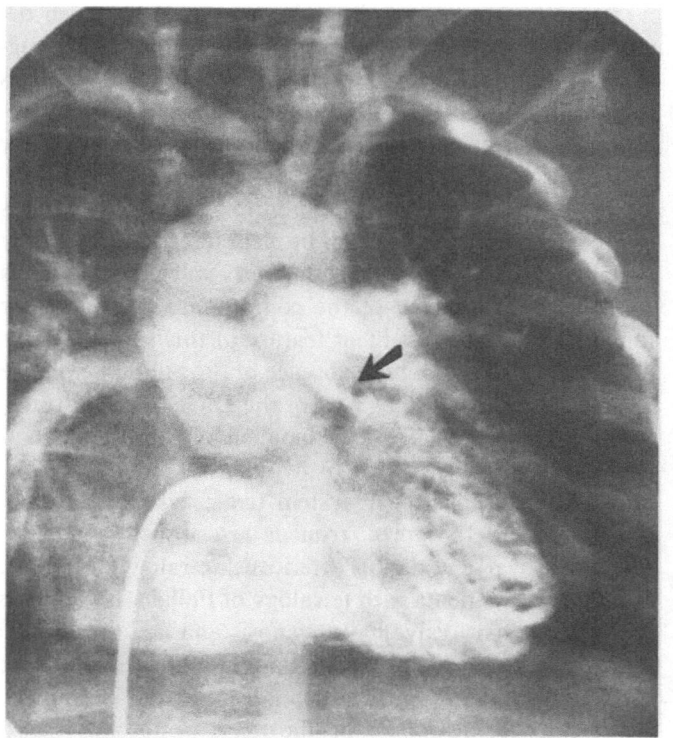

A

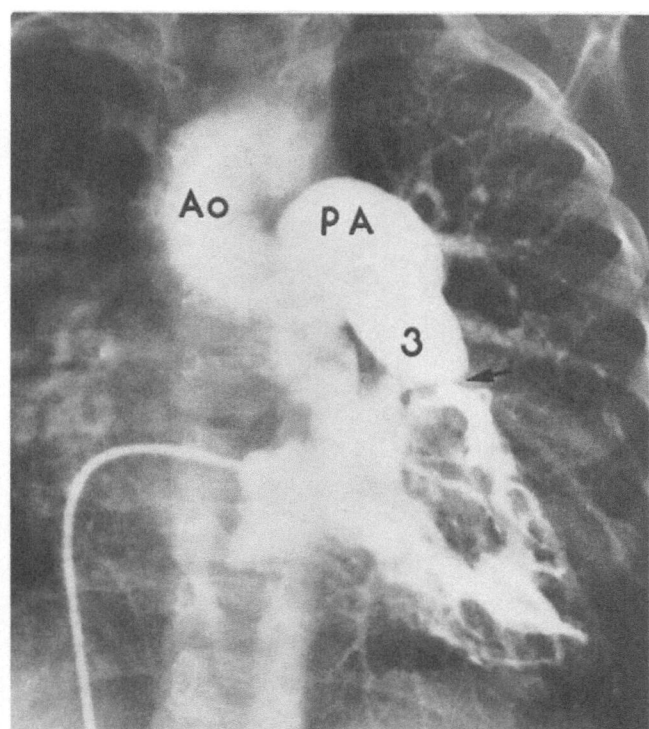

B

Fig. 7–160. *Infundibular pulmonic stenosis in two patients with tetralogy of Fallot.* **A** is the frontal view of a right ventriculogram in an 8-month-old boy showing severe infundibular pulmonic stenosis (*arrow*). **B** and **C** are frontal and lateral views of a right ventriculogram in the patient in Figure 7–154A showing stenosis of the os infundibuli with dilatation of the right ventricular outflow tract (third chamber, *3*). *Ao* = aorta; *PA* = pulmonary artery.

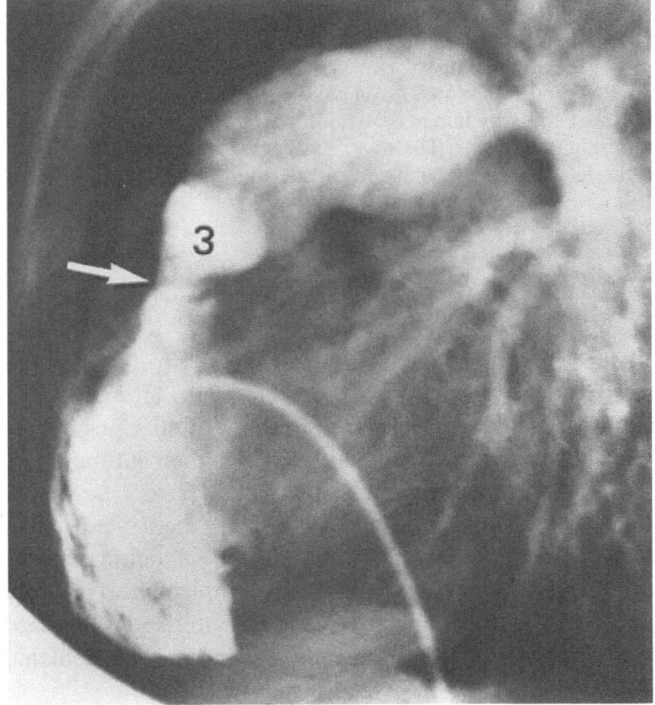

C

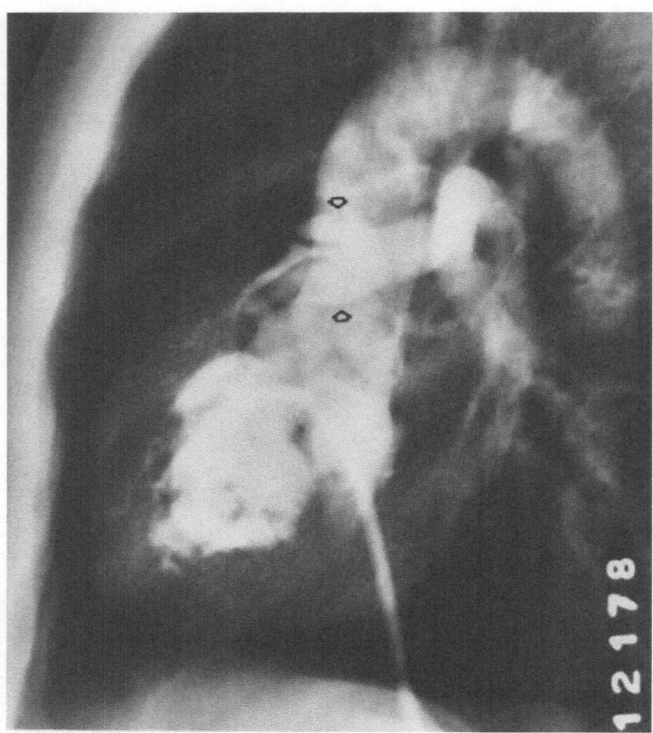

Fig. 7–161. *Lateral view of a right ventriculogram in a 1-year-old boy with tetralogy of Fallot.* The bicuspid pulmonary valve is reminiscent of Pac Man with the mouth open, the semilunar sinuses forming the disk (*arrows*) and the open valve leaflets forming the mouth. Below the valve a streak of contrast medium represents the tiny lumen of the outflow tract of the right ventricle (diffusely narrowed). The overriding aorta and the outflow tract of the left ventricle opacify from this site.

in presence of these associated features, while complete repair is delayed until later in childhood.

Postoperative Findings Pulmonary valve insufficiency occurs frequently after repair of tetralogy of Fallot and may result in chronic enlargement of the RV. Other postoperative findings include residual VSD, residual infundibular or valvar PS, stenosis of the pulmonary artery beyond a transanular patch and aneurysm of the right ventricular outflow tract (Fig. 7–163). Arrhythmias, including premature ventricular contractions and complete heart block, may occur immediately after surgery or may occur late postoperatively. The risk of infective endocarditis remains even after definitive repair of tetralogy of Fallot.

Tetralogy of Fallot with Absence of the Pulmonary Valve
This syndrome consists of absence of the pulmonary valve, stenosis of the pulmonary ring, ventricular septal defect and aneurysmal dilatation of the pulmonary arteries. Infundibular stenosis may also be present.

Absence of the pulmonary valve has been described in association with patent ductus arteriosus, atrial septal defect, double-outlet right ventricle, endocardial cushion defect, Marfan syndrome and ventricular septal defects without stenosis of the pulmonary ring.

Recently, absence of the pulmonic valve has been described with agenesis of the ductus arteriosus. It is suggested that massive dilatation of the pulmonary arteries may be due to obstruction to forward flow caused by absence of the ductal pathway from the pulmonary artery to the descending aorta.

Rabinovitch et al. reported multiple segmental arteries that compress the distal small bronchi in cases of tetralogy of Fallot with absence of the pulmonary valve. These vessels could account for part of the compromise of pulmonary function that is a prominent feature in this syndrome.

Tetralogy of Fallot with absence of the pulmonary valve has also been observed as part of the DiGeorge syndrome, which includes defective development of the thymus and parathyroid glands (aplasia or hypoplasia) and abnormalities of the cardiovascular system (e.g., right aortic arch, interruption of the aorta, truncus arteriosus, ventricular septal defect, patent ductus arteriosus, tetralogy of Fallot).

Clinically, patients with tetralogy of Fallot with absence of the pulmonary valve have cyanosis and a characteristic murmur of pulmonary regurgitation (late in onset after A_2, low pitched and of crescendo-decrescendo character). Respiratory distress may be the main symptom, caused by the hugely dilated pulmonary arteries compressing the bronchi, which results in lobar emphysema with or without mediastinal shift and herniation of the lung. RV hypertrophy is usually noted on electrocardiography.

Roentgenograms of the chest (Fig. 7–164) show moderate to marked cardiomegaly with large central pulmonary arteries and normal to diminished pulmonary vascularity. A right-sided aortic arch is often present. The lungs are hyperinflated (pattern of lobar emphysema) with or without atelectasis. Echocardiography demonstrates overriding of the aortic valve consistent with tetralogy of Fallot. In addition, dilatation of the RV and paradoxical motion of the interventricular septum result from the volume overload secondary to the pulmonic regurgitation. The massively dilated pulmonary arteries are evident in all views. Doppler echocardiography confirms the presence of pulmonary regurgitation. At catheterization the RV pressure is elevated to systemic levels. The direction of the shunt is determined by the pulmonary resistance, the size of the pulmonary ring, and the severity of narrowing of the infundibulum. Low diastolic pressure (wide pulse pressure) in the pulmonary artery is consistent with pulmonic regurgitation. At angiography the ventricular septal defect is demonstrated, together with overriding of the aorta. The pulmonary trunk and right pulmonary artery are aneurysmally dilated. The left pulmonary artery may be aneurysmally dilated, normal or small. Absence of the left pulmonary artery or anomalous origin of the left pulmonary artery from the ascending aorta (left hemitruncus) may also be observed (see Fig. 7–223). Unilateral or bilateral branch stenosis occurs on occasion. The outflow tract of the RV may be displaced to the left so that the right pulmonary artery runs horizontally over the top of the LA.

Numerous surgical procedures have been recommended

Fig. 7–162. *A systemic collateral vessel from the left subclavian artery supplies branches of both pulmonary arteries in a 14-year-old girl with severe tetralogy of Fallot (pseudotruncus). Retrograde filling has opacified the main pulmonary artery. In the frontal projection* **(A)** *the pulmonary branches arise from the main pulmonary artery, reminiscent of the wings of a flying bird. On the lateral view* **(B)** *the main pulmonary artery has the shape of a bird's beak pointing toward the right ventricular outflow tract. Most of the right lung and a significant portion of the left lung are not perfused by these vessels, necessitating the search for systemic collaterals.*

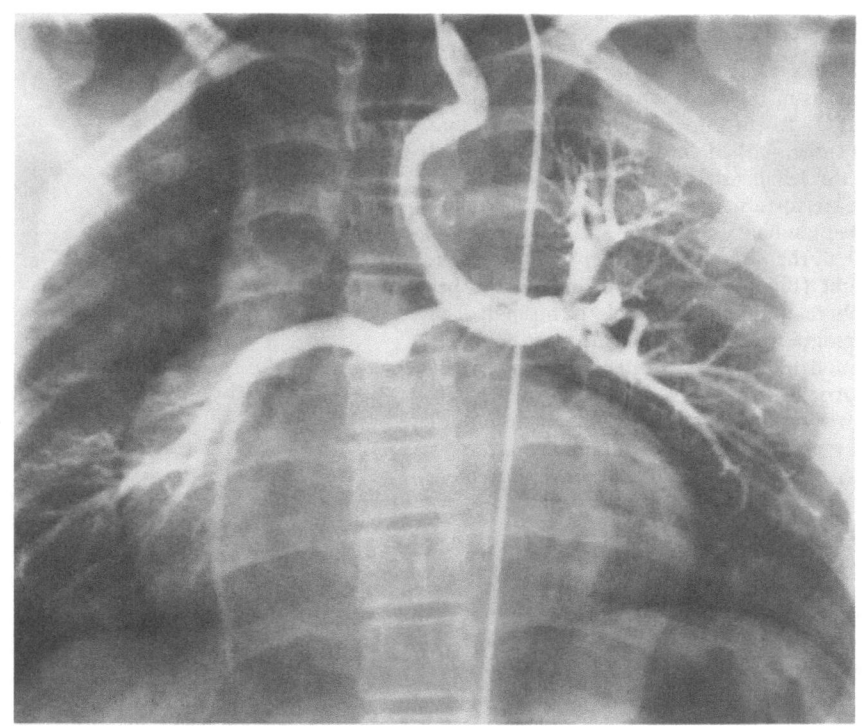

A

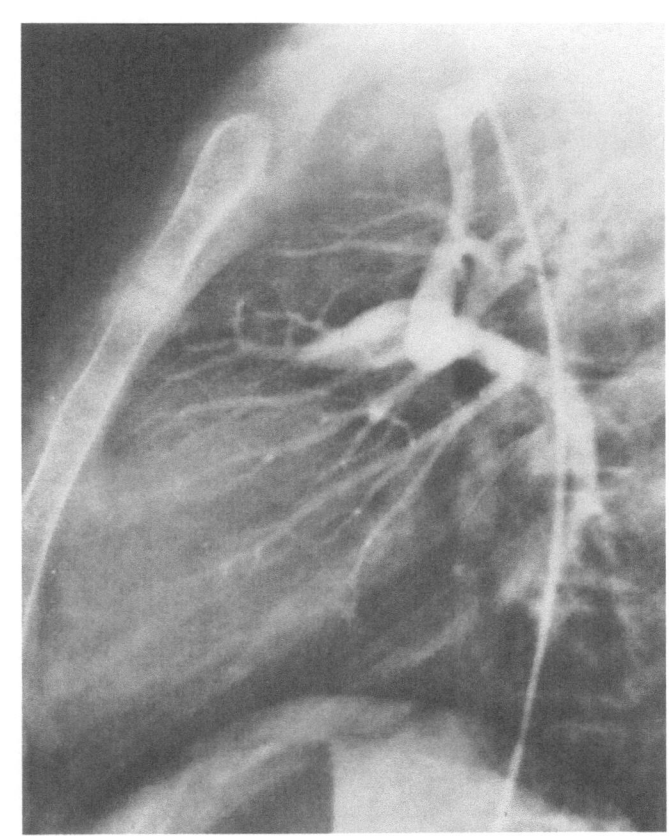

B

for infants with severe respiratory symptoms. At present the surgical results are not very encouraging.

Surgical treatment of small infants seeks to relieve respiratory symptoms by moving the dilated pulmonary arteries away from the bronchi. Plastic repairs of the aneurysmal pulmonary arteries and rerouting of the pulmonary arteries with or without suspension to the retrosternal fascia have been reported. Complete repair in older infants is similar to repair in tetralogy of Fallot. Insertion of a prosthetic pulmonary valve may improve the results. Lung function frequently remains compromised after palliative procedures and after complete repair of TOF with absence of the pulmonic valve. Persistence of pulmonary symptoms may be due to an increased number of segmental arteries that may obstruct the small distal bronchi. Obstruction of the small airways by multiple segmental vessels would not be relieved by decompression of the proximal pulmonary arteries.

Fig. 7–163. *Aneurysm of the right ventricular outflow tract after complete repair of tetralogy of Fallot using an outflow patch* (Same patient as in Figs. 7–154A, 7–158 and 7–160B and C). Roentgenograms of the chest (**A** and **B**) show marked cardiomegaly with bulging of the left heart border. On the lateral film the retrosternal clear space is obliterated. The pulmonary vessels are still enlarged, similar to the film obtained after the Waterston shunt (Fig. 7–158). The caliber of the peripheral pulmonary vessels is normal. The angiogram in the same patient (**C** and **D**) demonstrates marked dilatation of the right ventricle with a huge aneursym of the outflow tract and dilatation of the main pulmonary artery. The right pulmonary artery is narrowed at the site of the previous Waterston anastomosis.

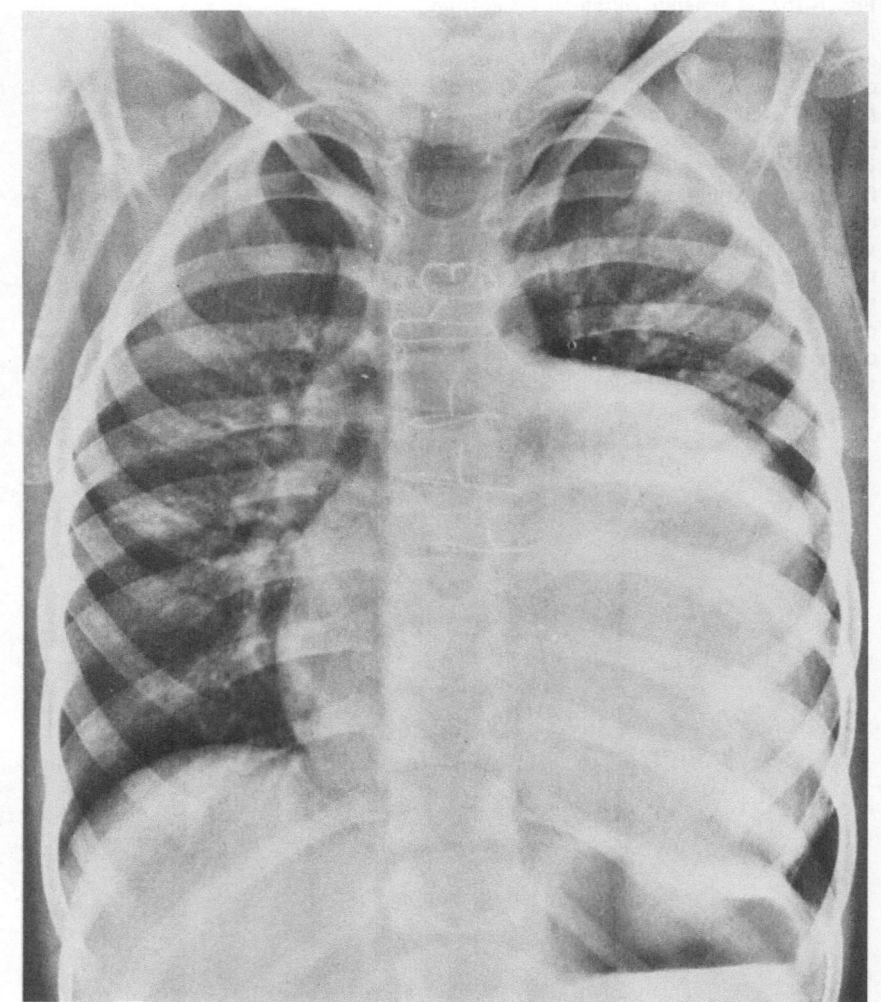

A

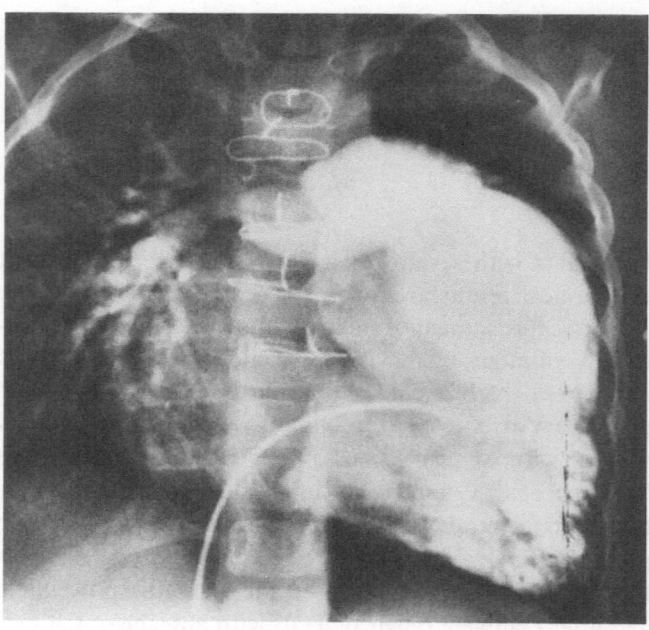

C

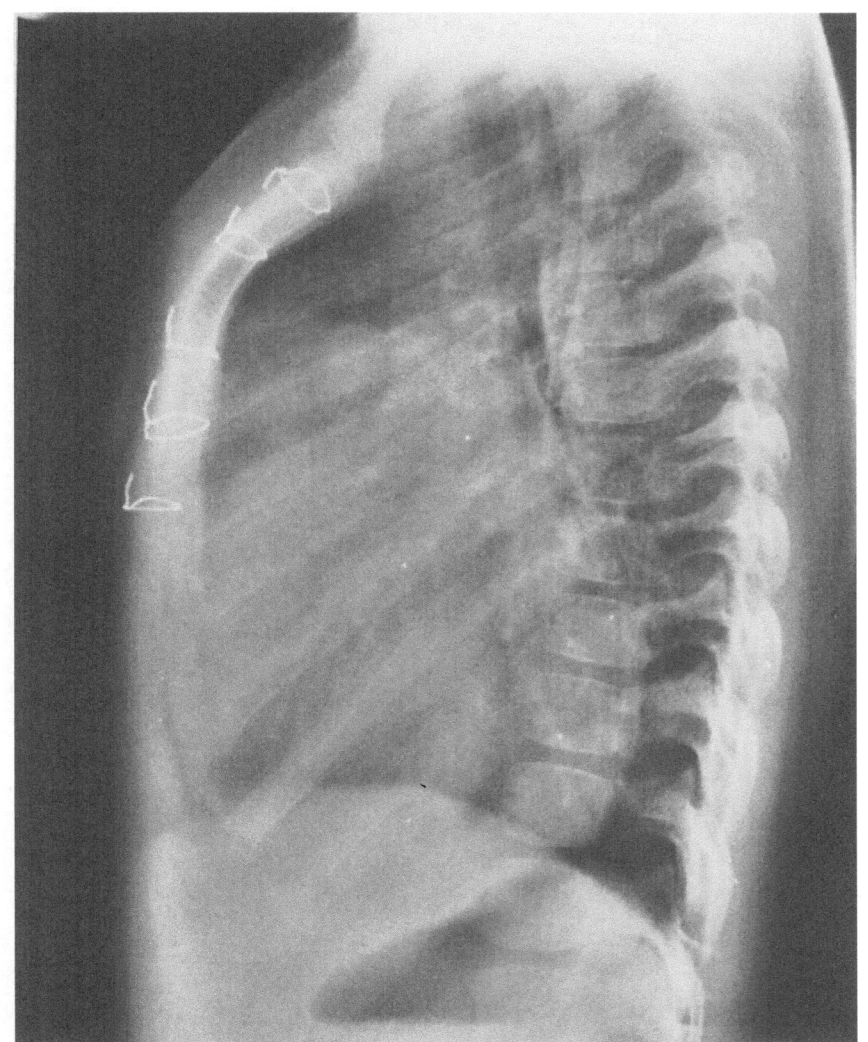

B

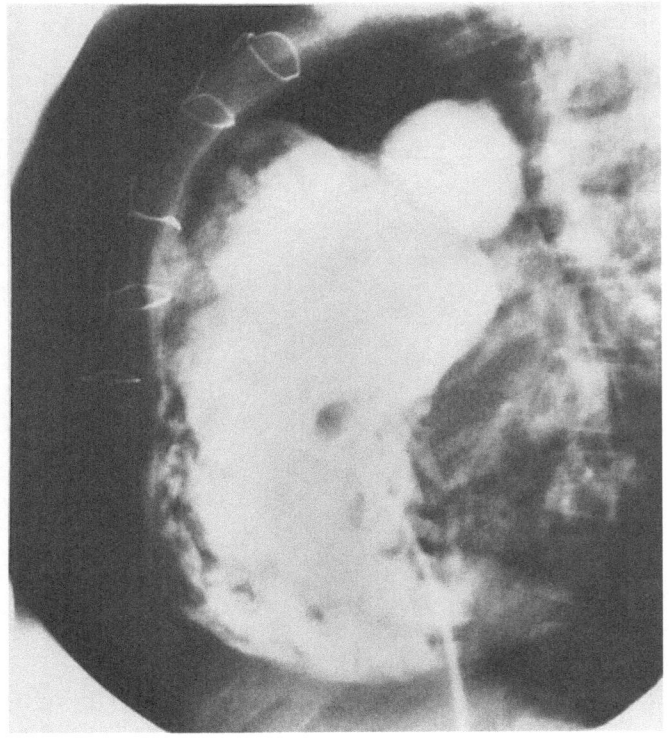

D

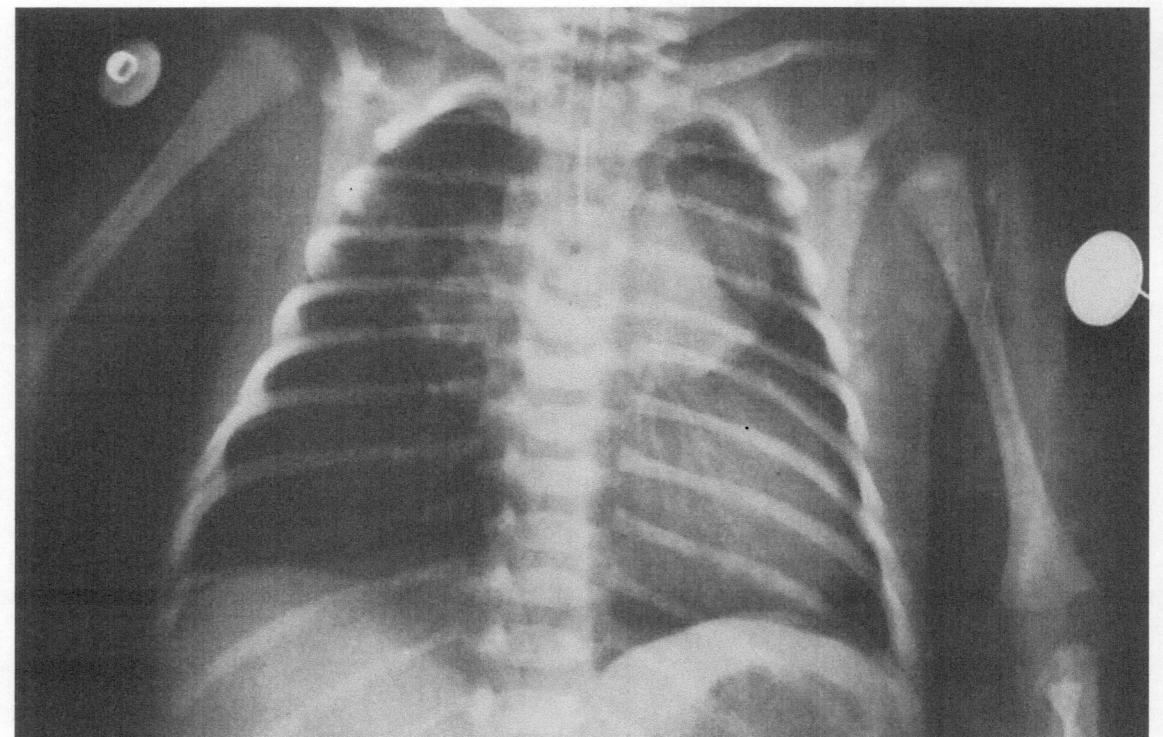

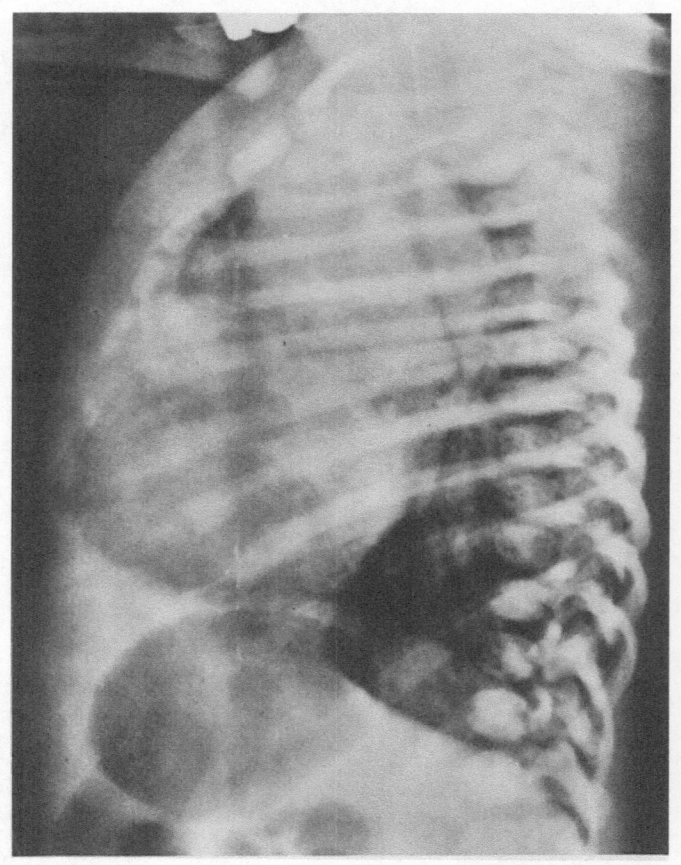

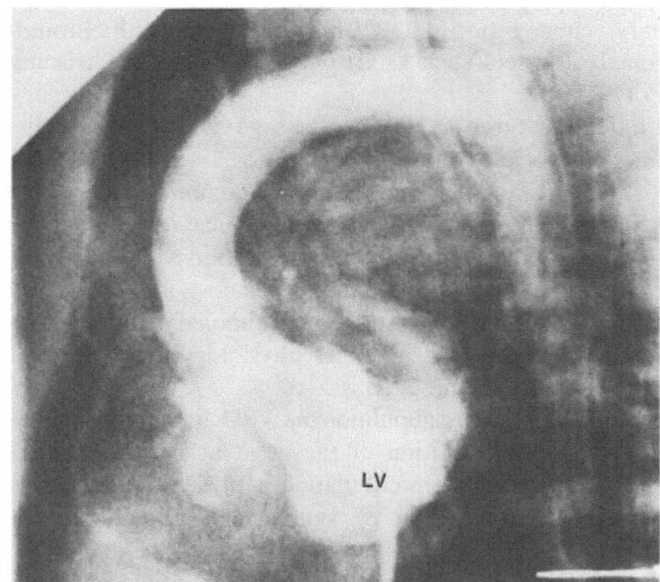

C

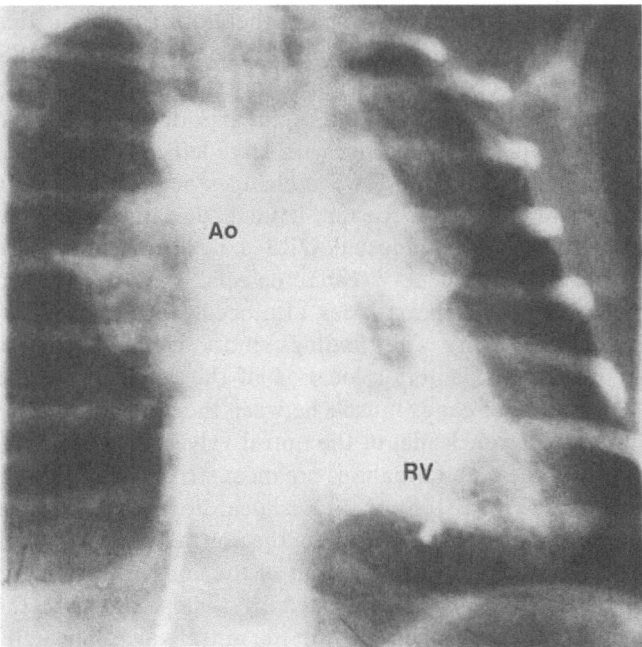

D

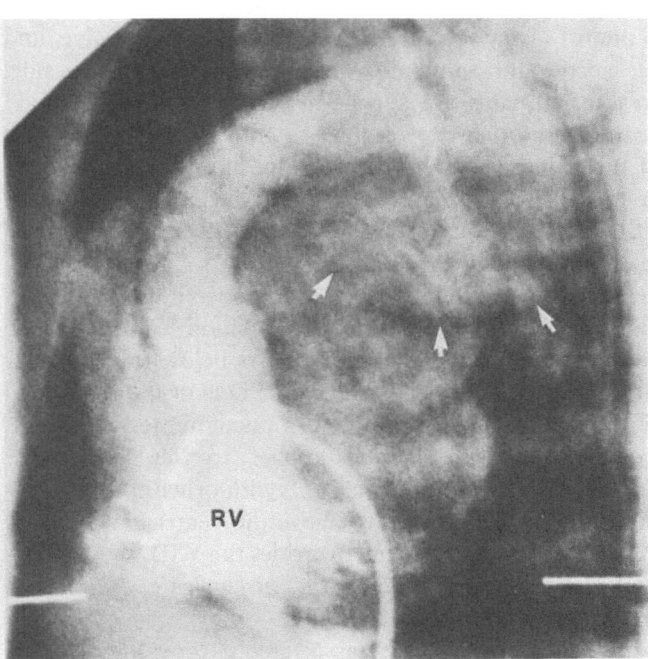

E

Fig. 7–164. *Tetralogy of Fallot with absence of the pulmonary valve in a newborn infant.* **A** and **B** are frontal and lateral roentgenograms of the chest; **C** lateral view of the left ventriculogram; **D** and **E** frontal and lateral views of the right ventriculogram. The roentgenograms of the chest (**A** and **B**) show cardiomegaly and pulmonary undercirculation. Two large hilar masses represent the massively dilated pulmonary arteries. On the lateral film the huge LPA simulates a superior mediastinal mass. The left ventriculogram (**C**) shows the retrodisplaced left ventricle (*LV*) with minimal filling of the right ventricle. The sweep of the aortic arch is markedly broadened by the dilated right pulmonary artery. (The venous catheter was directed by way of the inferior vena cava to the right atrium, then through the foramen ovale and left atrium to reach the LV). The frontal view of an injection into the right ventricle (*RV*) during systole (**D**) shows simultane- ous opacification of the pulmonary artery and aorta. The aortic arch (*Ao.*) is on the right. The outflow tract of the right ventricle is not stenotic; however, on motion ciné studies the pulmonary anulus was hypoplastic. The main pulmonary artery and proximal left pulmonary artery form one spherical density while the right pulmonary artery forms a second spherical density. Together they give the appearance of a dumbbell, in which the relatively narrow center is formed by the proximal portion of the right pulmonary artery surrounded by the aorta. On the lateral view of the right ventriculogram (**E**) the right pulmonary artery forms a circular density encircled by the aorta. The left pulmonary artery forms a second circular opacity somewhat higher, partially overlying the right pulmonary artery and the aortic arch (*arrows*). At autopsy absence of the leaflets of the pulmonary valve was confirmed.

Double-Outlet Right Ventricle

Double-outlet right ventricle (DORV) comprises an uncommon group of congenital heart defects in which both the aorta and the pulmonary artery originate from the RV. The outlet from the LV is by way of a ventricular septal defect (VSD) or, rarely, through an atrial septal defect if the ventricular septum is intact (see Fig. 7–169). DORV may be due to failure of resorption of the bulboventricular flange. Persistence of the flange prevents transfer of the posterior channel of the conus to the LV, leaving conus muscle interposed between the great vessels and the atrioventricular (A-V) valves. The resulting lack of fibrous continuity between the semilunar valves and the A-V valves is a hallmark of DORV. On occasion an elongated anterior leaflet of the mitral valve maintains tenuous fibrous continuity with the aortic valve; nevertheless, DORV is diagnosed because both great vessels arise above the RV. As the aortic and pulmonic valves are both above a conus, they are located at about the same height. The aortic valve is almost always to the right of the pulmonary valve, and the aortic and pulmonic valves are usually side by side. In unusual cases the aortic valve may be in a "normal" position. In other cases it may lie anterior and to the right of the pulmonic valve (dextromalposition). Rarely it may be to the left of the pulmonic valve (levomalposition). The VSD may be infracristal (Fallot type, subaortic), supracristal (Taussig-Bing type, subpulmonic) or intracristal (beneath both semilunar valves). Intracristal VSD is designated by some authors to be doubly committed or subaortic and subpulmonic. If the VSD occurs below the crista far from both great vessels, or if the VSD is of the A-V canal type, it may be called remote or noncommitted. The term *Taussig-Bing malformation* applies to the complex of DORV with a subpulmonic VSD, with or without overriding of the pulmonary valve above the ventricular septum. When the pulmonary trunk overrides the VSD, the designation *right ventricular aorta and biventricular pulmonary trunk* has been used.

The incidence of other associated cardiac and noncardiac malformations is high as well. Valvar pulmonic stenosis, infundibular pulmonic stenosis or both are often associated. Obstruction to systemic blood flow is also frequent (e.g., aortic valve stenosis or subaortic stenosis, coarctation or interruption of the aortic arch, tubular hypoplasia of the aortic arch) especially in Taussig-Bing hearts. Abnormalities of the atrioventricular valves (A-V valves) may also occur with DORV (e.g., endocardial cushion defects, mitral valve stenosis or atresia, parachute mitral valve, supravalvular mitral ring, straddling of left or right A-V valves or both, and atrioventricular septal malalignment, also called anular override). Presence of any of these abnormalities greatly influences the prognosis of patients with DORV.

DORV may also be part of the situs ambiguus syndrome (asplenia, polysplenia, anisosplenia). In these patients DORV is often associated with endocardial cushion defects, single ventricle and abnormalities of systemic and pulmonary venous return. DORV may also occur with chromosomal disorders such as trisomy E (16–18) and trisomy D (13–15).

Clinical Features DORV can be separated into three distinct categories:

1) DORV with subaortic, doubly committed or remote VSD without pulmonic stenosis has clinical features similar to a large VSD (pulmonary overcirculation with or without congestive heart failure). Although cyanosis is not clinically evident, desaturation is present. Pulmonary vascular obstructive disease (Eisenmenger physiology) may occur if the defect is left untreated.

2) DORV with subpulmonary VSD has the same features as D-transposition of the great arteries with VSD in that pulmonary overcirculation is present and cyanosis is evident. Eisenmenger physiology may also develop in this group.

3) DORV with PS presents with marked cyanosis and normal pulmonary vascularity or pulmonary undercirculation. The clinical appearance is therefore similar to that of tetralogy of Fallot (VSD plus PS) or D-TGA with PS.

The electrocardiogram in all forms of DORV usually shows RV hypertrophy and right axis deviation. Biventricular hypertrophy occurs with large left-to-right shunts. LV hypertrophy with T wave changes may occur with a restrictive VSD. On occasion, left axis deviation is present with DORV. This unusual QRS axis occurs in DORV with and without A-V canal defects. First-degree and higher degrees of heart block also occur with DORV.

Echocardiography The findings most characteristic of DORV are the anterior location of the aortic valve and the presence of conus muscle between the semilunar valves and the anterior leaflet of the mitral valve (fibrous discontinuity). These abnormalities are most striking on M-mode arc scans (Fig. 7–165) or 2-D echocardiography long axis view from the aortic valve to the mitral valve (Fig. 7–166). The anterior displacement of the aortic root relative to the mitral valve is indicated by a step-off where the aortic root should continue into the mitral valve. The anterior leaflet of the mitral valve (AML) appears distinctly posterior to the back wall of the aortic root. Conus muscle interposed between the aortic root and the AML is thicker than the wall of the aorta, and thickens during ventricular systole. It is important to appreciate that an elongated mitral valve in DORV may maintain tenuous fibrous continuity between the aortic root and the mitral valve, obscuring the M-mode findings.

On 2-D echocardiography the parasternal long axis view is optimum for defining the position of the semilunar valves relative to the LV, the conus and the mitral valve. Both great arteries appear anterior to the ventricular septum and are separated from the mitral valve by conus muscle. The only outlet from the LV is the VSD, if present. If the aorta is in front of the pulmonary artery (dextromalposition), then the LV, the VSD, the pulmonary valve and the aortic valve may all be lined up in order (from back

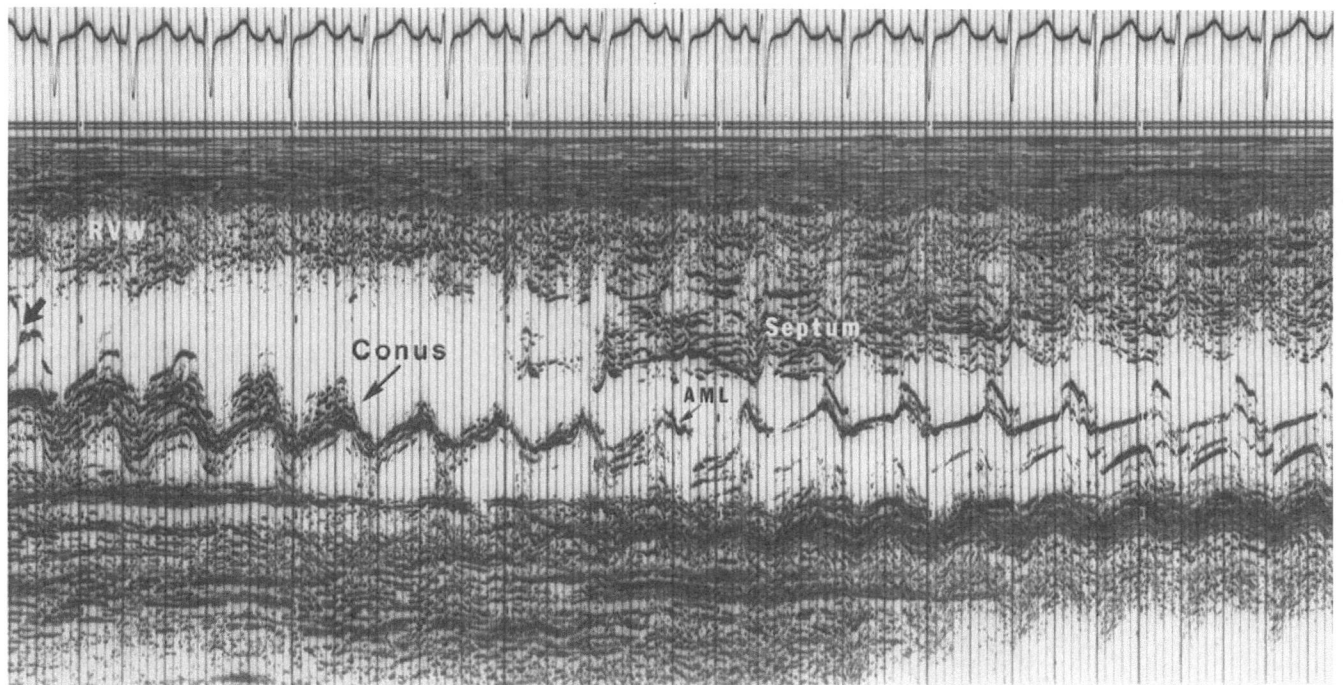

A

Fig. 7–165. *M-mode echocardiogram in double-outlet right ventricle.* **A** *is an arc scan from the aortic root to the left ventricle in a 3-month-old cyanotic infant.* **B** *is an M-mode echocardiogram through the pulmonary valve (pv).*

A The aortic valve (*arrow*) and root are far anterior, with no cardiac chamber anterior to the aortic root. Conus is represented by a thick mass of tissue continuous with the posterior wall of the aortic root. The right ventricular free wall (*RVW*) is thick in an area adjacent to the anterior wall of the aorta, suggesting the presence of conus muscle anteriorly. Further toward the apex lies the ventricular septum. The mitral valve (*AML*) appears within the left ventricle. Thus the aortic valve is far anterior, being separated from the mitral valve by conus muscle. **B** shows a smaller semilunar valve (most likely the pulmonary valve since pulmonary undercirculation was noted on plain films of the chest). This valve is situated toward the left and posterior to the aortic valve. The diagnosis must therefore be double-outlet right ventricle with dextromalposition (aorta toward the right and anterior) and pulmonic stenosis or imperforate pulmonary valve.

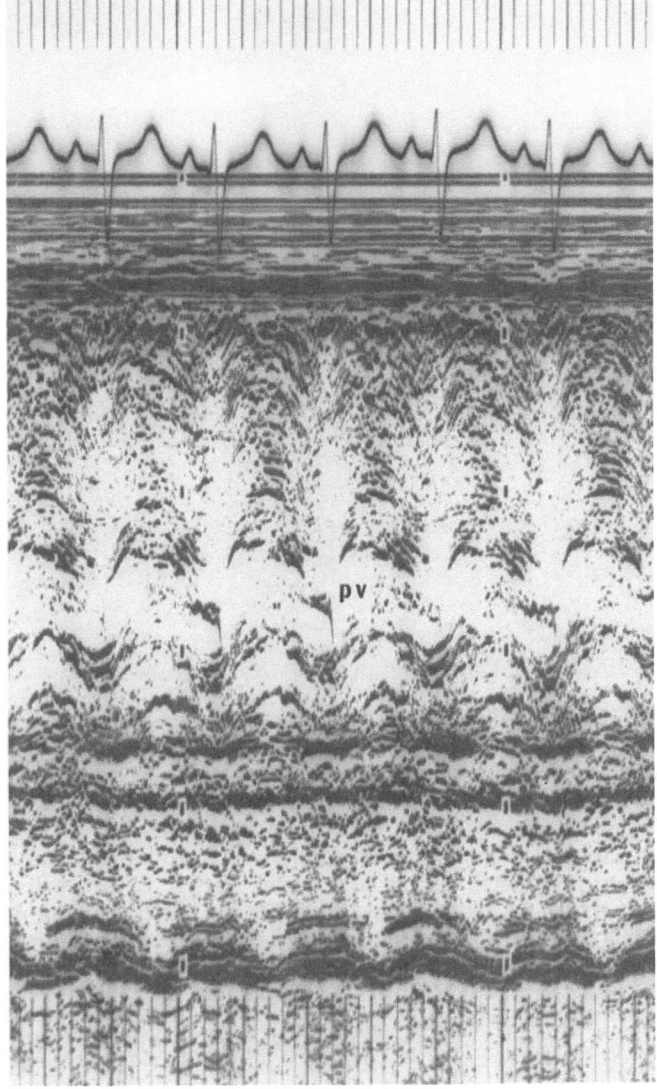

B

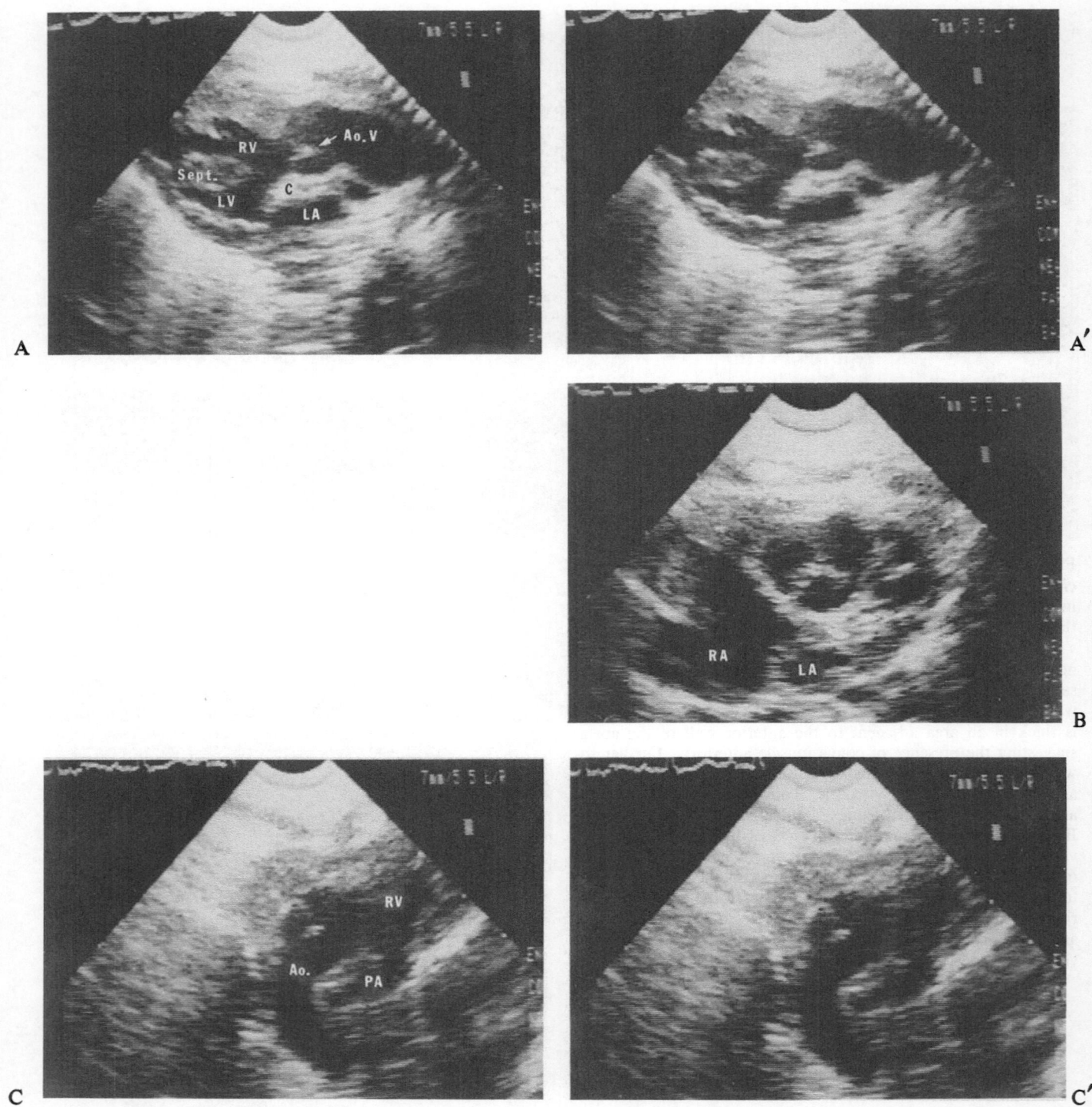

Fig. 7–166. *Two-dimensional echocardiograms in a newborn infant with double-outlet right ventricle and pulmonic stenosis.* **A** and **A′** are from a long-axis view in diastole. The aortic valve (*Ao.V*) arises entirely above the right ventricle (*RV*). Conus (*C*) is interposed between the aortic valve and the mitral valve. The left ventricle (*LV*) empties by way of the ventricular septal defect which is infracristal. The right pulmonary artery is the small circle between the aorta and the left atrium (*LA*). **B** is a parasternal short axis view of the semilunar valves. The aortic valve is toward the right (dextro-malposition). The three leaflets of the aortic valve form the "Mercedes Benz" sign. The pulmonic valve is bicuspid. **C** and **C′** represent a subxiphoid view of the right ventricle (*RV*). Both the aorta (*Ao.*) and the pulmonary artery (*PA*) arise above this ventricle. **D** is a pulsed Doppler study with the sample volume in the main pulmonary artery. Only systolic flow is identified rather than continuous flow. Thus, the ductus arteriosus is not patent. **E** is a repeat Doppler study after a surgical systemic to pulmonary artery shunt. Flow away from the transducer (antegrade flow) is present in the main pulmonary artery during systole, while reverse flow is present during diastole. This diastolic flow into the main pulmonary artery is evidence for patency of the shunt.

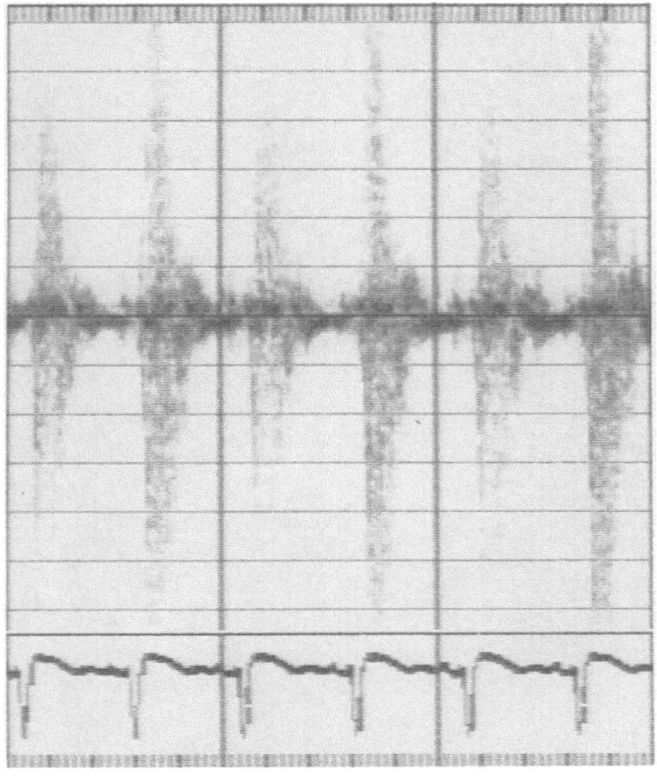

D

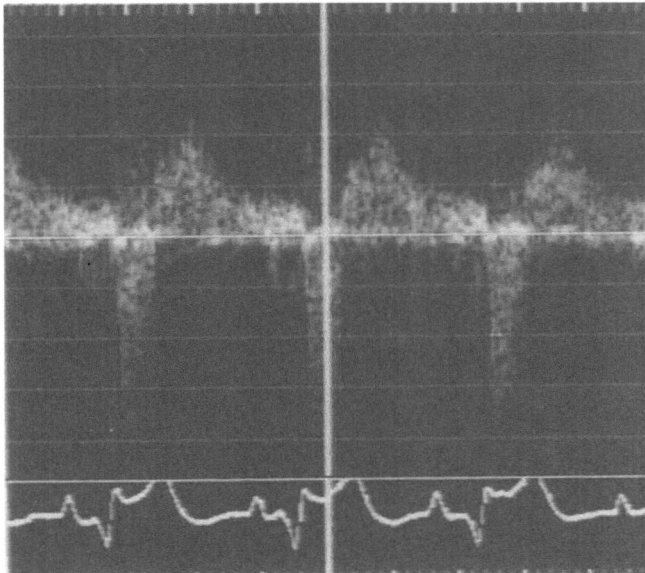

E

to front) in one image. If the great vessels are side by side, only one great vessel is imaged at a time, and a cross section at the level of the great vessels is necessary to define the spatial orientation of the great vessels. The four-chamber views (apex and subxiphoid) are helpful to identify associated defects such as A-V canal, mitral valve abnormalities or straddling of the A-V valves (anular override or abnormal chordal attachments or both). Imaging of the aortic arch and pulmonary trunk may demonstrate coarctation, hypoplasia or interruption of the aorta.

Radiological (Plain Film) Features Findings on roentgenograms of the chest are not characteristic (Fig. 7–167), depending on the presence or absence of pulmonic stenosis or associated malformations such as coarctation or mitral valvular disease. In the absence of pulmonic stenosis DORV may mimic a VSD with a large left-to-right shunt, or tetralogy of Fallot if pulmonic stenosis is present. Signs of left heart obstruction may be predominant in individuals with mitral valve abnormalities. A right aortic arch may be present.

Hemodynamics DORV should be suspected when the catheter easily enters both the aorta and the pulmonary artery from the RV, and the great vessels appear to be transposed (both great vessels are also entered from the RV in Tetralogy of Fallot, but the relationship is normal).

As with the clinical features, the hemodynamic data reflect the position of the VSD and presence or absence of pulmonic stenosis. A subpulmonic VSD results in oxygenated blood from the LV being directed into the pulmonary artery, thus leaving the aorta relatively desaturated. This type of VSD results in hemodynamics similar to complete transposition of the great arteries. A VSD in a location other than subpulmonic results in variable arterial oxygen saturation. In the absence of pulmonic stenosis or high pulmonary resistance a large oxygen step-up is identified in the RV; this step-up is carried out to the aorta. Thus the hemodynamics are those of a large VSD. In most cases of DORV, even without PS, venous admixture occurs in the ventricle, resulting in varying degrees of arterial desaturation. Pulmonic stenosis or high pulmonary vascular resistance lowers the systemic oxygen saturation further by reducing pulmonary blood flow. Pressure in the RV is equal to the aortic pressure unless aortic stenosis is present. Pressures in the LV and RV are also equal unless the VSD is restrictive or absent. Pulmonary artery pressure is equal to the ventricular pressure in the absence of pulmonic stenosis. Atrial level shunts are present with ASD, A-V communis and atresia of either A-V valve. Other hemodynamic alteration may occur in the presence of other associated defects.

Contrast Studies On angiography the aortic and pulmonic valves are usually side by side and at approximately the same level, with the aorta to the right of the pulmonary trunk. On occasion the aorta is to the right and anterior to the pulmonary trunk (dextromalposition); at other times the aorta is to the left and anterior to the pulmonary trunk (levomalposition). Both great vessels arise above the conus

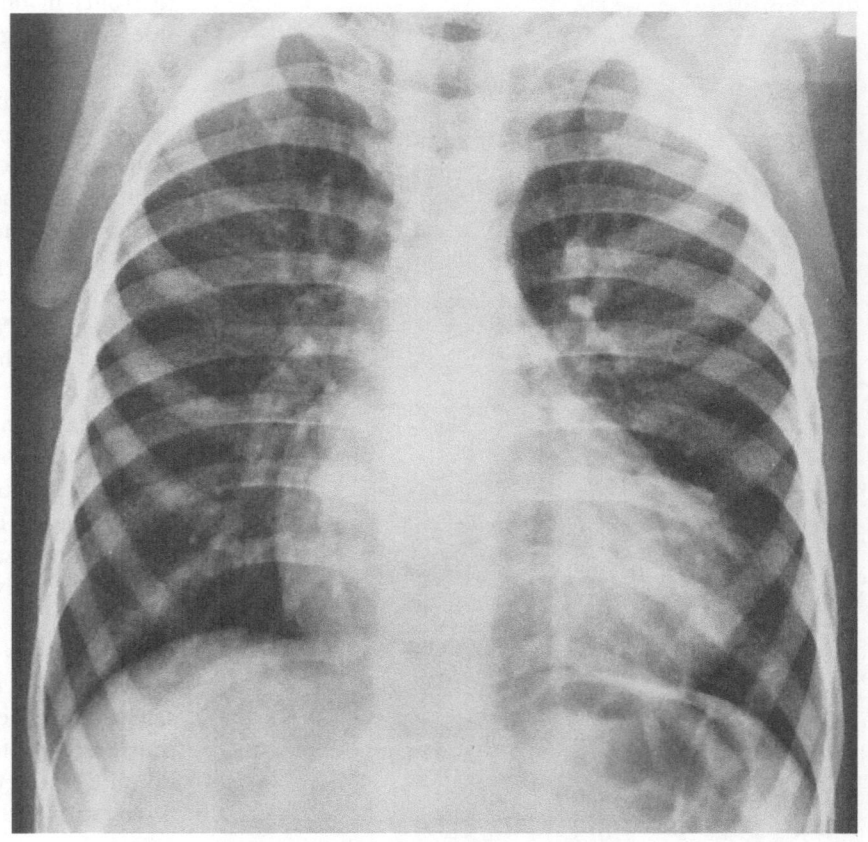

A

Fig. 7–167. *Radiological findings in a 3-year-old girl with double-outlet right ventricle and subpulmonic ventricular septal defect without pulmonic stenosis (Taussig-Bing Complex).* On the frontal roentgenogram of the chest **(A)** pulmonary overcirculation is present. The heart is enlarged with a rounded and uplifted apex, consistent with right ventricular enlargement. The aortic arch is on the left. The pulmonary artery segment is inconspicuous. Although the cardiac configuration is reminiscent of tetralogy of Fallot, the pulmonary overcirculation militates against this diagnosis. On the lateral film **(B)** the vascular pedicle is wide. On angiography **(C)** the left ventricle has no outlet other than the ventricular septal defect. Blood from the left ventricle tends to flow preferentially into the pulmonary artery, consistent with a subpulmonic ventricular septal defect. This diagnosis was confirmed at surgery. The right ventriculogram **(D)** shows the two great vessels arising from this chamber, with the aorta lying in front of the pulmonary artery.

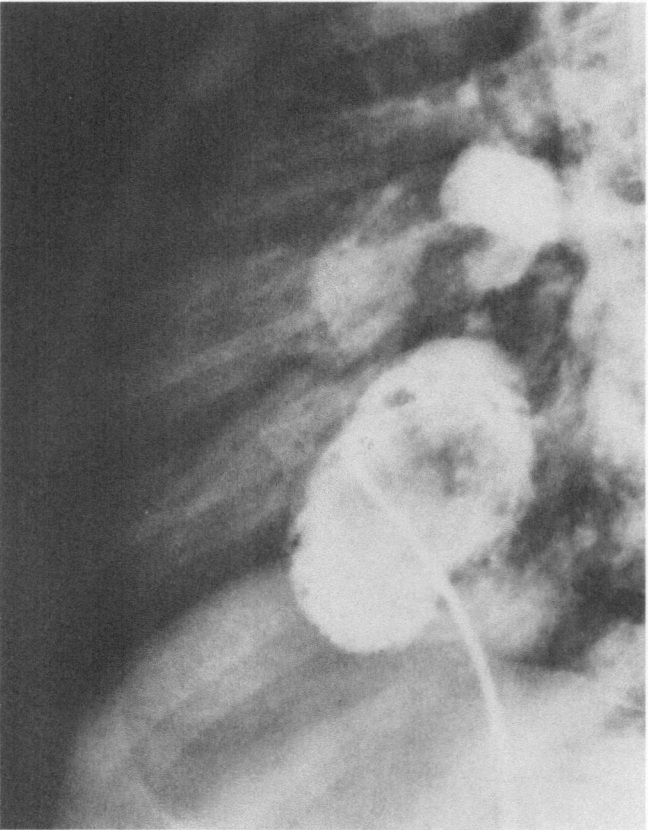

C

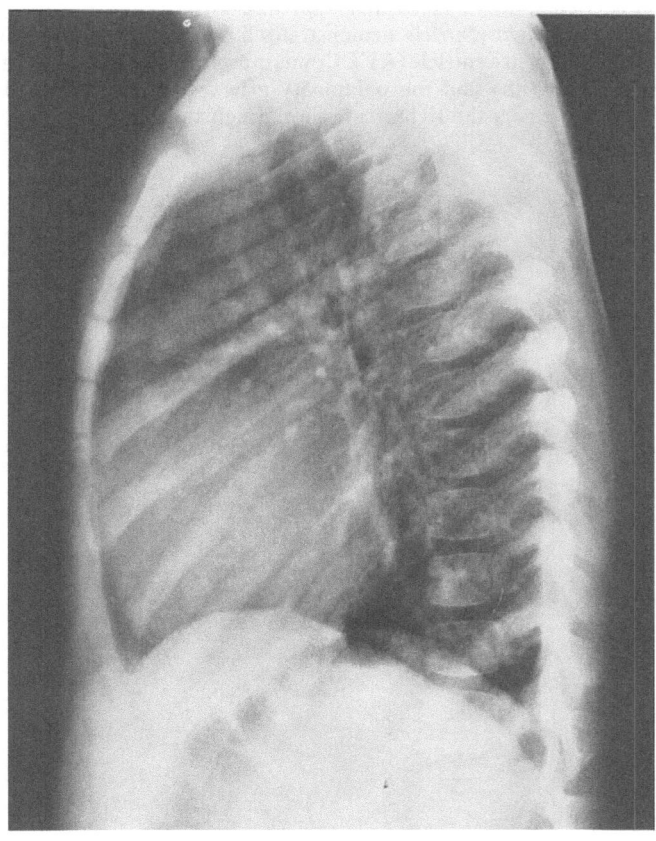

B

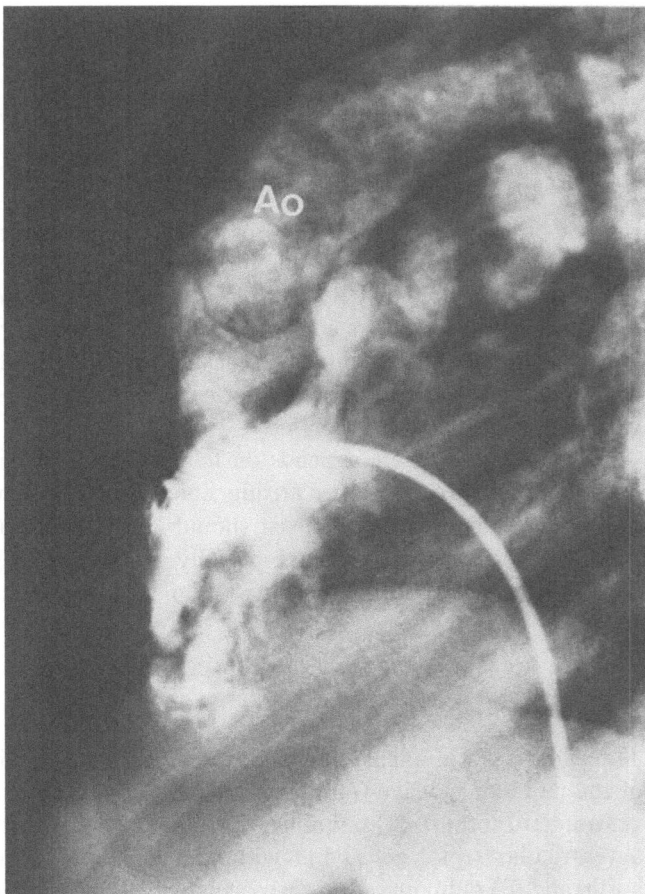

Ao

D

(Figs. 7–167d, 7–168, 7–169) thus, no great vessel arises from the LV (Fig. 7–167C). Mitral–semilunar valve fibrous continuity may rarely be observed. The location of the VSD and the presence of pulmonic stenosis are defined. Abnormalities of the mitral valve and other associated cardiovascular anomalies are delineated.

Treatment In DORV without PS medical treatment may be required for control of cardiac failure associated with a large left-to-right shunt. Paroxysmal hyperpnea and cyanosis ("tet spells", cyanotic spells) occurring in DORV with pulmonic stenosis are the same as those occurring with tetralogy of Fallot and are described under that heading. The acute episode is treated with oxygen, morphine and sodium bicarbonate. Palliative surgery involves pulmonary artery banding in patients with congestive heart failure secondary to left-to-right shunt or systemic-to-pulmonary anastomosis if pulmonic stenosis limits pulmonary blood flow severely. Corrective surgery involves incorporation of either great vessel and the VSD by a patch to direct LV blood into that great vessel. If the VSD is subaortic the patch surrounds the VSD and the aortic valve, creating a tunnel between the LV and the aorta, thus establishing a normal connection. A restrictive VSD may be enlarged with care to avoid the conduction system. If possible the pulmonary outflow tract is then widened by a patch. In many patients a conduit is necessary to reestablish communication between the RV and the pulmonary artery.

If the VSD is subpulmonic the patch can be placed to surround the VSD and the pulmonary valve. LV (oxygenated) blood then flows through the tunnel into the pulmonary artery, and the hemodynamics are those of complete transposition of the great vessels. An inflow procedure (Mustard or Senning) (Fig. 7–170) or an outflow procedure (Jatene, Kaye-Damus-Stansel or Aubert) is carried out at the same time to redirect the venous streams. Complex forms of DORV are repaired with combinations of patches and conduits or even with modifications of the Fontan procedure (atriopulmonary anastomosis).

Double-Outlet Left Ventricle

Double-outlet left ventricle (DOLV) is defined as an abnormal ventriculoarterial alignment in which both great arteries arise above or mostly above the anatomic LV. This definition includes hearts in which the aorta or the pulmonary artery override a VSD but is nevertheless related to (aligned with) the left ventricle. DOLV is a rare anomaly and may be extremely complex because of associated defects and malalignments. Nevertheless, many are repairable once the anatomy is understood.

The most frequent form is DOLV in situs solitus with normal ventricles (D-loop), D-malposition of the great arteries, subaortic VSD and pulmonic stenosis. On angiography this type may be mistaken for tetralogy of Fallot. In both the aorta overrides the ventricular septum. The difference is presence of the subpulmonic conus above the LV rather than the RV. The repair consists of closure of the

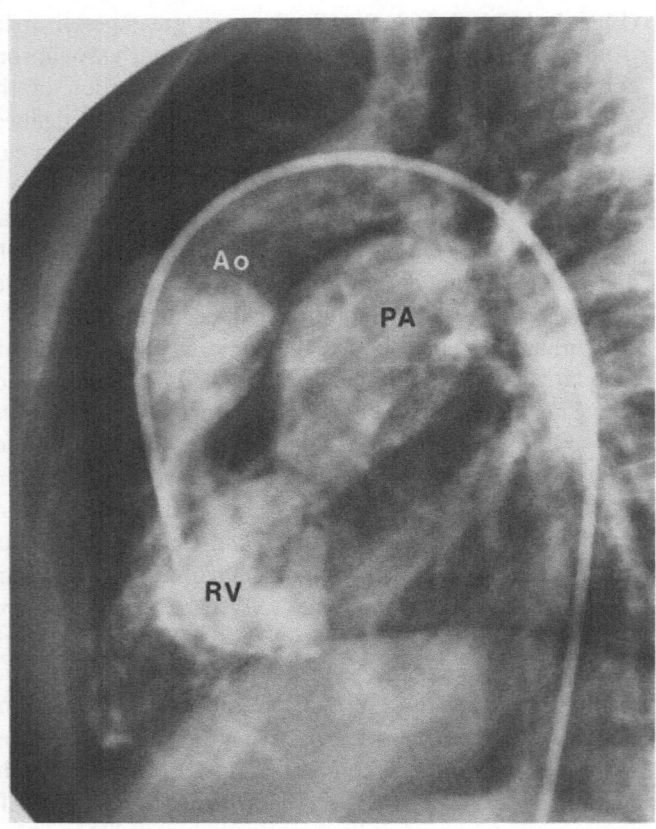

Fig. 7–168. *Right ventriculography in a 4-year-old girl with double-outlet right ventricle* demonstrates both great arteries to arise from the right ventricle (*RV*). Conus muscle is interposed beneath the aorta (*Ao*) and the pulmonary artery (*PA*). Note that the catheter enters the right ventricle through the aorta.

VSD leaving the aorta connected to the LV and insertion of a conduit connecting the RV to the pulmonary artery. In similar cases without pulmonic stenosis the VSD is closed in such a way as to attach the aorta to the RV. A Mustard or Senning procedure is performed at the same time to redirect the venous streams. DOLV has also been found with subpulmonic VSD (i.e., the pulmonic valve is closest to the VSD). This allows an intracardiac repair consisting of a patch which surrounds the VSD and the pulmonary valve. This results in attachment of the pulmonary artery to the right ventricle and normal blood flow. In a unique case of DOLV (Paul et al.) no VSD was present and the RV was hypoplastic with a blind outflow tract. The repair for this and other forms having no usable RV is a Fontan procedure (anastomosis of the right atrium to the main pulmonary artery). DOLV has also been reported with situs inversus; situs ambiguus (asplenia, polysplenia); with atrioventricular discordance; with tricuspid atresia; mitral atresia; straddling tricuspid valve; Ebstein anomaly; and with single ventricle. In DOLV with single ventricle both great arteries are aligned above or mostly above the main (LV) chamber rather than above the rudimentary outflow chamber. In all forms of DOLV the aorta may be anterior, posterior, right or left of the pulmonary artery. The subaortic and the subpulmonic conus may each be well developed, poorly developed, or absent. Aortic stenosis, pulmonic stenosis, stenosis of both outflow tracts, or no stenosis may be present. Hypoplastic ascending aorta and preductal coarctation of the aorta may be associated in cases with aortic stenosis.

Diagnosis during life depends on left ventriculography showing both great arteries arising above the LV. The knowledge that such defects exist should allow the astute radiologist to recognize them especially in the presence of other unusual abnormalities of position and alignment.

Pulmonary Atresia

Three forms of pulmonary atresia occur: (1) isolated atresia of the pulmonary valve (pulmonary atresia with an intact ventricular septum); (2) pulmonary atresia associated with a ventricular septal defect but without overriding of the aorta; and (3) pulmonary atresia associated with conotruncal malformations such as tetralogy of Fallot (pseudotruncus), double-outlet right ventricle and the various transposi-

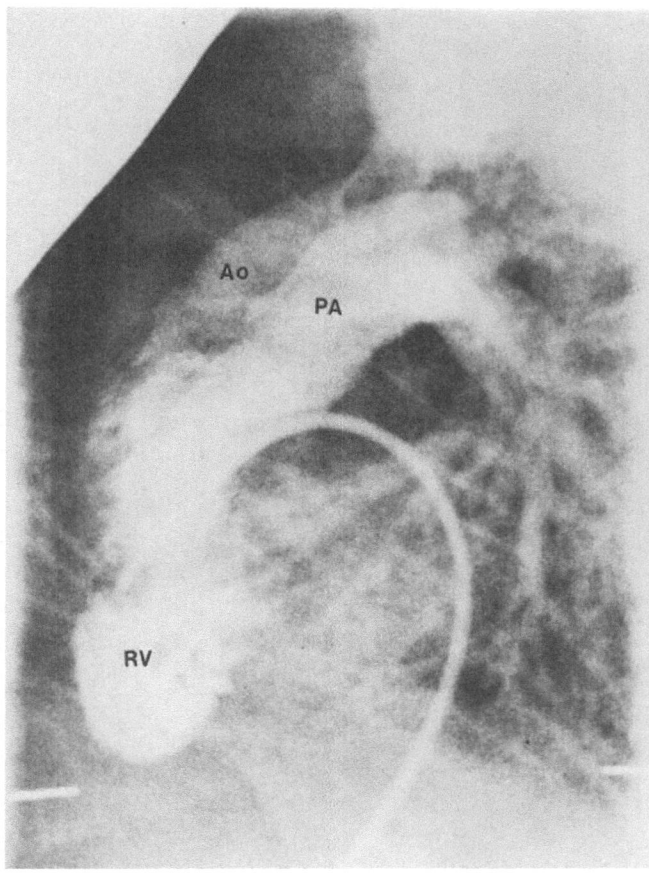

A

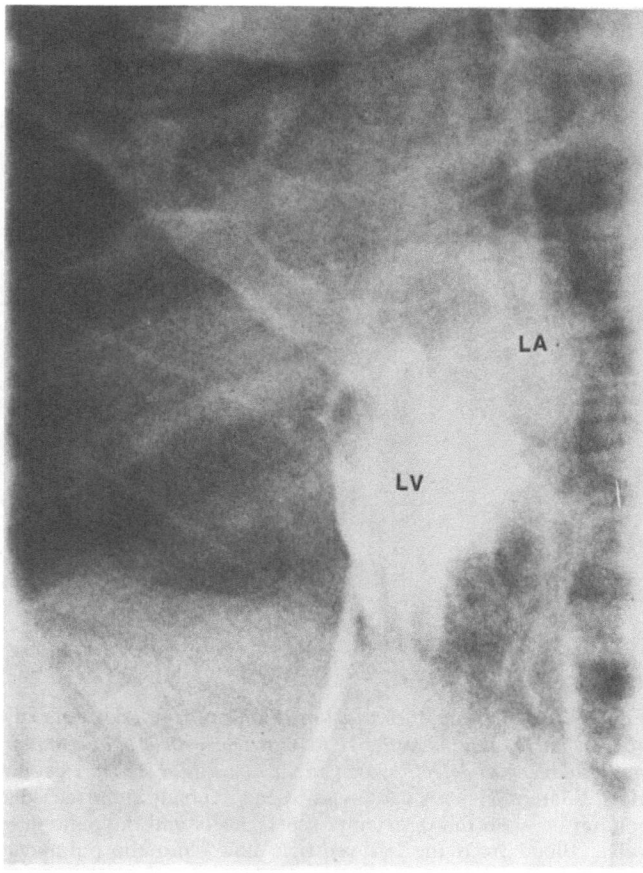

B

Fig. 7–169. *Double-outlet right ventricle with intact ventricular septum.* **A** Lateral view of the right ventriculogram showing both great vessels arising from the RV. The aortic valve is to the right and slightly anterior to the pulmonic valve. **B** The LAO view of the left ventriculogram shows no great vessel arising from the left ventricle (*LV*) and no VSD. The only exit from the LV is by way of the incompetent mitral valve (mitral insufficiency). The patient had a restrictive ASD, and a balloon septostomy was done at the time of cardiac catheterization. *LA* = left atrium; *Ao* = aorta; *PA* = pulmonary artery.

tion complexes including the cardiosplenic syndromes (situs ambiguus). Pulmonary atresia associated with conotruncal abnormalities is discussed in the corresponding sections on transpositions. Pulmonary atresia with a ventricular septal defect but without overriding of the aorta is similar clinically and physiologically to extreme tetralogy of Fallot (pseudotruncus) and is therefore discussed in that section.

Pulmonary Atresia with Intact Ventricular Septum

Isolated pulmonary atresia is an uncommon anomaly occurring in approximately 1%–3% of congenital heart defects. An interatrial communication is obligatory because of obstruction to forward flow by an imperforate or an atretic pulmonic valve in the presence of an intact ventricular septum. The size of the RV is variable. If the tricuspid valve is competent the RV is small and hypertrophied and the tricuspid ring tends to be small. Endocardial fibroelastosis may be present. Conversely, in cases with insufficiency of the tricuspid valve the RV may be normal or enlarged. In either case the tricuspid valve apparatus may be normal, or it may be grossly abnormal with fusion and shortening of the chordae tendineae. The tricuspid valve may be bicus-

pid or unicuspid. The leaflets may be dysplastic, or, rarely, muscular. The leaflets may be attached to a single papillary muscle (parachute tricuspid valve); they may be displaced downward into the RV cavity (Ebstein anomaly); or they may be absent. Diffuse or focal thinning of the right ventricular wall may be observed on occasion (Uhl disease). The RA varies in size, depending on the presence and severity of tricuspid insufficiency. It may be normal or moderately dilated if the tricuspid valve is competent, or it may be massively dilated in the presence of severe tricuspid regurgitation. The interatrial communication is usually a foramen ovale, but a true atrial septal defect may be present. The LA and LV are usually dilated. The aorta is large, and the lungs are perfused via a patent ductus arteriosus. Spontaneous closure of the ductus results in death, because perfusion of the lungs by systemic and bronchial vessels is inadequate. Intramyocardial sinusoids are often detected in patients with a competent tricuspid valve, these sinusoids anastomose with the coronary circulation, resulting in drainage into the aorta and coronary venous system. Bidirectional flow between aorta and sinusoids may be observed (See Fig. 7–174B and C).

Clinical Features Cyanosis, cyanotic spells and marked

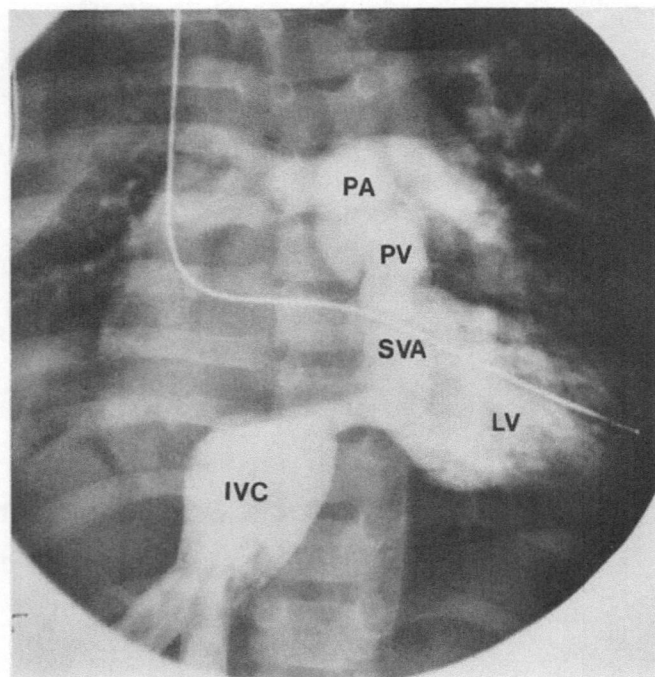

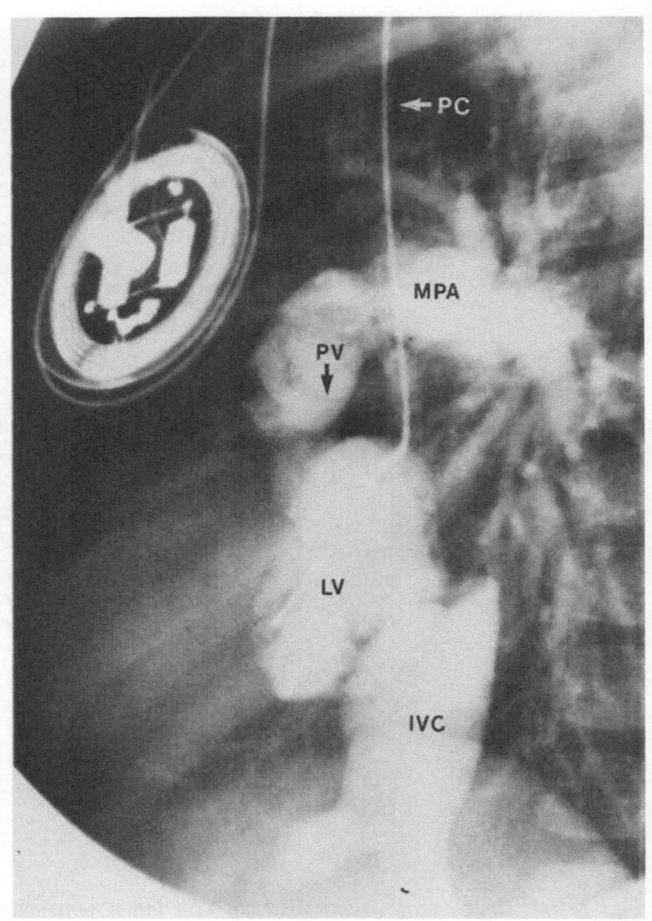

Fig. 7–170. *Injection of contrast medium in the inferior vena cava after repair of double-outlet right ventricle with a subpulmonary ventricular septal defect* (same patient as in Fig. 7–167). **A** Frontal view, **B** lateral view. A patch was placed to create an intracardiac conduit between the ventricular septal defect and the pulmonary valve. Blood from the left ventricle flows into the pulmonary artery, similar to D-transposition. A Mustard procedure was performed at the same time to redirect the systemic venous blood into the left ventricle and the pulmonary venous blood into the right ventricle. Note the presence of conus muscle interposed between the pulmonary valve and the left ventricle. The tip of the pacer catheter (*PC*) reaches the anatomical left ventricle via the superior vena cava and the systemic venous atrium.

IVC = inferior vena cava; *SVA* = systemic venous atrium; *LV* = left ventricle; *PA, MPA* = main pulmonary artery; *PV* = pulmonary valve.

right heart failure are prominent. The liver is large and shows a presystolic pulsation. A murmur of tricuspid regurgitation may be heard. Severe hypoxemia and metabolic acidosis may occur as the ductus closes. The electrocardiogram shows a normal axis in the frontal plane, while the RV forces are diminished or absent. Chest leads may show LV hypertrophy. With tricuspid insufficiency and RV enlargement right axis deviation is more likely.

Echocardiography M-mode echocardiography reveals a small RV cavity with a thick anterior RV wall and thick septum. The tricuspid valve is present but opens for only a very short time because of high RV diastolic pressure. In the presence of an imperforate pulmonic valve an echo resembling the opening of the pulmonary valve is identified on occasion, even though the pulmonary valve does not actually open. Two-dimensional echocardiography (Figs. 7–171 and 7–172) may help in visualizing the size of the RV and in assessing motion of the pulmonic valve or pulmonary diaphragm. Nevertheless, echocardiography is not totally reliable in determining whether the pulmonary valve is patent or imperforate. Absence of forward flow in the main pulmonary artery by Doppler echocardiography is evidence for pulmonary atresia.

Radiological (Plain Film) Features Although the pulmonary vascularity may be normal in the presence of a large ductus arteriosus, decreased pulmonary vascularity is the rule (bilateral undercirculation) (Fig. 7–173). The configuration of the heart is not specific. The heart may be of normal size (Fig. 7–174), moderately enlarged (Fig. 7–173) or markedly enlarged with massive dilatation of the RA (Fig. 7–175). The combination of severe undercirculation, concave pulmonary artery segment, rounded apex and aneurysmal dilatation of the RA in a sick cyanotic neonate are highly suggestive of pulmonary atresia with intact ventricular septum and tricuspid insufficiency (Fig. 7–175). Ebstein malformation in the neonatal period may have a similar appearance (see Fig. 1–6). The LA and LV are usually enlarged. The size of the RA and RV is dependent mainly on the presence and severity of tricuspid insufficiency. If the RV is small or diminutive, the LAO view may show flattening of the lower anterior border of the heart. The ascending aorta is large. The superior vena cava

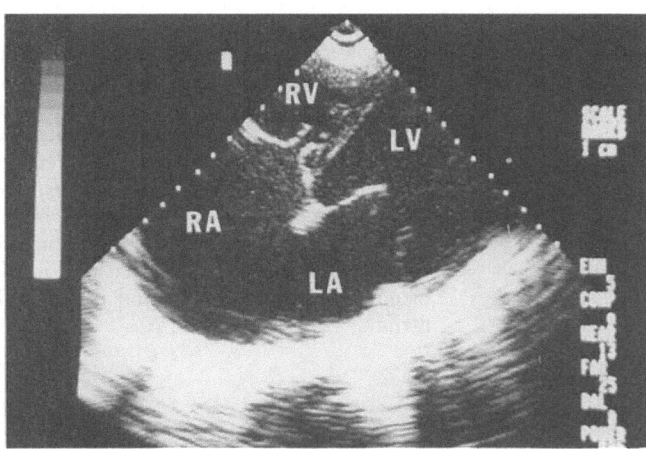

Fig. 7–171. *Imperforate pulmonic valve simulating tricuspid atresia in a 10-year-old boy.* Previous attempts to pass a cardiac catheter through the tricuspid valve or to demonstrate the right ventricle by injection of contrast agent into the right atrium had been unsuccessful. A previous Waterston anastomosis improved oxygenation, but resulted in chronic heart failure.

This apex 4-chamber view of a two-dimensional echocardiogram shows two atrioventricular valves and two ventricular cavities, the right ventricle (*RV*) being smaller than the left ventricle (*LV*). The right atrium (*RA*) and the left atrium (*LA*) are enlarged. (Same patient as Fig. 7–172 and 7–176.)

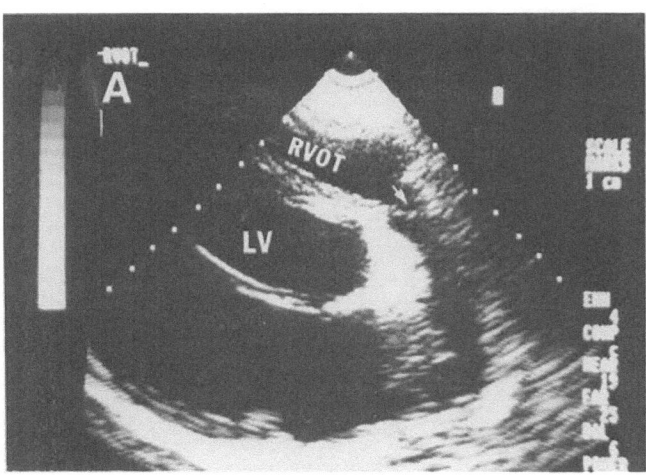

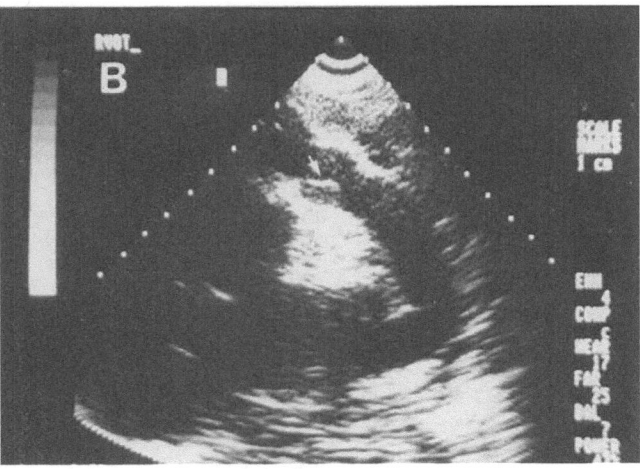

Fig. 7–172. *Same patient as Fig. 7–171 and 7–176.* The long axis view of the right ventricular outflow tract (*RVOT*) during systole (**A**) and diastole (**B**) show the well formed sinuses of Valsalva of the pulmonic valve as well as the poor motion of the valve itself. The valve domes during systole (**A**). *LV* = left ventricle.

may be displaced to the right by a pronounced curvature of the ascending aorta. A right aortic arch is unusual. Other diagnostic possibilities should be considered if the aortic arch is on the right.

Hemodynamics At catheterization the pulmonary artery cannot be entered. The RV systolic pressure is high. RA a waves may be peaked, while with tricuspid insufficiency large v waves are found in the RA. The left-sided pressures are normal. The systemic venous blood crosses at the atrial level, resulting in desaturation of the LA, LV and aorta.

Contrast Studies Angiocardiography shows atresia of the pulmonary valve with an intact ventricular septum. In true pulmonary atresia the RV outflow tract ends blindly, and no leaflets are outlined. If leaflets are outlined either from the right ventriculogram, or retrograde as the pulmonary artery fills from the ductus arteriosus, then imperforate pulmonary valve is present rather than pulmonary atresia. On occasion a tiny jet of contrast agent crosses a pinhole opening in the pulmonary valve. The size of the RV and RA will vary, depending on the function of the tricuspid valve (Fig. 7–173 to 7–175). The RV generally is markedly

hypertrophied. An atrial level right-to-left shunt is demonstrated. The LA and LV vary in size, but the LV is usually dilated, while the aorta is normal in size or dilated. The pulmonary arteries opacify by way of a patent ductus arteriosus. The main pulmonary artery fills in a retrograde manner, ending in a beaklike configuration at the site of atresia. On the other hand, the pulmonary sinuses of Valsalva will be outlined in a case of imperforate pulmonary valve (Fig. 7–176C). The pulmonary arteries are usually small. In the presence of a competent tricuspid valve, RV pressures are extremely high. In such cases myocardial sinusoids may communicate with the coronary circulation (Fig. 7–174B and C).

It is important to avoid a major pitfall that may lead to an erroneous diagnosis of tricuspid atresia in instances of pulmonary atresia with intact ventricular septum. Injection in the RA may fail to opacify the RV because of the high RV diastolic pressure. Faint opacification may not be apparent on cut film, but may be recognized on cine film because motion of the tricuspid valve is detected by this technique. The result of injection of contrast mate-

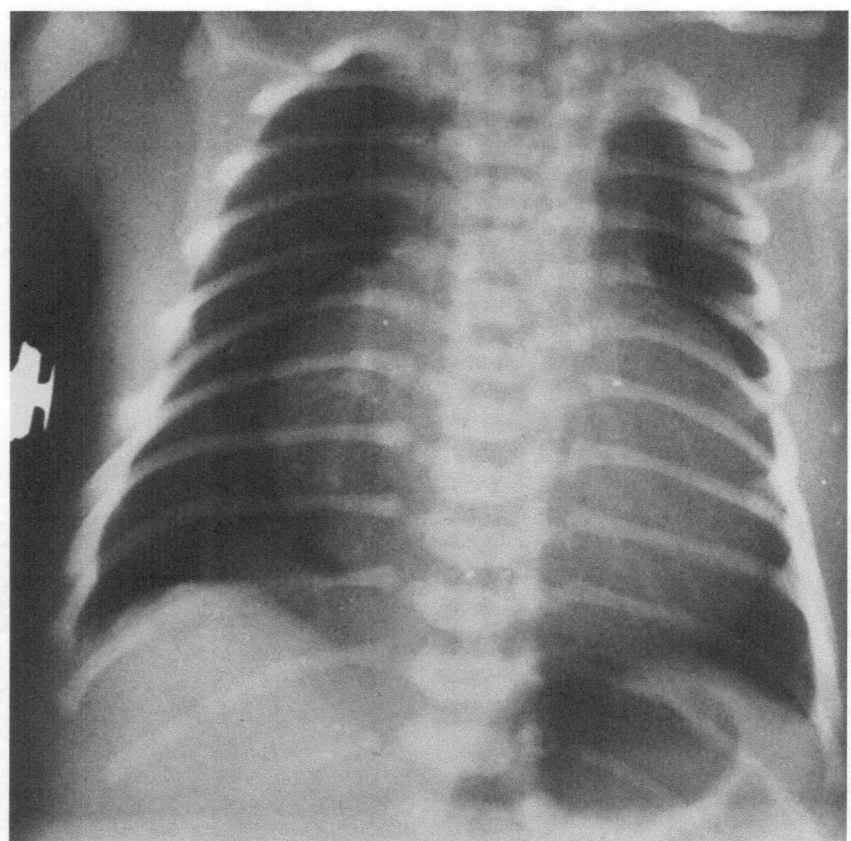

Fig. 7–173. *Pulmonary undercirculation in a 1-day-old boy with pulmonary atresia and intact ventricular septum.* On the frontal roentgenogram of the chest **(A)** cardiomegaly is present, with enlargement of the right atrium and ventricle. The right ventriculogram **(B)** demonstrates a large right ventricle with thick walls (RVH). The undersurface of the pulmonary valve is outlined, but no contrast material passes through (imperforate pulmonary valve). Tricuspid insufficiency results in opacification of the right atrium.

A

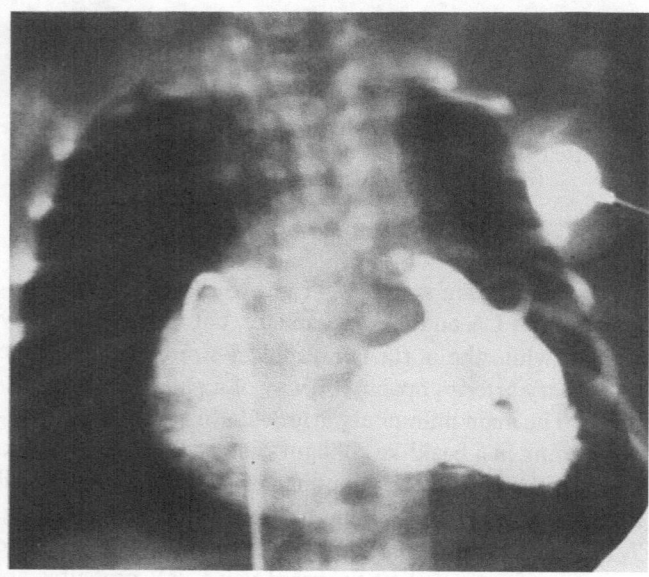

B

Fig. 7-174. *Normal-sized heart in a 25-day-old boy with pulmonary atresia and intact ventricular septum.* On the frontal roentgenogram of the chest (**A**) severe bilateral pulmonary undercirculation is present. The right ventriculogram (**B** and **C**) showed pulmonary atresia, a hypoplastic right ventricle (**RV**) with tricuspid stenosis and a competent tricuspid valve. The only exit of blood from the RV is by way of large sinusoids connecting the right ventricle to the coronary arteries. One sinusoid communicates by way of an extracardiac vessel with the left subclavian artery. Contrast from another sinusoid refluxes into the left sinus of Valsalva of the aorta. (*Continued*)

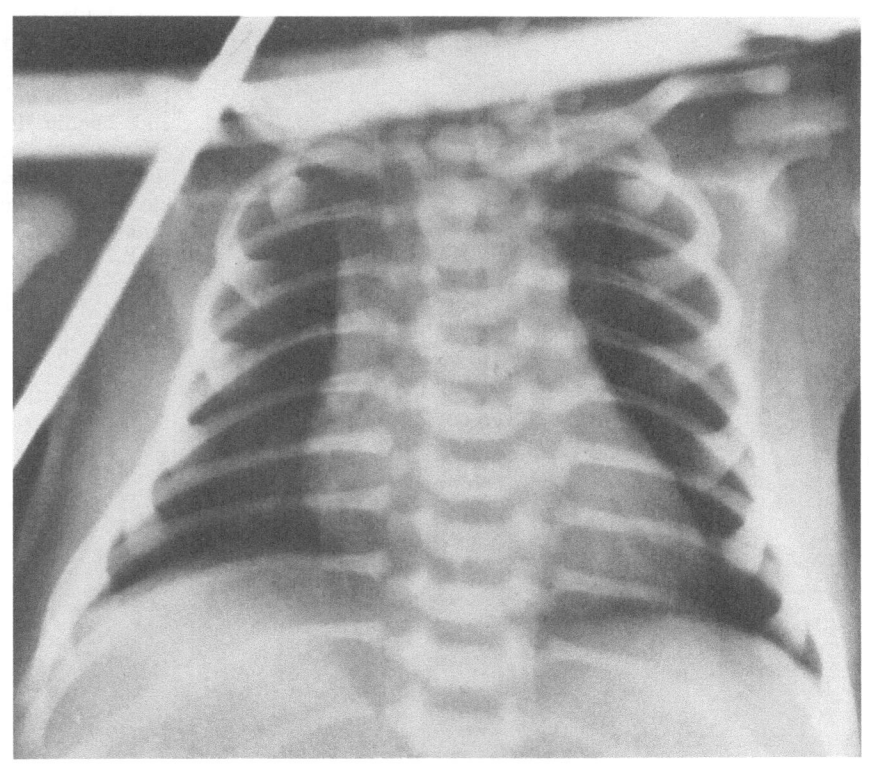

A

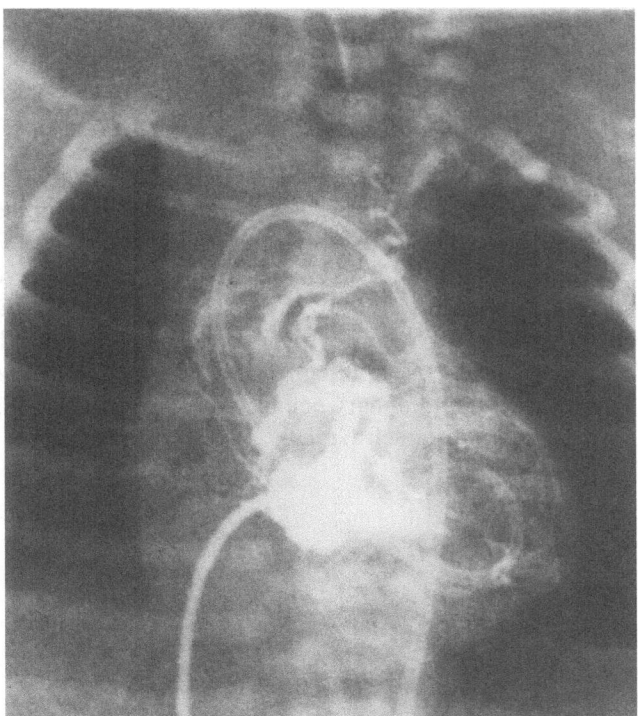

B

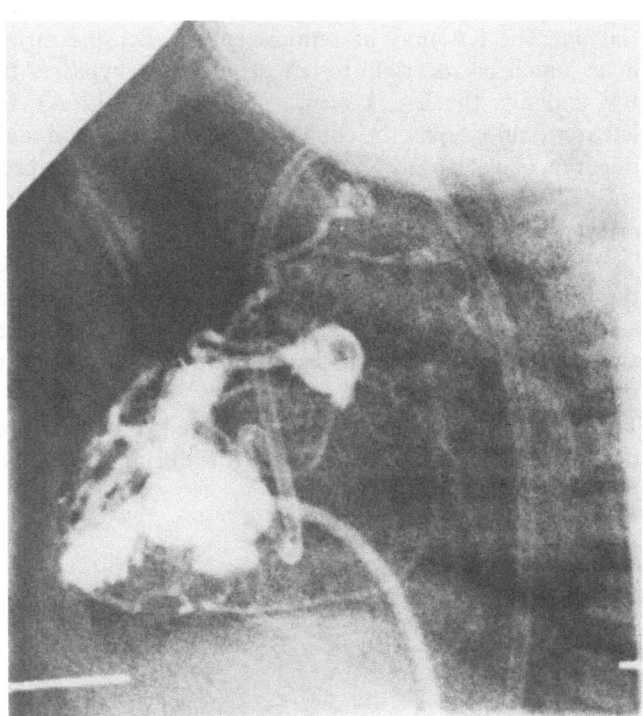

C

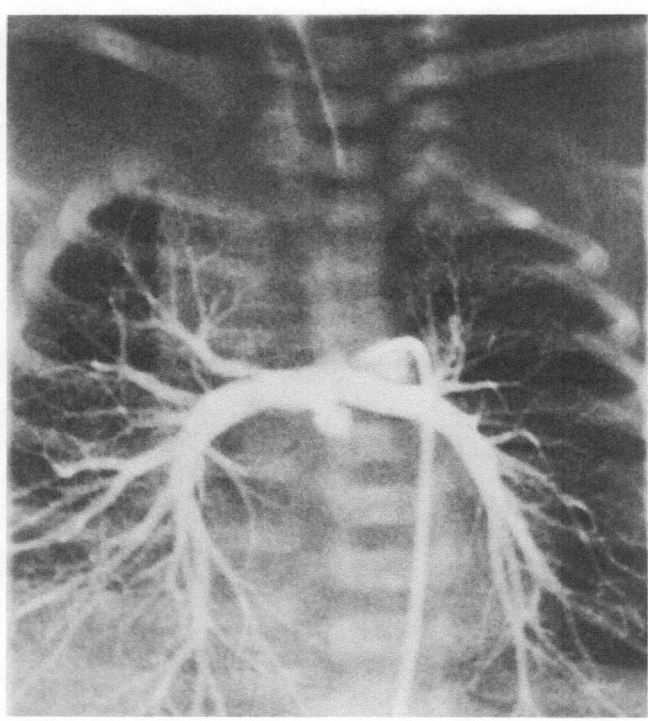

D

Fig. 7–174 (*Cont.*) **D** is a frontal view of an injection into the main pulmonary artery (the catheter passed through the patent ductus arteriosus). The main pulmonary artery ends blindly. The right and left pulmonary arteries are small. Obligatory right-to-left shunting occurred at the atrial level, and blood entered the lung by way of the ductus arteriosus.

rial into the RA may be reminiscent of tricuspid atresia in as much as the right-to-left atrial shunt bypasses the RV and fills the LA, LV and aorta (Fig. 7–176A). On left ventriculography the configuration of the LV and identification of a clear-cut ventricular septum indicate the presence of a RV cavity (Fig. 7–176B). The right coronary artery also outlines the surface of the RV cavity.

Thus a high index of suspicion should lead one to pursue the diagnosis of pulmonary atresia with intact ventricular septum in cases that resemble tricuspid atresia. Two-dimensional echocardiography is essential in the distinction of these two entities.

Treatment Initial management is directed toward correction of acid-base disturbances and toward increasing pul-

monary blood flow. Intravenous infusion of prostaglandin E_1 may dramatically improve oxygenation, by inducing ductal relaxation with resultant increase in pulmonary blood flow.

In infants with hypoplastic RV, balloon septostomy at catheterization is followed by surgical valvotomy combined with a systemic-to-pulmonary-artery shunt (Fig. 7–177). Subsequent growth of the RV has been demonstrated even in patients with extreme RV hypoplasia and endocardial fibroelastosis. In patients with inadequate growth of the RV, ultimate definitive repair is not possible. A Fontan procedure (atriopulmonary connection) may provide long-term palliation for such patients.

Fig. 7–175. *Massive cardiomegaly in a 1-day-old boy with pulmonary atresia, intact ventricular septum and massive tricuspid insufficiency.* On the frontal film of the chest **(A)** pulmonary undercirculation is observed. The right ventricle (*RV*) is enlarged, and the right atrium (*RA*) is aneurysmal in size. Ebstein malformation, congenital severe tricuspid insufficiency or cor triatriatum dexter may produce these radiological findings. The angiogram **(B)** demonstrates severe tricuspid insufficiency and an atretic pulmonary valve (*arrowhead*). The *arrows* outline the anulus of the tricuspid valve.

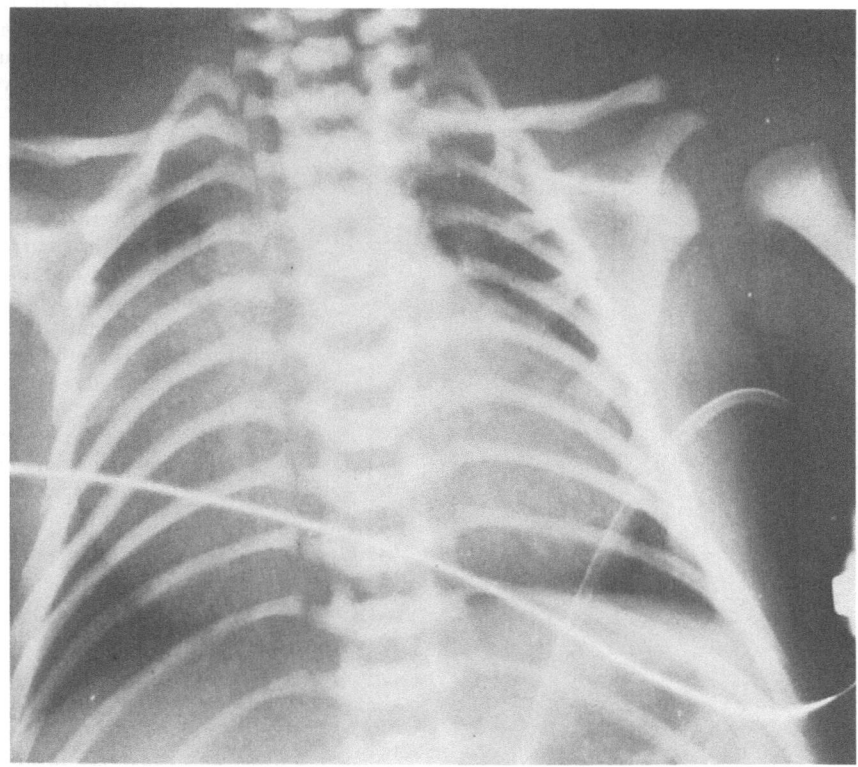

A

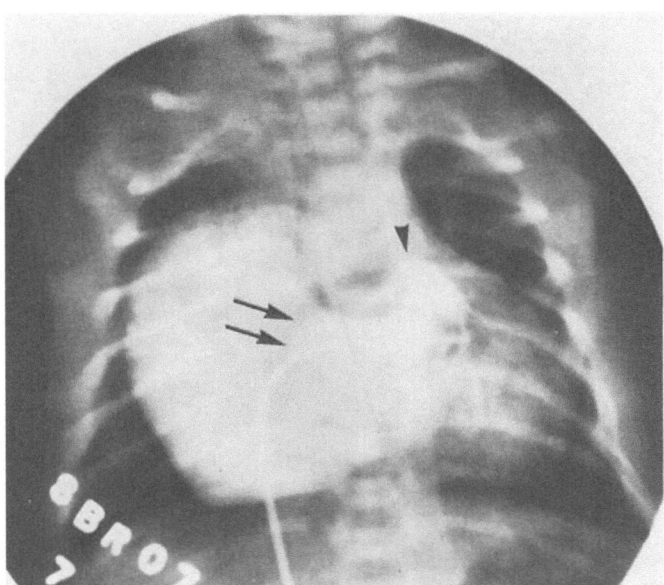

B

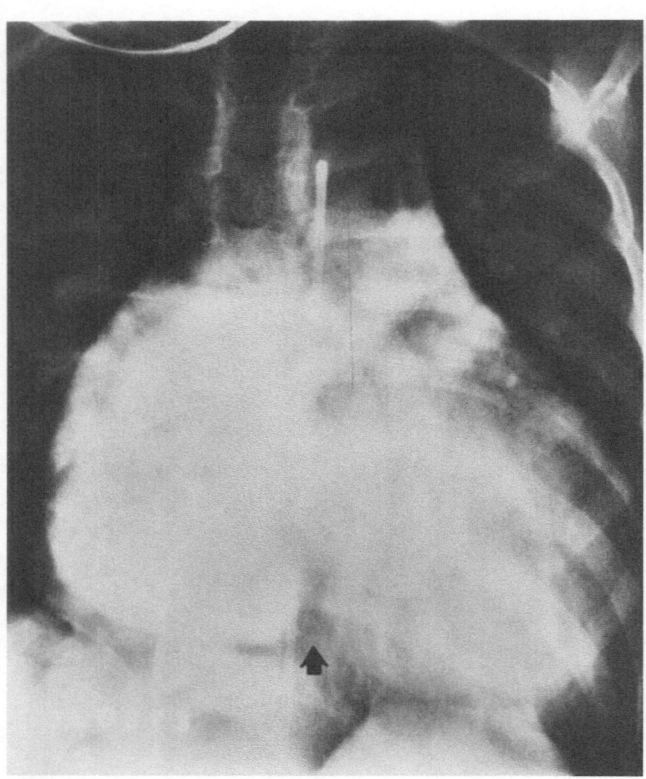

Fig. 7–176. *Imperforate pulmonary valve simulating tricuspid atresia (Same patient as in Figs. 7–171 and 7–172).* **A** An injection into the right atrium in the AP view; **B** left ventriculogram in the four-chamber view (LAO view with cranial tilt); **C** lateral view of an injection into the pulmonary artery through a Waterston anastomosis. In **A,** the right atrial injection, contrast medium from the dilated right atrium fills the left atrium and the left ventricle. The clear space (*arrow*) between the right atrium and the left ventricle corresponds to the location normally occupied by the right ventricle. This sequence simulated tricuspid atresia; however, a cineangiogram demonstrated a tricuspid valve. In **B** the left ventricle is enlarged and does not demonstrate a left-to-right shunt. The ventricular septum is clearly identified, indicating the presence of a right ventricle of significant size. The sweep of the coronary artery is also evidence for the presence of the right ventricle. The injection into the pulmonary artery by way of the Waterston anastomosis (**C**) demonstrates an imperforate pulmonary valve. The leaflets are thickened but mobile with no antegrade flow identified on this systolic frame.

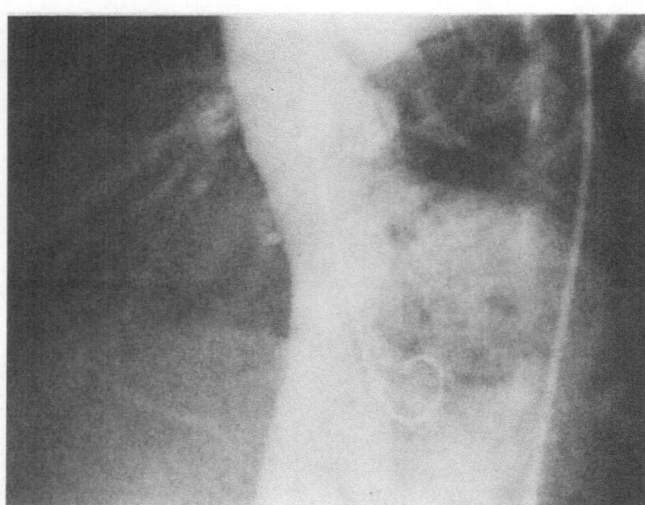

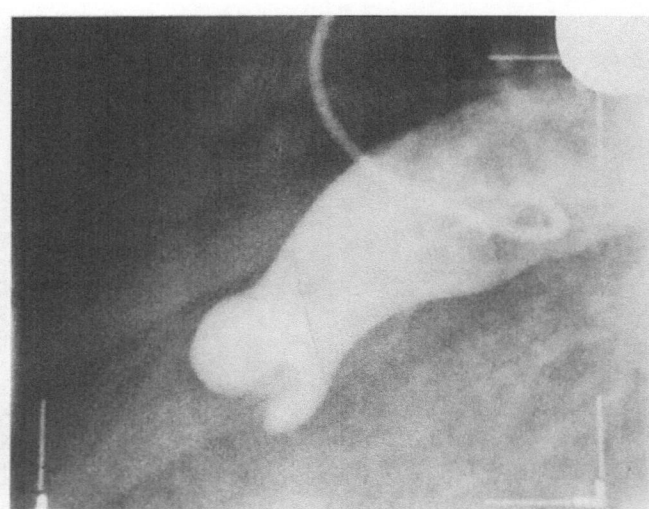

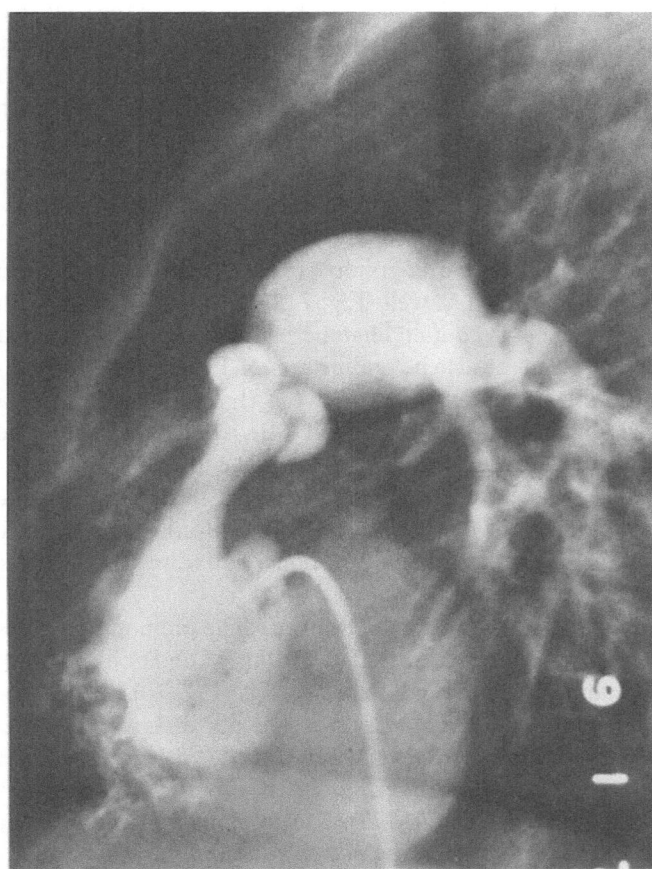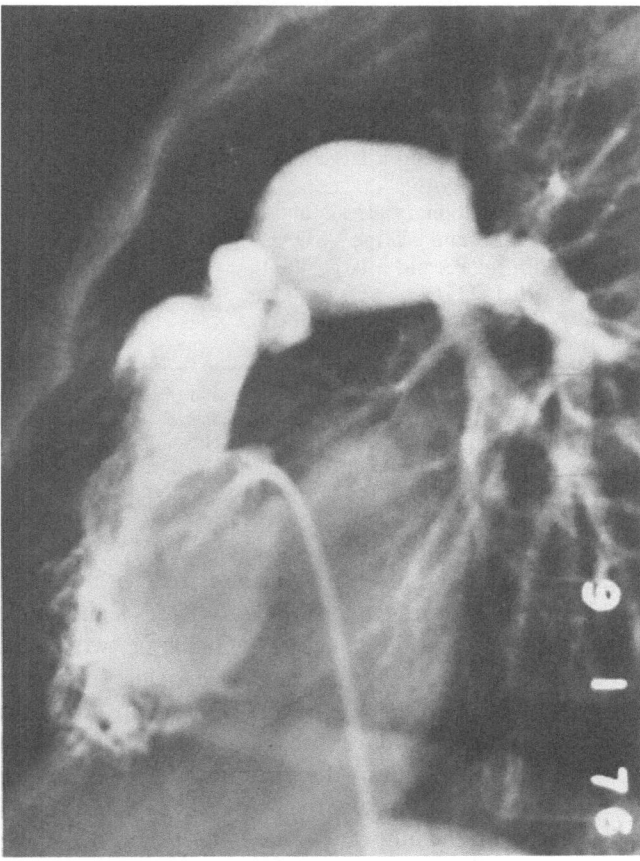

A   B

Fig. 7–177. *Radiological findings in an 8-year-old boy with pulmonary atresia and intact ventricular septum (postoperative pulmonary valvotomy and Blalock-Taussig anastomosis on the first day of life).* The right ventricle remains hypertrophied, but the cavity is of normal size. The enlarged right atrium is faintly opacified because of tricuspid insufficiency.

During systole (A) doming of the valve occurs. During diastole (B) the semilunar sinuses reconstitute. Poststenotic dilatation of the pulmonary artery is noted. Reconstitution of the sinuses indicates commissural fusion rather than a dysplastic valve. The peak systolic pressure gradient across the pulmonary valve was 30 mm Hg. The Blalock-Taussig anastomosis closed spontaneously.

Tricuspid Atresia

Tricuspid atresia (TA) is an uncommon but not rare (2%–3%) congenital anomaly, consisting of complete absence of the right atrioventricular (A-V) valve. The anomaly is usually associated with hypoplasia of the RV. This definition applies to cases with situs solitus and with A-V concordance; that is, when the morphological RA is right sided and the LA is left sided and the RA is in potential communication with the RV, while the LA communicates with the LV. This definition excludes single ventricle with atresia of the right-sided A-V valve. In single ventricle the RA is in potential communication with the main chamber.

In TA, systemic venous blood entering the RA is shunted through either an atrial septal defect or through a foramen ovale into the LA and then to the LV. Rarely the atrial septum is intact, and the interatrial communication is by way of the coronary sinus, which in turn connects with the LA through a perforation. Complete mixing of systemic venous and pulmonary venous blood in the LA results in arterial unsaturation. The blood reaches the lungs by way of associated heart defects (e.g., patent ductus arteriosus, ventricular septal defect). Diminution of pulmonary blood flow on serial roentgenograms of the chest and deterioration in systemic oxygen saturation may be due to spontaneous closure of a ventricular septal defect (VSD). In patients with TA and transposition of the great arteries, the blood reaches the systemic circulation via a large VSD or through a reversed patent ductus arteriosus or both. If the VSD closes in such instances, systemic blood flow is compromised. Classification of TA (Table 7–6) depends on the presence or absence of associated heart defects (i.e., transposition of the great arteries, pulmonic stenosis/atresia, VSD). Type I relates to TA associated with normally related great arteries; type II relates to TA with dextrotransposition of the great arteries (D-TGA) and type III relates to TA with levotransposition of the great arteries (L-TGA).

Cardiovascular abnormalities associated with TA include coarctation and interruption of the aorta, juxtaposition of the atrial appendages and patent ductus arteriosus, anomalies principally associated with type II TA.

Table 7–6. Classification of Tricuspid Atresia

I. Tricuspid atresia (TA) with normally related great vessels
    A. With pulmonary atresia and an intact ventricular septum
    B. With pulmonic stenosis (PS) and a small ventricular septal defect (VSD)
    C. With no PS and a large VSD
II. TA with D-TGA.
    A. With pulmonary atresia and a large VSD
    B. With PS and a large VSD
    C. With no PS and a large VSD
III. TA with L-TGA.
    A. With bulboventricular inversion
    B. With isolated bulbar inversion

* For details of type III TA see the text discussion of lesions only rarely encountered with tricuspid atresia. This classification does not include tricuspid atresia with double-outlet right ventricle and double-outlet left ventricle. Single ventricle with atresia of the right-sided atrioventricular valve is not a form of TA.

Lesions that are only rarely encountered with TA are double-outlet LV (with either D-TGA or L-TGA and single or double conus), and L-TGA. L-TGA is of two kinds: the common or classic form called ventricular inversion (bulboventricular inversion) and a rare form called isolated bulbar inversion. In bulboventricular inversion (also known as corrected transposition) the anatomical RV lies on the left side and the anatomical LV on the right side. In isolated bulbar inversion the inflow portions (sinuses) of the ventricles are normally placed, but the outflow portions are inverted, signifying that the anatomical LV has an infundibulum (conus) from which the aorta originates. The anatomical RV, on the other hand, lacks a conus (infundibulum), but gives origin to the pulmonary trunk. Because the A-V valves are part of the respective ventricular inflow portions (sinuses), the A-V valves are inverted in bulboventricular inversion and normally placed (noninverted) in isolated bulbar inversion. Thus, atresia of the left A-V valve occurs in TA with bulboventricular inversion, whereas the right A-V valve is atretic in TA with isolated bulbar inversion. For more complete details see specific articles listed in the bibliography.

TA is associated with extracardiac anomalies affecting the musculoskeletal and gastrointestinal system, and also occurs rarely with Down syndrome, asplenia, Christmas disease (hemophilia B) and cat-eye syndrome.

Clinical Features Children with TA and normally related great vessels are cyanotic from birth. Obstruction to pulmonary blood flow is caused by pulmonic stenosis or atresia. On the other hand, pulmonary overcirculation and even congestive heart failure are fairly common in TA with transposition of the great vessels. The electrocardiogram reveals LV hypertrophy with minimal RV forces. The axis is to the left at approximately −45°. In instances of TA with a VSD and large pulmonary blood flow and also in those with TGA the axis may be normal or even rightward. Enlargement of the RA suggests that the interatrial communication is inadequate.

Echocardiography The echocardiographic findings of TA

consist of a small RV, a large LV and atresia of the tricuspid valve. In place of the tricuspid valve is a highly reflective bar of tissue that may have motion on M-mode similar to that of a patent tricuspid valve (Fig. 7–178A), with no opening motion on 2-D echocardiography (Fig. 7–178C and D). In hypoplastic right-heart syndromes without tricuspid atresia (e.g., pulmonary atresia with intact ventricular septum) a small RV and a large LV are also demonstrated by echocardiography, but a functioning tricuspid valve is detected as well (Fig. 7–171). Single ventricle with a rudimentary outlet chamber and atresia of the right A-V valve may also be reminiscent of TA. Fibrous continuity will be demonstrated between the mitral valve and a semilunar valve in TA (Fig. 7–178B), whereas conus muscle will be interposed in cases of single ventricle. Two-dimensional echocardiography also may aid in determining the relationship of the great vessels and in estimating the size of the interatrial communication relative to the need for atrial septostomy.

Radiological (Plain Film) Features The pulmonary vascularity is usually decreased (pulmonary undercirculation), because of marked pulmonic stenosis (Fig. 7–179). Pulmonary flow may be increased in patients with a large VSD without pulmonic stenosis and in those with transposition of the great arteries. The heart is often enlarged, but it may be normal (Fig. 7–179). The pulmonary artery segment is flat or concave because of hypoplasia of the main pulmonary artery. The left upper heart border may be straightened or even convex in the presence of left-sided juxtaposition of the atrial appendages or LA dilatation with an enlarged LA appendage (Fig. 7–180). The aorta tends to be enlarged. On occasion a right aortic arch may be noted. The cardiac apex is usually rounded and is often elevated, simulating enlargement of the RV (Figs. 7–181 and 7–182). This appearance is brought about because in the absence of a RV of significant size, the LV assumes the position normally occupied by the RV. The RV itself is usually small, its size being best evaluated in the LAO and lateral views (Fig. 7–181B). An enlarged LV posteriorly in conjunction with a dilated RA and small RV situated anteriorly form a characteristic heart configuration.

Hemodynamics The findings at catheterization are determined by the associated defects. The RV cannot be entered directly from the RA. Oxygen saturations are equal in the superior and inferior venae cavae and RA; complete admixture of systemic and pulmonary venous blood occurs in the LA, resulting in identical saturations in the LV and systemic circulation. Pressure in the RA is greater than pressure in the LA. The venae cavae and RA pressure tracings show prominent a waves, while the LA, LV and aortic pressures are usually normal. In TA with normally related great vessels, pulmonary pressure and pulmonary blood flow are determined by the size of the VSD and severity of pulmonic stenosis. Usually the VSD is small and the pulmonary valve stenotic. Some infants are dependent on the ductus arteriosus for pulmonary blood flow. Thus, pulmonary flow and pressure are usually low. In

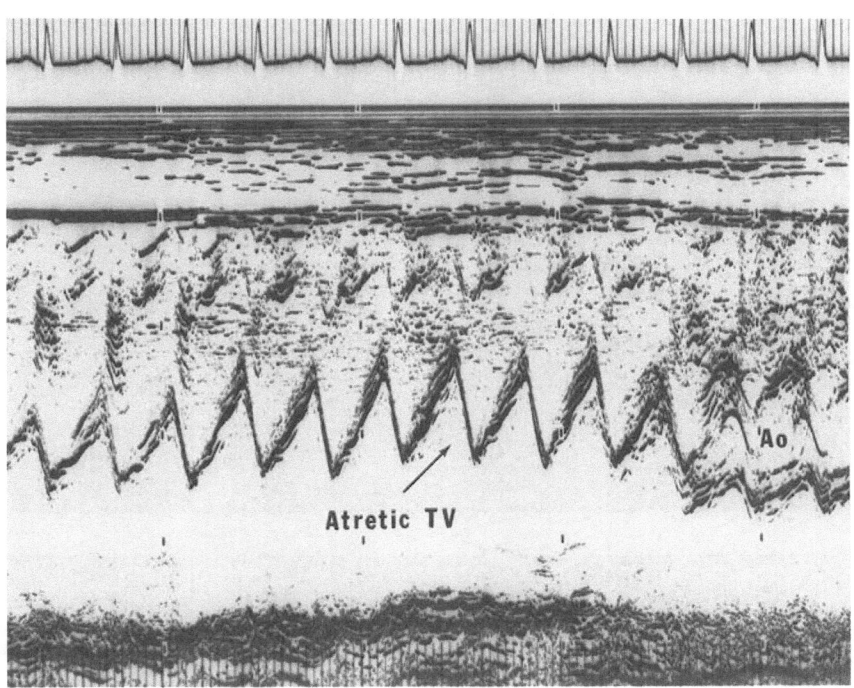

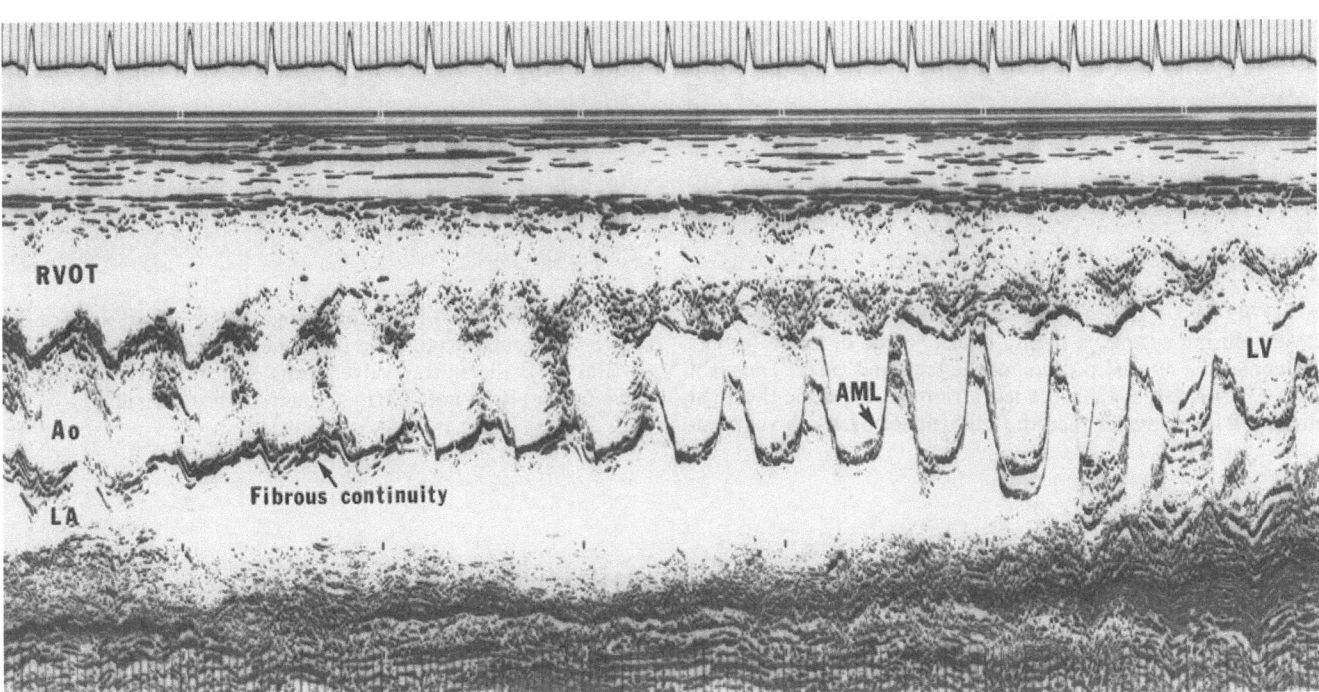

Fig. 7–178. *Echocardiography in a 3-year-old girl with tricuspid atresia and normally related great vessels.* **A** is an M-mode arc scan from the area of the atretic tricuspid valve (*Atretic TV*) to the aortic root (*Ao*). The motion of the atretic tricuspid valve is similar to the motion of a patent tricuspid valve. **B** is an M-mode arc scan from the aortic root to the mitral valve showing aortic-mitral fibrous continuity. A right ventricular outflow tract (*RVOT*) of significant size is present anteriorly. *Ao* = aorta; LA = left atrium; *AML* = anterior mitral leaflet; *LV* = left ventricle. (*Continued*)

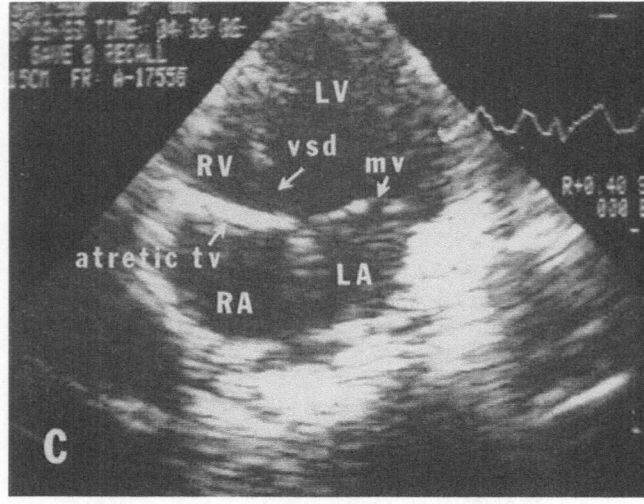 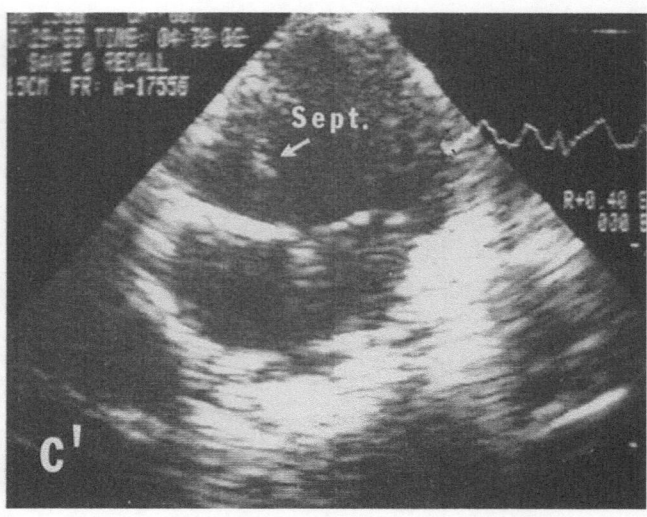

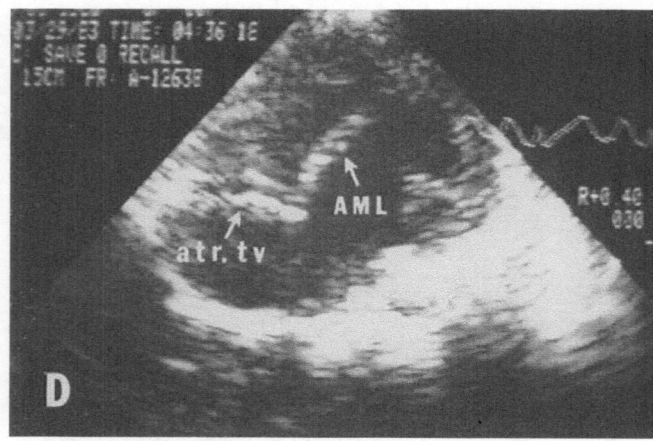 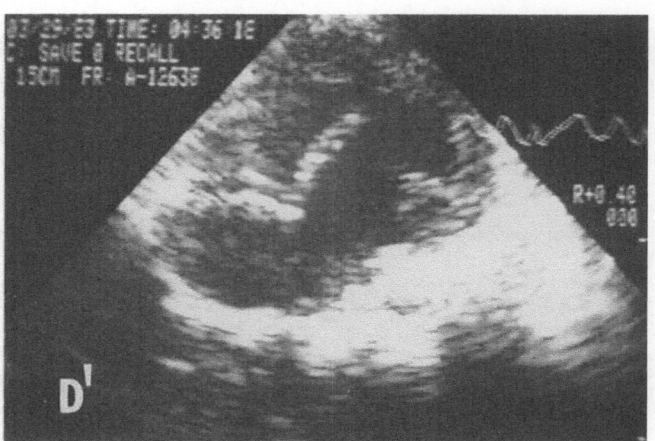

Fig. 7–178 (*Cont.*) In C and C′, representing an apex four-chamber view during systole, a highly reflective bar of tissue (*atretic tv*) occupies the normal position of the tricuspid valve. The right atrium (*RA*) is larger than the left atrium (*LA*), while the right ventricle (*RV*) is smaller than the left ventricle (*LV*). A ventricular septal defect (*vsd*) is demonstrated. *mv* = mitral valve; *Sept.* = interventricular septum. In the same apex view during diastole (**D** and **D′**), the mitral valve opens, but the atretic tricuspid valve (*atr.tv*) does not. *AML* = anterior mitral leaflet.

TA with TGA the pulmonary artery arises directly from the LV, often with little or no pulmonic stenosis. Pulmonary flow and pressure are high, and pulmonary resistance may be increased (Eisenmenger syndrome) in older infants and children with TA and TGA. Even a slight increase in pulmonary resistance constitutes a contraindication to a Fontan procedure (atriopulmonary connection).

Contrast Studies The RA angiogram demonstrates the atretic tricuspid valve and the interatrial communication. Rarely, if the foramen ovale is restrictive, an aneurysm of the atrial septum may occur. Opacification of the LA and LV with little or no opacification of the RV (by way of a VSD) results in a triangular filling defect between the contrast-medium–filled RA and the LV on the diaphragmatic border of the heart (Fig. 7–179B, 7–180B). Left ventriculography is valuable in determining the presence or absence of a VSD (Fig. 7–180C, 7–182). If a VSD is present the RV and pulmonary arteries are opacified.

The size of the RV, the size and function of the pulmonary valve and the anatomy of the pulmonary arteries are all important concerns relative to consideration of surgery. In the presence of transposition of the great arteries, subaortic stenosis may be caused by a restrictive VSD and may be accompanied by hypoplasia, coarctation or interruption of the aorta. Other associated cardiovascular malformations are also identified (e.g., juxtaposition of the atrial appendages, patent ductus arteriosus, persistent left superior vena cava). TA should be differentiated from other heart malformations causing hypoplasia of the right heart. Among these malformations are pulmonary atresia with intact ventricular septum, congenital tricuspid stenosis and congenital unguarded tricuspid orifice (absence of tricuspid valvular tissue). On occasion, Ebstein malformation, tumors of the right heart and isolated rheumatic tricuspid stenosis may cause tricuspid valve obstruction and a right-to-left interatrial shunt resulting in cyanosis.

Fig. 7–179. **A** *Plain film of the chest and* **B** *right atrial angiogram in a cyanotic 5-day-old boy with tricuspid atresia and normally related great arteries.* Marked pulmonary undercirculation is present. The size and configuration of the heart are normal. The angiogram shows the typical "tricuspid sequence"—that is, the right atrium, left atrium and left ventricle fill in that order. The right ventricle fills from the left ventricle through a ventricular septal defect, and the great vessels fill from their respective ventricles. A lucent triangle (clear window area, *arrow*) occupies the position of the inflow portion of the right ventricle. This sequence of filling of the cardiac chambers and the clear window area are considered characteristic of tricuspid atresia. These features are not pathognomonic, since they also may be encountered with other defects (e.g., pulmonary atresia or critical pulmonic stenosis with intact septum).

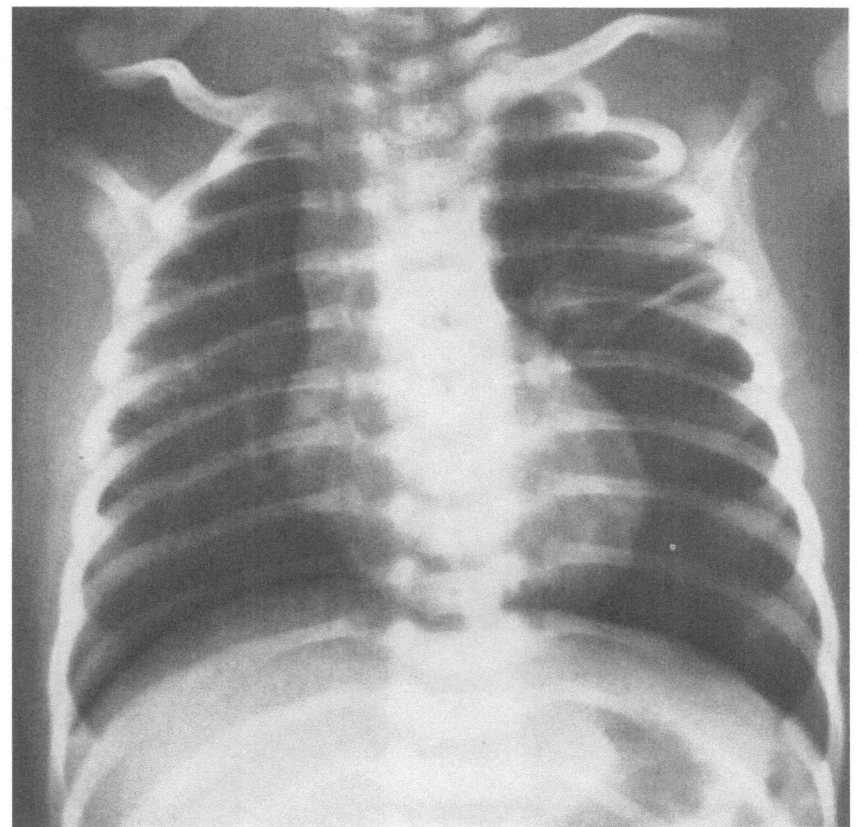

A

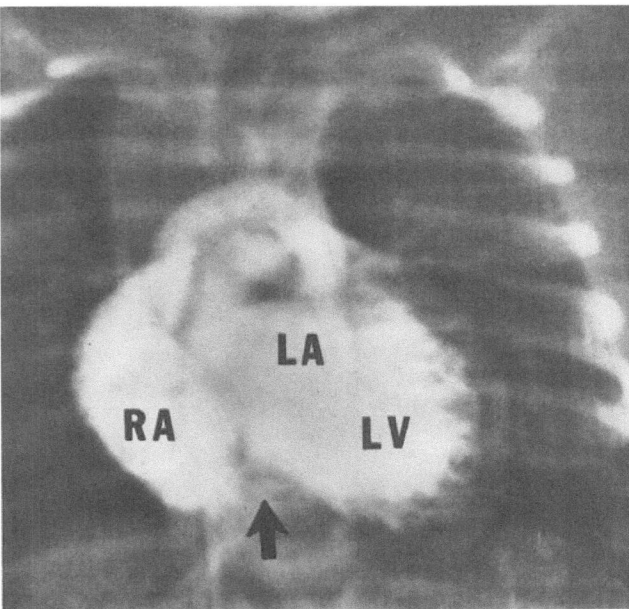

B

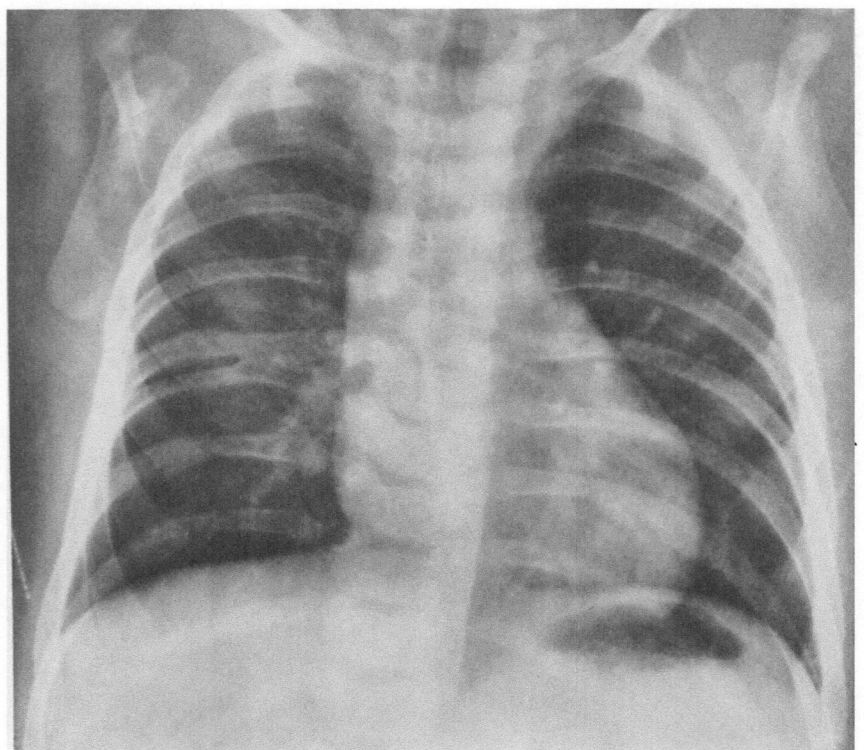

A

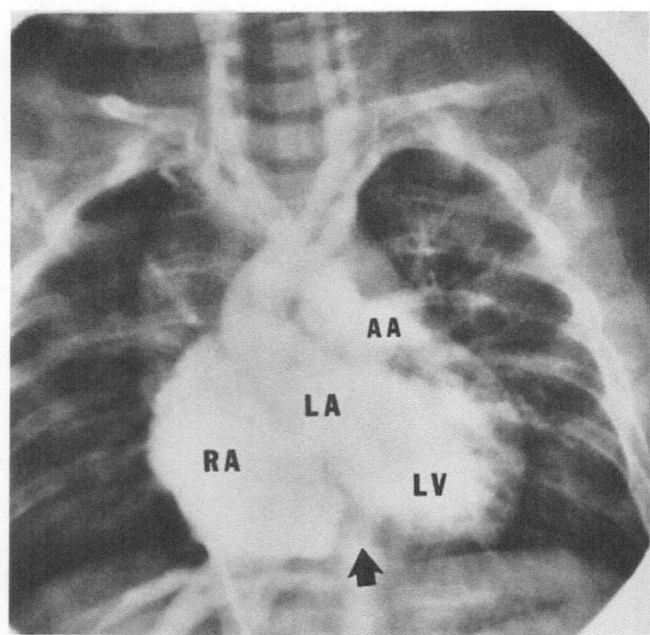

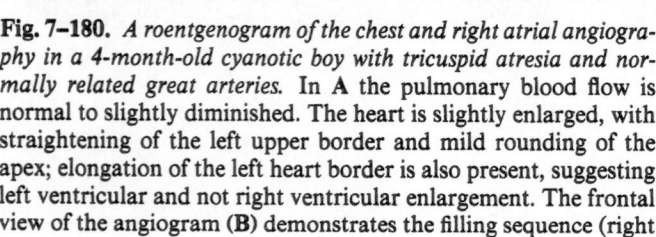

B

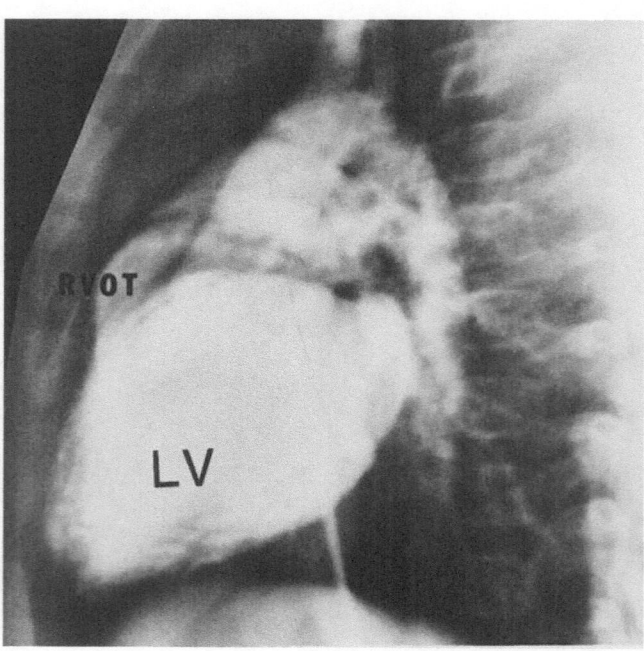

C

Fig. 7–180. *A roentgenogram of the chest and right atrial angiography in a 4-month-old cyanotic boy with tricuspid atresia and normally related great arteries.* In **A** the pulmonary blood flow is normal to slightly diminished. The heart is slightly enlarged, with straightening of the left upper border and mild rounding of the apex; elongation of the left heart border is also present, suggesting left ventricular and not right ventricular enlargement. The frontal view of the angiogram (**B**) demonstrates the filling sequence (right atrium, left atrium and left ventricle) and the triangular clear space (*arrow*) characteristic of tricuspid atresia. The left atrium (*LA*) is superimposed on the outflow tract of the left ventricle (*LV*), while the left atrial appendage (*AA*) contributes to straightening of the left heart border on the film of the chest. On the lateral view of the angiogram (**C**) the large left ventricle (*LV*) fills the right ventricle by way of a ventricular septal defect. *RVOT* = right ventricular outflow tract.

Fig. 7–181. *A roentgenogram of the chest in a cyanotic 1-day-old girl with tricuspid atresia (same patient as in Fig. 7–182).* In the frontal view (**A**) severe undercirculation is present. The heart is enlarged, and the apex is rounded and elevated, to an extent in excess of what is usually observed in tetralogy of Fallot. The pulmonary artery segment is concave. The right atrium appears normal. This type of cardiac configuration and pulmonary undercirculation with right axis deviation and right ventricular hypertrophy on the electrocardiogram are consistent with tetralogy of Fallot, critical pulmonic stenosis or other obstructive lesions of the right heart without hypoplasia of the right ventricle. When these findings on plain film are accompanied by left axis deviation tricuspid atresia should be considered instead. Even in the absence of an appropriate history the lateral roentgenogram (**B**) is helpful because it shows left ventricular enlargement, and not right ventricular enlargement. The lower retrosternal area is relatively lucent, corresponding to a small right ventricle.

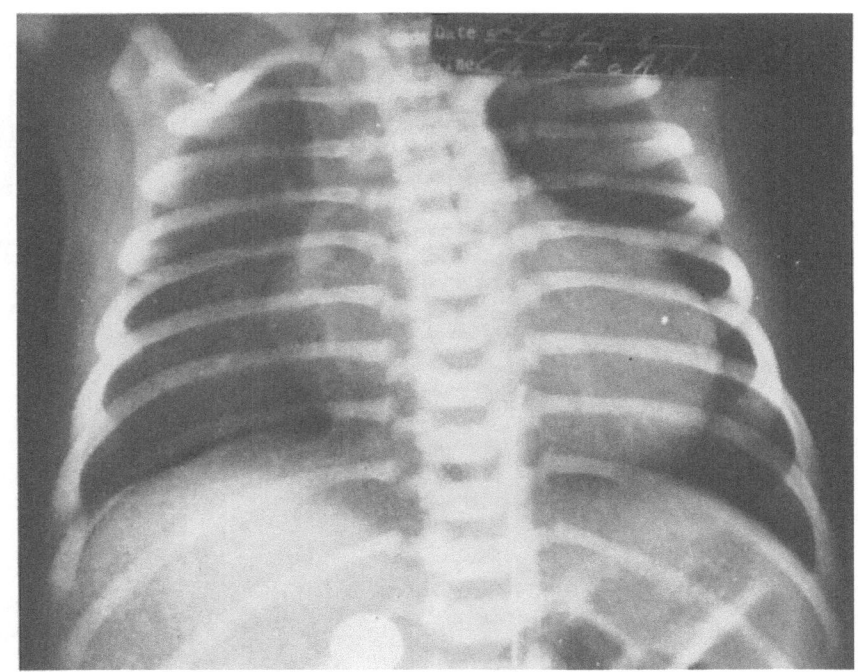

A

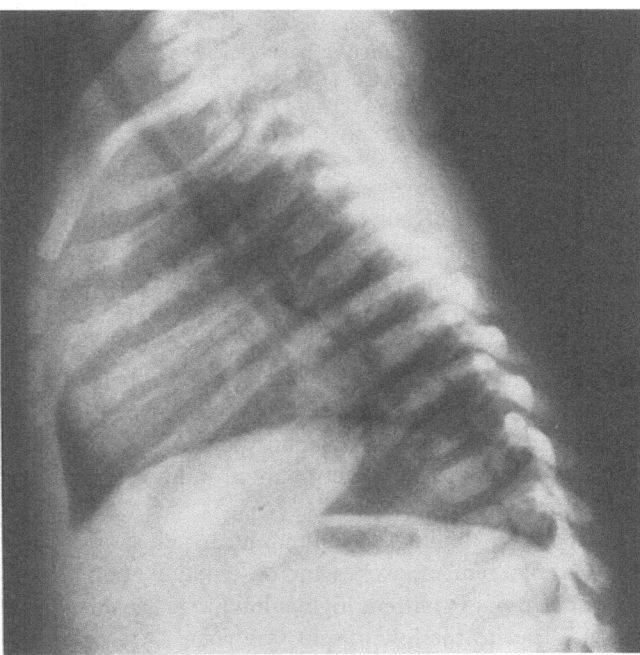

B

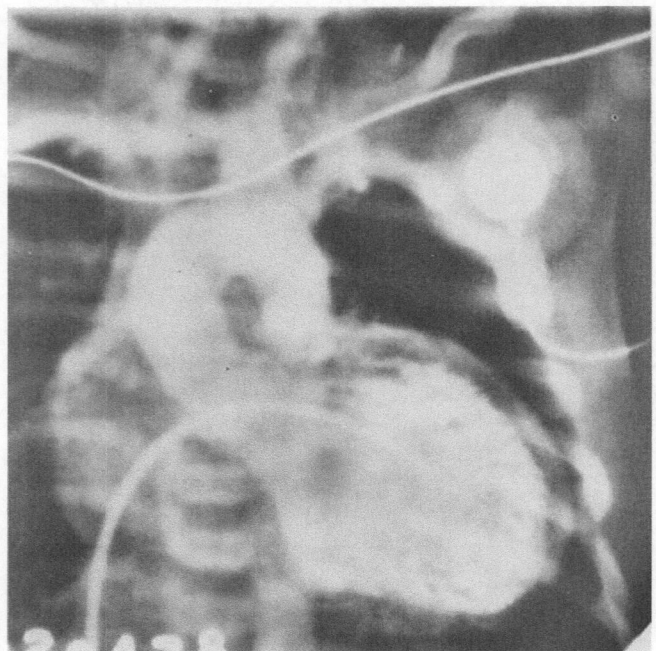 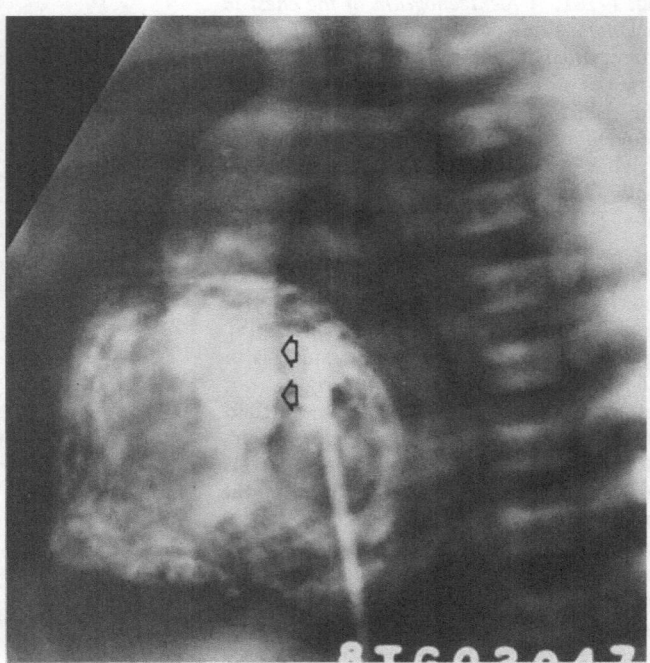

A   B

Fig. 7–182. *Left ventriculogram in a cyanotic 1-day-old girl with tricuspid atresia (same patient as in Fig. 7–181).* In the frontal view of the left ventriculogram (**A**) the large left ventricle accounts for the appearance of the cardiac apex on the plain film of the chest. The pulmonary arteries opacify faintly. In the lateral view (**B**) the left ventricle is markedly enlarged because all of the sys-temic and pulmonary venous blood flows through it. The septum appears intact (type IA, see Table 7–6). Fibrous continuity between the aortic and mitral valves is clearly demonstrated (*open arrows*), thus excluding single ventricle. The right atrial injection (not shown) demonstrated the typical filling sequence of tricuspid "atresia."

Treatment Balloon atrial septostomy during the initial cardiac catheterization procedure is recommended even if obstruction to emptying of the RA is not demonstrated. Prostaglandin E₁ is administered until palliative aorta-to-pulmonary shunts are created if pulmonary flow is inadequate. Pulmonary banding may be useful in cases in which pulmonary flow is excessive. A recent approach to total correction involves prosthetic connections of the RA directly to the RV outflow tract or main pulmonary artery (Fontan procedure).

Postoperative findings after Fontan procedures may include RA enlargement, ascites and obstruction at any level of the connection. Persistent high pulmonary vascular resistance will lead to the low output syndrome. Arrhythmias occurring after the Fontan procedure include sinus arrest and other atrial arrhythmias, as well as complete heart block, requiring a pacemaker.

Cor Triatriatum Dexter

This rare entity usually accompanies other forms of right-sided cardiac obstruction, but may occur as an isolated anomaly. It is characterized by an enlarged valve of the sinus venosus that separates the RA into an inflow portion and an outflow portion. The superior and inferior venae cavae enter the inflow chamber; blood flows from here through an opening in the membrane to reach the tricuspid valve. In the case reported by Verel et al., no pressure gradient was measured across the membrane. In contrast in the case of Nakano et al., surgical excision was required. Jones and Niles described a patient with tricuspid atresia and a large valve of the sinus venosus, which intermittently obstructed the foramen ovale and led to acute decompensation and, eventually, death. The case reported by Gerlis and Anderson included cor triatriatum dexter with imperforate Ebstein malformation of the tricuspid valve and atresia of the pulmonary valve.

Clinical features and radiological findings vary, depending on the severity of obstruction and associated defects. Isolated cor triatriatum dexter, with obstruction, produces enlargement of the RA, simulating Ebstein anomaly. Cardiac catheterization may reveal a right-to-left shunt at the atrial level, while on angiography the RA is divided into two chambers by a membrane.

Bibliography

Primary (Idiopathic) Pulmonary Hypertension

Edwards WD, Edwards JE (1977) Clinical primary pulmonary hypertension. Three pathologic types. Circulation 56:884–888

Goodman DJ, Harrison DC, Popp RL (1974) Echocardiographic features of primary pulmonary hypertension. Am J Cardiol 33:438–443

Ikram H, Maslowski AH, Nicholls MG, Espiner EA, Hull FTL (1982) Hemodynamic and hormonal effects of captopril in primary pulmonary hypertension. Br Heart J 48:541–555

Keane JF, Fyler DC, Nadas AS (1978) Hazards of cardiac catheterization in children with primary pulmonary vascular obstruction. Am Heart J 96:556–558

Klinke WP, Gilbert JAL (1980) Diazoxide in primary pulmonary hypertension. N Engl J Med 302:91–92

Lupi-Herrera E, Sandoval J, Seoane M, Bialostozky D (1982) The role of hydralazine therapy for pulmonary arterial hypertension of unknown cause. Circulation 65:645–650

Nagasaka Y, Akutsu H, Lee YS, Fujimoto S, Chikamori J (1978) Longterm favorable effect of oxygen administration on a patient with primary pulmonary hypertension. Chest 74:299–300

Rubin LJ, Graves BM, Reeves JT, Frosolono M, Handel F, Cato AE (1982) Prostacyclin-induced acute pulmonary vasodilatation in primary pulmonary hypertension. Circulation 66:334–337

Rubin LJ, Peter RH (1980) Oral hydralazine therapy for primary pulmonary hypertension. N Engl J Med 302:69–73

Shettigar UR, Hultgren HN, Specter M, Martin R, Davies DH (1976) Primary pulmonary hypertension. Favorable effect of isoproterenol. N Engl J Med 295:1414–1415

Wagenvoort CA, Wagenvoort N (1970) Primary pulmonary hypertension: A pathologic study of the lung vessels in 156 clinically diagnosed cases. Circulation 42:1163–1184

Wang SWS, Pohl JEF, Rowlands DJ, Wade EG (1978) Diazoxide in treatment of primary pulmonary hypertension. Br Heart J 40:572–574

Pulmonic Stenosis

Alday LE, Moreyra E (1973) Calcific pulmonary stenosis. Br Heart J 35:887–889

Caldwell RL, Weyman AE, Hurwitz RA, Girod DA, Feigenbaum H (1979) Right ventricular outflow tract assessment by cross-sectional echocardiography in tetralogy of Fallot. Circulation 59:395–402

Castaneda-Zuniga WR, Formanek A, Amplatz K (1977) Radiologic diagnosis of different types of pulmonary stenoses. Cardiovasc Radiol 1:2–14

Chen JTT, Robinson AE, Goodrich JK, Lester RG (1969) Uneven distribution of pulmonary blood flow between left and right lungs in isolated valvular pulmonary stenosis. Am J Roentgenol 107:343–350

Cooper LZ, Krugman S (1966) Diagnosis and management: Congenital rubella. Pediatrics 37:335–338

Davis GL, McAlister WH, Friedenbery MJ (1965) Congenital aortic stenosis due to failure of histogenesis of aortic valve (myxoid dysplasia). Am J Roentgenol 95:621–628

D'Cruz IA, Arcilla RA, Agustsson MH (1964) Dilatation of the pulmonary trunk in stenosis of the pulmonary valve and of the pulmonary arteries in children. Am Heart J 68:612–620

Deshmukh M, Guvenc S, Bentivoglio L, Goldberg H (1960) Idiopathic dilatation of the pulmonary artery. Circulation 21:710–716

Desilets DT, Marcano BA, Emmanouilides GC, Gyepes MT (1968) Severe pulmonary stenosis and atresia. Radiol Clin North Am 6:367–382

Forney WR, Robinson SJ, Pascoe DJ (1966) Congenital heart disease, deafness, and skeletal malformations: A new syndrome? J Pediatr 68:14–26

Gorlin RJ, Anderson RC, Blaw M (1969) Multiple lentigenes syndrome. Am J Dis Child 117:652–662

Gregg N (1941) Congenital cataract following German measles in the mother. Trans Ophthalmol Soc Aust 3:35–46

Hardy JB (1973) Clinical and developmental aspects of congenital rubella. Arch Otolaryngol 98:230–236

Holt RG, Gross R, Carlsson E (1978) Angiographic features of carcinoid heart disease. Radiology 127:601–605

Hurwitz LE, Roberts WC (1973) Quadricuspid semilunar valve. Am J Cardiol 31:623–626

Jeffery RF, Moller JH, Amplatz K (1972) The dysplastic pulmonary valve: A new roentgenographic entity. With a discussion of the anatomy and radiology of other types of valvular pulmonary stenosis. Am J Roentgenol 114:322–339

Kan JS, White RI Jr, Mitchell SE, Gardner TJ (1982) Percutaneous balloon valvuloplasty: A new method for treating congenital pulmonary valve stenosis. N Engl J Med 307:540–542

Keith A (1909) The Hunterian lecture on malformation on the heart. Lancet 70:52

Koletsky S (1941) Congenital bicuspid aortic valves. Arch Intern Med 67:129–156

Koretzky ED, Moller JH, Korns ME, Schwartz CJ, Edwards JE (1969) Congenital pulmonary stenosis resulting from dysplasia of valve. Circulation 40:43–53

Lange LW, Sahn DJ, Allen HD, Goldberg SJ (1979) Subxyphoid cross-sectional echocardiography in infants and children with congenital heart disease. Circulation 59:513–524

Linde LM, Turner SW, Sparkes RS (1973) Pulmonary valvular dysplasia. A cardiofacial syndrome. Br Heart J 35:301–304

McLoughlin TG, Krovitz LJ, Schiebler GL (1964) Heart diseases in the Laurence-Moon-Biedl-Bardet syndrome. A review and a report of 3 brothers. J Pediatr 65:388–399

Menser MA, Dods L, Harley JD (1967) A 25-year follow-up of congenital rubella. Lancet 2:1347–1350

Nadas AS, Fyler DC (1972) Pediatric cardiology, 3rd ed. Saunders, Philadelphia

Neiman HL, Mena E, Holt JE, Stern AM, Perry BL (1974) Neurofibromatosis and congenital heart disease. Am J Roentgenol 122:146–149

Orell SR, Karnell J. Wahlgreen F (1960) Malformation and multiple stenoses of the pulmonary arteries with pulmonary hypertension. Acta Radiol 54:449–459

Pepine CJ, Gessner IH, Feldman RL (1982) Percutaneous balloon valvuloplasty for pulmonic valve stenosis in the adult. Am J Cardiol 50:1442–1445

Phornphutkul C, Rosenthal A, Nadas AS (1973) Cardiomyopathy in Noonan's syndrome. Report of three cases. Br Heart J 35:99–102

Rao PS, Liebman J, Borkat G (1976) Right ventricular growth in a case of pulmonic stenosis with intact ventricular septum and hypoplastic right ventricle. Circulation 53:389–394

Riggs W, Jr (1970) Roentgen findings in Noonan's syndrome. Radiology 96:393–395

Robinson CD, Perry LW, Barlee A, Mella GW (1971) Smith-Lemli-Opitz syndrome with cardiovascular abnormality. Pediatrics 47:844–847

Rohde RA (1966) The chromosomes in heart disease. Clinical and cytogenetic studies of 68 cases. Circulation 34:484–502

Rowe RD (1963) Maternal rubella and pulmonary artery stenoses. Report of 11 cases. Pediatrics 32:180–185

Rowe RD (1966) Cardiovascular lesions in rubella (letter to the editor). J Pediatr 68:147

Summitt RL (1969) Turner syndrome and Noonan's syndrome. J Pediatr 75:730–731

Tang JS, Kauffman SL, Lunfield J (1971) Hypoplasia of the pulmonary arteries in infants with congenital rubella. Am J Cardiol 27:491–496

Taylor AI (1967) Patau's, Edwards' and Cri du Chat syndromes: A tabulated summary of current findings. Dev Med Child Neurol 9:78–86

Taylor AI (1968) Autosomal trisomy syndromes: A detailed study of 27 cases of Edwards' syndrome and 27 cases of Patau's syndrome. J Med Genet 5:227–252

Venables AW (1965) The syndrome of pulmonary stenosis complicating maternal rubella. Br Heart J 27:49–55

Wasserman MP, Varghese PJ, Rowe RD (1968) The evolution of pulmonary arterial stenosis associated with congenital rubella. Am Heart J 76:638–644

Williams JCP, Barratt-Boyes BG, Lowe JB (1963) Underdeveloped right ventricle and pulmonary stenosis. Am J Cardiol 11:458–468

Subvalvar Pulmonic Stenosis

Ehrenhaft JL, Theilen EO, Fisher J (1959) Ectopic tricuspid leaflet producing symptoms of infundibular pulmonic stenosis. Ann Surg 150:937–940

Fellows KE, Martin EC, Rosenthal A (1977) Angiocardiography of obstructing muscular bands of the right ventricle. Am J Roentgenol 128:249–256

Fisher CH, James AE Jr, Humphries JO, Forster J, White RI Jr (1971) Radiographic findings in anomalous muscle bundle of the right ventricle. An analysis of 15 cases. Radiology 101:35–43

Forster JW, Humphries JO (1971) Right ventricular anomalous muscle bundle. Clinical and laboratory presentation and natural history. Circulation 43:115–127

Goldberg SJ, Allen HD, Sahn DJ (1980) Pediatric and adolescent echocardiography, 2nd edn. Year Book, Chicago, pp 208–209

Hartmann AF Jr, Goldring D, Carlsson E (1964) Development of right ventricular obstruction by aberrant muscular bands. Circulation 30:679–685

Hartmann AF Jr, Goldring D, Ferguson TB, Burford TH, Smith CH, Kissane JM, Frech RS (1970) The course of children with the two-chambered right ventricle. J Thorac Cardiovasc Surg 60:72–83

Hartmann AF, Tsifutis AA, Arvidsson H, Goldring D (1962) The two-chambered right ventricle. Report of nine cases. Circulation 26:279–287

Heger JJ, Weyman AE (1979) A review of m-mode and cross-sectional echocardiographic findings of the pulmonary valve. J Clin Ultrasound 7:98–107

Hindle WV Jr, Engle MA, Hagstrom JW (1968) Anomalous right ventricular muscles: A clinicopathologic study. Am J Cardiol 21:487–495

Neufeld HN, Ongley PA, Edwards JE (1960) Combined congenital subaortic and infundibular pulmonary stenosis. Br Heart J 22:626–690

Pate JW, Ainger LE, Butterick OD (1964) A new form of right ventricular outflow obstruction. Case report. Am Heart J 68:249–251

Pate JW, Richardson RL Jr, Giles HH (1968) Accessory tricuspid leaflet producing right ventricular outflow obstruction. N Engl J Med 279:867–868

Patel R, Astley R (1973) Right ventricular obstruction due to anomalous muscle bands. Br Heart J 35:890–893

Idiopathic Dilatation of the Pulmonary Artery

Befeler B, Macleod C, Baum GL, Schwartz H (1967) Idiopathic dilatation of the pulmonary artery. Am J Med Sci 254:667–674

Deshmukh M, Guvenc S, Bentivoglio L, Goldberg H (1960) Idiopathic dilatation of the pulmonary artery. Circulation 21:710–716

Espino-Vela J (1959) Dilatacion idiopatica de la arteria pulmonar. In: Malformaciones cardiovasculares congenitas. Edition of Instituto Nacional de Cardiologia. Mexico, Chap 25, pp 353–359

Teitelbaum JE, Altman M (1978) Idiopathic dilatation of peripheral pulmonary arteries. Chest 73:241–242

Supravalvar Pulmonary Stenosis

Arvidsson H, Carlsson E, Hartmann A Jr, Tsifutis A, Crawford C (1961) Supravalvular stenoses of the pulmonary arteries. Report of 11 cases. Acta Radiol 56:466–480

Barrillon A, Havy G, Scebat L, Baragan J, Gerbaux A (1974) Congenital pressure gradients between main pulmonary artery and its primary branches. Br Heart J 36:669–675

Eldredge WJ, Tingelstad JB, Robertson LW, Mauck HP, McCue CM (1972) Observations on the natural history of pulmonary artery coarctations. Circulation 45:404–409

Smith WG (1958) Pulmonary hypertension and continuous murmur due to multiple peripheral stenoses of pulmonary arteries. Thorax 13:174

Tang JS, Kauffman SL, Lynfield J (1971) Hypoplasia of the pulmonary arteries in infants with congenital rubella. Am J Cardiol 27:491–496

Venables AW (1965) The syndrome of pulmonary stenosis complicating maternal rubella. Br Heart J 27:49–55

Stenosis of the Tricuspid Valve

Calleja HB, Hosier DM, Kissane RW (1960) Congenital tricuspid stenosis. The diagnostic value of cineangiocardiography and hepatic pulse tracing. Am J Cardiol 6:821–829

Hansing CE, Young WP, Rowe GG (1972) Cor triatriatum dexter. Persistent right sinus venosus valve. Am J Cardiol 30:559–564

Henriques U (1963) Isolated tricuspid stenosis. N Engl J Med 269:1267–1268

Lewis T (1944) Congenital tricuspid stenosis. Clin Sci 5:261–273

Schlesinger P, Benchimol CB, Lopes AS, Barbosa J, Jasbik W, Benchimol AB (1983) Isolated tricuspid stenosis: Report of a case submitted to valvar commissurotomy. Clin Cardiol 6:182–187

Accessory Tricuspid Valve Tissue

Ehrenhaft JL, Theilen EO, Fisher J (1959) Ectopic tricuspid leaflet producing symptoms of infundibular pulmonic stenosis. Ann Surg 150:937–940

Levy MJ, Lillehei CW, Elliot LP, Carey LS, Adams PJ Jr, Edwards JE (1963) Accessory valvular tissue causing subpulmonic stenosis in corrected transposition of the great arteries. Circulation 27:494–502

McLean LD, Culligan JA, Kane DJ (1963) Subaortic stenosis due to accessory tissue on mitral valve. J Thoracic Cardiovasc Surg 45:382–388

Pate JW, Richardson RL Jr, Giles HH (1968) Accessory tricuspid leaflet producing right ventricular outflow obstruction. N Engl J Med 279:868–869

Ebstein Anomaly of the Tricuspid Valve

Aaron BL, Mills M, Lower RR (1976) Congenital tricuspid insufficiency. Definition and review. Chest 69:637–641

Amplatz K, Lester RG, Schiebler GL, Adams P Jr, Anderson RC (1959) The roentgenologic features of Ebstein's anomaly of the tricuspid valve. Am J Roentgenol 81:788–794

Andersen KR, Zuberbuhler JR, Anderson RH, Becker AE, Lie JT (1979) Morphologic spectrum of Ebstein's anomaly of the heart. A review. Mayo Clin Proc 54:174–180

Bialostozky D, Horwitz S, Espino-Vela J (1972) Ebstein's malformation of the tricuspid valve: A review of 65 cases. Am J Cardiol 29:826–836

Blount SG, McCord MC, Gelb IJ (1957) Ebstein's anomaly. Circulation 15:210–224

Boucek RJ Jr, Graham TP Jr, Morgan JP, Atwood GF, Boerth RC (1976) Spontaneous resolution of massive congenital tricuspid insufficiency. Circulation 54:795–800

Bucciarelli RL, Nelson RM, Egan II, Eitzman DV, Gessner IH (1977) Transient tricuspid insufficiency of the newborn: A form of myocardial dysfunction in stressed newborns. Pediatrics 59:330–337

Danielson GK (1982) Ebstein's anomaly: Editorial comments and personal observations. Ann Thorac Surg 34:396–400

Danielson GK, Maloney, JD, Devloo RAE (1979) Surgical repair of Ebstein's anomaly. Mayo Clin Proc 54:185–192

Ellis K, Griffiths SP, Burris JO, Ramsay GC, Fleming RJ (1964) Ebstein's anomaly of the tricuspid valve. Angiocardiographic considerations. Am J Roentgenol 92:1338–1352

Fabian CE, Mundt WP, Abrams HL (1966) Ebstein's anomaly. The direct demonstration of contractile synchrony between the two parts of the right ventricle. Invest Radiol 1:63–68

Farooki ZQ, Henry JG, Green EW (1976) Echocardiographic spectrum of Ebstein's anomaly of the tricuspid valve. Circulation 53:63–68

Genton E, Blount SG Jr (1967) The spectrum of Ebstein's anomaly. Am Heart J 73:395–425

Gerlis LM, Anderson RH (1976) Cor triatriatum dexter with imperforate Ebstein's anomaly. Br Heart J 38:108–111

Giuliani ER, Fuster V, Brandenburg RO, Mair DD (1979) Ebstein's anomaly. The clinical features and natural history of Ebstein's anomaly of the tricuspid valve. Mayo Clin Proc 54:163–173

Hanson DJ, Rosenbaum HD (1964) Posterior cardiac prominence in Ebstein's anomaly simulating mitral disease. Am J Roentgenol 92:1331–1337

Hernandez FA, Rochkind R, Cooper HR (1958) The intracavitary electrocardiogram in the diagnosis of Ebstein's anomaly. Am J Cardiol 1:181–190

Hipona FA, Arthachinta S (1964) Ebstein's anomaly of the tricuspid valve. A report of 16 cases and review of the literature. Prog Cardiovasc Dis 7:434–448

Hirschklau MJ, Sahn DJ, Hagan AD, Williams DE, Friedman WF (1977) Cross-sectional echocardiographic features of Ebstein's anomaly of the tricuspid valve. Am J Cardiol 40:400–404

Huhta JC, Edwards WD, Tajik AJ, Mair DD, Puga FJ, Ritter DG (1982) Pulmonary atresia with intact ventricular septum, Ebstein's anomaly of hypoplastic tricuspid valve, and double-chamber right ventricle. Two-dimensional echocardiographic-anatomic correlation. Mayo Clin Proc 27:515–519

Kastor JA, Goldreyer BN, Josephson ME, Perloff JK, Scharf DL, Manchester JH, Shelbourne JC, Hirshfeld JW Jr (1975) Electrophysiologic characteristics of Ebstein's anomaly of the tricuspid valve. Circulation 52:987–995

Kerber RE, Marcus ML, Wolfson PM (1975) Demonstration of Ebstein's anomaly by simultaneous catheter-tip localization of the tricuspid valve and right coronary artery visualization: A new method. Chest 68:99–102

Lundstrom NR (1973) Echocardiography in the diagnosis of Ebstein's anomaly of the tricuspid valve. Circulation 47:597–605

Matsumoto M, Matsuo H, Nagata S, Hamanaka Y, Fujita T, Kawashima Y, Nimura Y, Abe H (1976) Visualization of Ebstein's anomaly of the tricuspid valve by two-dimensional and standard echocardiography. Circulation 53:69–79

Milner S, Meyer RA, Venables AW, Korfhagen J, Kaplan S (1976) Mitral and tricuspid valve closure in congenital heart disease. Circulation 53:513–518

Ports TA, Silverman NH, Schiller NB (1978) Two-dimensional echocardiographic assessment of Ebstein's anomaly. Circulation 58:336–343

Rebolledo JR (1967) Ebstein's anomaly with right aortic arch. Review of the cardiovascular defects associated with Ebstein's malformation of the tricuspid valve. J Pediatr 71:66–69

Roberts WC, Glancy DL, Seningen RP, Maron BJ, Epstein SE (1976) Prolapse of the mitral valve (floppy valve) associated with Ebstein's anomaly of the tricuspid valve. Am J Cardiol 38:377–382

Ruschhaupt DG, Bharati S, Lev M (1976) Mitral valve malformation of Ebstein type in absence of corrected transposition. Am J Cardiol 38:109–112

Sodi-Pallares D, Testelli MR (1964) Electrocardiography in the diagnosis of congenital heart disease. Heart Bull 13:24–30

Tajik AJ, Gau GT, Giuliani ER, Ritter DG, Schattenberg TT (1973) Echocardiogram in Ebstein's anomaly with Wolff-Parkinson-White preexcitation syndrome, type B. Circulation 47:813–818

Watson H (1974) Natural history of Ebstein's anomaly of tricuspid valve in childhood and adolescence. An international cooperative study of 505 cases. Br Heart J 36:417–427

Westaby S, Karp RB, Kirklin JW, Waldo AL, Blackstone EH (1982) Surgical treatment in Ebstein's malformation. Ann Thorac Surg 34:388–395

Tetralogy of Fallot

Benrey J, Leachman RD, Cooley DA, Klima T, Lufschanowski R (1976) Supravalvular mitral stenosis associated with tetralogy of Fallot. Am J Cardiol 37:111–114

Blalock A (1948) Surgical procedures employed and anatomic variations encountered in the treatment of congenital pulmonic stenosis. Surg Gynecol Obstet 87:385–409

Brock RC (1952) Seminars on congenital heart disease. Congenital pulmonary stenosis. Am J Med 12:706–719

Castaneda AR, Williams RG, Rosenthal A, Sade RM (1976) Tetralogy of Fallot: Primary repair in infancy. In: Langford Kidd BS, Rowe RD (eds): The child with congenital heart disease. Futura Publishing Co., Mount Kisco, NY, pp 63–69

Cooley DA, Hallman GL (1966) Intrapericardial aortic-right pulmonary arterial anastomosis. Surg Gyncol Obstet 122:1084–1086

Engle MA (1976) Cyanotic congenital heart disease. Am J Cardiol 37:283–308

Fallot A (1941) Contribution to the pathologic anatomy of Morbus Caeruleus (translated summary) In: Willins, Keys (eds): Cardiac classics. Mosby, St. Louis, pp 689–690

Gasul BM, Dillo RF, Urla V, Hait G (1957) Ventricular septal defects. Their natural transformation into those with infundibular stenosis or into cyanotic or noncyanotic type of tetralogy of Fallot. JAMA 164:847–853

Goor DA, Lillehei CW, Edwards JE (1971) Ventricular septal defects and pulmonic stenosis with and without dextroposition. Anatomic features and embryologic implications. Chest 60:117–128

Henry WL, Maron BJ, Griffith JM, Redwood DR, Epstein SE (1975) Differential diagnosis of anomalies of the great arteries by real-time two-dimensional echocardiography. Circulation 51:283–291

Hipona FA, Bloom DL (1965) Postoperative aneurysm of the right ventricle. Am J Roentgenol 95:642–654

Hipona FA, Crummy AB (1964) Congenital pericardial defect associated with tetralogy of Fallot. Herniation of normal lung into the pericardial cavity. Circulation 29:132–135

Honey M, Chamberlain DA, Howard J (1983) The effect of beta-sympathetic blockade on arterial oxygen saturation in Fallot's tetralogy. Circulation 30:501–510

Johns TNP, Williams GR, Blalock A (1953) Original communications. The anatomy of pulmonary stenosis and atresia with comments on surgical therapy. Surgery 33:161–172

Knight L, Edwards JE (1974) Right aortic arch. Types and associated cardiac anomalies. Circulation 50:1047–1051

Lev M, Eckner FAO (1964) The pathologic anatomy of tetralogy of Fallot and its variations. Chest 45:251–261

Levin AR, Boineau JP, Spach MS, Canent RV Jr, Capp MP, Anderson PA (1966) Ventricular pressure-flow dynamics in tetralogy of Fallot. Circulation 34:4–13

Lillehei CW, Cohen M, Warden HE, Read RL, Aust JB, DeWall RA, Varco RL (1955) Direct vision intracardiac surgical correction of the tetralogy of Fallot, pentalogy of Fallot, and pulmonary atresia defects. Report of first 10 cases. Ann Surg 142:418–445

Lillehei CW, Cohen M, Warden HE, Read RC, DeWall RA, Aust JB, Varco RL (1955) Direct vision intracardiac surgery by means of controlled cross circulation or continuous arterial reservoir perfusion for correction of ventricular septal defects, atrioventricularis communis, isolated infundibular pulmonic stenosis and tetralogy of Fallot. In: Lam CRE (ed) Henry Ford Hospital International Symposium on Cardiovascular Surgery. Saunders, Philadelphia

McManus BM, Waller BF, Jones M, Epstein SE, Roberts WC

(1982) The case for preoperative coronary angiography in patients with tetralogy of Fallot and other complex congenital heart diseases. Am Heart J 103:451–456

Meyer R, Bloom K, Schwartz D, Kaplan S (1973) Mitral flutter without aortic incompetence. Circulation 48:IV-81 (abstract)

Miller RA, Lev M, Paul MH (1962) Congenital absence of the pulmonary valve. The clinical syndrome of tetralogy of Fallot with pulmonary regurgitation. Circulation 26:266–278

Mitchell SC, Korones SB, Berendes HW (1971) Congenital heart disease in 56,109 births. Incidence and natural history. Circulation 43:323–331

Murphy JD, Freed MD, Keane JF, Norwood WI, Castaneda AR, Nadas AS (1980) Hemodynamic results after intracardiac repair of tetralogy of Fallot by deep hypothermia and cardiopulmonary bypass. Circulation 62 (suppl 1): 1–174

Nagao GI, Daoud GI, McAdams J, Schwartz DC, Kaplan S (1967) Cardiovascular anomalies associated with tetralogy of Fallot. Am J Cardiol 20:206–215

Ober WB, Moore TE (1955) Congenital cardiac malformations in the neonatal period. N Engl J Med 253:271–275

Payne WS, Kirklin JW (1961) Late complications after plastic reconstruction of outflow tract in tetralogy of Fallot. Ann Surg 154:53–57

Ponce FE, Williams LC, Webb HM, Riopel DA, Hohn AR (1973) Propranolol palliation of tetralogy of Fallot: Experience with long-term drug treatment in pediatric patients. Pediatrics 52:100–108

Potts WJ, Smith S, Gibson S (1946) Anastomosis of the aorta to a pulmonary artery. Certain types in congenital heart disease. JAMA 132:627–631

Rao BNS, Anderson RC, Edwards JE (1971) Anatomic variations in the tetralogy of Fallot. Am Heart J 81:361–371

Rastelli GC, Ongley PA, Davis GD, Kirklin JW (1965) Surgical repair for pulmonary valve atresia with coronary pulmonary artery fistula. Report of a case. Mayo Clin Proc 40:521–527

Saphir O, Lev M (1941) The tetralogy of Eisenmenger. Am Heart J 21:31–46

Stewart JR, Kincaid OW, Titus JL (1974) Right aortic arch: Plain film diagnosis and significance. Am J Roentgenol 97:377–389

Velasquez G, Nath PH, Castaneda-Zuniga WR, Amplatz K, Formanek A (1980) Aberrant left subclavian artery in tetralogy of Fallot Am J Cardiol 45:811–818

Waterston DJ (1962) Treatment of Fallot's tetralogy in children under 1 year of age. Rozhl Chir 41:181–183

Tetralogy of Fallot with Absence of the Pulmonary Valve

Anselmi G, Munoz S, Espino-Vela J, Perez Soto J, Villegas M, Monroy G (1960) Agenesis de las valvulas sigmoideas pulmonares: presentacion de dos casos y revision de la literatura. Arch Inst Cardiol Mex 30:409–427

Calder AL, Brandt PWT, Barratt-Boyes BG, Neutze JM (1980) Variant of tetralogy of Fallot with absent pulmonary valve leaflets and origin of one pulmonary artery from the ascending aorta. Am J Cardiol 46:106–116

Emmanouilides GC, Thanopoulos B, Siassi B, Fishbein M (1976) "Agenesis" of ductus arteriosus associated with the syndrome of tetralogy of Fallot and absent pulmonary valve. Am J Cardiol 37:403–409

Fontana ME, Wooley CF (1978) The murmur of pulmonic regurgitation in tetralogy of Fallot with absent pulmonic valve. Circulation 57:986–990

Ilbawi MN, Idriss FS, Muster AJ, Wessel HU, Paul MH, DeLeon SY (1981) Tetralogy of Fallot with absent pulmonary valve. Should valve insertion be part of the intracardiac repair? J Thorac Cardiovasc Surg 81:906–915

Lakier JB, Stanger P, Heymann MA, Hoffman JIE, Rudolph AM (1974) Tetralogy of Fallot with absent pulmonary valve. Natural history and hemodynamic considerations. Circulation 50:167–175

Macartney FJ, Miller GAH (1970) Congenital absence of the pulmonary valve. Br Heart J 32:483–490

Osman MZ, Meng CCl, Girdany BR (1969) Congenital absence of the pulmonary valve: Report of eight cases with review of the literature. Am J Roentgenol 106:58–69

Pernot C, Hoeffel JC, Henry M, Worms AM, Stehlin H, Louis JP (1972) Radiological patterns of congenital absence of the pulmonary valve in infants. Radiology 102:619–622

Pinsky WW, Nihill MR, Mullins CE, Harrison G, McNamara DG (1978) The absent pulmonary valve syndrome. Considerations of management. Circulation 57:159–162

Rabinovitch M, Grady S, David I, Van Praagh R, Sauer U, Buhlmeyer K, Castaneda AR, Reid L, Silva DK (1982) Compression of intrapulmonary bronchi by abnormally branching pulmonary arteries associated with absent pulmonary valves. Am J Cardiol 50:804–813

Rose JS, Levin DC, Goldstein S, Laster W (1974) Congenital absence of the pulmonary valve associated with congenital aplasia of the thymus (DiGeorge's syndrome). Am J Roentgenol 122:97–102

Smith RD, DuShane JW, Edwards JE (1983) Congenital insufficiency of the pulmonary valve, including a case of fetal cardiac failure. Circulation 20:554–560

Double-Outlet Right Ventricle

Ainger LE (1965) Double-outlet right ventricle: Intact ventricular septum, mitral stenosis, and blind left ventricle. Am Heart J 70:521–525

Baron MG (1971) Angiographic differentiation between tetralogy of Fallot and double-outlet right ventricle—relationship of mitral and aortic valves. Circulation 43:451–455

Carey LS, Edwards JE (1965) Roentgenographic features in cases with origin of both great vessels from the right ventricle without pulmonary stenosis. Am J Roentgenol 93:269–297

Davachi F, Moller JH, Edwards JE (1968) Origin of both great vessels from right ventricle with intact ventricular septum. Am Heart J 75:790–794

Elliott LP, Adams P Jr, Levy MJ, Edwards JE (1963) Right ventricular aorta and biventricular pulmonary trunk, an uncommon form of transposition. Am Heart J 66:478–484

Hagler DJ, Tajik AJ, Seward JB, Mair DD, Ritter DG (1981) Double-outlet right ventricle: Wide-angle two-dimensional echocardiographic observations. Circulation 63:419–428

Hallermann FJ, Kincaid OW, Ritter DG, Titus JL (1970) Mitral-semilunar valve relationships in the angiography of cardiac malformations. Radiology 94:63–68

Lincoln C, Anderson, RH, Shinebourne EA, English TAH, Wilkinson JL (1975) Double outlet right ventricle with l-malposition of the aorta. Br Heart J 37:453–463

Pacifico AD, Kirklin JW, Bargeron LM, Jr (1973) Complex congenital malformations: Surgical treatment of double-outlet right ventricle and double-outlet left ventricle. In: Kirklin JW (ed) Advances in cardiovascular surgery. Grune & Stratton, New York, p 57

Perloff JK, Urschell CW, Roberts WC, Caulfield WH Jr (1968) Aneurysmal dilatation of the coronary arteries in cyanotic congenital cardiac disease. Report of a 40 year old patient with the Taussig-Bing complex. Am J Med 45:802–810

Rogers TR, Hagstrom WC, Engle MA (1965) Origin of both great vessels from the right ventricle associated with the trisomy–18 syndrome. Circulation 32:802–807

Rogoff JH, Anthony W (1966) Double-outlet right ventricle with pulmonary valve atresia. Report on a patient surviving to age 25. Am Heart J 72:259–264

Smith DW (1963) The no. 18 trisomy and D_1 trisomy syndromes. Pediatr Clin North Am 10:389–407

Sondheimer HM, Freedom RM, Olley PM (1977) Double outlet right ventricle: Clinical spectrum and prognosis. Am J Cardiol 39:709–714

Sridaromont S, Feldt RH, Ritter DG, Davis GD, Edwards JE (1976) Double outlet right ventricle: Hemodynamic and anatomic correlations. Am J Cardiol 38:85–94

Sridaromont S, Ritter DG, Feldt RH, Davis GD, Edwards JE (1978) Double-outlet right ventricle. Anatomic and angiocardiographic correlations. Mayo Clin Proc 53:555–577

Taussig HB, Bing RJ (1949) Complete transposition of the aorta and a levoposition of the pulmonary artery. Clinical, physiological, and pathological findings. Am Heart J 37:551–559

Van Praagh R (1968) What is the Taussig-Bing malformation? Circulation 38:445–449

Wilcox BR, Ho SY, Macartney FJ, Becker AE, Gerlis LM, Anderson RH (1981) Surgical anatomy of double-outlet right ventricle with situs solitus and atrioventricular concordance. J Thorac Cardiovasc Surg 82:405–417

Yeh HC, Wolf BS, Steinfield L, Baron MG (1977) Echocardiography of double outlet right ventricle: New diagnostic criteria. Radiology 123:435–439

Zamora R, Moller JH, Edwards JE (1975) Double-outlet right ventricle. Anatomic types and associated anomalies. Chest 68:672–677

Double-Outlet Left Ventricle

Bharati S, Lev M, Stewart R, McAllister HA, Kirklin JW (1978) The morpholigic spectrum of double outlet left ventricle and its surgical significance. Circulation 58:558–565

Fontan F, Mounico FB, Baudet E, Siminneau S, Gordo J, Goufrant P (1971) "Correction" de l'atrésie triscupidènne: Rapport de deux cas "corrigés" par l'utilisation d'une technique chirurgicale nouvelle. Ann Chir Thorac Cardiovas 10:39–47

Katasi T, Takeuchi S, Katsumoto K, Fukuda T, Morishita M, Inoue T (1979) Surgical correction of double outlet left ventricle associated with hypoplastic right ventricle: Direct anastomosis of right atrial appendage and pulmonary artery. Circulation J (Japan) 43:768–774

Kerr AR, Barcia A, Bargeron LM, Kirklin JW (1971) Double-outlet left ventricle with ventricular septal defect and pulmonary stenosis: Report of surgical repair. Am Heart J 81:688–693

Kinsley RH, Levin SE, O'Donovan TG (1979) Transposition of the great arteries associated with a double left ventricular outflow tract. Br Heart J 42:483–486

Kirklin JW, Pacifico AD, Bargeron LM, Soto B (1973) Cardiac

repair in anatomically corrected malposition of the great arteries. Circulation 48:153–159

Murphy DA, Gillis DA, Sridhara KS (1981) Intraventricular repair of double-outlet left ventricle. Ann Thorac Surg 31:364–369

Otero Coto E, Quero-Jimenez M, Castaneda AR, Rufilanchas JJ, Deverall PB (1979) Double outlet from chambers of left ventricular morphology. Br Heart J 42:15–21

Paul MH, Sinha SN, Muster AJ, Cole RB, Van Praagh R (1970) Double outlet left ventricle. Report of an autopsy case with an intact ventricular septum and consideration of its developmental implications. Circulation 41:129–139

Rivera R, Infantes C, Gil de la Pena M (1980) Double outlet left ventricle. Report of a case with intraventricular surgical repair. J Cardiovasc Surg 21:361–366

Stegmann T, Oster H, Bissenden J, Kallfelz HC, Oelert H (1979) Surgical treatment of double-outlet left ventricle in 2 patients with D-position and L-position of the aorta. Ann Thorac Surg 27:121–129

Urban AE, Anderson RH, Stark J (1977) Double outlet left ventricle associated with situs inversus and atrioventricular concordance. Am Heart J 94:91–95

Van Praagh R, Weinberg PM (1983) Double outlet left ventricle. In Adams FH, Emmanouidides GC (eds): Moss's heart disease in infants, children and adolescents, 3rd ed. Williams & Wilkins, Baltimore, pp 370–385

Vaseenon T, Diehl AM, Mattioli L (1978) Tricuspid atresia with double-outlet left ventricle and bilateral conus. Chest 74:676–680

Villani M, Lipsombe S, Ross DN (1979) Double outlet left ventricle: How should we repair it? Anatomical details and report of two successful surgical cases. J Cardiovasc Surg 20:413–418

Pulmonary Atresia

Bharati S, Paul MH, Idriss FS, Potkin RT, Lev M (1975) The surgical anatomy of pulmonary atresia with ventricular septal defect: Pseudotruncus. J Thorac Cardiovasc Surg 69:713–721

Blake HA, Manion WC, Mattingly TW, Baroldi A (1964) Coronary artery anomalies. Circulation 30:927–940

Caddell JL, Whittemore R (1963) Pulmonary atresia with dilated right ventricle. A case with congenital atrial flutter. Am J Cardiol 12:254–262

Cole RB, Muster AJ, Lev M, Paul MH (1968) Pulmonary atresia with intact ventricular septum. Am J Cardiol 21:23–31

deLeval M, Bull C, Stark J, Anderson RH, Taylor JFN, Macartney FJ (1982) Pulmonary atresia and intact ventricular septum: Surgical management based on a revised classification. Circulation 66:272–280

Elliott LP, Adams P Jr, Edwards JE (1963) Pulmonary atresia with intact ventricular septum. Br Heart J 25:489–501

Ellis K, Casarella WJ, Hayes CJ, Gersony WM, Bowman FO, Jr., Malm JR (1972) Pulmonary atresia with intact ventricular septum. New developments in diagnosis and treatment. Am J Roentgenol 116:501–513

Finegold MJ, Klein KM (1971) Anastomotic coronary vessels in hypoplasia of the right ventricle. Am Heart J 82:678–683

Godman MJ, Tham P, Langford KBS (1974) Echocardiography in the evaluation of the cyanotic newborn infant. Br Heart J 36:154–166

Greenwold WE, DuShane JW, Burchell HB, Bruwer A, Edwards JE (1956) Congenital pulmonary atresia with intact ventricular septum: Two anatomic types. Circulation 14:945–946

Hagler DJ (1976) The utilization of echocardiography in the differential diagnosis of cyanosis in the neonate. Mayo Clin Proc 51:143–154

Heymann MA, Rudolph AM (1977) Ductus arteriosus dilatation by prostaglandin E_1 in infants with pulmonary atresia. Pediatrics 59:325–329

Kieffer SA, Carey LS (1963) Radiological aspects of pulmonary atresia with intact ventricular septum. Br Heart J 25:655–662

Kieffer SA, Carey LS (1963) Roentgen evaluation of pulmonary atresia with intact ventricular septum. Am J Roentgenol 89:999–1011

Kiely B, Morales F, Rosenblum D (1963) Pulmonary atresia with intact ventricular septum. Pediatrics 32:841–854

Kugel MA (1931) Congenital heart disease. A clinical and pathological study of two cases of truncus solitarius aorticus (pulmonary atresia). Am Heart J 7:262–273

Lewis BS, Amitai N, Simcha A, Merin G, Gotsman M (1979) Echocardiographic diagnosis of pulmonary atresia with intact ventricular septum. Am Heart J 97:92–95

Olley PM (1975) Non-surgical palliation of congenital heart malformations. N Engl J Med 292:1292–1294

Olley PM, Coceani F, Bodach E (1976) E-type prostaglandins. A new emergency therapy for certain cyanotic congenital heart malformations. Circulation 53:728–731

Rudolph AM, Heymann MA, Fishman N, Lakier JB (1975) Formalin infiltration of the ductus arteriosus. A method for palliation of infants with selected congenital cardiac lesions. N Engl J Med 292:1263–1268

Sissman NJ, Abrams HL (1965) Bidirectional shunting in a coronary artery-right ventricular fistula associated with pulmonary atresia and an intact ventricular septum. Circulation 32:582–588

Trusler GA, Yamamoto N, Williams WG, Izukawa T, Rowe RD, Mustard WT (1976) Surgical treatment of pulmonary atresia with intact ventricular septum. Br Heart J 38:957–960

Uhl HSM (1952) A previously undescribed congenital malformation of the heart: Almost total absence of the myocardium of the right ventricle. Bull Johns Hopkins Hosp 91:197–209

Van Praagh R, Ando M, Van Praagh S, Lenno A, Hougen TJ, Novak G, Gastreiter AR (1976) Pulmonary atresia: Anatomic considerations. In: Ed (Langford Kidd BS, Rowe RD (eds)). The child with congenital heart disease. Futura Publishing Co., Mount Kisco, NY, pp 103–134

Venables AW (1964) The patterns of pulmonary circulation in pulmonary atresia. Br Heart J 26:760–769

Zuberbuhler JR, Anderson RH (1979) Morphological variations in pulmonary atresia with intact ventricular septum. Br Heart J 41:281–288

Tricuspid Atresia

Anderson RH, Wilkinson JL, Gerlis LM, Smith A, Becker AE (1977) Atresia of the right atrioventricular orifice. Br Heart J 39:414–428

Astley R, Oldham JS, Parsons C (1953) Congenital tricuspid atresia. Br Heart J 15:287–297

Beppu S, Nimura Y, Tamai M, Nagata S, Matsuo H, Kawashima Y, Kozuka T, Sakakibara H (1978) Two-dimensional echocardiography in diagnosing tricuspid atresia. Differentiation from other hypoplastic right heart syndromes and common atrioventricular canal. Br Heart J 40:1174–1183

Davis WH, Jordaan FR, Snyman HW (1959) Case Reports. Persistent left superior vena cava draining into the left atrium, as an isolated anomaly. Am Heart J 57:616–622

Dimich I, Goldfinger P, Steinfeld L, Sukban SB (1973) Congenital tricuspid stenosis. Am J Cardiol 31:89–92

Edwards JE, Burchell HB (1949) Congenital tricuspid atresia: A classification. Med Clin North Am 33:1177–1197

Freedom RM, Gerald PS (1973) Congenital cardiac disease and the "cat eye" syndrome. Am J Dis Child 126:16–18

Freedom RM, Rowe RD (1976) Aneurysm of the atrial septum in tricuspid atresia. Diagnosis during life and therapy. Am J Cardiol 38:265–267

Fyler DC, Buckley LP, Hellenbrand WE, Cohn HE, Kirklin JW, Nadas AS (1980) Report of the New England Regional Infant Cardiac Program. Pediatrics 65:375–461

Gale AW, Danielson GK, McGoon DC, Wallace RB, Mair DD (1980) Fontan procedure for tricuspid atresia. Circulation 62:91–96

Kanjuh VI, Stevenson JE, Amplatz K, Edwards JE (1964) Congenitally unguarded tricuspid orifice with coexistent pulmonary atresia. Circulation 30:911–917

Lawson R, Rullman D, Brodeur M, Starr A (1975) Tricuspid atresia with Christmas disease (hemophilia B). Report of a case. J Thorac Cardiovasc Surg 69:585–588

Marcano BA, Riemenschneider TA, Ruttenberg HD, Goldberg SJ, Gyepes M (1969) Tricuspid atresia with increased pulmonary blood flow. An analysis of 13 cases. Circulation 40:399–410

Marder SN, Seaman WB, Scott WG (1953) Roentgenologic considerations in the diagnosis of congenital tricuspid atresia. Radiology 61:174–182

Melhuish BPP, Van Praagh R (1968) Juxtaposition of the atrial appendages. A sign of severe cyanotic congenital heart disease. Br Heart J 30:269–284

Morgan JR, Forker AD, Coates JR, Myers WS (1971) Isolated tricuspid stenosis. Circulation 44:729–732

Neal WA, Knight L, Blieden L, Bessinger FB Jr, Edwards JE (1975) Clinical pathologic conference. Am Heart J 89:514–520

Patel R, Fox K, Taylor JFN, Graham GR (1978) Tricuspid atresia. Clinical course in 62 cases (1967–1974). Br Heart J 40:1408–1414

Rao PS (1977) Natural history of the ventricular septal defect in tricuspid atresia and its surgical implications. Br Heart J 39:276–288

Rao PS, Jue KL, Jones JI, Ruttenberg HD (1973) Ebstein's malformation of the tricuspid valve with atresia. Differentiation from isolated tricuspid atresia. Am J Cardiol 32:1004–1009

Rose AG, Beckman CB, Edwards JE (1974) Communication between coronary sinus and left atrium. Br Heart J 36:182–185

Salazar E, Benavides P, Contreras R, Espina-Vela J (1965) Congenital mitral and tricuspid stenoses. Am J Cardiol 16:758–764

Takahashi O, Eshaghpour E, Kotler MN (1979) Tricuspid and pulmonic valve echoes in tricuspid and pulmonary atresia. Chest 76:437–440

Tandon R, Edwards JE (1974) Tricuspid atresia. A re-evaluation and classification. J Thorac Cardiovasc Surg 67:530–542

Tandon R, Marin-Garcia J, Moller JH, Edwards JE (1974) Tricuspid atresia with l-transposition. Am Heart J 88:417–424

Tuchman H, Brown JF, Huston JH, Weinstein AB, Rowe GG, Crumpton CW (1956) Superior vena cava draining into left atrium. Another cause for left ventricular hypertrophy with cyanotic congenital heart disease. Am J Med 21:481–484

Vaseenon T, Diehl AM, Mattioli L (1978) Tricuspid atresia with double-outlet left ventricle and bilateral conus. Chest 74:676–679

Wittenborg MH, Neuhauser EBD, Sprunt WH (1951) Roentgenographic findings in congenital tricuspid atresia with hypoplasia of the right ventricle. Am J Roentgenol 66:712–727

Cor Triatriatum Dexter

Gerlis LM, Anderson RH (1976) Cor triatriatum dexter with imperforate Ebstein's anomaly. Br Heart J 38:108–111

Hansing CE, Young WP, Rowe GG (1972) Cor triatriatum dexter. Persistent right sinus venosus valve. Am J Cardiol 30:559–564

Hausdorf G, Gravinghoff L, Sieg K, Keck EW (1985) Pitfalls in the diagnosis of tricuspid atresia: Report of a new angiocardiographic sign. Clin Cardiol 8:189–198

Jones RN, Niles NR (1968) Spinnaker formation of sinus venosus valve. Case report of a fatal anomaly in a 10-year-old boy. Circulation 38:468–473

Kauffman SL, Andersen DH (1963) Persistent venous valves, maldevelopment of the right heart, and coronary artery-ventricular communications. Am Heart J 66:664–669

Nakano S, Kawashima Y, Miyamoto T, Kitamura S, Manabe H (1974) Supravalvular tricuspid stenosis resulting from persistent right sinus venosus valve. A report of successful correction. Ann Thorac Surg 17:591–595

Runcie J (1968) A complicated case of cor triatriatum dexter. Br Heart J 30:729–731

Verel D, Pilcher J, Hynes DM (1970) Cor triatriatum dexter. Br Heart J 32:714–716

Chapter 7, Section 4
Left Heart Obstruction

In this section are included congenital defects that limit flow of blood through the left heart (Table 7–7). These are presented in reverse anatomical sequence, starting with coarctation and pseudocoarctation of the aorta, and progressing proximally to include supravalvular aortic stenosis and disorders of the aortic valve, left ventricle (LV), mitral valve and left atrium (LA). Although aortic regurgitation and aortico-left ventricular tunnel are not considered obstructive lesions, they are included here because they interfere with forward flow through the left side of the heart.

Congenital bicuspid aortic valve is not considered in this section, but is included in the chapter entitled Valvular Heart Disease. The major reason for this decision deals with the fact that patients with this disorder usually present clinically during adult life at about the same time as do individuals with rheumatic and degenerative diseases of the aortic valve.

Aortic atresia and hypoplastic left heart syndrome are discussed as a single group because their clinical presentations are similar.

Coarctation of the Aorta

Coarctation of the aorta consists of a discrete, localized narrowing of the aorta that usually occurs between the aortic arch and the descending aorta. Coarctation of the aorta accounts for 7%–8% of all congenital heart defects. In infants with congestive heart failure the incidence of coarctation, especially in association with other disorders, is much higher; accounting for 17% of all babies who died with congenital heart defects in one large series. The sex ratio is approximately 2:1 with male predominance.

Pathologically, coarctation of the aorta consists of an eccentric, ridgelike infolding of the media of the aortic wall with intimal proliferation resulting in eccentric narrowing of the aorta, usually opposite the aortic insertion of the ligamentum arteriosum or ductus arteriosus (juxtaductal) or immediately distal to the ductus (postductal). Juxtaductal and postductal coarctation have identical manifestations, differing only slightly in their appearance on angiography. Juxtaductal coarctation is the most frequent type of coarctation at all ages and is also called the adult type. Preductal coarctation is less common, and occurs in symptomatic neonates, usually in association with tubular hypoplasia of the aortic isthmus (i.e., that part of the aorta between the left subclavian artery and the ductus arteriosus) or of the entire aorta (infantile coarctation). Preductal coarctation of the aorta with tubular hypoplasia

Table 7–7. Congenital Abnormalities Causing Left Heart Obstruction*

A. Isolated lesions
    Coarctation and Pseudocoarctation
    Aortic stenosis
      Supravalvar
      Valvar
      Subvalvar (membranous, fibrous tunnel, muscular)
    Aortic insufficiency†
    Aortico-left ventricular tunnel†
    Congenital absence of the aortic valve†
    Mitral stenosis (valvar, supravalvar)
      Accessory mitral valve tissue
      Parachute mitral valve
      Anomalous mitral arcade
      Supravalvar mitral ring
    Cor triatriatum
    Stenosis, atresia, or agenesis of pulmonary veins
B. Combined lesions
    Coarctation with:
      Patent ductus arteriosus
      Ventricular septal defect
      Atrial septal defect
      Tubular hypoplasia of aorta
      Bicuspid aortic valve
      Subaortic stenosis
      Endocardial cushion defect
      Single ventricle
      Endocardial fibroelastosis
      Hypoplastic left heart syndrome
      Shone syndrome
      Double-outlet right ventricle
    Biventricular origin of pulmonary trunk with subaortic stenosis (Becu complex)

---

* Normal pulmonary vasculature or pulmonary venous hypertension; no cyanosis except in newborns.
† Although these entities do not represent an anatomical obstruction, aortic insufficiency interferes with forward flow and therefore, for the purpose of classification, we include them in this group.

of the ascending aorta and aortic arch usually is associated with aortic atresia or hypoplastic left heart syndrome. With preductal coarctation, right ventricular blood flows through the ductus arteriosus into the descending aorta as long as the ductus remains patent. Coarctation may also occur in the abdominal aorta. Multiple coarctations of the aorta have also been reported. Tubular hypoplasia without a focal coarctation may be found on occasion in seriously ill newborns. The clinical manifestations will be similar to those associated with coarctation of the aorta.

In older children with coarctation of the aorta the external wall of the aorta is indented in the region of the focal thickening. The descending aorta is often widened just distal to the coarctation. In infants the external appearance of the aorta does not always reflect the infolding (R. W. M. Frater, personal communication). A jet lesion caused by flow through the constriction may be observed in the upper portion of the descending aorta. Left ventricular hypertrophy and subendocardial fibrosis develop in response to the hypertension caused by the afterload lesion. Formation of collateral circulation to the lower body is roughly proportional to the severity of the constriction. The subclavian and the internal mammary arteries are the main sources of collateral flow.

Associated Cardiac Defects The incidence of associated congenital malformations is high, bicuspid aortic valve being the most frequently encountered lesion in older children and adults (up to 85%). The valve is rarely stenotic. Ventricular septal defect and patent ductus arteriosus are the most commonly associated cardiac disorders in infants. One type of ventricular septal defect occurring with coarctation of the aorta is a malalignment ventricular septal defect with displacement of the conus tissue into the LV outflow tract causing LV outflow tract obstruction. Other forms of subaortic obstruction and atrial septal defects also occur. Less frequent are anomalies of the mitral valve and malposition of the great arteries, with or without single ventricle. Coarctation may also be part of the Shone syndrome (coarctation, aortic stenosis, subaortic diaphragm, parachute mitral valve and supravalvar mitral ring). Endocardial fibroelastosis may be observed in children with isolated coarctation of the aorta (Table 7–7). Studies in animal fetuses and the frequent association with intracardiac defects have led to the hypothesis that coarctation may be secondary to a decrease in aortic blood flow during fetal development. The right ventricle (RV) is enlarged because during fetal life it supplies the descending aorta by way of the ductus arteriosus. The LV and the aortic arch remain small because flow of blood through these is impaired. Thus, RV hypertrophy, patent ductus arteriosus, hypoplasia of the LV and tubular hypoplasia of the aortic arch may be associated with coarctation of the aorta in infants.

Tracheoesophageal fistula and cystic disorders of the kidneys are the most commonly associated extracardiac lesions. Gonadal dysgenesis (XO Turner syndrome) often occurs with coarctation of the aorta. Conversely, in Marfan syndrome coarctation is uncommon. The subclavian steal syndrome may be observed in children with coarctation if either subclavian artery is stenotic or atretic. The right subclavian artery may have an anomalous origin from the descending aorta below the coarctation. The most important complications of coarctation are (1) heart failure in neonates, (2) subarachnoid hemorrhage secondary to ruptured berry aneurysms of the circle of Willis, (3) dissection of the aorta, (4) infective endocarditis and mycotic aneurysm.

Clinical Features Coarctation of the aorta has two distinct clinical presentations. In infancy, coarctation often is responsible for severe congestive heart failure. Older children and adults are generally asymptomatic, and the defect is discovered during an evaluation for hypertension. These two clinical entities are described separately.

As indicated, coarctation of the aorta in infancy produces congestive heart failure, especially in the presence of significant associated disorders. Symptoms usually appear within the first week of life. Rarely the clinical presentation is delayed. This delay may be caused by patency of the aortic end of the ductus arteriosus that maintains an adequate lumen of the aorta in spite of the infolding of tissue opposite the ductus. Tachypnea and loss of appetite are the first manifestations to appear, followed by pallor and diaphoresis on exertion. On physical examination the extremities are cool with the pulses normal or increased in the arms and weak or absent in the legs. The blood pressure in the arms may or may not be increased. The blood pressure in the legs is lower and is nonpulsatile, resulting in difficulty measuring it by noninvasive techniques. A RV heave is palpated, and a gallop is usually heard. Murmurs occur in babies with associated intracardiac defects such as PDA with left-to-right shunt or aortic stenosis. The liver and spleen may be enlarged.

The electrocardiogram in infants with coarctation of the aorta may reflect the associated defect (e.g., single ventricle, atrioventricular canal) or may show RV hypertrophy, as a result of the role of the RV during fetal life in assuming most of the fetal cardiac output. Acidosis may supervene as a result of the low cardiac output. Babies with isolated coarctation of the aorta may respond to digoxin and diuretics, and may be managed without surgery. In the presence of associated cardiac defects, symptoms are usually refractory to medical management, so that surgical intervention is mandatory.

The clinical manifestations of coarctation of the aorta in children and adults are quite different from those occurring in infants. Beyond infancy, symptoms are usually absent. Weakness or atrophy of the legs (on occasion associated with claudication) are subtle findings that may be elicited on diligent examination, but are not the presenting complaint in many instances. On occasion, absence of femoral pulses calls attention to the problem, but usually this is discovered during search for the etiology of hypertension. It is important to note that coarctation of the aorta does not necessarily produce a murmur. If a murmur is heard it can frequently be attributed to an associated cardiac disorder. Thus, continuous murmurs may be present with coarctation, but they are usually due to coexisting patent ductus arteriosus rather than collateral flow. Aortic clicks are also heard and are likely to be associated with abnormalities of the aortic valve, although some authors suggest that dilatation of the ascending aorta and hypertension may produce a click. With valvar or subvalvar aortic stenosis, systolic ejection murmurs and thrills may be heard. Mitral valve abnormalities cause characteristic findings of mitral insufficiency, mitral stenosis or both. The pulse in the right arm is bounding, and blood pressure in that extremity is increased. The pulse and pressure in the left arm may be increased, depending on where the coarctation is relative to the origin of the left subclavian artery. Pulses in the legs may be palpable, but weak. In older children and adults a radial-femoral lag will be recognized if the right radial pulse and the femoral pulse are palpated simultaneously. Blood pressure in the legs is lower than that in the arm or may be unobtainable. Rarely pulsation or bruits or both will be identified over the left scapula due to flow in collateral vessels. The electrocardiogram may be normal or may show left ventricular hypertrophy.

Echocardiography Two-dimensional echocardiography can demonstrate the coarctation from the suprasternal notch (Fig. 7–183). Tubular hypoplasia of the aorta may also be recognized and interruption of the aortic arch excluded. A combined approach, using M-mode and 2-D echocardiography, is helpful in identifying associated abnormalities. Recognition of tubular hypoplasia of the aorta, together with an associated defect (e.g., ventricular septal defect or ventricular septal defect with subaortic stenosis, aortic stenosis, mitral valve disease, left ventricular dysfunction, single ventricle), should lead to consideration of early surgical intervention, since symptoms in such cases are often refractory to medical therapy. Echocardiography is most helpful in excluding hypoplastic left heart syndrome, in which the clinical presentation may be similar to that of coarctation. Doppler echocardiography shows decreased systolic pulsations in the descending aorta as well as diastolic augmentation of blood flow (Fig. 2–49). Associated VSD, PDA and stenosis or insufficiency of either the aortic or mitral valve are also assessed.

Radiological (Plain Film) Features Two principal radiological presentations occur in infants with coarctation of the aorta. With the symptomatic juxtaductal (uncomplicated) coarctation (Fig. 7–184), the pulmonary vasculature shows signs of congestive heart failure, and the heart is of normal size or moderately enlarged. In most such cases the configuration of the heart and aorta are not characteristic. The findings are similar to those occurring with other forms of left heart obstruction (e.g., hypoplastic left heart syndrome, severe aortic stenosis, mitral stenosis).

In preductal coarctation (with associated defects) the pulmonary pattern usually shows a combination of overcirculation and pulmonary venous hypertension (congestive heart failure) (Fig. 7–185). The heart is enlarged with dilatation of the right atrium (RA) and RV. The main pulmonary artery is large, and the aorta is inconspicuous.

The radiological findings in older children and adults may be divided into two categories, the classical features and the more subtle manifestations. With the full-blown picture of coarctation of the aorta the pulmonary vascularity is normal. The heart is not enlarged, but the LV may be prominent and the ascending aorta dilated. The classic "three sign" is observed on the frontal and left anterior oblique projections (Fig. 7–186). The upper convexity is usually formed by a dilated left subclavian artery, but, on occasion, represents the aortic knob. The lower convexity is formed by the dilated proximal descending aorta with the indentation representing the site of coarctation.

On the barium esophagogram the reverse three sign (or E sign) is caused by pressure on the esophagus by the convexities just described. Aneurysmal dilatation and calcification of the subclavian arteries may be present (Fig. 7–187A). *Rib notching* usually affects the lower margins of the fourth through the eighth ribs (posterior segments) and is usually bilateral (Fig. 7–187B and C). Unilateral, right-sided rib notching occurs if the coarctation involves the origin of the left subclavian artery so that low pressure in that vessel prevents it from being a source of collaterals. Unilateral left-sided rib notching results if the right subclavian artery has an anomalous origin from the descending aorta below the coarctation. Retrosternal scalloping is due to erosion by dilated internal mammary arteries. It should be stressed that rib notching also occurs with other disorders that enlarge the intercostal arteries, veins or nerves. Commonly mentioned but rarely observed is unilateral rib notching on the ipsilateral side of a Blalock-Taussig shunt for cyanotic congenital heart disease. Unilateral absence of a pulmonary artery may also result in unilateral rib notching.

Although the features just described are stressed as diagnostic for coarctation, in most cases findings are more subtle and the radiologist should be alert to them. The first of these is discontinuity between the aortic arch and the descending aorta (Fig. 7–187A and 7–188A). The second is an inconspicuous aortic arch with a dilated descending aorta. On occasion the only clue might be a dilated ascending aorta that may simulate aortic valvular disease. Another subtle clue is a dilated left subclavian artery that may even simulate a high cervical arch.

Hemodynamics in Infants In infants with congestive heart failure the foramen ovale is often found to be sealed (premature closure); thus no atrial shunt will occur, and entry of the venous catheter into the left heart will be prevented. If the foramen ovale is patent a left-to-right shunt may be detected at the atrial level, reflecting an atrial septal defect or incompetence of the flap of the foramen ovale in the presence of high left atrial pressure (congestive heart failure). An additional shunt at the ventricular level may indicate a ventricular septal defect. A shunt may occur at the ductal level if the ductus is shunting from left to right. In some cases the ductus shunts from right to left, causing desaturation in the descending aorta. Pressures in the RV and pulmonary artery are increased, usually to systemic levels. Pressure in the LA is elevated secondary to left heart failure. Left ventricular pressure may or may not be increased. The descending aorta is usually reached by a catheter from the RV by way of the ductus arteriosus. Pressure in the descending aorta is damped if the ductus is partly closed. During infusion of prostaglandin E_1 or during periods of hypoxia and acidosis, the ductus may widen so that pressures in the aorta, the pulmonary artery and the descending aorta are all equal.

Hemodynamics in Children and Adults If the right heart is catheterized in asymptomatic children and adults with isolated coarctation of the aorta, no oxygen "step-up" is detected, and right heart pressures, including pulmonary wedge pressure, generally are normal. Pressures in the LV and ascending aorta are increased. Pressure in the descending aorta is lower and has a narrow pulse pressure. Additional gradients across the outflow tract of the LV and the aortic valve should be sought to exclude other stenotic lesions (e.g., valvar and subvalvar aortic stenosis).

Contrast Studies The preferred location for the initial angiogram in a symptomatic infant with coarctation of the aorta is the LV if that chamber can be reached via the foramen ovale. The injected contrast agent will delineate the anatomical features of the aortic arch and site of coarctation and will identify intracardiac defects as well. In addition, LV size and function are assessed. If the LV cannot be reached, then the venous catheter is directed from the pulmonary artery through the ductus into the descending aorta. The coarctation, the ductus and, on occasion, the transverse arch and isthmus can be delineated by injection of contrast medium in this location (Fig. 7–185). As an alternative, the levophase, after injection into the RV or main pulmonary artery, may opacify the LV, the aortic arch and the coarctation. Presence or absence of ventricular septal defect may also be determined from the levophase. Digital subtraction techniques may enhance the images so that a peripheral injection of contrast material may be sufficient to demonstrate the anatomical defects.

For asymptomatic children and adults with characteristic findings of coarctation of the aorta but no evidence of significant associated defects, left ventriculography (Fig. 7–186 B and C) or aortography is adequate to delineate the anatomical features. In the authors' experience the aortic root usually can be reached retrograde from the femoral artery, even though femoral pulses may be weak or absent. No complications have occurred with this approach. If the femoral artery cannot be entered, the right brachial approach may be necessary. In many children a venous catheter can be directed across the foramen ovale and into the LV. An angiogram obtained from that position will be adequate for diagnosis. The levophase, after injection into the main pulmonary artery, will also provide adequate images if the other approaches are not feasible.

The information that may be obtained from the angiogram is (1) location of the coarctation relative to the left subclavian artery and the ductus arteriosus (if visualized); (2) size of the left subclavian artery (important if a prosthetic graft from the left subclavian artery to the descending aorta is to be considered; (3) source and size of collateral vessels; (4) presence or absence of other anomalies of the branches of the aorta (e.g., anomalous origin of the right subclavian artery); (5) presence or absence of aneurysmal dilatation of the ascending aorta, left subclavian artery, ductus diverticulum or collateral vessels and (6) abnormalities of the aortic valve.

In children or in adults with evidence of additional cardiac abnormalities a left ventriculogram should be recorded as the initial angiogram. If visualization of the coarctation is not adequate, an aortogram becomes necessary.

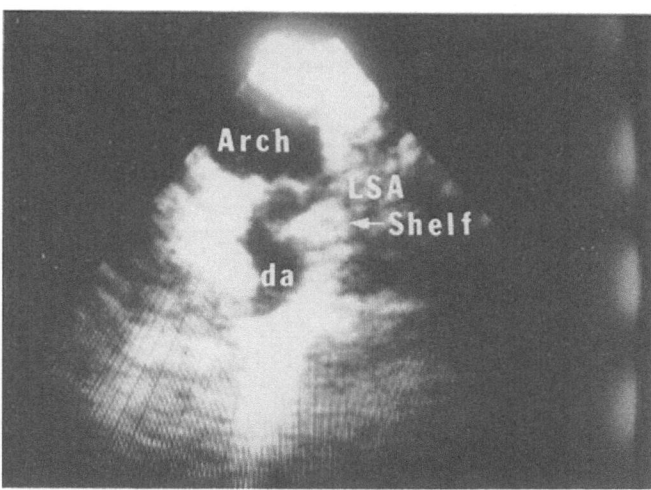

Fig. 7–183. *Two-dimensional echocardiogram from the suprasternal notch in a 10-year-old boy with coarctation of the aorta.* The posterior infolding (*Shelf*) that constitutes the coarctation appears as a highly reflective wedge of tissue protruding into the lumen of the aorta. The isthmus, the segment of the aorta between the left subclavian artery (*LSA*) and the coarctation, is narrow. *Arch* = aortic arch; *da* = descending aorta beyond the coarctation.

Treatment In children and adults, hypertension secondary to coarctation is extremely difficult to treat without surgical intervention. In symptomatic infants, intensive therapy for congestive heart failure may reduce the symptoms to the point that surgical procedures can be delayed. If heart failure is not rapidly controlled, however, operation is urgent, since acidosis and death can supervene suddenly in these infants. In very young babies, prostaglandin E_1 will dilate the ductus so that the RV can perfuse the lower body temporarily until diagnostic studies and an operation can be performed.

Repair of coarctation was first reported by Crafoord and Nylin and by Gross and Hufnagel in 1945. The technique described was excision of the coarcted segment and reanastomosis. This procedure generally is satisfactory in older children and adults if the narrow segment is short and if the individual has reached nearly full growth. In infants this operation has not been satisfactory, because it does not solve the problem of tubular hypoplasia. In addition, the circumferential scar necessitates a secondary repair as the child outgrows the anastomotic site.

Newer techniques for repair of coarctation in infancy constitute attempts to circumvent these problems. Large prosthetic roof patches may be applied over the coarcted segment, or the coarctation may be bypassed with a large tubular prosthetic graft from the left subclavian artery to the descending aorta (Fig. 7–188 A and B). The left subclavian artery of the affected infant may also be used as a patch, so that the entire circumference of the anastomotic site is living tissue.

In some cases, coarctation and associated intracardiac defects such as VSD can be repaired in one stage during deep hypothermia and circulatory arrest. In other instances, two-stage repair is chosen in infants. During the

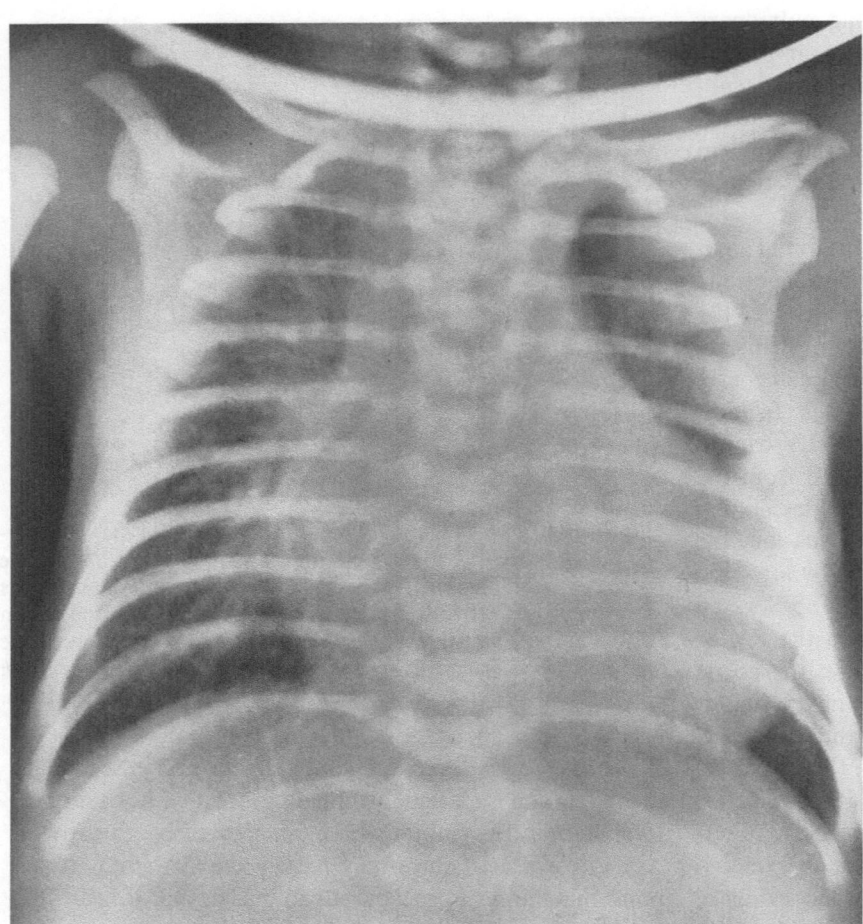

Fig. 7–184 *Coarctation of the aorta and congestive heart failure in a 1-month-old girl.* **A** Frontal roentgenogram of the chest; **B** and **C** frontal and lateral views of the left ventriculogram. **A** Pulmonary venous hypertension and cardiomegaly are present. **B** and **C** The left ventricle is enlarged and hypertrophied. A juxtaductal coarctation is present, with hypoplasia of part of the aortic arch. The ductus was probe patent; however, no flow through the ductus was demonstrated. The ascending aorta is dilated. Note that the venous catheter passed through the right atrium, the foramen ovale and the left atrium to reach the left ventricle. The left subclavian artery arises at the site of the coarctation.

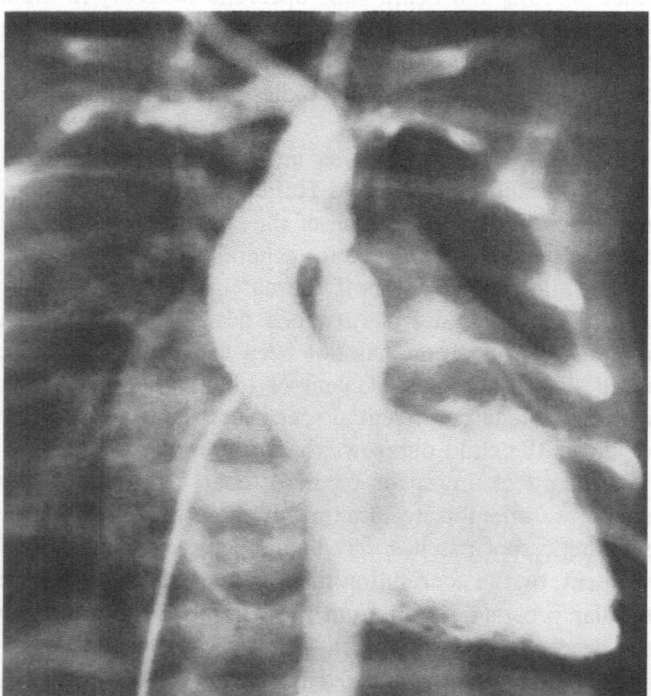

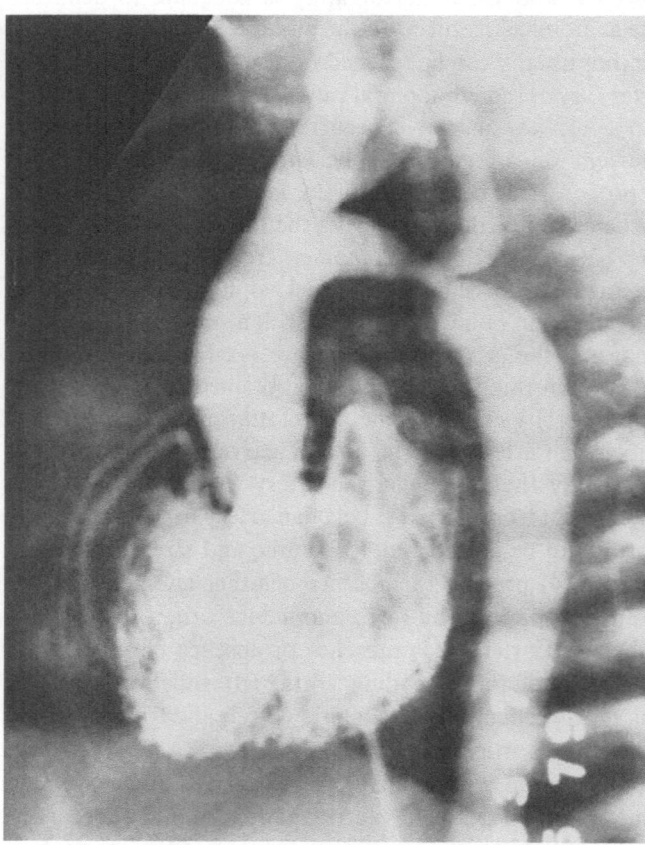

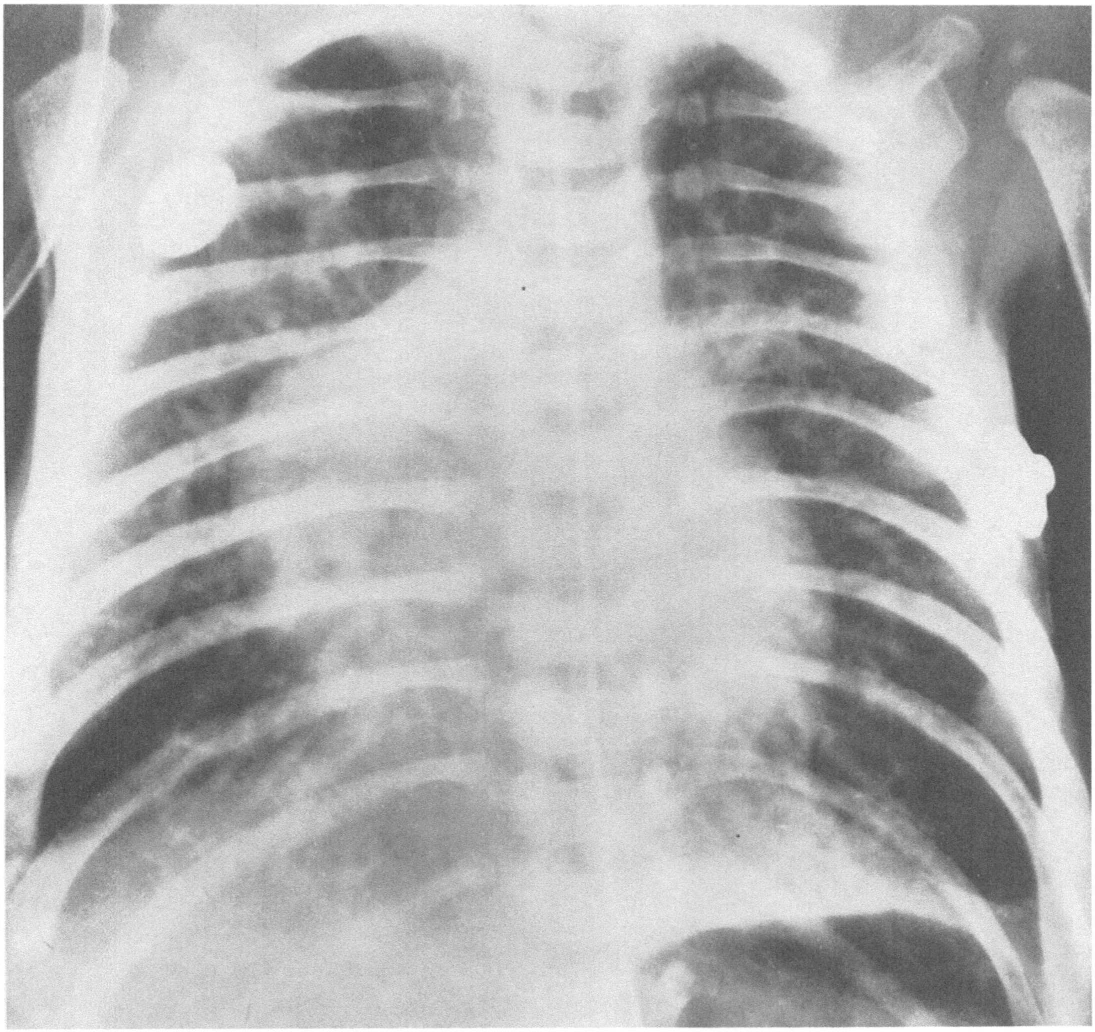

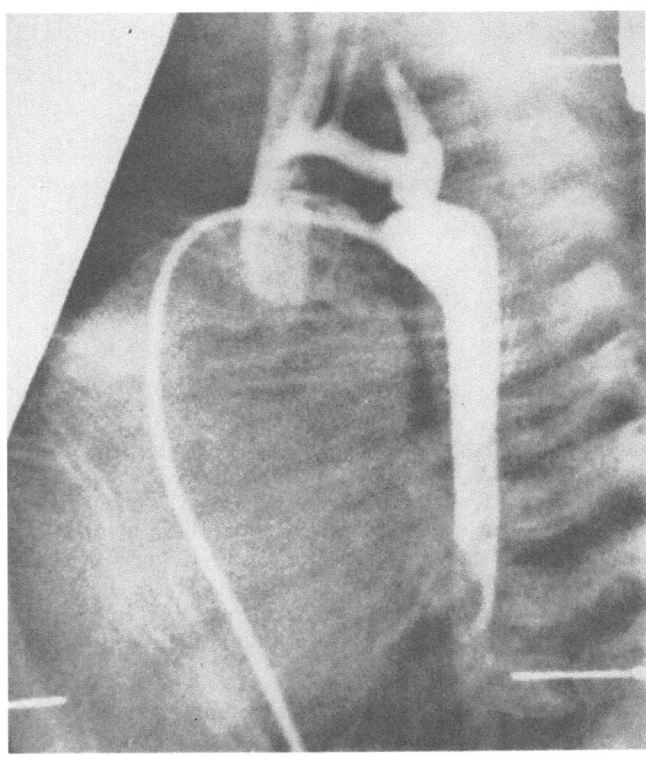

A

Fig. 7–185. *Preductal coarctation, a hypoplastic aortic isthmus and a ventricular septal defect in a 3-month-old boy.* **A** frontal film of the chest; **B** angiogram.

A Cardiomegaly is present, with enlargement of the right atrium and right ventricle. A combination of pulmonary venous hypertension and pulmonary overcirculation is present. The pulmonary venous hypertension pattern predominates. **B** The venous catheter was directed through the right atrium, right ventricle, pulmonary artery and ductus arteriosus into the proximal portion of the descending aorta. The distal end of the ductus, the coarctation, the aortic arch and the aortic root are all opacified from the proximal portion of the descending aorta. The coarctation is preductal; the isthmus of the aorta and the transverse arch are hypoplastic. The aortic root and the ascending aorta are normal in size. At cardiac catheterization an atrial level left-to-right shunt was demonstrated, probably brought about by high left atrial pressure causing incompetence of the flap of the foramen ovale rather than an actual atrial septal defect.

B

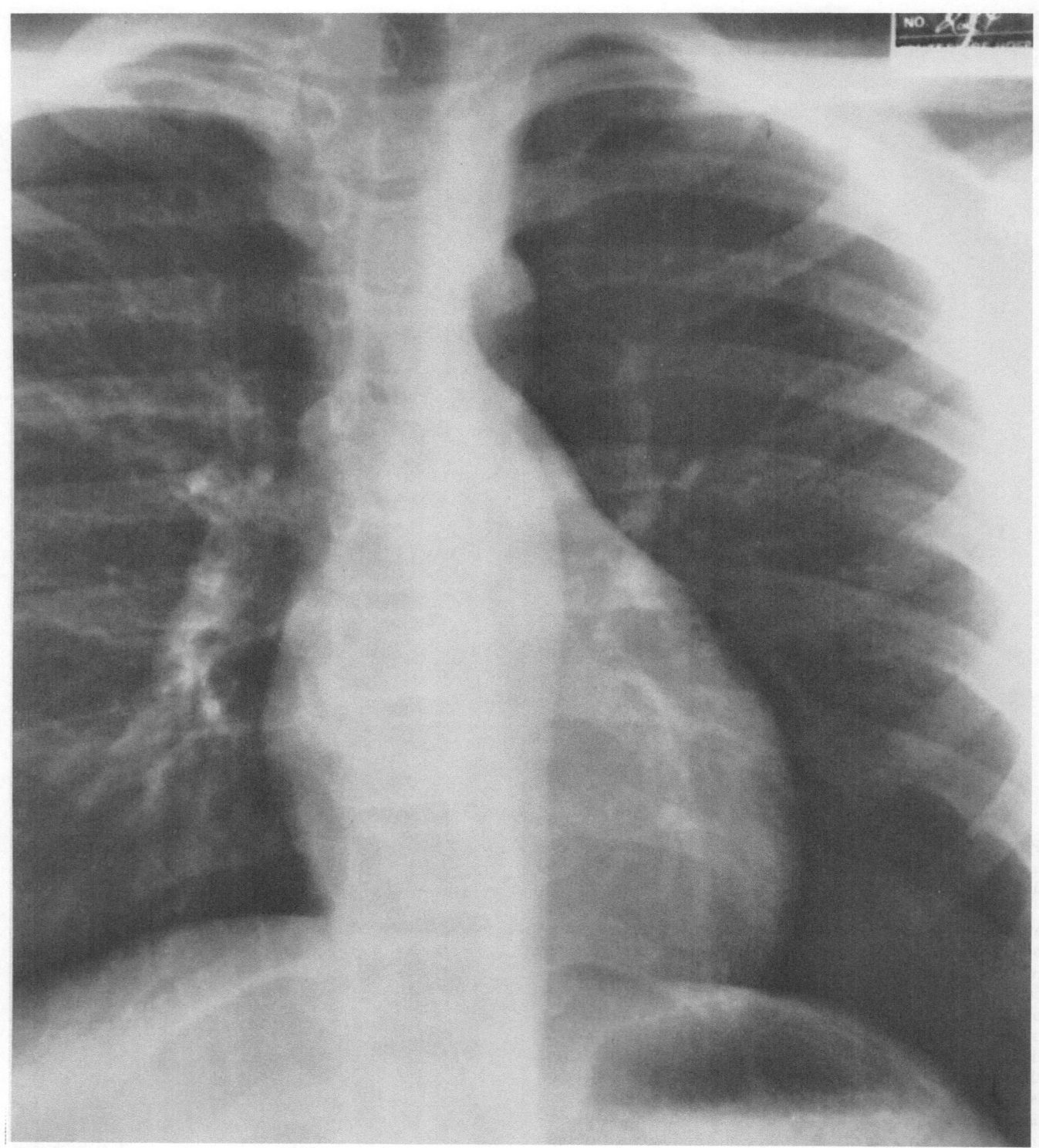

A

Fig. 7–186. *Coarctation of the aorta in a 10-year-old boy.* **A** Frontal roentgenogram of the chest; **B** and **C** left ventriculogram.

A The heart is of normal size. Pulmonary vasculature is normal. The two convexities along the left upper heart border constitute the "three sign." The upper convexity is the aortic arch; the lower convexity is the descending aorta. The indentation between the convexities represents the coarctation of the aorta. **B** and **C** are the frontal and lateral views of the left ventriculogram.

The ascending aorta is mildly dilated while the arch and the brachiocephalic vessels are normal in size. A small patent ductus arteriosus is present. The coarctation (*arrow*) is slightly distal to the ductus (postductal). The internal mammary arteries are dilated, serving as a source of collateral vessels. Note the anterior leaflet of the mitral valve (*arrowheads*) in fibrous continuity with the aortic valve.

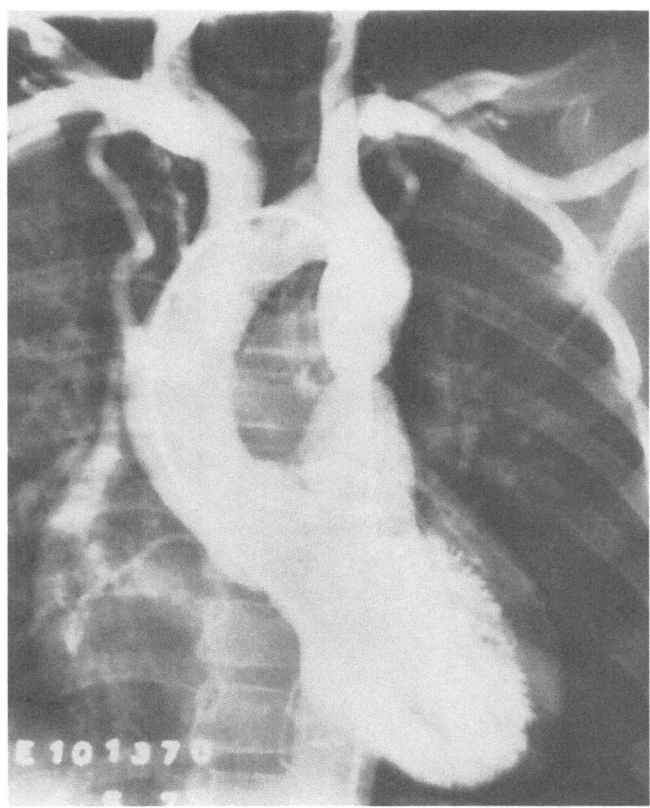

B

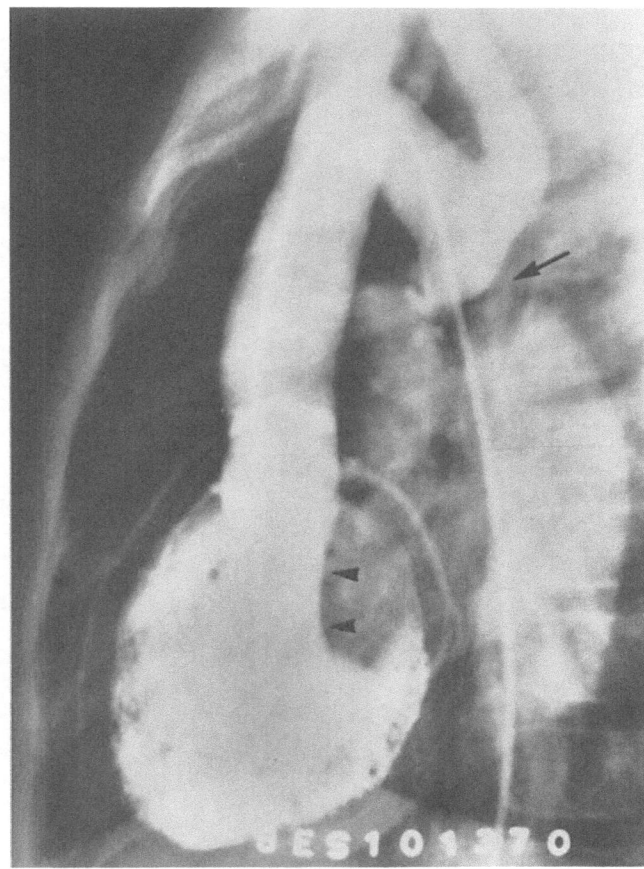

C

first stage the coarctation is repaired, the ductus ligated and the main pulmonary artery banded if necessary. Heart failure can then be managed medically, and an open surgical procedure can be delayed. Later in infancy the band is removed and the intracardiac defect repaired.

Postoperative Findings Complications of surgical intervention include paraplegia, paradoxical hypertension, mesenteric arteritis, recurrent laryngeal nerve palsy, paralysis of the left hemidiaphragm (injury to the phrenic nerve), local bleeding and development of an aneurysm or pseudoaneurysm of the aorta at the site of the repair.

Paraplegia is the most feared complication and may be due to compromise of the circulation to the spinal cord.

Paradoxical hypertension often follows release of the cross-clamp after repair of coarctation; immediately upon release the blood pressure falls, but then rises rapidly to equal or excede the pressure in the ascending aorta prior to the repair. This paradoxical hypertension is thought to contribute to the etiology of mesenteric arteritis. The mechanism of paradoxical hypertension is thought to relate initially to activation of the sympathetic nervous system and is followed in a few days by a rise in plasma renin. This form of hypertension responds to reserpine and to alpha-methyldopa, which block the sympathetic nervous system, and to a combination of propranolol and vasodilators (e.g., diazoxide, nitroprusside, hydralazine). Inhibitors of angiotensin-converting enzyme (e.g., captopril) have also been successful in reducing blood pressure.

In children and adults, mesenteric arteritis may occur 1 to 2 weeks after repair of coarctation, resulting in ileus, ischemia or gangrene of the small bowel, usually requiring laparotomy. This complication is believed to occur as a result of mesenteric ischemia during aortic cross-clamping or as a result of high pressure and pulsatile flow to mesenteric arterioles that have adapted to low pressure and nonpulsatile flow.

After the patient's recovery from the surgical procedure, blood pressures in arms and legs are measured at rest and with exercise. If a marked pressure difference occurs during rest or during exercise, angiography is indicated to assess the site of repair looking for residual or recurrent narrowing. A repeat surgical procedure may be necessary. Some adults continue to have systemic hypertension after adequate repair of coarctation. Strokes are frequent in these individuals, often secondary to berry aneurysms.

Recently balloon angioplasty has been performed on unoperated coarctations and on repaired coarctations with residual gradients. Although initial reduction in pressure gradient has been obtained in some patients, the role of this new technique will be determined by further experience and longer follow-up. Although no significant morbidity or mortality has been reported in children or adults after balloon angioplasty a small number of neonates with coarctation and patent ductus arteriosus have died after the procedure, some associated with rupture of the aorta at the site of the ductus. Prophylaxis against infective endo-

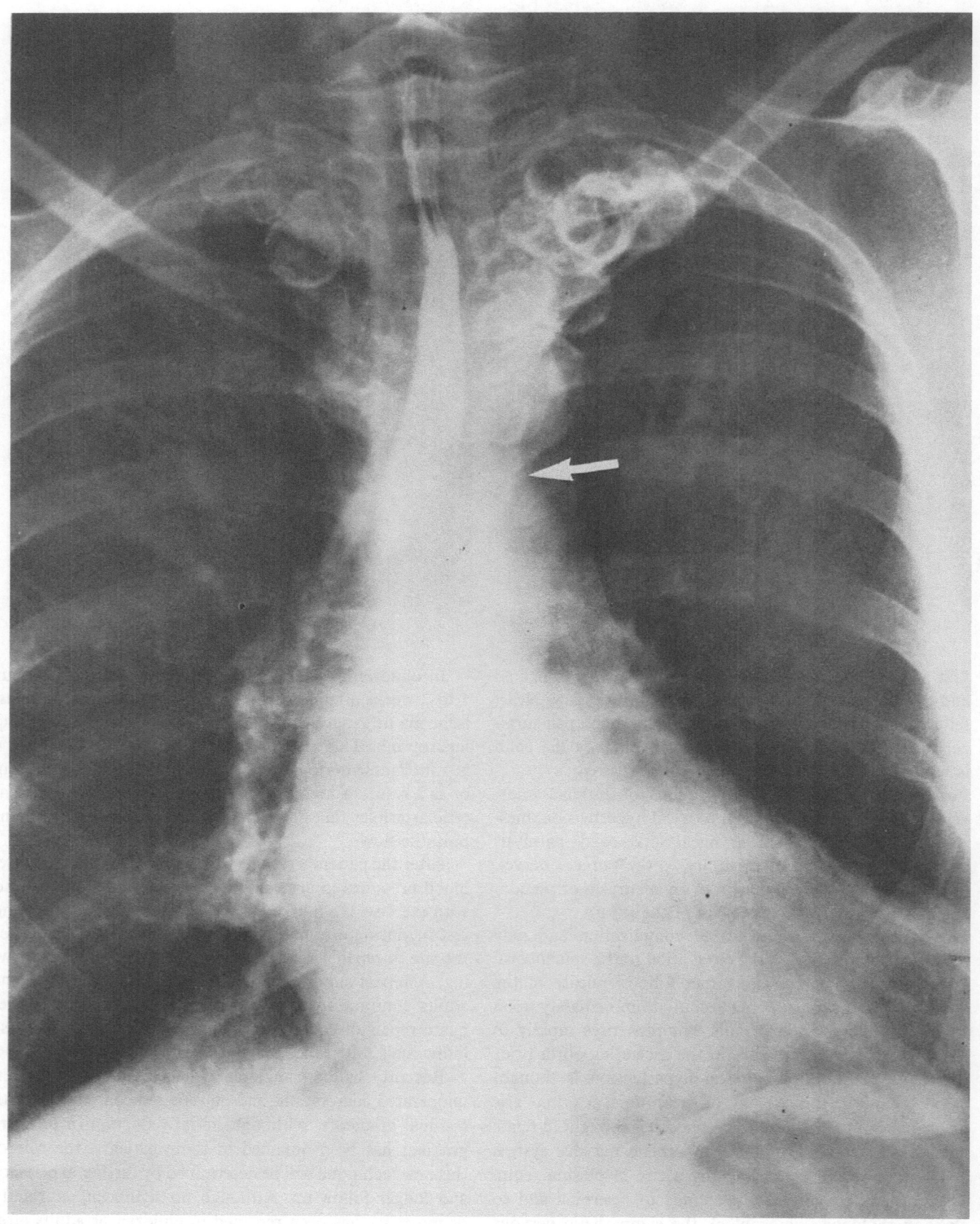

A

Fig. 7–187. *Films of the chest and ribs in adults with coarctation of the aorta.* **A** In this woman extensive calcification is present in aneurysms of the subclavian arteries. The *arrow* points to dis- continuity between the aortic arch and the descending aorta. **B** and **C** The heart is normal in size in this adult. Mild pulmonary venous hypertension is present. Bilateral rib notching is evident.

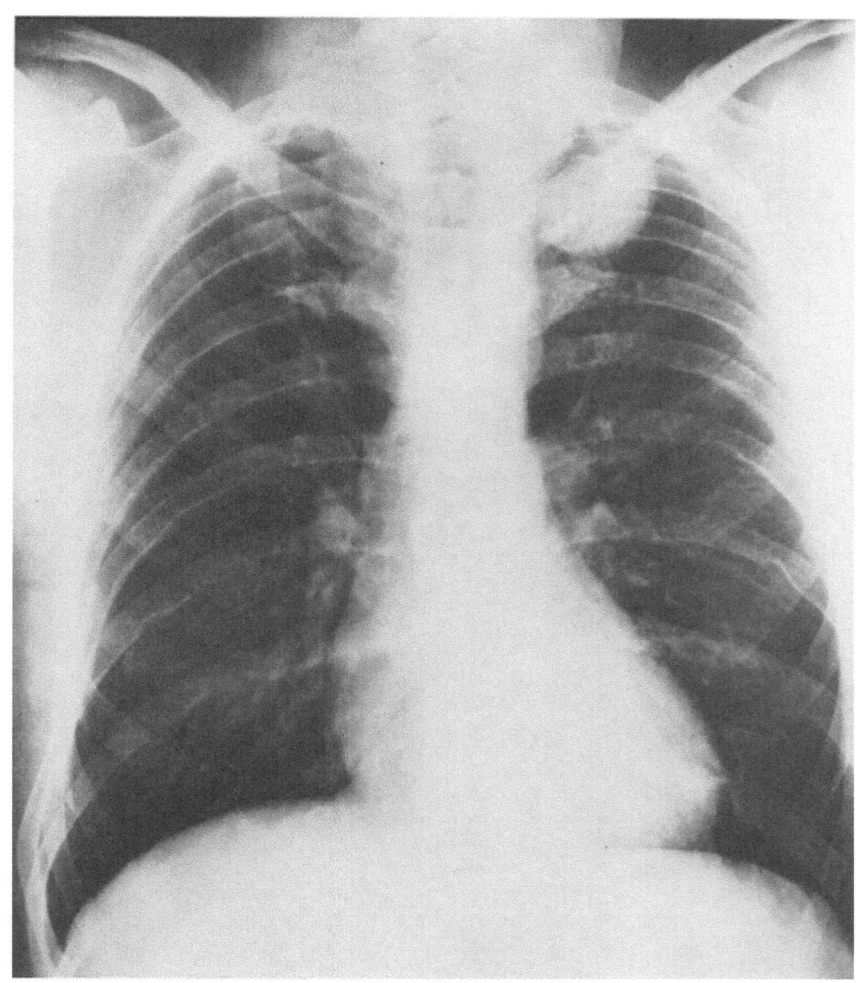

B

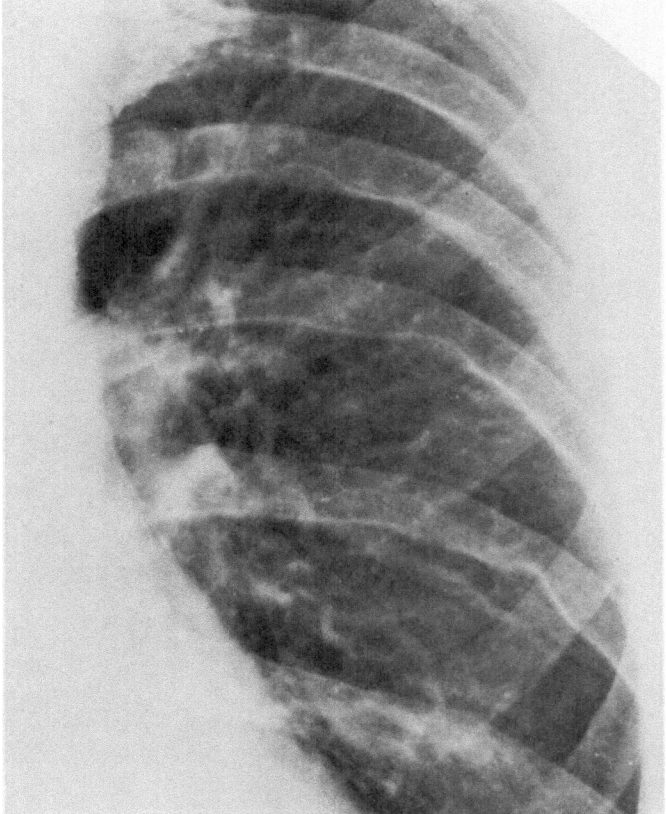

C

The mass in the left apex (**B**) represents aneurysmal dilatation of the left subclavian artery with calcification of its wall. The cone-down view (**C**) shows the rib notching. This patient had a subarachnoid hemorrhage, secondary to a berry aneurysm in the circle of Willis.

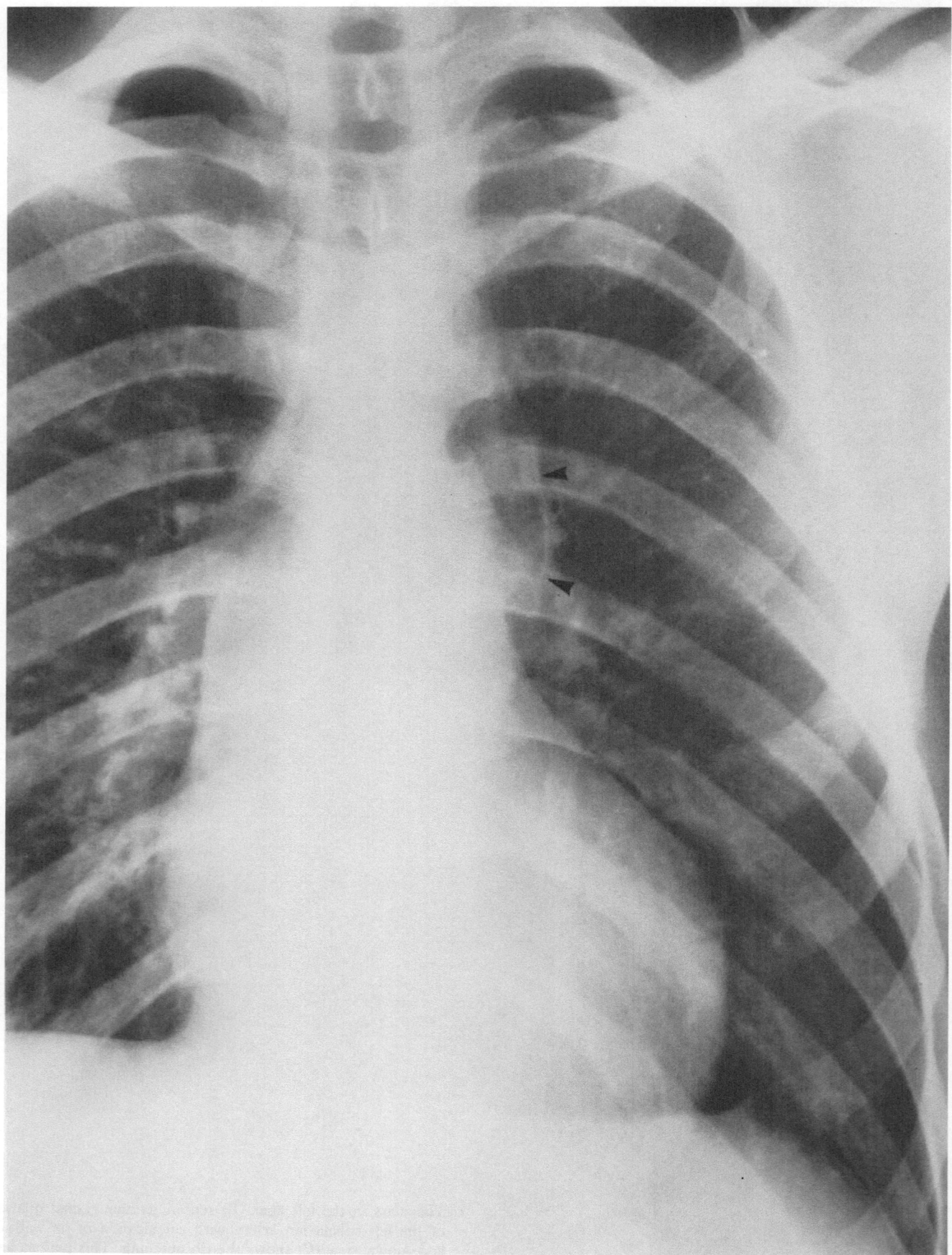

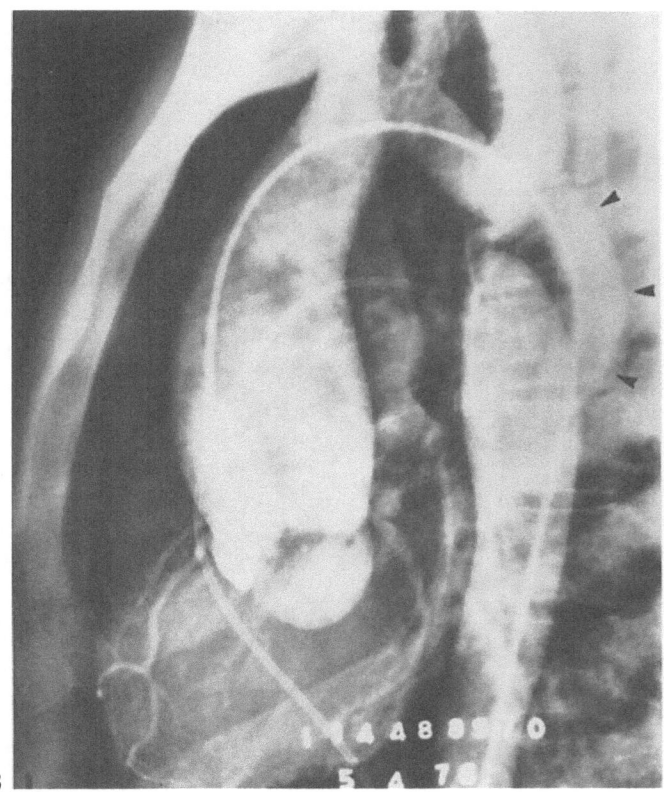

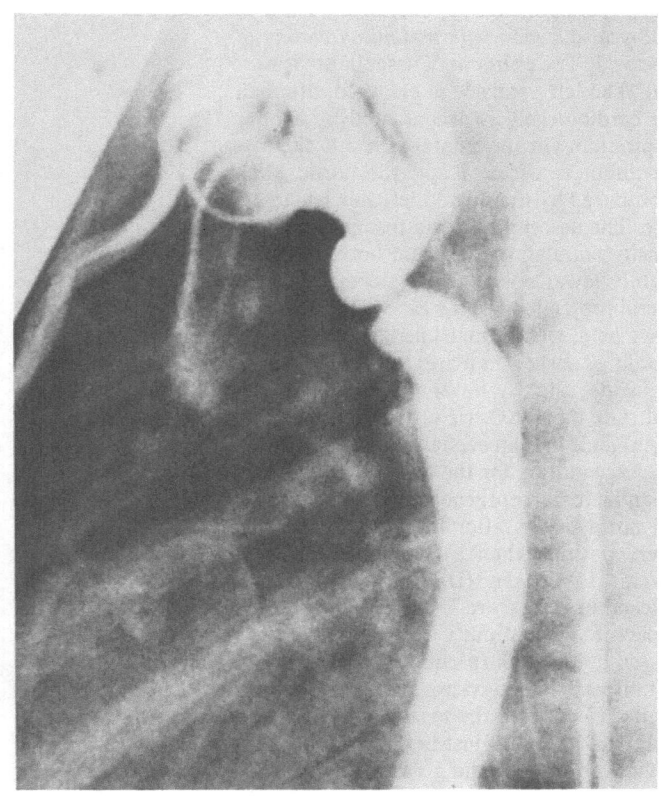

B

C

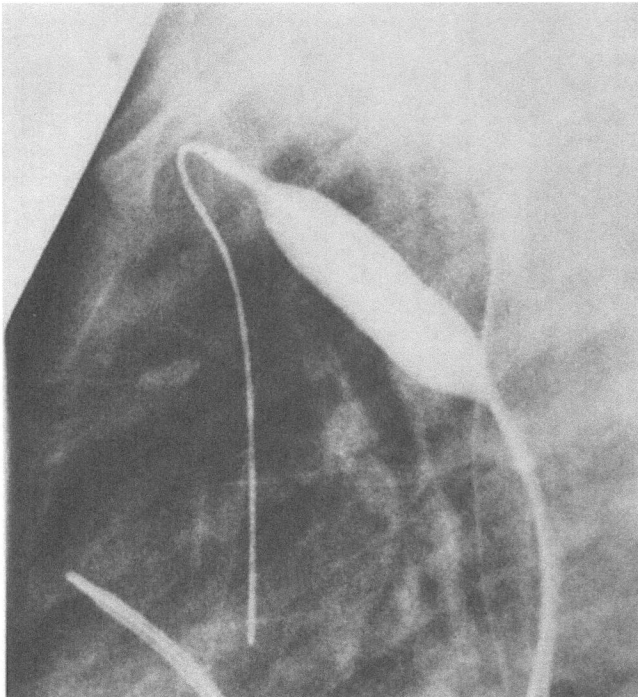

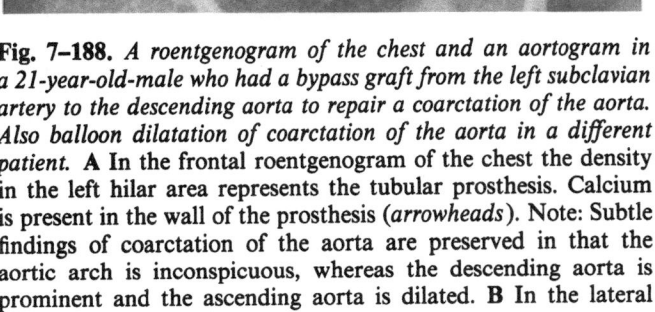

D

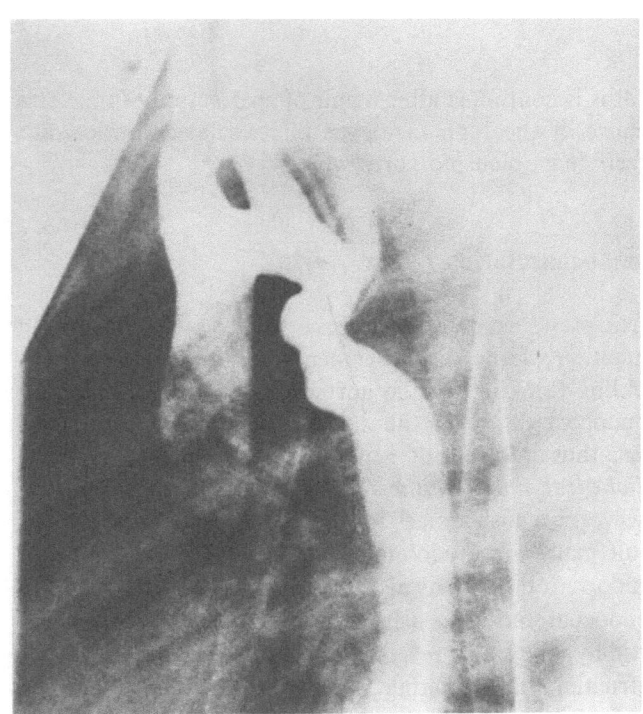

E

Fig. 7–188. *A roentgenogram of the chest and an aortogram in a 21-year-old-male who had a bypass graft from the left subclavian artery to the descending aorta to repair a coarctation of the aorta. Also balloon dilatation of coarctation of the aorta in a different patient.* **A** In the frontal roentgenogram of the chest the density in the left hilar area represents the tubular prosthesis. Calcium is present in the wall of the prosthesis (*arrowheads*). Note: Subtle findings of coarctation of the aorta are preserved in that the aortic arch is inconspicuous, whereas the descending aorta is prominent and the ascending aorta is dilated. **B** In the lateral view of the aortogram the aortic valve is bicuspid and the ascending aorta is dilated. The coarctation and tubular prosthesis (*arrowheads*) are evident. The aortic isthmus is hypoplastic.

C, D, and **E** are frames from a different patient. In **C** a lateral view of the aortogram shows severe coarctation of the aorta. **D** shows the position of a balloon angioplasty catheter inflated in the coarctation. The tip of the guide wire is in the left ventricle. **E** is a frame from the aortogram after angioplasty. The coarctation has been dilated. No intimal tear is demonstrated.

Fig. 7–189. *Roentgenograms of the chest in a 68-year-old man with pseudocoarctation of the aorta.* The pulmonary vasculature is normal. The left ventricle is enlarged although the cardiomegaly is accentuated by a poor inspiration. On the frontal view (**A**) the mediastinum is widened and the aortic knob is obscured by the dilated left subclavian artery. The descending aorta forms a spheroid density simulating an aortic arch, but in a slightly lower position than normal. On the lateral projection (**B**) the ascending aorta appears as a mediastinal mass, while the descending aorta simulates an aortic arch, again in a slightly lower position than normal. On the RAO view (**C**) the ascending aorta and brachiocephalic vessels form a mass accounting for the density on the frontal and lateral roentgenograms. The descending aorta begins after the "kink" but in a lower position than a normal aortic arch. On the LAO view (**D**) the ascending and descending aorta are both prominent. The apparent discontinuity between them is caused by the kink (pseudocoarctation). The frontal and lateral views of the aortogram (**E** and **F**) confirm the location of the aortic arch with a "kink" just beyond the left subclavian artery and the area of dilatation of the descending aorta.

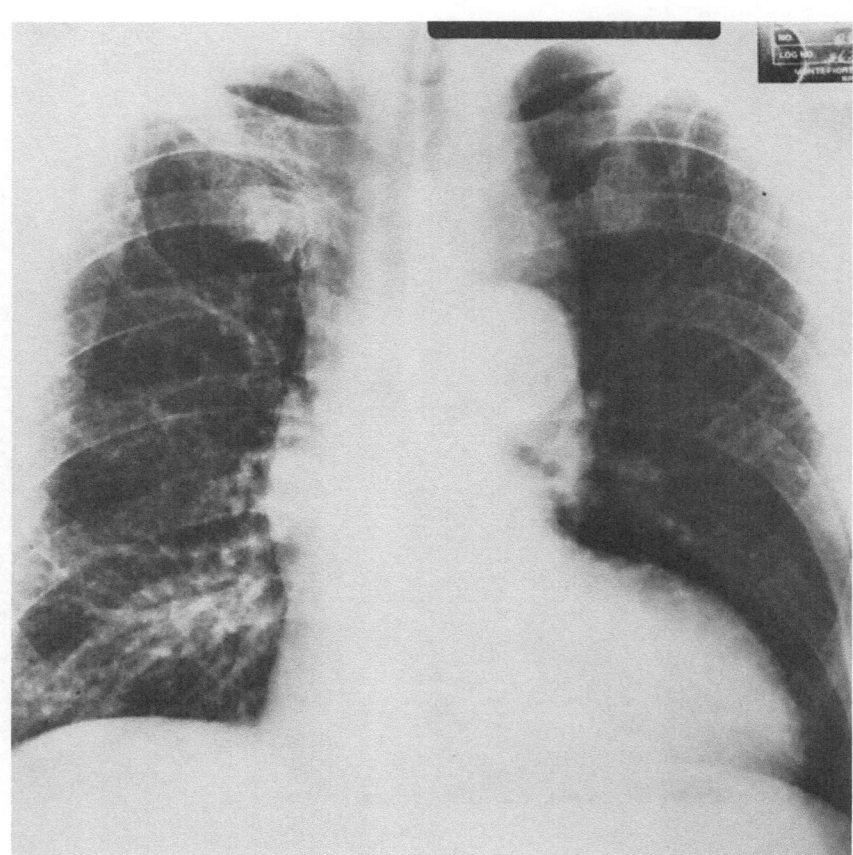

A

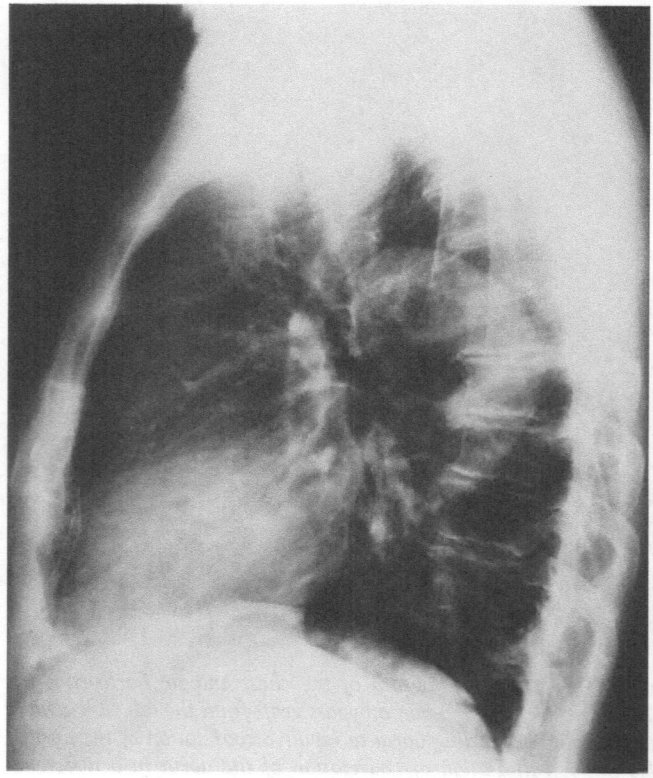

B

carditis is continued after repair of coarctation of the aorta because of the high incidence of associated intracardiac defects (e.g., bicuspid aortic valve).

Pseudocoarctation of the Aorta

Aortic pseudocoarctation is characterized by tortuosity and elongation of the distal segment of the aortic arch and buckling (kinking) of the aorta at the site of the ductus. Pseudocoarctation of the aorta usually causes no symptoms; thus it does not generally require treatment. The *radiological manifestations* may be a cause for concern, however, because a mass is observed on films of the chest. Adult males are predominantly affected (Fig. 7–189), but pseudocoarctation may also occur in children (Fig. 7–190). Pseudocoarctation is usually not obstructive. Associated aortic hypoplasia or severe kinking of the aorta may cause obstruction, necessitating surgical repair. An aneurysm may form in the descending aorta distal to the pseudocoarctation. The left subclavian artery may originate at or below the aortic kink. The authors have observed two cases of an aberrant right subclavian artery arising from the descending aorta just below the aortic kink. Pseudocoarctation of the aorta may also be associated with other cardiac anomalies similar to those occurring with juxtaductal coarctation (e.g., bicuspid aortic valve). Pseudocoarctation may be observed in Turner syndrome, Noonan syndrome and Hurler syndrome. On roentgenograms of the chest

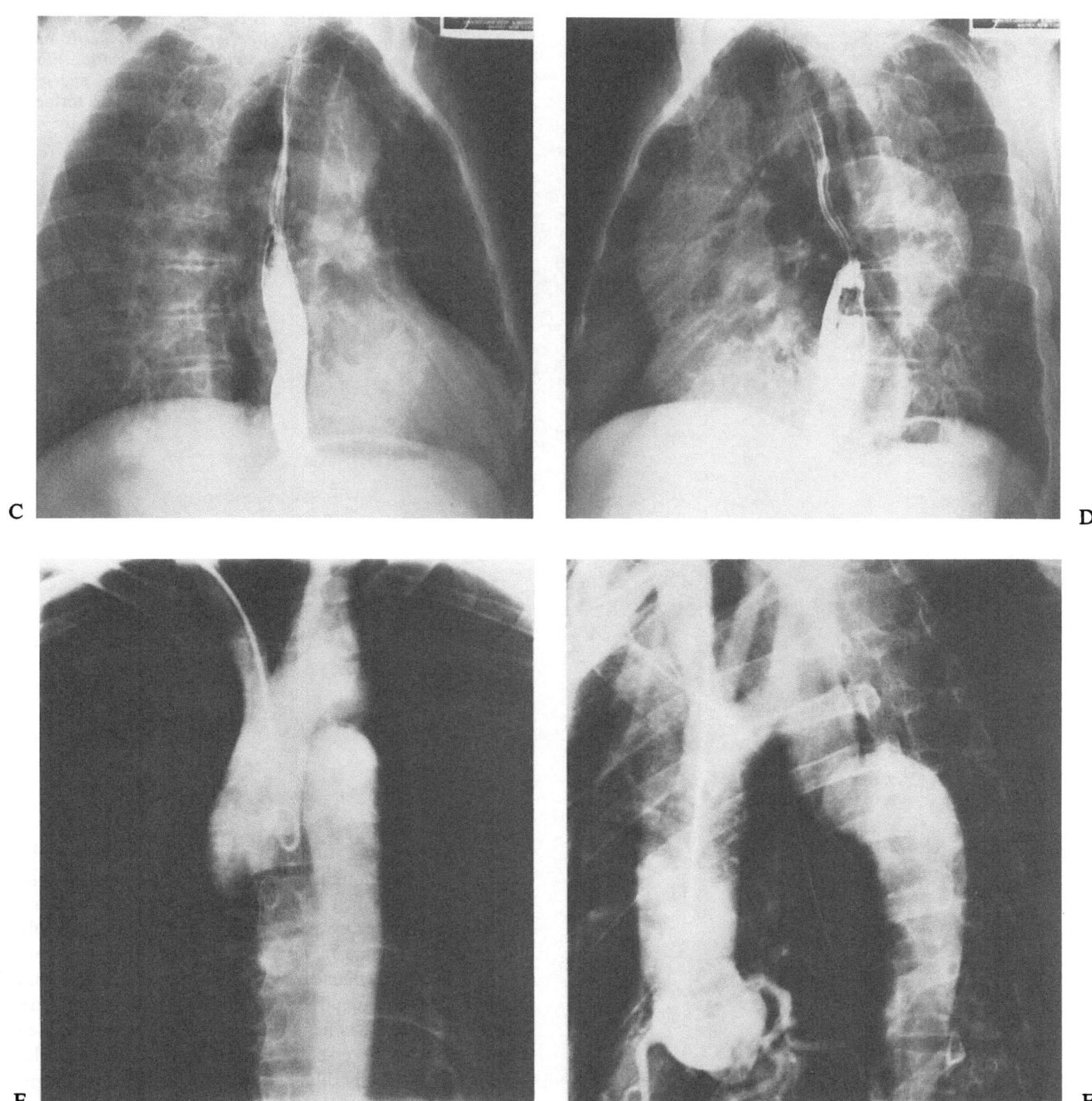

C

D

E

F

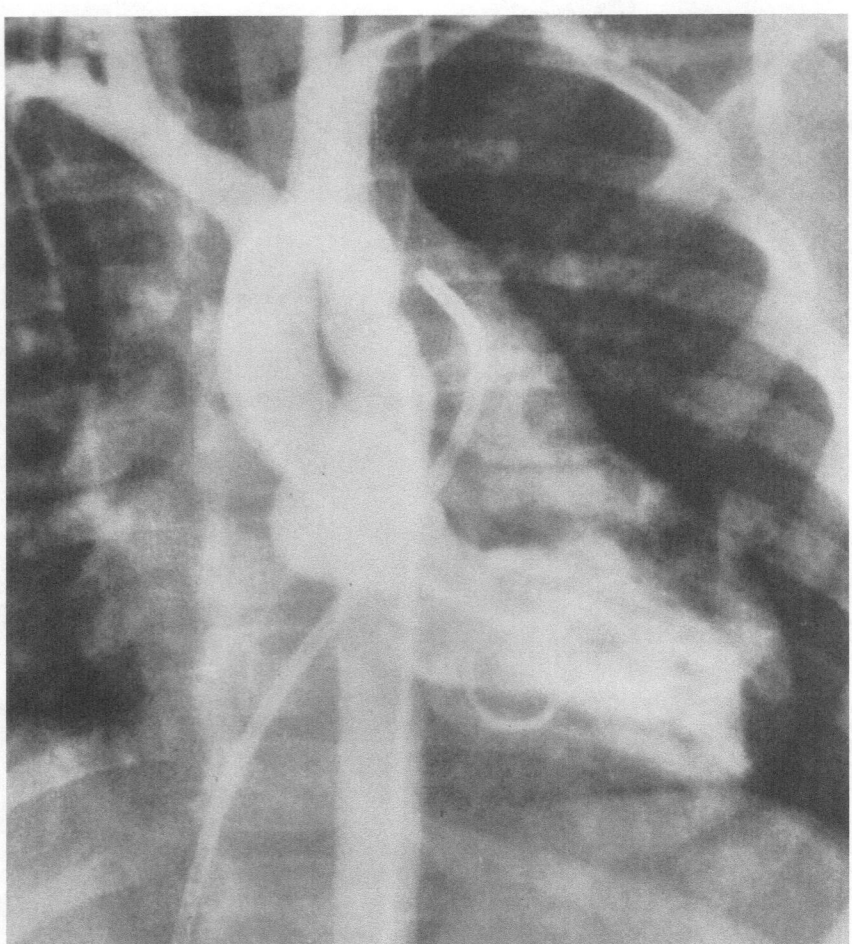

A

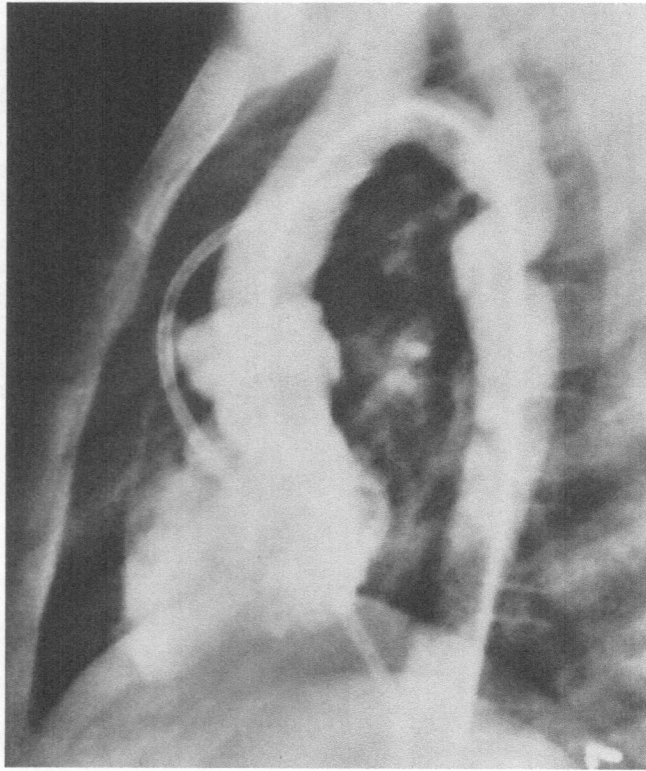

B

Fig. 7–190. A-B *A left ventriculogram in a 4-year-old girl with a bicuspid aortic valve and pseudocoarctation of the aorta.* Blood pressures were equal in the arms and legs. The angiogram shows an elongated tortuous distal aortic arch with a "kink" at the site of the ductus arteriosus.

the elongated aortic arch may widen the left side of the superior mediastinum, simulating a mediastinal mass. The descending aorta just distal to the aortic kink is dense and dilated, producing a convexity that may be mistakenly interpreted as the aortic arch. The lateral and LAO views are very helpful in delineating the characteristic aortic kink or indentation of pseudocoarctation (figure of three sign). The barium-filled esophagus may be indented by the dilated aortic segments (reversed three or E sign). The left subclavian artery is usually dilated and contributes to the widening of the left side of the superior mediastinum. Notching of the ribs will not occur, since the pseudocoarctation is not obstructed.

Echocardiography will identify associated anomalies of the aortic valve, LV or mitral valve. The view of the aorta from the suprasternal notch may delineate the kink in the aorta. The kink may simulate the posterior shelf, occurring in true coarctation of the aorta.

At *catheterization,* difficulty in passing the catheter across the site of pseudocoarctation may be caused by tortuosity of the aorta in this area. No pressure gradient, or at most a mild pressure gradient, may be encountered.

On *angiography,* pseudocoarctation of the aorta appears as a marked kink of the aorta at the site of the ligamentum arteriosum. Pseudocoarctation must be distinguished from true coarctation and from cervical aortic arch.

Aortico-Left Ventricular Tunnel

This rare congenital abnormality is characterized by an anomalous communication between the aorta and left ventricle. The communication starts above the right semilunar sinus of Valsalva near the commissure between the right and the noncoronary sinuses. The communication courses behind the RV outflow tract and pierces the interventricular septum to end in the LV below the right aortic cusp. The tunnel or duct may be aneurysmal and may partially obstruct the RV outflow tract. Histologically the proximal end of the tunnel resembles the aortic wall, containing elastic fibers. The distal end of the tunnel wall is composed of collagen and endothelial lining, suggesting that the tunnel probably represents an anomalous vessel. The aortico-left ventricular tunnel is, on occasion, associated with other cardiac defects. Among these, lesions of the aortic valve are the most common (e.g., bicuspid valve, dysplastic valve).

These infants present with a high-intensity, continuous murmur and evidence of LV hypertrophy by electrocardiography. The peripheral arterial pulses are bounding. Heart failure often develops in the first year of life.

M-mode echocardiography shows a dilated hyperkinetic LV, flutter of the mitral valve and early closure of the mitral valve, all of which may also occur with aortic regurgitation. Two-dimensional echocardiography may actually delineate the tunnel. The LV end of the tunnel may resemble a ventricular septal defect; however, echocardiographic contrast fails to pass through the opening from RV to LV, even though clinical evidence of elevated RV pressure is present. Careful scanning from multiple positions on the chest and in the suprasternal notch may delineate the course of the tunnel and its opening into the aorta.

Roentgenograms of the chest show cardiomegaly with LV enlargement and marked dilatation of the ascending aorta. In the lateral view of the chest the ascending aorta may obliterate the restrosternal clear space. The barium esophagogram may show an anterior indentation, also caused by the dilated aorta.

On aortography marked dilatation of the aorta is present with immediate filling of the LV through the tunnel. The aortic end of the tunnel opens above the aortic valve near the right coronary artery and enters the LV below the right coronary cusp. These anatomical features are best demonstrated in the LAO view. The tunnel may form an aneurysm that projects anteriorly and toward the left to encircle and compress the pulmonary trunk.

On left ventriculography two outlets are noted between the LV and the aorta. One outlet is the aortic valve, and the other, the tunnel, which is anterior and to the right of the aortic valve. Again the lateral and LAO views (standard and angulated) are most helpful. Failure of the RV

to opacify excludes ventricular septal defect with aortic insufficiency or rupture of a sinus of Valsalva into the right ventricle with aortic insufficiency. Demonstration of two coronary arteries, separate from the tunnel, excludes coronary arteriovenous fistula.

Aortico-left ventricular tunnel results in deformity of the aortic valve and aortic insufficiency, if untreated. Sudden death may occur during medical treatment. Early surgical intervention, even in infancy, is therefore recommended. Repair consists of a patch or direct suture in the aortic end of the tunnel.

Congenital Aortic Insufficiency due to Absence of a Cusp of the Aortic Valve

Congenital absence of the leaflets of the aortic valve is extremely rare. The authors have encountered a neonate in whom the non-coronary cusp was absent and only a ridge was present. Two other cusps were present. A recent report describes another case of fetal aortic insufficiency in which all three cusps of the aortic valve were absent.

In the case identified by the authors the deformity of the aortic valve was associated with a large infracristal ventricular septal defect extending into the inlet portion of the ventricular septum. The membranous portion of the ventricular septum and the membranous portion of the atrioventricular septum were partially intact and were larger than normal. Valvar pulmonic stenosis was also present. The ductus arteriosus was widely patent. In the patient described by Bierman, et al. multiple anomalies were associated (i.e., polysplenia, with absence of the right superior vena cava and anomalous drainage of the left superior vena cava into the right atrium; azygos continuation of the inferior vena cava with drainage into the left superior vena cava; A–V communis with a hypoplastic left ventricle; hypoplastic mitral valve; double-outlet right ventricle; double aortic arch with hypoplastic left arch). In addition, malrotation of the midgut was present without obstruction. Doppler echocardiography allowed prenatal diagnosis of the aortic insufficiency. Clinically both babies had systolic and diastolic murmurs as well as progressive congestive heart failure, leading to death during the first few days of life.

Echocardiography in the case identified by the authors revealed a dilated aorta with hyperdynamic pulsations. The motions of the aortic leaflets were indistinct. Both ventricles were dilated. The location of the ventricular septal defect was identified on 2-dimensional echocardiography.

Roentgenograms of the chest (Fig. 7–191) showed pronounced bilateral pulmonary undercirculation with marked generalized cardiomegaly.

At angiography a large patent ductus arteriosus was present with bidirectional shunting. The injection in the ductus arteriosus opacified not only the descending aorta but also the ascending aorta and the left ventricle (due to severe aortic insufficiency). Injection in the left ventricle demonstrated a markedly dilated hypokinetic left ven-

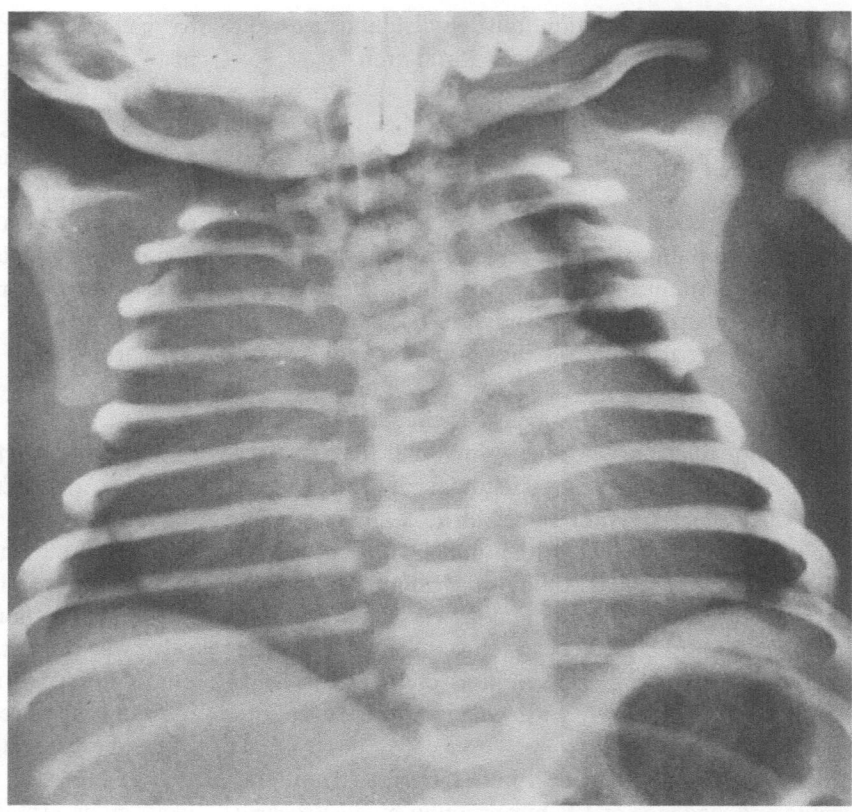

A

tricle with a left-to-right shunt through the ventricular septal defect. The aortic anulus was mildly hypoplastic. The ascending and descending aorta were markedly dilated, reminiscent of the dilatation of the main pulmonary artery occurring with tetralogy of Fallot with absence of the pulmonary valve. The pulmonic valve was thickened.

Supravalvular Aortic Stenosis (Williams Syndrome)

The anatomical features of this lesion are variable, ranging from a simple membranous diaphragm above the aortic valve to hypoplasia of the entire aorta. The usual form (coarctation of the supravalvar aorta) is characterized by a circular narrowing of the aorta just distal to the coronary ostia. Williams et al. suggested that the combination of mental retardation, a characteristic (elfin) facies and supravalvular aortic stenosis may constitute a new syndrome. The typical facies consists of a full face, broad forehead, heavy cheeks, wide mouth, prominent lips and ears and pointed chin. Some affected individuals also have strabismus, hernia and dental abnormalities; sexual precocity may be present in the females. Features of Marfan syndrome may also occur in some patients with Williams syndrome. The findings in Williams syndrome are reminiscent of a syndrome associated with neonatal hypervitaminosis D and hypercalcemia (the neonatal hypercalcemic syndrome). It

has been suggested that Williams syndrome may be a chronic form of this entity even though neonatal hypercalcemia has not been recognized in many patients with supravalvar aortic stenosis.

Peripheral pulmonary artery stenosis is another commonly associated disorder of Williams syndrome. Other anomalies include postductal coarctation of the aorta and stenosis of the branches of the aortic arch.

Clinical Features The cardiac findings may be indistinguishable from those of valvar or subvalvar obstruction. Supravalvar aortic stenosis may be suspected if the murmur and thrill are transmitted strongly to the neck and if there is no systolic ejection click.

Echocardiography Two-dimensional echocardiography shows narrowing of the aorta just above the sinuses of Valsalva. The enlargement of the coronary arteries may be recognized. Doppler study from the suprasternal notch may demonstrate the site of the pressure difference.

Radiological (Plain Film) Features Dilatation of the aorta is uncommon in this anomaly. The ascending aorta and aortic arch are often inconspicuous, producing the "empty vascular pedicle." This feature, together with clinical evidence of aortic stenosis, should alert the radiologist to consider the diagnosis of supravalvular aortic stenosis. Multiple pulmonary artery branch stenosis may be diagnosed on plain films by the "sausagization" sign (stenosis of a pulmonary artery branch followed by poststenotic dilatation; see Fig. 7–144). Signs of pulmonary venous hypertension may be present.

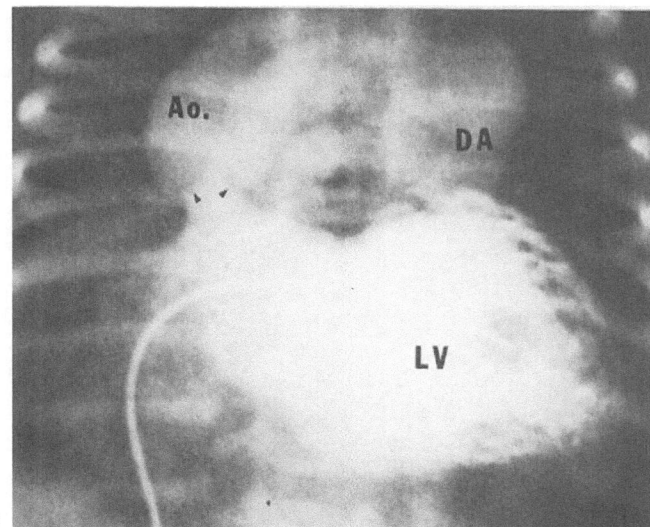

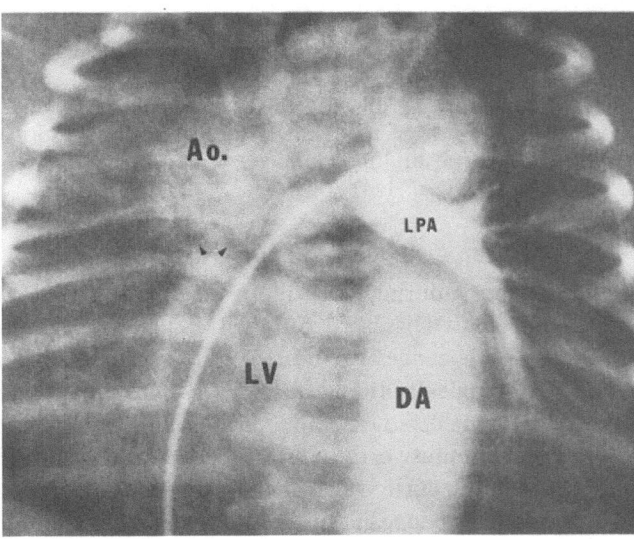

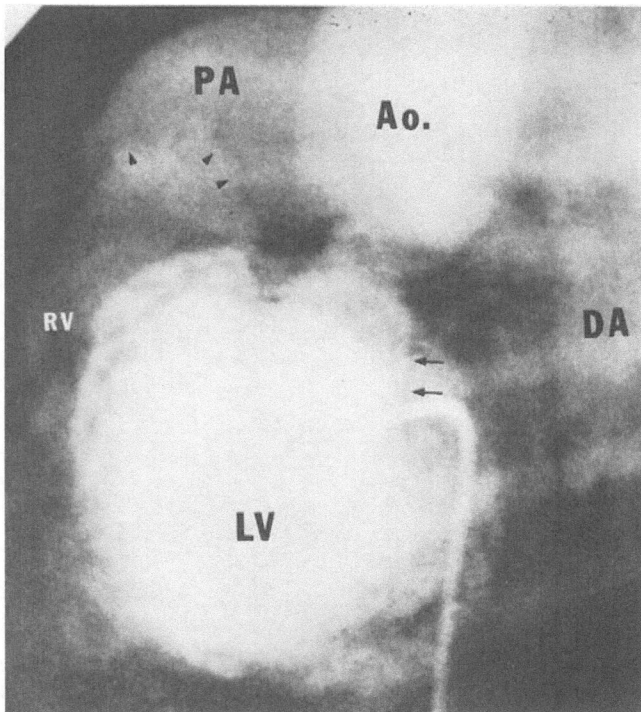

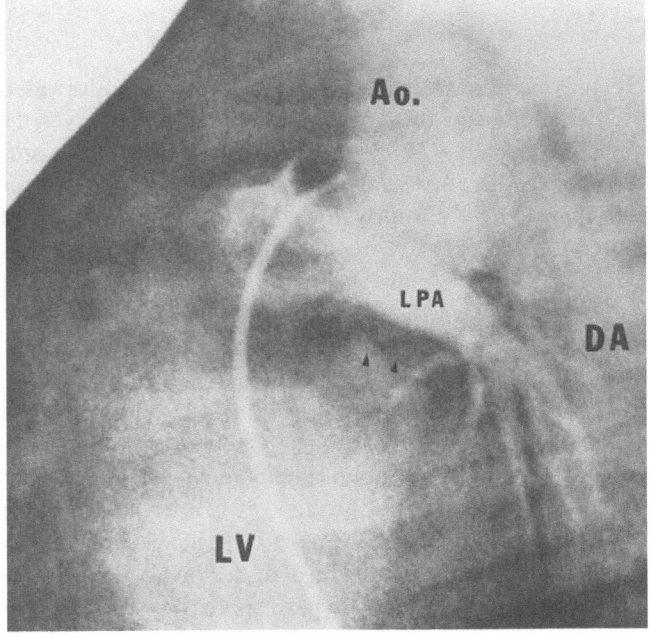

Fig. 7–191. *Radiographic findings in a 1 day old baby with congenital absence of the aortic valve.* The frontal film of the chest (**A**) shows massive cardiomegaly and severe pulmonary undercirculation. The frontal and lateral views of the left ventriculogram (**B** and **C**) show a dilated and hypokinetic left ventricle (*LV*) with mild hypoplasia of the aortic anulus (*arrowheads* in **B**, unlabeled in **C**). The ascending aorta (*Ao.*) and descending aorta (*DA*) are markedly dilated. The right ventricle (*RV*) and pulmonary artery (*PA*) are opacified by way of the VSD. The main pulmonary artery forms a double density superimposed on the ascending aorta in the frontal view. The aorta and pulmonary artery are separated in the lateral view so that the full width of each vessel can be appreciated. The thickened pulmonic valve is indicated by *arrowheads* in **C**. Note that mitral to aortic fibrous continuity is present. The *arrows* in **C** point to the anterior leaflet of the mitral valve. After injection in the patent ductus arteriosus (**D** and **E**) the dilated descending aorta opacifies. Contrast also flows retrograde into the ascending aorta and the LV due to severe aortic regurgitation. The mildly thickened cusps of the aortic valve are indicated by arrowheads in **E**. *LPA* = left pulmonary artery.

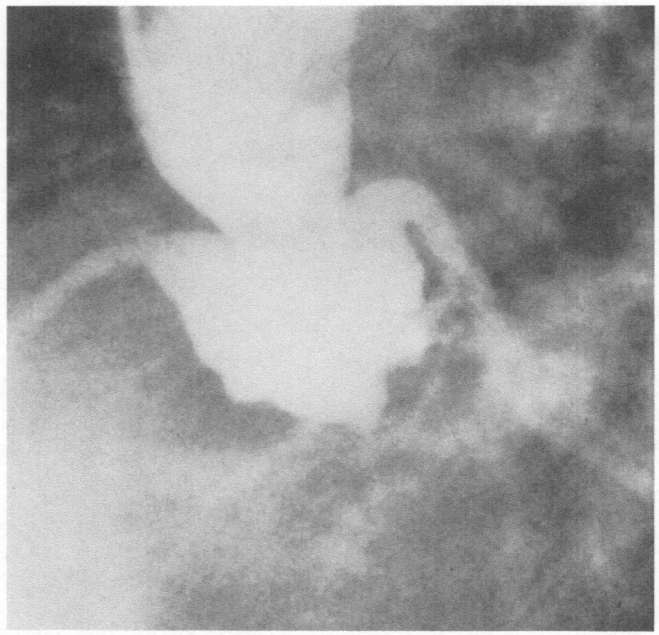
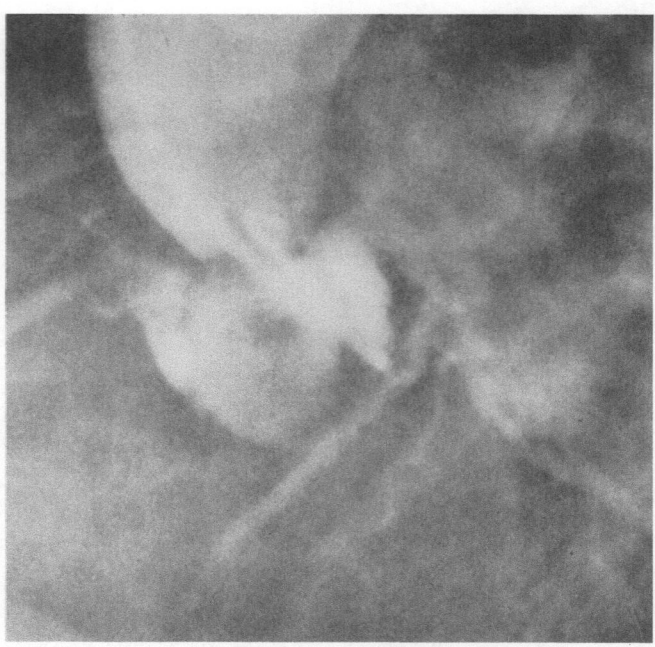

Fig. 7-192. *Cine aortogram in a 19-year-old girl with supravalvular aortic stenosis (Williams syndrome).* **A** diastolic frame; **B** systolic frame. Localized narrowing is present just above the coronary ostia, but the aorta is normal beyond the stenosis. The coronary arteries are not dilated. During systole the leaflets open incompletely, because of tethering of the leaflets to the orifice of the stenotic area. Multiple pulmonary branch stenoses were also present (see Fig. 7-144).

Hemodynamics The pressure tracings on withdrawal of the catheter from the LV show three distinct curves: (1) high LV pressure, (2) followed by equally high aortic pressure above the aortic valve but proximal to the stenosis, and then (3) by abruptly lower systolic pressure, which represents the pressure in the aorta distal to the stenosis. **Contrast Studies** Angiocardiography is helpful in localizing the area of stenosis, characterized by a ringlike narrowing of the ascending aorta immediately above the origins of the coronary arteries or a tubular narrowing of the ascending aorta and aortic arch (Fig. 7-192). The coronary arteries are dilated and tortuous. Rarely the coronary ostia are narrowed by the stenotic ring. Some degree of hypoplasia of the aorta distal to the stenosis is a frequent finding. The aortic valve is usually normal (trileaflet). Tethering of the aortic cusps to the area of supravalvular stenosis has been noted. The LV is hypertrophied. Associated (unilateral or bilateral) multiple pulmonary artery branch stenosis may be recognized on pulmonary angiography. Stenosis of the origins of the brachiocephalic vessels together with hypoplasia of these vessels has been described. **Treatment** Treatment consists of excision of a discrete membrane, application of a patch to widen a short segment of stenosis or insertion of a tubular prosthesis to replace a long segment of stenosis.

Critical Valvar Aortic Stenosis in Infancy

The most common anatomical defect causing valvar aortic stenosis is a bicuspid aortic valve. The usual presentation of aortic stenosis during adult life is discussed in Chapter 5, Valvular Heart Disease. Aortic valve stenosis may also be present with congestive heart failure in the newborn period. Pathologically the valve may be bicuspid with severe stenosis, unicuspid (acommissural or unicommissural) or tricuspid (diminutive, dysplastic or with cuspal inequalities). A dysplastic aortic valve consists of thickened leaflets with myxomatous deposits in the sinuses of Valsalva. The anulus may be small or normal in size. An aortic valve with four or more cusps occurs exceptionally and, on occasion, may be stenotic. In the presence of aortic stenosis in a newborn the LV may be small, secondary to decreased flow during fetal life, or large, secondary to fetal valvular cardiomyopathy. Endocardial fibroelastosis may develop secondary to high left ventricular diastolic pressure that prevents adequate perfusion to the endocardium. For similar reasons subendocardial ischemia and subendocardial infarction may occur in the newborn period, further compromising cardiac output.

Symptoms of severe heart failure due to critical aortic stenosis occur almost immediately after birth. This is in contrast to left-to-right shunts, which may not become clinically significant until 3 to 6 weeks after birth. Pallor and mottling accompany cyanosis because of venous desaturation. Tachypnea, dyspnea and râles are present on auscultation of the lungs. The heart is enlarged with a RV heave. The liver and spleen are enlarged. The extremeties are cool and pale, and all the pulses are weak. The blood gases show normal or slightly decreased oxygenation, with metabolic acidosis secondary to low cardiac output. The electrocardiogram may demonstrate LV hypertrophy with strain

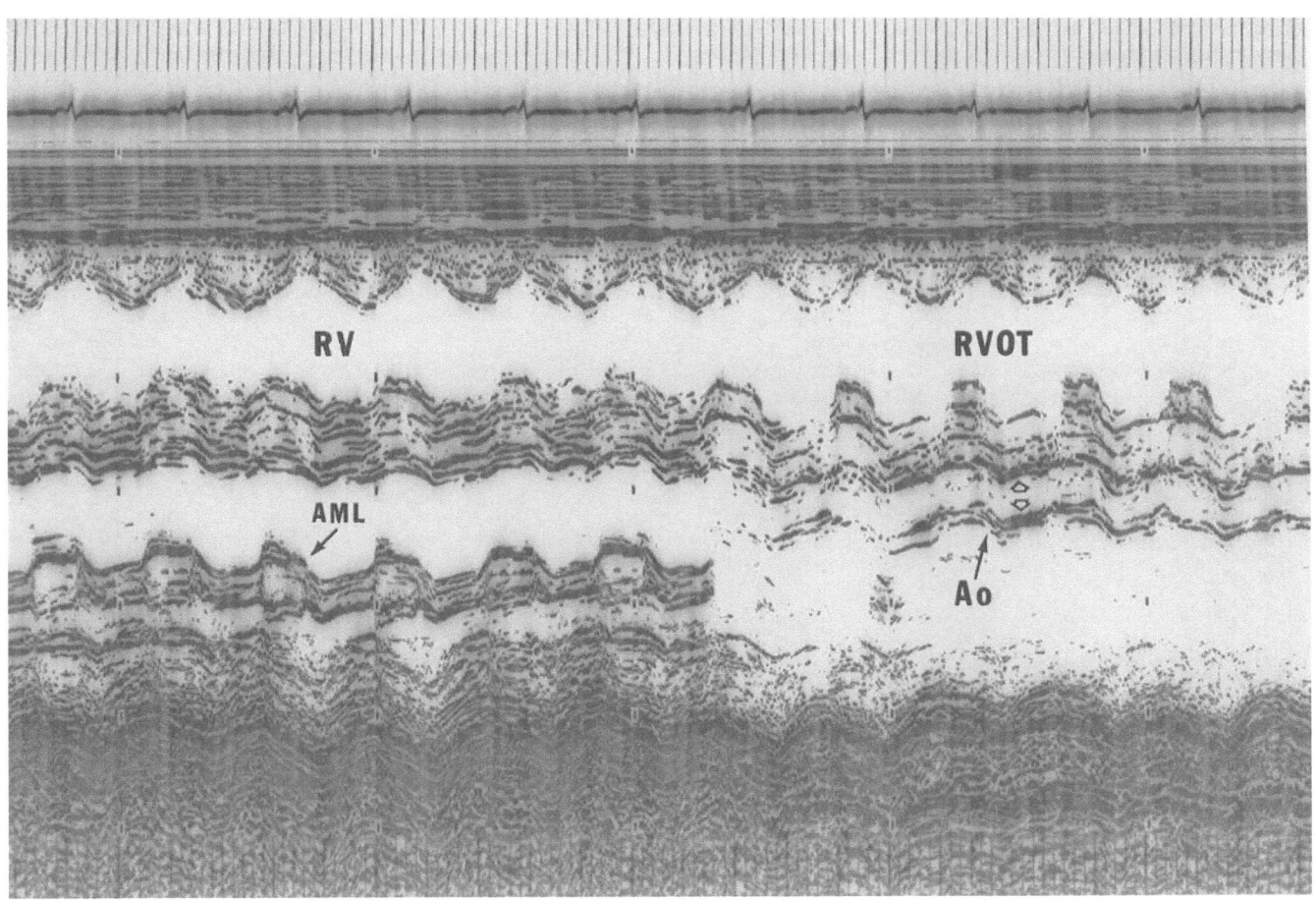

Fig. 7–193. *M-mode echocardiogram in a 1-day-old boy with severe congestive heart failure due to critical valvar aortic stenosis.* This arc scan from the left ventricle to the aortic root shows the free wall of the left ventricle and the septum to be hypertrophied (left ventricular wall = 0.6 cm, septum = 0.9 cm). The excursion of the mitral valve is reduced because of elevation of the left ventricular diastolic pressure. No subaortic narrowing is present, but the orifice of the aortic valve is small (*open arrows*). The left atrium is enlarged.

(negative T waves in V_6) or may show RV hypertrophy, inasmuch as the RV has been supplying a larger than normal share of the combined cardiac output during fetal life.

Echocardiography (Fig. 7–193) indicates a normal or slightly small diameter of the aortic root. If the diameter of the aortic root is less than 0.5 cm, then aortic atresia rather than aortic stenosis is suspected. Motion of the leaflets of the aortic valve may occur in both aortic stenosis and aortic atresia. The LV may be dilated and hypocontractile or hypoplastic with relatively thick walls. An end-diastolic diameter of the LV on M-mode echocardiography less than 1.3 cm or a cross-sectional area of the LV on 2-D echocardiography less than 1.6 cm² indicates a hypoplastic LV, which presages a poor prognosis after surgery. The LA has a large diameter. The RV and pulmonary artery may be dilated because of excessive RV output prior to birth or because of a left-to-right shunt at the atrial level. The motion of the pulmonary valve and the pulmonary systolic time intervals are consistent with pulmonary hypertension. Doppler echocardiography shows a flow disturbance in the ascending aorta and a greater than normal velocity corresponding to the pressure difference across the valve.

The *roentgenograms of the chest* (Fig. 7–194A) demonstrate evidence of pulmonary venous hypertension with the heart being mildly to markedly enlarged.

At *cardiac catheterization* a step-up in oxygen saturation may be detected in the RA. The pressures in the RV and pulmonary artery are increased. LA pressure and LV end-diastolic pressure also are increased. The systolic pressure in the LV may be normal or increased. Aortic pressures are lower than LV pressures and are damped unless the ductus arteriosus is open. Pressure in the aorta may be equal to that in the pulmonary artery in the presence of a widely patent ductus arteriosus.

A *left ventriculogram* from a venous approach by way of the foramen ovale is the preferred method to identify critical aortic stenosis (Fig. 7–194B–C). The function of the LV will be assessed, and associated defects, such as ventricular septal defect and deformities of the mitral valve, will be demonstrated.

Treatment of congestive heart failure with digoxin, dopamine and diuretics will reduce the risk of cardiac catheterization and a surgical procedure. Prostaglandin E_1 is given to open the ductus so the RV can supply blood to the aorta and thereby relieve the acidosis. Medical treat-

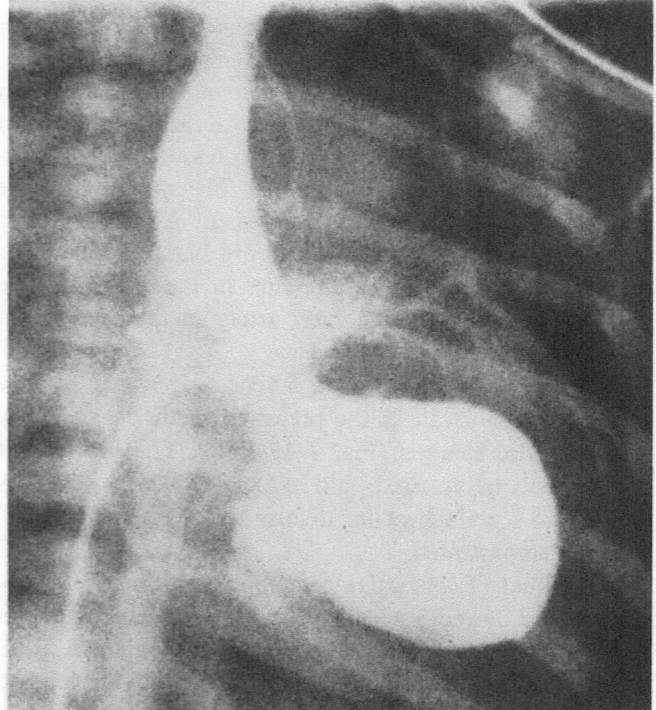

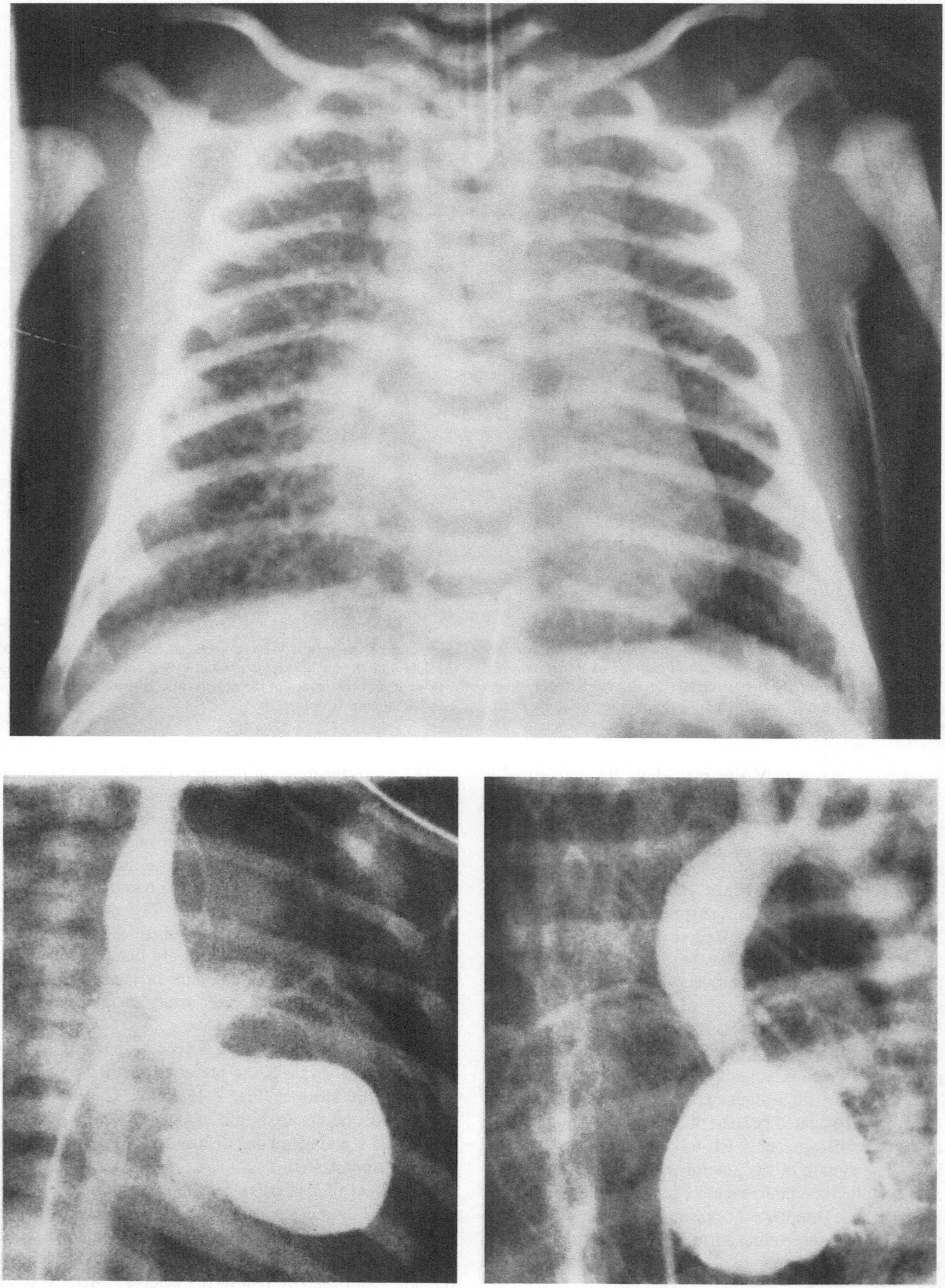

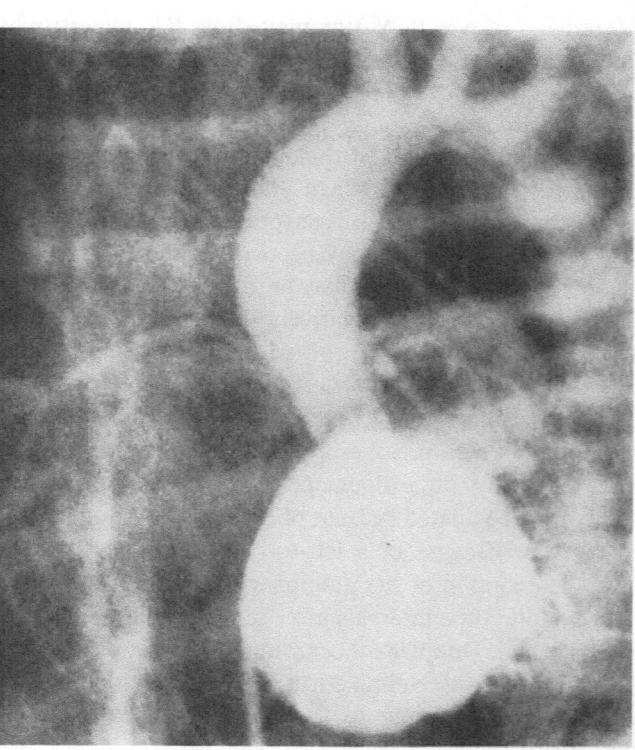

◄ **Fig. 7–194.** *Roentgenogram of the chest in a 1-day-old boy with critical aortic stenosis* (**A**) *and left ventriculogram in a 1-month-old boy with critical aortic stenosis and severe congestive heart failure* (**B–C**). **A** The heart is mildly enlarged. The lungs show a reticulated pattern consistent with severe pulmonary venous hypertension. **B** The RAO view shows a dilated ventricle with thick walls. The left ventricle shows severe global hypokinesis with minimal change in size between diastole and systole. **C** The LAO view during systole shows the aortic valve to be thickened and domed. The aortic arch and isthmus are narrow.

ment may provide transient improvement, but usually not long-term survival in critical aortic stenosis.

Surgical treatment consists of valvotomy, with success depending on the finding of a valve whose orifice can be improved without causing severe aortic insufficiency. In neonates with critical aortic stenosis the aortic valve is seldom repairable, resulting in a very low incidence of survival. Poor LV function also contributes to high operative mortality.

Subaortic Stenosis

Entities that produce obstruction of the outflow tract of the left ventricle (LVOT) include idiopathic hypertrophic cardiomyopathy, discrete membranous subaortic stenosis, subaortic fibrous tunnel and, rarely, malattachment or adherence of the anterior leaflet of the mitral valve to the ventricular septum associated with accessory endocardial cushion tissue (mitral).

In individuals with endocardial cushion defects subaortic stenosis may be caused by tethering of the mitral component of the common anterior leaflet to the top of the ventricular septum, by an abnormal position of the papillary muscles in the LVOT or by hypoplasia of the LVOT. Discrete membranous subaortic stenosis can also occur with endocardial cushion defect. In infants, obstruction of the LVOT may be caused by a malalignment type of ventricular septal defect with deviation of the conus septum into the LVOT (Becu syndrome). Overriding of the pulmonary valve above the ventricular septum is also part of the Becu syndrome. This syndrome is usually associated with coarctation of the aorta, aortic atresia or interruption of the aortic arch. Moulaert et al. suggest that the muscle mass in the LVOT in Becu syndrome represents the anterolateral muscle bundle of the LV rather than a deviated conus muscle. The muscle mass usually results in severe stenosis.

Some infants of diabetic mothers have a transient form of hypertrophic cardiomyopathy causing obstruction of the LVOT. In patients with single ventricle and a subaortic chamber the conus muscle or a restrictive bulboventricular foramen (ventricular septal defect) may produce subaortic stenosis. The subaortic conus may also be obstructive in instances of levotransposition of the great arteries.

In this chapter, discrete membranous subaortic stenosis and fibrous subaortic tunnel are discussed. Idiopathic hypertrophic cardiomyopathy and transient hypertrophic car-

diomyopathy are included in Chapter 6, Cardiomyopathy. The malalignment type of ventricular septal defect (Becu syndrome) is described with ventricular septal defect. Subaortic stenosis with endocardial cushion defect is addressed in the discussion of endocardial cushion defects. Subaortic stenosis caused by a subaortic conus is considered in the section on single ventricle and transposition.

Discrete Membranous Subaortic Stenosis and Fibrous Subaortic Tunnel

Discrete membranous subaortic stenosis (DMSS) and fibrous tunnel subaortic stenosis comprise approximately 16% of cases of congenital obstruction of the LVOT. DMSS is a congenital obstructing lesion of the LVOT, located just below the aortic valve or within 2 cm below it. The obstructing lesion varies from a fibrous membrane (web), less than 1 mm thick, to diffuse, fibrous or fibromuscular narrowing (tunnel-like obstruction). The severity of the obstruction differs from case to case and is frequently progressive. The aortic valve is deformed and thickened, perhaps because of a jet or turbulence from the subaortic narrowing. Aortic insufficiency is frequently present. Relatives of affected individuals with DMSS have a high incidence of LV obstruction (13%). The incidence of infective endocarditis is also high (13%). DMSS is frequently associated with other congenital heart lesions, such as coarctation of the aorta, mitral valve deformity, ventricular septal and endocardial cushion defect. DMSS is also part of the Shone syndrome. It is important to diagnose DMSS in the presence of other defects so that LVOT obstruction will not be neglected when surgical therapy is undertaken. DMSS should also be sought in patients suspected of having idiopathic hypertrophic cardiomyopathy, since the membrane may be the cause of stenosis, with the hypertrophy being secondary.

On examination a systolic ejection murmur is heard at the right upper sternal border or at the left midsternal border with radiation to the neck. Absence of an ejection click in the presence of this murmur of aortic stenosis should suggest a form of aortic stenosis other than valvular. The murmur of aortic regurgitation may be evident. Peripheral pulses are normal unless stenosis is severe. The electrocardiogram may be normal or may reflect LV hypertrophy. A LV pattern of strain (T wave changes) correlates with severe obstruction.

On M-mode echocardiography the membrane appears as an echodense structure attached to the left side of the ventricular septum just below the aortic valve. The LVOT may be narrowed. The aortic valve shows flutter and early systolic closure (Fig. 7–195). On 2-D echocardiography the fibrous diaphragm is attached to the ventricular septum and to the mitral valve (anterior leaflet), protruding into the LVOT (Fig. 7–195). See also Fig. 7–71, which illustrates a similar formation in the LVOT in dextrotransposition of the great arteries (D-TGA). Pulsed Doppler echocardiography from the apex window may define the level of stenosis within the LVOT. The flow disturbance and in-

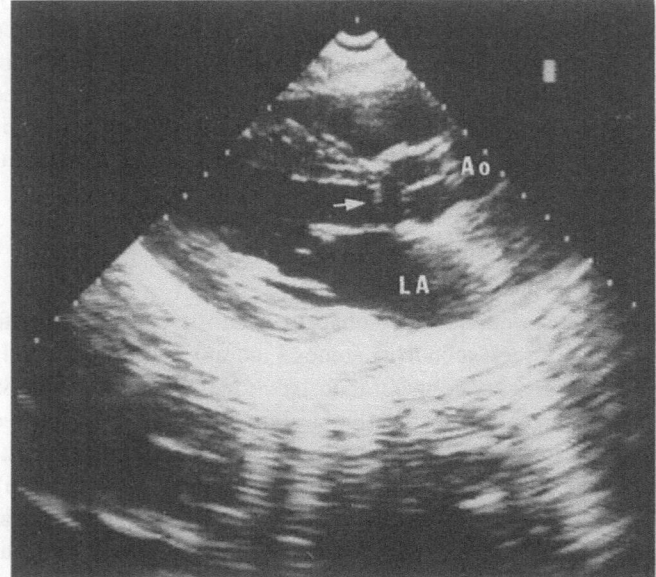

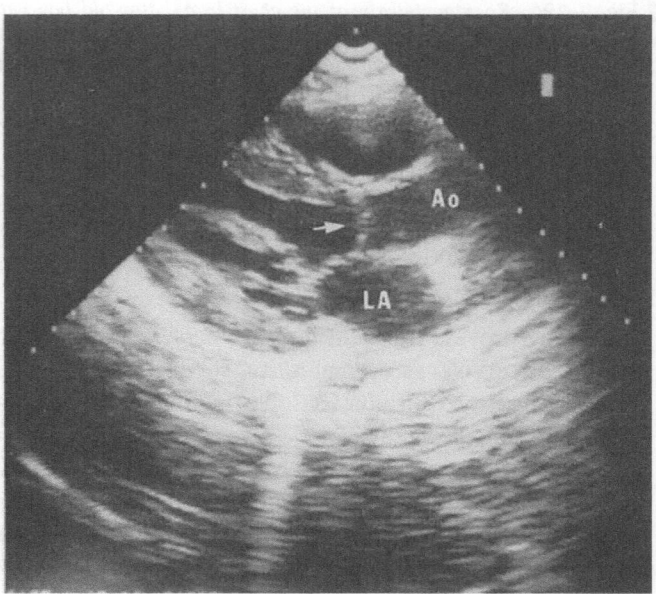

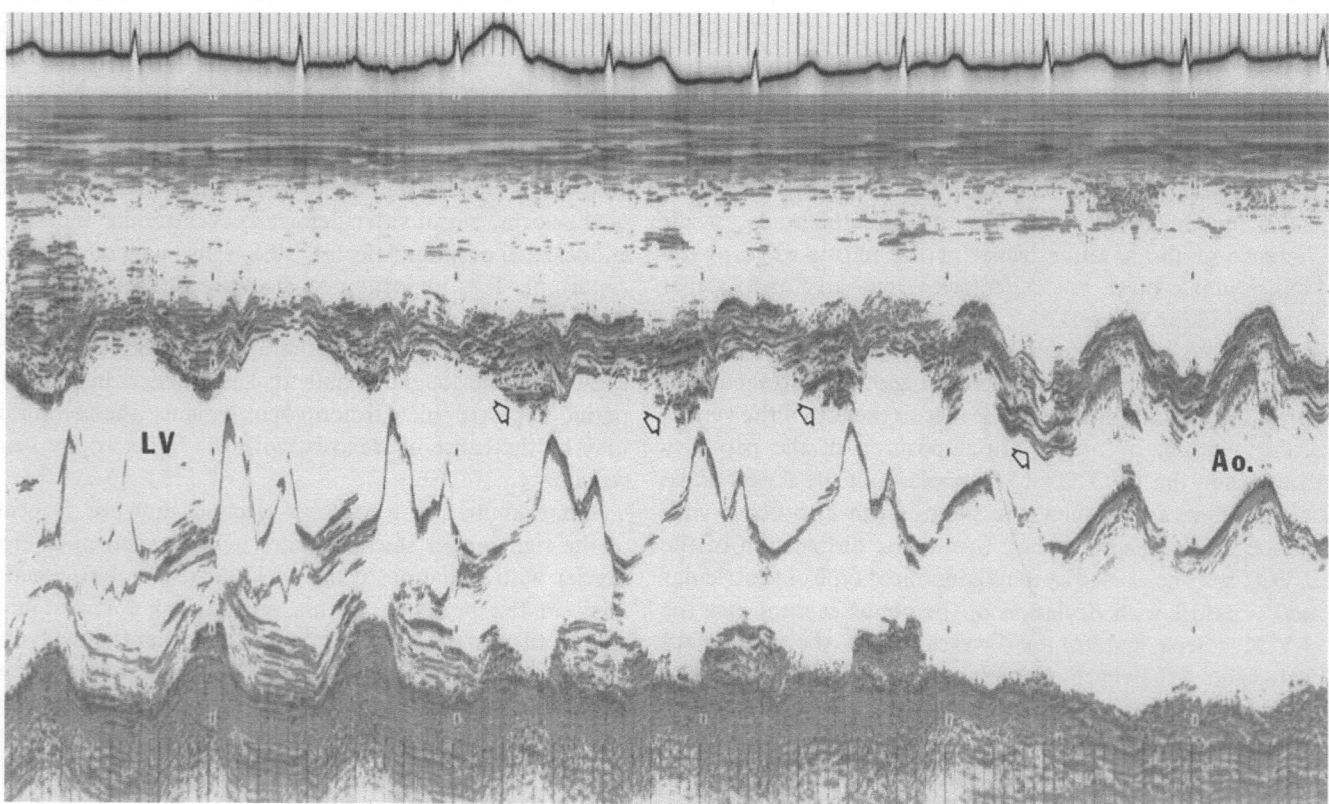

A

B

C

Fig. 7–195. *Two-dimensional echocardiograms in a 10-year-old boy with discrete membranous subaortic stenosis. During diastole* **(A)** the membrane is represented by a narrow line (*arrow*) across the left ventricular outflow tract approximately three mm. below the aortic valve. The aortic leaflets are not thickened. The line of coaptation of the aortic leaflets forms a linear density rather than a dot within the aortic root. This appearance is caused by a slight obliquity of the angle of the transducer. During systole **(B)** the membrane (*arrow*) curves toward the aorta while the aortic leaflets open completely so that only their attachments are perceptible. **C** is an M-mode arc scan from the left ventricle (*LV*) to the aorta (*Ao.*) in another 10-year-old boy with the same diagnosis. The subaortic membrane (*open arrows*) appears as an echo-dense structure attached to the left side of the ventricular septum. The left ventricle contracts normally. The septum and left ventricular free wall are not thickened. **D** The M-mode tracing of the aortic valve shows early systolic closure (*ESC*) and marked systolic flutter, representing signs of subaortic stenosis. The valve is symmetrical with a normal excursion. **E** A systolic ejection murmur (*SEM*) without a systolic ejection click is recorded on the phonocardiogram, and systolic shudder (*open arrow*) is present on the carotid pulse tracing. Absence of a systolic ejection click in a patient with a shudder on the carotid tracing should lead to the likely possibility of aortic stenosis at a level other than the aortic valve (e.g., subvalvar, supravalvar). S_1 = first heart sound; S_2 = second heart sound.

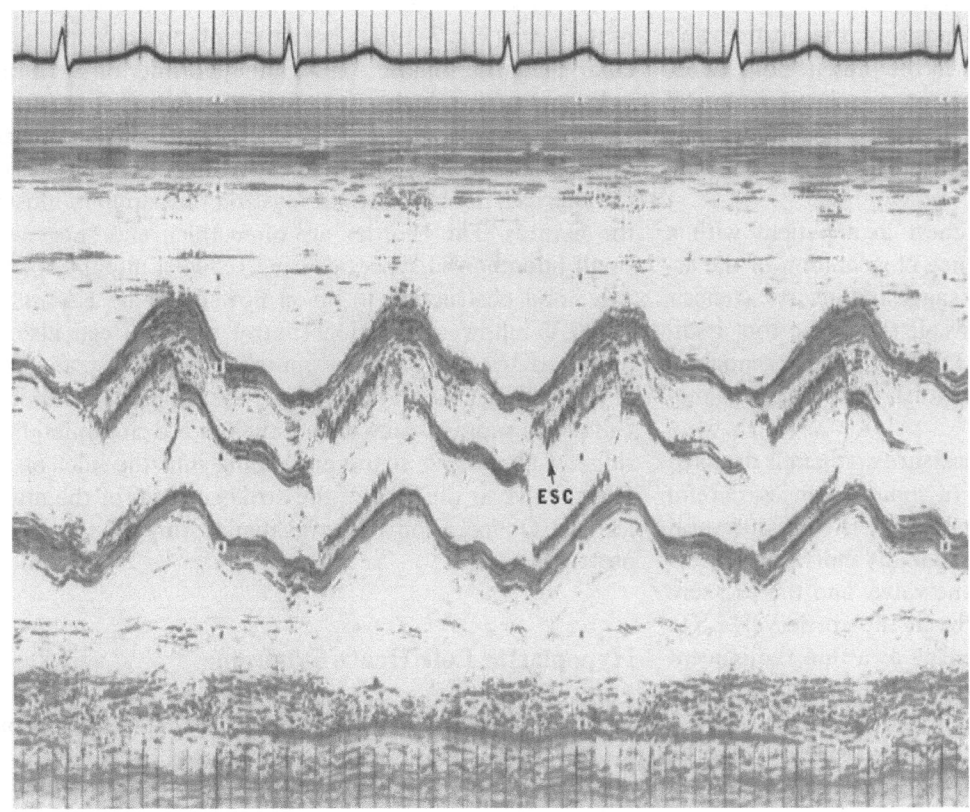

D

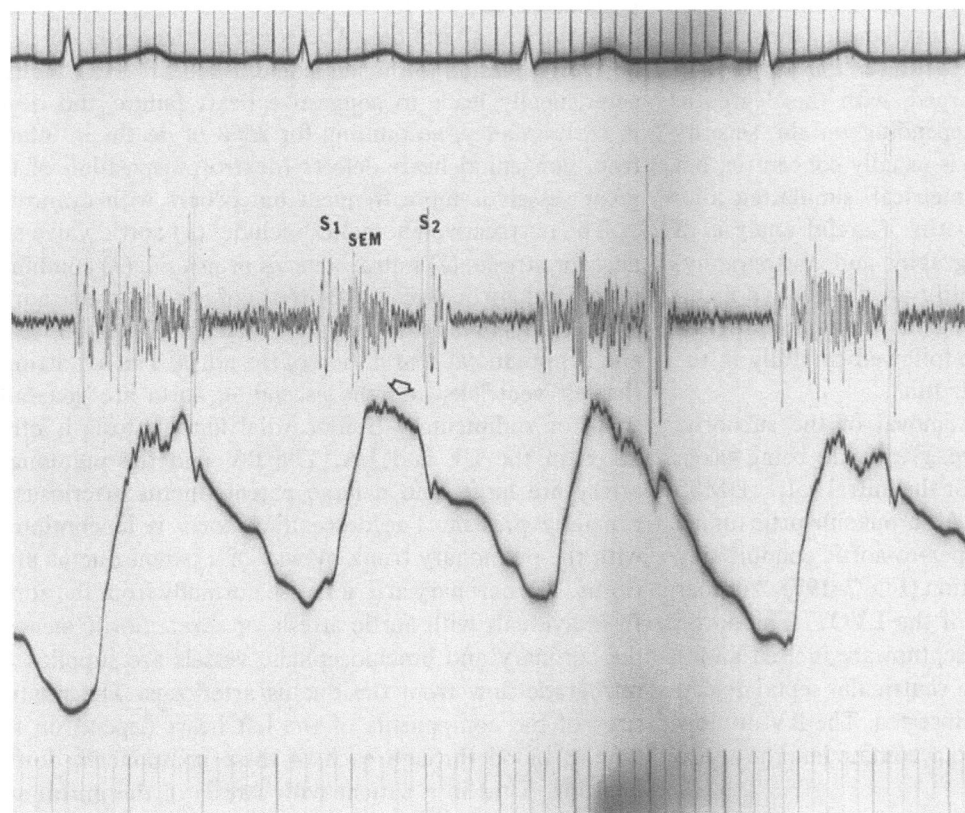

E

creased velocity associated with subaortic stenosis will extend into the aorta so that stenosis of the aortic valve may not be detected by Doppler in the presence of DMSS. Aortic insufficiency is an important associated finding if present and may be detected by Doppler echocardiography in patients without the characteristic diastolic decrescendo murmur.

On roentgenograms of the chest in a patient with a murmur of aortic stenosis, absence of dilatation of the ascending aorta (see Fig. 7–197A) suggests subaortic stenosis rather than valvar aortic stenosis. If the aortic root is dilated in a patient with isolated DMSS the roentgenogram of the chest will not help to distinguish valvar aortic stenosis from DMSS.

At cardiac catheterization a pressure gradient is detected between the LV and the aorta. In some instances, careful withdrawal of the catheter may localize the pressure gradient just below the aortic valve. In many individuals, however, the membrane is close to the valve, and the pressure gradient may falsely appear to be at the aortic valve. On left ventriculography DMSS appears as a thin radiolucent line (Fig. 7–196), as a polypoid filling defect or as diffuse narrowing of the outflow tract. In some instances, DMSS is delineated on the standard frontal and lateral or in the LAO and RAO views. If DMSS is suspected but not visible in these standard projections, a LAO view with cranial angulation will usually demonstrate the membrane (Fig. 7–196C). In the presence of aortic insufficiency the regurgitant stream may outline the obstructing lesion during aortography. The LV may be enlarged, with the degree of hypertrophy of this chamber depending on the severity of the obstruction. Hypertrophy is usually concentric, but in severe cases it may be asymmetrical, simulating idiopathic hypertrophic cardiomyopathy. Careful analysis of the angiograms (left ventriculography and aortography) usually will be sufficient to identify an obstructive membrane. Cases with small gradients may tend to progress in severity, and patients must be followed carefully in the event surgery is needed at a later time.

Surgical treatment involves removal of the subaortic membrane or fibrous excrescence, great care being taken not to damage the bundle of His or the mitral valve. DMSS may recur after surgical removal. A fibrous subaortic tunnel is difficult to repair, and an LV apex-to-aortic conduit may be required to bypass the obstruction (Fig. 7–197). Another method involves reconstruction of the LVOT. The aortic valve and subaortic ventricular septum are incised and a patch placed to close the resulting ventricular septal defect, while a prosthetic aortic valve is inserted. The RV outflow tract is then widened by a patch to accommodate the aortic valve that encroaches into it.

Shone Syndrome

This syndrome is a developmental complex consisting of multiple defects producing obstruction of the left heart.

The four defects that coexist frequently are coarctation of the aorta (Fig. 7–196), discrete membranous or fibromuscular subaortic stenosis, parachute deformity of the mitral valve and supravalvular ring of the LA. In parachute mitral valve the chordae tendineae converge on a single papillary muscle. The leaflets resemble the canopy of a parachute, the chordae, its shrouds or strings and the papillary muscle, the harness. The chordae are often thick and short with small interchordal spaces causing reduced mobility of the valve and obstruction to blood flow from the LA to the LV. LV inflow obstruction (mitral stenosis) can also be produced by two papillary muscles being close together or fused so that the chordae converge as in parachute mitral valve. The supravalvular ring of the LA is a circumferential ridge of connective tissue protruding into the inlet of the mitral valve at the base of the atrial surfaces of the mitral leaflets. On occasion a supravalvular ring of the LA is obstructive.

Hypoplastic Left Heart Syndrome

Hypoplastic left heart syndrome (HLHS) is the second most frequent defect of the heart reported in the first week of life (Fyler) and is the most common cause of cardiac failure in the first week of life (Lambert et al.). It encompasses several pathological entities related by their pathophysiological alterations. The common denominator is an obstructive lesion to the left side of the heart. HLHS characteristically leads to congestive heart failure and death in early infancy, accounting for 25% of deaths in infants from congenital heart defects (dextrotransposition of the great vessels is more frequent but occurs with cyanosis).

The obstructive anomalies include: (1) aortic valve stenosis or atresia, (2) mitral stenosis or atresia, (3) combined mitral and aortic atresia, (4) atresia of the transverse aortic arch, (5) hypoplasia of the aortic arch (tubular hypoplasia) and (6) preductal coarctation of the aorta. The left atrium, the left ventricle, and the ascending aorta are generally small or rudimentary. Endocardial fibroelastosis is often noted in the LV and LA. The RV and the pulmonary artery are large, and a large patent ductus arteriosus is generally present. The descending aorta is in continuity with the pulmonary trunk by way of a patent ductus arteriosus. The coronary arteries arise normally from the aorta. In individuals with aortic atresia or severe aortic stenosis the coronary and brachiocephalic vessels are supplied by retrograde flow from the ductus arteriosus. The relative sizes of the components of the left heart depend on the flow of blood through each of these components during fetal life. Thus in a patient with atresia of the mitral and aortic valves the LV will be vestigial. Conversely, with mitral atresia, a ventricular septal defect and a patent aortic valve, the LV may be of significant size. The LA is almost always small. If the mitral valve is atretic and no interatrial communication is present an alternate route for pulmonary venous flow may be present. These routes include anoma-

Fig. 7–196. *Left ventriculography in a 4-year-old girl with discrete membranous sub-aortic stenosis.* The membrane is approximately 1 mm below the aortic valve. **A** On the frontal view the membrane (*open arrows*) forms two indentations in the left ventricular outflow tract. **B** On the lateral view the attachment of the membrane to the ventricular septum is visualized (*open arrow*). **C** On the LAO view with cranial tilt (four-chamber view) the membrane extends across the left ventricular outflow tract (*arrows*). The aortic valve is thickened. The left ventricle is hypertrophied, and only a single large posterior papillary muscle (*m*) is identified. The anterior papillary muscle is absent. The identification of a single papillary muscle is consistent with a parachute mitral valve. Other significant findings are coarctation of the aorta and a hypoplastic aortic arch. The combination of coarctation of the aorta, discrete membranous subaortic stenosis and single papillary muscle (parachute mitral valve) constitutes the Shone syndrome.

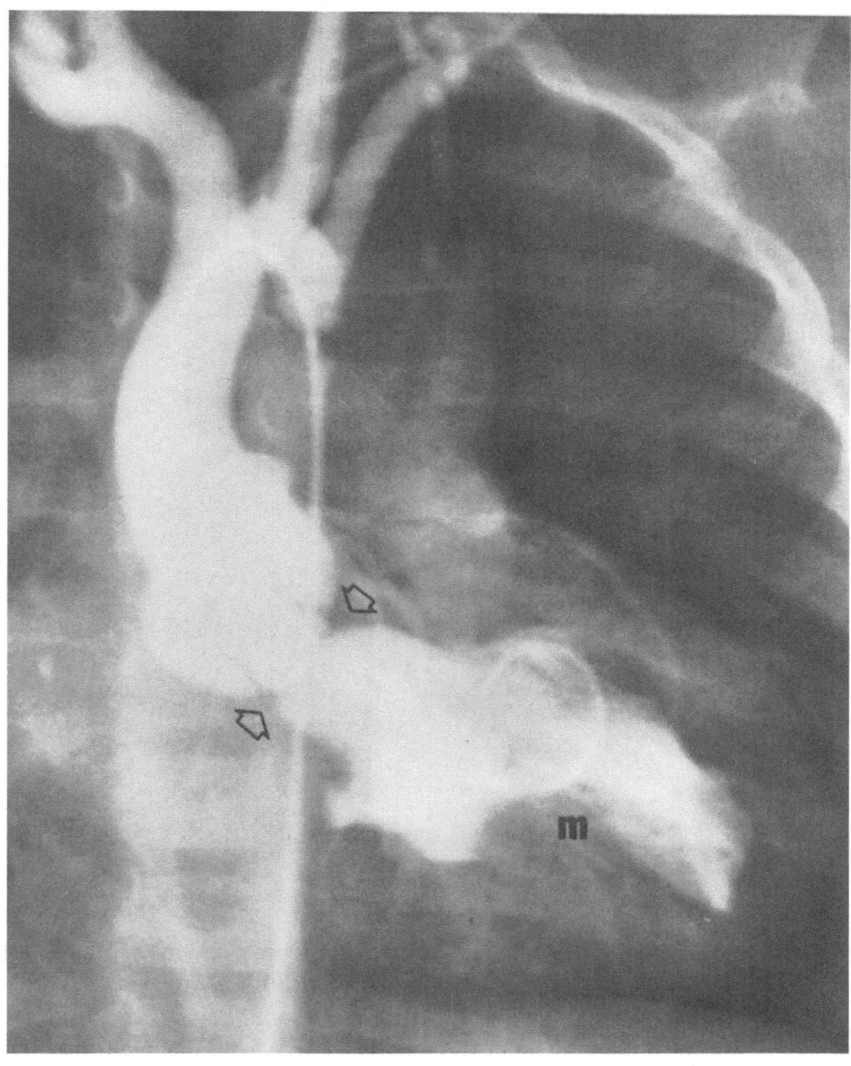

A

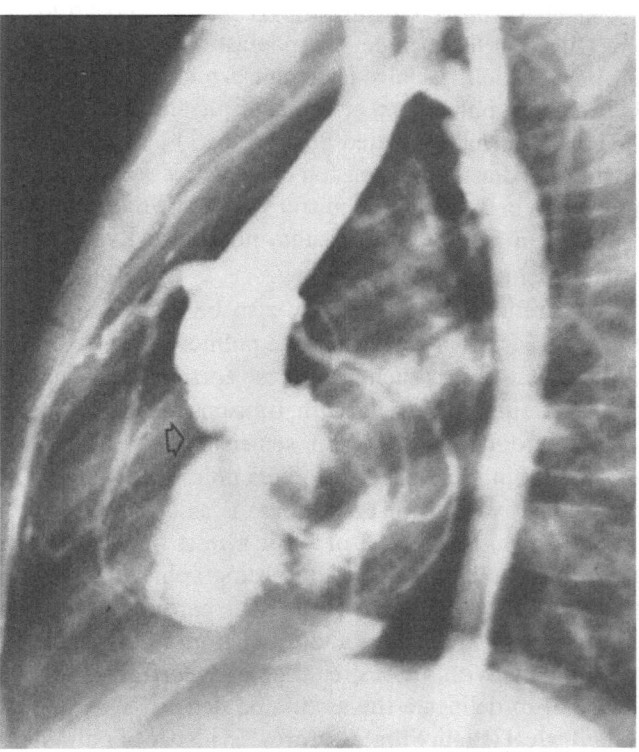

B

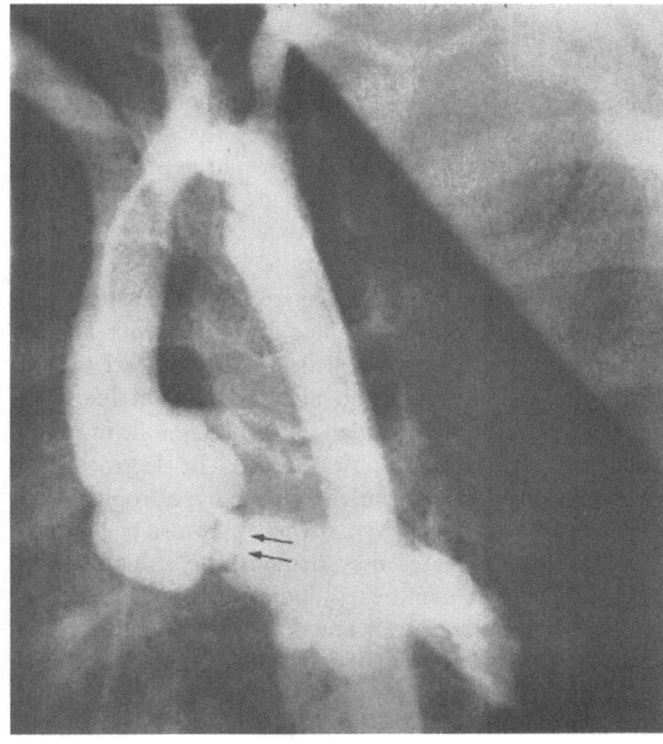

C

Fig. 7–197. *A roentgenogram of the chest and left ventriculogram in an 8-year-old boy after apicoaortic conduit for fibrous subaortic tunnel.* **A** and **B** Frontal and lateral films of the chest; **C** and **D** frontal (systole) and lateral (diastole) frames of the left ventriculogram. In **A** the heart is enlarged with prominence of the left ventricle and mild left atrial enlargement. The ascending aorta is not dilated. A dense tubular area in the left hemithorax represents the conduit connecting the apex of the heart to the descending aorta. The ring represents the site of the porcine valve. In the lateral film (**B**) the conduit is not well delineated. The prosthetic valve ring is posterior. **C** and **D** The left ventriculogram outlines the course and sites of anastomosis of the conduit.

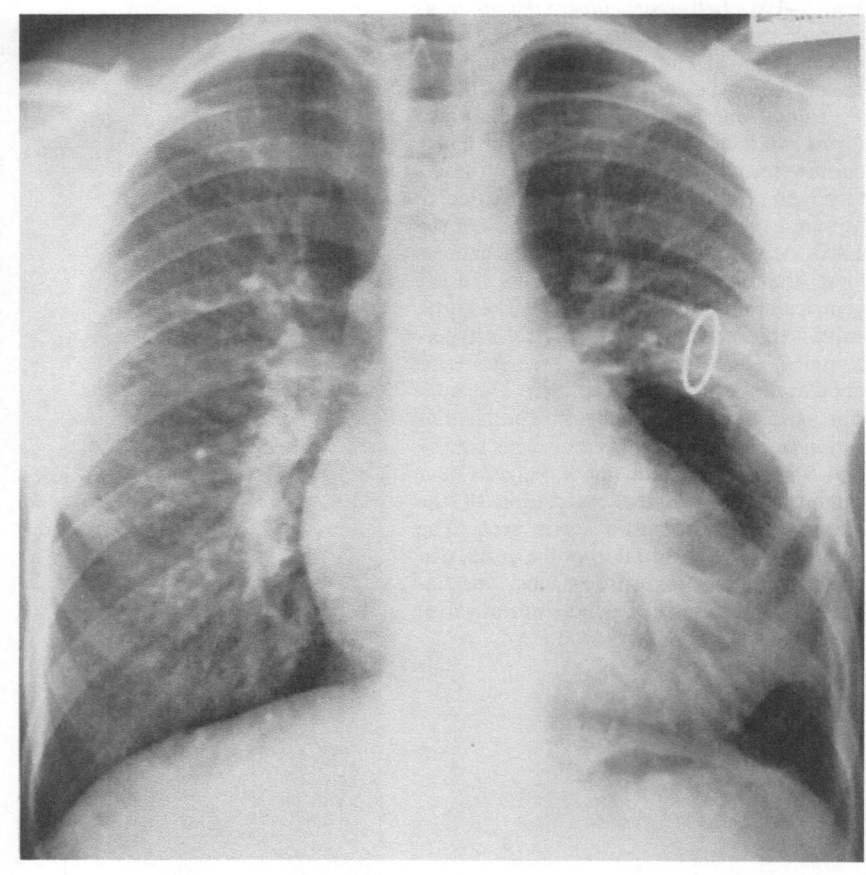

A

lous pulmonary venous drainage, a vertical vein from the LA to the left innominate vein, a channel connecting a pulmonary and a systemic vein and a fenestration of the coronary sinus into the LA, permitting blood to flow from the LA through the coronary sinus into the RA.

Premature closure of the foramen ovale, with consequent absence of the physiological right-to-left fetal shunt, has been postulated as the pathogenetic mechanism of this syndrome. It is also believed that this syndrome results from a large ductus arteriosus that reduces the flow of blood to the LV and ascending aorta. It would appear that impaired growth of the left side of the heart might result from any abnormality tending to reduce flow to or through this side of the heart during early fetal life.

Clinical Features Males are affected more frequently than females in a ratio of 3:2. Almost all infants with HLHS develop cyanosis, tachypnea and congestive heart failure during the first few hours to first few days of life. The peripheral pulses are weak or absent, and a systolic murmur usually is heard at the left sternal border. The electrocardiogram shows right axis deviation and RV hypertrophy, with decreased LV forces. RA hypertrophy may also be present. Analysis of blood gases may demonstrate a higher pO_2 in the right arm than in the left, indicating that the ascending aorta is perfused in an antegrade direction from the LV while the aortic arch is perfused by the RV via the ductus. Profound metabolic acidosis is common.

Echocardiography Echocardiography is extremely helpful in distinguishing the hypoplastic left heart syndrome from defects such as critical aortic stenosis, severe coarctation of the aorta, myocarditis and cardiomyopathy. These last named may have similar clinical presentation but can be salvaged by conventional medical or surgical treatment.

The characteristic features of HLHS on echocardiography (Fig. 7–198) include a hypoplastic aortic root in its normal location (usually less than 5 mm in diameter), a dilated main pulmonary artery anterior and to the left of the aorta (normally related great arteries) and a large RV cavity. The diastolic dimension of the LV is small, measuring 10 mm or less, and the mitral valve shows an excursion of less than 5 mm. On occasion, no LV cavity or mitral valve is demonstrated.

An atretic aortic valve may also be recognized in an abnormal location, anterior to the pulmonary valve or side by side with it. In such instances, aortic atresia may be part of a single ventricle with transposition of the great vessels or double-outlet right ventricle. Two A-V valves are present in these affected infants unless A-V communis or atresia of one of the A-V valves is associated.

Until recently, all cases of aortic atresia were considered uniformly fatal, and the echocardiographic diagnosis of aortic atresia eliminated the need for cardiac catheterization. Now that palliation and correction are available for some infants with HLHS, cardiac catheterization may be indicated to delineate the associated defects.

Radiological (Plain Film) Features Evidence of pulmonary

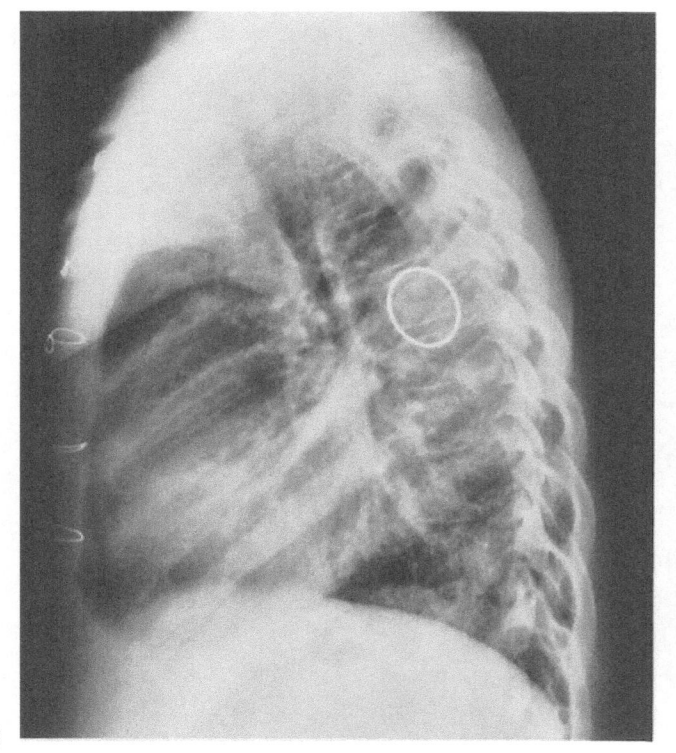

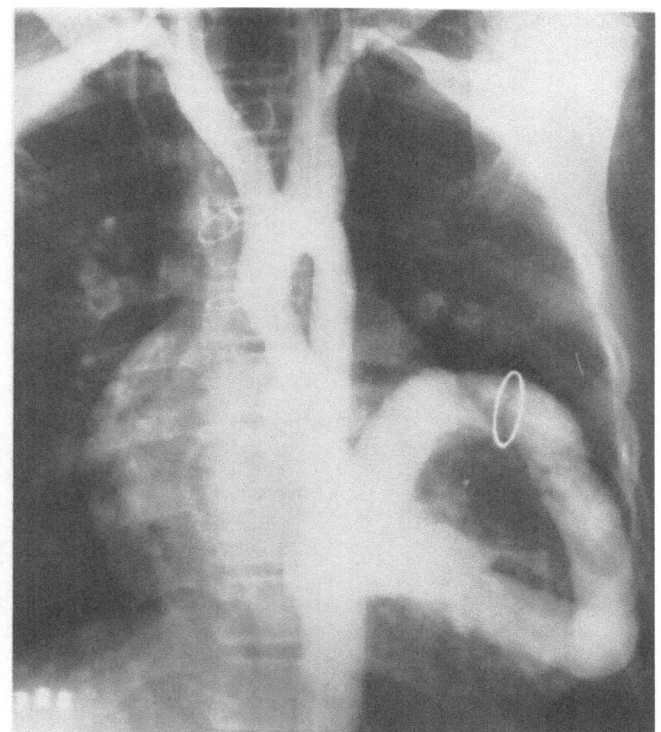

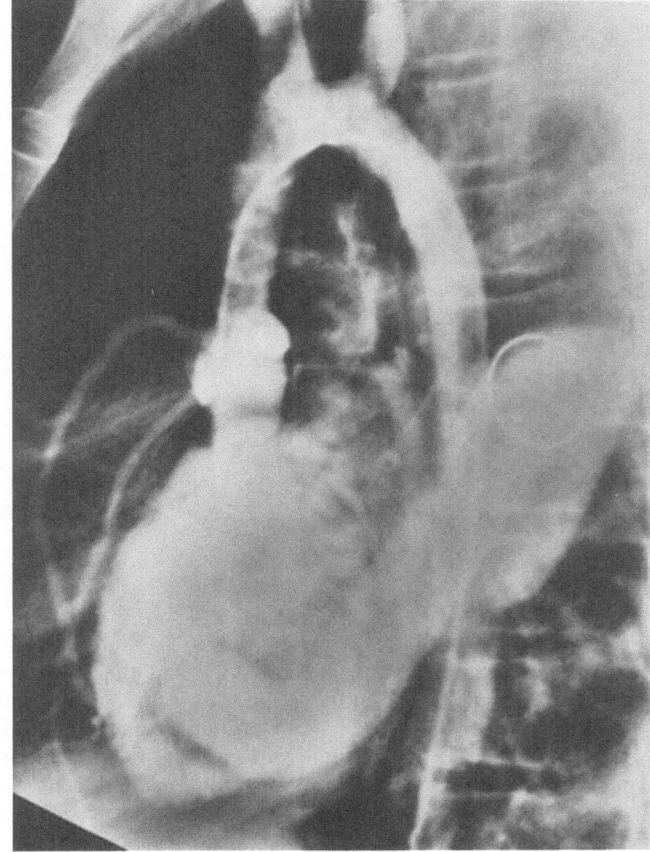

B

C

D

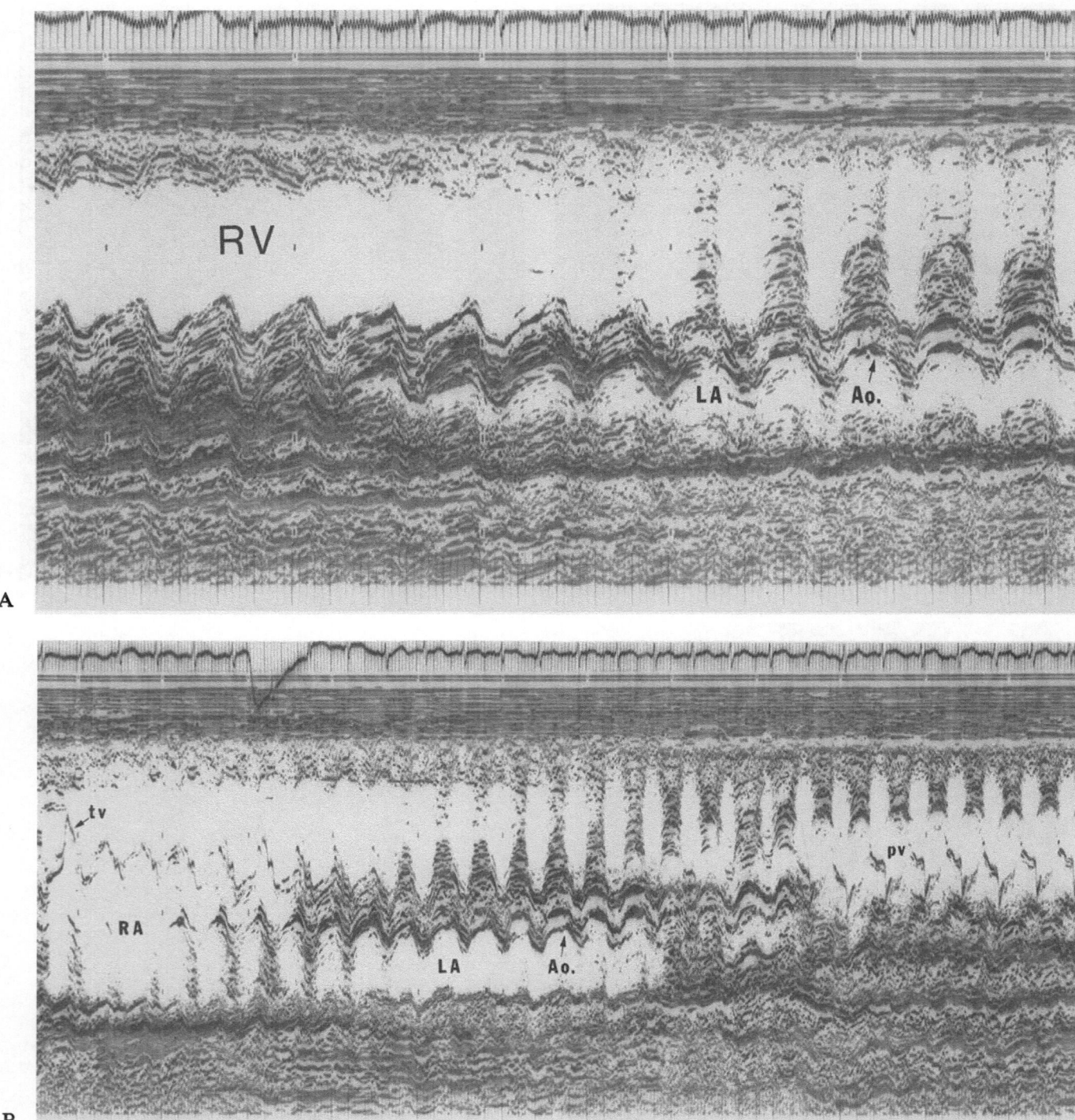

Fig. 7–198. *M-mode echocardiograms in hypoplastic left heart syndrome.* **A** Arc scan from the right ventricle to the hypoplastic aorta; **B** arc scan from the tricuspid valve to the pulmonary valve in the same patient; **C** right and left ventricle in another patient. **A** shows no left ventricular cavity posterior to the right ventricle. The right ventricle (*RV*) is dilated. The hypoplastic aorta (*Ao.*) is in its normal position. *LA* = left atrium. In **B** the operator has noted that the tricuspid valve (*tv*) is inferior and to the right of the aortic root (*Ao.*), and the pulmonary valve (*pv*) is superior and to the left of the aortic root (normally related great arteries). *RA* = right atrium; *LA* = left atrium. In **C** the left ventricular diastolic dimension (*LVDD*) is 4 mm, and the mitral valve excursion is less than 5 mm, both consistent with a hypoplastic left ventricle. *RV* = right ventricle; *LVPW* = posterior wall of left ventricle. The 10 mm marks are indicated. (*Continued*)

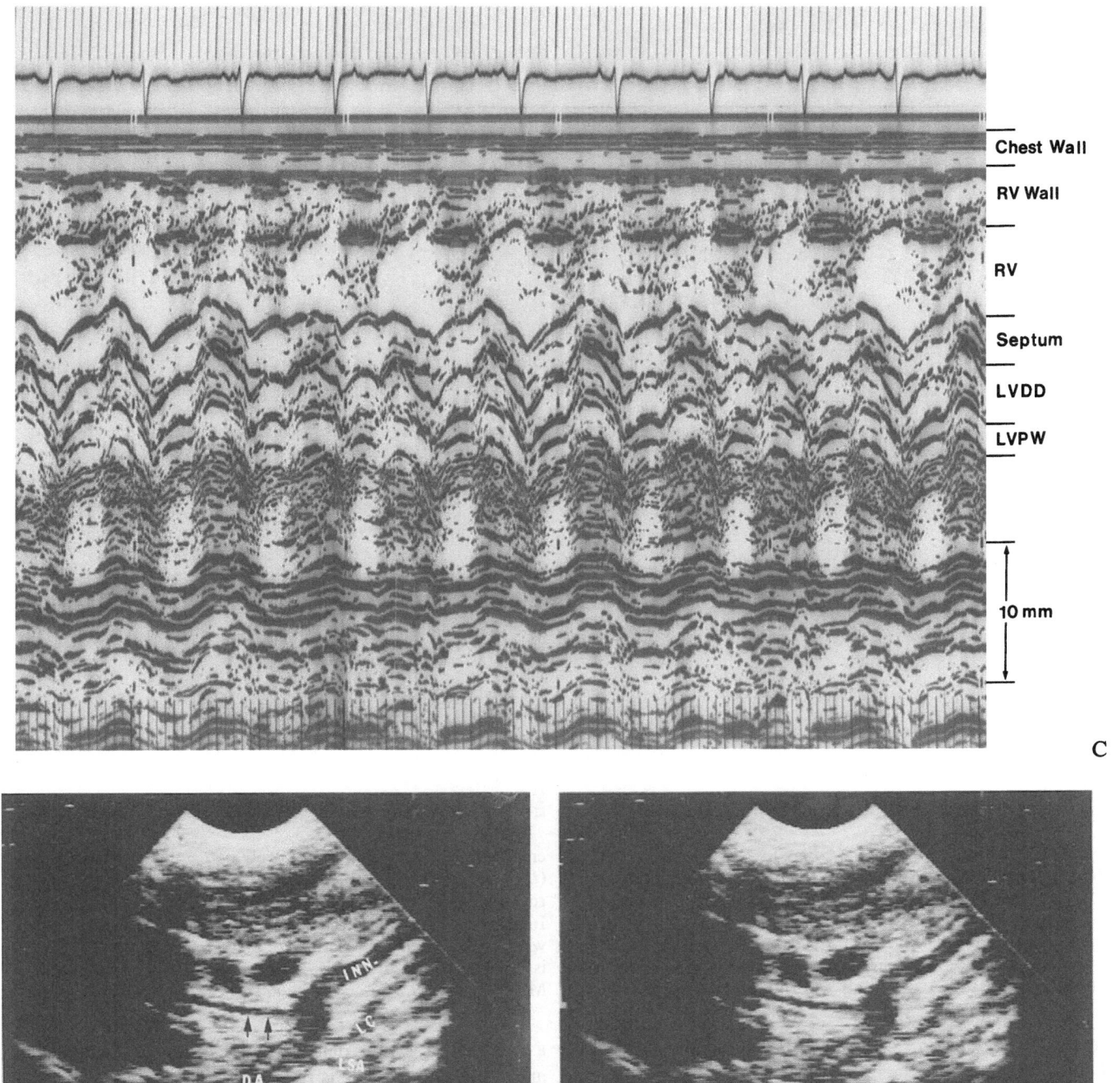

Chest Wall

RV Wall

RV

Septum

LVDD

LVPW

10 mm

C

D

D'

Fig. 7–198 *(Cont.)*. *Two-dimensional echocardiogram in a 2-day-old baby with hypoplastic left heart syndrome (HLHS).* In **D** and **D'**, a parasternal long axis view, the hypoplastic ascending aorta *(arrows)* is in continuity with the aortic arch, which has a greater caliber. The innominate artery (INN.) is the first branch of the aorta. The left common carotid artery *(LC)* and the left subclavian artery *(LSA)* are also present in this plane. The descending aorta *(DA)* continues inferiorly. *(Continued)*

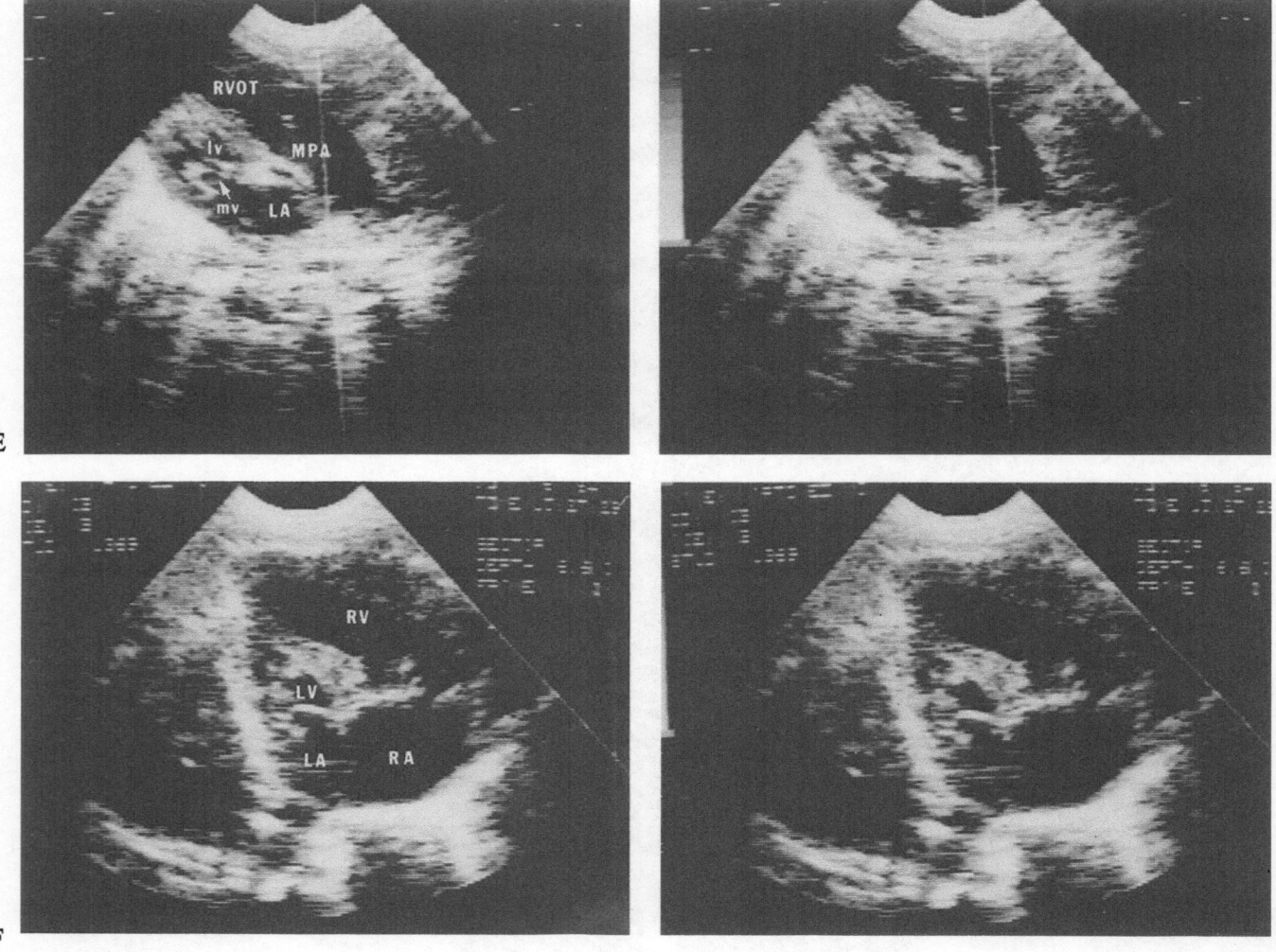

Fig. 7–198 (*Cont.*). In **E** and **E′**, a parasternal long axis view, the right ventricular outflow tract (*RVOT*) and the hypoplastic left ventricle (*lv*) are visualized. The narrow lumen of the ascending aorta is delineated between the main pulmonary artery (*MPA*) and the left atrium (*LA*) as it arises from the left ventricle. *mv* = mitral valve. **F** and **F′** are from an apex four-chamber view. The left ventricle (*LV*) is small and the right ventricle (*RV*) is enlarged. The atrial septum is barely perceptible. The left atrium (*LA*) is small. (Note: the right-left orientation of this image is reversed compared to other four-chamber views in this book.) In some patients with HLHS the left ventricle is atretic. In patients with no LV cavity the finding of a hypoplastic ascending aorta is the key to the diagnosis. (**D-F** courtesy of Henry Issenberg, M.D., Bronx, N.Y.)

venous hypertension constitutes the usual pattern (Figs. 7–199, 7–200), but associated increased pulmonary vascularity (pulmonary overcirculation) also may be present. The heart usually is moderately to markedly enlarged. The combination of cardiomegaly, marked dilatation of the pulmonary artery and a pattern of congestive heart failure is characteristic of the hypoplastic left heart syndrome.

These characteristic findings should be distinguished from those in sick infants with total anomalous pulmonary venous return with obstruction and from those in infants with cor triatriatum in whom the heart tends to be normal in size. The respiratory distress syndrome may closely simulate any of the entities just named. The heart in these infants is mildly to moderately enlarged with a ground-glass appearance of the lungs. The clinical features together with the findings on echocardiography are essential in distinguishing these entities from each other.

Hemodynamics This description refers to HLHS without a ventricular septal defect. The LA and LV are small, and the foramen ovale is restrictive, preventing exit of pulmonary venous blood from the LA. The only source of systemic blood flow is the ductus arteriosus. Prior to cardiac catheterization of a patient with HLHS an infusion of prostaglandin E_1 is begun in order to prevent closure of the ductus arteriosus so that systemic blood flow is maintained. At the time of cardiac catheterization a left-to-right shunt (oxygen step-up) is encountered in the RA, which allows mixing of the two venous streams in the RA (venous admixture). Oxygen saturation is equal in the RV, pulmonary artery, and aorta. Pressure in the RV, pulmonary artery, and aorta are also identical. If the LA can be entered via the foramen ovale the pressure in that chamber will be found to be elevated. Systemic and pulmonary blood flow are determined by the relative resistances of the two circuits.

Contrast Studies In classic hypoplastic left heart syndrome

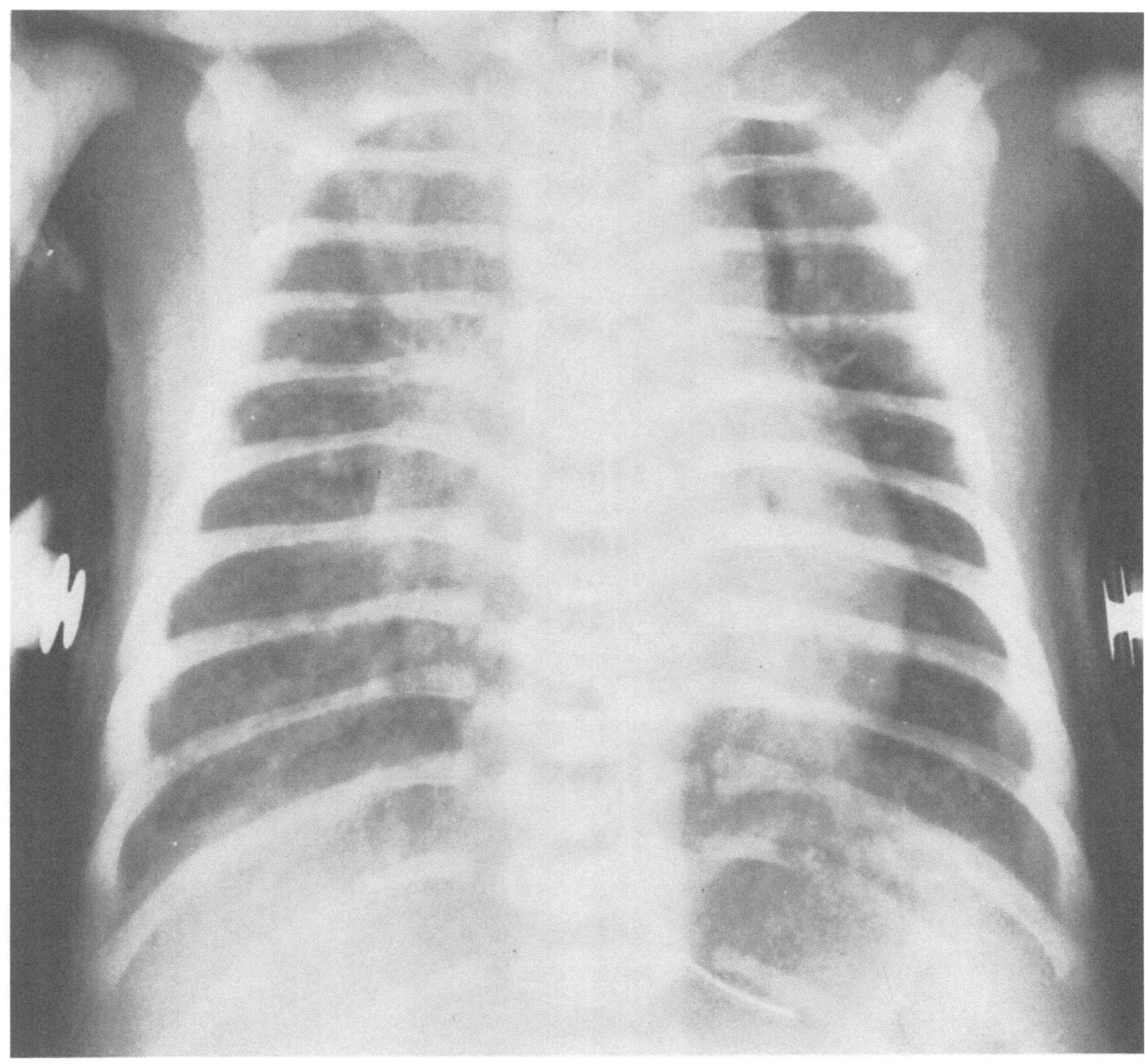

A

Fig. 7–199. *Plain film and angiocardiographic studies in a 5-day-old boy with hypoplastic left heart syndrome.* In **A** mild to moderate cardiomegaly is present. The configuration of the heart is not characteristic. The right atrium and right ventricle are enlarged. Widening of the mediastinum might be mistakenly interpreted as total anomalous pulmonary venous return of the supracardiac type. The left-sided widening of the mediastinum is due to dilatation of the main pulmonary artery, whereas the widening on the right is probably due to enlargement of the superior vena cava. The pulmonary arteries are tortuous and are observed on end (*dotted appearance*). This pattern often occurs with pulmonary venous hypertension, with or without pulmonary overcirculation. (*Continued*)

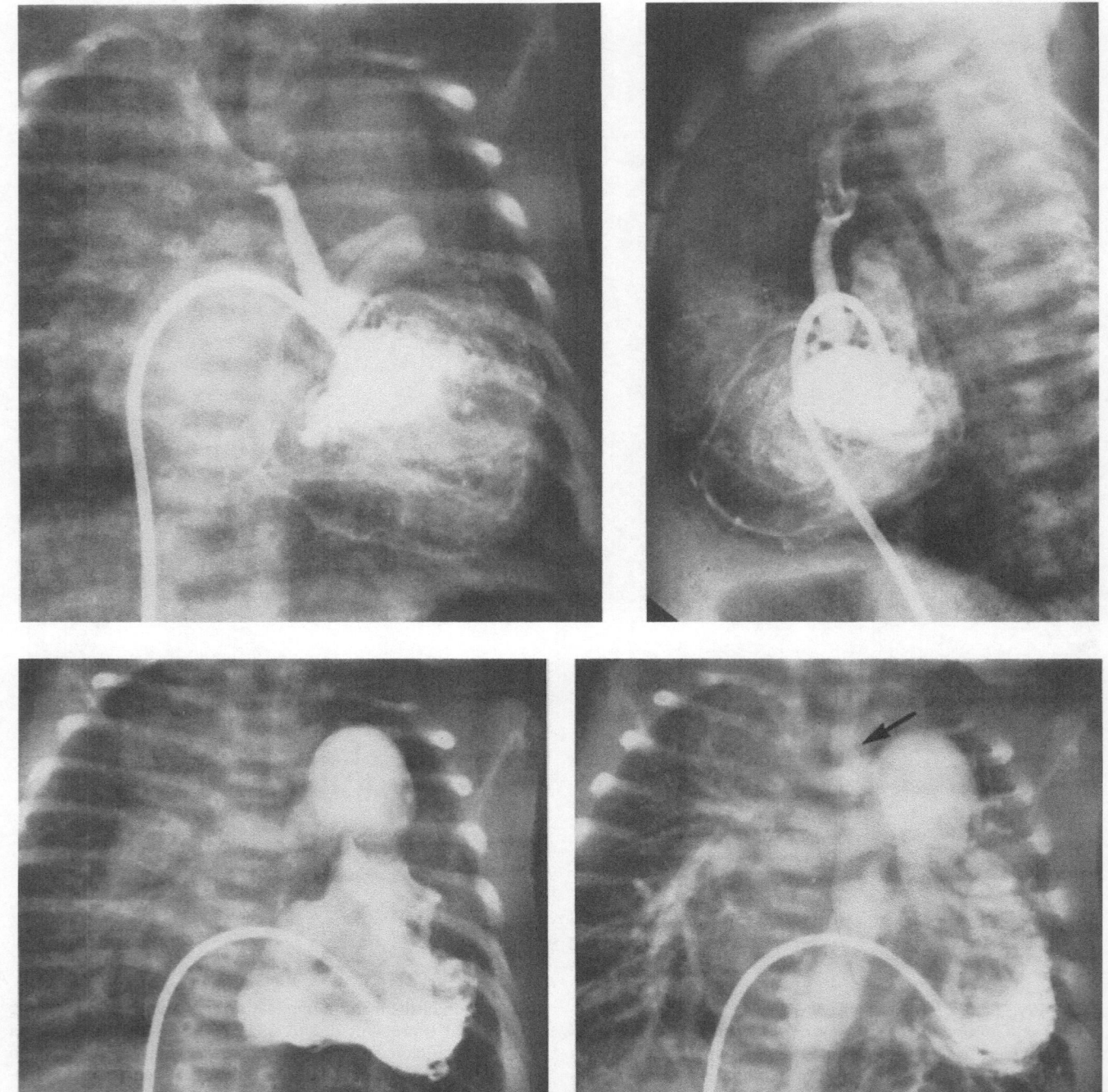

B

C

D

E

Fig. 7–199 (*Cont.*). In **B** and **C** the venous catheter reaches the left ventricle from the right atrium across the atrial septum, left atrium, and mitral valve. The left ventriculogram demonstrates a hypoplastic left ventricle with a very thick wall. Small collections of contrast medium surrounding the cavity of the left ventricle represent myocardial sinusoids. The ascending aorta is diffusely narrowed (tubular hypoplasia). The sinuses of Valsalva are small but well formed, and the coronary arteries arise normally. The arch and brachiocephalic vessels do not fill from the left ventricle,

but are opacified retrogradely from the ductus arteriosus. **D** and **E** are frames from the right ventriculogram. The venous catheter was withdrawn to the right atrium and then advanced across the tricuspid valve to the right ventricle. The right ventricle and pulmonary artery are dilated, with the pulmonary artery projecting almost to the apex of the left hemithorax. In **E**, a later frame, the brachiocephalic vessels (*arrow*) and the descending aorta fill from the main pulmonary artery via the ductus arteriosus.

Fig. 7–200. *Roentgenogram of the chest in a neonate with hypoplastic left heart syndrome.* The heart is mildly to moderately enlarged. Pulmonary edema is present, producing an appearance similar to the ground-glass appearance occurring with idiopathic respiratory distress syndrome.

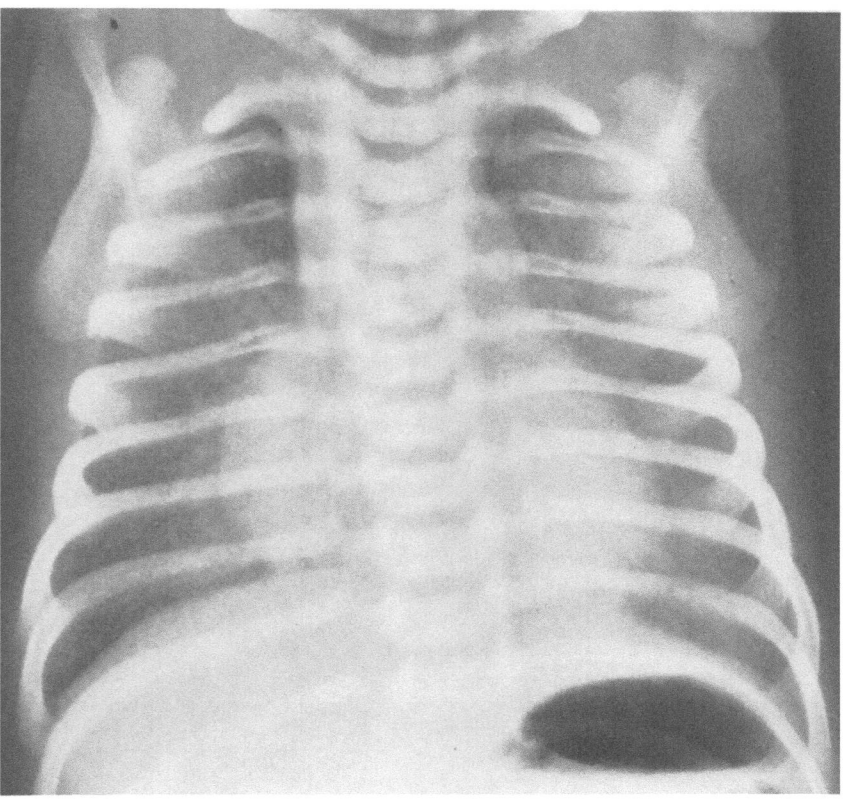

with atresia of the aortic valve, atresia of the mitral valve and a vestigial LV, injection of contrast medium into the large RV will demonstrate a massively dilated pulmonary trunk that fills dilated pulmonary branches and is connected to the descending aorta by way of a ductus arteriosus. When the ductus is fully open and maintains the same diameter as the descending aorta, an erroneous diagnosis of truncus arteriosus may be entertained, although in HLHS the coronary arteries do not arise above the pulmonary valve. (In truncus arteriosus the coronary arteries, pulmonary arteries, brachiocephalic vessels and descending aorta all arise from the truncus.) In HLHS, retrograde flow fills the aortic arch and the brachiocephalic vessels (Fig. 7–199D and E). The ascending aorta also fills in a retrograde direction with blood ending in the coronary vessels. The pulmonary branches are dilated, but the peripheral pulmonary vessels are constricted, secondary to increased arteriolar resistance. The pulmonary veins drain normally into a small LA. Pulmonary venous blood then crosses an atrial septal defect or stretched foramen ovale into a dilated RA, finally recirculating through the lungs. Injection into the LV will reveal a diminutive chamber with thick walls and numerous myocardial sinusoids (Fig. 7–199B and C).

Important variations include mitral atresia with ventricular septal defect, in which the LV fills from the RV, resulting in a LV of significant size. The aorta fills from the LV, and the size of the aorta is variable. A patent ductus arteriosus fills the brachiocephalic vessels in varying

degrees, depending on the volume of antegrade flow through the aortic valve.

In some patients, severe coarctation of the aorta (Fig. 7–201) or interrupted arch is part of the complex of HLHS. In interrupted arch the ductus does not fill the ascending aorta, and injection into the LA or LV may be necessary to assess the size of the ascending aorta.

Treatment Infants with this group of defects, left untreated, as a general rule do not survive beyond infancy, death usually occurring within a few days. Medical palliation with prostaglandin E_1 maintains patency of the ductus. At the same time, treatment of acidosis and congestive heart failure may allow time for diagnostic studies and surgical palliation. Surgical approaches involve anastomosis of the RV to the aorta, using a tubular prosthesis between the pulmonary artery and the aortic arch or between a ventriculotomy incision and the descending aorta. The pulmonary branches or the main pulmonary artery are banded, and the atrial septal defect is enlarged, if necessary, thus producing a univentricular heart.

Norwood et al. achieve a similar result by another procedure. The main pulmonary artery is transected and the distal vessel oversewn. The ascending aorta is anastomosed to the proximal portion of the main pulmonary artery. The ductus arteriosus is ligated, and the flow of blood into the lungs is reestablished by use of a shunt from the aorta to the distal portion of the pulmonary artery. The atrial septal defect is enlarged, if necessary. In the second stage of this procedure the pulmonary and systemic circula-

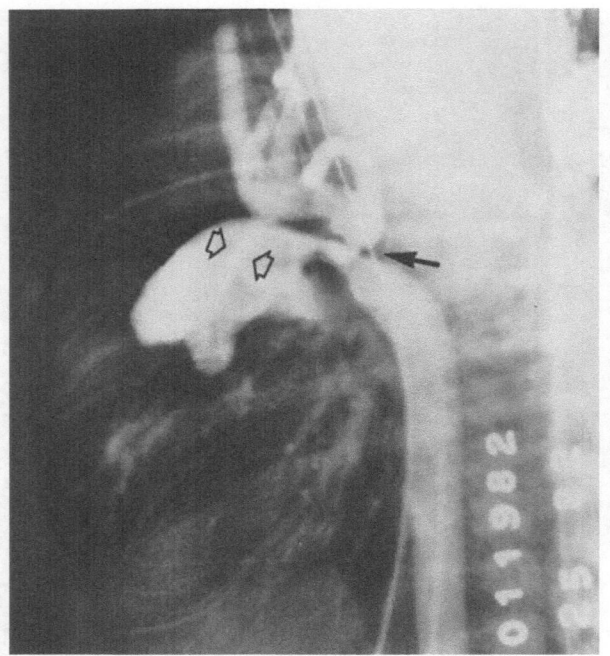

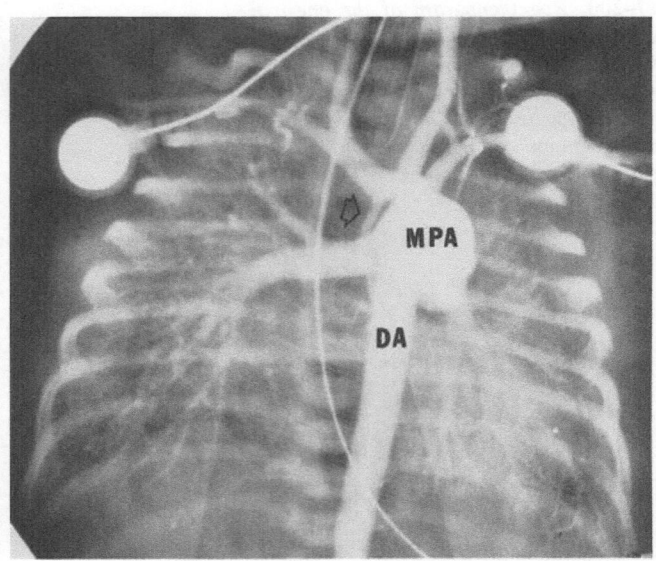

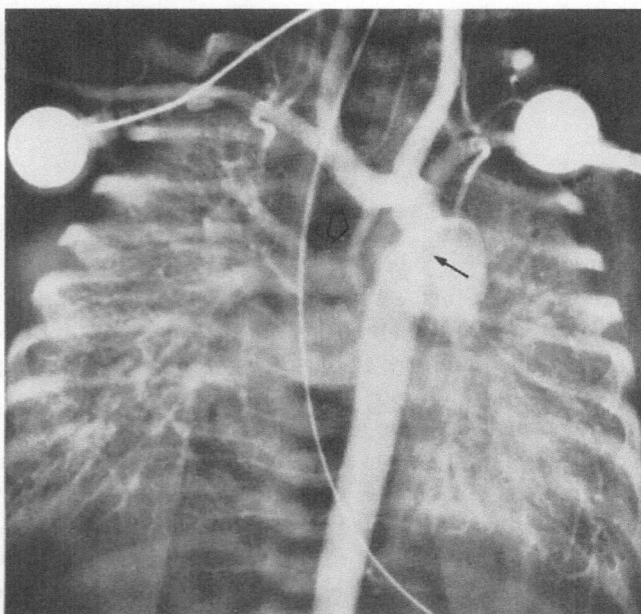

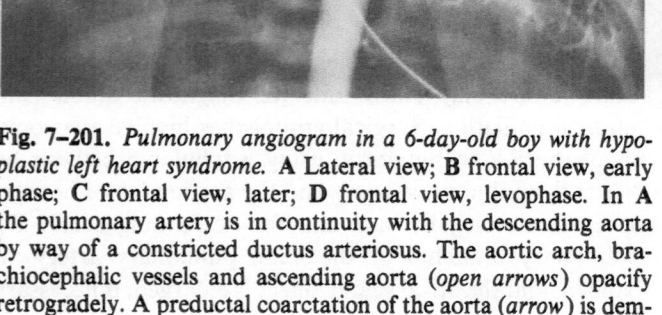

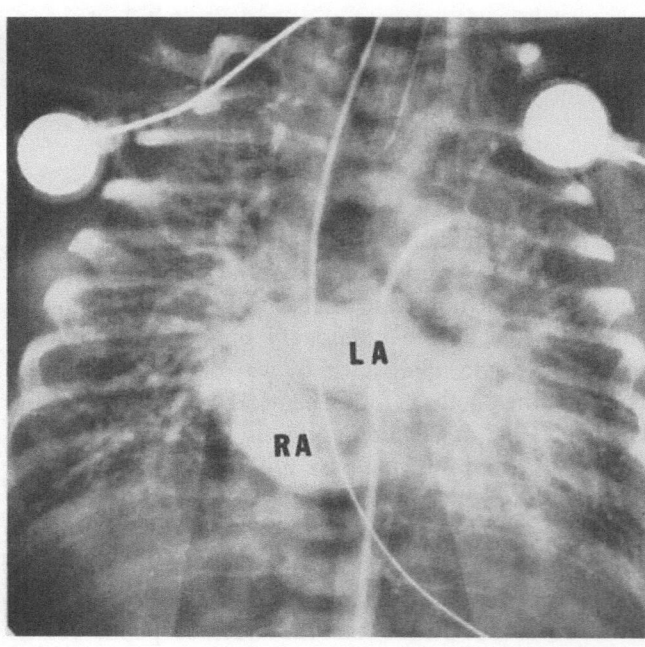

Fig. 7–201. *Pulmonary angiogram in a 6-day-old boy with hypoplastic left heart syndrome.* **A** Lateral view; **B** frontal view, early phase; **C** frontal view, later; **D** frontal view, levophase. In **A** the pulmonary artery is in continuity with the descending aorta by way of a constricted ductus arteriosus. The aortic arch, brachiocephalic vessels and ascending aorta (*open arrows*) opacify retrogradely. A preductal coarctation of the aorta (*arrow*) is demonstrated. In **B** and **C** the main pulmonary artery (*MPA*) fills the descending aorta (*DA*). Tubular hypoplasia of the ascending aorta is better appreciated (*open arrows*). The aortic arch is also smaller than normal. The coarctation is noted in **C** (*small arrow*). In **D** the left atrium (*LA*) is small, and the right atrium (*RA*) is opacified by way of a left-to-right shunt across the atrial septum.

tions are separated by closing the atrial septal defect and connecting the RA to the pulmonary arteries (Fontan procedure), as is accomplished with tricuspid atresia and some forms of single ventricle.

Congenital Mitral Stenosis

Congenital mitral stenosis (MS) may affect any or all of the components of the apparatus of the mitral valve (leaflets, chordae tendineae, papillary muscles, anulus and adjacent supravalvar and infravalvar regions). Congenital MS is a rare malformation, occurring in only 0.6% of autopsied patients with congenital heart disease and in 0.21%–0.42% of a general series. A male predilection, with a 2.2:1 ratio, has been noted.

Congenital MS includes a large variety of anomalies, such as hypoplasia of all components of the mitral valve without sclerosis, supravalvar mitral stenosis (supravalvar left atrial ring), accessory tissue of the mitral valve, congenital commissural mitral stenosis, short chordae tendineae, anomalous mitral arcade (direct insertion of leaflets onto papillary muscles), anomalous position of the papillary muscles and single papillary muscle (parachute mitral valve). Combinations of these occur frequently. The incidence of associated cardiovascular defects is high (in 74% of affected individuals) consisting of ventricular septal defect, patent ductus arteriosus, coarctation of the aorta and aortic stenosis. More infrequently tetralogy of Fallot, pulmonic stenosis and atrial septal defect may be observed. MS due to supravalvar left atrial ring and parachute mitral valve is also part of the Shone syndrome. The incidence of associated noncardiac anomalies is also high—37%. The most frequent are genitourinary tract abnormalities and cystic ovaries with accessory lobation of the lungs (Collins-Nakai et al.).

Clinical Features Symptoms appear early in life—before 1 month of age in about one third of the infants and before 1 year in about three fourths of the group. Dyspnea, cough, difficulty in feeding, frequent respiratory infections and failure to thrive are common. On examination, diastolic murmurs are frequently but not invariably present. A loud S_1, a loud P_2 and an opening snap are also heard on auscultation, but not in all patients. Many neonates have stigmata relative to the associated defects that obscure the findings of mitral stenosis (e.g., ventricular septal defect, patent ductus arteriosus, coarctation of the aorta, atrial level left-to-right shunt). The classic murmur-sound-snap complex is unusual. The electrocardiogram shows RV hypertrophy, right axis deviation and RA and LA enlargement. Associated cardiac anomalies alter this electrocardiographic pattern.

Echocardiography (Fig. 7–202A) The E-F slope (diastolic closure rate) of the anterior mitral leaflet is reduced (less than 25 mm per second in a term newborn infant). A diminished opening excursion (D-E) of the mitral valve suggests hypoplasia of this valve (deficient tissue of the leaflets or short chordae tendineae) or hypoplasia of the LV or both. Anterior motion of the posterior leaflet of the mitral valve during diastole suggests chordal fusion. A single papillary muscle of a parachute mitral valve may be observed on 2-D echocardiography. Additional echoes in the LA may be due to a supravalvular left atrial ring. The diameter of the LA is usually increased. Doppler echocardiography shows a flow disturbance and an increased velocity just inside the mitral valve.

Radiological (Plain Film) Features Pulmonary venous hypertension of varying degrees may be present but may be obscured by overcirculation in the presence of large left-to-right shunts or pneumonia. The size of the heart may be normal or considerably increased with right ventricular enlargement. The LA generally is enlarged. The radiological features are usually modified by the associated anomalies.

Hemodynamics At cardiac catheterization the hemodynamic features may be similar to those occurring with rheumatic mitral stenosis. Cardiac catheterization is useful in assessing the severity of the associated cardiac lesions.

Contrast Studies Left ventriculography delineates the apparatus of the mitral valve, the pathological features of the LV (Fig. 7–202B) and the associated malformations (e.g., ventricular septal defect, aortic stenosis, coarctation). Pulmonary or LA injections are useful in distinguishing congenital MS from other causes of pulmonary venous hypertension, especially cor triatriatum and supravalvular ring of the LA.

Treatment Medical treatment with diuretics and rest may be adequate for mild to moderate MS. Surgical intervention is indicated if the MS is severe or if a supravalvular left atrial ring is identified. Resection of a supravalvular ring, in which the operative mortality is low, usually results in relief of the obstruction. Surgical repair of a congenitally stenotic mitral valve, on the other hand, is accompanied by high mortality and often does not relieve the obstruction completely. Replacement of the mitral valve in infants also is associated with high operative mortality, as well as significant late morbidity. Thus it is important to differentiate stenosis of the mitral valve from supravalvular ring, since treatment of the two disorders differs.

Cor Triatriatum

This rare congenital anomaly is reported in 0.4% of autopsies in cases of congenital heart defects (Jegier et al). Most varieties of cor triatriatum can be explained as failure of incorporation of the common pulmonary vein into the back wall of the LA. The typical form consists of a posterior chamber (accessory chamber) that receives the pulmonary veins and communicates with the LA through a restrictive opening.

Variations of cor triatriatum include communication of the posterior chamber to the RA by way of an abnormal communication between the posterior chamber and the

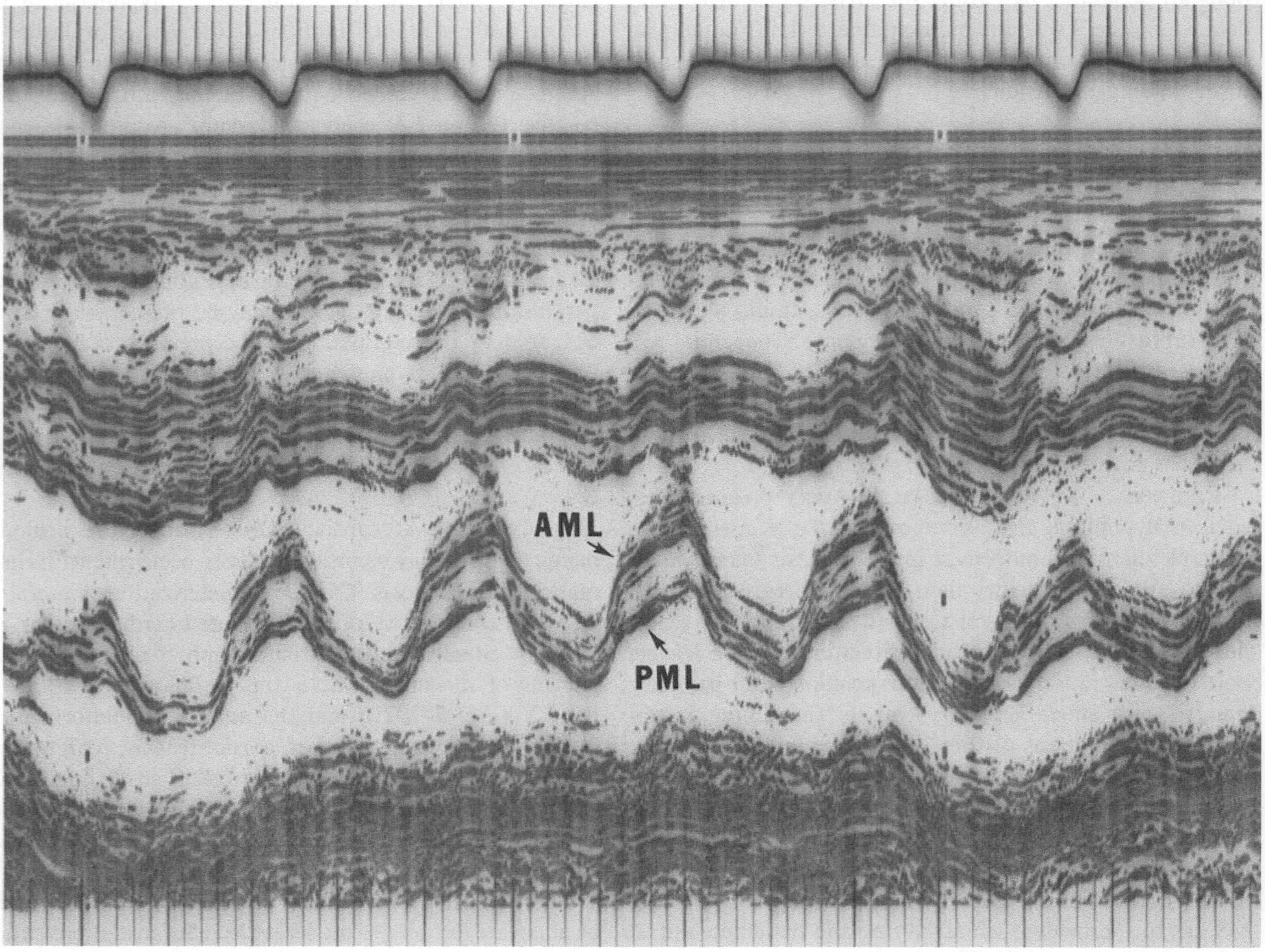

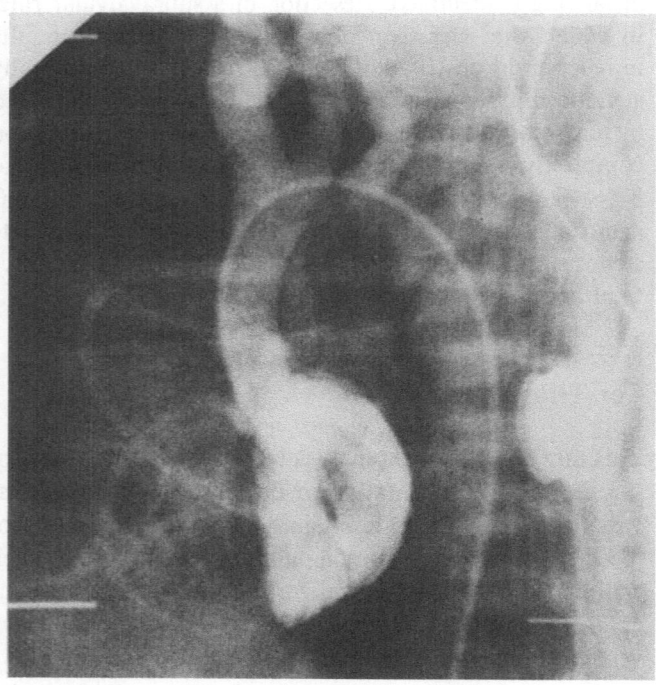

A

B

Fig. 7–202. A *M-mode echocardiogram through the mitral valve in a 2-day-old boy with congenital mitral stenosis.* The D to E excursion of the valve is mildly reduced, and the leaflets separate only minimally during diastole. **B** is a lateral view of the left ventriculogram during diastole. The left ventricle is of normal size and is markedly retrodisplaced by a dilated right ventricle. The ventricular contractions were poor. Only the interventricular septum and the posterolateral wall showed normal contractions. The orifice of the mitral valve appears as a narrow ovoid lucency when unopacified blood is entering the LV during diastole. At autopsy the mitral valve anulus was hypoplastic, but the leaflets were well formed and were not thickened. *AML* = anterior mitral leaflet; *PML* = posterior mitral leaflet.

RA, a vertical vein from the posterior chamber to the left innominate vein or a common pulmonary vein to the portal vein. On occasion, the posterior chamber receives only two pulmonary veins with the other pulmonary veins connecting normally to the LA or by way of anomalous connections to the RA (unilateral cor triatriatum). In other instances the posterior chamber may fail to communicate with the LA, resulting in the pulmonary venous blood returning entirely through anomalous venous connections or through an abnormal communication to the RA. An additional right-to-left shunt at the atrial level is obligatory for survival in patients with cor triatriatum. Cor triatriatum is usually not associated with other cardiac or noncardiac anomalies. In some adults the intraatrial membrane may calcify. Thrombus may form in the posterior chamber. Complex forms of cor triatriatum may demonstrate the physiological parameters of total anomalous pulmonary venous return. The usual form of cor triatriatum causes obstruction to pulmonary venous return, so that the physiological features are similar to those of mitral stenosis.

The age at presentation and the severity of symptoms are determined by the degree of pulmonary venous obstruction. Presentation may occur in childhood or adult life with dyspnea on exercise and a history of multiple pulmonary infections.

On physical examination a RV heave and a loud second sound are characteristic. The murmur may be a soft systolic ejection murmur, a diastolic flow rumble or even a continuous murmur.

On M-mode *echocardiography,* the intraatrial membrane appears as an extra echoreflective layer behind the mitral valve, which may on occasion move in a manner similar to a stenotic mitral valve. If obstruction is severe the RV will be dilated and signs of high pulmonary resistance will be present (e.g., abnormal RV systolic time intervals). An additional finding is a diastolic flutter of the mitral leaflets. Two-dimensional echocardiography may show the diaphragm separating the posterior from the anterior chamber. Transesophageal 2-D echocardiography has been determined to be more sensitive than transthoracic 2-D echocardiography (Schluter et al.).

The roentgenogram of the chest (Fig. 7–203A) shows pulmonary venous hypertension. The heart is often normal in size, or the pulmonary artery, RV, and RA may be enlarged. In contrast to mitral valve disease the LA is not enlarged in patients with cor triatriatum.

Other defects which must be considered in patients with pulmonary venous hypertension and normal heart size are total anomalous pulmonary venous return below the diaphragm (infants), congenital mitral stenosis, left atrial myxoma, supravalvar mitral stenosis, ball valve thrombus, and obstruction of the pulmonary veins by tumor, thrombus, membrane (web) or mediastinal fibrosis.

At *cardiac catheterization* in symptomatic patients, pres-

Fig. 7–203. *Radiological findings in a 17-month-old girl with cor triatriatum.*

The frontal film of the chest **(A)** shows severe pulmonary venous hypertension (pulmonary edema) without cardiomegaly. Any congenital obstruction to the left side of the heart may produce these features. The heart is normal in size, lending evidence to the diagnosis of congenital mitral stenosis, cor triatriatum, left atrial tumor or stenosis of the pulmonary veins. Total anomalous pulmonary venous drainage with obstruction (infradiaphragmatic) may present this appearance but is unlikely at this age. (*Continued*)

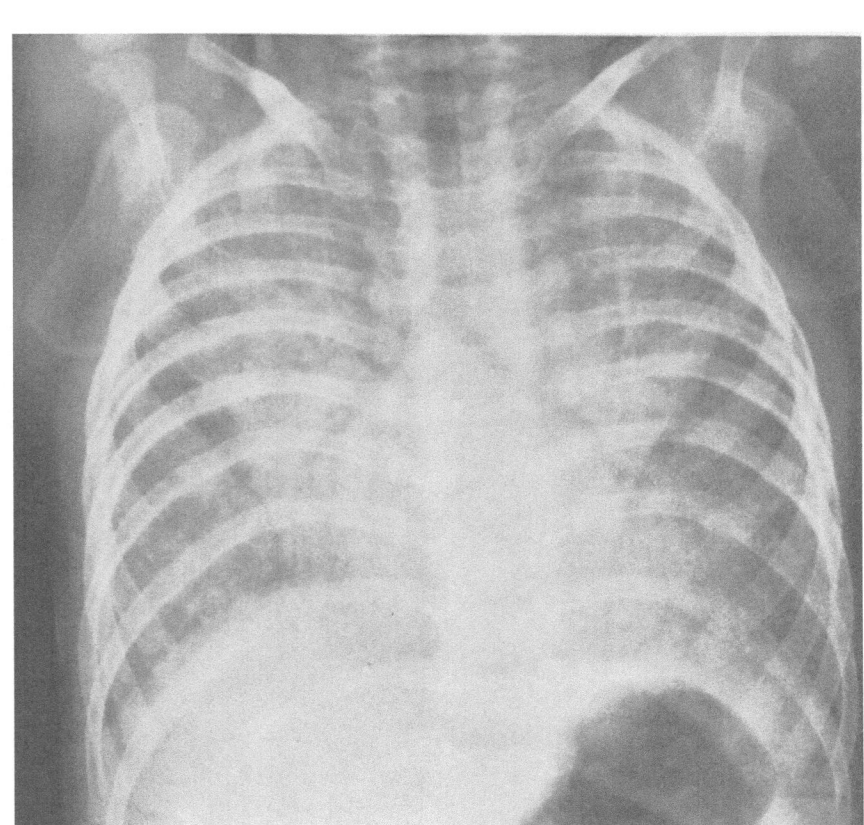

A

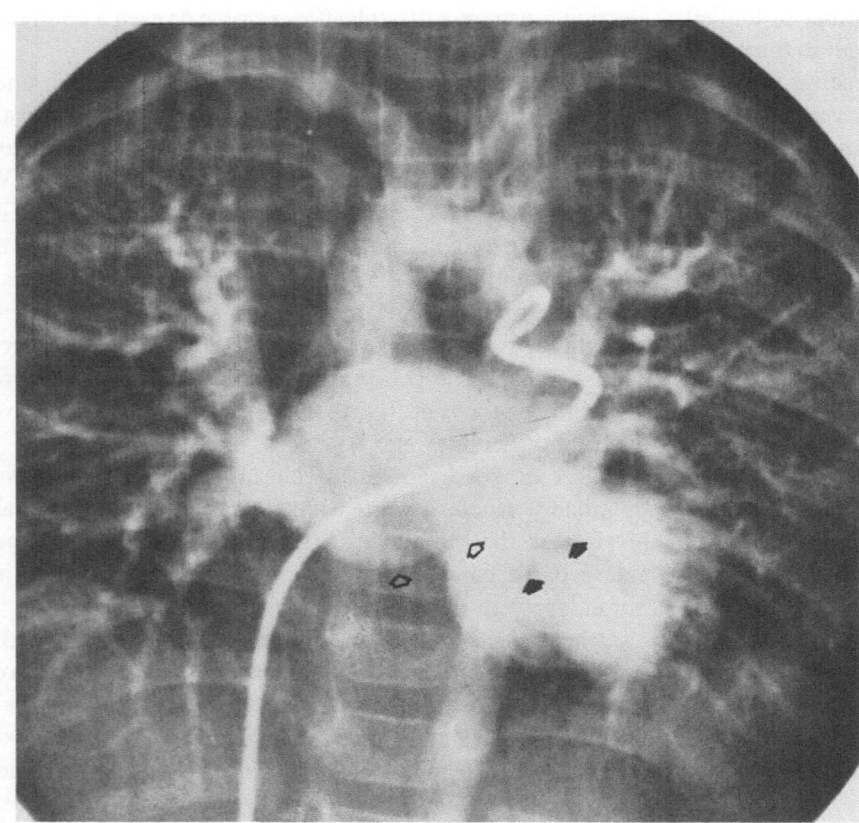

B

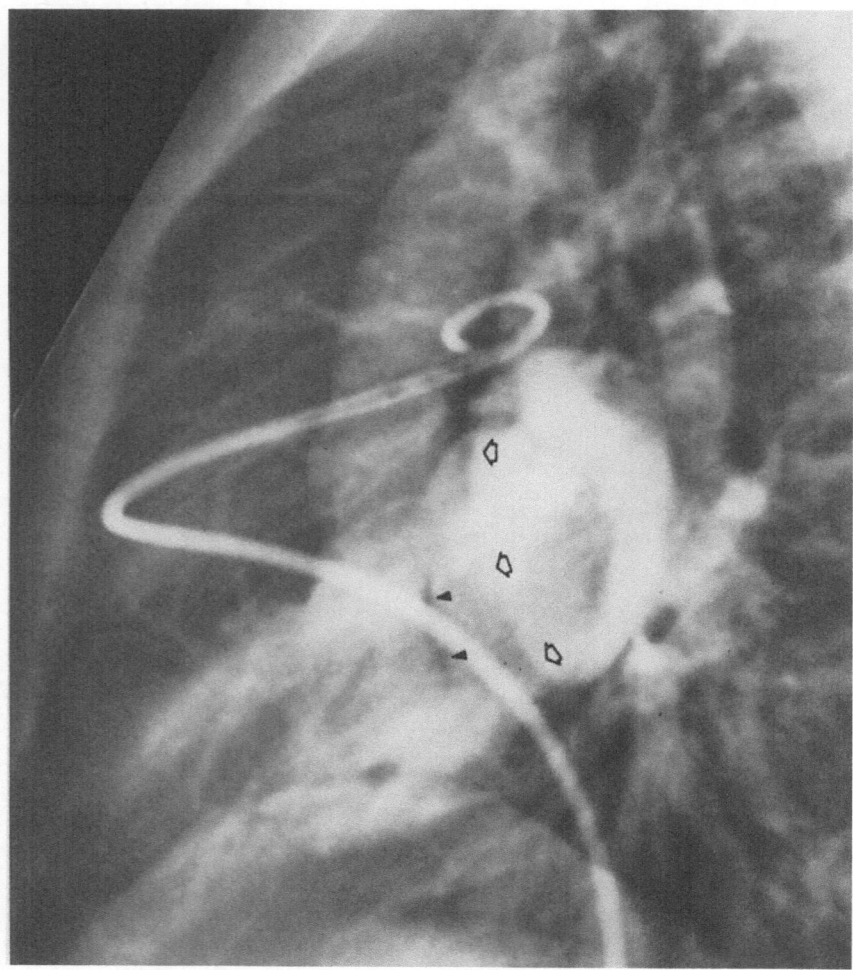

C

Fig. 7–203 (*Cont.*). The frontal and lateral views of the levophase of the pulmonary angiogram (**B** and **C**) show two left atrial chambers, a posterior chamber (high-pressure chamber, *open arrows*) and an anterior chamber (low pressure chamber, *closed arrows*). The obstructive membrane is represented by a curved line between the chambers. In the lateral view the mitral valve (*arrowheads*) forms the anterior extent of the low-pressure chamber. Each atrial chamber can be distinguished by following its outline, starting from the arrows and arrowheads.

sures in the RV and pulmonary artery are increased, and the pulmonary capillary wedge pressure will be higher than the LV diastolic pressure. If the venous catheter passes through the foramen ovale into the low pressure anterior chamber (true LA) then the distinction between cor triatriatum and stenosis or atresia of the pulmonary veins may not be appreciated. If the catheter enters the posterior chamber, which has a high pressure, the differential diagnosis includes cor triatriatum and mitral stenosis. Pulmonary angiography (Fig. 7–203B and C) is definitive in the diagnosis of cor triatriatum. The posterior chamber fills from the pulmonary veins, and a thin membrane separates this chamber from the anterior chamber. The left atrial appendage is part of the chamber with a low pressure (anterior chamber). This last-named feature distinguishes cor triatriatum from supravalvular left atrial ring, which occurs below the left atrial appendage so that this structure becomes part of the chamber with high pressure.

Surgical *treatment* consists of excision of the obstructing membrane in an uncomplicated case. In others, additional procedures may be necessary such as ligation of the vertical vein or redirection of anomalous pulmonary veins.

Bibliography

Coarctation of the Aorta and Pseudocoarctation of the Aorta

Bahabozorgui S, Nemir P Jr (1966) Coarctation of the abdominal aorta. Am J Surg 111:224–229

Baron MG (1971) Radiologic notes in cardiology. Obscuration of the aortic knob in coarctation of the aorta. Circulation 43:311–316

Becker AE, Becker MJ, Edwards JE (1970) Anomalies associated with coarctation of aorta. Particular reference to infancy. Circulation 41:1067–1075

Becu LM, Tauxe WN, DuShane JW, Edwards JE (1955) A complex of congenital cardiac anomalies: Ventricular septal defect, biventricular origin of the pulmonary trunk, and subaortic stenosis. Am Heart J 50:901–911

Björk L, Friedman R (1965) Routine roentgenographic diagnosis of coarctation of the aorta in the child. Am J Roentgenol 95:636–641

Boone ML, Swenson BE, Felson B (1964) Rib notching: Its many causes. Am J Roentgenol 91:1075–1088

Casta A, Conti VR, Talabi A, Brouhard BH (1982) Effective use of captopril in postoperative paradoxical hypertension of coarctation of aorta. Clin Cardiol 5:551–553

Cheitlin MD, Robinowitz M, McAllister H, Hoffman JIE, Bharati S, Lev M (1980) The distribution of fibrosis in the left ventricle in congenital aortic stenosis and coarctation of the aorta. Circulation 62:823–830

Clagett OT, Kirklin JW, Edwards JE (1954) Anatomic variations and pathologic changes in coarctation of the aorta. A study of 124 cases. Surg Gynecol Obstet 98:103–114

Crafoord C, Nylin G (1945) Congenital coarctation of the aorta and its surgical treatment. J Thorac Surg 14:347–361

d'Abreau AL, Aldridge GV, Astley AR, Jones MAC (1961) Coarctation of the aorta proximal to both subclavian arteries producing reversible papilloedema. Br J Surg 48:525–527

Edwards JE (1961) The congenital bicuspid aortic valve (editorial). Circulation 23:485–488

Edwards JE (1973) Aneurysms of the thoracic aorta complicating coarctation. Circulation 48:195–201

Edwards JE, Christensen NA, Clagett OT, McDonald JR (1948) Pathologic considerations in coarctation of the aorta. Proc Mayo Clin 23:324–333

Edwards JE, Clagett OT, Drake RL, Christensen NA (1948) The collateral circulation in coarctation of the aorta. Proc Mayo Clin 23:333–343

Eiken M (1959) Coarctation of the aorta. Atypical localization central to the origin of the innominate artery. Acta Med Scand 165:235–238

Eldridge R (1964) Coarctation in the Marfan syndrome. Arch Intern Med 113:342–349

Figley MM (1954) Accessory roentgen signs of coarctation of the aorta. Radiology 62:671–686

Garman JE, Hinson RE, Eyler WR (1965) Coarctation of the aorta in infancy: Detection on chest radiography. Radiology 85:418–422

Gross RE, Hufnagel CA (1945) Coarctation of the aorta. Experimental studies regarding its surgical correction. N Engl J Med 233:287

Heymann MA, Berman W Jr, Rudolph AM, Whitman V (1979) Dilatation of the ductus arteriosus by prostaglandin E₁ in aortic arch abnormalities. Circulation 59:169–173

Izukawa T, Mulholland HC, Rowe RD, Cooke DH, Bloom KR, Trusler GA, Williams WG, Chance GW (1979) Structural heart disease in the newborn. Changing profile: Comparison of 1975 with 1965. Arch Dis Child 54:281–285

Konar NR, Chaudhury DCR, Basu AK (1955) Clinical reports. A case of coarctation of aorta in an unusual site. Am Heart J 49:275–280

Lababidi Z (1983) Neonatal transluminal balloon coarctation angioplasty. Am Heart J 106:752–753

de Lezo JS, Fernandez R, Sancho M, et al (1984) Percutaneous transluminal angioplasty for aortic isthmic coarctation in infancy. Am J Cardiol 54:1147–1149

Lock JE, Bass JL, Amplatz K, Fuhman BP, Castaneda-Zuniga WR (1983) Balloon dilatation angioplasty of coarctations in infants and children. Circulation 68:109–116

Lock JE, Castaneda-Zuniga WR, Bass JL, Foker JE, Amplatz K, Anderson RW (1982) Balloon dilatation of excised aortic coarctation. Radiology 143:689–691

Martin EC, Diamon NG, Casarella WJ (1980) Percutaneous transluminal angioplasty in non-atherosclerotic disease. Radiology 135:27–33

Martin EC, Strafford MA, Gersony WM (1981) Initial detection of coarctation of the aorta: An opportunity for the radiologist. Am J Roentgenol 137:1015–1017

Moulaert AJ, Bruins CC, Oppenheimer-Dekker A (1976) Anomalies of the aortic arch and ventricular septal defects. Circulation 53:1011–1015

Nora JJ, Torres FG, Sinha AK, McNamara DG (1970) Characteristic cardiovascular anomalies of XO Turner syndrome, XX and XY phenotype and XO/XX Turner mosaic. Am J Cardiol 25:639–641

Odman P (1953) The appearance of internal mammary arteries in coarctation of the aorta. Acta Radiol 39:47–56

Reifenstein GH, Levine SA, Gross RE (1947) Coarctation of the aorta. A review of 104 autopsied cases of the "adult type," 2 years of age or older. Am Heart J 33:146–168

Rocchini AP, Rosenthal A, Barger AC, Castaneda AR, Nadas AS (1976) Pathogenesis of paradoxical hypertension after coarctation resection. Circulation 54:382–387

Schumacker HB, Nahrwold DL, King H, Waldhausen JA (1968) Coarctation of the aorta. Current Progress in Surgery. Year Book, Chicago

Shaher RM, Patterson P, Stranahan A, Older T, Farina M, Bishop M (1972) Congenital pulmonary and subclavian arteries steal syndrome. Am Heart J 84:103–109

Shone JD, Sellers RD, Anderson RC, Adams P Jr, Lillihei CW, Edwards JE (1963) The developmental complex of "parachute mitral valve," supravalvular ring of left atrium, subaortic stenosis, and coarctation of aorta. Am J Cardiol 11:714–725

Sinha SN, Kardatzke ML, Cole RB, Muster AJ, Wessel HU, Paul MH (1969) Coarctation of the aorta in infancy. Circulation 40:385–398

Sos T, Sniderman KW, Rettek-Sos B, Strupp A, Alonso DR (1979) Percutaneous transluminal dilatation of coarctation of thoracic aorta postmortem. Lancet 2:970–971

Spach MS, Serwer GA, Anderson PAW, Canent RV Jr, Levin AR (1980) Pulsatile aortopulmonary pressure-flow dynamics of patent ductus arteriosus in patients with various hemodynamic states. Ciruclation 61:110–122

Subramanian AR (1972) Coarctation or interruption of aorta proximal to origin of both subclavian arteries. Report of three cases presenting in infancy. Br Heart J 34:1225–1226

Talner NS, Berman MA (1975) Postnatal development of obstruction in coarctation of the aorta: Role of the ductus arteriosus. Pediatrics 56:4

Taylor DG, Grainger RG, Matthews HL, Thornton AJ, Verel D (1966) Suprarenal abdominal aortic obstruction. Br J Surg 53:195–198

Wilkins L, Fleishmann W (1944) Ovarian agenesis; pathology, associated clinical symptoms and the bearing on the theories of sex differentiation. J Clin Endocrinol Metab 4:357–375

Williams GW, Shindo G, Trusler GA, Dishe MR, Olley PM (1980) Results of repair of coarctation of the aorta during infancy. J Thorac Cardiovasc Surg 79:603–608

Wing JP, Findlay WA, Sahn DJ, McDonald G, Allen HD, Goldberg SJ (1978) Serial echocardiographic profiles in infants and children with coarctation of the aorta. Am J Cardiol 41:1270–1277

Yen HO S, Anderson RH (1979) Coarctation, tubular hypoplasia and the ductus arteriosus. Histological study of 35 specimens. Br Heart J 41:268–274

Zaroff LI, Kreel I, Sobel HJ, Baronofsky ID (1959) Multiple and infraductal coarctations of the aorta. Circulation 20:910–917

Aortico-Left Ventricular Tunnel

Levy MJ, Lillehei CW, Anderson RC, Amplatz K, Edwards JE (1963) Aortico-left ventricular tunnel. Circulation 27:841–853

Levy MJ, Schachner A, Blieden LC (1982) Aortico-left ventricu-

lar tunnel: Collective review. J Thorac Cardiovasc Surg 84:102–109

Llorens R, Arcas R, Herreros J, Dela Fuente A, Barriuso C, Casillas JA, Enriquez A (1982) Aortico-left ventricular tunnel: A case report and review of the literature. Tex Heart Inst J 9:169–175

Morgan RI, Mazur JH (1963) Congenital aneurysm of aortic root with fistula to left ventricle: A case report with autopsy findings. Circulation 28:589–594

Turley K, Silverman NH, Teitel D, Mavroudis C, Snider R, Rudolph A (1982) Repair of aortico-left ventricular tunnel in the neonate: Surgical, anatomic and echocardiographic considerations. Circulation 65:1015–1020

Villani M, Tiraboschi R, Marino A, DeTommasi M, Velitti F, Giani PC, Parenzan L (1980) Aortico-left ventricular tunnel in infancy. Scan J Thor Cardiovasc Surg 14:169–175

Supravalvular Aortic Stenosis

Anti AV, Wiltse HE, Rowe RD (1967) Pathogenesis of the supravalvular aortic stenosis syndrome. J Pediatr 71:431–441

Beuren AJ, Schulze C, Eberle P, Harmjanz D, Apitz J (1964) The syndrome of supravalvular aortic stenosis, peripheral pulmonary stenosis, mental retardation and similar facial appearance. Am J Cardiol 13:471–483

DoValle PV, Barcia A, Bargeron LM Jr, Karp RB (1969) Angiographic study of supravalvular aortic stenosis and associated lesions. Report of five cases and review of literature. Ann Radiol (Paris) 12:779–796

Eisenberg R, Young D, Jacobson B, Bioto A (1964) Familial supravalvular aortic stenosis. Am J Dis Child 108:341–347

Garcia RE, Friedman WF, Kaback MM (1964) Idiopathic hypercalcemia and supravalvular aortic stenosis. Documentation of a new syndrome. N Engl J Med 271:117–120

Jones KL, Smith DW (1975) The Williams elfin facies syndrome. J Pediatr 86:718–723

Morrow AG, Waldhausen JA, Peters RL, Bloodwell RD, Braunwald E (1959) Supravalvular aortic stenosis. Clinical, hemodynamic and pathologic observations. Circulation 20:1003–1010

Rastelli GC, McGoon DC, Ongley PA, Mankin HT, Kirklin JW (1966) Surgical treatment of supravalvular aortic steosis. Report of 16 cases and review of literature. J Thorac Cardiovasc Surg 51:873–882

Underhill WC, Tredway JB, DiAngelo GJ, Baay JEW (1971) Familial supravalvular aortic stenosis. Am J Cardiol 27:560–656

Weisz D, Hartmann AF Jr, Weldon CS (1976) Results of surgery for congenital supravalvular aortic stenosis. Am J Cardiol 37:73–77

Williams JCP, Barratt-Boyes BJ, Lowe JB (1961) Supravalvular aortic stenosis. Circulation 24:1311–1318

Critical Valvar Aortic Stenosis in Infancy

Bharati S, Lev M (1973) Congenital polyvalvular disease. Circulation 47:575–586

Broderick TW, Higgins CB, Guthaner DF, Friedman WF, Stevenson JG, French JW (1978) Critical aortic stenosis in neonates. Radiology 129:393–399

Burnell RM, Ghadiale PE, Joseph MC, Paneth M (1970) Management of critical valvular outflow obstruction in neonates. Thorax 25:116–119

Davis GL, McAlister WH, Friedenberg MM (1965) Congenital

aortic stenosis due to failure of histogenesis of the aortic valve (myxoid dysplasia). Am J Roentgenol 95:621–628

Freed M, Rosenthal A, Plauth WH Jr (1973) Development of subaortic stenosis after pulmonary artery banding. Circulation 47 and 48, suppl 3, pp 7, 10

Keane JF, Bernhard WF, Nadas AS (1975) Aortic stenosis surgery in infancy. Circulation 52:1138–1143

Lakier JB, Lewis AB, Heymann MA, Stanger P, Hoffman JIE, Rudolph AM (1974) Isolated aortic stenosis of the neonate: Natural history and hemodynamic considerations. Circulation 50:801–808

Latson LA, Cheatham JP, Gutgesell HP (1981) Relocation of the echocardiographic estimate of left ventricular size to mortality in infants with severe left ventricular outflow obstruction. Am J Cardiol 48:887–891

McCall I (1958) Pericarditis due to a mycotic aneurysm in subacute bacterial endocarditis. Report of a case affecting congenitally stenosed quadricuspid aortic valve. Guy's Hosp Rep 107:34–47

Moller JH, Nakib A, Eliot RS, Edwards JE (1966) Symptomatic congenital aortic stenosis in the first year of life. J Pediatr 69:728–734

Reeve R Jr, Robinson SJ (1964) Hypoplastic anulus—an unusual type of aortic stenosis: A report of three cases in children. Dis Chest 45:99–102

Roberts WC (1970) The congenitally bicuspid aortic valve. A study of 85 autopsy patients. Am J Cardiol 26:72–83

Roberts WC (1970) The structure of the aortic valve in clinically isolated aortic stenosis. An autopsy study of 162 patients over 15 years of age. Circulation 42:91–97

Roberts WC (1973) Valvular, subvalvular and supravalvular aortic stenosis. Cardiovasc Clin 5:97–126

Subaortic Stenosis

Bjornstad PG, Rastan H, Kentel J, Bueren AJ, Koncz J (1979) Aortoventriculoplasty for tunnel subaortic stenosis and other obstructions of the left ventricular outflow tract. Circulation 60:59–69

Deutsch V, Shem-Tov A, Yahini JH, Neufeld HN (1971) Subaortic stenosis (discrete form). Classification and angiocardiographic features. Radiology 101:275–286

Edwards JE (1965) Pathology of left ventricular outflow tract obstruction. Circulation 31:586–599

Ergin MA, Cooper R, LaCorte M, Golinko R, Griepp RB (1981) Experience with left ventricular apicoaortic conduits for complicated left ventricular outflow obstruction in children and young adults. Ann Thorac Surg 32:369–376

Fisher DJ, Snider AR, Silverman NH, Stanger P (1982) Ventricular septal defects with discrete subaortic stenosis. Pediatr Cardiol 2:265–269

Freedom RM, Culham JAG, Rowe RD (1977) Angiocardiography of subaortic obstruction in infancy. Am J Roentgenol 129:813–824

Katz NM, Buckley MJ, Liberthson RR (1977) Discrete membranous subaortic stenosis. Report of 31 patients, review of the literature, and delineation of management. Circulation 56:1034–1038

Kelly DT, Wulfsberg E, Rowe RD (1972) Discrete subaortic stenosis. Circulation 46:309–322

Misbach GA, Turley K, Ullyot DJ, Ebert PA (1982) Left ventri-

cular outflow enlargement by the Konno procedure. J Thorac Cardiovasc Surg 84:696–703

Neufeld EA, Muster AJ, Paul MH, Idriss FS, Riker WL (1976) Discrete subvalvular aortic stenosis in childhood. Study of 51 patients. Am J Cardiol 38:53–61

Piccoli GP, Ho SY, Wilkinson JL, Macartney FJ, Gerlis LM, Anderson RH (1982) Left-sided obstructive lesions in atrioventricular septal defects. An anatomic study. J Thorac Cardiovasc Surg 83:453–460

Schneeweiss A, Motro M, Shem-Tov A, Blieden LC, Neufeld HN (1983) Discrete subaortic stenosis associated with congenital valvular aortic stenosis—A diagnostic challenge. Am Heart J 106:55–59

Sellers RD, Lillehei CW, Edwards JE (1964) Subaortic stenosis caused by anomalies of the atrioventricular valves. J Thorac Cardiovasc Surg 48:289–302

Shem-Tov A, Schneeweiss A, Motro M, Neufeld HN (1982) Clinical presentation and natural history of mild discrete subaortic stenosis: Follow-up of 1–17 years. Circulation 66:509–512

Shore DF, Smallhorn J, Stark J, Lincoln C, Deheval MR (1982) Left ventricular outflow tract obstruction coexisting with ventricular septal defect. Br Heart J 48:421–427

Vered Z, Schneeweiss A, Meltzer RS, Neufeld HN (1983) Echocardiographic assessment of left ventricular outflow tract obstruction. Am Heart J 106:177–181

Discrete Membranous Subaortic Stenosis and Fibrous Subaortic Tunnel

Freed MD, Rosenthal A, Plauth WH Jr, Nadas AS (1973) Development of subaortic stenosis after pulmonary artery banding. Circulation 48:111–7–10

Freedom RM, Dische MR (1976) The angiocardiographic appearance of the endocardial cushion defect in selected transposition and malposition complexes. Acta Cardiol 31:287–299

Gutgesell HP, Mullins CE, Gillette PC, Speer M, Rudolph AJ, McNamara DG (1976) Transient hypertrophic subaortic stenosis in infants of diabetic mothers. J Pediatr 89:120–125

Jue KL, Edwards JE (1976) Anomalous attachment of mitral valve causing subaortic atresia. Observations in a case with other cardiac anomalies and multiple spleens. Circulation 35:928–932

Lauer RM, DuShane JW, Edwards JE (1960) Obstruction of left ventricular outlet in association with ventricular septal defect. Circulation 22:110–125

MacLean LD, Culligan JA, Kane DJ (1963) Subaortic stenosis due to accessory tissue of the mitral valve. J Thorac Cardiovasc Surg 45:382–388

Moulaert AJ, Oppenheimer-Dekker AJE (1976) Anterolateral muscle bundle of the left ventricle, bulboventricular flange and subaortic stenosis. Am J Cardiol 37:78–81

Neufeld HN, Ongley PA, Swan HJC, Burgert EO Jr, Edwards JE (1961) Biventricular origin of the pulmonary trunk with subaortic stenosis above the ventricular septal defect. Am Heart J 61:189–198

Reder RF, Dimich I, Steinfeld L, Litwak RS (1977) Left ventricle to aorta valved conduit for relief of diffuse left ventricular outflow tract obstruction. Am J Cardiol 39:1068–1072

Sellers RD, Lillehei CW, Edwards JE (1964) Subaortic stenosis caused by anomalies of the atrioventricular valves. J Thorac Cardiovasc Surg 48:289–302

Shone JD, Sellers RD, Anderson RC, Adams P Jr, Lillehei CW,

Edwards JE (1963) The developmental complex of "parachute mitral valve," supravalvular ring of left atrium, subaortic stenosis, and coarctation of aorta. Am J Cardiol 11:714–725

Van Praagh R, Corwin RD, Dahlquist AH Jr, Freedom RM, Mattioli L, Nebesar RA (1970) Tetralogy of Fallot with severe left ventricular outflow tract obstruction due to anomalous attachment of the mitral valve of the ventricular septum. Am J Cardiol 26:93–101

Hypoplastic Left Heart Syndrome

Bass JL, Ben-Shachar G, Edwards JE (1980) Comparison of M mode echocardiography and pathologic findings in the hypoplastic left heart syndrome. Am J Cardiol 45:79–86

Chesler E, Joffe HS, Vecht R, Beck W, Schrire (1970) Ultrasound cardiography in single ventricle and the hypoplastic left and right heart syndromes. Circulation 42:123–129

Eliot RS, Shone JD, Kanjuh VI, Ruttenberg HD, Carey LS, Edwards JE (1965) Mitral atresia. A study of 32 cases. Am Heart J 70:6–22

Farooki ZQ, Henry JG, Green EW (1976) Echocardiographic spectrum of the hypoplastic left heart syndrome. A clinicopathologic correlation in 19 newborns. Am J Cardiol 38:337–343

Folger GM Jr, Saied A (1973) A new roentgenographic sign of hypoplastic left heart. Chest 64:298–302

Fontan F, Baudet E (1971) Surgical repair of tricuspid atresia. Thorax 26:240–248

Freedom RM, Culham JAG, Rowe RD (1981) Left atrial-coronary sinus fenestration (partially unroofed coronary sinus): Morphological and angiographic observations. Br Heart J 46:63–68

Freedom RM, Williams WG, Dische MR, Rowe RD (1976) Anatomic variants in aortic atresia. Potential candidates for ventriculo-aortic reconstitution. Br Heart J 38:821–826

Fyler DC (1980) Report of the New England regional infant cardiac program. Pediatrics 65:376–461

Grant CA, Robertson B (1972) Microangiography of the pulmonary arterial system in "hypoplastic left heart syndrome." Circulation 45:382–388

Haworth SG, Reid L (1977) Quantitative structural study of pulmonary circulation in the newborn with aortic atresia, stenosis, or coarctation. Thorax 32:121–128

Lambert EC, Canent RV, Hohn AR (1966) Congenital cardiac anomalies in the newborn. A review of conditions causing death or severe distress in the first month of life. Pediatrics 37:343–351

Lambert EC, Tingelstad JB, Hohn AR (1966) Diagnosis and management of congenital heart disease in the first week of life. Pediatr Clin North Am 13:943–982

Lang P, Norwood WI (1983) Hemodynamic assessment after palliative surgery of hypoplastic left heart syndrome. Circulation 68:104–108

Latson LA, Cheatham JP, Gutgesell HP (1981) Relation of the echocardiographic estimate of left ventricular size to mortality in infants with severe left ventricular outflow obstruction. Am J Cardiol 48:887–891

Lev M (1952) Pathologic anatomy and interrelationship of hypoplasia of the aortic tract complexes. Lab Invest 1:61–70

Lev M, Arcilla R, Rimoldi HJA, Licata R, Gasul BM (1963) Premature narrowing or closure of the foramen ovale. Am Heart J 65:638–647

Lumb G, Dawkins WA (1960) Congenital atresia of mitral and aortic valves with vestigal left ventricle (three cases) Am Heart J 60:378–387

Lundstrum NR (1972) Ultrasound cardiographic studies of the mitral valve region in young infants with mitral atresia, mitral stenosis, hypoplasia of the left ventricle and cor triatriatum. Circulation 45:324–334

Meyer RA, Kaplan S (1972) Echocardiography in the diagnosis of hypoplasia of the left to right ventricle in the neonate. Circulation 41:55–64

Miller GAH (1971) Aortic atresia. Diagnostic cardiac catheterization in first week of life. Br Heart J 33:367–369

Neumann MP, Heidelberger KP, Dick M, Rosenthal A (1980) Pulmonary vascular changes associated with hypoplastic left ventricle syndrome. Pediatr Cardiol 1:301–306

Noonan JA, Nadas AS (1958) The hypoplastic left heart syndrome. An analysis of 101 cases. Pediatr Clin North Am 5:1029–1056

Norwood WI, Kirlin JK, Sanders SP (1980) Hypoplastic left heart syndrome: Experience with palliative surgery. Am J Cardiol 45:87–91

Norwood WI, Lang P, Hansen DD (1983) Physiologic repair of aortic atresia–hypoplastic left heart syndrome. N Engl J Med 308:23–26

Roberts WC, Perry LW, Chandra RS, Myers GE, Shapiro SR, Scott LP (1976) Aortic valve atresia: A new classification based on necropsy study of 73 cases. Am J Cardiol 37:753–756

Saied A, Folger GM Jr (1972) Hypoplastic left heart syndrome. Clinicopathologic and hemodynamic correlation. Am J Cardiol 29:190–198

Unger FM, Tuuri DT, Schatzman ER, Cavanaugh DJ, Johnson GF, Beekman R (1983) Real-time ultrasonic diagnosis of valvular aortic atresia and other hypoplastic left heart syndromes. RadioGraphics 3:679–709

Von Reuden TJ, Knight L, Moller JH, Edwards JE (1975) Coarctation of the aorta associated with aortic valvular atresia. Circulation 59:951–954

Watson DG, Rowe RD (1962) Aortic-valve atresia. Report of 43 cases. JAMA 179:14–18

Congential Mitral Stenosis

Collins-Nakai RL, Rosenthal A, Castaneda AR, Bernhard WF, Nadas AS (1977) Congenital mitral stenosis. A review of 20 years' experience. Circulation 56:1039–1047

Driscoll DJ, Gutgesell HP, McNamara DG (1978) Echocardiographic features of congenital mitral stenosis. Am J Cardiol 42:259–266

Glancy DL, Roberts WC (1976) Congenital obstructive lesions involving the major pulmonary veins, left atrium or mitral valve: A clinical, laboratory, and morphologic survey. Cathet Cardiovasc Diagn 2:215–252

LaCorte M, Harada K, Williams RG (1976) Echocardiographic features of congenital left ventricular inflow obstruction. Circulation 54:562–566

Lundstrom NR (1976) Value of echocardiography in diagnosis of congenital mitral stenosis. Br Heart J 38:534–535

Shone JD, Sellers RD, Anderson RC, Adams P Jr, Lillehei CW, Edwards JE (1963) The developmental complex of "parachute mitral valve," supravalvular ring of left atrium, subaortic stenosis, and coarctation of aorta. Am J Cardiol 11:714–725

Cor Triatriatum

Arciniegas E, Farooki ZQ, Hakimi M, Perry BL, Green EW

(1981) Surgical treatment of cor triatriatum. Ann Thorac Surg 32:571–577

Canedo MI, Stefanouros MA, Frank MJ, Moore HV, Cundey DW (1977) Echocardiographic features of cor triatriatum, Am J Cardiol 40:615–619

Jacobstein MD, Hirshfeld SS (1982) Concealed left atrial membrane: Pitfalls in the diagnosis of cor triatriatum and supravalve mitral ring. Am J Cardiol 49:780–786

Jegier W, Gibbons JE, Wiglesworth FW (1963) Cor triatriatum: Clinical, hemodynamic and pathologic studies: Surgical correction in early life. Pediatrics 31:255–267

Kelley MJ, Glanz S, Hellenbrand WE, Taunt KA, Berman MA (1977) Diagnosis of cor triatriatum by echocardiography. Radiology 123:159–160

McLoughlin MJ (1970) Cor triatriatum sinister. The role of radiology in the diagnosis of this rare, but curable anomaly. Clin Radiol 21:287–296

Schluter M, Langenstein BA, Thier W, Schmiegel W, Krebber H, Kalmar P, Hanrath P (1983) Transesophageal two-dimensional echocardiography in the diagnosis of cor triatriatum in the adult. J Am Coll Cardiol 2:1011–1015

Van Praagh R, Corsini I (1969) Cor triatriatum: Pathologic anatomy and a consideration of morphogenesis based on 13 postmortem cases and a study of normal development of the pulmonary vein and atrial septum in 83 human embryos. Am Heart J 78:379–405

Chapter 7 Section 5
Abnormalities of the Great Vessels

Abnormalities of the aortic arch and pulmonary arteries are not necessarily symptomatic. The lesions causing symptoms may be categorized into three groups: vascular rings causing stridor or dysphagia, interruptions of the aortic arch causing congestive heart failure, and associated intracardiac disorders causing cyanosis or congestive heart failure.

A vascular ring consists of a combination of vascular structures, in continuity, that encircle the esophagus and trachea. This congenital abnormality occurs in cases of double aortic arch, left aortic arch with right descending aorta and right ductus arteriosus, and with right aortic arch and left ductus arteriosus or ligamentum arteriosum. A vascular ring may also result from anomalous origin of a pulmonary artery (pulmonary sling) or rarely from an anomalous connection between the right pulmonary artery and the thoracic aorta (ductus sling).

Two concepts are helpful in understanding these and other abnormalities of the great vessels. The first is the theoretical double aortic arch system described by Edwards (Fig. 7–204) and the concept of single and double atresia or interruption (break) defined by Garti et al. (Fig. 7–205). The hypothetical double aortic arch (Fig. 7–204B, 7–205A) consists of the ascending aorta and the two arches, each with a common carotid artery, a subclavian artery and a ductus arteriosus. The arches join posteriorly to form the descending aorta. The esophagus and trachea are present inside the ring formed by the hypothetical double arch system. If no break or regression occurs, then a double aortic arch results. A break in the right aortic arch posterior to the right ductus, and regression of the right ductus arteriosus result in a normal human aortic arch (Figs. 7–204, 7–205). Breaks elsewhere result in all varieties of right aortic arch, interruption of the aorta and other abnormalities of the aortic arch described subsequently in this section.

Also included in this section is hemitruncus, which may result from abnormal migration of the sixth branchial arch, resulting in ectopic origin of either pulmonary artery from the ascending aorta. Table 7–8 lists congenital abnormalities of the great vessels.

Double Aortic Arch

Double aortic arch is a rare anomaly that usually occurs without intracardiac defects, resulting from persistence of all components of the hypothetical double aortic arch. One or both ducti may be patent (Fig. 7–205A). Both arches may be of equal size, or one, usually the left, may be hypoplastic or atretic. The vascular structures surround the trachea and esophagus.

Table 7–8. Abnormalities of the Great Vessels*

I. Double aortic arch†
II. Right aortic arch
    A. Right arch with mirror-image branching
        1) With ductus arising from innominate artery
        2) With ductus arising from aortic diverticulum†
    B. Right aortic arch with aberrant left subclavian artery
        1) With ductus from left subclavian artery†
        2) With left-sided descending aorta and with ductus from left subclavian artery†
    C. Right aortic arch with aberrant innominate artery and left ductus†
    D. Right aortic arch with isolation of left subclavian artery or innominate artery
III. Left aortic arch
    A. Left aortic arch with normal branching
        1) With left ductus (normal)
        2) With right ductus from aortic diverticulum†
    B. Left aortic arch with aberrant right subclavian artery
        1) With left-sided ductus
        2) With right ductus arising from aberrant right subclavian artery†
        3) With right ductus and right-sided descending aorta†
    C. Left aortic arch with isolation of the right subclavian artery
    D. Left aortic arch with anomalous origin of the innominate or left common carotid artery (bicarotid origin)
    E. Single brachiocephalic trunk arising from the aortic arch
IV. Cervical aortic arch
V. Interruption of the aortic arch
    A. Distal to the left subclavian artery
    B. Between the left common carotid and left subclavian arteries
    C. Between the innominate and left common carotid arteries
VI. Slings
    A. Pulmonary artery sling
    B. Ductus arteriosus sling
VII. Anomalous origin of one pulmonary artery from the ascending aorta (hemitruncus)
    A. Right hemitruncus
    B. Left hemitruncus (variant of tetralogy of Fallot)

* Pulmonary vascularity is normal unless associated defects are present.
† Lesions that constitute vascular rings.

Fig. 7–204. *Development of the normal aortic arch and its* ▶ *branches.* A represents the basic Rathke diagram showing six pairs of branchial arches that form between the dorsal aortae and the ventral aortae. The seventh (intersegmental) branches eventually become the subclavian arteries. **B** shows regression of the first, second and fifth arches (*dotted lines* on the left of the picture). The intersegmental arteries migrate up from the descending aorta to the dorsal arch, eventually moving proximal to the sixth arch (*dotted arrow*). The truncoaortic sac divides into the aorta and the main pulmonary artery. At the same time the ostia of the sixth arches migrate to attach to the main pulmonary artery. The right and left pulmonary arteries are outgrowths

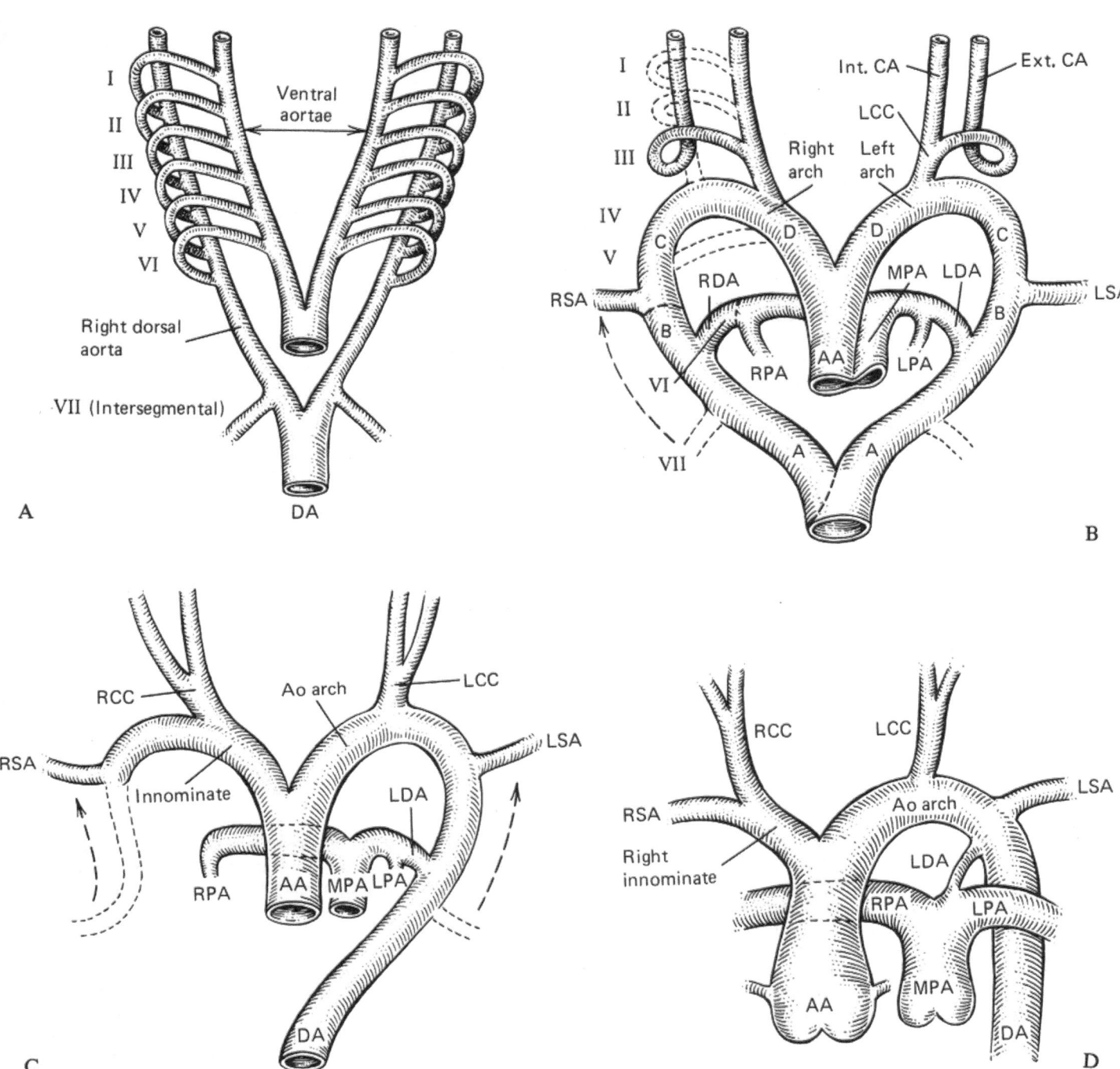

from the sixth arches, which penetrate the developing lung buds. Thus the proximal portions of the sixth arches become the right and left pulmonary arteries, while the distal sixth arches become the right and the left ductus arteriosus. The right ductus arteriosus normally disappears, as does the right aortic arch between the right subclavian artery and the descending aorta (*area demarcated by dashed lines*). **B** also illustrates the hypothetical double aortic arch of Edwards. In addition, the letters *A, B, C, D* in **B** correspond to those in Fig. 7–205. These letters denote the locations of breaks in the hypothetical double aortic arch, which result in normal and abnormal development of the aortic arch and pulmonary arteries (e.g., double aortic arch, right aortic arch, vascular rings, interruption of the aortic arch). **C** shows the results of all the normal regressions. The aortic arch is formed from the ventral aorta, the fourth branchial arch and the left dorsal aorta. The innominate artery is derived from the right ventral aorta, while the right subclavian artery develops from the fourth

branchial arch, the proximal segment of the dorsal aorta, and the right seventh intersegmental artery. The pulmonary arteries represent the proximal portion of the sixth arches, while the ductus arteriosus is derived from the distal portion of the left sixth arch. **D** represents an image similar to **C**, but drawn to approximate the normal appearance of the great vessels.

AA = ascending aorta; *DA* = descending aorta; *Ext. CA* = external carotid artery; *Int. CA* = internal carotid artery; *LCC* = left common carotid artery; *LDA* = left ductus arteriosus; *LPA* = left pulmonary artery; *LSA* = left subclavian artery; *MPA* = main pulmonary artery; *RCC* = right common carotid artery; *RDA* = right ductus arteriosus; *RPA* = right pulmonary artery; *RSA* = right subclavian artery. Modified from Langman J, (1969) Medical embryology human development—normal and abnormal, 2nd ed., p. 216. Copyright The Williams and Wilkins Co., Baltimore, Maryland.

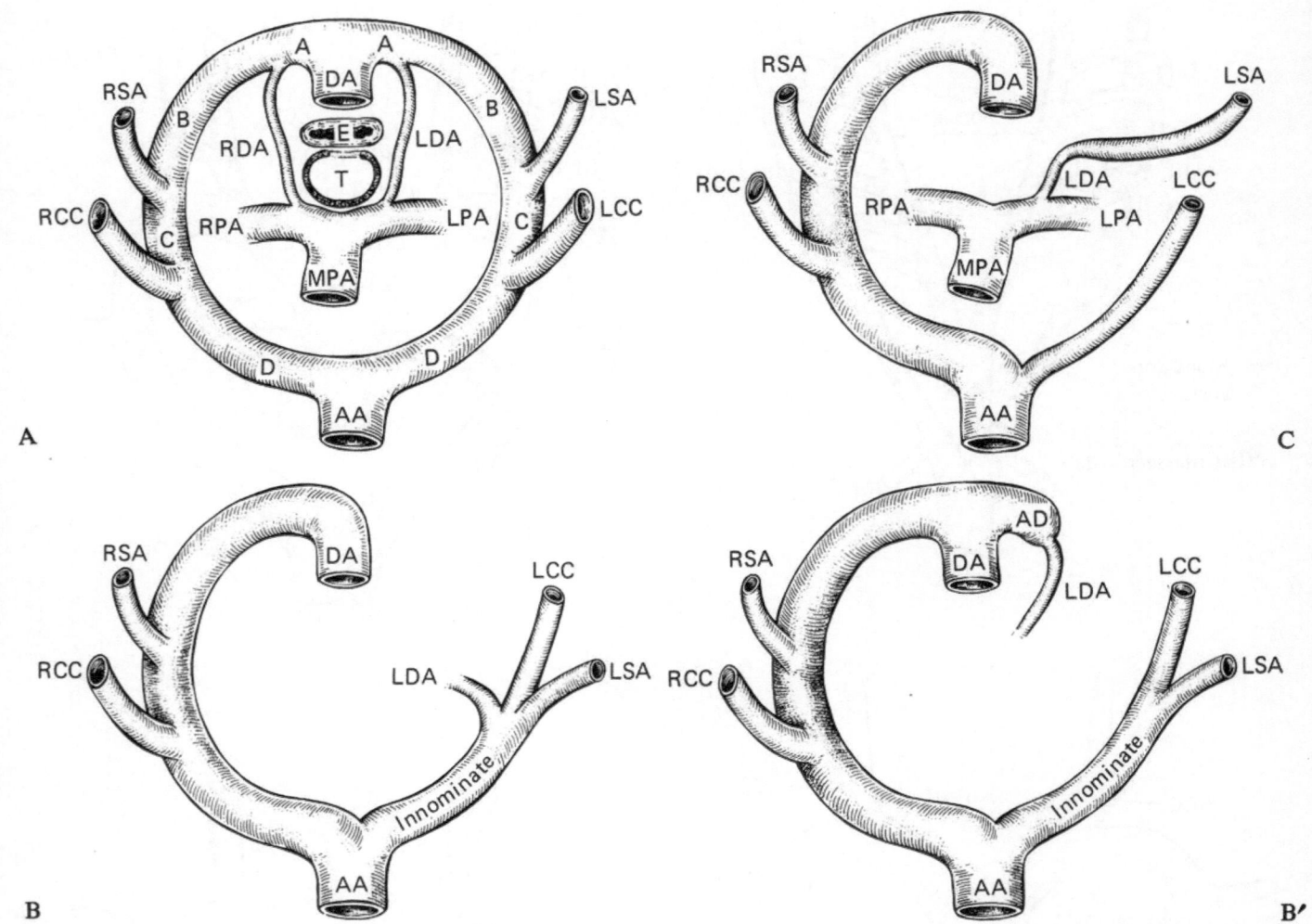

Fig. 7–205. *The hypothetical embryologic double aortic arch.* **A** Double aortic arch results from persistence of all structures with no breaks or interruptions (portions may be hypoplastic or atretic). Single or multiple interruptions (breaks) at various positions (*A,B,C,D*) explain the normal aortic arch as well as the reported anomalies of the aortic arch. The development of unreported anomalies is predicted. As an example, a break in the right aortic arch at position *A* results in a normal left aortic arch, whereas a break in the left arch at position *A* results in a right aortic arch with mirror-image branching (**B**). The ductus remains attached to the innominate artery. A break in the left arch at *B* results in the rare form of right aortic arch with mirror-image branching and left ductus (**B′**). A break in the right arch at *B* results in the rarely encountered left arch with normal branching and right ductus arteriosus. Both anomalies represent vascular rings. Of incidental significance is the aortic diverticulum formed from portion *A*. A break at *C* on the left results in a right aortic arch with aberrant left subclavian artery. If the left ductus persists a vascular ring results. A break at *C* on the right results in a left aortic arch with an aberrant right subclavian artery. Persistence of a right ductus arteriosus would complete the vascular ring.

A break at *D* on the left is rare and results in right aortic arch with aberrant left innominate artery. Of the anomalies resulting from two interruptions, isolation of a subclavian artery is the most common. The breaks occur at *A* and *C* so that the subclavian artery has no connection to the aorta, but is attached by way of the ductus arteriosus to the pulmonary artery (**C**).

AA = ascending aorta; *AD* = aortic diverticulum; *DA* = descending aorta; *LCC* = left common carotid artery; *LDA* = left ductus arteriosus; *LPA* = left pulmonary artery; *LSA* = left subclavian artery; *MPA* = main pulmonary artery; *RCC* = right common carotid artery; *RDA* = right ductus arteriosus; *RPA* = right pulmonary artery; *RSA* = right subclavian artery; *T* = trachea; *E* = esophagus.

Stridor and dysphagia usually begin in infancy; although rare, asymptomatic cases have been reported in adults. Recurrent pulmonary infections are common and may obscure the diagnosis. On physical examination the airway sounds are easily audible. The heart is not enlarged, no murmur is present, and the pulses generally are normal. The electrocardiogram is normal. The typical finding on plain films in older children and adults is the presence of bilateral aortic arches indenting the trachea (Fig. 7–206). The right arch is usually larger and higher than the left, occurring at or above the level of the azygos vein. The aorta usually descends on the right. On the lateral film the trachea may be indented by the posterior component of the ring.

In symptomatic infants these characteristic findings are rarely present, and even identification of the right aortic arch may be difficult. Useful clues when the right-sided aortic arch is not evident consist of a slight indentation of the trachea on the right side and a right-sided descending aorta (Figs. 7–207, 7–208). This radiological pattern in an infant with respiratory difficulty should lead to the suspicion of double aortic arch or another form of vascular ring.

In all age groups the barium esophagogram shows bilateral and posterior indentations at the level of the aortic arches. Usually the right-sided indentation is higher than the left-sided indentation. The retroesophageal portion of the aorta is a continuation of the left arch, which courses obliquely down from left to right to join the right arch. The proximal two thirds of the thoracic aorta descend on the right and then cross the midline to enter the aortic hiatus on the left.

Computerized axial tomography, magnetic resonance imaging, digital angiography and 2-D echocardiography all have the potential for demonstrating this anomaly if both arches are patent. On angiography, studies of the aortic arch are diagnostic even though one arch is atretic (Fig. 7–207). Compound axial views may be of assistance in exposing the small arch encircling the esophagus and in defining the origins of the brachiocephalic vessels.

Right Aortic Arch

Right aortic arch represents persistence of the right fourth arch with a break in the left. It is classified according to the pattern of branching of the brachiocephalic vessels. The two most common patterns are right aortic arch with mirror-image branching and right aortic arch with aberrant left subclavian artery. Either may be associated with a vascular ring.

Fig. 7–206. *Double aortic arch in an adult.* A PA film of the chest with barium-filled esophagus demonstrates the classic findings in an asymptomatic adult. The right arch is larger and higher than the left. The trachea is indented on the right, and the esophagus is indented on both sides. The aorta descends on the right side. (*Continued*)

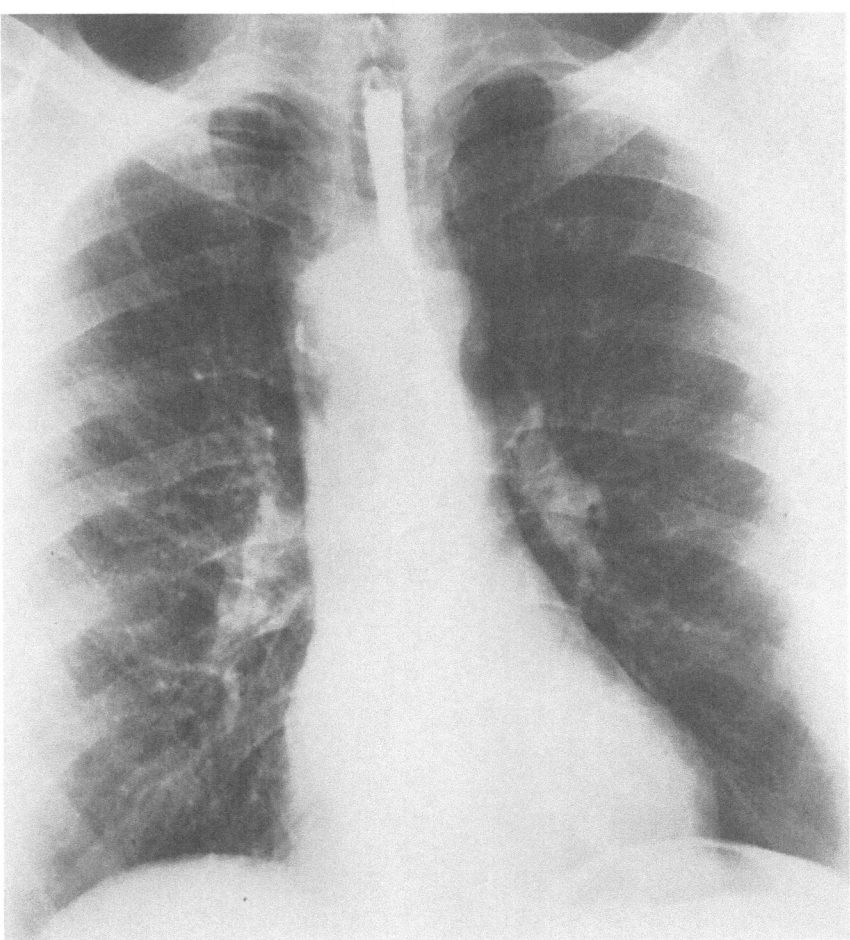

A

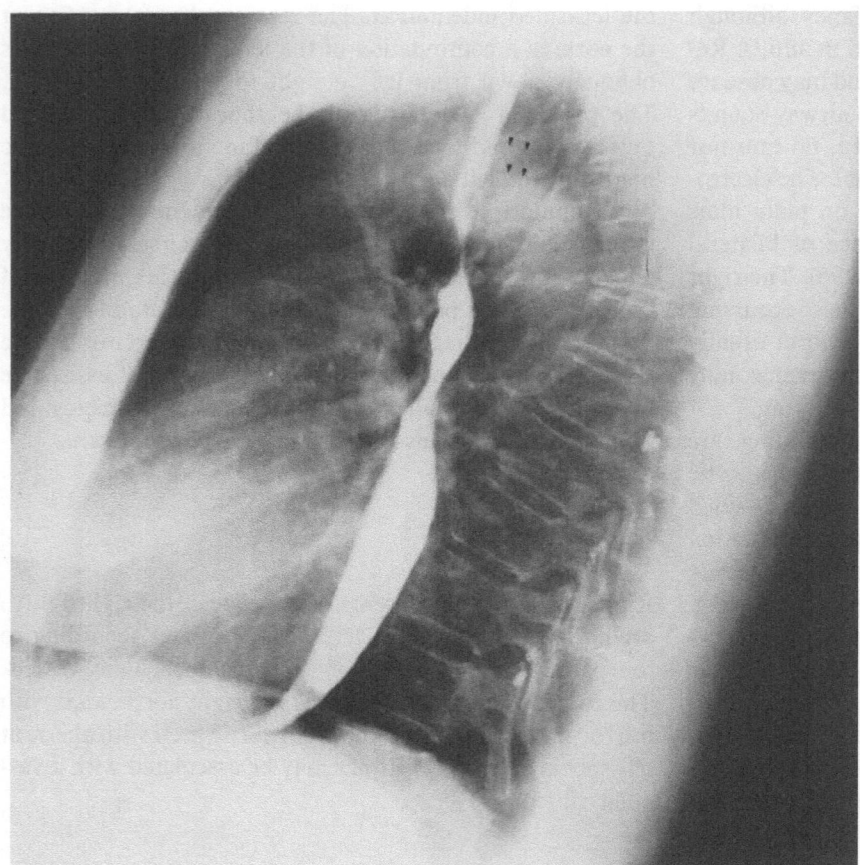

Fig. 7–206 (*Cont.*). The lateral projection (**B**) shows mild posterior indentation of the trachea and esophagus. Both arches are outlined (*arrowheads*), the left being smaller and appearing sharper in this lateral film. A "coned" view of the arches in the right anterior oblique projection (**C**) demonstrates the indentation of the trachea on the right and the descent of the right arch as it joins the left arch posteriorly to form the descending aorta (*arrows*).

B

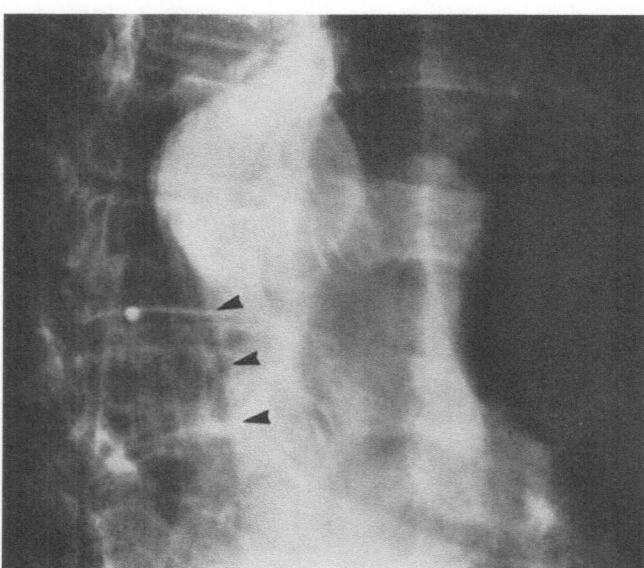

C

Fig. 7–207. *Double aortic arch in a 6-month-old boy with stridor.* **A** The frontal film shows the usual presentation in this age group in which the right arch may be difficult to appreciate until subtle clues are considered. Here the presence of the right-sided descending aorta (*arrowheads*) should suggest the correct diagnosis. **B** The lateral film shows narrowing of the trachea. (*Continued*)

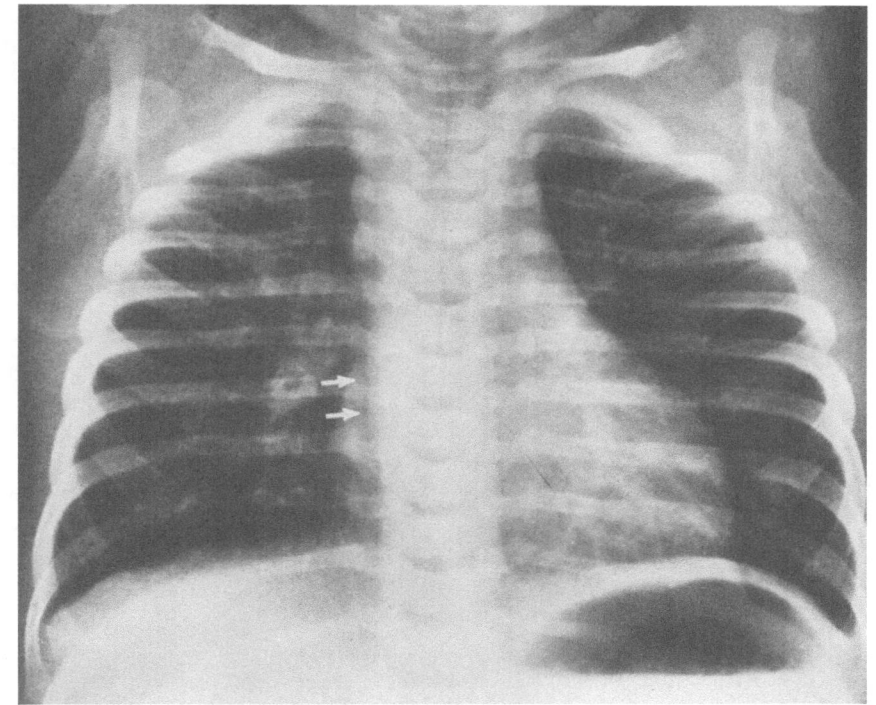

A

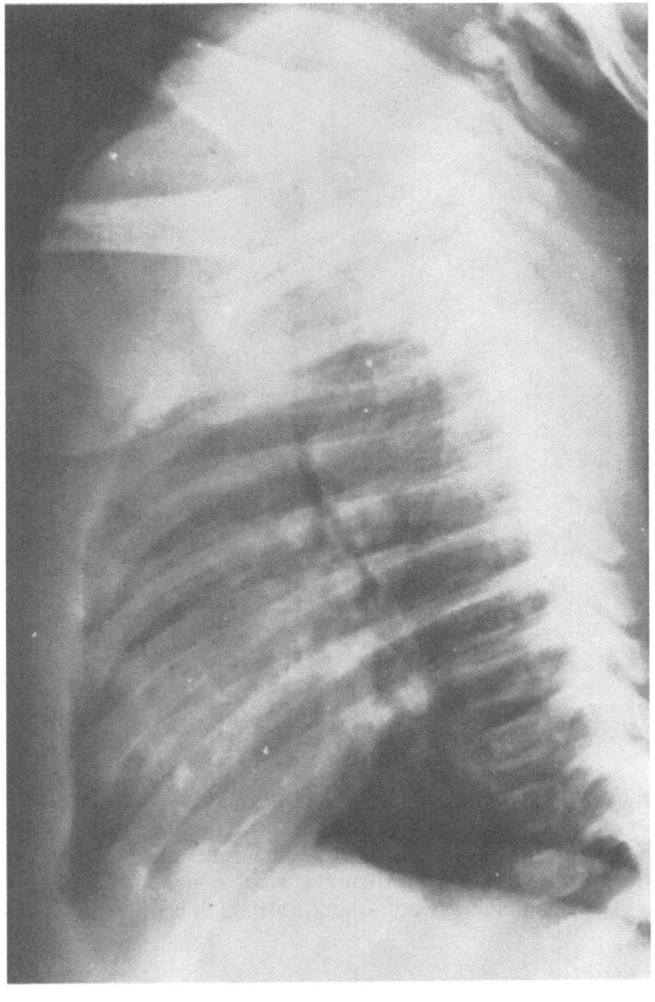

B

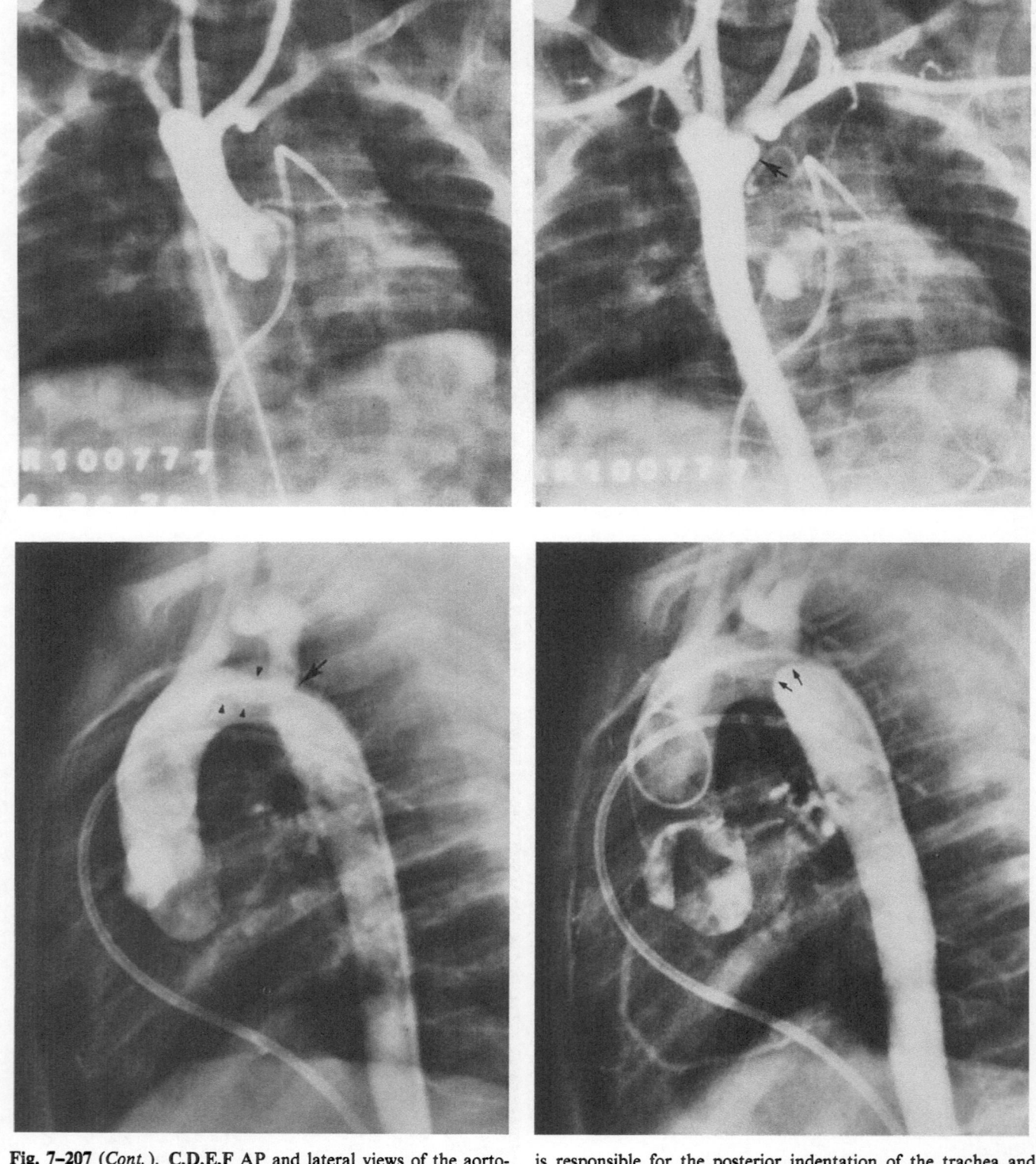

Fig. 7–207 (*Cont.*). **C,D,E,F** AP and lateral views of the aortogram. **C** The ascending aorta and both arches, each giving off a carotid and a subclavian artery. **D** The right-sided descending aorta and a large aortic diverticulum, which represents the posterior segment of the left aortic arch (*arrow*). This diverticulum is responsible for the posterior indentation of the trachea and esophagus. **E** The left aortic arch (*arrowheads*) and atresia of the left arch (*arrow*) just beyond the left subclavian artery. **F** Aortic diverticulum (*arrows*).

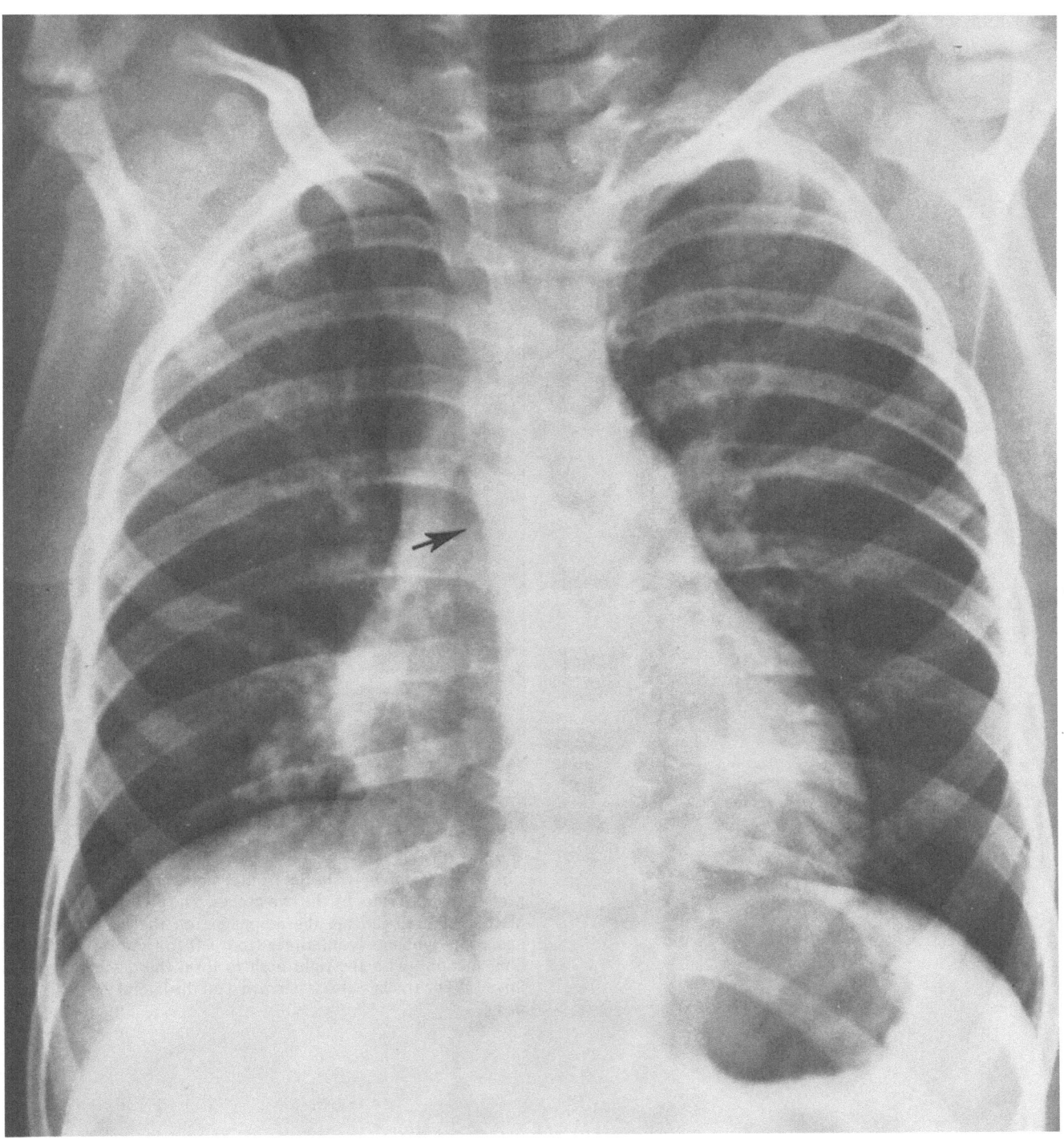

A

Fig. 7–208. *Double aortic arch in a 2-year-old child with stridor and dysphagia.* **A** Frontal roentgenogram of the chest; **B** and **C** AP and lateral views of the barium esophagogram. **D** Left ventriculogram; **E** lateral film of selective opacification of the left arch. **A** The signs of the right aortic arch are less obvious than those occurring in adults and older children. Clues to the diagnosis include the following: (1) There is widening of the superior me-diastinum and slight indentation of the trachea on the right; (2) the left arch is not conspicuous; (3) the right-sided descending aorta is outlined sharply (*arrow*). In many infants visualization of the right-sided descending aorta is the only clue to the diagnosis of right aortic arch. In a child with stridor and dysphagia, signs of a right arch should suggest a double aortic arch or other vascu-lar ring. (*Continued*)

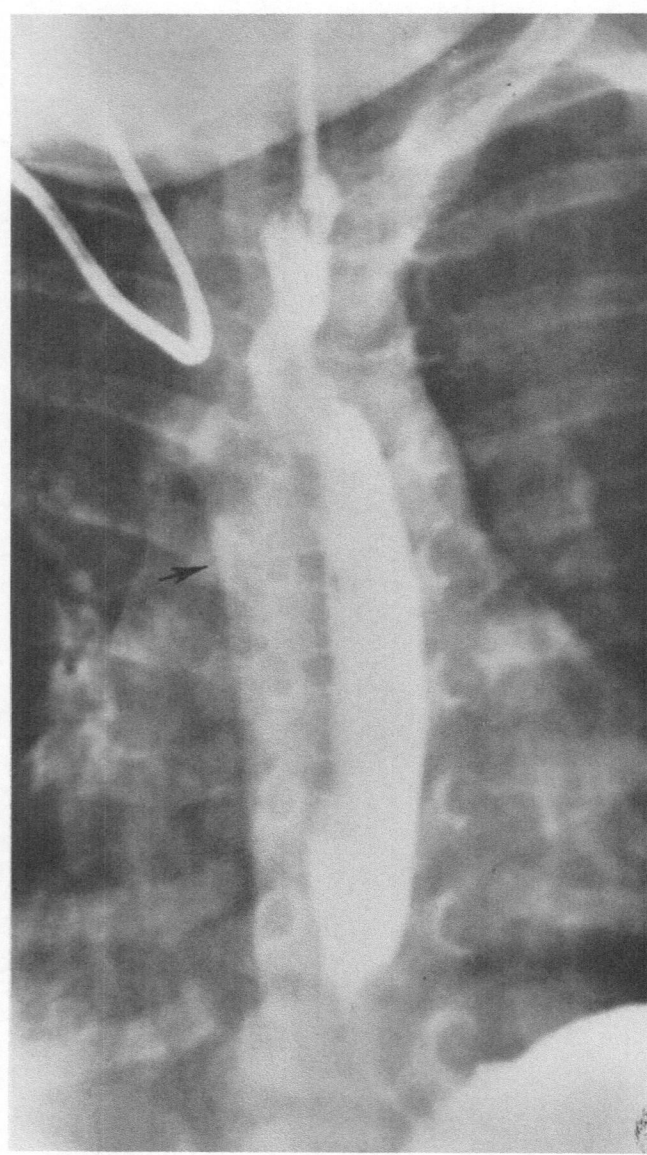

B

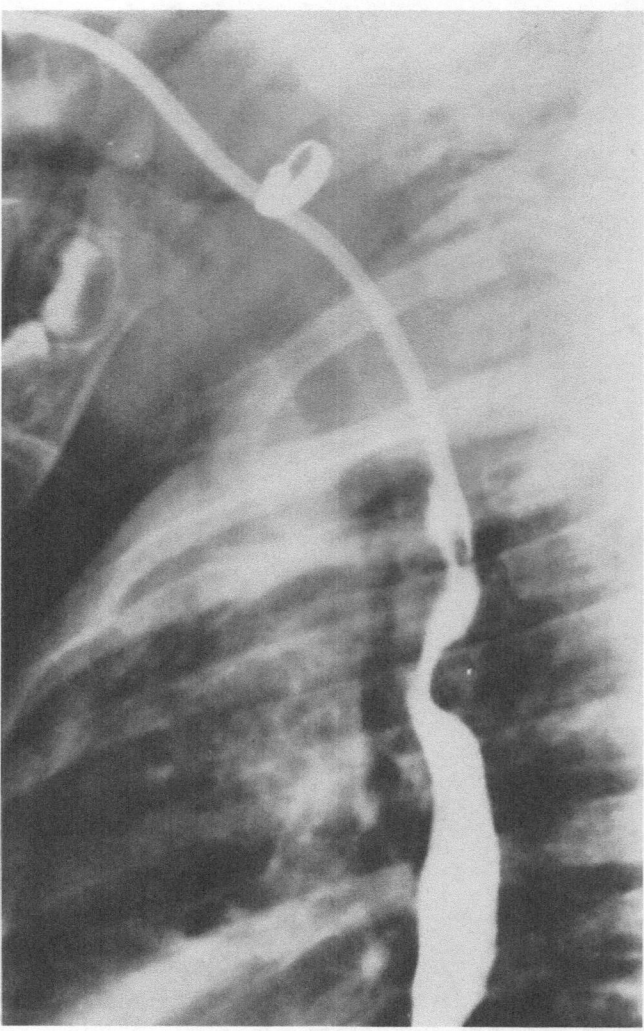

C

Fig. 7–208 (*Cont.*). **B** On the frontal view the esophagus is compressed on both sides by the two arches. The posterior component of the left arch indents the esophagus on the lateral view (**C**) and courses obliquely inferiorly from left to right on the frontal film, merging with the right arch to form the descending aorta (*arrow*). The trachea also is narrowed on the lateral view. (*Continued*)

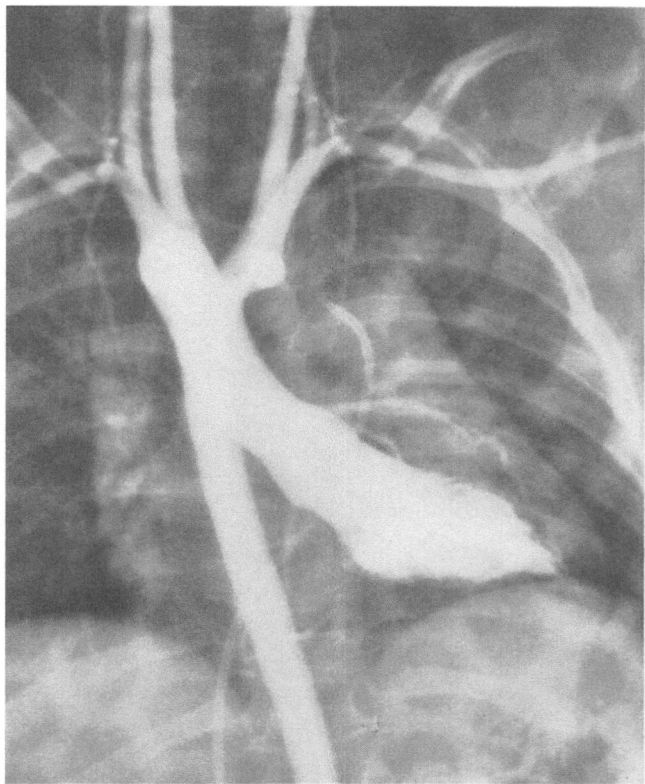

D

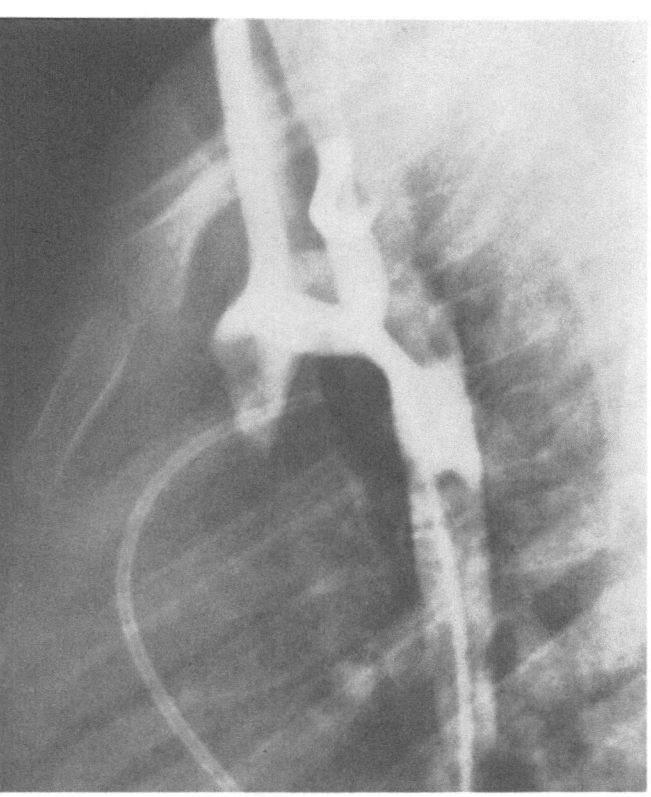

E

Fig. 7–208 (*Cont.*). **D** Two patent aortic arches are shown; each gives off a carotid and a subclavian artery. The right aortic arch is larger and higher than the left. The aorta descends on the right, then crosses the midline and enters the aortic hiatus.

E The left arch is hypoplastic, particularly the posterior segment. The branches of the left arch, the left common carotid artery and the left subclavian artery, are delineated.

Right Aortic Arch with Mirror-Image Branching

The usual form of right aortic arch with mirror-image branching (Figs. 7–205B and 7–209) represents a break in the left aortic arch between the left ductus arteriosus and the descending aorta (position A on the left, Fig. 7–205A). The first branch of the right arch is the left innominate artery; the second branch is the right common carotid; and the last branch is the right subclavian artery. The ductus arteriosus is attached to the left innominate artery anterior to the esophagus. No vascular ring is present. The aorta descends on the right, then crosses the midline to enter the aortic hiatus of the diaphragm. This form of right aortic arch is almost always associated with cyanotic congenital heart defects, usually tetralogy of Fallot and its variants. Other cyanotic defects such as truncus arteriosus, transposition of the great vessels, pulmonary atresia and tricuspid atresia are also associated.

The rare form of right aortic arch with mirror-image branching represents a break in the left arch between the left subclavian artery and the left ductus arteriosus (position B, Fig. 7–205A). The branching is the same as in the previous form of right arch; however, the ductus is attached to an aortic diverticulum that originates from the proximal descending aorta and passes behind the esophagus. A vascular ring is present. This rare form of right aortic arch with mirror-image branching is not associated with cyanotic heart defects.

In most individuals with a right aortic arch the aorta descends on the right; rarely the aorta encircles the esophagus and descends on the left.

On plain films in older children and adults a right aortic arch with mirror-image branching indents the trachea and esophagus on the right side (Fig. 7–209). The aorta usually descends on the right side. In infants a right-sided aortic arch may be difficult to identify; however, an indentation of the trachea on the right or a right-sided descending aorta is the most reliable sign of right aortic arch when the aortic arch is not conspicuous.

Barium swallow in individuals with a right aortic arch and mirror-image branching will show indentation on the right side of the esophagus. A posterior indentation will be present only in the rare form with a retroesophageal aortic diverticulum and left-sided ductus (vascular ring). Aortography (Fig. 7–209B and C) or digital angiography is definitive for the diagnosis of right aortic arch.

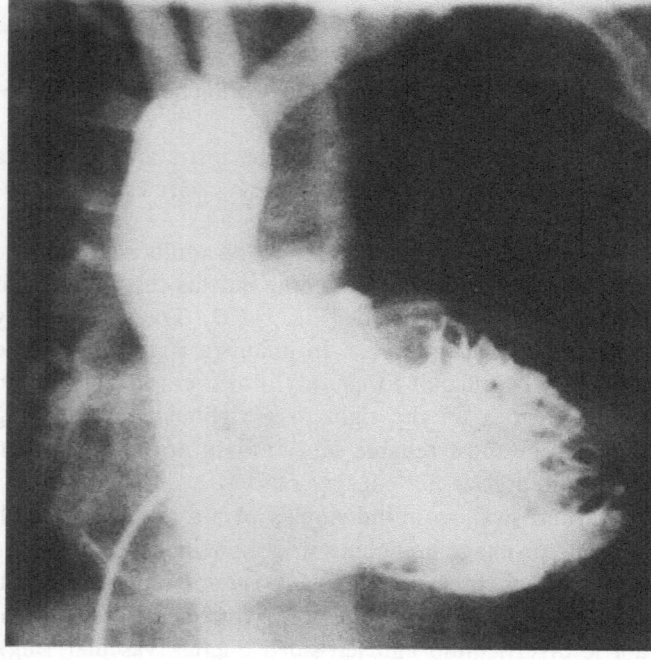

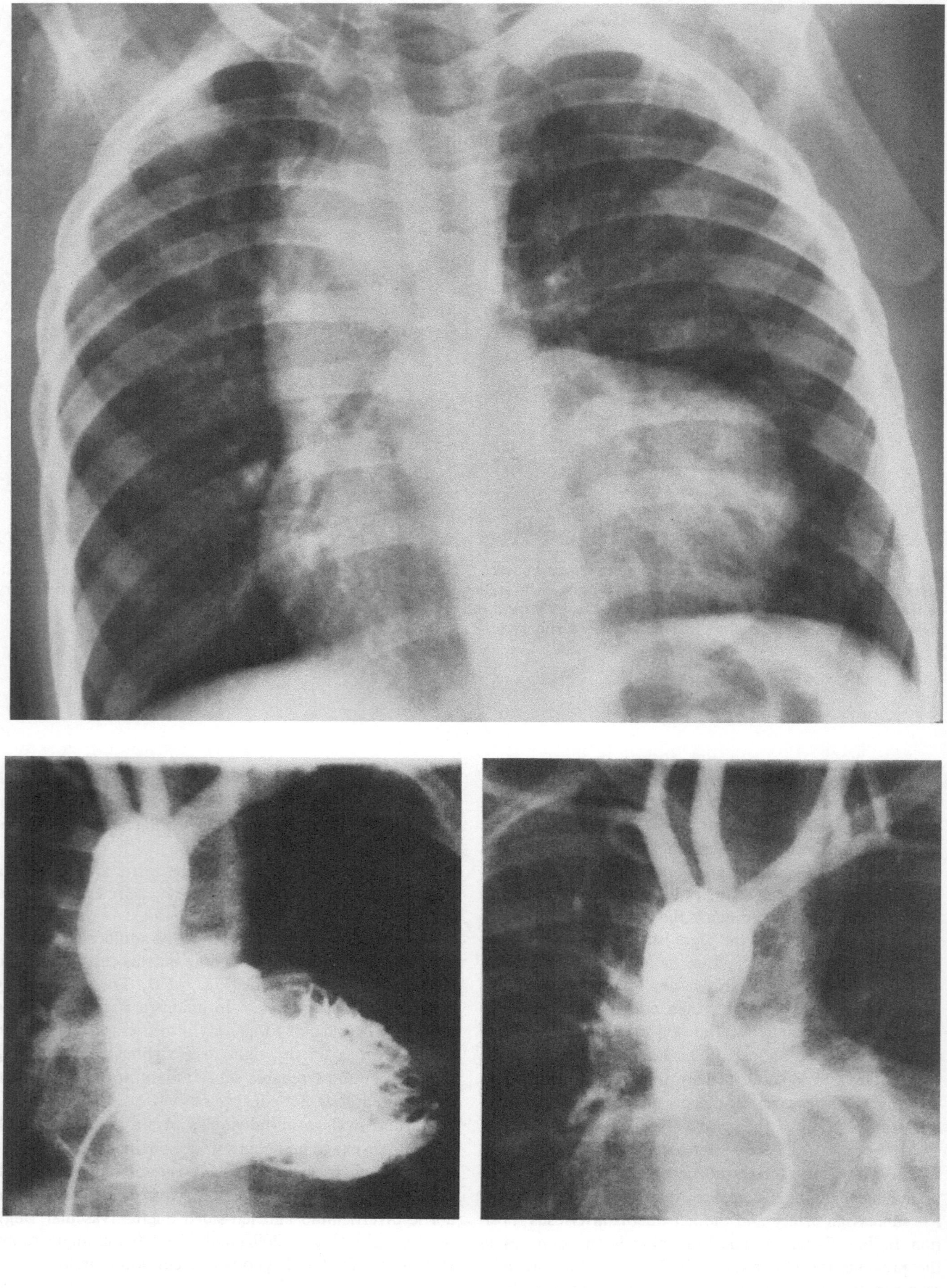

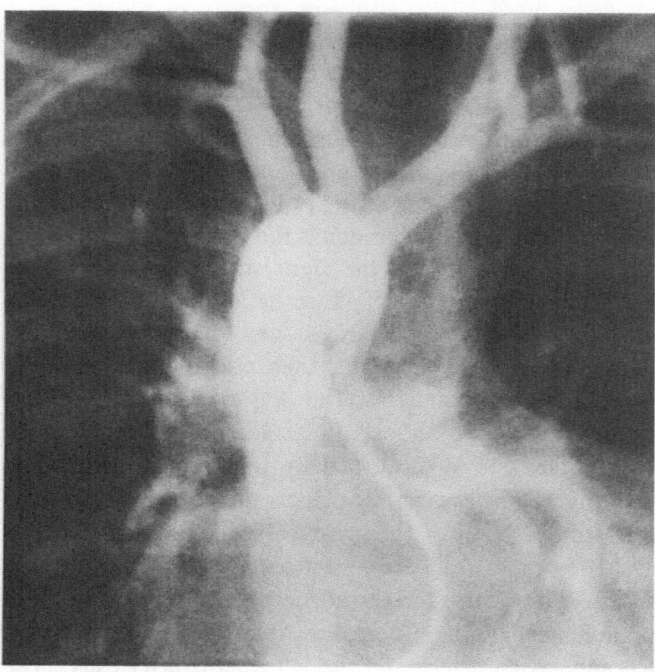

A

B

C

◀ **Fig. 7–209.** *Right aortic arch with mirror-image branching in a 19-month-old-girl with tetralogy of Fallot.* The roentgenogram of the chest (**A**) shows the characteristic boot-shaped heart (coeur en sabot). The superior mediastinum is widened on the right by the dilated ascending aorta. The aortic arch indents the trachea on the right, and the thoracic aorta descends on the right. **B** The right ventriculogram in the same patient shows atresia of the pulmonary valve and an aorta being filled by a right-to-left shunt through the VSD. The aortic arch is right sided with mirror image branching. **C** The aortogram also shows the right aortic arch with mirror image branching. The first branch is the left innominate artery. The second branch is the right common carotid artery, and the third branch is the right subclavian artery. In this patient the innominate artery gives off the left common carotid artery, the thyrocervical trunk, the vertebral artery, and the internal mammary artery.

Right Aortic Arch with Aberrant Left Subclavian Artery

Right aortic arch with aberrant left subclavian artery (Fig. 7–210) is not associated with cyanotic congenital heart defects. It is usually an incidental finding in asymptomatic adults. The theoretical break occurs in the left aortic arch between the left common carotid and the left subclavian artery (position C in the left arch, Fig. 7–205A). The first branch of the right aortic arch is the left common carotid artery. The second branch is the right common carotid artery, and the third is the right subclavian artery. The

fourth branch is the left subclavian artery, which originates from the proximal descending aorta and passes obliquely superiorly behind the esophagus.

Some patients have a large retroesophageal diverticulum from which the left subclavian artery arises. The posterior indentation of the esophagus (Fig. 7–210B) may be produced either by the aberrant left subclavian artery or by the aortic diverticulum. The ductus arteriosus is on the left, arising from the aortic diverticulum if present, or from the left subclavian artery. This combination of a right aortic arch and left ductus arteriosus forms a vascular ring; nevertheless, most individuals with this anomaly do not have symptoms of vascular ring because the ring remains relatively loose.

In a few patients with a right aortic arch, aberrant left subclavian artery and left ductus, the aorta encircles the trachea and esophagus and descends on the left. These are more likely to exhibit symptoms of vascular ring.

Right Aortic Arch with Aberrant Left Innominate Artery

Right aortic arch with an aberrant left innominate artery is rare. It represents a break in the primitive left aortic arch proximal to the left carotid artery (position D on the left, Fig. 7–205A). The first branch of the right aortic arch is the right common carotid artery; the second is

A

Fig. 7–210. *Right aortic arch with aberrant left subclavian artery noted incidentally during evaluation for scoliosis.* The right-sided aortic arch and the right-sided descending aorta are clearly recognized on the frontal view (**A**). The left subclavian artery passes obliquely and superiorly behind the esophagus, creating an oblique indentation in the barium column on the frontal view and a posterior indentation on the lateral film (**B**).

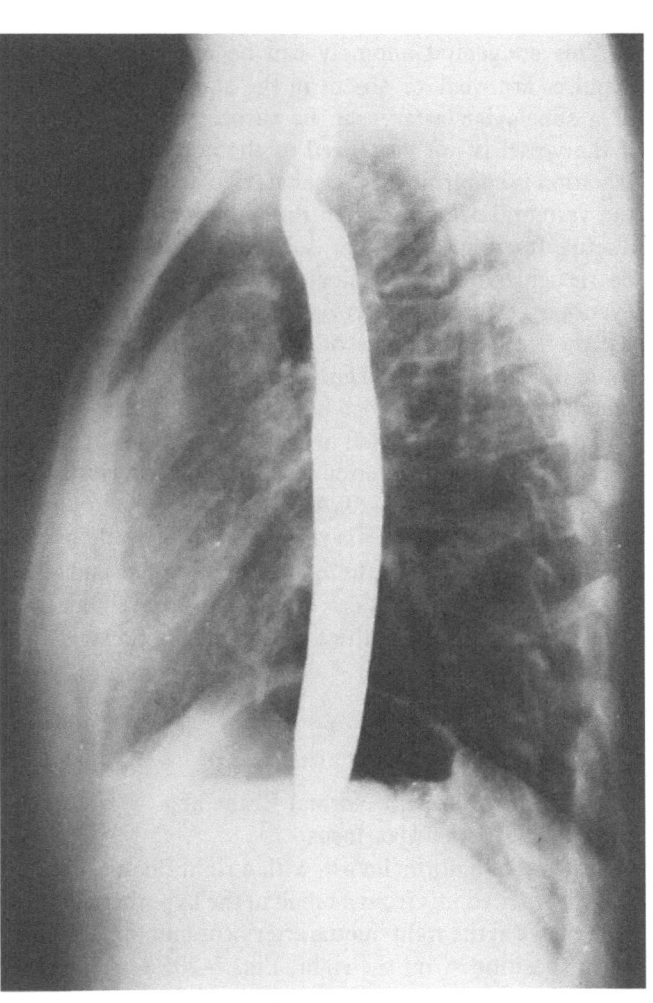

B

the right subclavian artery. The last branch, the innominate artery, passes behind the esophagus and gives off the left subclavian and the left common carotid arteries. The left ductus arises from the innominate artery and forms a vascular ring. Again this vascular ring may or may not be symptomatic.

Isolation of a Subclavian Artery

Isolation of a subclavian artery (Fig. 7–205C) results theoretically from two breaks in the primitive aortic arch system that leave the subclavian artery and the ductus arteriosus separated from the rest of the system (positions A and C in either arch, Fig. 7–205A). This anomaly occurs on the side opposite the aortic arch, being more common with a right arch so that the left subclavian artery is most often involved. The ductus may be patent or atretic.

If the ductus is atretic the subclavian artery receives its blood supply by way of the vertebral arteries and the circle of Willis, resulting in a subclavian steal. If the ductus is patent and pulmonary pressure is low, blood from the vertebral artery will flow to the arm as well as through the ductus arteriosus into the pulmonary circulation; thus a left-to-right shunt results in addition to a subclavian steal. If pulmonary pressure is elevated, blood will flow from the pulmonary artery through the ductus arteriosus into the arm, resulting in a right-to-left shunt and differential cyanosis, the affected arm being blue.

This congenital anomaly can be recognized clinically if pulses are weak or absent in the affected arm. Isolation of a subclavian artery can be suspected on angiography if the vessel is not visualized as the aortic arch opacifies. Isolation is confirmed if the subclavian artery fills late from the vertebral artery or from the pulmonary artery via the ductus. It is important that isolation of a subclavian artery be recognized either clinically or angiographically in all cyanotic cardiac disorders so that an operating surgeon will not attempt the use of an isolated subclavian artery to construct a Blalock-Taussig shunt. *Isolation of the left innominate artery* has also been reported. This occurs secondary to breaks in the left arch anterior to the left common carotid artery and posterior to the ductus arteriosus (positions A and D, Fig. 7–205A).

The interested reader is referred to the article by Garti et al., which presents the concepts of single and double breaks of the hypothetical double aortic arch, describes some of the unusual entities and predicts others.

Left Aortic Arch

Left Aortic Arch with Normal Branching and Right Ductus Arteriosus

Consisting of a normal aorta with a right ductus arteriosus this disorder results from a break in the hypothetical double arch between the right ductus arteriosus and the descending aorta (position A on the right, Fig. 7–205A). This abnormality differs from normal, in that the right ductus persists,

being attached to the innominate artery and thereby producing no vascular ring. If the break in the hypothetical double arch occurs anterior to the right ductus (position B on the right, Fig. 7–205A) the ductus will remain attached to an aortic diverticulum (if present) or to the proximal segment of the descending aorta to complete a vascular ring. In some cases reported with vascular ring the aortic arch encircled the esophagus and trachea and descended on the right (Fig. 7–211). This last anomaly, encountered rarely, is important, because it represents an example of a vascular ring with a left-sided aortic arch.

Left Aortic Arch with Aberrant Right Subclavian Artery

Three distinct patterns exist: (1) with left ductus arteriosus and left-sided descending aorta (Figs. 7–212, 7–213A), (2) with right ductus arteriosus and left-sided descending aorta (Fig. 7–213B), (3) with right ductus arteriosus and right-sided descending aorta (Fig. 7–213C).

Any of these three complexes may be associated with an aortic diverticulum. The most common form is left aortic arch with an aberrant right subclavian artery and a left ductus arteriosus, which has an incidence varying from 0.4% to 2.0% of all congenital heart defects. Embryologically, left aortic arch with aberrant right subclavian artery results from a break in the right aortic arch between the common carotid and subclavian arteries (position C on the right, Fig. 7–205A). The right ductus also disappears. The aberrant right subclavian artery arises as the last branch of the aortic arch or proximal descending aorta and ascends obliquely and superiorly behind the esophagus to reach the right arm. This form is usually recognized incidentally during the performance of a gastrointestinal examination or on obtaining a cardiac series. An aberrant right subclavian artery has also been encountered among the anomalies associated with tetralogy of Fallot, patent ductus arteriosus, coarctation and pseudocoarctation of the aorta and ventricular septal defect. The major roentgenographic finding is an oblique indentation on the posterior aspect of the barium-filled esophagus above the aortic arch, extending upward and to the right. Cine fluorography with barium swallow may show the pulsations of the aberrant vessel.

This anomaly generally is asymptomatic, but occasionally it may be responsible for severe symptoms. Klinkhamer described children with respiratory symptoms but no dysphagia and found that the combination of an aberrant right subclavian artery and common origin of the carotid arteries (bicarotid trunk), or abnormal juxtaposition of the carotid vessels, was associated with anterior tracheal compression.

If an aberrant right subclavian artery is associated with coarctation of the aorta it may arise above, at or below the coarctation. If the aberrant artery arises at or below the site of the coarctation, the blood pressure in the right arm will be low. On angiography, subclavian steal may be encountered.

Rarely a right ductus arteriosus may persist, arising from an aberrant right subclavian artery or from an aortic

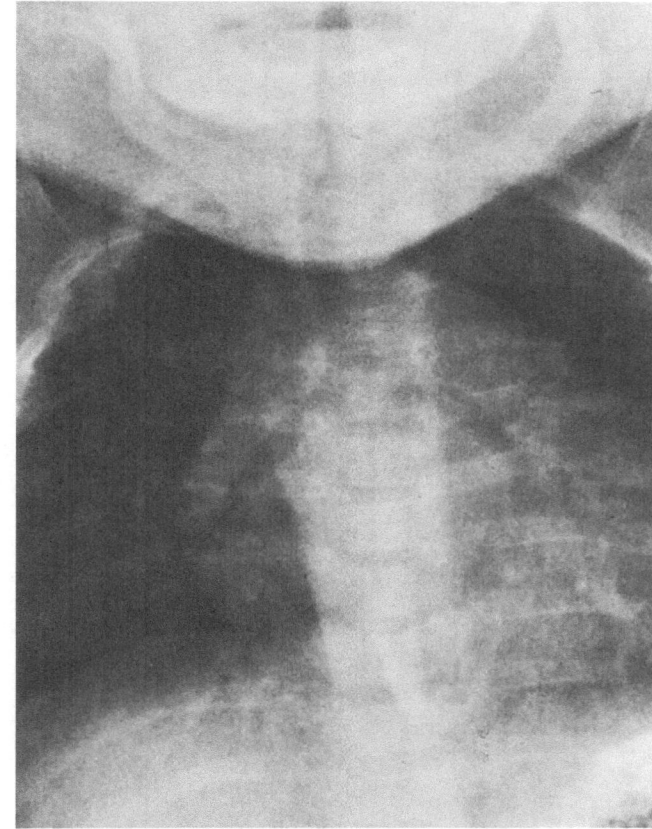

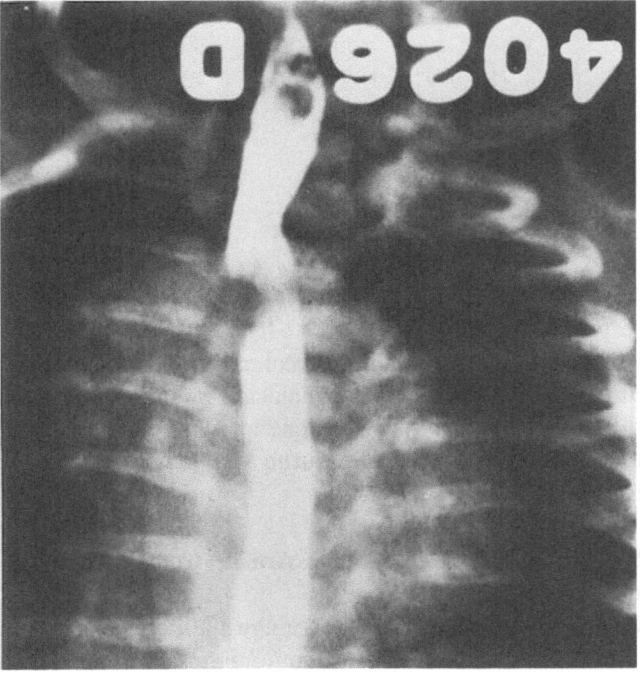

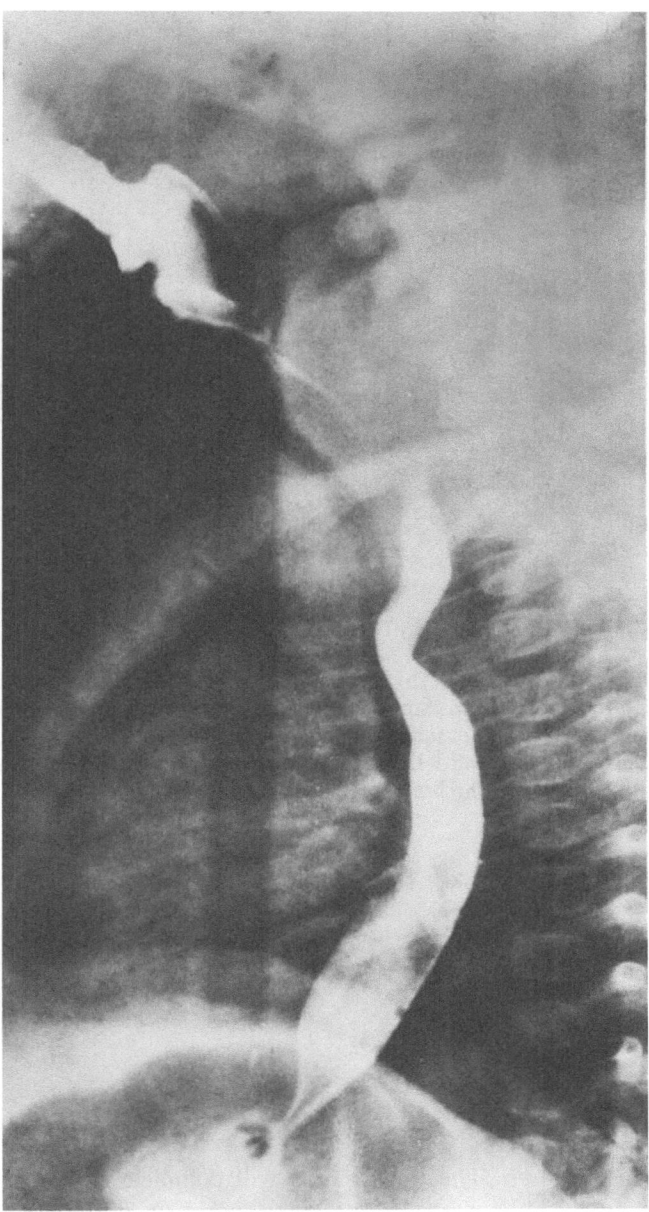

Fig. 7–211. *Left aortic arch with a right-sided descending aorta, normal brachiocephalic branching and a right ductus arteriosus arising from the descending aorta (vascular ring).* This 2½ month old girl had minimal stridor and dysphagia. **A** Frontal roentgenogram of the chest. **B–C** Frontal and lateral views of the barium esophagogram. **D–E** Frontal and lateral views of the left ventriculogram. In **A** the aortic arch is not clearly defined and no indentation is present on either side of the trachea. The descending aorta is on the right. In **B** the esophagus is indented on both sides, more on the right. An oblique indentation runs inferiorly and from left to right. In **C** a large posterior indentation is present in the esophagus. The trachea is also narrowed. (*Continued*)

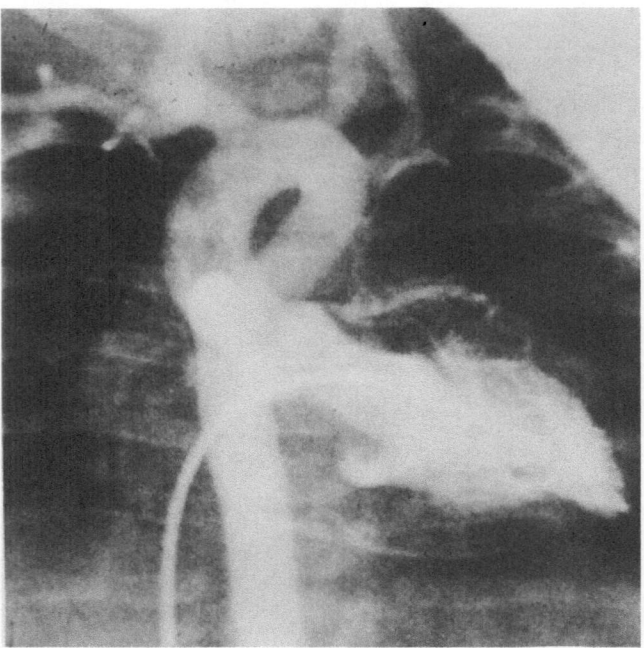

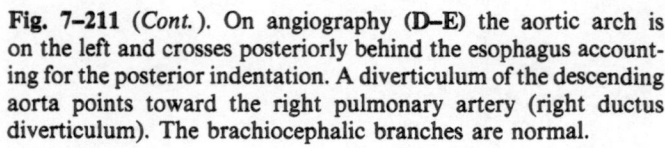

D

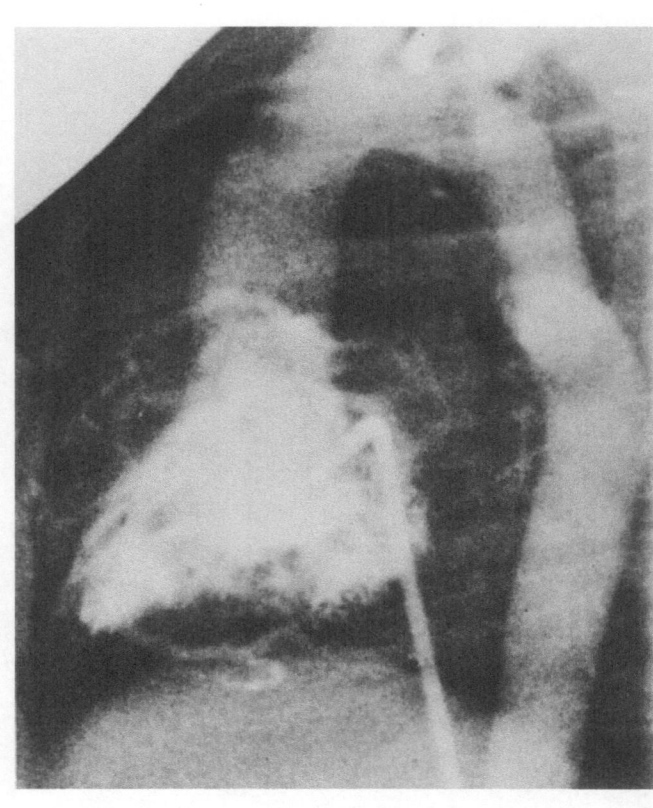

E

Fig. 7–211 (*Cont.*). On angiography (**D–E**) the aortic arch is on the left and crosses posteriorly behind the esophagus accounting for the posterior indentation. A diverticulum of the descending aorta points toward the right pulmonary artery (right ductus diverticulum). The brachiocephalic branches are normal.

diverticulum. The ductus thus will complete a vascular ring, which may or may not cause symptoms of dysphagia or obstruction to the airway. On occasion the aorta encircles the esophagus and trachea and descends on the right, resulting in a posterior indentation in the esophagus. The indentation may be horizontal, or it may be oriented obliquely downward toward the right. With an aortic diverticulum and with a right-sided descending aorta, the indentation is large.

Left Aortic Arch with Anomalous Origin of the Innominate or Left Common Carotid Artery (Bicarotid Origin)

Reported by Gross and by Klinkhamer, this entity is an unusual cause of dysphagia or dyspnea. The first two branches of the aorta arise very close together, or the innominate artery arises distal to its normal origin, thus enveloping the trachea anteriorly.

According to Gross and Klinkhamer the diagnosis is suggested by anterior compression of the trachea noted on a lateral roentgenogram of the chest or by tracheoscopy. The diagnosis of bicarotid origin is especially likely if the

narrowing is relatively constant during all phases of the respiratory cycle.

In contradistinction, if tracheal narrowing varies greatly during respiration, tracheomalacia is considered more likely. Klinkhamer reported relief of symptoms secondary to bicarotid origin after suturing the innominate artery to the sternum.

Single Brachiocephalic Trunk Arising from the Aortic Arch

Unless associated with other abnormalities of the aortic arch this rare anomaly is asymptomatic. The carotid and subclavian arteries may arise independently from the common trunk or from an "innominate" vessel on each side. In the case illustrated in Fig. 7–214 coarctation of the aorta was associated, and there was a ligament between the left subclavian artery and the proximal descending aorta. The case reported by McDowell et al. was discovered during carotid artery angiography for cerebral ischemia due to atherosclerosis.

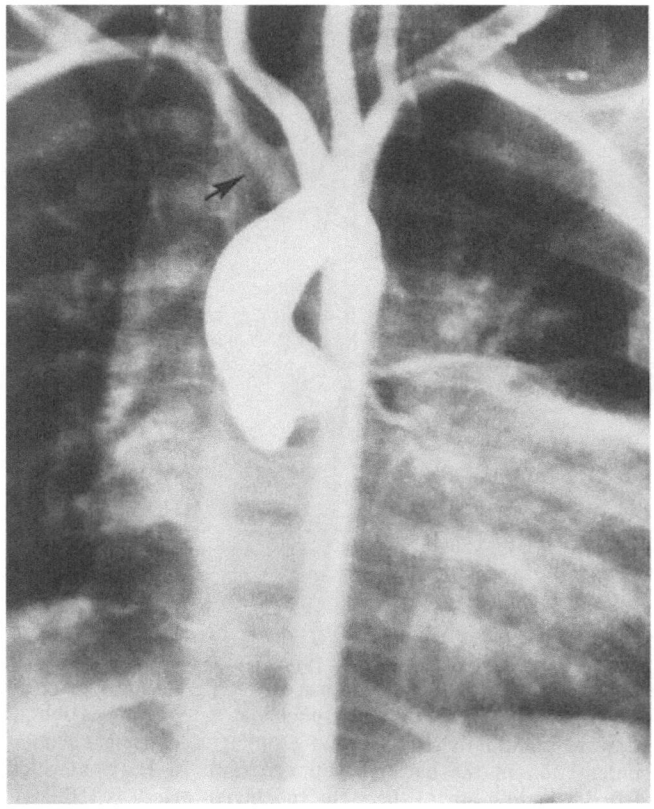

A

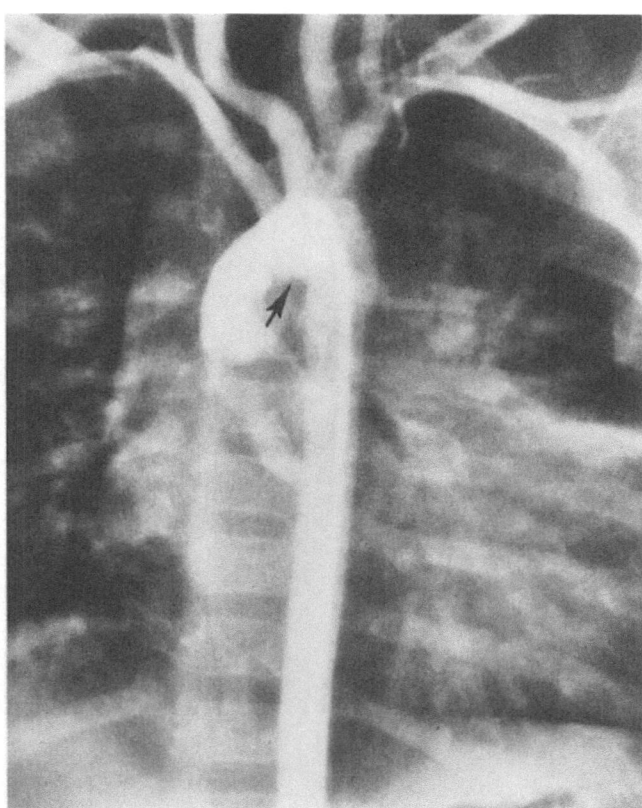

B

Fig. 7–212. *Aberrant right subclavian artery discovered incidentally during evaluation for ventricular septal defect in a 2-year-old girl.* On injection into the aortic root **(A)** four separate brachiocephalic vessels are opacified. The right subclavian artery is only faintly filled *(arrow)*. As the descending aorta fills during systole **(B)** the right subclavian artery fills more densely. In this frame the origin of the right subclavian artery from the descending aorta is demonstrated *(arrow)*. On the lateral projection **(C)** the aberrant right subclavian artery *(arrow)* is the fourth branch of the aortic arch. A closing patent ductus arteriosus is also noted *(open arrow)*.

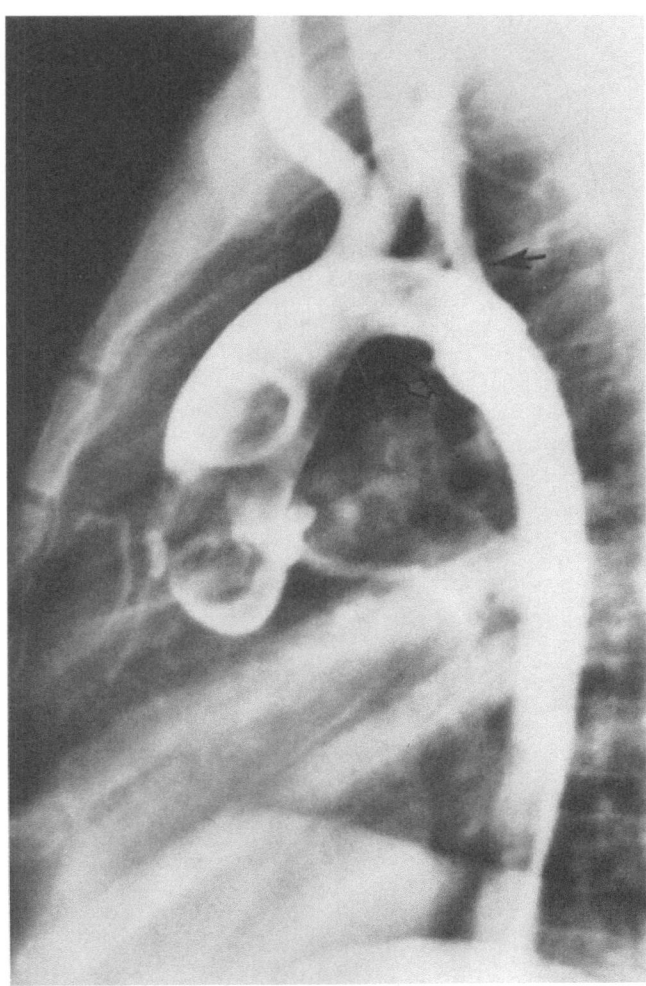

C

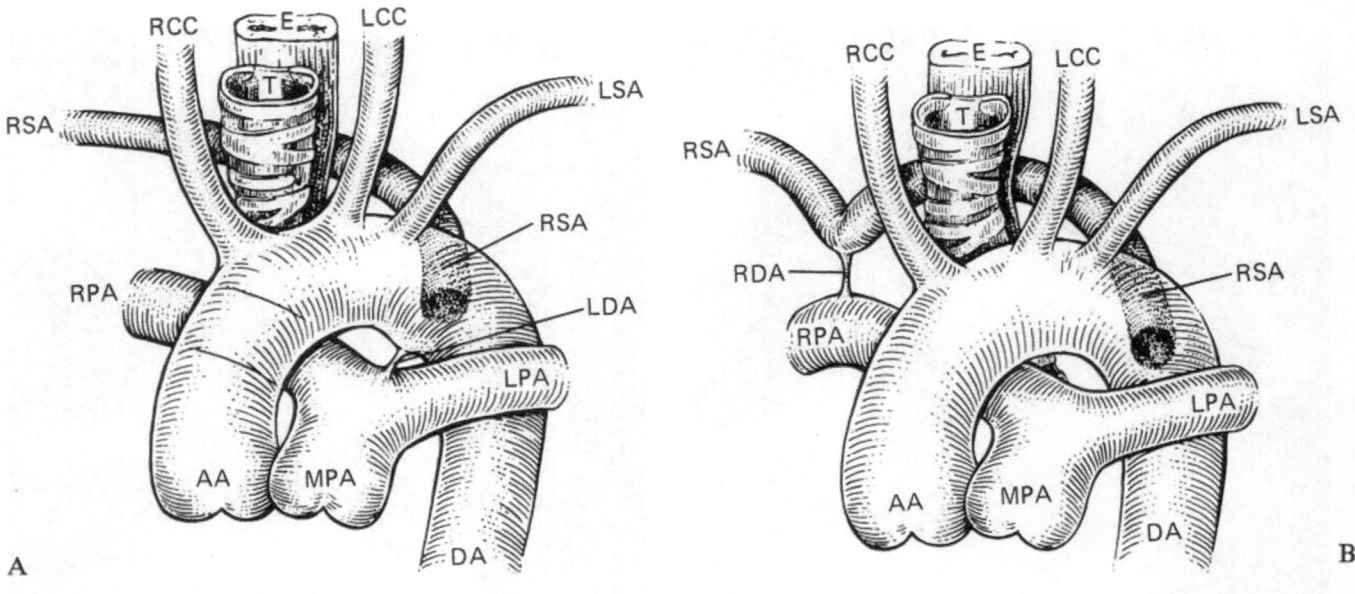

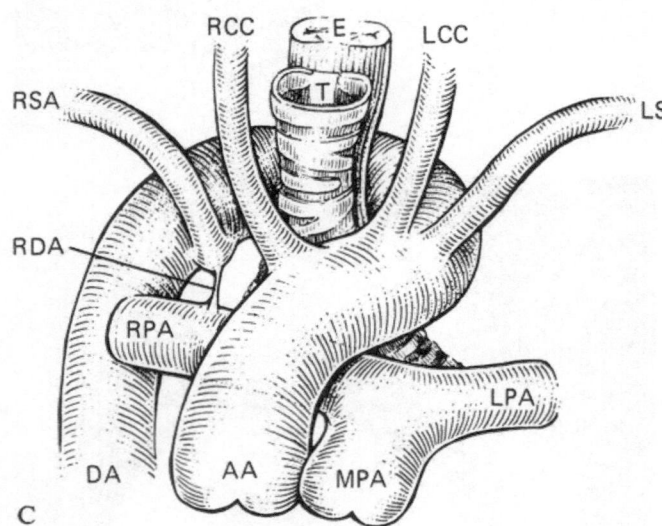

Fig. 7–213. *Three varieties of left aortic arch with aberrant right subclavian artery.* In all three types the right subclavian artery arises from the descending aorta. In **A** (left ductus arteriosus, left descending aorta) the right subclavian artery courses obliquely upward behind the trachea and esophagus, causing an oblique indentation in the barium esophagogram. In **B** (right ductus, left descending aorta) the right subclavian artery is tethered to the pulmonary artery by a ductus or ductus ligament, forming a vascular ring. In **C** (right ductus, right descending aorta) the aortic arch encircles the trachea and esophagus, producing a large indentation. The right ductus arteriosus is attached to the aorta near the aberrant right subclavian artery, creating a vascular ring. Modified from Stewart JR, et al. (1964) An atlas of vascular rings and related malformations of the aortic arch system. Thomas, Springfield, Ill., p 64.

AA = ascending aorta; *DA* = descending aorta; *LCC* = left common carotid artery; *LDA* = left ductus arteriosus; *LPA* = left pulmonary artery; *LSA* = left subclavian artery; *MPA* = main pulmonary artery; *RCC* = right common carotid artery; *RDA* = right ductus arteriosus; *RPA* = right pulmonary artery; *RSA* = right subclavian artery; *T* = trachea; *E* = esophagus.

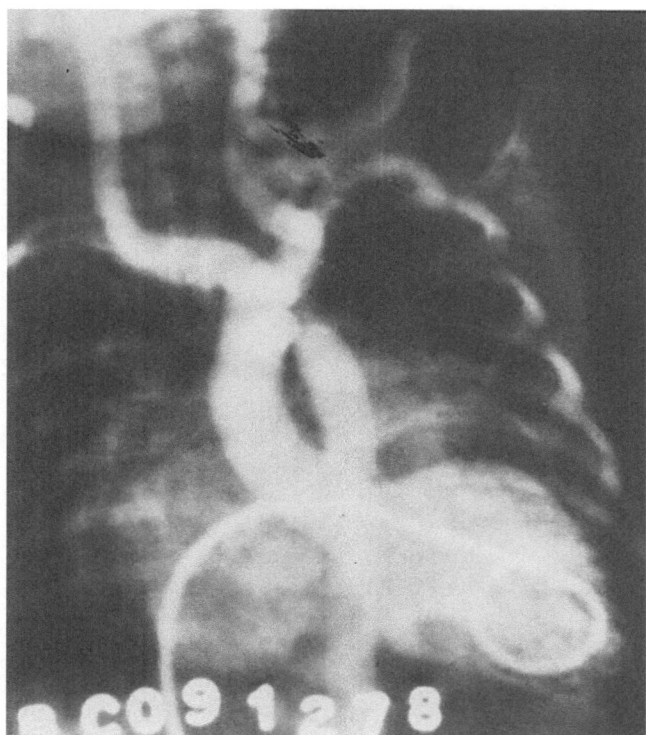

A

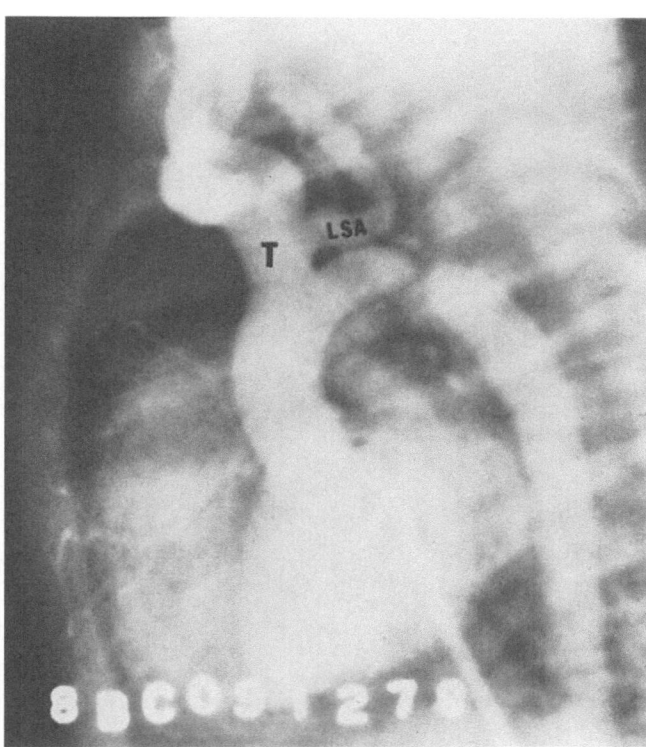

B

Fig. 7–214. *Single arterial trunk from the aortic arch in an infant with coarctation of the aorta.* The frontal projection of the left ventriculogram (**A**) demonstrates mitral insufficiency and a shunt at the atrial level. Coarctation of the aorta is delineated. The lateral film of the same angiogram (**B**) demonstrates the common arterial trunk (*T*) arising from the aorta. The left subclavian artery (*LSA*) is retracted posteriorly by a ligament noted at surgery to be attached to the proximal portion of the descending aorta. The right subclavian and the right common carotid arteries arise from an innominate-like vessel.

Cervical Aortic Arch

Cervical aortic arch is a rare, frequently asymptomatic, congenital anomaly in which the aortic arch lies high in the superior mediastinum on either side (Figs. 7–215 and 7–216), on occasion extending into the soft tissues of the neck. Variability of the origins of the branches of the aorta provides evidence for various hypotheses relating to the embryogenesis of the anomaly, although no single hypothesis explains all cases. The typical patient has a supraclavicular, pulsating mass on either side of the neck. Affected children may also have vascular rings as part of the cervical arch. Some children have symptoms of compression of the airway, even though a vascular ring is not present.

Moncada et al., and Shuford and Sybers have described the plain film findings of cervical aortic arch. These findings pertain primarily to right cervical aortic arch with a left-sided descending aorta and include nonspecific widening of the mediastinum, absence of the aortic knob, an oblique cutoff of the tracheal air column at the level of the thoracic inlet on the frontal view, and anterior displacement of the trachea on the lateral projection. The trachea is displaced and its air column obliterated by the retroesophageal segment of the aortic arch. In addition the authors of this work have noted a high takeoff of the descending aorta which is specific for a right cervical aortic arch with a left-sided descent (Fig. 7–215A). The barium swallow shows anterior displacement of the esophagus by the retroesophageal portion of the aortic arch.

In the authors' cases with left cervical aortic arch (Fig.

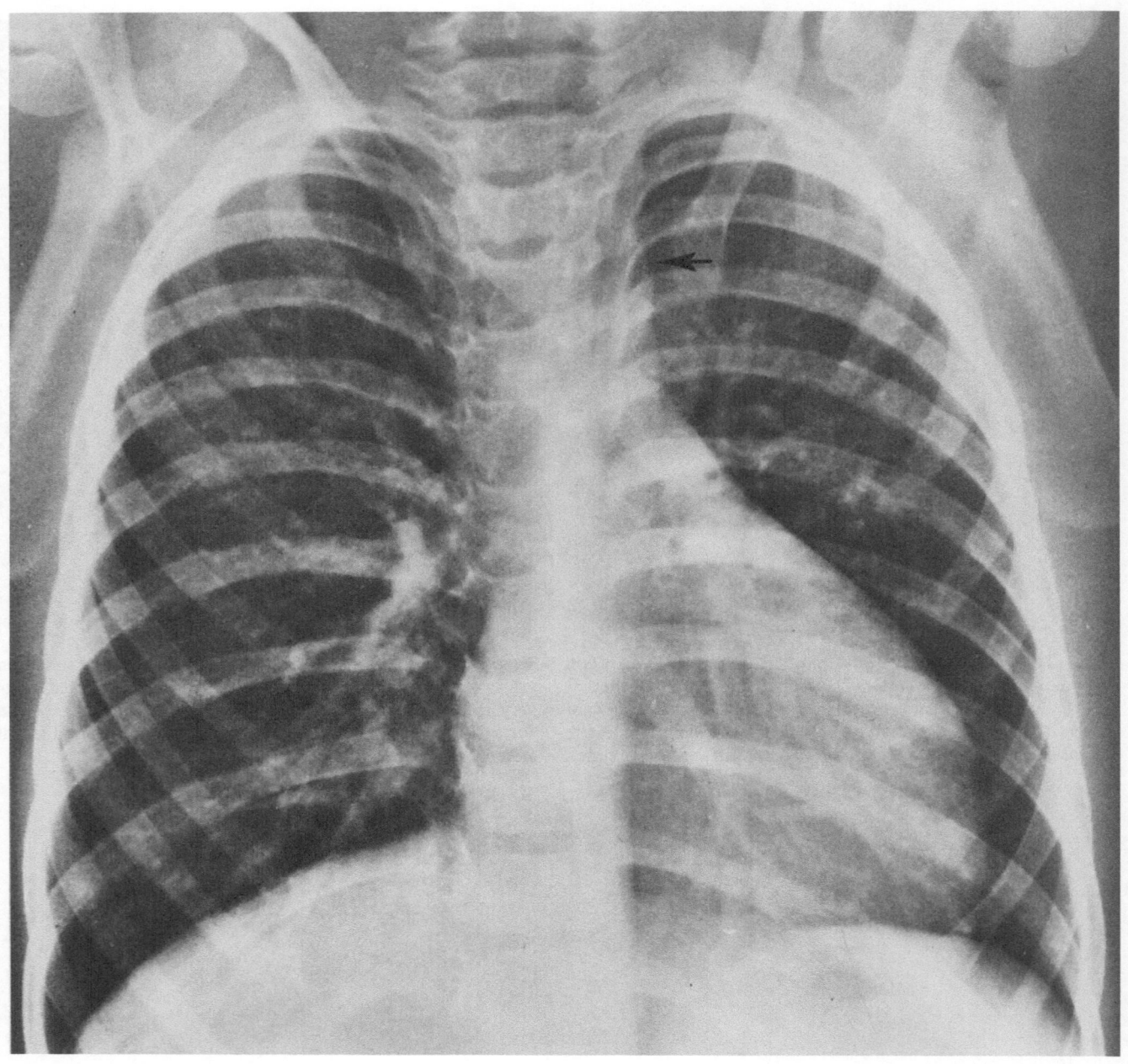

A

Fig. 7–215. *Right-sided cervical aortic arch in a 4-year-old boy with clinical findings of aortic stenosis.* The frontal roentgenogram of the chest (**A**) shows mild cardiomegaly with left ventricular enlargement. The superior mediastinum is widened by a right-sided cervical aortic arch. The trachea is obliterated by the posterior portion of the arch as it crosses to the left. The descending aorta starts high in the superior mediastinum (*arrow*). (*Continued*)

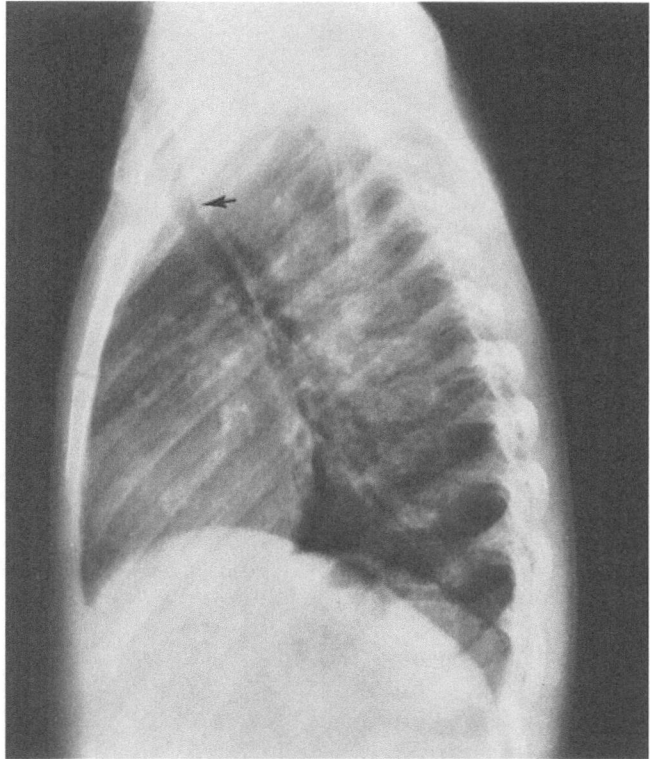

B

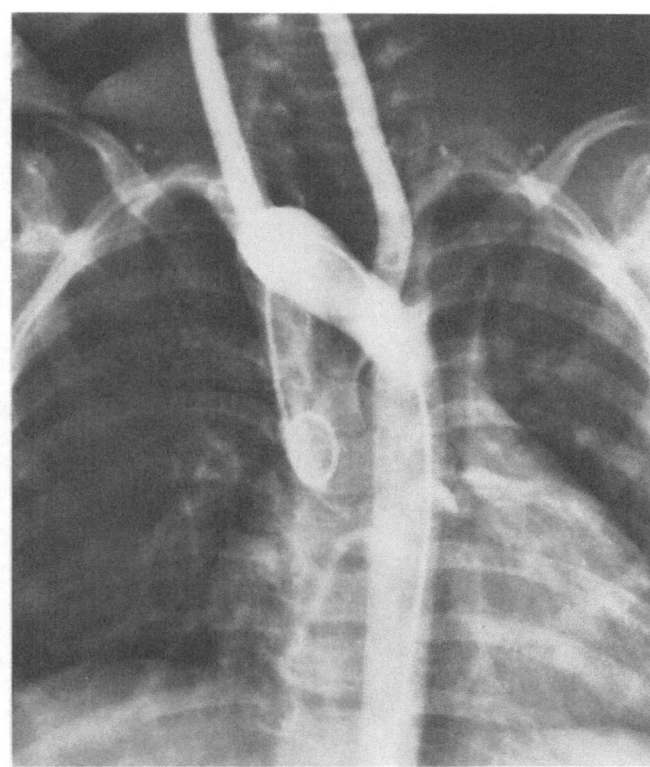

C

Fig. 7–215 (*Cont.*). On the lateral view (**B**) the trachea is displaced anteriorly by a density representing the aortic arch (*arrow*). The aortogram (**C**) demonstrates a right cervical arch that curves posteriorly behind the trachea and esophagus and descends on the left. The four brachiocephalic vessels that arise separately are the left common carotid artery, the right common carotid artery, the right subclavian artery and the left subclavian artery, which arises from the descending aorta. A bicuspid aortic valve was also noted (not shown).

7–216A) the most prominent roentgenographic feature is widening of the mediastinum by the aortic arch (aortic knob) which is in the apex of the left hemithorax. Continuity between the aortic arch and the descending aorta differentiates cervical aortic arch from other causes of widening of the mediastinum. The density of the ascending and descending aorta partially obliterates the carina and the proximal portion of the left main bronchus. The trachea is not deviated.

The barium swallow in patients with left cervical aortic arch shows that the esophagus is not indented but follows the course of the descending aorta in all views.

The two-dimensional echocardiogram from the suprasternal notch (Fig. 7–216B) shows the high position of the aortic arch and an acute angle formed between the aortic arch and the descending aorta. The branching may also be delineated. Doppler studies confirm the normal flow patterns.

On aortography (Figs. 7–215C, 7–217) the arch and the branching of the brachiocephalic vessels are delineated. Branching may be normal or mirror-image in type. The common carotid artery on the ipsilateral side with the arch may be absent, the internal and external carotid arteries arising separately from the aorta. The subclavian artery on the side opposite the arch often has an anomalous origin from the descending aorta. If the site of origin is stenotic, subclavian steal may result. Angiography will also delineate other congenital anomalies such as tetralogy of Fallot and bicuspid aortic valve.

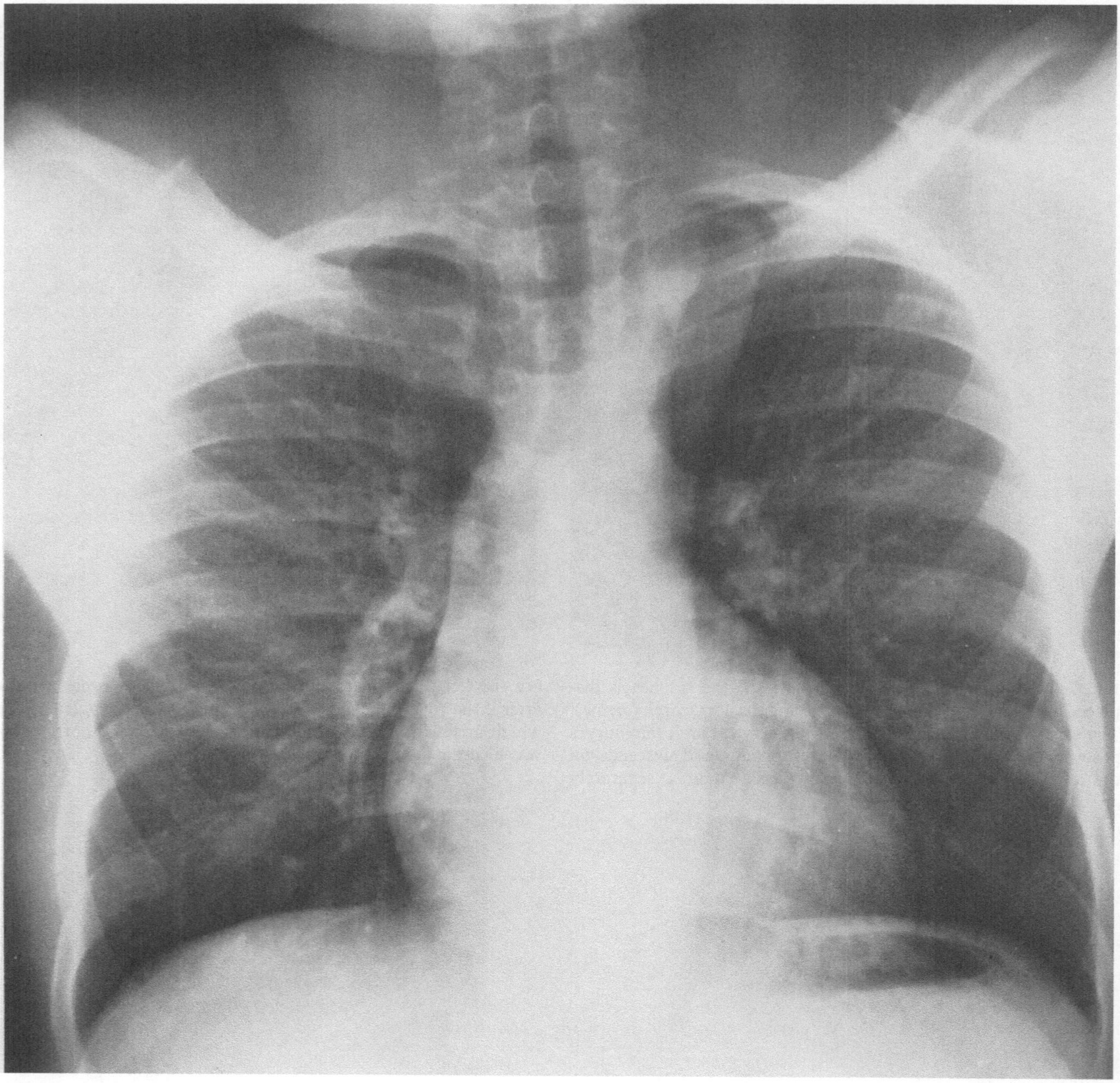

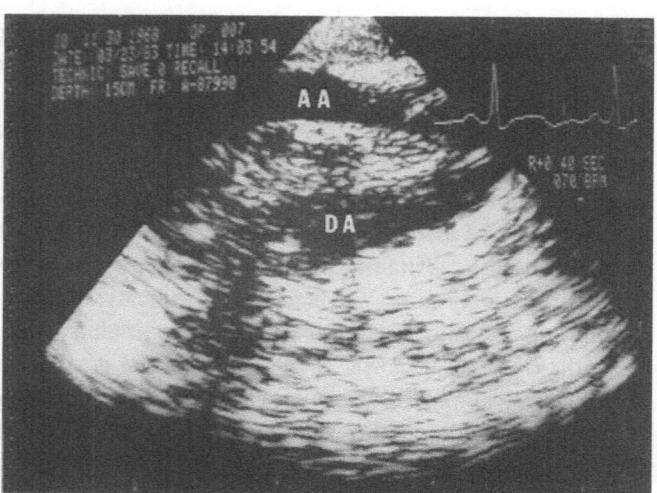

A

B

Fig. 7–216. *Left-sided cervical aortic arch in a 12-year-old boy with a pulsating mass in the left side of the neck.* **A** The frontal roentgenogram of the chest shows widening of the superior mediastinum. The aortic arch is high in the left thoracic apex. The descending aorta begins higher than usual. The carina and left main bronchus are partially obliterated by the ascending and descending portions of the aorta and by the esophagus. The trachea is not deviated. On the barium esophagogram (not shown) the esophagus followed the course of the descending aorta in all views. **B** The two-dimensional echocardiogram from the suprasternal notch demonstrates the high position of the aortic arch (*AA*) and the acute angle between the aortic arch and the descending aorta (*DA*). Aortography was not considered essential for diagnosis in this patient.

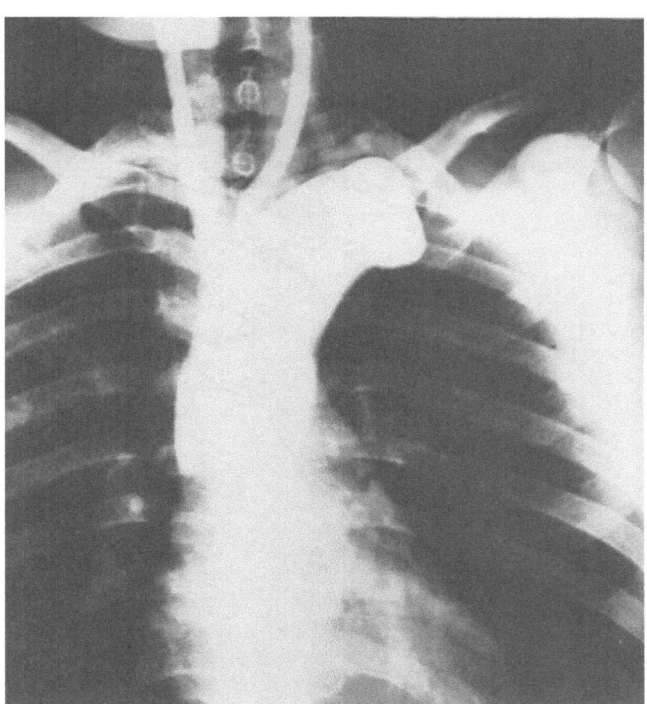

Fig. 7–217. *Aortography in an adult with left-sided cervical aortic arch.* The roentgenogram of the chest (not shown) demonstrated a soft tissue density in the left apex, which was in continuity with the descending aorta. The high position of the arch is demonstrated. The brachiocephalic vessels (not shown) arose in this order: (1) right common carotid, (2) left common carotid, (3) left subclavian, (4) right subclavian artery (aberrant). Courtesy of Alfred Kurtz, M.D., Jefferson Hospital Medical Center, Philadelphia, Pennsylvania.

Interruption of the Aortic Arch (Steidele Complex)

Interruption of the aortic arch is a rarely encountered cardiovascular malformation occurring in less than 1% of all congenital heart defects. It is characterized by failure of connection between the ascending and the descending aorta. The descending aorta receives blood from the pulmonary artery by way of the ductus arteriosus during fetal life and until the ductus closes after birth (Fig. 7–218).

Interruption of the aortic arch should be distinguished from atresia of the aortic arch, which is also a very rare anomaly. Interruption of the aortic arch is characterized by complete absence of tissue connecting the arch and the descending aorta, whereas atresia of the aortic arch has a fibrous band between the aortic arch and the descending aorta. Interruption of the aortic arch usually occurs between the left common carotid artery and the left subclavian artery (45%; type B, Figs. 7–218, 7–219), between the left subclavian artery and the ductus arteriosus (42%; type A, Fig. 7–218) or between the innominate and left common carotid arteries (4%; type C, Fig. 7–218). Variations of these three types occur when the right subclavian artery arises from the proximal segment of the descending aorta (aberrant right subclavian artery) or from the right ductus (isolation of the right subclavian artery). Physiologi-

cally, interruption of the aortic arch resembles severe coarctation of the aorta proximal to the ductus arteriosus (preductal coarctation). In both disorders the ascending aorta is supplied by the LV and the descending aorta by the RV through the ductus.

Interruption of the aortic arch invariably is associated with a patent ductus arteriosus and almost always with a ventricular septal defect. Another defect frequently associated with interruption of the aortic arch is absence of the subpulmonary infundibulum. An atrial septal defect is not uncommon. Among other associated cardiovascular abnormalities are the hypoplastic left heart syndrome, transposition of the great vessels and aortic stenosis.

The ventricular septal defect and the characteristic subaortic stenosis in some patients with interruption of the aortic arch appear to be the result of malalignment of the infundibular septum and septal band (trabecula septomarginalis), with posterior and leftward deviation of the conal or infundibular septum. The ventricular septal defect is often subpulmonary in location. Prolapse of an aortic cusp may be observed, and the pulmonary artery may override the interventricular septum. A combination of all these cardiac disorders associated with interruption of the aortic arch constitutes the Becu complex. The Becu complex should be differentiated from the Taussig-Bing complex, a form of double-outlet RV in which the pulmonary artery overrides the ventricular septum. In the Becu complex the aorta arises from the LV, and the great vessels are related normally, whereas in the Taussig-Bing complex the aorta arises from the RV and is anterior to the pulmonary artery.

Interruption of the aortic arch has been sporadically reported in association with truncus arteriosus and with aorticopulmonary septal defects (aorticopulmonary window). In the latter, the ventricular septum is commonly intact. The DiGeorge syndrome (third and fourth pharyngeal pouch syndrome) consists of underdevelopment of the thymus and parathyroid glands, together with abnormalities of the conotruncus (e.g., truncus arteriosus, tetralogy of Fallot) and aortic arch (e.g., right aortic arch, interrupted aorta). Although patients with DiGeorge syndrome have hypocalcemia and a deficit in cellular immunity (T-cell deficiency) the initial symptoms often are related to the severe congenital cardiac defects.

Clinical Features Most infants with interruption of the aortic arch have generalized cyanosis and congestive heart failure. If pulses are absent in the legs the clinical picture may be indistinguishable from severe coarctation of the aorta. If the pulses are weak in the arms as well, the presentation is like that observed in the hypoplastic left heart syndrome. A clue to the diagnosis of interrupted arch is the presence of bounding pulses in the carotid arteries with weak pulses elsewhere. Differential cyanosis is a rare finding. The electrocardiogram, while not specific, usually shows RA and RV hypertrophy.

Echocardiography Echocardiography is helpful in delineating the nature of the intracardiac abnormalities. Two-dimensional echocardiography, with the probe in the suprasternal region, may outline the interrupted arch. The ascending aorta may be small and has a vertical course, rather than curving posteriorly as is normal. The descending aorta is continuous with the ductus arteriosus.

Radiological (Plain Film) Features Films of the chest may show overcirculation or pulmonary venous hypertension or both, with enlargement of the right side of the heart and marked prominence of the pulmonary artery segment. A trachea positioned in the midline, not deviated by the crossing of the aorta, and absence of the normal aortic impression on the barium-filled esophagus are helpful signs, particularly in an individual with poor pulses or absence of pulses in the extremities and bounding carotid pulses.

Hemodynamics In the neonatal period if these defects are suspected clinically and by echocardiography, an infusion of prostaglandin E_1 is begun prior to cardiac catheterization in order to maintain patency of the ductus arteriosus, which is the only source of blood flow to the descending aorta. Usually a left-to-right shunt (oxygen step-up) is encountered in the RA due to elevation of LA pressure and stretching of the foramen ovale (congestive heart failure). If a ventricular septal defect is present, a left-to-right shunt is encountered in the RV as well. Pressure in the RV, the pulmonary artery, and the descending aorta are equal if the ductus is widely patent. The LV is normally saturated; whereas the descending aorta has a lower oxygen content because its source of supply is the ductus arteriosus. Desaturation in the descending aorta may not be severe, as the blood in the right side of the heart is fairly well saturated due to the atrial and ventricular left-to-right shunts.

Contrast Studies Angiocardiography is essential in demonstrating the site of interruption and associated anomalies (e.g., ventricular septal defect commonly with a left-to-right shunt and an obligatory right-to-left ductus shunt). The ascending aorta may be small. A subclavian steal may be present when one or both subclavian arteries arise from the descending aorta and the ductus is partially or completely closed, producing lower pressure in the descending aorta than in the ascending aorta.

An important clue to the distinction among interrupted arch, severe coarctation, hypoplasia of the aortic isthmus, and aortic atresia, is the curve of the ascending aorta. With coarctation and aortic atresia, the aorta curves posteriorly and leftward toward the transverse arch. With aortic interruption, the ascending aorta follows a relatively straight vertical course toward the brachiocephalic vessels. Only type A (beyond the left subclavian artery) may have a slight curve, which is not the normal curve of the aorta.

Treatment Prostaglandin E_1 may temporarily open the ductus arteriosus in infants with no blood flow to the lower body. Surgical intervention consists of interposition of a tubular prosthetic graft to establish continuity between the ascending and descending aorta. The ductus arteriosus is closed as well. The ventricular septal defect may be closed at the same time, or a pulmonary artery band may be placed to control the left-to-right shunt through the ventricular septal defect.

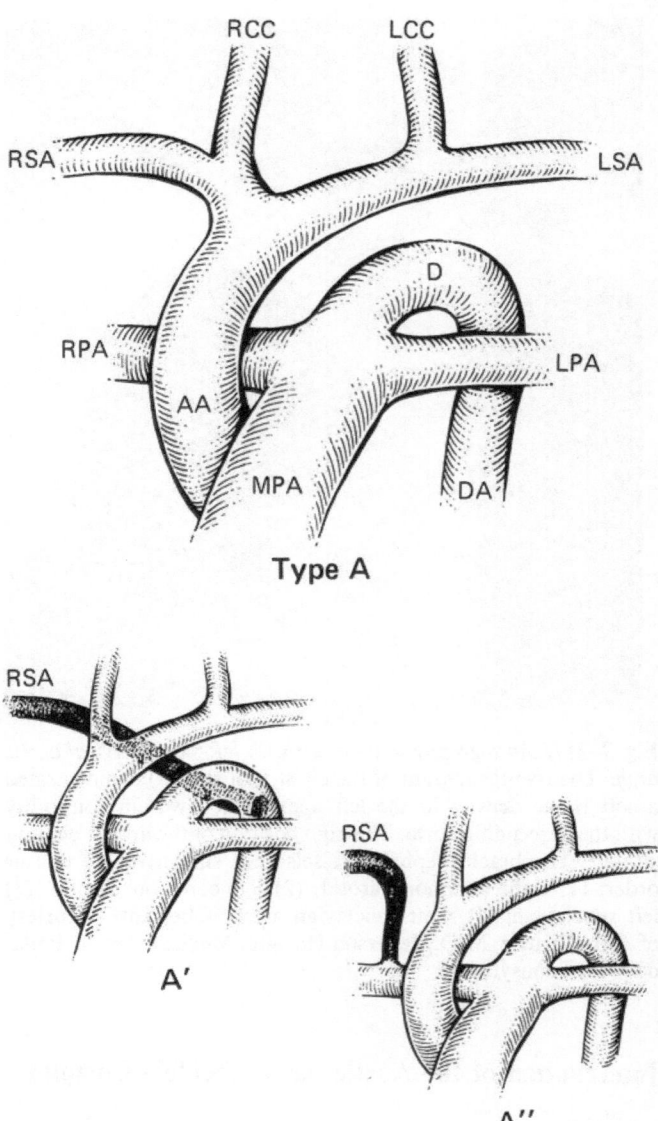

Fig. 7-218. *The types of interrupted aortic arch.* All forms of interrupted arch have in common discontinuity between the ascending aorta and the descending aorta. The pulmonary artery is in continuity with the descending aorta by way of the ductus arteriosus. In type A the interruption occurs beyond the left subclavian artery; in type B, between the left common carotid and the left subclavian artery; in type C, between the innominate artery and the left common carotid artery. In each of the three types the right subclavian artery (*RSA*) may arise normally from

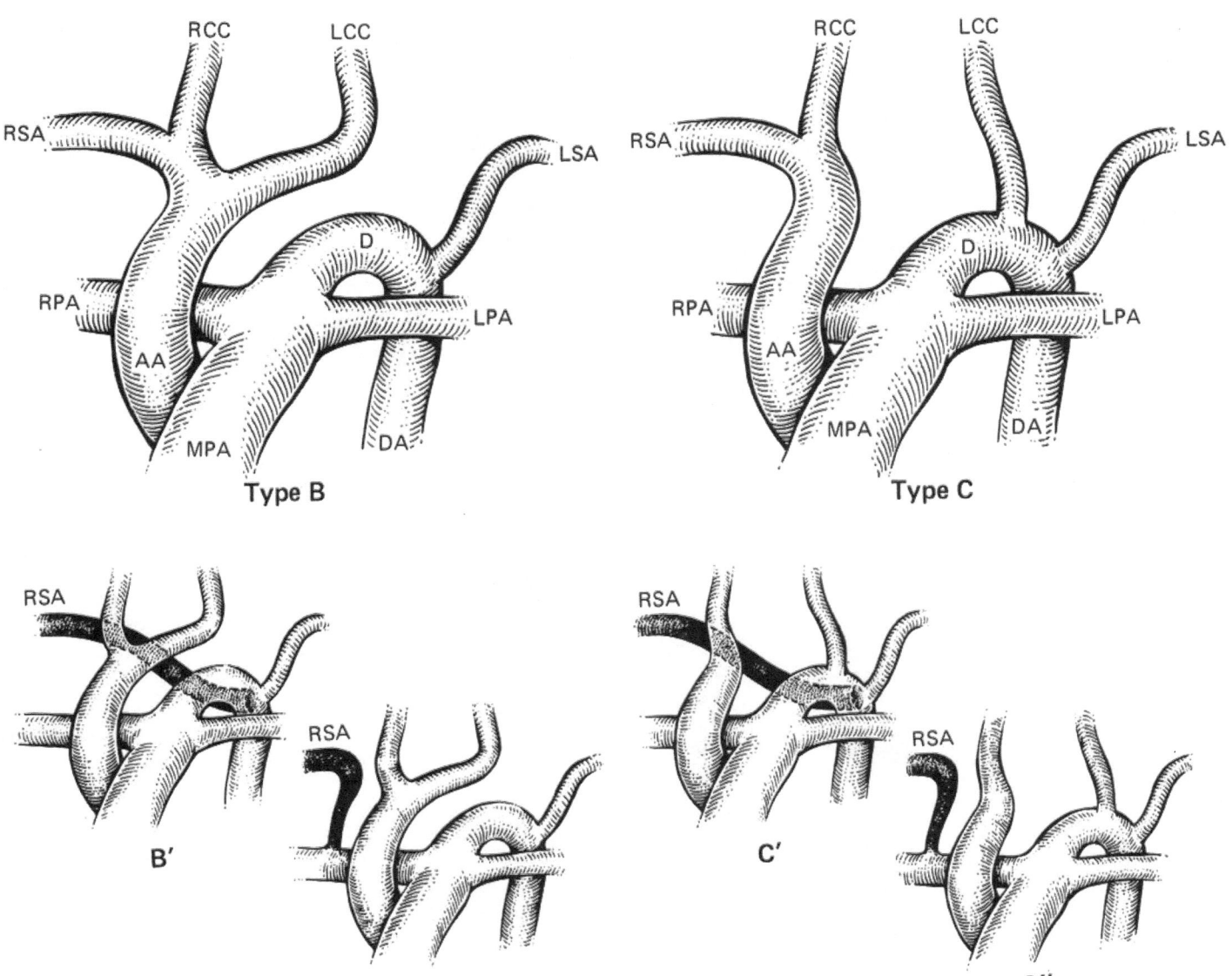

Type B

Type C

B'

B''

C'

C''

the innominate artery (types A, B and C) or may arise aberrantly from the proximal segment of the descending aorta (A', B' and C') or from the right pulmonary artery by way of a right ductus arteriosus (A", B" and C").

AA = ascending aorta; *D* = ductus arteriosus; *DA* = descending aorta; *LCC* = left common carotid artery; *LPA* = left pulmonary artery; *LSA* = left subclavian artery; *MPA* = main pulmonary artery; *RCC* = right common carotid artery; *RPA* = right pulmonary artery; *RSA* = right subclavian artery.

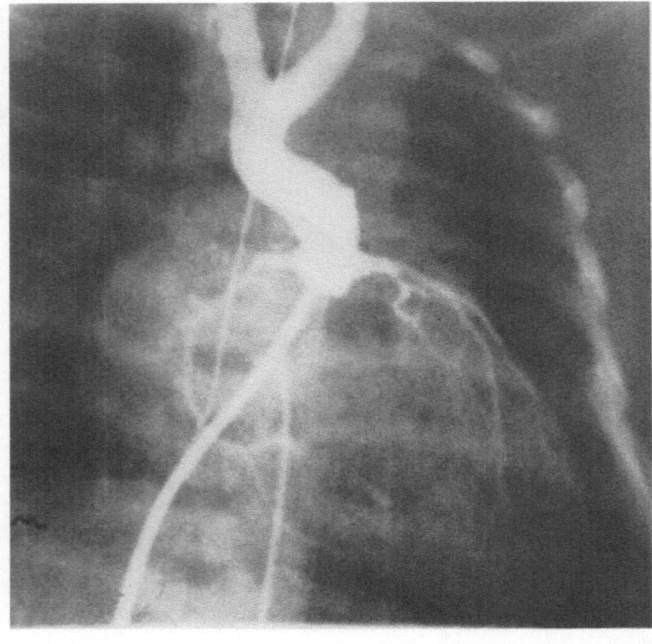

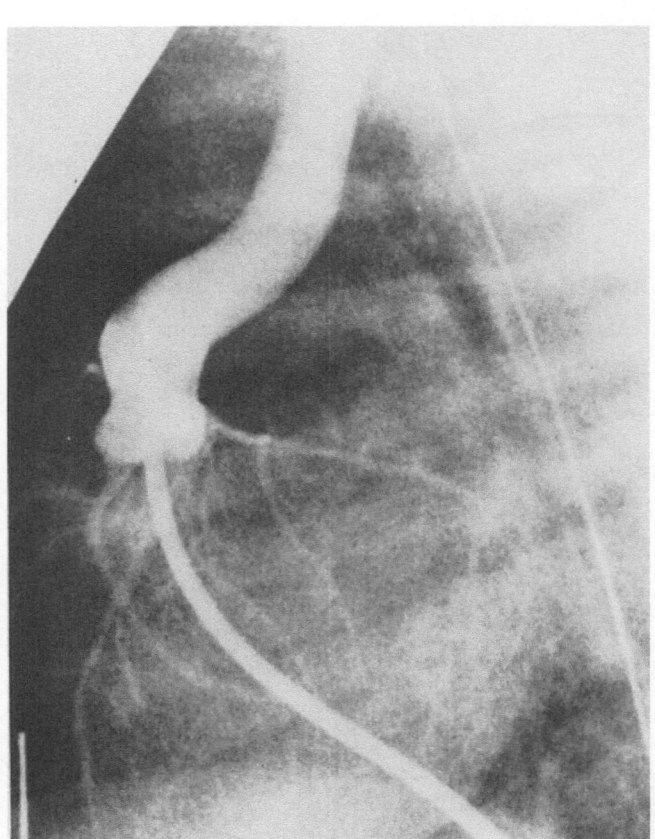

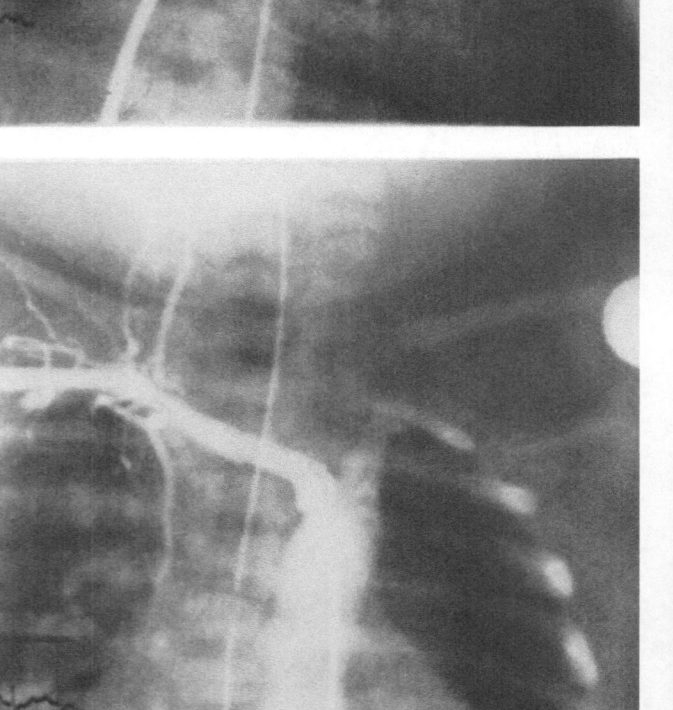

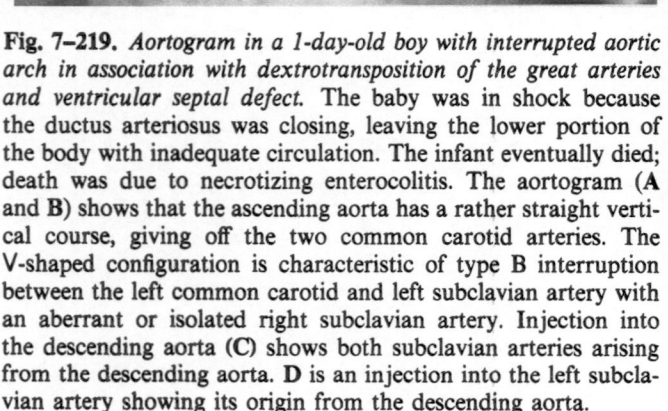

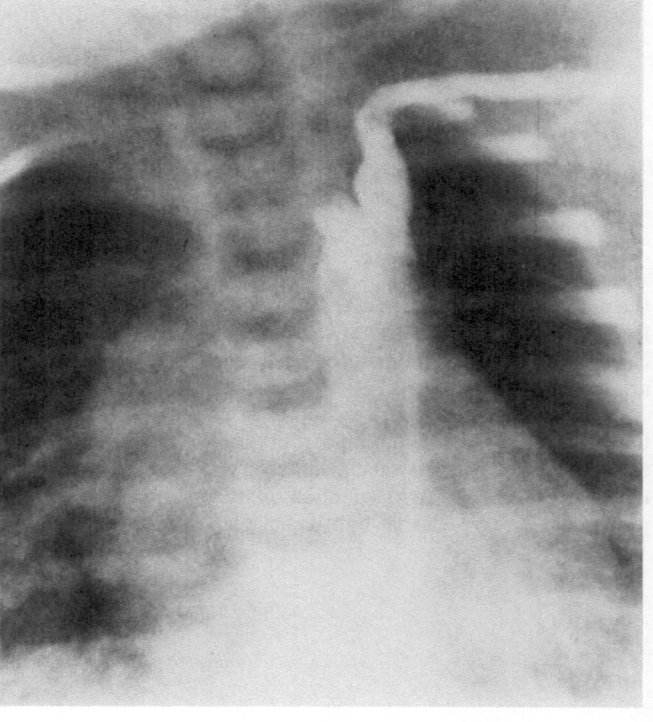

Fig. 7–219. *Aortogram in a 1-day-old boy with interrupted aortic arch in association with dextrotransposition of the great arteries and ventricular septal defect.* The baby was in shock because the ductus arteriosus was closing, leaving the lower portion of the body with inadequate circulation. The infant eventually died; death was due to necrotizing enterocolitis. The aortogram (**A** and **B**) shows that the ascending aorta has a rather straight vertical course, giving off the two common carotid arteries. The V-shaped configuration is characteristic of type B interruption between the left common carotid and left subclavian artery with an aberrant or isolated right subclavian artery. Injection into the descending aorta (**C**) shows both subclavian arteries arising from the descending aorta. **D** is an injection into the left subclavian artery showing its origin from the descending aorta.

Fig. 7–220. A *Diagram of a pulmonary sling.*
The left pulmonary artery (*LPA*) arises from
the right pulmonary artery (*RPA*) and passes
between the esophagus (*E*) and trachea (*T*)
to enter the left lung. *MPA* = main pulmonary artery. (*Continued*)

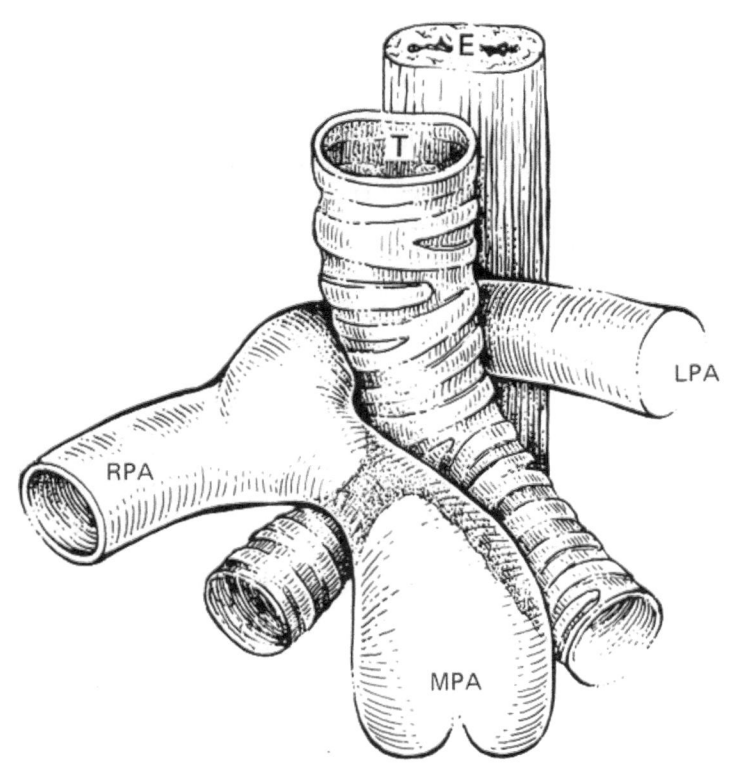

A

Pulmonary Artery Sling

Pulmonary artery sling (aberrant left pulmonary artery)
is an uncommon anomaly in which the left pulmonary
artery arises from the proximal portion of the right main
pulmonary artery. The aberrant left pulmonary artery then
courses between the esophagus and trachea to enter the
left lung (Fig. 7–220A). A pulmonary sling usually occurs
as an isolated anomaly. However, cardiovascular, tracheoesophageal and gastrointestinal anomalies may be noted.
Cardiovascular anomalies include ventricular septal defect,
atrial septal defect, patent ductus arteriosus, tetralogy of
Fallot, single ventricle and persistent left superior vena
cava. The ductus (or ligamentum arteriosum), if present,
connects the proximal descending aorta to the main pulmonary artery rather than to the aberrant left pulmonary
artery. The aberrant left pulmonary artery causes compression of the trachea and right main bronchus, resulting in
respiratory symptoms in the neonatal period. Stridor associated with a pulmonary sling is said to be most evident
on expiration, while stridor associated with other vascular
rings is more evident on inspiration. Dysphagia is unusual
with a pulmonary sling.

Radiographic findings include indentation of the distal
trachea and proximal right main bronchus on the frontal
view and a soft-tissue mass interposed between the trachea
and esophagus on the lateral film (Fig. 7–220B-C). The
trachea is narrow on the lateral projection. The barium
esophagogram exhibits an anterior pressure defect (Fig.
7–220C). A similar anterior indentation on the barium-
filled esophagus may also be present in ductus arteriosus
sling. Rarely an aberrant subclavian artery may course
between the trachea and the esophagus. Right-sided or
left-sided lobar emphysema is often observed during early
infancy. Atelectasis and infection are also found. An
opaque right or left upper lobe, due to retained fetal pulmonary fluid, may be the only radiographic finding in neonates.

The pulmonary arteriogram demonstrates the origin of
the left pulmonary artery from an elongated main pulmonary trunk.

At surgery the aberrant vessel is divided and anastomosed to the main pulmonary artery or brought forward
and reanastomosed to the original stump anterior to the
trachea. An interposing graft or conduit may be needed.
Surgical results have been uniformly poor. However,
Campbell et al. have reported a 24-year follow-up of the
first patient operated on for this anomaly.

Fig. 7–220 (*Cont.*). **B–C** *Pulmonary sling in an infant in severe respiratory distress.* The lateral roentgenogram (**B**) of the chest shows a dense mass interposed between the trachea and the air-filled esophagus. The barium esophagogram (**C**) confirms the plain film findings. The esophagus is indented anteriorly by the aberrant pulmonary artery. The baby died before further studies or a surgical procedure could be performed.

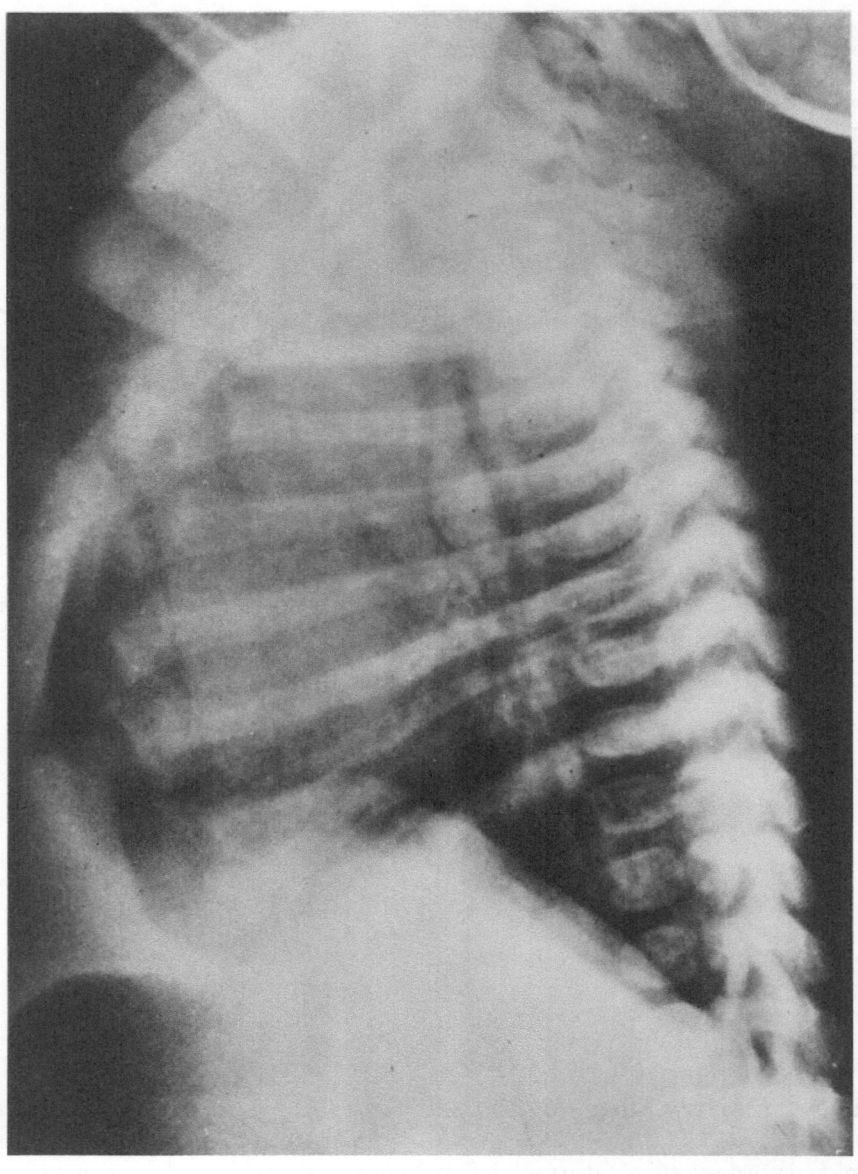

B

Ductus Arteriosus Sling

Ductus arteriosus sling consists of an abnormal vessel connecting the right main pulmonary artery and the isthmic portion of the thoracic aorta. The vessel passes between the trachea and the esophagus, causing airway compression (Fig. 7–221). The unusual course may represent persistence of a primitive connection between the primary pulmonary arteries that has been identified in 8-mm embryos connecting to the aorta by way of the most dorsal segment of the ductus arteriosus. Binet et al. reported a patient who also had an aberrant right subclavian artery.

The clinical presentation is similar to that reported with pulmonary sling. The barium esophagogram shows a mass between the trachea and esophagus.

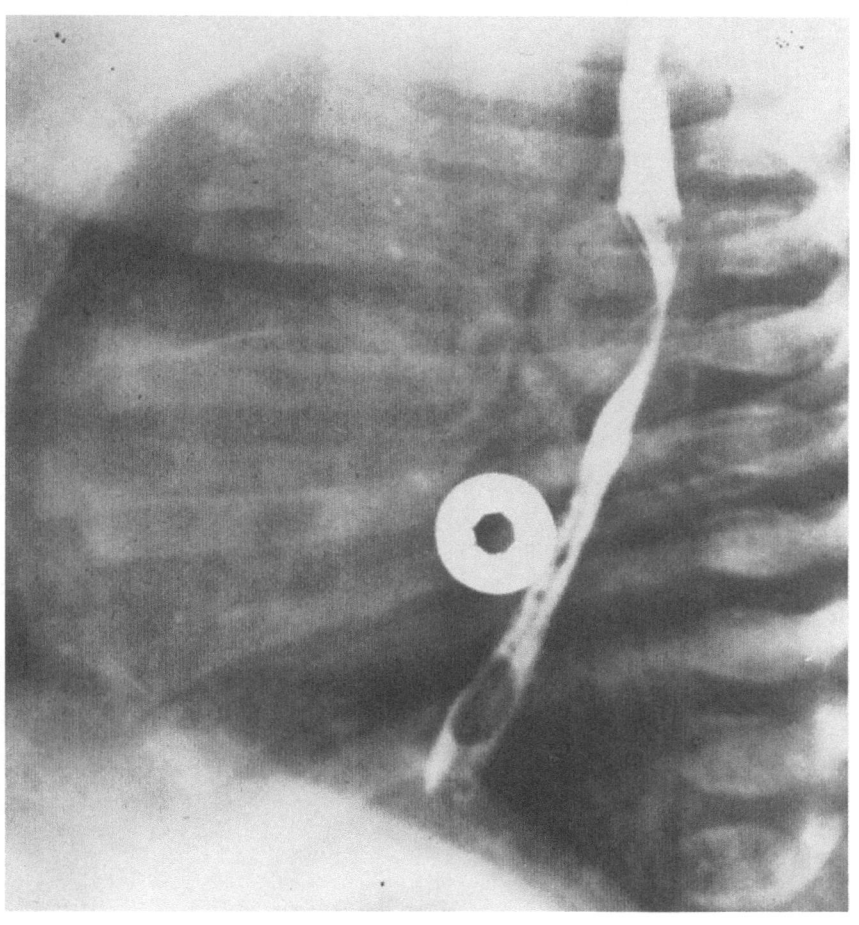

C

Fig. 7–221. *A ductus arteriosus sling.* The ductus arteriosus sling (*DS*) arises from the right pulmonary artery (*RPA*), passes between the trachea (*T*) and esophagus (*E*) and attaches to the isthmic portion of the aorta. In this drawing the other brachiocephalic vessels have been eliminated for clarity. *LPA* = left pulmonary artery; *MPA* = main pulmonary artery; *Ao* = aorta; *RSA* = right subclavian artery; *RB* = right bronchus; *LB* = left bronchus. In the case described by Binet et al. there was also an aberrant right subclavian artery.

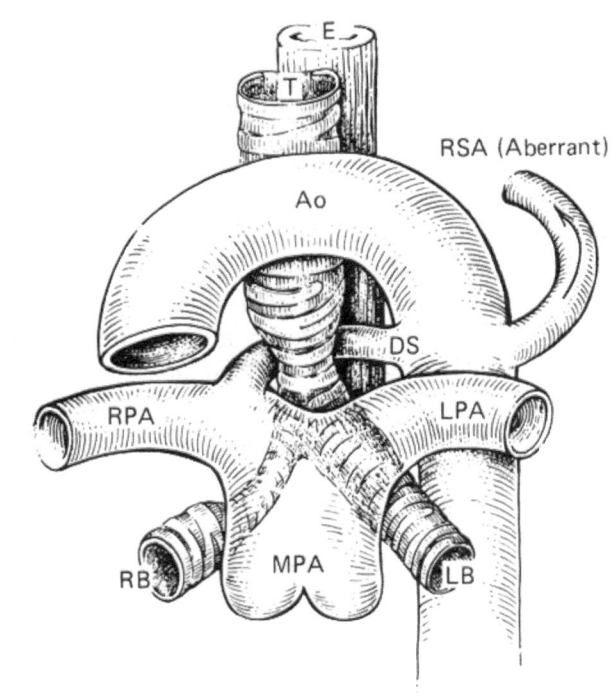

Aortography will demonstrate patency of the abnormal vessel with the unusual course described here. At surgery the anomalous vessel may be divided at both ends. The indentation in the trachea may persist thereafter so that stridor may not resolve for some time.

Fig. 7-222. *Anomalous origin of the right pulmonary artery from the aorta (right hemitruncus).* **A** Mild cardiomegaly is present with unilateral, right-sided pulmonary overcirculation. The lateral projection **(B)** is from the same patient 7 years later. The large right pulmonary artery is reflected as a circular structure anterior to the trachea. The posterior view of a pulmonary perfusion scan **(C)**, using ^{131}I-MAA (macroaggregated albumin human serum tagged with ^{131}I) demonstrates perfusion of the left lung only, with no perfusion to the right lung. This occurs because venous blood enters the left lung, while the right lung receives its blood supply from the aorta. Left ventriculography in the frontal view **(D)** demonstrates the origin of the right pulmonary artery from the posterior wall of the ascending aorta, accounting for the unilateral pulmonary overcirculation on the plain film of the chest. The second catheter is the venous catheter, which traverses the right atrium and right ventricle to enter the main pulmonary artery. *(Continued)*

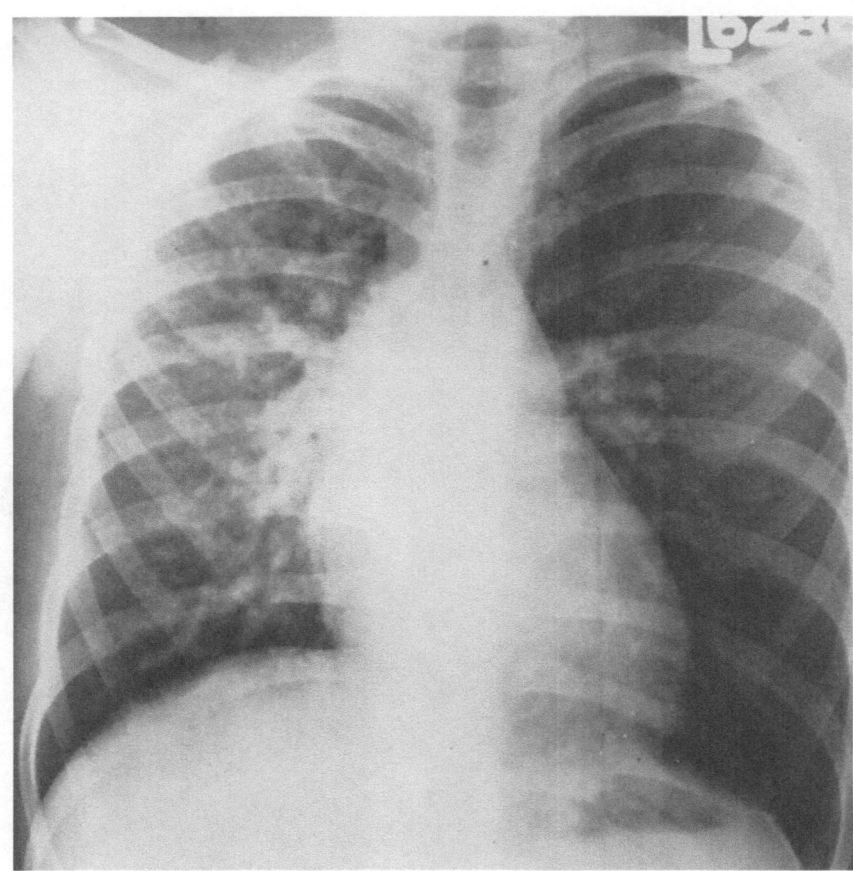

A

Anomalous Origin of One Pulmonary Artery from the Ascending Aorta (Hemitruncus)

Ectopic origin of the right or left pulmonary artery from the aorta (so-called hemitruncus) is a rare cardiovascular malformation. It is probably the result of faulty septation of the truncus with dorsal rotation of the left or right truncoconal ridge causing the ipsilateral sixth arch to be incorporated into the ascending aorta. Flow patterns in the affected fetus are thought to favor persistence of the contralateral fourth arch. Thus the aortic arch is found on the side opposite the ectopic pulmonary artery.

Anomalous origin of the right pulmonary artery (A-RPA) is by far the most common variety (Fig. 7-222). It is almost always associated with a patent ductus arteriosus, but rarely with an aorticopulmonary window; however, it usually presents without a defect in the ventricular septum. Anomalous origin of the left pulmonary artery (A-LPA) usually occurs as part of complex tetralogy of Fallot (Fig. 7-223) with right aortic arch and rarely with right ductus arteriosus.

Clinical Features Respiratory distress, congestive heart failure and cyanosis are the predominant clinical manifestations. The electrocardiogram usually shows right ventricular hypertrophy or combined hypertrophy. Signs of severe pulmonary hypertension and pulmonary vascular disease usually appear early if therapy is not instituted.

Radiological (Plain Film) Features The characteristic findings in patients without additional defects are overcircula-

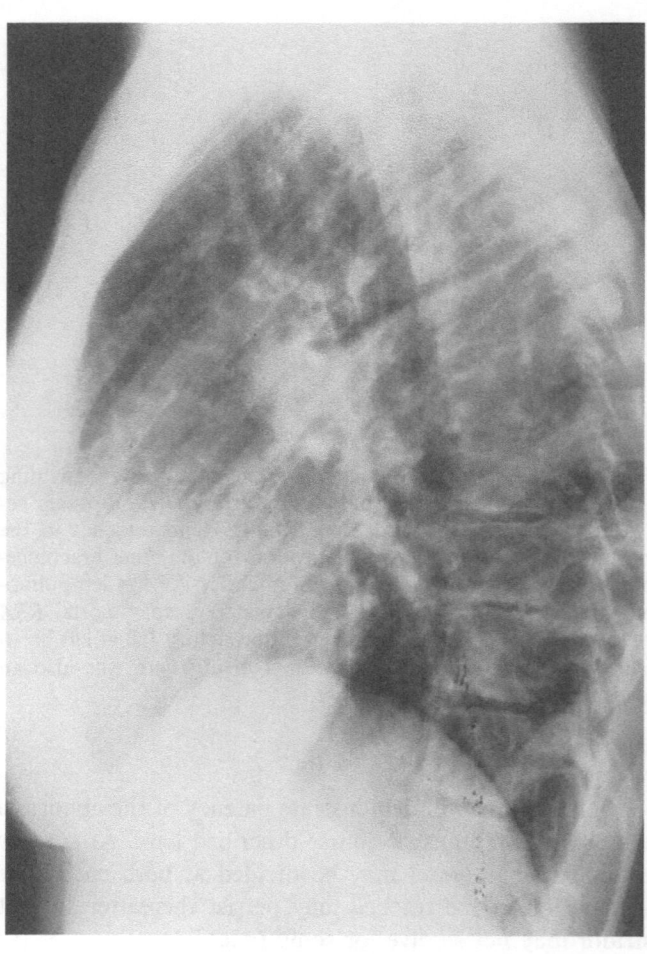

B

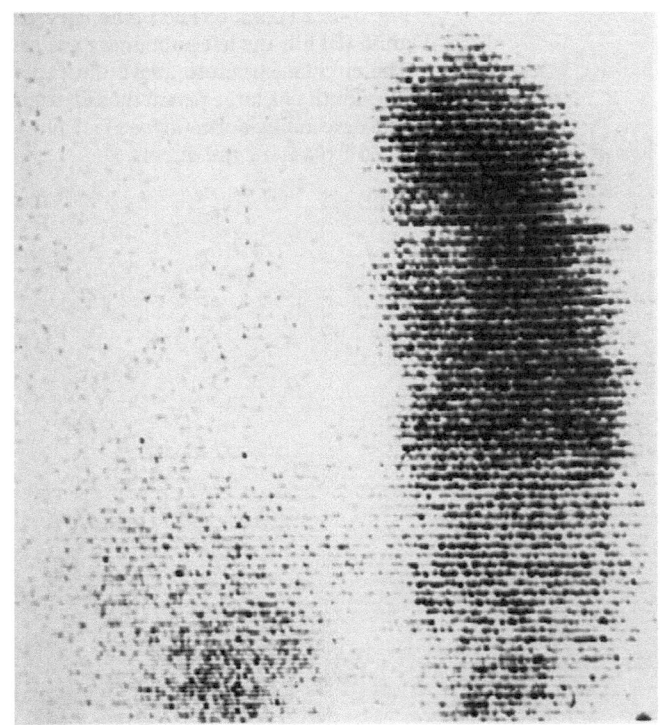

C

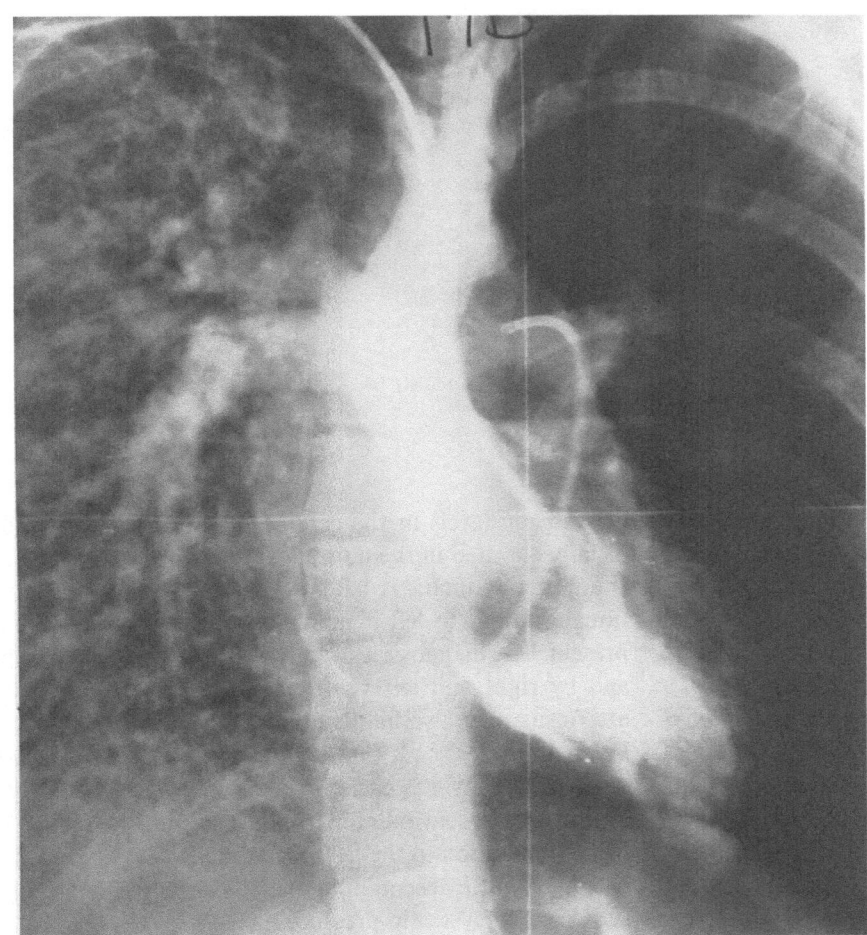

D

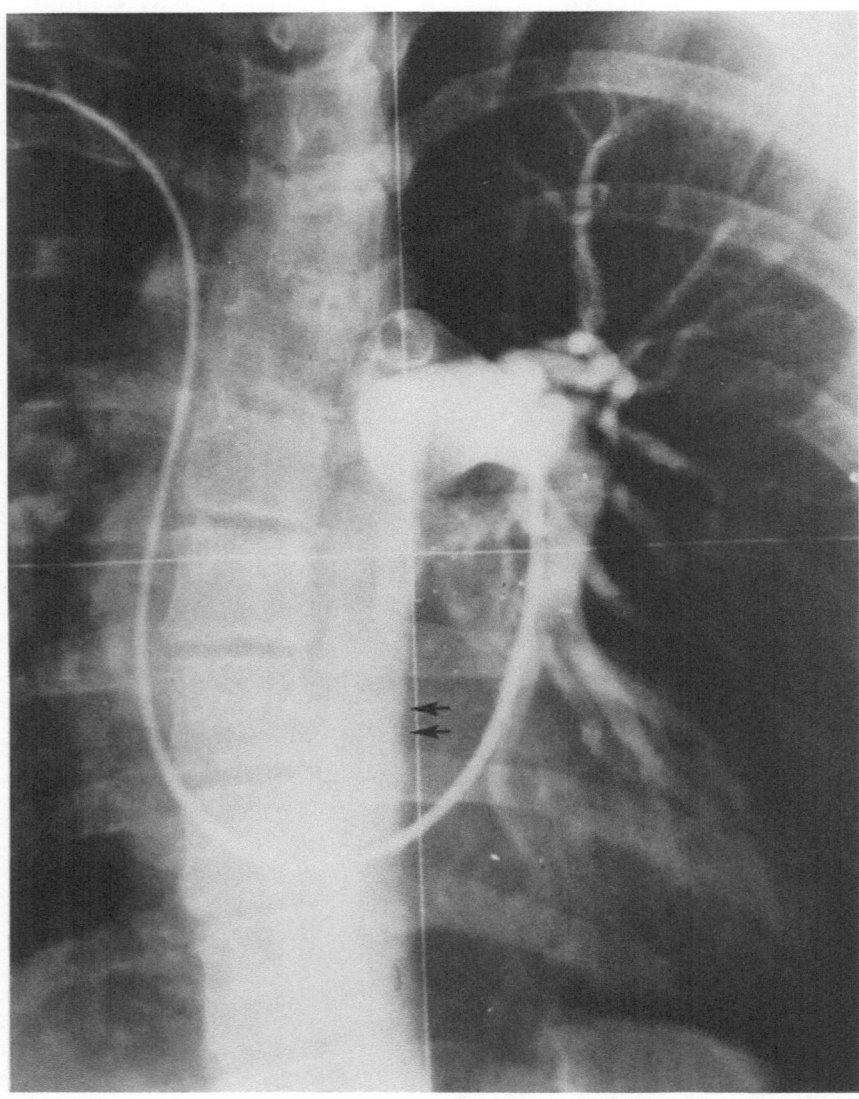

Fig. 7–222 (*Cont.*). The pulmonary arteriogram (**E**) fills the left pulmonary artery only. The circular structure above the catheter is the mouth of a large patent ductus arteriosus. The descending aorta (*arrows*) is faintly opacified by way of the ductus.

E

tion, which is marked on the side of the ectopic pulmonary artery (unilateral overcirculation pattern). The heart is enlarged, but its configuration is usually not specific. A pulmonary perfusion scan reveals the apparent paradox of absence of uptake in the overly perfused lung and normal or increased uptake in the contralateral lung (Fig. 7–222C).

In one of the authors' patients a pattern of lobar emphysema of the right lower lobe and predominant overcirculation on the left with marked cardiomegaly and a right-sided aortic arch led to the suspicion of A-LPA with tetralogy of Fallot and absence of pulmonary valve (Fig. 7–223A). The lobar emphysema pattern was caused by a huge right pulmonary artery compressing the bronchus.

Hemodynamics and Contrast Studies in Patients with A-RPA At catheterization only one pulmonary artery can be entered from the RV, and the lung supplied by this artery receives the entire systemic venous return. The opposite lung receives blood from the aorta. The pressure is

at systemic levels in the ectopic pulmonary artery and is usually elevated in the normally arising artery as well. The shunt at the ductus is left to right, but it may be bidirectional or right to left if pulmonary artery hypertension is present. The diagnosis is usually established by aortography and by right and left ventriculography. A patent ductus arteriosus may also be identified.

Hemodynamics and Contrast Studies in Patients with A-LPA A-LPA is generally associated with tetralogy of Fallot with absent pulmonary valve or other complex defects. In addition to the hemodynamic findings of tetralogy of Fallot with absent pulmonary valve, the left lung is subjected to systemic pressure.

Treatment Reimplantation of the ectopic pulmonary artery to the main pulmonary trunk with or without a tubular graft has been performed with good results in some patients. A fixed increase of pulmonary vascular resistance is a contraindication to corrective surgery.

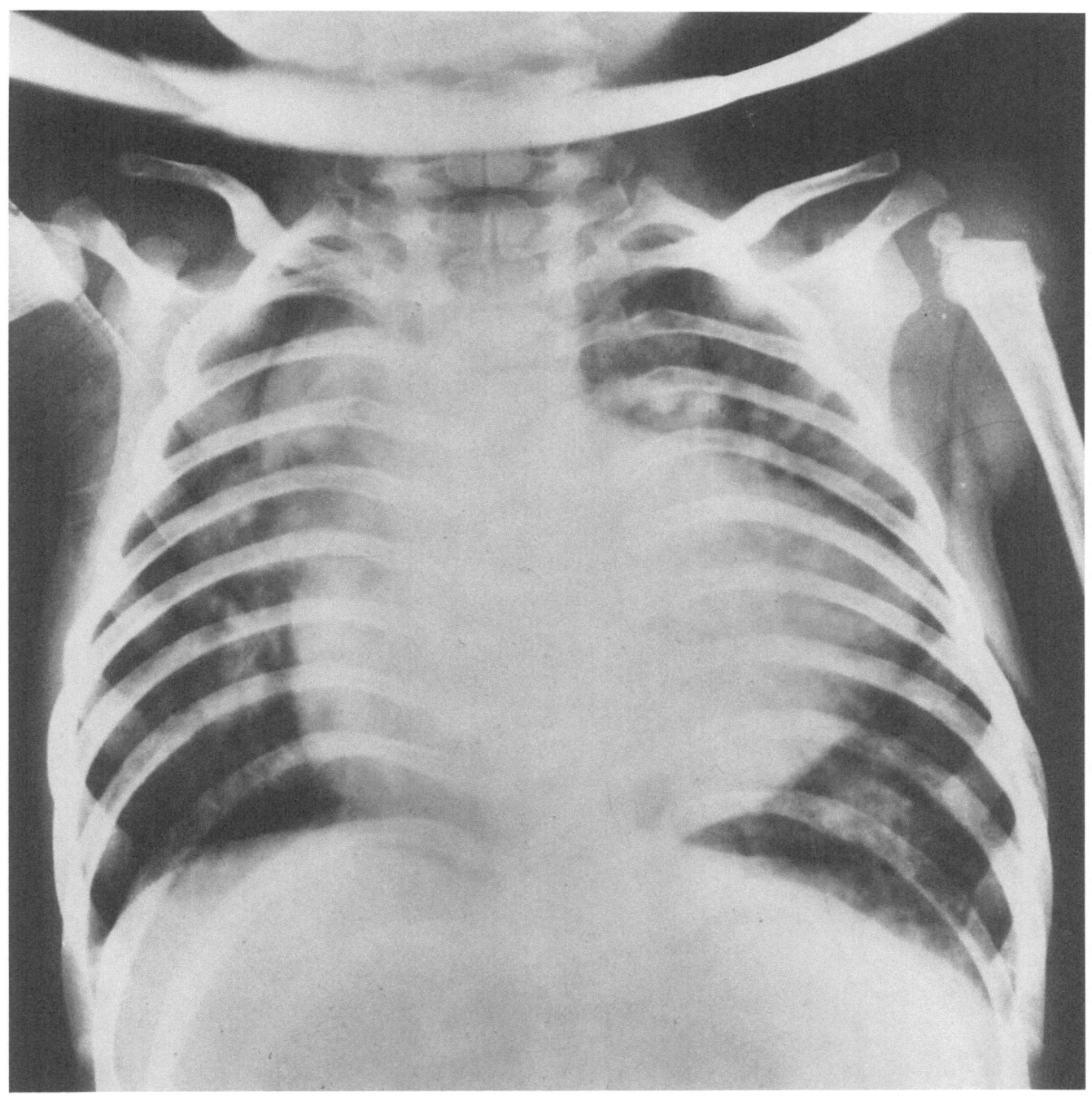

A

Fig. 7–223. *Anomalous origin of the left pulmonary artery from the aorta (left hemitruncus) in association with tetralogy of Fallot and absence of the pulmonary valve in an 8-month-old boy. A frontal film of the chest (A) shows marked cardiomegaly with a right aortic arch. The apex is uplifted, and the main pulmonary* artery segment is concave. Pulmonary overcirculation is present bilaterally. The right lower lobe is relatively underperfused. Marked enlargement of the right-sided chambers is also evident in the lateral projection **(B).** *(Continued)*

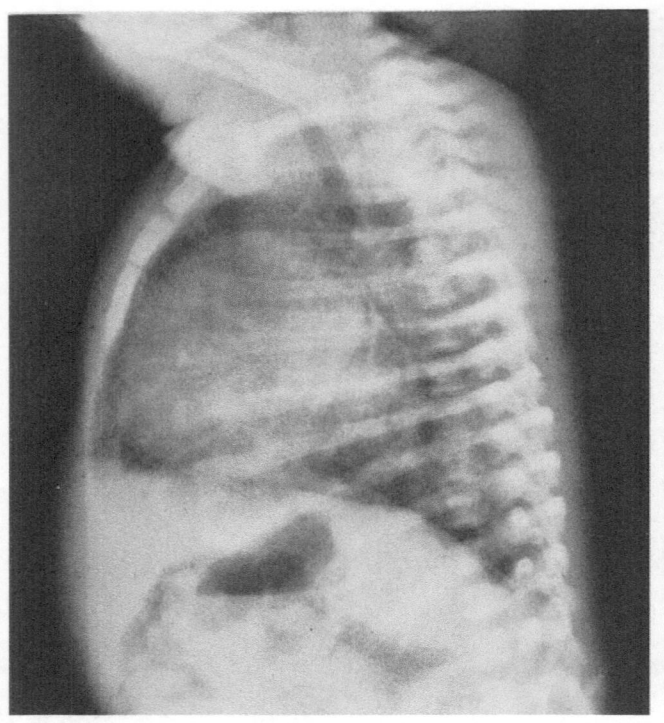

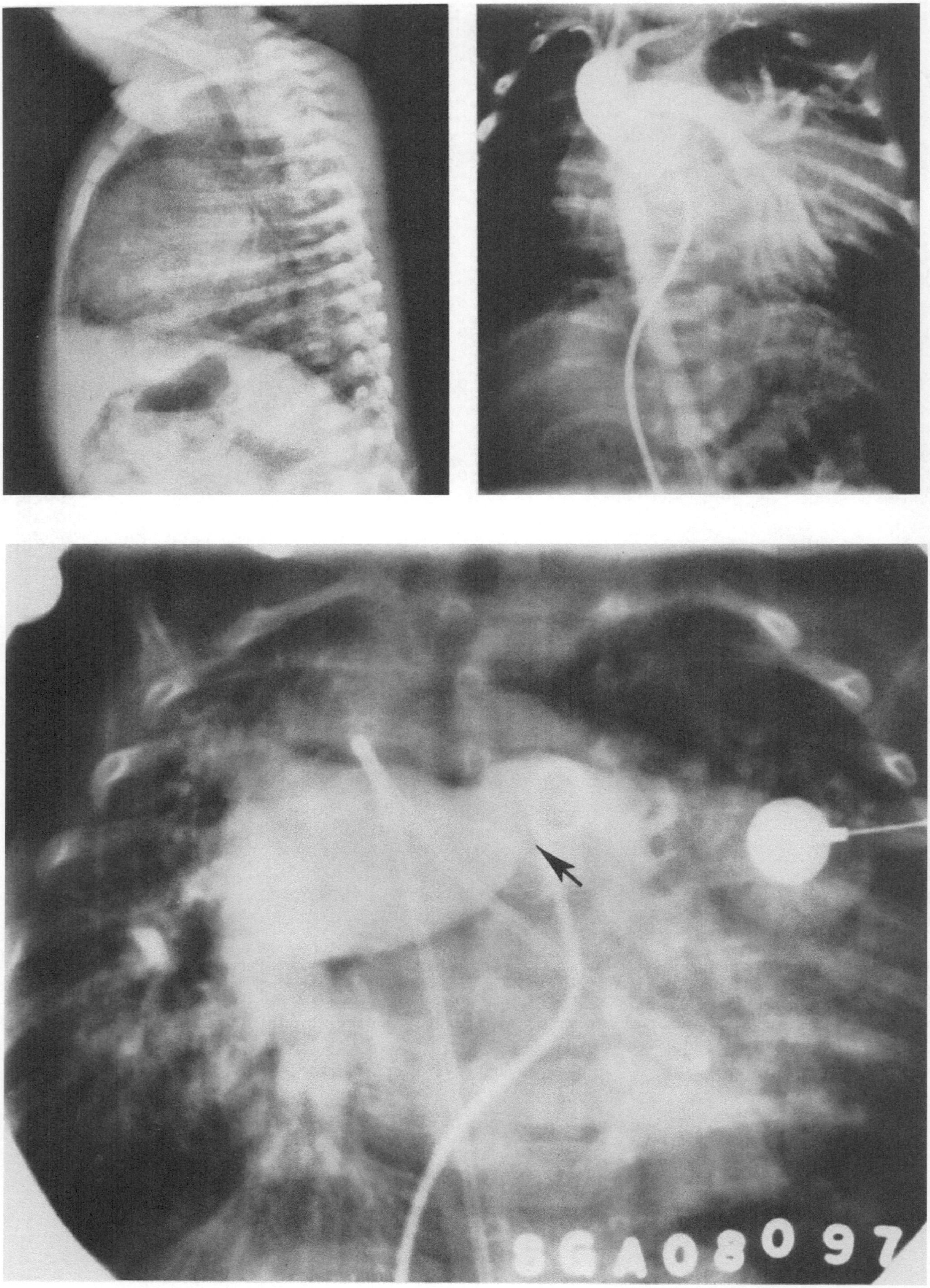

B

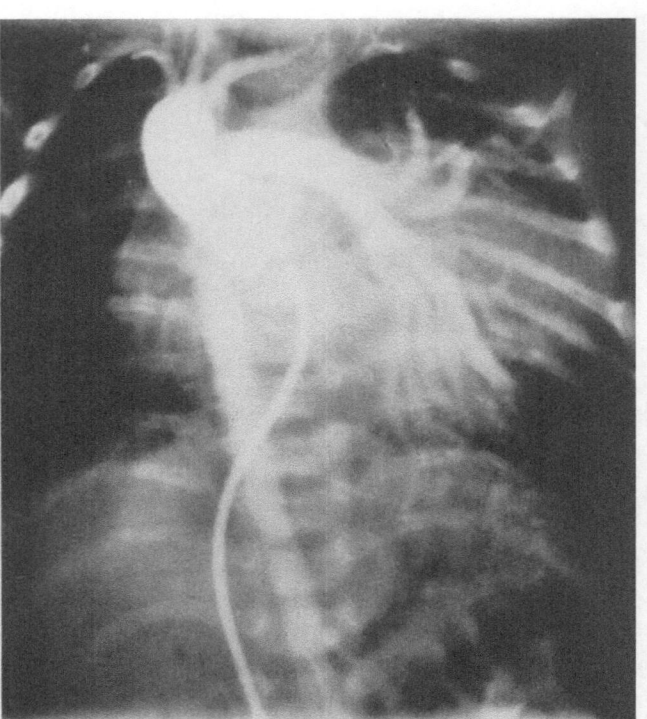

C

D

Fig. 7–223 (*Cont.*). The aortogram (**C**) demonstrates the origin of the left pulmonary artery from the ascending aorta. The aortic arch is on the right with mirror-image branching. The catheter has passed from the right atrium to the right ventricle, and then into the overriding aorta. When the catheter can be passed easily from the right ventricle into the aorta, transposition of the great arteries, atrioventricular canal, double-outlet right ventricle or overriding of the aorta should be considered (see also Fig. 7–219). A late film of the right ventriculogram (**D**) shows an aneurysmally dilated right pulmonary artery with no filling of the left pulmonary artery. The pulmonary anulus (*arrow*) is hypoplastic, with absence of the pulmonary valve (pulmonary regurgitation was noted on pulmonary cine angiography). The base of the right lung is hyperlucent because the enlarged right pulmonary artery compresses the right bronchus, resulting in lobar emphysema. The catheter tip is in the pulmonary outflow tract. The second catheter is a retrograde catheter, the tip of which is in the left ventricle. The lateral projection of the left ventriculogram (**E**) shows the aorta (*Ao*) overriding the ventricular septum. The dilated right pulmonary artery (*rpa*) is under the aortic arch. The catheter entered the right atrium and was directed across the foramen ovale, and through the left atrium to enter the left ventricle (*LV*). *RV* = right ventricle.

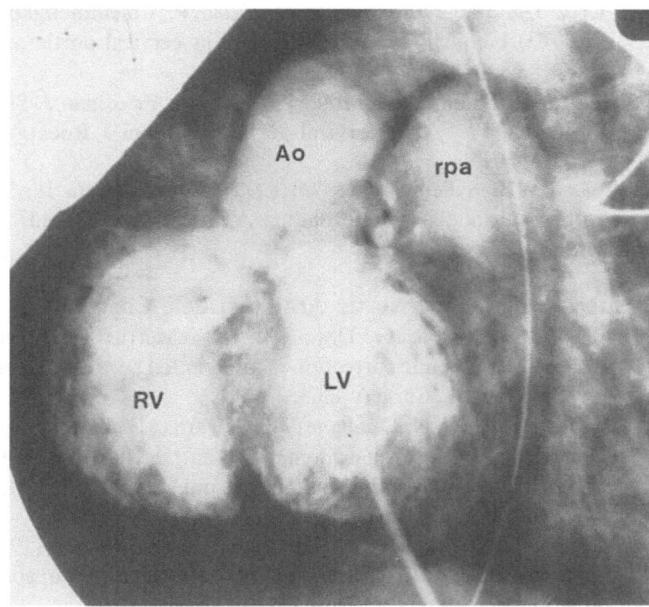

E

Bibliography

Abnormalities of the Great Vessels

Binet JP, Langlois J (1977) Aortic arch anomalies in children and infants. J Thorac Cardiovasc Surg 73:248–252

Congdon ED (1922) Transformation of the aortic arch system during the development of the human embryo. Contrib Embryol 14:47–110

Edwards JE (1948) Anomalies of the derivatives of the aortic arch system. Med Clin North Am 32:925–949

Shuford WH, Sybers RG (1974) The aortic arch and its malformations. With emphasis on the angiographic features. Thomas, Springfield, Ill

Stewart JR, Kincaid OW, Edwards JE (1964) An atlas of vascular rings and related malformations of the aortic arch system. Thomas, Springfield, Ill

Tonkin IL, Elliot LP, Bargeron LM (1980) Concomitant axial cineangiography and barium esophagography in the evaluation of vascular rings. Radiology 135:69–76

Warden HD (1961) Esophageal obstruction due to aberrant intercostal artery. Report of a case. Arch Surg 83:749–751

Double Aortic Arch

Higashino SM, Ruttenberg HD (1968) Double aortic arch associated with complete transposition of the great vessels. Br Heart J 30:579–581

Sahn DJ, Valdes-Cruz LM, Ovitt TW, Pond G, Mammana R, Goldberg SJ, Allen HD, Copeland JG (1982) Two dimensional echocardiography and intravenous digital video subtraction angiography for diagnosis and evaluation of double aortic arch. Am J Cardio 50:342–346

Right Aortic Arch

Berman W, Yabek SM, Dillon T, Neal JF, Akl B, Burstein J (1981) Vascular ring due to left aortic arch and right descending aorta. Circulation 63:458–460

D'Cruz IA, Cantez T, Namin EP, Licata R, Hastreiter AR (1966) Right-sided aorta. II. Right aortic arch, right descending aorta, and associated anomalies. Br Heart J 28:725–739

Felson B, Palayew MJ (1963) The two types of right aortic arch. Radiology 81:745–759

Garti IJ, Aygen MM, Vidne B, Levy MJ (1973) Right aortic arch with mirror-image branching causing vascular ring. A new classification of the right aortic arch patterns. Br J Radiol 46:115–119

Grollman JH Jr, Bedynek JL, Henderson HS, Hall RJ (1968) Right aortic arch with an aberrant retroesophageal innominate artery: Angiographic diagnosis. Radiology 90:782–783

Hastreiter AR, D'Cruz IA, Cantez T (1966) Right-sided aorta. I. Occurrence of right aortic arch in various types of congenital heart disease. Br Heart J 28:722–725

Knight L, Edwards JE (1974) Right aortic arch types and associated cardiac anomalies. Circulation 50:1047–1051

Leonardi HK, Naggar CZ, Ellis H Jr (1980) Dysphagia due to aortic arch anomaly. Diagnostic and therapeutic considerations. Arch Surg 115:1229–1232

Mustard WT, Trimble AW, Trusler GA (1962) Mediastinal vascular anomalies causing tracheal and esophageal compression and obstruction in childhood. Can Med Assoc J 87:1301–1305

Shuford WH, Sybers RG, Edwards FK (1970) The three types of right aortic arch. Am J Roentgenol 109:64–74

Stewart JR, Kincaid OW, Titus JL (1966) Right aortic arch: Plain film diagnosis and significance. Am J Roentgenol 97:377–389

Left Aortic Arch with Normal Branching and Right Ductus Arteriosus

Heim de Balsac R (1960) Left aortic arch (posterior or circumflex type) with right descending aorta. Am J Cardiol 5:546–550

Heinrich WD, Perez-Tamayo R (1956) Left aortic arch and right descending aorta: Case report. Am J Roentgenol 76:762–777

Paul RN (1948) A new anomaly of the aorta: Left aortic arch with right descending aorta. J Pediatr 32:19–29

Stewart JR, Kincaid OW, Edwards JE (1964) An atlas of vascular rings and related malformations of the aortic arch system. Thomas, Springfield, Ill.

Left Aortic Arch with Aberrant Right Subclavian Artery

Beaubout JW, Stewart JR, Kincaid OW (1964) Aberrant right subclavian artery. Dispute of commonly accepted concepts. Am J Roentgenol 92:855–864

Bosniak MA (1964) An analysis of some anatomic roentgenologic aspects of the branchiocephalic vessels. Am J Roentgenol 91:1222–1231

Felson B, Cohen S, Courter SR, McGuire J (1950) Anomalous right subclavian artery. Radiology 54:340–349

Klinkhamer A (1966) Aberrant right subclavian artery. Clinical and roentgenographic aspects. Am J Roentgenol 97:438–446

Left Aortic Arch with Right Descending Aorta

Berman W Jr, Yabek SM, Dillon T, Neal JF, Aki B, Burstein J (1981) Vascular ring due to left aortic arch and right descending aorta. Circulation 63:458–460

Left Aortic Arch with Anomalous Origin of the Innominate or Left Common Carotid Artery (Bicarotid Origin)

Berdon WE, Baker DH, Bordiuk J, Mellins R (1969) Innominate artery compression of the trachea in infants with stridor and apnea. Method of roentgen diagnosis and criteria for surgical treatment. Radiology 92:272–278

Felson B, Cohen S, Courter SR, McGuire J (1950) Anomalous right subclavian artery. Radiology 54:340–349

Gross RE (1955) Arterial malformations which cause compression of the trachea or esophagus. Circulation 11:124–134

Klinkhamer AC (1966) Aberrant right subclavian artery. Clinical and roentgenographic aspects. Am J. Roentgenol 97:438–446

Single Brachiocephalic Trunk Arising from the Aortic Arch

McDowell DE, Grant MA, Gustafson RA (1980) Single arterial trunk arising from the aortic arch. Circulation 62:181–182

Nizankowski C, Rajchel Z, Ziolkowski M (1975) Abnormal origin of arteries from the aortic arch in man. Folia Morphol 34:109–116

Cervical Aortic Arch

D'Cruz IA, Stanley A, Vitullo D, Desai P, Chiemmongkoltip P (1983) Noninvasive diagnosis of right cervical aortic arch. Chest 83:820–822

Moncada R, Shannon M, Miller R, White H, Friedman J, Shufford WH (1975) The cervical aortic arch. Am J Roentgenol 125:591–601

Shuford WH, Sybers RG (1974) Cervical aortic arch. In: The aortic arch and its malformations. Thomas, Springfield, Ill., pp 145–188

Interruption of the Aortic Arch (Steidele Complex)

Bailey LL, Jacobson JG, Doroshow RW, Merritt WH, Petry EL (1981) Anatomic correction of interrupted aortic arch complex in neonates. Surgery 89:553–557

Becu LM, Tauxe WN, DuShane JW, Edwards JE (1955) A complex of congenital cardiac anomalies: Ventricular septal defect, biventricular origin of the pulmonary trunk, and subaortic stenosis. Am Heart J 50:901–911

Berman W Jr, Heyman MA, Whitman V, Rudolph AM (1979) Dilatation of the ductus arteriosus by prostaglandin E, in aortic arch abnormalities. Circulation 59:169–173

Conley ME, Beckwith JB, Mancer JFK, Tenckhoft L (1979) The spectrum of the DiGeorge syndrome. J Pediatr 94:883–890

Finley JP, Collins GF, de Chadarevian JP, Williams RL (1977) DiGeorge syndrome presenting as severe congenital heart disease in the newborn. Can Med Assoc J 116:635–637

Garcia OL, Hernandez FA, Tamer D, Poole C, Gelband H, Castellanos AW (1979) Congenital bilateral subclavian steal. Ductus-dependent symptoms in interrupted aortic arch associated with ventricular septal defect. Am J Cardiol 44:101–104

Jaffee RB (1975) Complete interruption of the aortic arch. I. Characteristic radiographic findings in 21 patients. Circulation 52:714–721

Jaffee RB (1976) Complete interruption of the aortic arch. Circulation 53:161–168

Lie JT (1967) The malformation complex of the arch of the aorta—Steidele's complex. Am Heart J 73:615–625

Moes CAF, Freedom RM (1980) Aortic arch interruption with truncus arteriosus or aorticopulmonary septal defect. Am J Roentgenol 135:1011–1016

Moller JH, Edwards JE (1965) Interruption of aortic arch. Anatomic patterns and associated cardiac malformations. Am J Roentgenol 95:557–572

Moulton AL, Bowman FO Jr (1981) Primary definitive repair of type B interrupted aortic arch, ventricular septal defect, and patent ductus arteriosus. J Thorac Cardiovasc Surg 82:501–510

Neye-Bock S, Fellows KE (1980) Aortic arch interruption in infancy: Radio and angiographic features. Am J Roentgenol 135:1005–1010

Ober WB, Moore TEJ (1955) Congenital cardiac malformations in the neonatal period: An autopsy study. N Engl J Med 253:271–275

Riggs TW, Berry TE, Aziz KU, Paul MH (1982) Two-dimensional echocardiographic features of interruption of the aortic arch. Am J Cardiol 50:1385–1390

Takashina T, Ishikura Y, Yamane K, Yorifuji S, Iwasaki T, Yoshida Y, Takeshita I, Oka K (1972) The congenital cardiovascular anomalies of the interruption of the aorta—Steidele's complex. Am Heart H 83:93–99

Zahka KG, Roland MA, Cutilleta AF, Gardner TJ, Donahoo JS, Kidd L (1980) Management of aortic arch interruption with prostaglandin E, infusion and microporous expanded polytetrafluoroethylene grafts. Am J Cardiol 46:1001–1005

Pulmonary Artery Sling

Campbell CD, Wernly JA, Koltip PC, Vitullo D, Replogle RL (1980) Aberrant left pulmonary artery (pulmonary artery sling): Successful repair and 24 year follow-up report. Am J Cardiol 45:316–320

Gumbiner CH, Mullins CE, McNamara DG (1980) Pulmonary artery sling. Am J Cardiol 45:311–315

Koopot R, Nikaido H, Idriss FS (1975) Surgical management of anomalous left pulmonary artery causing tracheo-bronchial obstruction: Pulmonary sling. J Thorac Cardiovasc Surg 69:239–246

Park CD, Waldhauser JH, Friedman S, Aberdeen E, Johnson J (1971) Tracheal compression by the great arteries in the mediastinum: Report of 39 cases. Arch Surg 103:626–632

Pernot C, Hoeffel JC, Henry M, Worms AM, Stehlin H, Louis JP (1972) Radiologic patterns of congenital absence of the pulmonary valve in infants. Radiology 102:619–622

Said RM, Rosenthal A, Fellows K, Castaneda AR (1975) Pulmonary artery sling. J Thorac Cardiovasc Surg 69:333–346

Tonkin IL, Elliot LP, Bargeron LM Jr (1980) Concomitant axial cineangiography and barium esophagography in the evaluation of vascular rings. Radiology 135:69–76

Williams RG, Jaffe RB, Condon VR, Nixon GW (1979) Unusual features of pulmonary sling. Am J Roentgenol 133:1065–1069

Wittenborg MH, Tantiwongse T, Rosenberg BF (1956) Anomalous course of left pulmonary artery with respiratory obstruction. Radiology 67:339–345

Ductus Arteriosus Sling

Binet JP, Conso JF, Losay J, Narcy PH, Raynaud EJ, Beaufils FR, Dor C, Bruniaux J (1978) Ductus arteriosus sling: Report of a newly recognized anomaly and its surgical correction. Thorax 33:72–75

Anomalous Origin of One Pulmonary Artery from the Ascending Aorta (Hemitruncus)

Cucci CE, Doyle EF, Lewis EW Jr (1964) Absence of a primary division of the pulmonary trunk. An ontogenetic theory. Circulation 29:124–131

Gula G, Chew C, Radley-Smith R, Yacoub M (1978) Anomalous origin of the right pulmonary artery from the ascending aorta associated with aortopulmonary window. Thorax 33:265–269

Herbert WH, Rohman M, Farnsworth P, Swamy S (1973) Anomalous origin of left pulmonary artery from ascending aorta, right aortic arch and right patent ductus arteriosus. Chest 63:459–461

Keane JF, Maltz D, Bernhard WF, Corwin RD, Nadas AS (1974) Anomalous origin of one pulmonary artery from the ascending aorta. Diagnostic, physiological and surgical considerations. Circulation 50:588–594

Weintraub RA, Fabian CE, Adams DF (1966) Ectopic origin of one pulmonary artery from the ascending aorta. Radiology 86:666–676

Chapter 7 Section 6
Abnormalities of Visceroatrial Situs

Diagnosis of the visceroatrial situs (position and morphology of the atria) is of paramount importance in the analysis of complex congenital cardiac defects. The Latin term *situs solitus* (SS) is used to indicate normal position of the viscera, including the cardiac atria. The mirror-image presentation of the normal visceroatrial morphology and relationships is termed *situs inversus* (SI). Thus there are two normal or determinate types of situs. In SS the morphological right atrium (*RA*) is on the right side and the morphological left atrium (*LA*) is on the left side. The liver, the spleen and other noncardiac viscera are also in normal position. In SI the morphological RA is on the left side of the morphological LA, which is right sided. The liver, spleen and other noncardiac viscera also have a mirror-image relationship. The immotile cilia syndrome on occasion is associated with situs inversus (Kartagener triad of SI, sinusitis and bronchiectasis). Table 7–9 is a list of abnormalities of visceroatrial situs.

Anatomically the morphological RA is identified by the crista terminalis and the limbus of the fossa ovalis. On angiography the RA is identified by the RA appendage, which is a broad, triangular structure with a wide orifice and coarse pectinate muscles. The RA and LA have no distinctive appearance on roentgenograms of the chest; however, their respective positions correspond to the thoracic situs. The RA is under the right main-stem bronchus and right pulmonary artery. The LA is under the left main-stem bronchus and left pulmonary artery. Therefore, analysis of the pattern of branching of the tracheobronchial tree and the central pulmonary arteries permits a prediction concerning the locations of the cardiac atria (Figs. 7–224, 7–225). In SS the right lung has three lobes, and the right main bronchus has a relatively vertical course. Its first branch, the upper lobe bronchus or eparterial bronchus, lies above the right pulmonary artery. The eparterial bronchus arises almost immediately after the tracheal bifurcation and travels initially in a horizontal direction, appearing on end in the lateral view. Thus the right bronchus is recognized on the frontal view because of its short course, proximal to the first branch. The morphological right pulmonary artery arises at a right angle from the pulmonary trunk, appearing in the lateral projection as a dense sphere of varying size in front of the proximal left main bronchus.

The left lung has two lobes. The left main bronchus is called hyparterial because it is situated beneath the morphological left pulmonary artery. An anatomical left main bronchus is recognized on the frontal radiograph of the chest by its longer course and more distal bifurcation. The left upper-lobe bronchus is directed in a more horizontal plane, thus being visualized on end on the lateral film of the chest as a round lucent area a variable distance below

Table 7–9. Abnormalities of Visceroatrial Situs*

Situs inversus totalis (may have no heart defect)
Levoisomerism (polysplenia syndrome)
Dextroisomerism (asplenia syndrome)
M-anisosplenia (third syndrome)
F-anisosplenia (fourth syndrome)
Thoracoabdominal discordance

* Pulmonary vascular pattern reflects the presence or absence of pulmonic stenosis or atresia

the right upper lobe bronchus. The proximal portion of the morphological left pulmonary artery is above the left bronchus, and its distal segment curves behind the left bronchus, being visible on the lateral film as a dense tube curving posteriorly and inferiorly. This anatomical configuration is in contrast to the dense sphere cast by the right pulmonary artery.

When the morphological right bronchus and right pulmonary artery are on the right and the morphological left bronchus and pulmonary artery are on the left, SS is present. A mirror-image relationship of the bronchi and pulmonary arteries indicates SI. These anatomical arrangements predict the location of the RA and LA. In SS the RA is on the right side and below the eparterial bronchus, while

Fig. 7–224. *The two types of normal (determinate) situs: situs solitus and situs inversus.* The pattern of branching of the tracheobronchial tree defines the thoracic situs and corresponds to the position of the cardiac atria. The right bronchus is recognized by its short, relatively vertical course before the first branch (the eparterial branch), while the left bronchus has a longer, more horizontal course and is slightly concave. The right atrium is under the right main bronchus (eparterial), and the left atrium is under the left main bronchus (hyparterial). In situs solitus the anatomical right main-stem bronchus and right atrium are on the right, while in situs inversus the anatomical right bronchus and right atrium are on the left. The apex of the heart usually is on the left in situs solitus and on the right in situs inversus. Other locations of the apex are associated with an increased incidence of congenital abnormalities of the heart. Situs solitus with mesoversion often has no cardiac abnormality, and if an abnormality is present it is likely to be L-TGA. SS with dextroversion tends to be associated with complex cyanotic defects (pulmonary stenosis or atresia or tricuspid atresia). Similarly *situs inversus* with dextroversion and *situs inversus* with mesoversion are associated with relatively less complex defects while *situs inversus* with levoversion is associated with more complex defects. A normal heart is unlikely in individuals with situs solitus and dextroversion or situs inversus with levoversion. Although this diagram depicts atrioventricular concordance (left atrium connected to left ventricle, right atrium connected to right ventricle) it is important to note that the ventricles may be concordant or discordant. Thus the tracheobronchial tree predicts the position of the atria but not of the ventricles.

SS = situs solitus; *SI* = situs inversus; *RA* = right atrium; *LA* = left atrium; *RV* = right ventricle; *LV* = left ventricle.

Situs Solitus

Situs Inversus

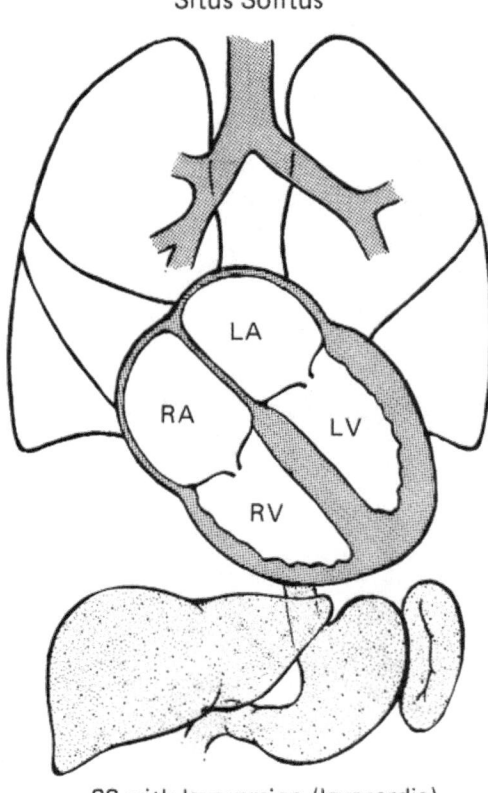

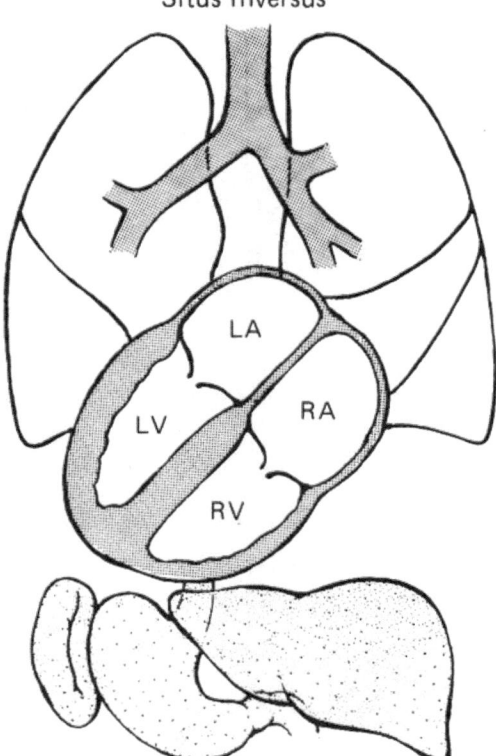

SS with levoversion (levocardia)
(Normal)

SI with dextroversion (dextrocardia)
(Mirror image of normal)

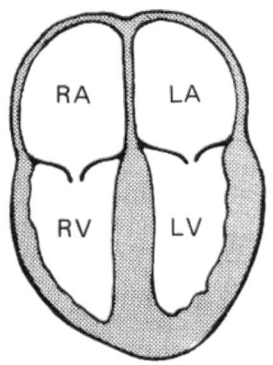

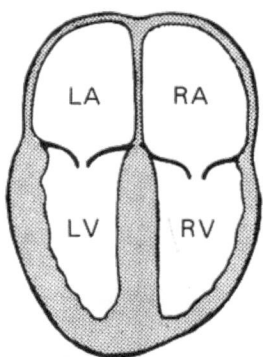

SS with mesoversion (mesocardia)

SI with mesoversion (mesocardia)

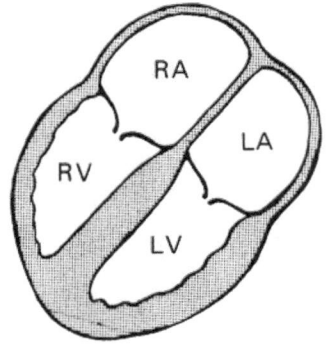

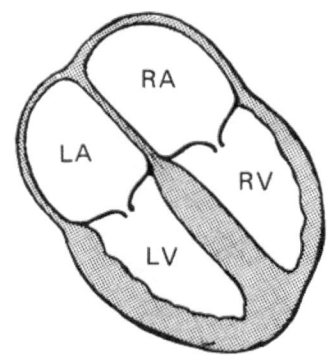

SS with dextroversion (dextrocardia)

SI with levoversion (levocardia)

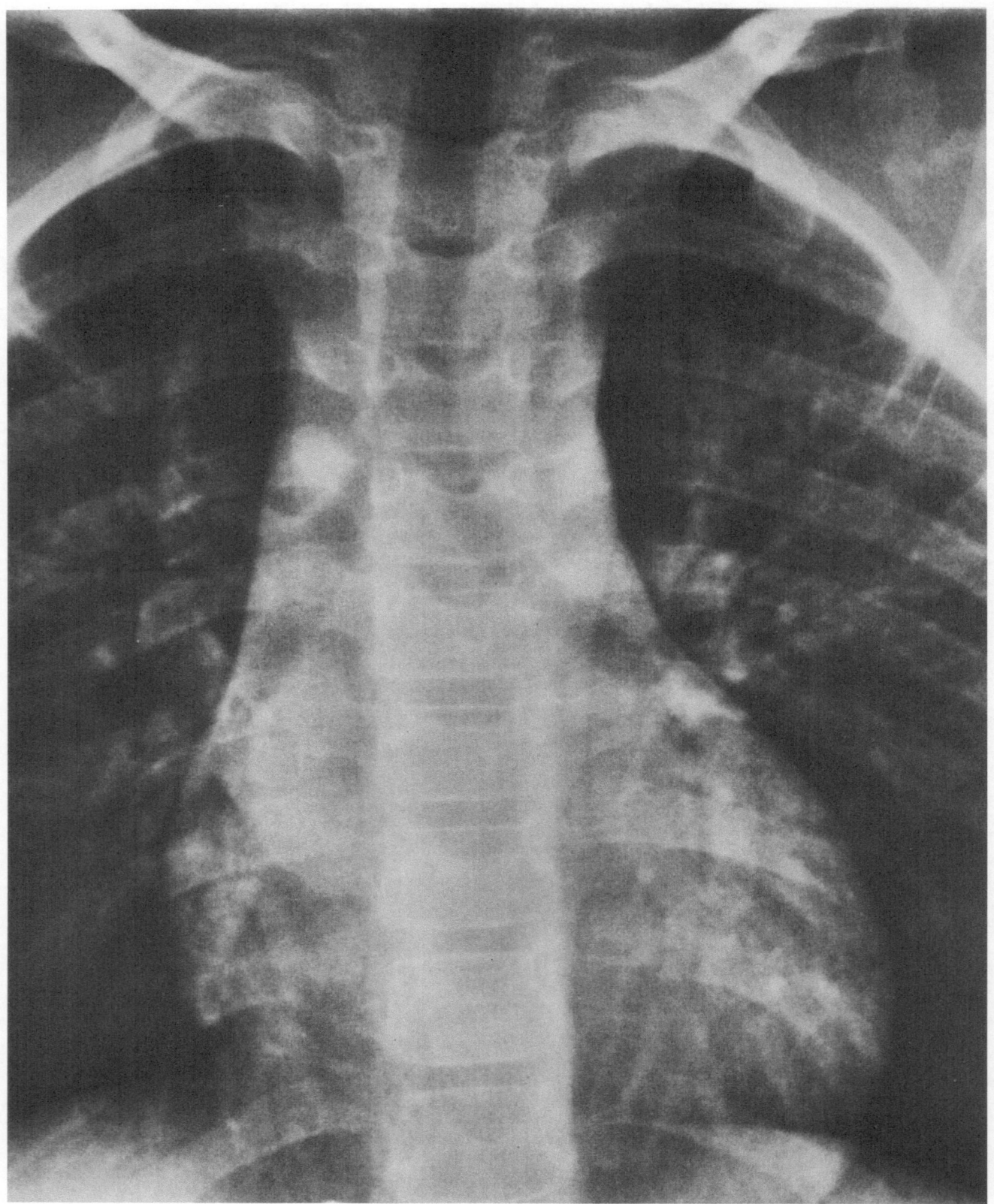

Fig. 7–225. *The tracheobronchial tree with situs solitus.* The right bronchus has a short, relatively vertical course. The first branch, the eparterial branch, runs above the right pulmonary artery. The left bronchus has a longer more horizontal course and is slightly concave, coursing beneath the left pulmonary artery (hyparterial). These findings define the thoracic situs as situs solitus and predict the locations of the cardiac atria. Thus the right atrium is beneath the right bronchus, and the left atrium is beneath the left bronchus.

in SI the anatomical RA is on the left. In this regard it is important to understand that the configuration of the tracheobronchial tree predicts only the position of the atria (visceroatrial situs) and not that of the ventricles or the great arteries. The ventricles may be concordant or discordant. Concordance means normal connection, that is, the RA connects with the right ventricle (RV), and the LA connects with the left ventricle (LV). Discordance indicates abnormal connection, the RA being connected to the anatomical LV, while the LA is connected to the RV (ventricular inversion). The location of the cardiac apex (ventricular mass) is also independent of the position of the atria (Fig. 7–224). The cardiac apex is usually left sided in SS; however, it may be located on the right (dextroversion) or in the midline (mesoversion). On the other hand, in SI the cardiac apex is usually right sided, but it can be left sided (levoversion) or midline (mesoversion). The terms *dextroversion, mesoversion* and *levoversion* (Fig. 7–224) specifically indicate the position of the cardiac apex when this structure is not in its usual location for the corresponding visceroatrial situs (e.g., SS with mesoversion or dextroversion; SI with mesoversion or levoversion). The incidence of cyanotic congenital heart disease is higher in patients with SS and dextroversion and in SI with levoversion. Patients with SS and mesoversion (Fig. 7–226) usually have a normal heart, but on occasion may have levotransposition (L-TGA) of the great arteries. SS with dextroversion (Fig. 7–227) is associated with complex cyanotic cardiac abnormalities, and only rarely is the heart normal. Similarly, SI with mesoversion (Fig. 7–228) is associated with relatively less complex defects, and SI with levoversion (Fig. 7–229) is associated with more complex defects.

The terms *dextrocardia, mesocardia* and *levocardia* indicate the position of the heart within the thorax without consideration of the visceralatrial situs. These terms have been used interchangeably with *dextroversion, mesoversion* and *levoversion*. Therefore the type of visceroatrial situs should be stated when either terminology is used.

It is usual for patients with thoracic SS (atrial SS) to have concordant abdominal situs (e.g., abdominal SS, left-sided gastric air bubble and right-sided liver). On occasion a discordant thoracoabdominal situs is identified, indicating that the situs of the thorax and the situs of the abdomen are different. Thoracoabdominal discordance has been reported with no cardiac malformations; however, cardiac abnormalities are not infrequently encountered in this group of individuals. As examples, in instances of thoracic SS solitus and abdominal SI, tetralogy of Fallot and stigmata of asplenia (Howell-Jolly bodies) have been identified. The authors have studied a patient with this type of situs who also had ostium primum atrial septal defect (Fig. 7–230). In addition, thoracic SI may be associated with abdominal situs indeterminus (stomach and liver on same side) (Fig. 7–229).

Failure of lateralization of the thoracic and abdominal viscera into a pattern of either SS or SI results in a symmetrical visceral configuration (isomerism), with duplica-

tion of either left- or right-sided structures, termed situs ambiguus (also referred to as indeterminate situs or heterotaxy syndrome) (Fig. 7–231). This configuration frequently is associated with splenic abnormalities and with major malformations in the cardiovascular system (see Table 7–10).

Asplenia

Situs ambiguus with dextroisomerism or bilateral right-sidedness (asplenia syndrome or Ivemark syndrome) (Figs. 7–231, 7–232) results in duplication of the right-sided structures—that is, bilateral right lungs (trilobed) with bilateral eparterial bronchi, common atrium with anatomical characteristics suggesting bilateral RA (bilateral crista terminalis and sinus node), two superior venae cavae, hepatic symmetry and a left- or right-sided stomach (Figs. 7–231 and 7–232). Absence of the spleen is associated with the presence of Heinz or Howell-Jolly bodies in the peripheral blood smear.

Among the cardiovascular abnormalities observed in the asplenia syndrome are: (1) bilateral superior venae cavae, (2) common atrium or a large atrial septal defect, (3) single ventricle or a large ventricular septal defect, (4) A-V communis (atrioventricular canal), (5) transposition of the great arteries, (6) anomalous pulmonary venous return (either supracardiac or infracardiac), (7) cardiac malposition, (8) midline crossing of the inferior vena cava just below the diaphragm to enter the systemic venous atrium, (9) a common course of the inferior vena cava and abdominal aorta and (10) severe pulmonic stenosis or atresia often accompanying any of the foregoing (Fig. 7–232, Table 7–10).

Structural anomalies of the gastrointestinal and genitourinary systems include malrotation of the gut, agenesis of the gallbladder, annular pancreas, imperforate anus, horseshoe kidney and ureteral and urethral valves (Table 7–10).

It should be stressed that absence of the spleen results in frequent life-threatening infections.

Polysplenia

Bilateral left-sidedness (levoisomerism, polysplenia) is characterized by bilateral left lungs (bilobed, absence of the minor fissure) with bilateral hyparterial bronchi (Fig. 7–233) and a common atrium with anatomical characteristics suggestive of bilateral left atria (LA isomerism). The liver is symmetrical, and the stomach may be on either side. Multiple spleens are present, but no Heinz or Howell-Jolly bodies are found on peripheral blood smears. (Howell-Jolly bodies have also been identified in individuals with a normal spleen or with polysplenia. Such patients are considered to have functional hyposplenia.)

Cardiovascular anomalies associated with polysplenia include: (1) anomalous systemic venous connections (bilat-

(Continued on page 634)

Table 7–10. Asplenia, Polysplenia and Related Syndromes (*Situs Ambiguus*)

I. ASPLENIA

Bilateral right sidedness—males affected twice as commonly as females. More severe anomalies than polysplenia—poor prognosis. Associated with cyanosis.

A. Cardiac Anomalies
  1. Common atrium or large atrial septal defect
  2. If two atria, both resemble right atrium in configuration of atrial appendage and presence of sinoatrial node
  3. Absent coronary sinus (approx. 80%)
  4. Atrioventricularis communis (A-V communis)
  5. Anomalous pulmonary venous return (usually total)
  6. Bilateral superior venae cavae (approx. 50%)
  7. Single ventricle or large VSD
  8. Dextrocardia (approx. 50%)
  9. Pulmonary atresia or severe stenosis
  10. Dextro- or levotransposition of great vessels (D-TGA, L-TGA)

Rarely, double outlet right ventricle, hypoplastic left heart, single coronary artery.

B. Noncardiac Anomalies
  1. Bilateral eparterial bronchi—bilateral right lung with three or more lobes in each lung
  2. No spleen—Howell Jolly bodies on peripheral smear
  3. Transverse or symmetric liver
  4. Abdominal heterotaxy
  5. Genitourinary abnormalities, i.e., horseshoe kidney, hydroureter (approx. 15%)
  6. Fused or horseshoe adrenals
  7. Malrotations of the bowel
  8. Susceptibility to sepsis (21%)

C. Findings on roentgenograms of the chest
  1. Pulmonary vascularity undercirculated
  2. Bilateral eparterial bronchi
  3. Malposition of the heart
  4. Transverse liver

D. Liver spleen scan showing no spleen

II. POLYSPLENIA

Splenic tissue divided into two or more spleens of nearly equal size so that total splenic mass approximates that of a normal spleen. Slight female predominance. Bilateral left sidedness. Milder course—approximately 25% with no significant cardiac anomaly.

A. Cardiac Anomalies
  1. Azygos continuation of inferior vena cava
  2. Atrial septal defect or endocardial cushion defect
  3. Bilateral left atria
  4. Anomalous pulmonary venous return (usually partial with each lung returning blood to its ipsilateral atrium)
  5. Pulmonic stenosis—not severe (33%)
  6. Ventricular septal defect
  7. Double outlet right venticle (15–25%)
  8. Dextrocardia (approx. 50%)
  9. Malpositions of the great vessels, single ventricle, single atrium—all quite rare

B. Noncardiac Anomalies
  1. Bilateral hyparterial bronchi—bilateral left lung with two lobes in each lung
  2. Two or more spleens
  3. Transverse or symmetric liver
  4. Abdominal heterotaxy
  5. Gall bladder abnormalities (including biliary atresia)
  6. Genitourinary abnormalities (approx. 15%)

C. Findings on roentgenograms of the chest
  1. Pulmonary vascularity normal or overcirculated
  2. Bilateral hyparterial bronchi
  3. Malposition of the heart
  4. Azygos arch—smooth rounded prominence at upper right or left base of heart
  5. Transverse liver
  6. Absent IVC on lateral projection

D. Liver spleen scan showing multiple spleens

III. ANISOSPLENIA

Variant described by Landing consisting of congenital heart disease, symmetrical pulmonary lobation, and abnormality of the spleen but not typical of polysplenia. Spleen described as bifurcated—consisting of one or more large main spleens and one or more accessory spleens. Occasionally associated with bronchopulmonary-atrial discordance

A. M-Anisosplenia (Males, Third Syndrome)
  1. Bilateral eparterial bronchi—resembling a mild form of asplenia
  2. Total anomalous pulmonary venous return
  3. Pulmonary stenosis
  4. Atrioventricularis communis (A-V communis)
  5. Bilateral superior venae cavae
  6. Right aortic arch
  7. Relatively normal abdominal visceral situs

B. F-Anisosplenia (Females, Fourth Syndrome)
  1. Bilateral hyparterial bronchi—resembling a severe form of polysplenia
  2. Abnormalities of the great veins—bilateral superior venae cavae, azygos continuation of the inferior vena cava
  3. Double-outlet right ventricle
  4. Abnormalities of situs of the abdominal viscera

This table was prepared by Joel Rakow, M.D., during his rotation in Cardiac Radiology at Montefiore Medical Center, Bronx, N.Y.

References:
Landing, et al. (1971) Am J Cardiol 28:456–462
Moerman, et al. (1982) Clinical Genetics 22:143–147
Moss (1983) Heart Disease in Infants, Children, and Adolescents, 3rd ed. pp 341–349
Rose et al. (1975) Br Heart J 37:840–852
Shinohara et al.: (1982) Acta Pathol (Jpn) 32(3):505–511
Waldman JD, Rosenthal A, Smith AL, Shurin S, Nadas AS (1977) Sepsis and congenital asplenia. J. Pediat . 90:555–559.

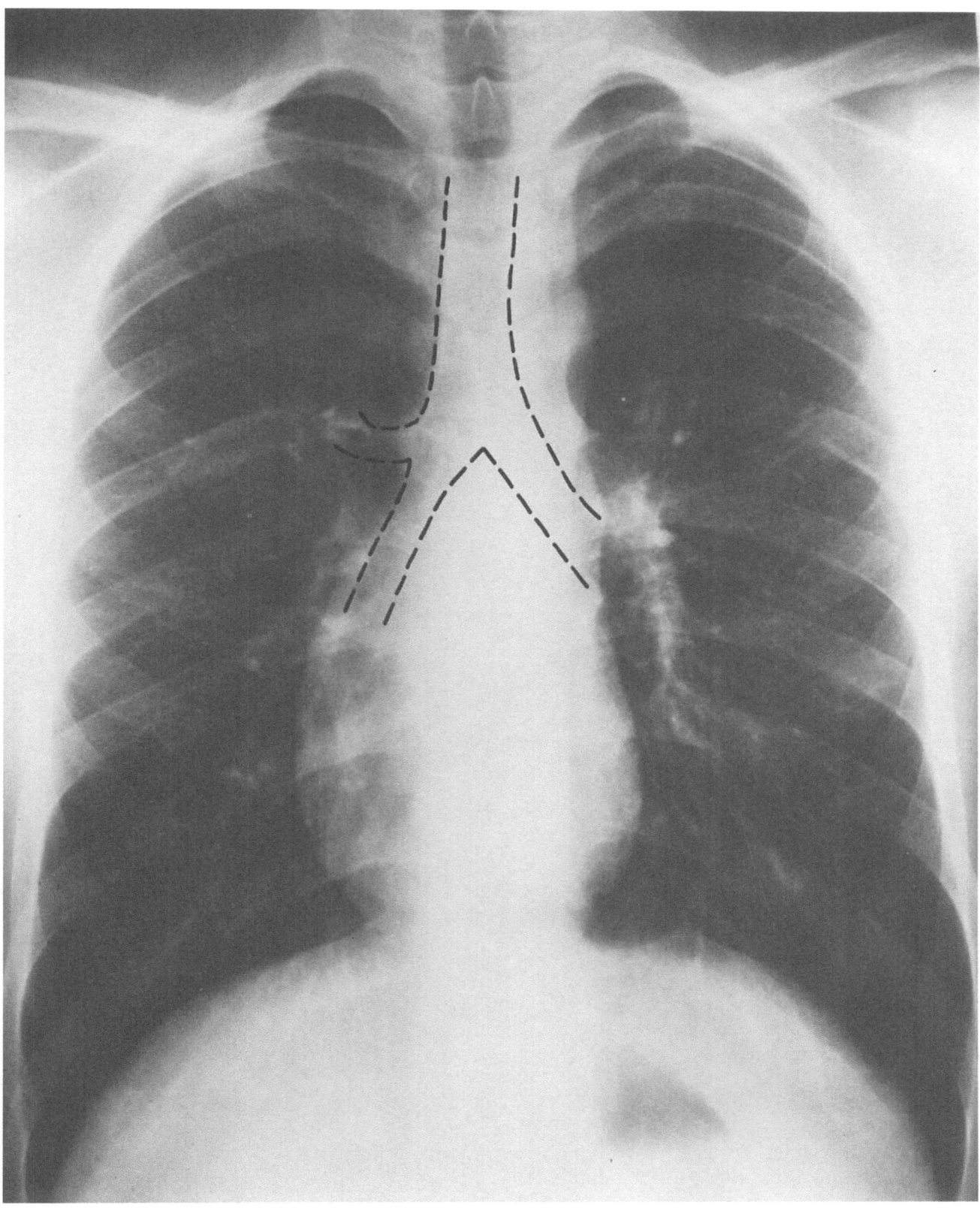

Fig. 7–226. *Situs solitus and mesoversion* (mesocardia). The epar-terial bronchus is on the right, and the hyparterial bronchus is on the left. No cardiac abnormality is present in this patient.

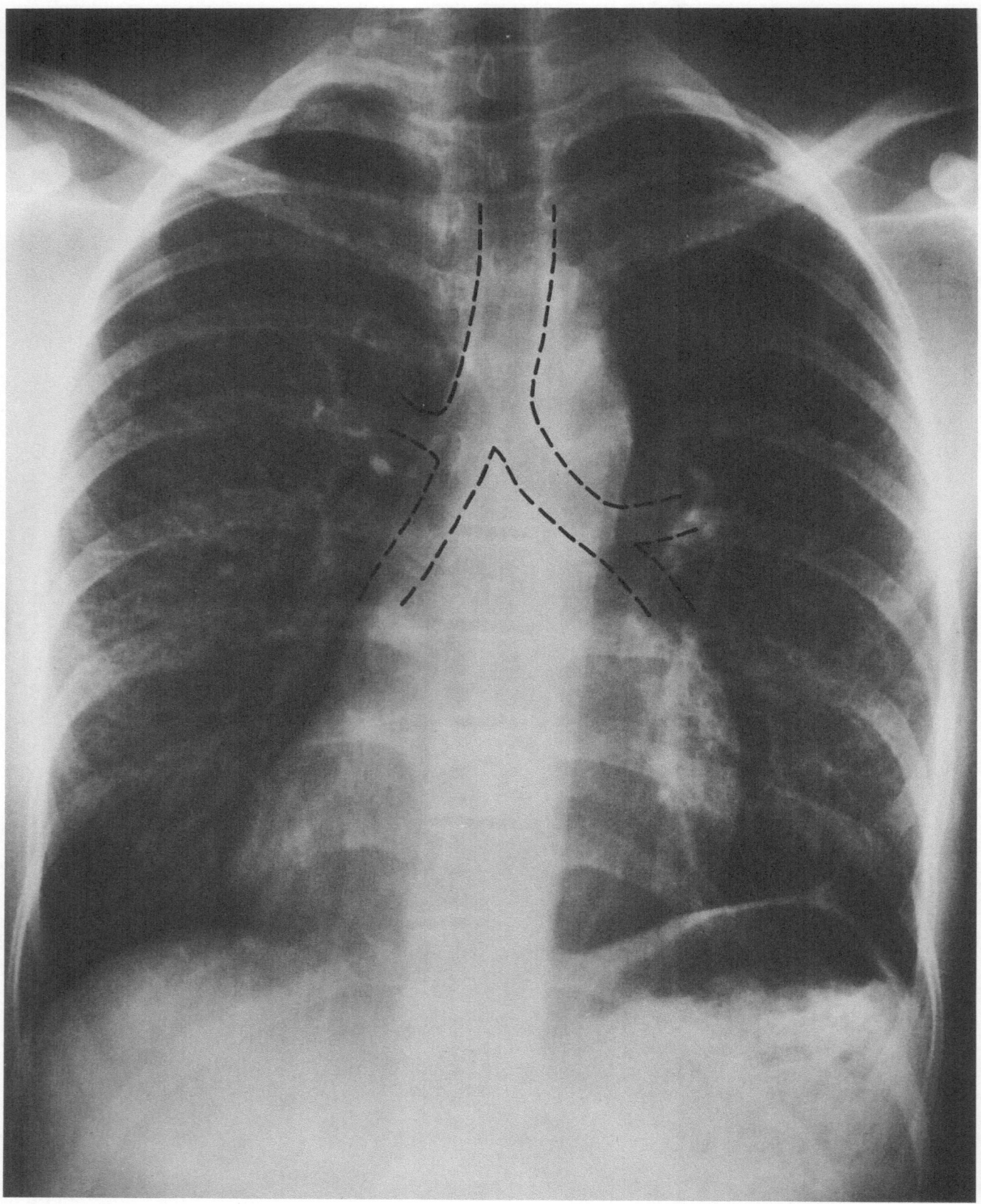

Fig. 7–227. *Situs solitus with dextroversion (dextrocardia).* The eparterial bronchus on the right and the hyparterial bronchus on the left define the thoracic situs as solitus and predict the locations of the atria. This patient has L-TGA (ventricular inver-sion) with atresia of the right atrioventricular valve and severe pulmonic stenosis. Thus the ventricles are not concordant, demon-strating that the structural anatomy of the tracheobronchial tree does not predict the location of the ventricles.

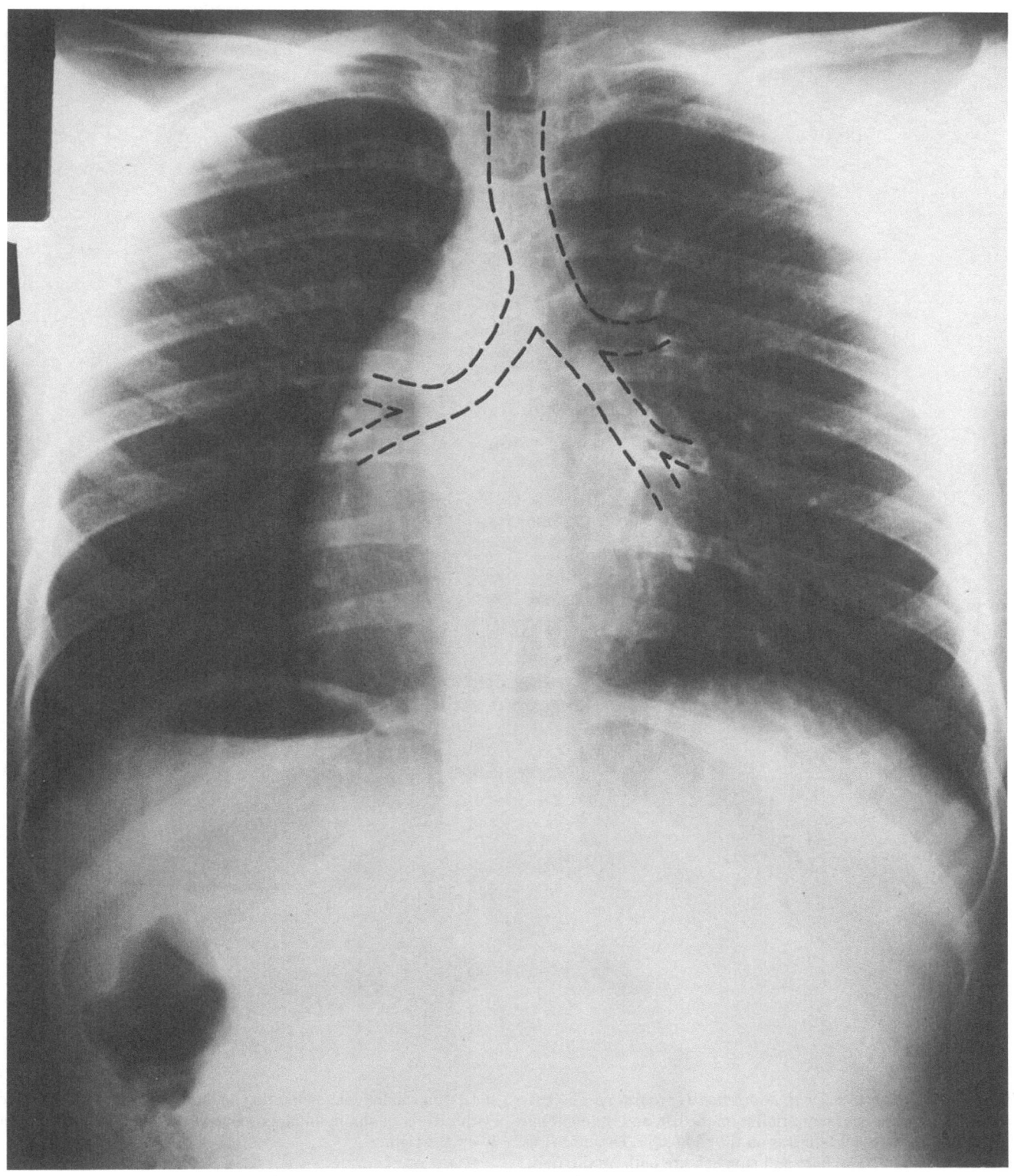

Fig. 7–228. *Situs inversus with mesoversion* (*mesocardia*). The eparterial bronchus (anatomical right bronchus) is on the left, and the hyparterial bronchus is on the right. The apex is in the midline. This 12 year old boy had no intracardiac defect.

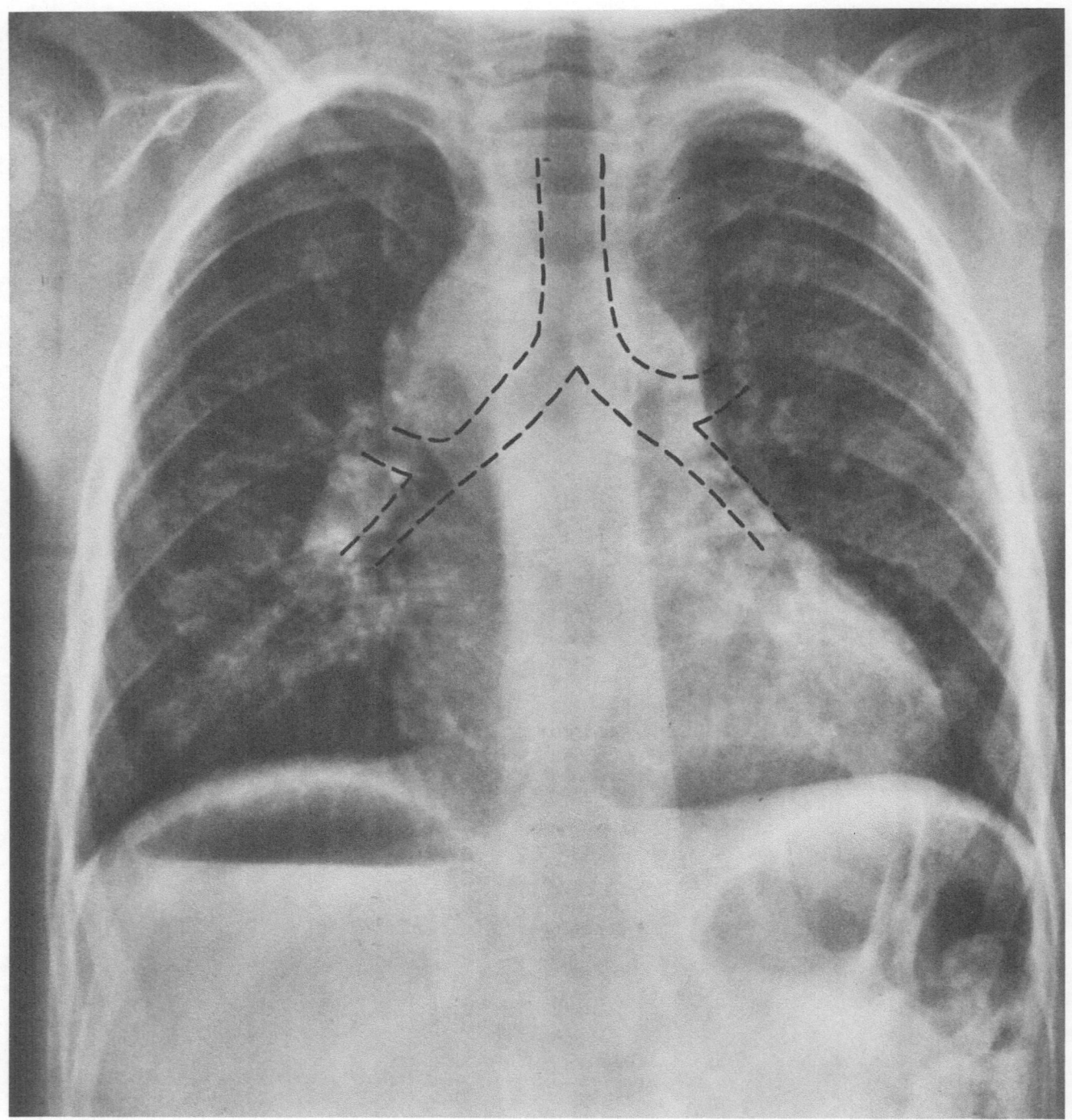

Fig. 7–229. *Situs inversus with levoversion (levocardia).* The anatomical right bronchus (eparterial) is on the left, and the anatomical left bronchus (hyparterial) is on the right side. Thoracic situs inversus is present. The liver and stomach are both on the right, indicating abdominal heterotaxy. Double-outlet right ventricle with atresia of the pulmonary valve is present. The aortic arch is on the right.

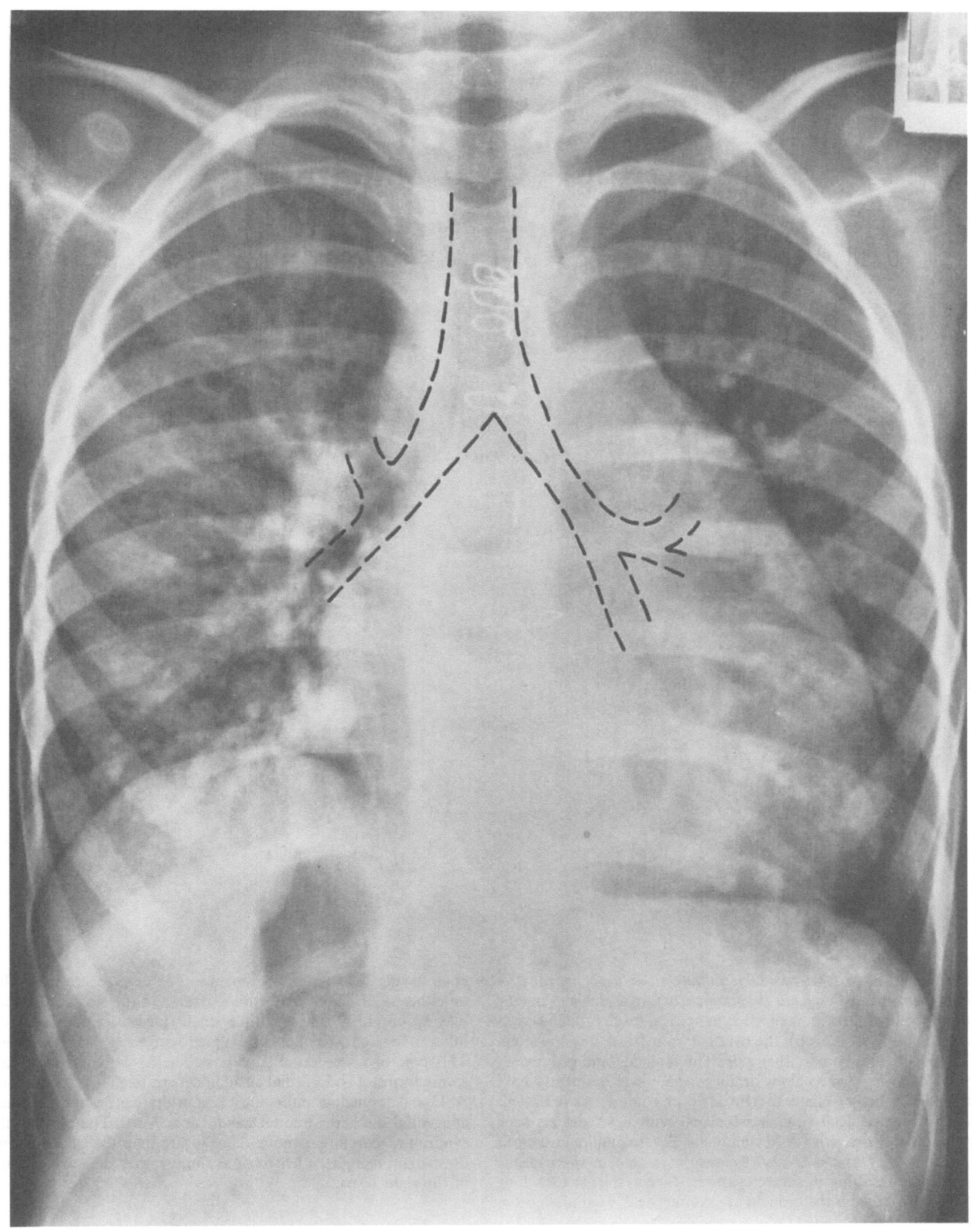

Fig. 7–230. *Thoracoabdominal discordance.* The configuration of the tracheobronchial tree indicates situs solitus, while the positions of the liver, stomach and spleen are reversed (abdominal situs inversus). Pulmonary overcirculation is present. An atrial septal defect of the endocardial cushion type was found.

Asplenia

Polysplenia

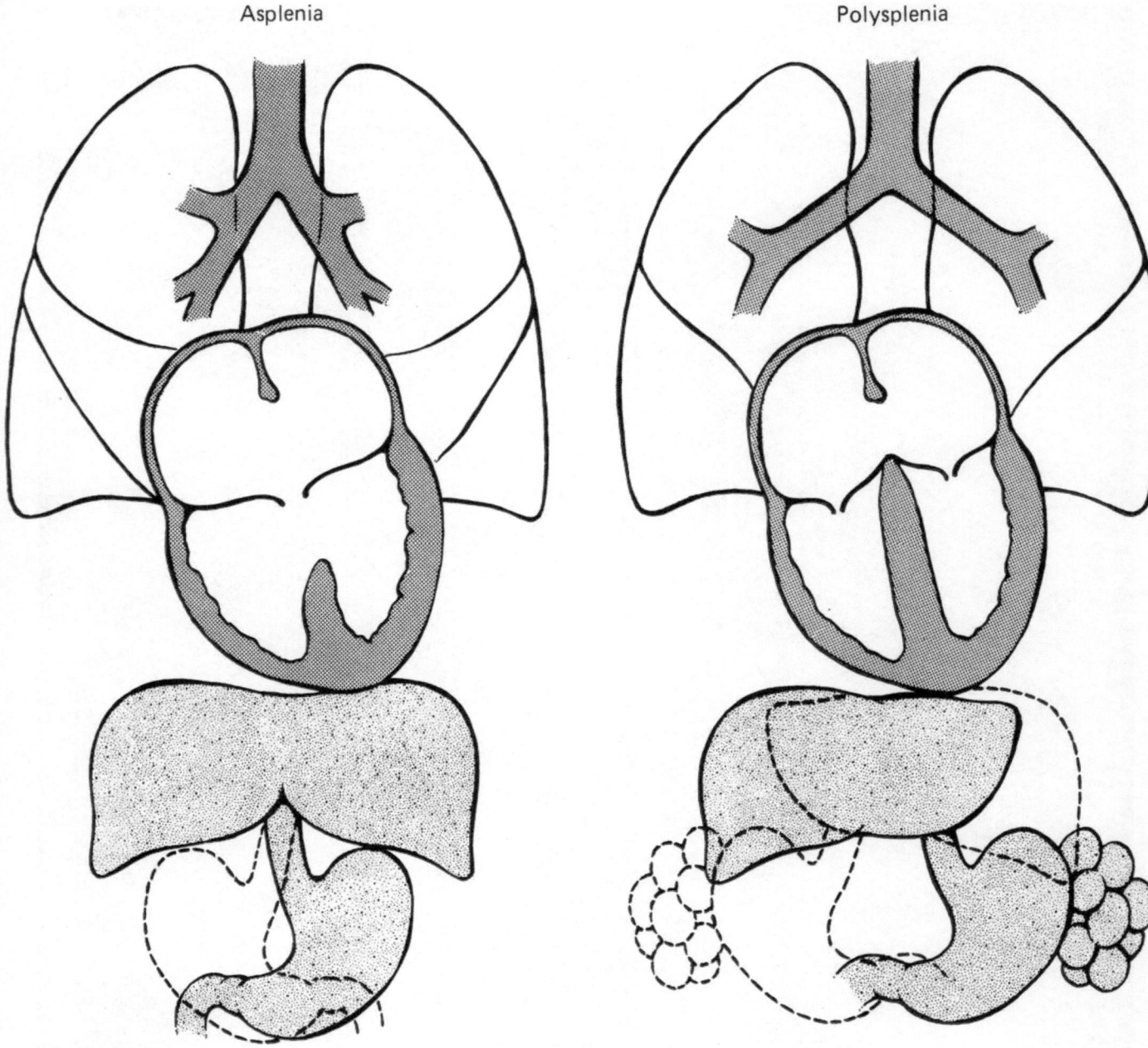

Fig. 7–231. *Two types of indeterminate situs: asplenia (dextro-isomerism) and polysplenia (levoisomerism).* In asplenia each lung has three lobes, the bronchi are symmetrical (each bronchus having an eparterial branch), the liver is symmetrical, and the stomach bubble can be on either side. The systemic and pulmonary veins often have anomalous drainage. The atria frequently have the appearance of bilateral right atria or common atrium. This type of visceroatrial situs is associated with heart defects such as single ventricle with A-V communis. Severe pulmonic stenosis or pulmonary atresia is also frequently present in the asplenia syndrome resulting in severe cyanosis. In polysplenia each lung has two lobes, and the bronchi are symmetrical, each main bron-chus having a hyparterial bronchus. The cardiac apex may be on either side. The liver is symmetrical, and the stomach bubble may be on either side. Multiple small spleens are present. The inferior vena cava is often interrupted with azygos continuation. This type of visceroatrial situs is associated with relatively less severe forms of endocardial cushion defects (e.g., ostium primum ASD) and anomalous pulmonary venous drainage as well as other congenital disorders (see text and Table 7–10). The polysplenia syndrome, therefore, is noted later in life than the asplenia syndrome and includes a left-to-right shunt rather than obstruction of the right heart.

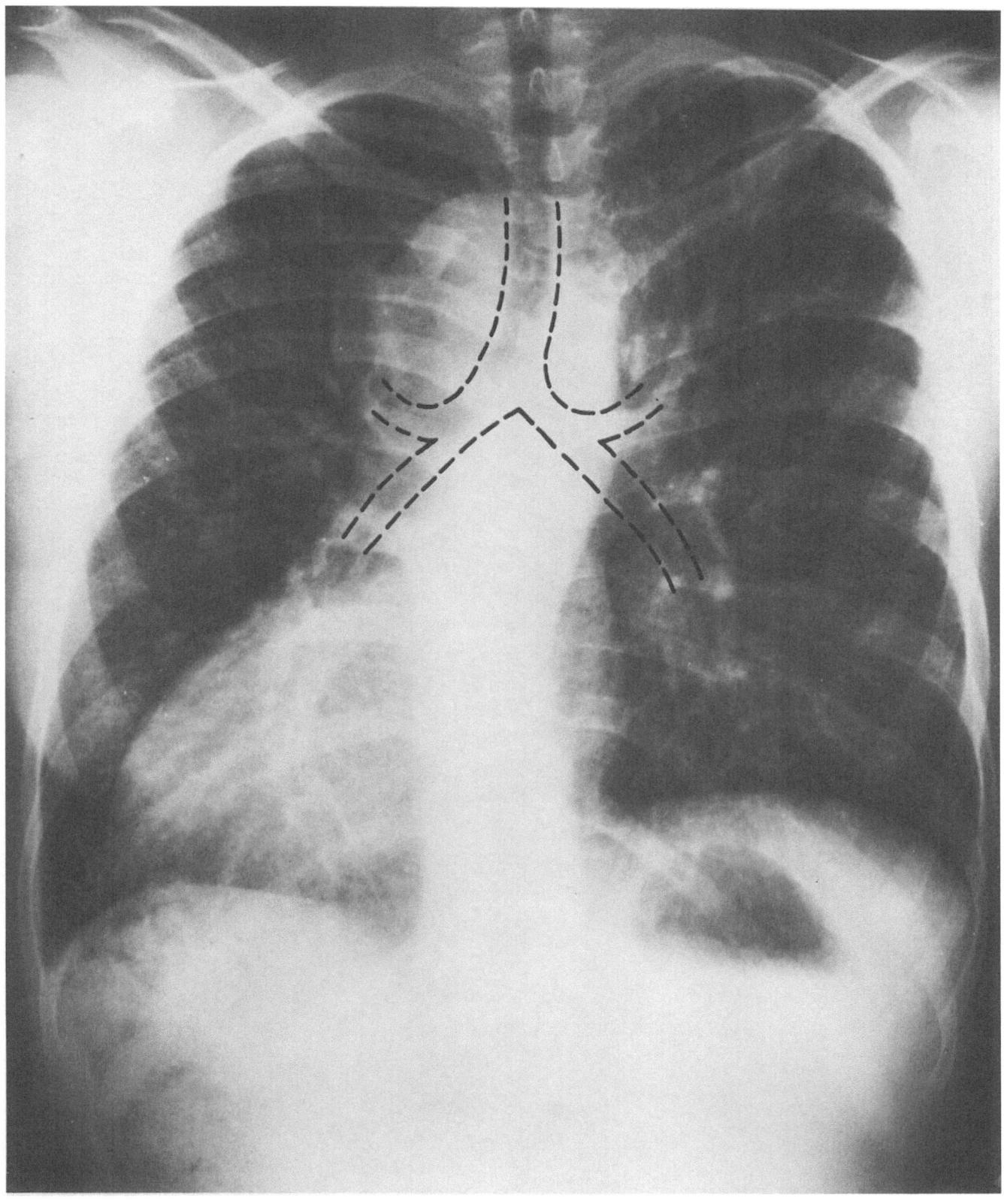

A

Fig. 7–232. *Asplenia syndrome in a 14-year-old girl.* The frontal roentgenogram of the chest (**A**) shows bilateral eparterial bronchi (dextroisomerism). The cardiac apex is on the right (dextrocardia). The liver is symmetrical, and the stomach bubble is on the left. On the lateral projection (**B**) a dense area representing the right pulmonary artery is present, but none is apparent in the position of the left pulmonary artery. Widening of the superior mediastinum in the frontal view (**A**) and a dense mass anterior to the trachea on the lateral view (**B**) is consistent with total anomalous pulmonary venous drainage of the supracardiac type. Bilateral pulmonary undercirculation indicates right heart obstruction. An additional finding is dextroscoliosis. (*Continued*)

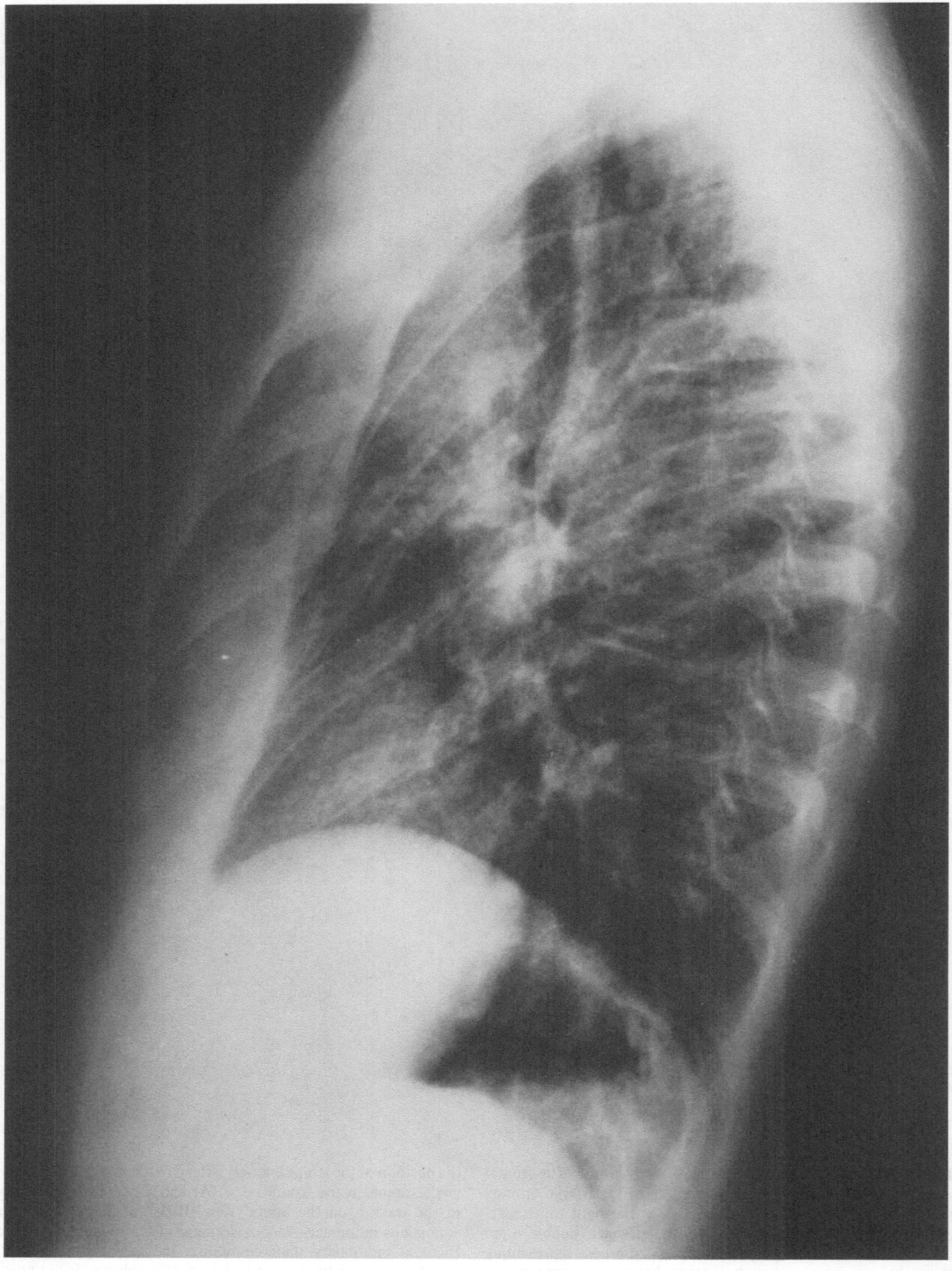

B

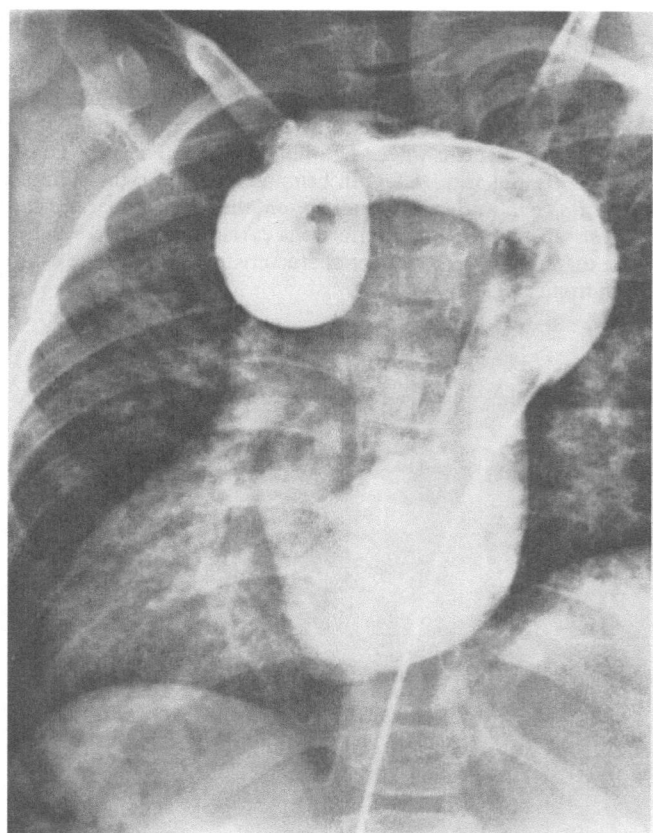

C

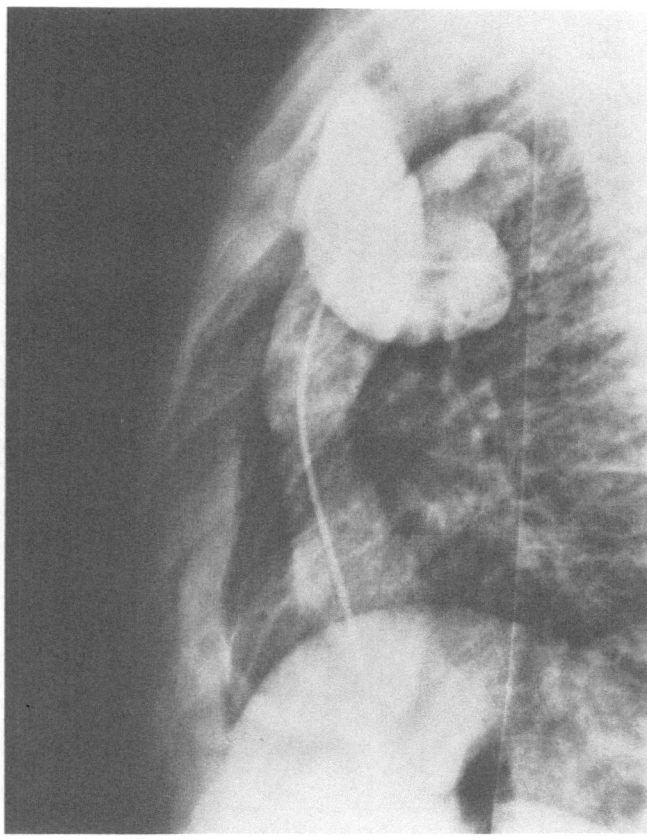

D

Fig. 7–232 (*Cont.*). *In* **C** and **D** a catheter has been advanced from the right-sided inferior vena cava across the midline to enter a common atrium and thence into an anomalous pulmonary vein to demonstrate total anomalous pulmonary venous return. The anomalous pulmonary vein accounts for widening of the superior mediastinum in the frontal projection and the dense mass anterior to the trachea on the lateral projection. The abnormal course of the inferior vena cava is characteristic of the asplenia syndrome. In **E** and **F** a venous catheter has been advanced to the ventricle. (*Continued*)

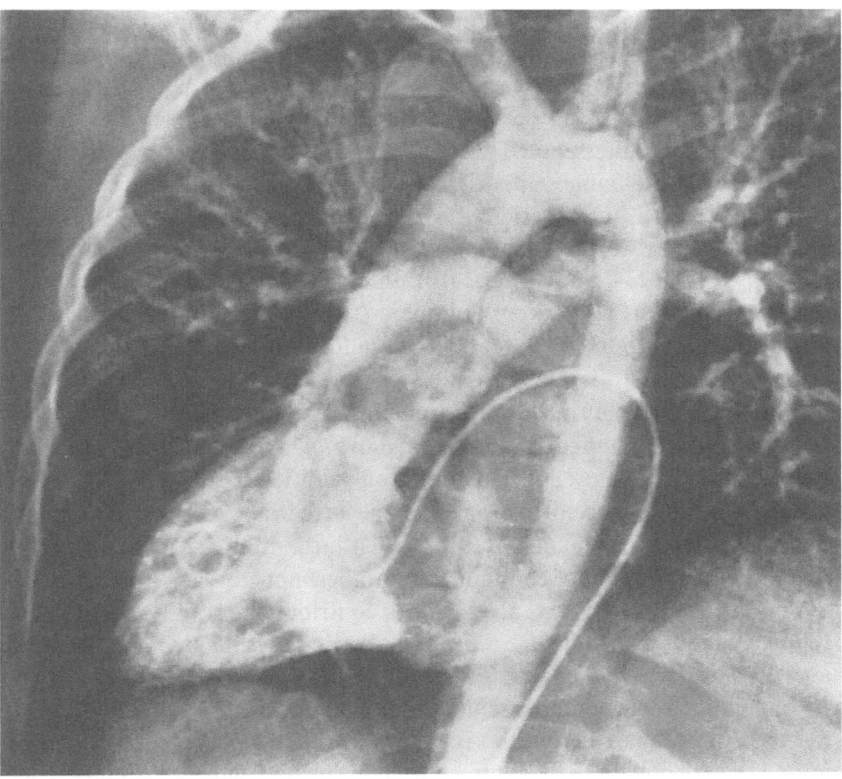

E

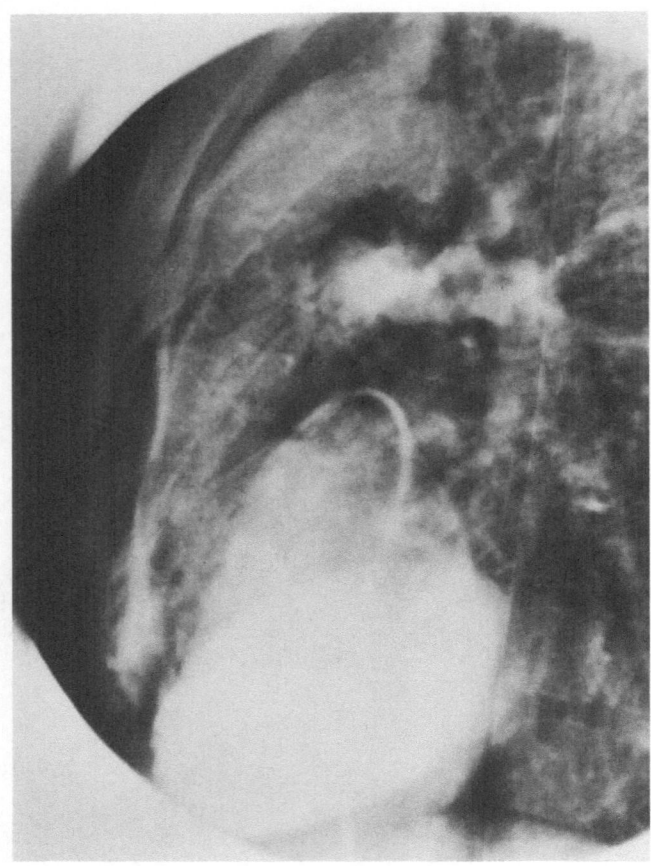

F

Fig. 7–232 (*Cont.*). A single ventricle of the left ventricular type with A-V communis and a rudimentary outlet chamber is demonstrated. Both great vessels arise from the outlet chamber with dextromalposition of the great arteries. On cine ventriculography, no conus tissue separated the aortic from the pulmonary valve. Pulmonic stenosis was caused by compression of the pulmonary valve by the aortic valve. The pulmonary arteries are identical on the frontal view (**E**), both being anatomical right pulmonary arteries, confirming the findings on the roentgenogram of the chest. Observe that the inferior vena cava overlaps the aorta below the diaphragm in **E**, another characteristic feature of the asplenia syndrome.

eral superior venae cavae) and interruption of the inferior vena cava with azygos continuation, (2) anomalous pulmonary venous return (partial or total of the cardiac variety), (3) common atrium, (4) primum or secundum atrial septal defect, (5) ventricular septal defect, often of the endocardial cushion type, (6) double-outlet right ventricle, (7) left-sided obstructive lesions (coarctation of aorta, subaortic stenosis, hypoplastic left heart syndrome), (8) cardiac malposition (Figs. 7–233, 7–234, and Table 7–10). In contrast to asplenia, transpositions and severe pulmonic stenosis are rare, although the authors have found that mild to moderate pulmonic stenosis often is present.

Although the polysplenia syndrome is a well-defined entity in which anomalies of the cardiovascular system usually dominate the clinical picture, an additional subgroup of cases of polysplenia has been reported in which no congenital cardiac anomalies are identified. Malrotations of the bowel are common, and other noncardiac anomalies such as biliary atresia also contribute to the relatively high mortality in individuals with polysplenia and no cardiac defect (Table 7–10).

In summary, the cardiovascular complications of asplenia tend to occur earlier, with severe cyanosis and pulmonary undercirculation, in contrast to polysplenia, which presents later and is characterized by pulmonary overcirculation on plain films.

Anisosplenia

Anisosplenia, another group of defects with situs ambiguus (isomerism) is characterized by a symmetrical visceral configuration and splenic abnormalities with a bifid spleen (one or two large spleens with multiple accessory spleens). Two complexes have been described: M-anisosplenia or "third syndrome" and F-anisosplenia or "fourth syndrome."

M-anisosplenia consists of bilateral right lungs, bilateral eparterial bronchi, anomalous pulmonary venous return, bilateral superior venae cavae, atrioventricularis communis, pulmonic stenosis, dextrocardia and right aortic arch. M-anisosplenia has a striking male preponderance.

F-anisosplenia is associated with bilateral left lungs, bilateral hyparterial bronchi, bilateral superior venae cavae, abnormal inferior caval pattern, dextrocardia, double-outlet right ventricle, left aortic arch, and malrotation. F-anisosplenia has a marked predilection for females.

Fig. 7–233. *Polysplenia syndrome in a 2-year-old boy.* On the PA film of the chest **(A)** cardiomegaly and pulmonary overcirculation are present. The bronchi are both hyparterial (levoisomerism). Hilar density on the lateral view represents the two anatomical left pulmonary arteries. The cardiac apex is on the left (levocardia), and the stomach bubble on the right, but it is obscured by the colon in this film. The liver is symmetrical. On the lateral view **(B)** the stomach is posterior; no inferior vena cava is identified. Individuals with polysplenia often have left-to-right shunts (pulmonary overcirculation), whereas those with asplenia are more likely to have pulmonary undercirculation due to obstruction of the right side of the heart. This patient has interruption of the inferior vena cava with azygos continuation. (*Continued*)

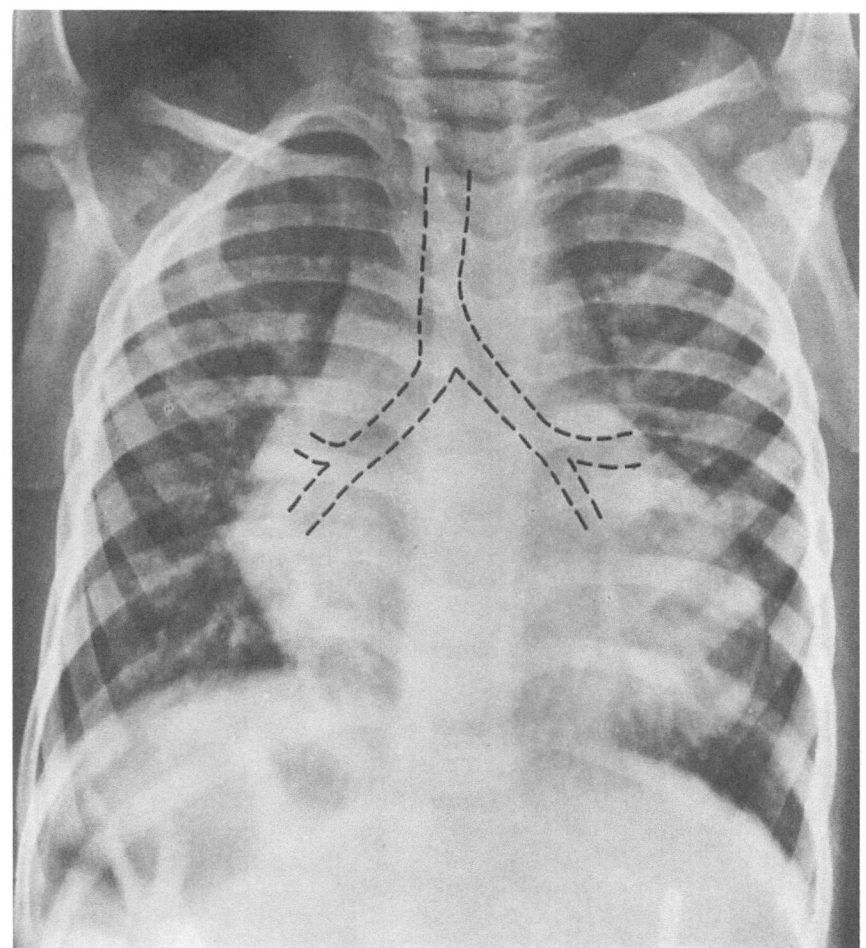

A

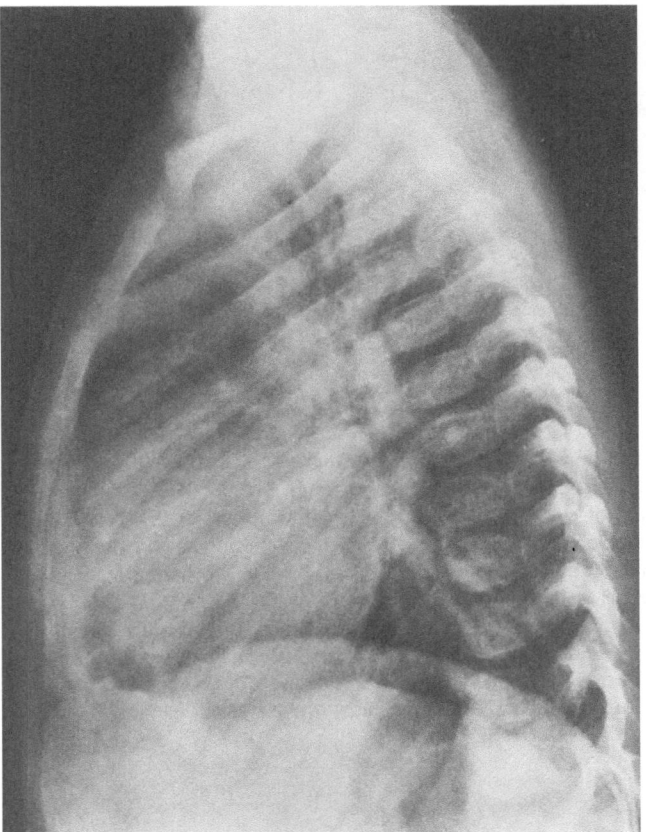

B

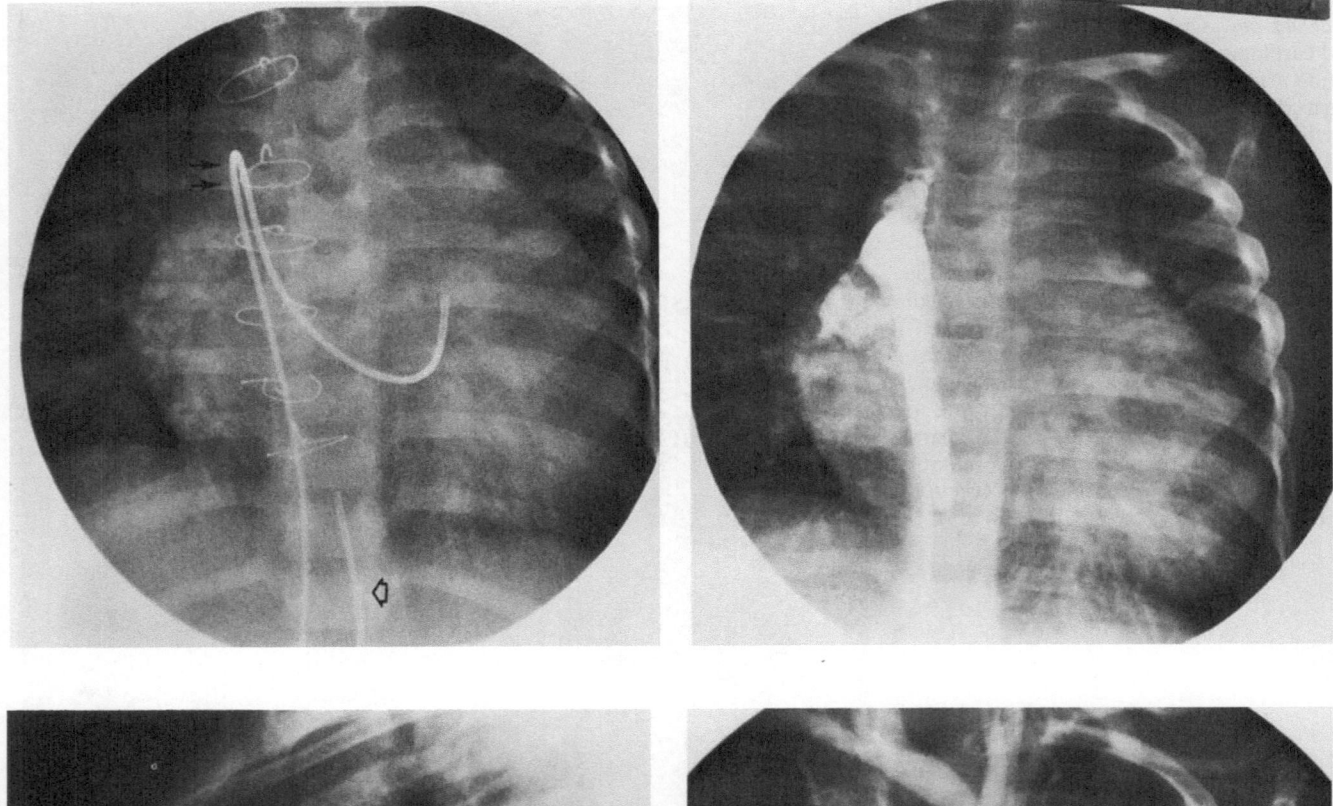

C

D

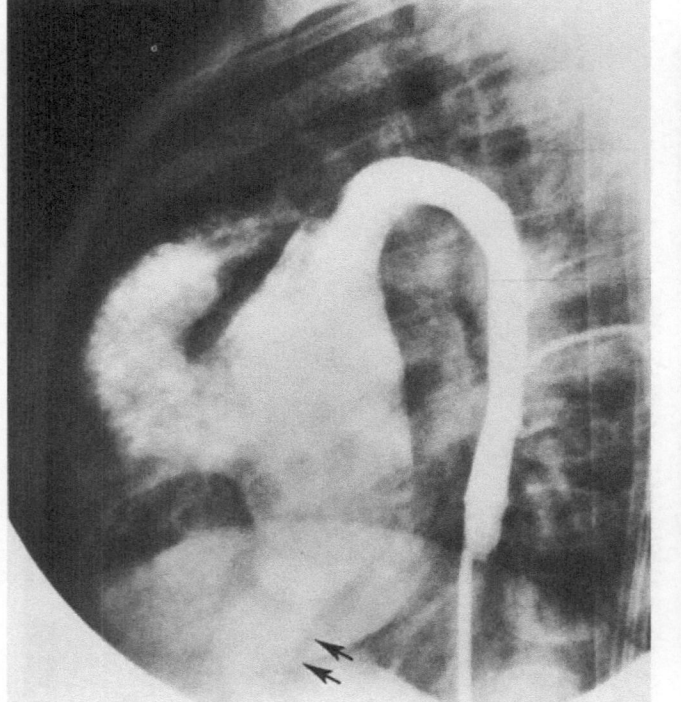
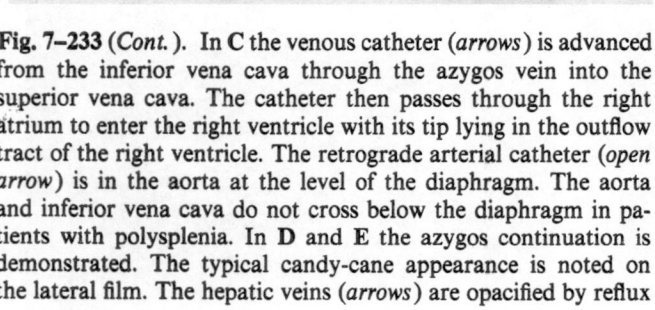

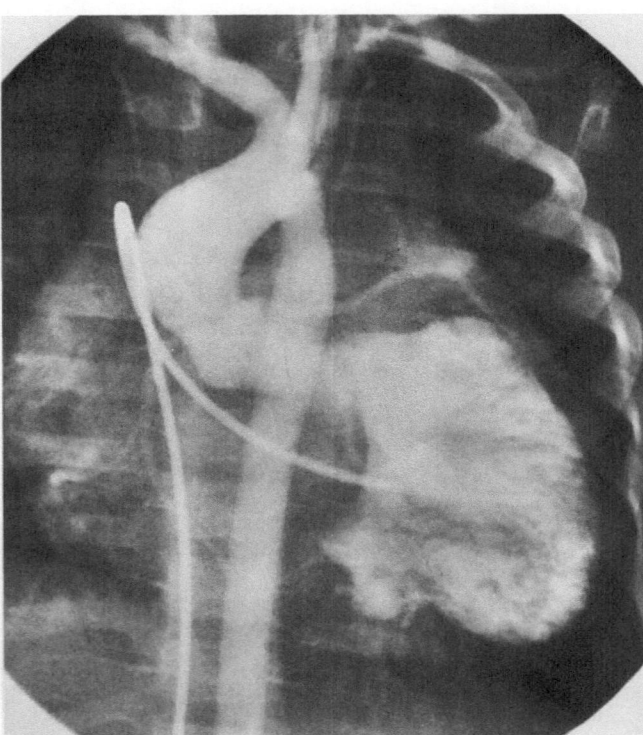

E

F

Fig. 7–233 (*Cont.*). In **C** the venous catheter (*arrows*) is advanced from the inferior vena cava through the azygos vein into the superior vena cava. The catheter then passes through the right atrium to enter the right ventricle with its tip lying in the outflow tract of the right ventricle. The retrograde arterial catheter (*open arrow*) is in the aorta at the level of the diaphragm. The aorta and inferior vena cava do not cross below the diaphragm in patients with polysplenia. In **D** and **E** the azygos continuation is demonstrated. The typical candy-cane appearance is noted on the lateral film. The hepatic veins (*arrows*) are opacified by reflux from the right atrium. In some individuals the hepatic veins may simulate the density of the inferior vena cava on the lateral film of the chest. In **F** the venous catheter has been advanced from the right atrium across the atrial septal defect through the left atrium and into the left ventricle. The typical gooseneck deformity of an endocardial cushion defect is demonstrated. An ostium primum atrial septal defect is present. The M-mode echocardiogram also demonstrated the equivalent of a gooseneck deformity (Fig. 7–8). (*Continued*)

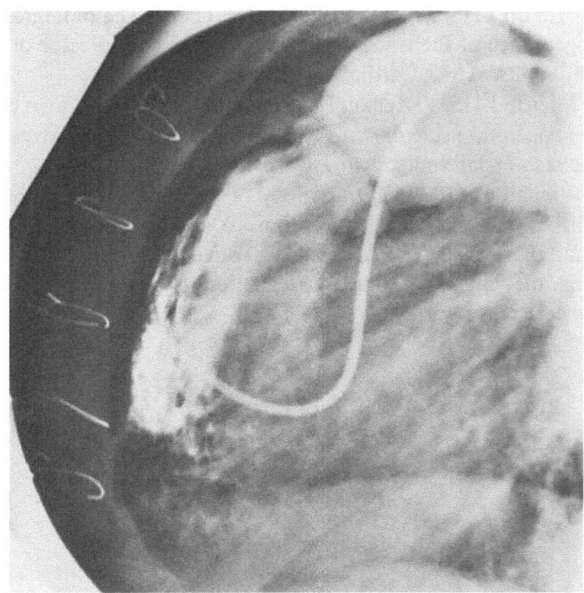

G

Fig. 7–233 (*Cont.*). The right ventriculogram after surgery for atrial septal defect (**G**) shows thickening and doming of the pulmonary valve, with poststenotic dilatation of the pulmonary artery consistent with valvar pulmonic stenosis.

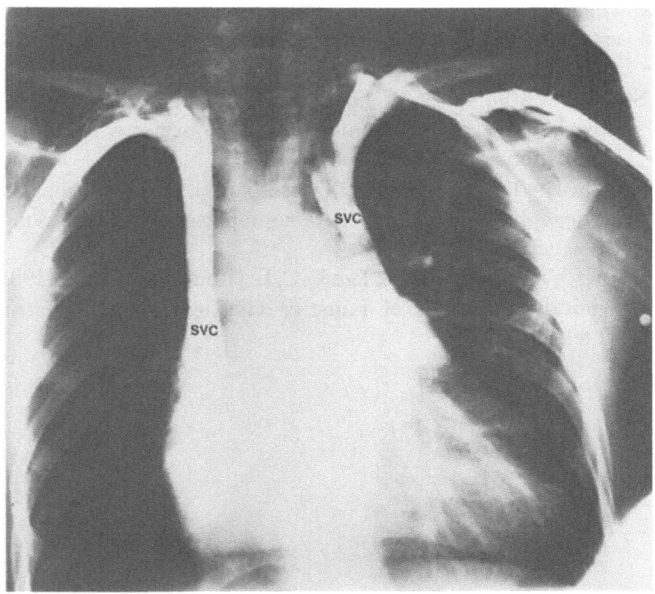

Fig. 7–234. *Polysplenia syndrome in a 16-year-old boy.* Simultaneous injections into the antecubital veins demonstrate bilateral superior venae cavae (*SVC*). The left superior vena cava drains directly into the left atrium.

Bibliography

Brandt HM, Liebelow AA (1968) Right pulmonary isomerism associated with venous, splenic and other anomalies. Lab Invest 7:469–504

Chacko KA (1982) Isolated atrial inversion (letter). Am Heart J 104:885 (See also reply to the letter)

Chandra RS (1974) Biliary atresia and other structural anomalies in the congenital polysplenia syndrome. J Pediatr 85:649–655

Diener KA (1962) Agenesis of the spleen. Presentation of a case without congenital defects of the heart. Bol Med Hosp Infant Mex 19:711–715

Elliot LP, Cramer GC, Amplatz K (1966) The anomalous relationship of the inferior vena cava and abnormal aorta as a specific sign of asplenia. Radiology 87:859–863

Elliot LP, Jue KL, Amplatz K (1966) A roentgen classification of cardiac malpositions. Invest Radiol 1:17–28

Espino-Vela J (1978) Septal defect in transposition of great arteries (letter). Am J Cardiol 42:692

Freedom RM (1972) The asplenia syndrome: A review of significant extracardiac structural abnormalities in 29 necropsied patients. J Pediatr 81:1130–1133

Hastreiter AR, Rodriquez-Caronel A (1968) Discordant situs of thoracic and abdominal viscera. Am J Cardiol 22:111–118

Ivemark BI (1955) Implications of agenesis of the spleen on the pathogenesis of cono-truncus anomalies in childhood; an analysis of the heart malformations in the splenic agenesis syndrome, with fourteen new cases. Acta Paediat Scand 44 (suppl 104)

Landing BH (1975) Syndromes of congenital heart disease with tracheobranchial anomalies. Am J Roentgenol 123:679–686

Landing BH, Lawrence TK, Payne VC, Wells TR (1971) Bronchial anatomy in syndromes with abnormal visceral situs, abnormal spleen and congenital heart disease. Am J Cardiol 28:456–462

Lane EJ Jr, Whalen JP (1969) A new sign of left atrial enlargement: Posterior displacement of the left bronchial tree. Radiology 93:279–284

Loosekoot TG (1973) Mirror image dextrocardia with situs solitus of the abdominal organs and a normal heart. Eur J Cardiol 1:49–54

Lucas RV Jr, Neufeld HN, Lester RG, Edwards JE (1962) The symmetrical liver as a roentgen sign of asplenia. Circulation 25:973–975

Moller JH, Nakib MD, Anderson RC, Edwards JE (1967) Congenital heart disease associated with polysplenia. Circulation 36:789–799

Murphy JW, Mitchell WA: (1957) Congenital absence of the spleen. Pediatrics 20:253–256

Partridge J (1979) The radiological evaluation of atrial situs. Clin Radiol 30:95–103

Salazar J, Martinez F, Valero MI, Casado de Frias E (1976) Polysplenia with left ventricular hypoplasia and partial anomalous pulmonary venous connection. Acta Cardiol 31:483–490

Soto B, Pacifico AD, Souza AR, Bargeron LM Jr, Ermocilla R, Tonkin IL (1978) Identification of thoracic isomerism from the plain chest radiograph. Am J Roentgenol 131:995–1002

Spindola-Franco H, Siegelman SS (1969) Segmental agenesis of inferior vena cava with azygos substitution. Angiographic findings. Ann Thorac Surg 8:458–463

Stanger P, Benassi RC, Korns ME, Jul KL, Edwards JE (1968)

Diagrammatic portrayal of variations in cardiac structure. Reference to transposition, dextrocardia and the concept of four normal hearts. Circulation 37 (suppl 4):16

Stanger P, Rudolph AM, Edwards JE (1977) Cardiac malpositions. An overview based on study of 65 necropsy specimens. Circulation 56:159–172

Tonkin IL, Tonkin AK (1982) Visceroatrial situs abnormalities. Sonographic and computed tomographic appearance. Am J Roentgenol 138:509–515

Turner JAP, Corkey CWB, Lee JYC, Levison H, Sturgess J (1981) Clinical expressions of immotile cilia syndrome. Pediatrics 67:805–810

Van Mierop LHS, Eisen S, Schiebler GL (1970) The radiographic appearance of the tracheobronchial tree as an indicator of visceral situs. Am J Cardiol 26:432–435

Van Mierop LHS, Patterson PR, Reynolds RW (1964) Two cases of congenital asplenia with isomerism of the cardiac atria and the sino-atrial nodes. Am J Cardiol 13:407–414

Van Praagh R (1977) Terminology of congenital heart disease. Glossary and commentary (editorial). Circulation 56:139–143

Yarnal JR, Golish JA, Ahmad M, Tomashefski JF (1982) The immotile cilia syndrome. Explanation for many a clinical-mystery. Postgrad Med 71:195–217

8 Neoplasms of the Heart

Neoplasms of the heart may be divided into primary (benign or malignant) and secondary (metastatic). Primary cardiac neoplasms are rare, but may occur at any age. The majority are benign, the most common being the myxoma, which develops as a polypoid mass usually arising from the left atrium (LA). Sarcoma and rhabdomyoma are the second and third most common primary neoplasms of the heart. Other rare benign neoplasms (hamartoma, fibroma, fibromyxoma, lymphangioendothelioma) and malignant neoplasms (lymphosarcoma, fibrosarcoma, leiomyosarcoma and rhabdomyosarcoma) have been reported. Cardiac neoplasms are further classified by their location in and around the heart (e.g., intracavitary, myocardial or intramural, pericardial). The myxoma, the polypoid fibroma and the sarcoma arise from the endocardium (intracavitary tumors), whereas the rhabdomyoma and myocardial fibroma originate from the myocardium (intramural tumors). Neoplasms of pericardial origin are mesothelioma, lipoma, pericardial fibroma and angioma. Teratoma may also occur within the pericardium.

Bronchogenic cyst, large metastatic lymph nodes, inflammatory lymph nodes and other extracardiac mediastinal masses that are contiguous with the heart may produce plain film findings identical to those occurring with pericardial neoplasms. The echocardiographic and angiographic findings with large vegetations, free-floating thrombi and cysts of the valves may be indistinguishable from those associated with intracardiac tumors. Endomyocardial fibrosis may also simulate a cardiac neoplasm clinically and on roentgenograms of the chest; however, echocardiography and angiocardiography are most helpful in distinguishing endomyocardial fibrosis from a neoplasm.

Because benign intracavitary cardiac neoplasms are amenable to surgery, their prompt diagnosis on echocardiography, plain films and angiocardiography is of utmost importance.

Clinical Features

The most common intracardiac neoplasm is the myxoma. This lesion may be sessile or pedunculated. The usual site of attachment is the fossa ovalis, most commonly in the LA and next in the right atrium (RA). This neoplasm is considered to be benign; however, on rare occasions myxoma may recur locally or metastasize. A myxoma may become large enough to cause mitral or tricuspid stenosis or incompetence and may also fragment and embolize. Infective endocarditis can develop on an intracardiac myxoma. Systemic symptoms of fever and loss of weight, as well as immunological and hematological abnormalities, may also develop in individuals with a noninfected myxoma. A clue to the diagnosis of a pedunculated mass may be a change in symptoms or physical findings with a change in position of the patient. As an example, dyspnea or a diastolic murmur of mitral stenosis or both may disappear if the patient changes to a supine position. Another characteristic sign is the tumor "plop" occurring in early diastole, with timing similar to that of an S_3 or opening snap.

RA neoplasms may produce tricuspid obstruction, resulting in peripheral edema, hepatomegaly and ascites. The tricuspid murmur and the tumor plop are similar to the murmur and gallop heard with Ebstein anomaly of the tricuspid valve. On occasion, neoplasms of the right side of the heart are associated with multiple pulmonary emboli and pulmonary hypertension without cardiac symptoms or signs.

The most common intracardiac neoplasm in childhood is rhabdomyoma. This tumor, often multiple, invariably arises within the ventricles, originating from the ventricular septum in the vicinity of the crista supraventricularis. The major clinical manifestation is obstruction to flow of blood. If the tumor is not large enough to interfere with cardiac function the affected individual may be asymptomatic. The obstruction may occur at the inlet or outlet of either ventricle, causing clinical findings of subaortic stenosis or infundibular pulmonic stenosis, mitral stenosis or mitral atresia.

In some series, more than 50% of individuals with intracardiac rhabdomyomas have tuberous sclerosis.

Other benign intracardiac neoplasms present in a manner similar to myxoma or rhabdomyoma, causing obstruction or valvular insufficiency, depending on location. See Table 8–1 for a list of neoplasms reported to occur within the heart and pericardium.

Pericardial neoplasms (e.g., hemangioma, lymphangioma) usually produce no signs or symptoms, generally occurring with pericardial effusion with or without tamponade. On occasion a pericardial tumor is large enough to compress the heart directly, causing cardiac tamponade. Pericardial neoplasms may also be present with abnormalities of the cardiac contour, which are identical to those produced by pericardial cysts and diverticula. A pericardial cyst usually occurs at the right cardiophrenic angle, but may be present in other locations as well; thus, pericardial neoplasms and other pericardial masses may be difficult to distinguish one from the other.

Metastases to the endocardium, myocardium and pericardium have all been observed. Most often these are asymptomatic and are discovered at autopsy. Intramyocardial masses may produce arrhythmias or, if sufficiently large, may interfere with myocardial function. Only rarely does a metastatic tumor in the endocardium behave as an intracardiac mass. Most metastatic tumors invade the heart by direct extension from the lungs. Other neoplasms that invade the pericardium and myocardium include carcinoma of the breast, esophagus, pancreas and bronchus, as well as melanoma and lymphoma.

Echocardiography

Echocardiography has become of paramount importance in the detection of intracardiac neoplasms. A pedunculated mass is recognized on M-mode by its characteristic motion. A sessile tumor produces thickening or extra layers within the heart (Fig. 8–1). A pedunculated LA mass is identified on M-mode as a line or shadow that moves anteriorly behind the anterior mitral leaflet as it opens during diastole (Fig. 8–2). The mass may or may not be defined as it reenters the LA during systole. A large neoplasm can present as a cloud of echoes or a dense multilayered area that appears to fill the mitral orifice during diastole. On occasion a mass is homogeneous, being poorly visualized as a consequence. RA myxoma produces similar findings related to the tricuspid valve (Fig. 8–3).

On 2-D echocardiography the size and shape of a pedunculated mass are optimally delineated. Although sessile tumors of the atrium are best visualized by 2-D echocardiography, even by this technique they may be difficult to distinguish from organized thrombus. A clue to the differential diagnosis is that an atrial myxoma usually attaches near the foramen ovale, whereas atrial thrombus may adhere to the LA wall. In addition, most atrial thrombi occur in association with severe mitral stenosis (rarely does an atrial myxoma occur in a patient with mitral stenosis).

TABLE 8–1. Primary and Metastatic Neoplasms of the Heart

I. Benign Intracavitary Neoplasms
  A. Myxoma
  B. Rhabdomyoma (probably hamartoma)
  C. Fibroma (probably hamartoma)
  D. Lipoma (including hibernoma, fibrolipoma, myolipoma)
  E. Lipomatous hypertrophy (atrial septum)
  F. Papillary tumor (heart valve)
  G. Cystic tumor

II. Malignant Intracavitary Neoplasms
  A. Sarcoma
    1. Fibrosarcoma
    2. Angiosarcoma
    3. Rhabdomyosarcoma
    4. Mesothelial sarcoma
    5. Kaposi sarcoma
    6. Liposarcoma
    7. Extraskeletal osteosarcoma
    8. Leiomyosarcoma
  B. Primary lymphoma
  C. Malignant fibrous histiocytoma

III. Benign Myocardial (Mural) Neoplasms
  A. Rhabdomyoma
  B. Fibroma
  C. Bronchogenic cyst (developmental)
  D. Lymphangioma
  E. Neurofibroma
  F. Neurofibroma as part of neurofibromatosis

IV. Malignant Myocardial (Mural) Neoplasms
  A. Sarcoma
    1. Rhabdomyosarcoma
    2. Angiosarcoma
    3. Fibrosarcoma
    4. Lymphoma, lymphosarcoma, Hodgkin disease

V. Benign Pericardial Neoplasms
  A. Vascular tumors (hemangioma, lymphangioma, lymphangioendothelioma)
  B. Lipoma
  C. Leiomyofibroma
  D. Fibroma
  E. Mesothelioma
  F. Thymoma
  G. Dermoid
  H. Teratoma
  I. Hamartoma

VI. Malignant Pericardial Neoplasms
  A. Sarcomas (all types)
  B. Malignant tumor of the nerve sheath
  C. Malignant teratoma
  D. Synovial sarcoma
  E. Lymphoma

VII. Metastatic Cardiac Neoplasms
  A. Intracavitary (very rare)
    1. Bronchogenic
    2. Lymphoma
    3. Ovarian
  B. Myocardial (mostly microscopic)
    1. Any primary focus
  C. Pericardial (by direct invasion)
    1. Lung
    2. Breast
    3. Pancreas
    4. Esophagus
    5. Lymphoma
    6. Melanoma

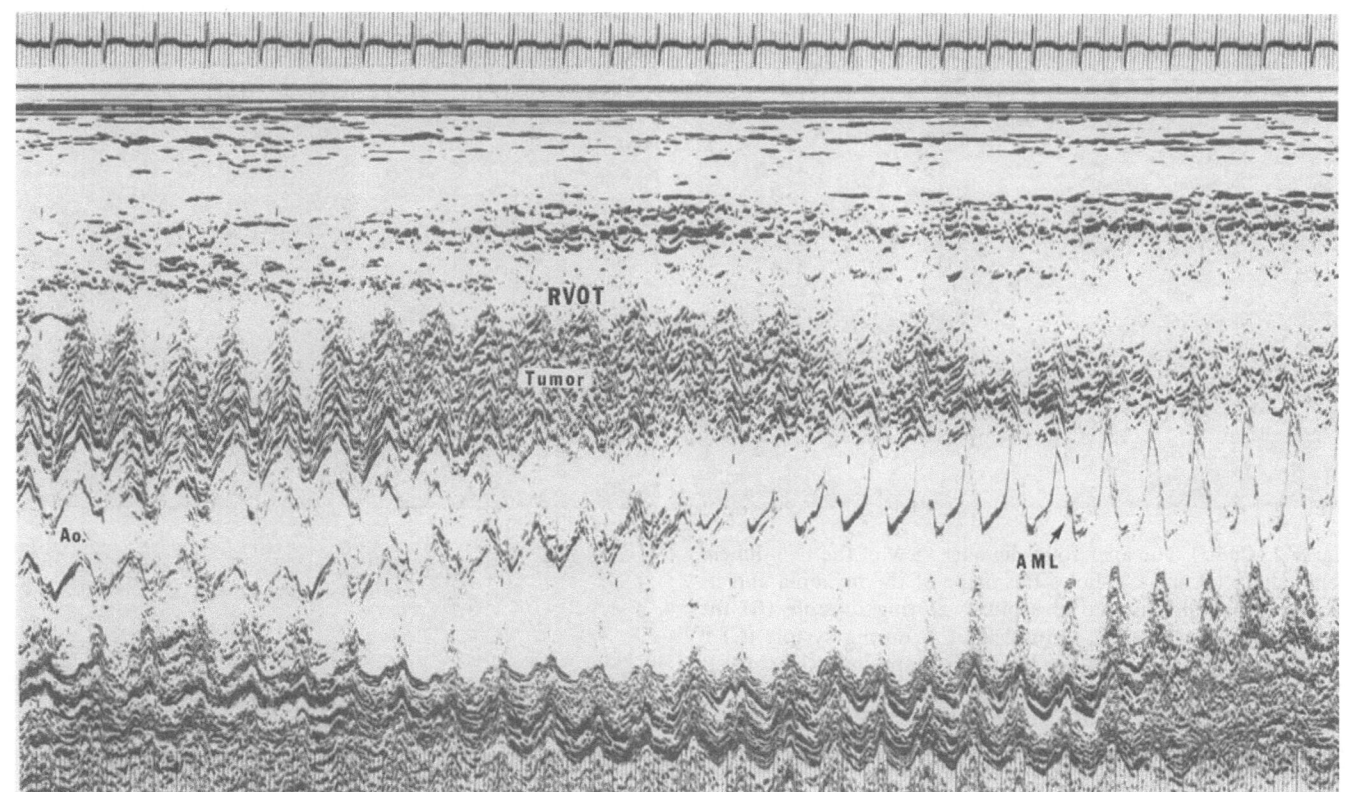

Fig. 8–1. *Rhabdomyoma arising from the crista supraventricularis in a newborn infant.* The M-mode arc scan from the aortic valve (*Ao.*) to the mitral valve (*AML*) showed a large mass in the right ventricular outflow tract (*RVOT*) that moved with the ventricular septum. At surgery a large rhabdomyoma was present, attached broadly to the crista supraventricularis.

The chest film and angiogram are illustrated in Fig. 1–14. Computerized tomography of the head showed intracranial calcifications characteristic of tuberous sclerosis.

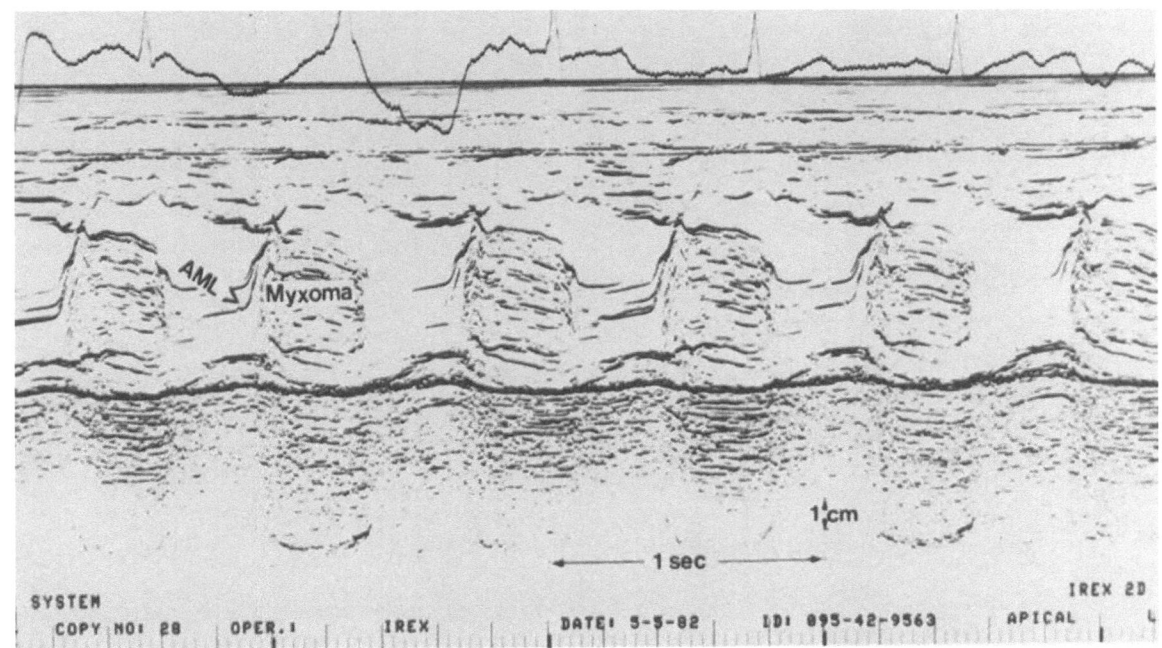

A

Fig. 8–2. *Left atrial myxoma.* The M-mode tracing (**A**) shows a mass with multiple echo interfaces behind the anterior leaflet of the mitral valve (*AML*). During diastole the mass moves anteriorly into the left ventricle. During systole it moves back toward the left atrium, out of the plane of the M-mode image. (*Continued*)

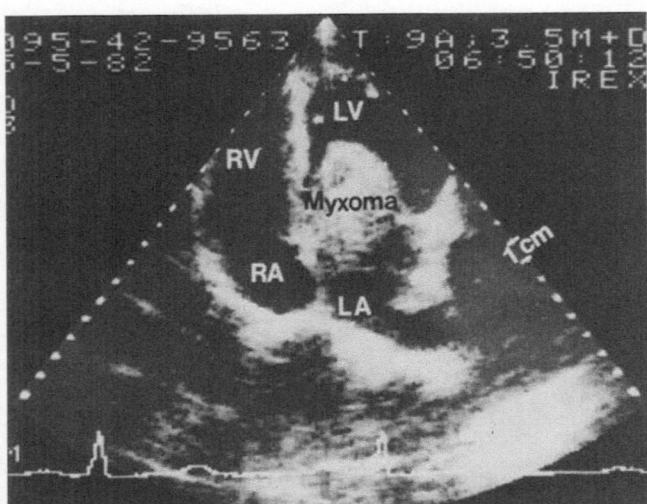

B

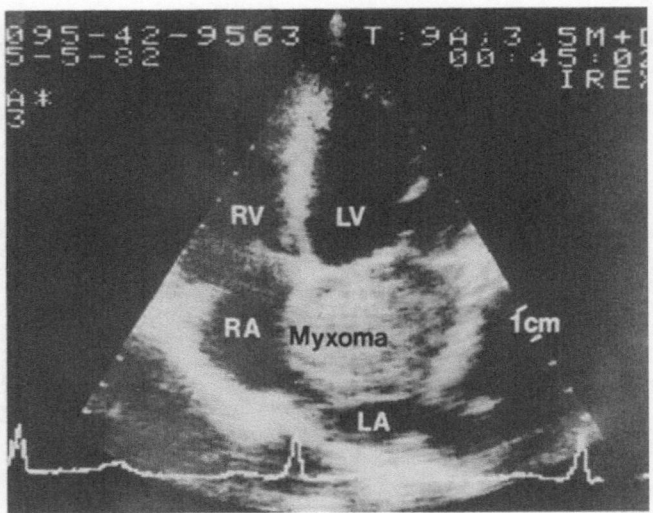

C

Fig. 8–2 (*Cont.*) The apex four-chamber view of the two-dimensional study (**B** and **C**) shows the shape of the myxoma and its attachment to the interatrial septum. During diastole (**B**) the mass moves into the left ventricle (*LV*); during systole (**C**) it returns to the left atrium (*LA*). The surgical specimen (**D**) consists of the atrial myxoma which was removed in-toto with its attachment to the atrial septum. *RA* = right atrium; *RV* = right ventricle. (Courtesy of M. Rosoff, M.D., Montefiore Medical Center, Bronx, N.Y.)

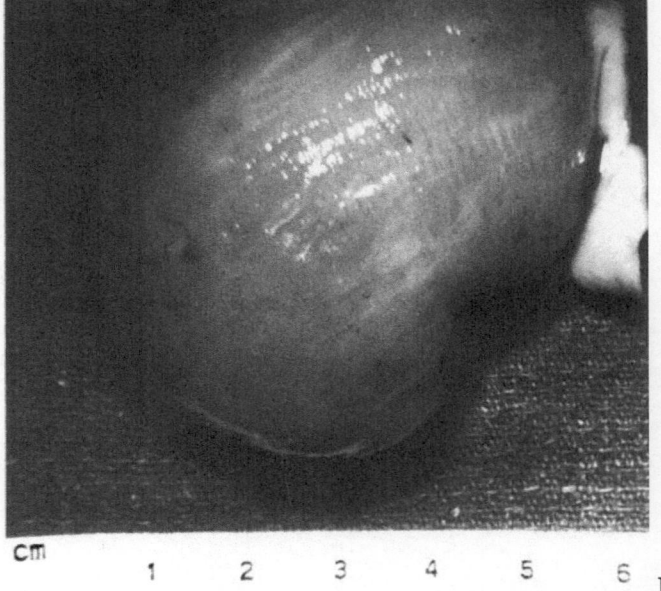

D

Fig. 8–3. *Right atrial myxoma causing obstruction of the tricuspid valve.* The PA roentgenogram of the chest (**A**) shows dilatation of the superior vena cava and pulmonary undercirculation. The M-mode echocardiogram (**B**) demonstrates a mass in the area of the tricuspid valve that moves posteriorly during ventricular systole and anteriorly during diastole. (*Continued*)

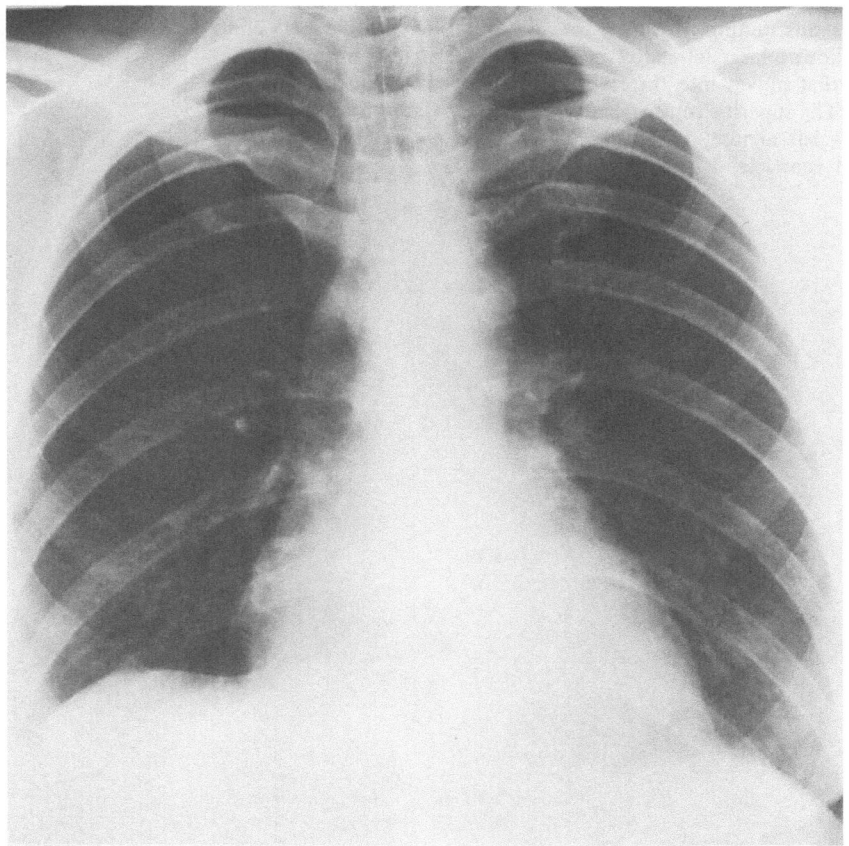

A

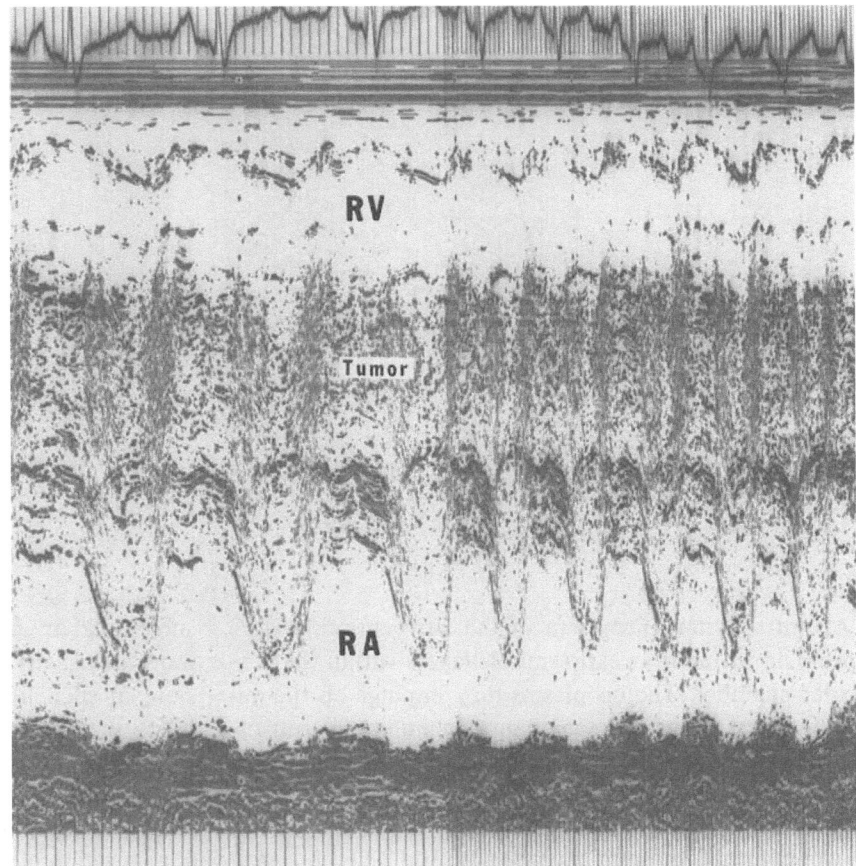

B

Fig. 8–3 (*Cont.*) The two-dimensional echocardiogram (**C**) confirms this finding. Injection into the superior vena cava (**D** and **E**) shows a large lobulated mass in the right atrium during systole (**D**) that moves into the right ventricular cavity during diastole (**E**). The superior vena cava and the inferior vena cava are dilated. *la* = left atrium; *lv* = left ventricle; *ra* = right atrium; *rv* = right ventricle; *T* = tumor.

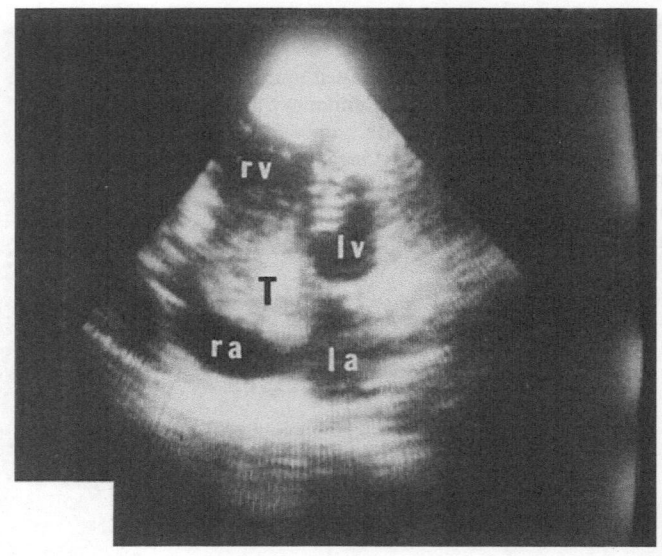

C

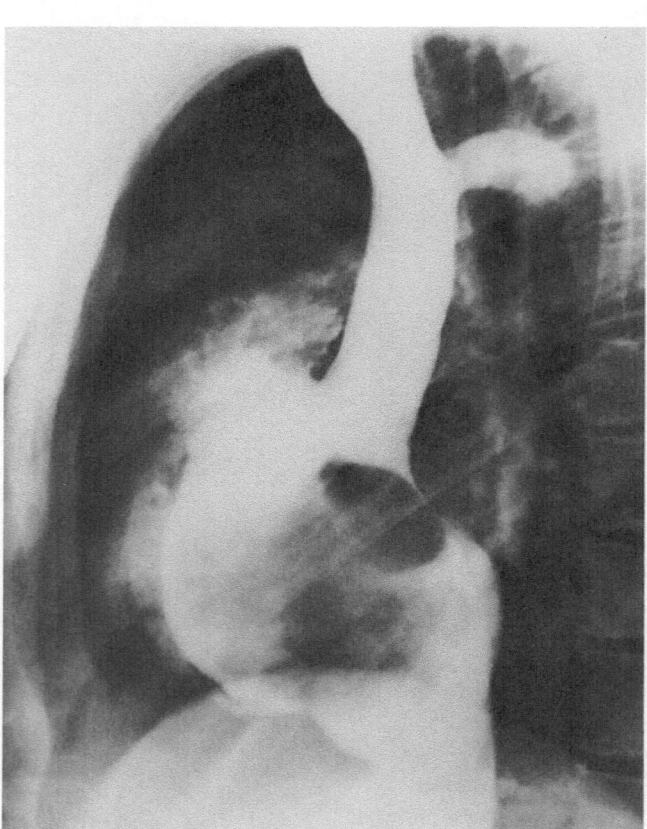

D

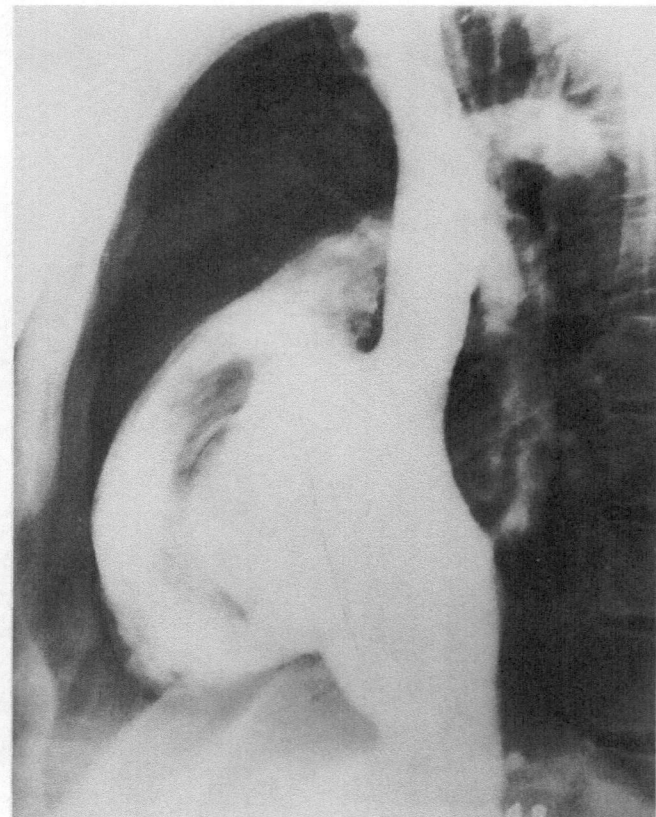

E

An intracavitary neoplasm of the left ventricule (LV) appears on M-mode as extra muscle layers within the ventricular chamber. The neoplasms may impinge on the mitral valve, restricting its opening motion, and may protrude into the LV outflow tract during systole. As with atrial tumors, 2-D echocardiography is superior in delineating intracavitary LV tumors.

Intramyocardial tumors may be noted on 2-D echocardiography as noncontractile nodules within the myocardium. Interatrial lipoma (lipomatous hypertrophy of the atrial septum) occurs as a thickened interatrial septum on the

subxiphoid or apex four-chamber view. Intrapericardial tumors are usually associated with significant pericardial effusion; in such instances the tumor mass, adjacent to the heart, may or may not be visualized.

Radiological (Plain Film) Features
The cardiac silhouette may be normal or enlarged. The configuration of the heart may be bizarre, or it may mimic such entities as pericardial effusion, ventricular aneurysm and pericardial cyst. On occasion a neoplasm of the heart may simulate specific chamber enlargement in one pro-

Fig. 8–4. *Pericardial neoplasm simulating right atrial enlargement.* The frontal projection (**A**) shows pronounced rounding of the lower segment of the right heart border. A shelf (shoulder) configuration is present on the LAO view (**B**). The superior vena cava is not dilated. The absence of dilatation militates against an intracavitary tumor with obstruction. Also noted incidentally is an old fracture of the left seventh rib posteriorly.

An injection into the superior vena cava (**C**) filled the right atrium, suggesting strongly that the tumor was outside the heart. Cine films demonstrated a smooth inner wall of the right atrium rather than an irregular surface as would be anticipated with a neoplasm of the heart.

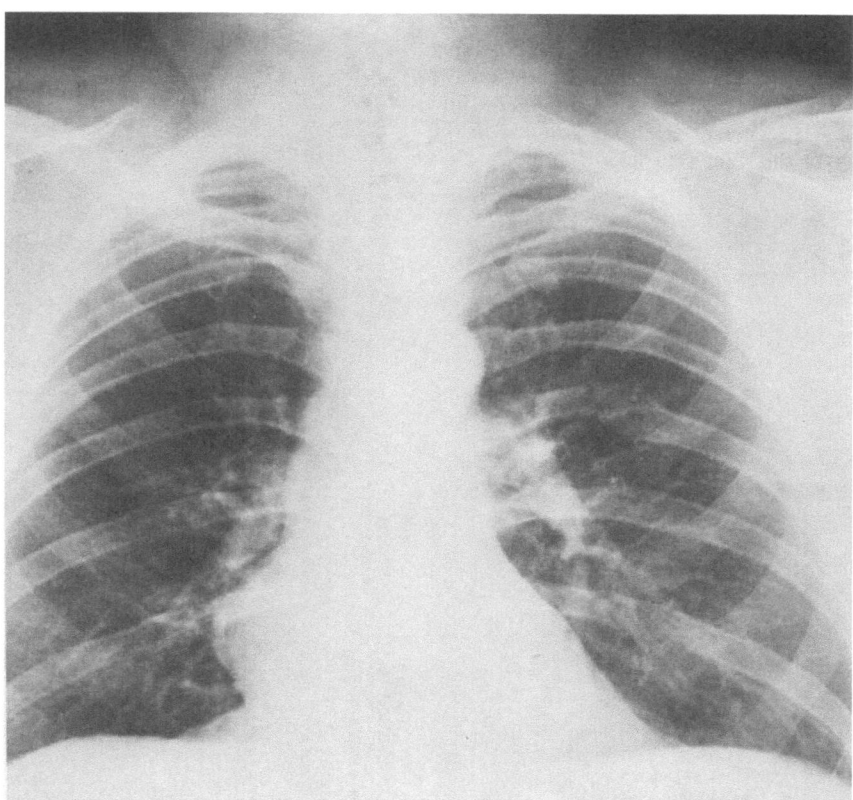

A

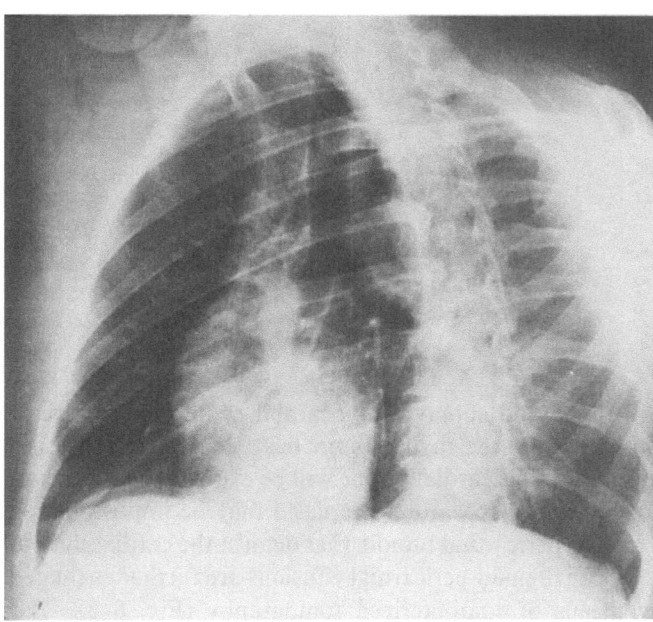

B

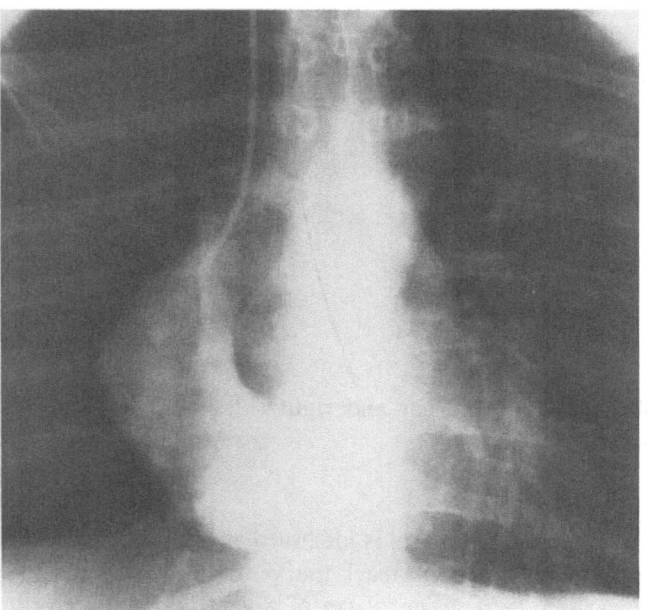

C

jection while other views indicate a mass rather than chamber enlargement. In other cases the configuration projected by the tumor may be indistinguishable from specific chamber enlargement (Fig. 8–4).

In cases of LA myxoma the cardiac silhouette may completely mimic rheumatic mitral stenosis, with enlargement of the LA and right ventricle (RV) and pulmonary venous hypertension (Fig. 8–5). RA myxoma may cause signs of tricuspid stenosis (enlargement of the RA, superior vena cava, azygos vein and inferior vena cava; Fig. 8–3). RV obstruction is reflected in pulmonary undercirculation (Fig.

8–3). On occasion, calcification of the neoplasm is present that is distinct from valvular calcification (Fig. 8–5). However, the calcification pattern may be difficult to distinguish from that associated with calcified thrombus.

Other types of neoplasm cause similar features, depending on their size and configuration and on the hemodynamic alterations they may produce.

Hemodynamics

The hemodynamic alterations reflect the size and position of the neoplasm. Tamponade as well as inflow and outflow

Fig. 8–5. *Calcified left atrial myxoma causing severe pulmonary venous hypertension.* The calcification is not as apparent on the frontal view **(A)** as it is on the lateral film **(B)**. A pacemaker electrode is noted in the apex of the right ventricle.

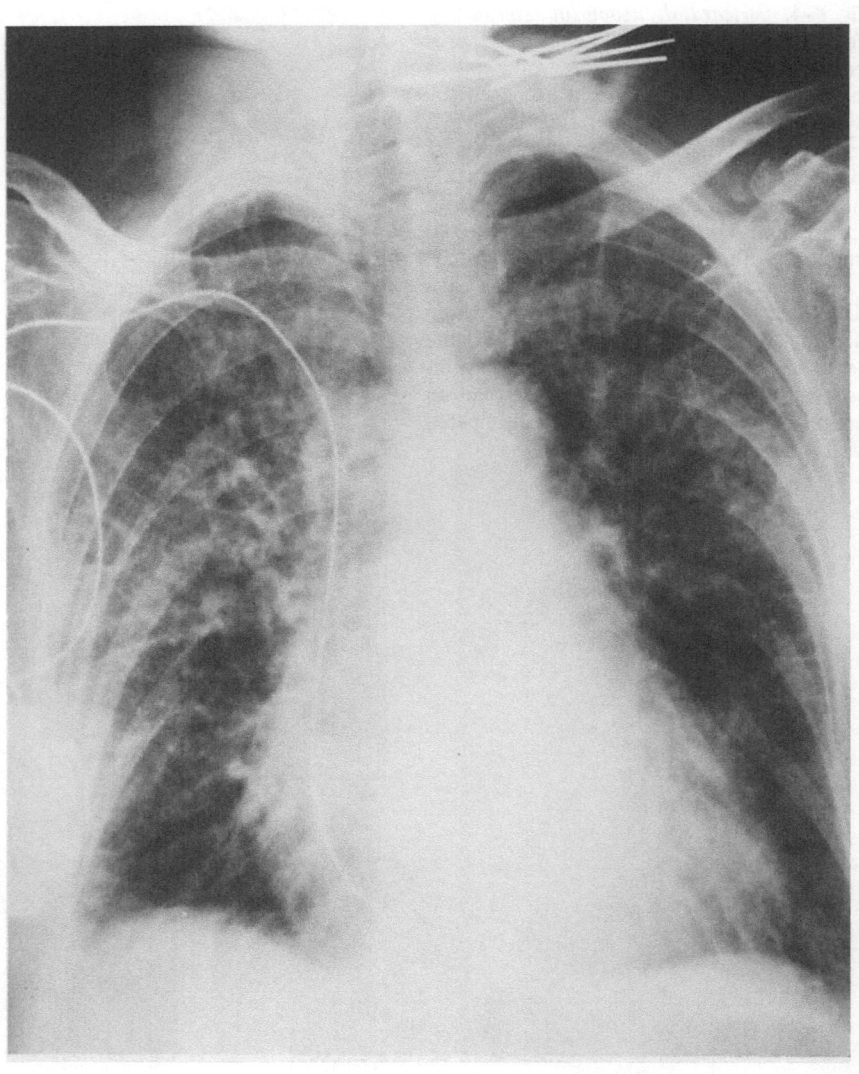

A

obstruction of the left and right sides of the heart may occur.

Contrast Studies

An intraatrial neoplasm is identified as a filling defect that may prolapse and obstruct the ventricle during diastole (Figs. 8–3, 8–6). A neoplasm of a ventricle may deform, displace and obstruct the ventricular chamber.

Coronary arteriography is often useful in defining the blood supply to the tumor. In this connection the authors have identified intracavity myxomas incidentally during aortography and coronary arteriography (Fig. 8–7). Increased vascular supply to an interatrial mass is evidence for myxoma rather than thrombus. Of course an organized thrombus attached to the wall of the atrium on occasion may also have blood vessels entering it. Coronary arteriography is also useful in distinguishing a myocardial from a pericardial neoplasm. Coronary vessels will not be present within most pericardial neoplasms, whereas the branches

will drape and supply a myocardial neoplasm. Obviously if invasion of the myocardium has taken place, parasitic supply to a pericardial tumor will be evident and differentiation from a myocardial neoplasm may be impossible.

Large pericardial tumors that deform the cardiac silhouette or malignant pericardial effusions are further evaluated by means of computerized tomography (Fig. 8–8). This technique may determine the density of the mass (water density is evidence in favor of a cyst), or it may delineate a communication between the mass and the pericardial cavity. Presence of such a communication is consistent with the diagnosis of a diverticulum (see also Fig. 9–10).

Treatment

Myxomas of all types and some rhabdomyomas can be excised surgically. Benign pericardial neoplasms are also amenable to excision. Pericardial cysts sometimes cannot be differentiated from neoplasms and must be surgically explored.

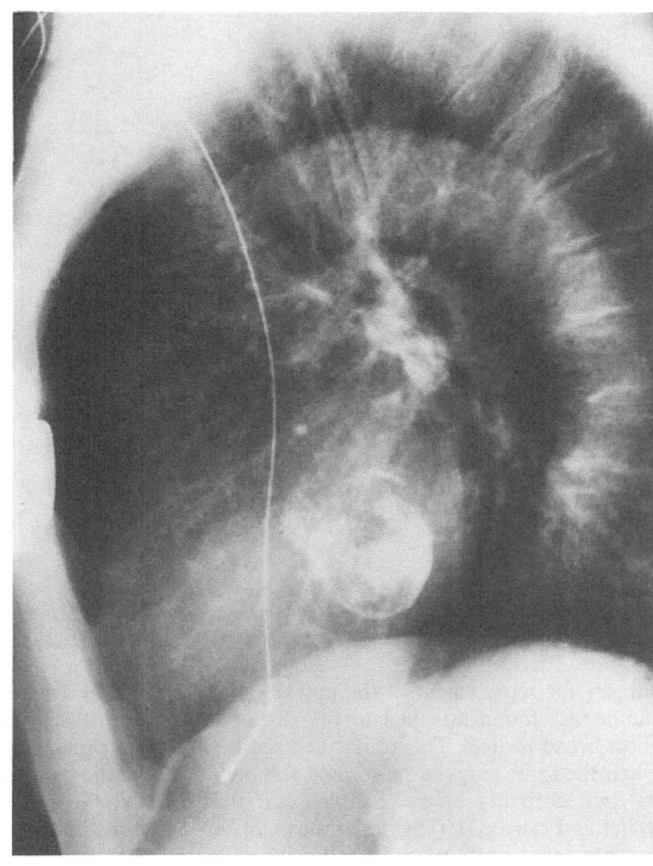

B

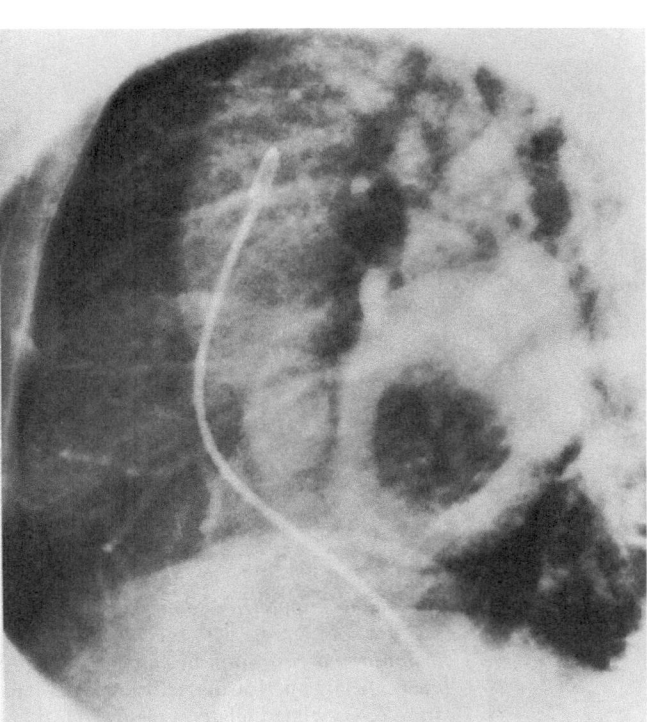

A

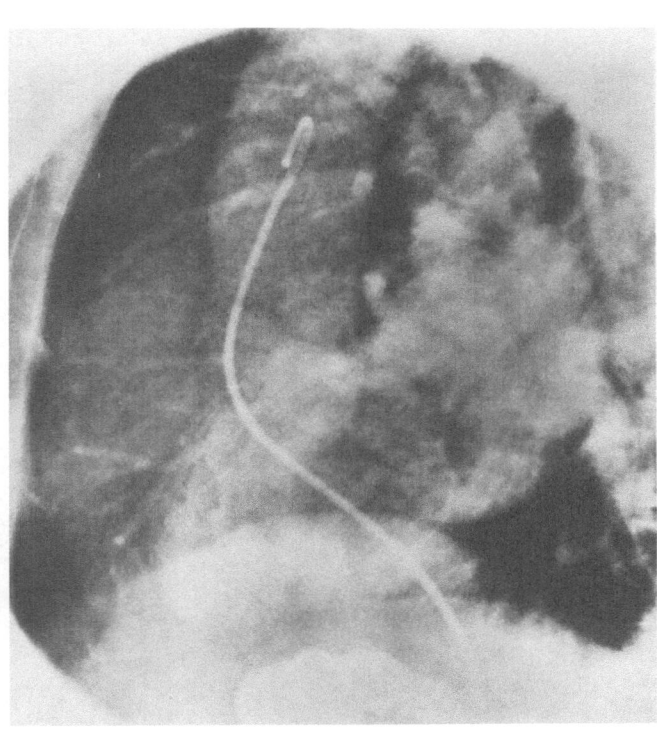

B

Fig. 8–6. *Left atrial myxoma.* The levophase after injection into the main pulmonary artery shows a large filling defect in the left atrium during systole (**A**), which prolapses into the left ventricle during diastole (**B**).

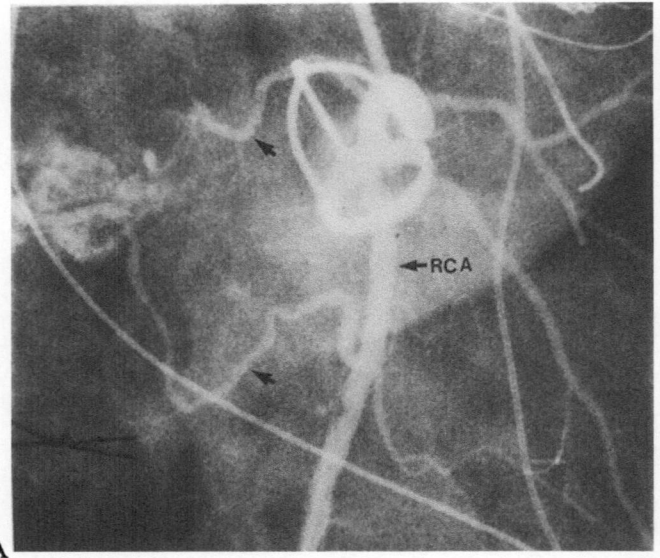

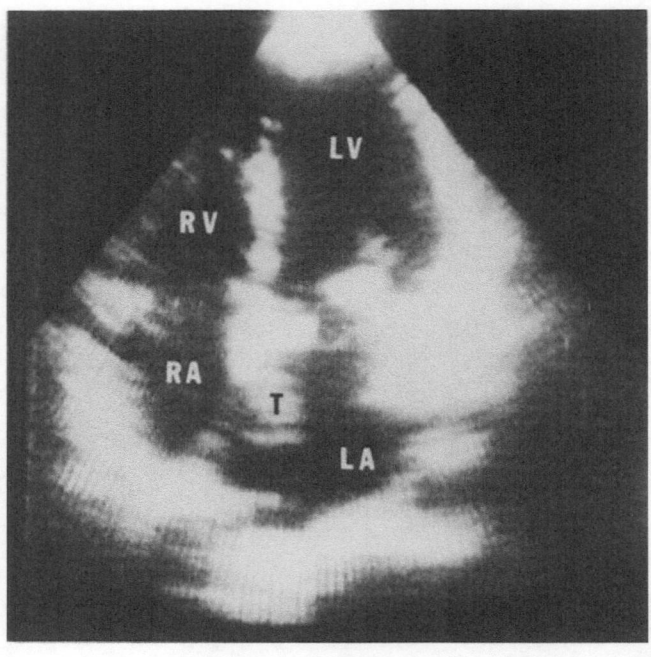

Fig. 8–7. *Left atrial myxoma discovered incidentally during aortography in a 68-year-old woman with rheumatic heart disease.* Eight years previously she had had replacement of her aortic valve and open commissurotomy of the mitral valve. The left ventriculogram showed severe mitral insufficiency. The tumor blush was discovered after an aortogram (not shown). The right coronary angiogram (A) delineates the vessels leading to the tumor (*arrow*). Subsequent to the angiographic studies the two-dimensional echocardiogram was performed. The apex four chamber view (B) shows a small tumor (*T*) in the left atrium (*LA*) near the fossa ovalis. The mitral valve is thicker than normal. At surgery for replacement of the mitral valve a 2 × 2.5 × 2.5 cm tumor was found attached to the rim of the fossa ovalis by a short broad pedicle. This tumor had not been present previously when the same surgeon performed the previous operation. *RCA* = right coronary artery. Shapiro MR, Cohen MV, Grose R, Spindola-Franco, H (1983) Diagnosis of left atrial myxoma by coronary angiography 8 years following open mitral commissurotomy. Am Heart J 105:325–327.

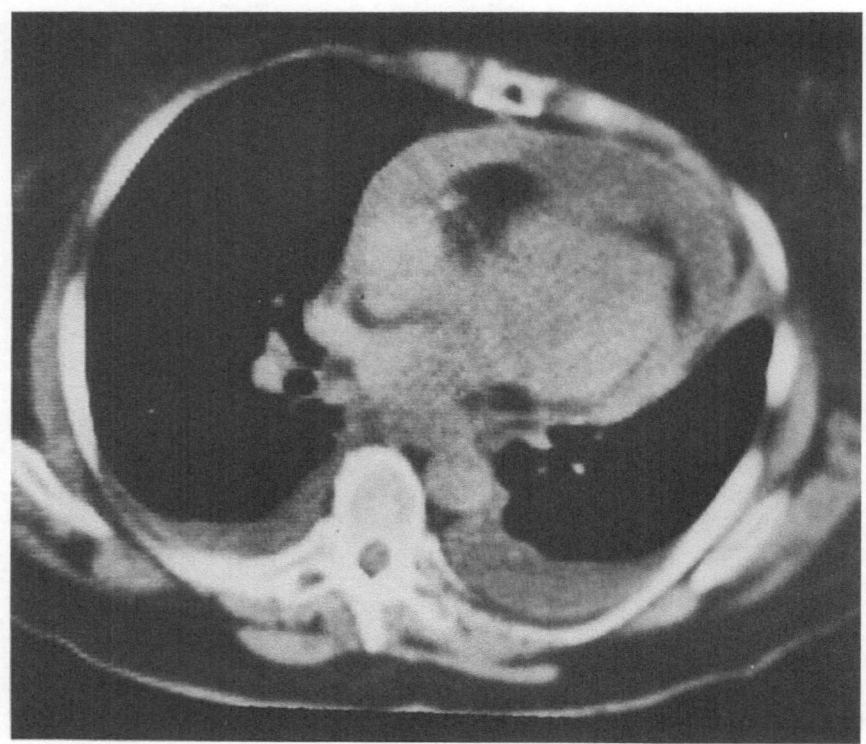

Fig. 8–8. *Computerized tomography (CT) in a 60-year-old female with metastatic involvement of the pericardium by carcinoma of the breast.* A large pericardial effusion is demonstrated. Associated bilateral pleural effusions are also noted. (Courtesy of David Frager, M.D., Montefiore Medical Center, Bronx, New York.)

Bibliography

Abrams HL, Adams DF, Grant HA (1971) The radiology of tumors of the heart. Radiol Clin North Am 9:299–326

Batchelir TM, Maun ME (1945) Congenital glycogenic tumors of the heart. Arch Pathol 39:67–73

Berry CL, Keeling J, Hilton C (1969) Teratomata in infancy and childhood: A review of 91 cases. J Pathol 98:241–252

Bjork VO, Bjork L (1965) Left ventricular myxoma. Thorax 20:534–536

Davis GD, Kincaid OW, Hallermann FJ (1969) Roentgen aspects of cardiac tumors. Semin Roentgenol 4:384–394

Duncan WJ, Rowe RD, Freedom RM, Izukawa T, Olley PM (1982) Space-occupying lesions of the myocardium: Role of two-dimensional echocardiography in detection of cardiac tumors in children. Am Heart J 104:780–785

Feigen DS, Fenoglio JJ, Maj MC McAllister HA, Madewall JE (1977) Pericardial cysts: A radiologic-pathologic correlation and review. Radiology 125:15–20

Fenoglio JJ Jr, Maj MC McAllister HA Jr, Ferrans VJ (1976) Cardiac rhabdomyoma: A clinicopathologic and electron microscopic study. Am J Cardiol 38:241–251

Goldberg HP, Steinberg I (1955) Primary tumors of the heart. Circulation 11:963–970

Hannah H, Eisemann G, Hiazczynskyj R, Winsky M, Cohen L (1982) Invasive atrial myxoma: Documentation of malignant potential of cardiac myxomas. Am Heart J 104:881–883

Magarey FR (1949) On the mode of formation of Lambl's excrescences and their relation to chronic thickening of the mitral valve. J Pathol 61:203–208

Mazer MS, Harrigan PR (1982) Left ventricular myxoma: M-mode and two-dimensional echocardiographic features. Am Heart J 104:875–877

McAllister HA Jr (1979) Primary tumors and cysts of the heart and pericardium. Curr Probl Cardiol 4:1–51

Morgan DL, Palazola J, Reed W, Bell HH, Kindred LH, Beauchamp GD (1977) Left heart myxomas. Am J Cardiol 40:611–614

Nasser WK, Davis RH, Dillon JC, Tavel ME, Helmen CH, Feigenbaum H, Fisch C (1972) Atrial myxoma. I. Clinical and pathologic features in nine cases. Am Heart J 83:694–704

Nasser WK, Davis RH, Dillon JC, Tavel ME, Helmen CH, Feigenbaum H, Fisch C (1972) Atrial myxoma. II. Phonocardiographic, echocardiographic, hemodynamic, and angiographic features in nine cases. Am Heart J 83:810–824

Pomerance A (1961) Papillary "tumours" of the heart valves. J Pathol 81:135–140

Read RC, White HJ, Murphy ML, Williams D, Sun CN, Flanagan WH (1974) The malignant potentiality of left atrial myxoma. J Thorac Cardiovasc Surg 68:857–867

Selzer A, Sakai FJ, Popper RW (1972) Protean clinical manifestations of primary tumors of the heart. Am J Med 52:9–18

Shapiro MR, Cohen MV, Grose R, Spindola-Franco H (1983) Diagnosis of left atrial myxoma by coronary angiography eight years following open mitral commissurotomy. Am Heart J 105:325–327

Spindola-Franco H, Bjork L, Berger M (1975) Intracavitary metastasis to the left ventricle: An angiocardiographic diagnosis. Br J Radiol 48:649–651

Steinberg I, Miscall L, Redo SF, Goldberg HP (1964) Angiocardiography in diagnosis of cardiac tumors. Am J Roentgenol 91:364–370

Wychulis AR, Connolly DC, McGoon DC (1971) Pericardial cysts, tumors, and fat necrosis. J Thorac Cardiovasc Surg 62:294–300

9 Diseases of the Pericardium

The pericardium is a thin fibroserous sac that surrounds the heart and the proximal portions of the great vessels. It is composed of an external layer of dense fibrous tissue (fibrous pericardium) and an inner serous layer (serous pericardium).

The serous pericardium has two layers: the visceral pericardium (epicardium) and the parietal pericardium. The visceral pericardium forms the outer layer of the heart, while the parietal pericardium forms the inner surface of the fibrous pericardium. The pericardial cavity is a potential space between the parietal and visceral pericardium. The pericardial surfaces are moistened with a watery fluid to allow for freedom of movement of the heart. The pericardial sac normally contains approximately 15–20 ml of fluid.

The fibrous pericardium is closed superiorly by attachments to the great vessels. It invests the ascending aorta for approximately one-half the distance from the aortic valve to the origin of the innominate artery, and invests the pulmonary trunk to a point just below its bifurcation. The investments of the inferior vena cava and pulmonary veins are short, while that of the superior vena cava is more extensive. Attachments to the manubrium and xiphoid process (superior and inferior pericardiosternal ligaments), spine (pericardiovertebral ligament), diaphragm (pericardiophrenic ligament) and pleura stabilize the pericardium within the mediastinum. The attachment between the pleura and the fibrous pericardium is loose, permitting the phrenic nerve and adjacent blood vessels to run between the pleura and pericardium. Near the apex of the heart the fibrous pericardium is separated from the mediastinal pleura by fatty tissue (pericardial fat pad); other fatty accumulations occur on the right side anterior to the inferior vena cava. These pericardial fat pads on occasion may simulate cardiomegaly on radiological studies.

The normal pericardium is usually not visualized on standard posteroanterior and lateral films of the chest. On occasion the presence of sufficient subepicardial fat may result in the pericardium becoming visible on standard roentgenograms (Kremens). The pericardium is noted, particularly at the apex, as a fine (approximately 2mm) dense line or curved line closely paralleling the subepicardial fat layer. The pericardium may become visible if it is calcified or if studied in the presence of air in the pericardial cavity. The subepicardial fat layer is often helpful in the recognition of pericardial effusion (see Pericardial Effusion and Cardiac Tamponade immediately following).

Pericardial disease may be asymptomatic. Often, however, the patient has fever, chest pain and the clinical features of acute cardiac tamponade or chronic cardiac constriction. Symptoms of restrictive cardiomyopathy are similar to those of constrictive pericarditis, and differentiation may be difficult. Table 9–1 lists causes of pericardial disease.

Pericardial Effusion and Cardiac Tamponade

Pericardial effusion is an accumulation of fluid in the pericardial cavity that may be caused by inflammatory or noninflammatory disturbances. The inflammatory processes include pericarditis of unknown etiology (also called nonspecific or acute benign), lupus erythematosus, acute rheumatic fever and specific infective disorders (virus, bacteria, tuberculosis, protozoa or fungus). Noninflammatory processes that may cause pericardial effusion include uremia, heart failure, myxedema, disease of the liver and neoplastic processes. If accumulation of fluid in the pericardium is slow, or if it is small, then cardiac decompensation will not occur.

Clinical Features
Pain in the chest and fever are common with pericardial effusion due to an inflammatory process. The pain is often relieved by leaning forward. On physical examination the heart sounds may be muffled. A triphasic friction rub may be present. Bacterial pericarditis usually results in spiking

Table 9–1. Causes of Pericardial Disease

I. Infective
   A. Viral (nonspecific)
   B. Bacterial (e.g., *Staphylococcus, Hemophilus influenzae*)
   C. Tuberculous
   D. Fungal
   E. Protozoal
II. Neoplastic
   A. Primary
      Rhabdomyosarcoma
      Teratoma
      Fibroma
      Leiomyofibroma
      Lipoma
      Angioma
   B. Metastatic
      Breast
      Lung
      Kidney
      Other
   C. Myelolymphoproliferative malignant neoplasms
III. Immunological (hypersensitivity or autoimmunity)
   A. Rheumatic fever
   B. Systemic lupus erythematosus
   C. Rheumatoid arthritis
   D. Scleroderma
   E. Periarteritis nodosa
   F. Dermatomyositis
   G. Dressler syndrome
   H. Kawasaki disease
   I. Postpericardiotomy syndrome
IV. Iatrogenic and traumatic
   A. Blunt or penetrating trauma to chest
   B. Percutaneous puncture of left ventricle
   C. Cardiac perforation by catheter or on implantation of pacemaker (not necessarily hemorrhagic)
IV. Hemopericardium
   A. Dissecting aneurysm of aorta
   B. Myocardial rupture
   C. Blunt or penetrating trauma to chest
   D. Anticoagulant therapy
   E. Iatrogenic during cardiac catheterization or implantation of pacemaker
VI. Metabolic
   A. Myxedema
   B. Uremia
VII. Physical agents
   A. Radiation
   B. Asbestosis
VIII. Circulatory
   A. Congestive heart failure
   B. Cardiomyopathy
IX. Effect of drugs
   A. Procainamide
   B. Cromolyn sodium
   C. Hydralazine
   D. Dantrolene
   E. Methysergide
X. Thymic cyst
XI. Hereditary
   A. Mulibrey nanism (mulibrey dwarf)

fevers, leukocytosis and an abnormal differential white blood cell count. Pericardial effusions secondary to noninflammatory processes may be asymptomatic, even though they may become large. Large collections of fluid may be asymptomatic because the pericardium can stretch gradually to accomodate them.

Cardiac tamponade results from rapid accumulation of fluid that compresses the heart and impairs diastolic filling. Compression of the heart also forces it to contract from a smaller volume so that systolic function is adversely affected. Pulsus paradoxus is characteristic of cardiac tamponade, consisting of accentuation of the normal decrease in blood pressure during inspiration. Normally the blood pressure decreases 3 or 4 mm during inspiration. Pulsus paradoxus is present when the pressure varies more than 10 mm Hg with respirations. Pulsus paradoxus is caused by acceleration of flow into the right ventricle (RV) during inspiration, shifting the ventricular septum toward the left ventricle (LV). Expansion of the right-sided chambers also displaces pericardial fluid. Internal compression due to the shift of the septum and external compression due to the displacement of pericardial fluid impair LV filling and acutely reduce LV output. Inspiration also increases capacitance of the pulmonary vessels, resulting in "pooling" of blood in the lungs and further reduction in filling of the LV. Intrapleural pressure is also reduced during inspiration. This reduction in pressure contributes directly to reduction in the arterial pressure.

Patients with pericardial tamponade are dyspneic with distended neck veins and poor peripheral blood flow. The cardiac impulse is faint or not palpable; however, the area of cardiac dullness is larger than normal. Heart sounds may be reduced in intensity. A pericardial "knock" may be evident. The electrocardiogram may show ST segment and T wave changes. The PR segment may also show deviation, and the QRS voltage may be reduced in all leads. Electrical alternans, a rhythmic change in QRS axis, occurs with large pericardial effusions and may result from oscillations of the heart within the fluid.

Echocardiography

Echocardiography is the most sensitive and specific method for recognition of pericardial effusion. Fluid surrounding the heart appears as an echo-free space between the visceral and parietal pericardium. Often fluid in the pericardial cavity is somewhat reflective and may not be recognized at normal gain settings. Reducing the output or the gain settings will demonstrate the space between the two layers of pericardium. On M-mode echocardiography a small effusion appears as a separation during systole only (Fig. 9–1). Moderate effusions show separation between the pericardial layers during systole and diastole (Fig. 9–2). Large pericardial effusions may be present anteriorly as well (Fig. 9–3). On arc scans from the aorta to the LV a pericardial effusion is present behind the ventricle, but is usually not present behind the left atrium (LA). Fibrous adhesions may be recognized as intermittent echo-dense structures

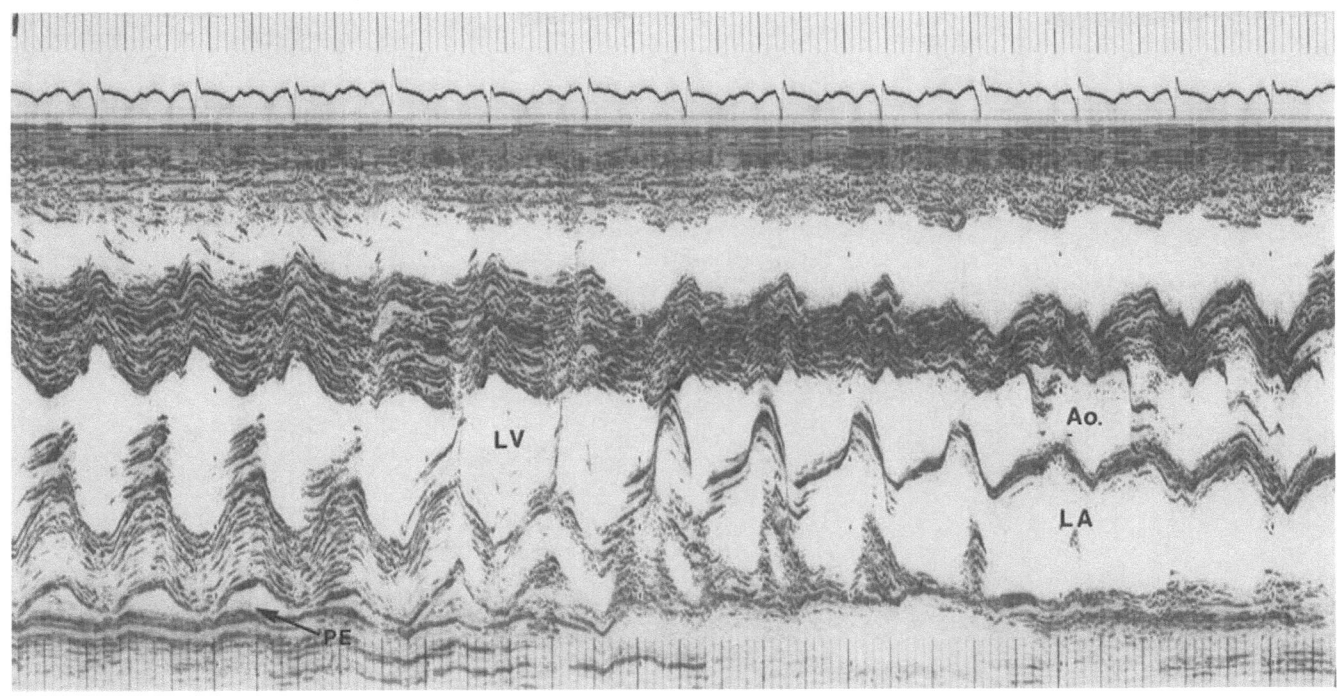

Fig. 9–1. *Small pericardial effusion.* M-mode arc scan from the left ventricle (*LV*) to the aorta (*Ao.*) in a 3-year-old boy with hypertrophic cardiomyopathy and a small pericardial effusion. The effusion (*PE*) appears as an echo-free space behind the left ventricle during systole only. No effusion is present anterior to the heart or behind the left atrium (*LA*).

within the pericardial cavity (Fig. 9–2). With a large pericardial effusion (Fig. 9–3) the heart swings within the fluid as it contracts. The septum may move paradoxically anteriorly during systole; alternately, the mitral valve may have a posterior motion during systole, suggesting mitral prolapse. On 2-D echocardiography (Fig. 9–4), fluid is present around the ventricles and behind the right atrium (RA), but little or no fluid is present behind the LA. Fibrous strands may undulate within the pericardial cavity or may extend from the visceral to the parietal pericardium. Two-dimensional scanning may identify a loculated pericardial effusion in areas other than behind the heart. An echo-free space anterior to the heart, without signs of effusion elsewhere, may be pericardial fat.

Pleural effusion must be differentiated from pericardial effusion. If pericardial and pleural effusions coexist the pericardium is delineated with fluid on both sides of this structure (Fig. 9–4). Pericardial fluid separates the heart and the descending aorta, whereas pleural fluid is not present between these two structures (Fig. 9–4).

Cardiac tamponade is not diagnosed by echocardiography with certainty; however, in the presence of the clinical features described in the foregoing, echocardiographic findings that suggest tamponade are (1) signs of large pericardial effusion; (2) signs of increased RV volume and reduction in LV volume and output with inspiration (these correlate with pulsus paradoxus); (3) signs of diastolic compression of the RA and LA; (4) presence of a notch in the motion of the RV epicardium during isovolumic contraction; (5) coarse oscillation of the LV free wall; and (6) dilatation of the pulmonary veins, inferior vena cava and superior vena cava.

Radiological (Plain Film) Features

Cardiomegaly secondary to pericardial effusion may be difficult to differentiate from enlargement of the cardiac chambers. Even the classic water-bottle configuration (Fig. 9–5) is not specific for effusion. On occasion, a loculated pericardial effusion may simulate chamber enlargement (e.g., RA, LV). A helpful finding in the diagnosis of pericardial effusion is abnormal separation of the subepicardial fat from the mediastinal fat on the lateral projection (Fig. 9–6). (Normally the subepicardial fat is located less than 1 cm behind the mediastinal layer, and the pericardium between them is no more than 2 mm thick.) Acute hemopericardium during cardiac catheterization is recognized by observation of a sudden separation of the subepicardial fat from the left heart border on the frontal or RAO view. The fat is highly radiolucent, surrounding the apex and anterolateral wall in the shape of a horseshoe and even merging with the atrioventricular groove, which crosses the base of the heart. Moments later, sudden deterioration may occur secondary to cardiac tamponade. Therefore radiologists and cardiologists should be on the alert for this finding, as prompt recognition may be lifesaving.

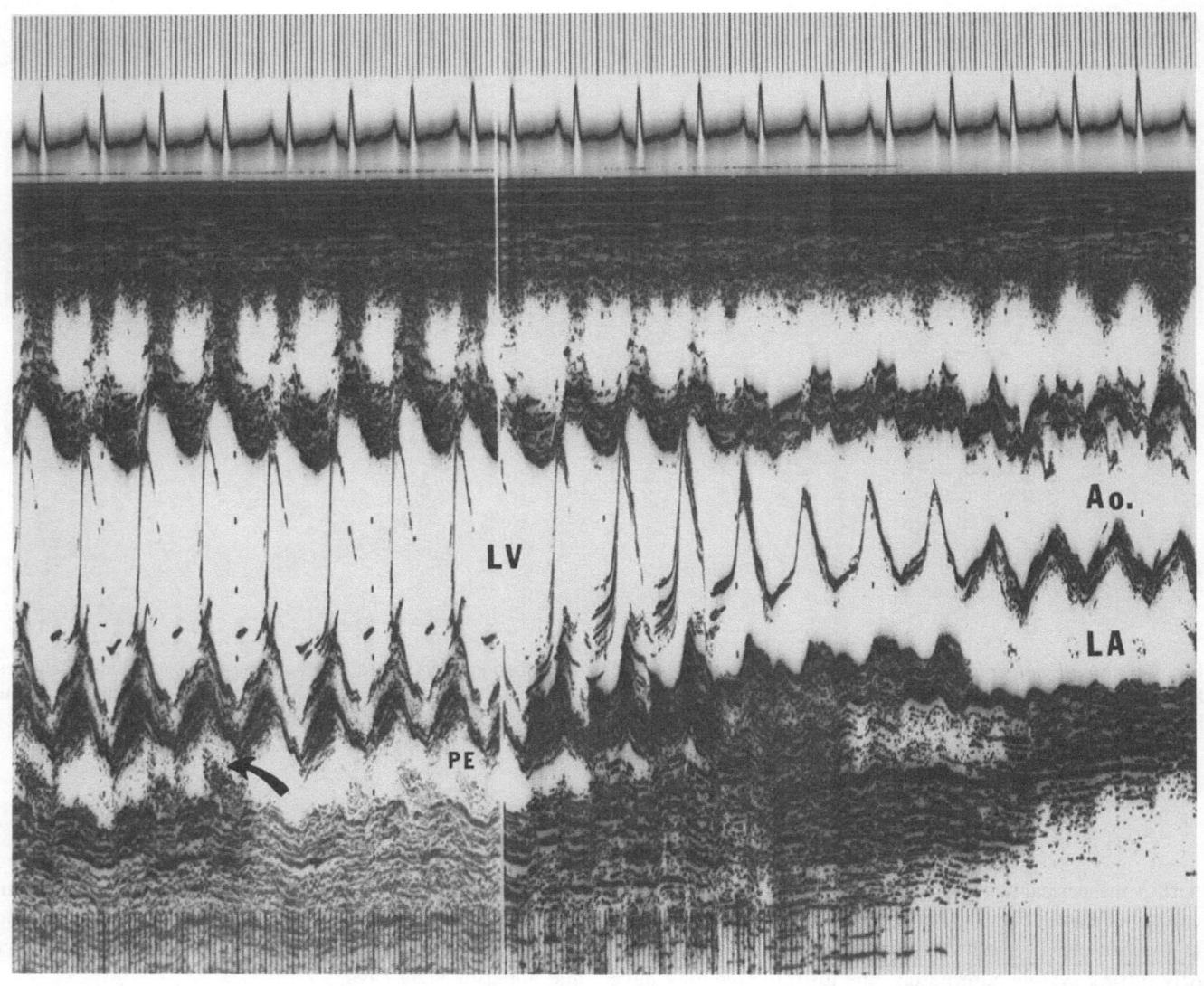

Fig. 9–2. *Moderate pericardial effusion.* An M-mode arc scan from the left ventrical (*LV*) to the aortic root (*Ao.*) in a 10-year-old boy with acute rheumatic fever shows moderate pericardial effusion (*PE*). The echo-free space persists throughout systole and diastole. Fibrous strands appear as intermittent, echo-dense structures within the pericardial space (*arrow*). Again, no effusion is present anterior to the heart or behind the left atrium (*LA*).

Hemodynamics

Since all chambers are constricted by the pericardium, all have the same (elevated) diastolic pressure (Fig. 9–7A). The a wave and the x descent are prominent, but the y descent of the atrial curve and the early diastolic dip of the ventricular curve are not present. Pulsus paradoxus correlates with an increase in right-sided systolic pressures and a reduction of left-sided systolic pressures during inspiration (Fig. 9–7B). LV filling and LV stroke volume are reduced.

Contrast Studies

During ventriculography in the presence of a large pericardial effusion, the heart may oscillate within the pericardial cavity. On both ventriculography and coronary arteriography the left heart border, as defined by the coronary arter-ies, is separated from the pericardial border by pericardial fluid.

Historically, pericardial effusions were diagnosed by instillation of carbon dioxide into an antecubital vein. A left lateral decubitus projection demonstrated separation between the carbon dioxide in the RA and the pericardium. Nuclear blood pool scanning has also proved effective. Echocardiography has now superseded both of these methods for diagnosing pericardial effusion.

Recently computerized tomography and magnetic resonance imaging (MRI) have proved to be highly sensitive and specific for detection of pericardial fluid. MRI is particularly helpful in identifying the type of fluid present (exudate, transudate, pus, blood).

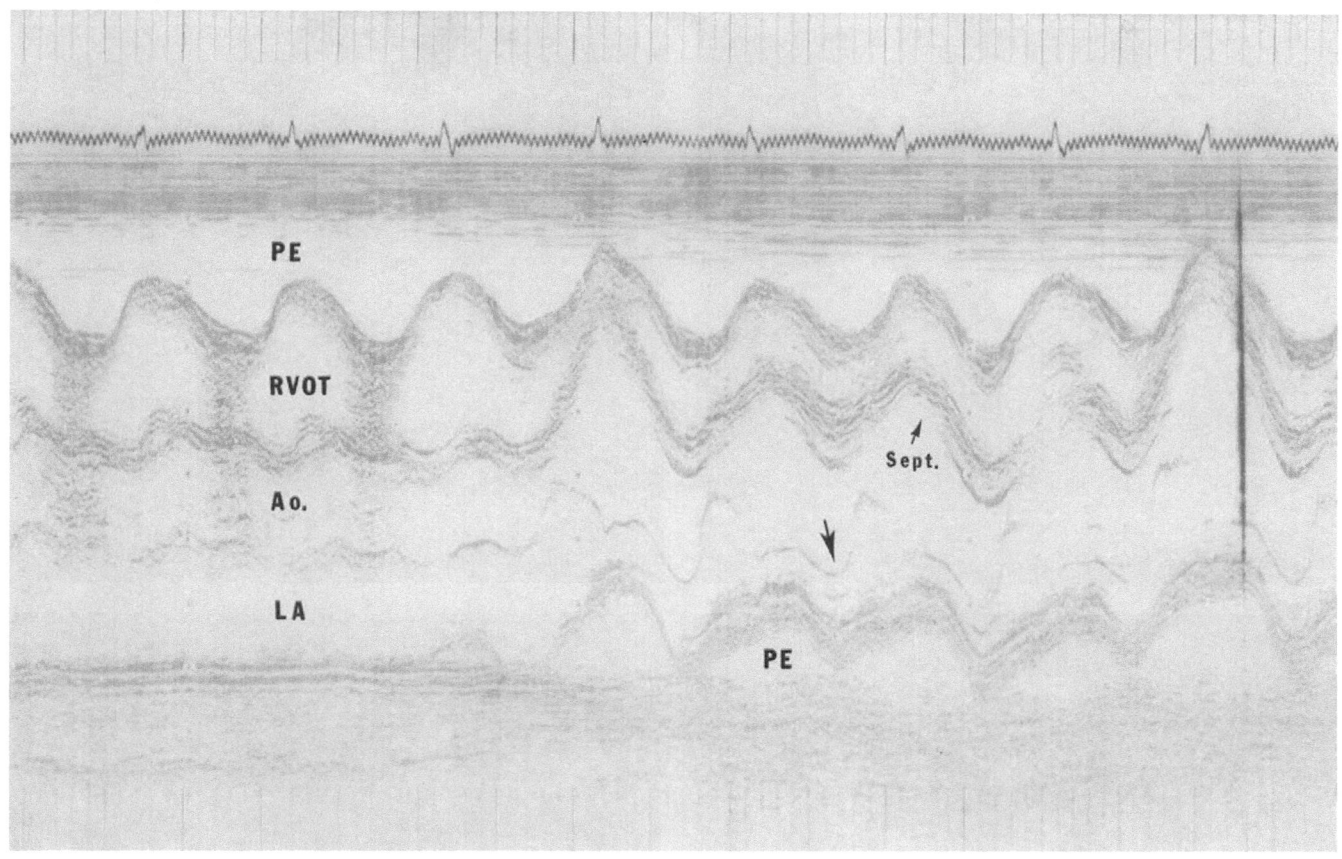

Fig. 9–3. *Large pericardial effusion.* An M-mode arc scan from the aorta (*Ao.*) to the left ventricle in a 16-year-old girl with a large pericardial effusion (*PE*), secondary to acute nonspecific pericarditis.

The echo-free space is present anteriorly and posteriorly. The heart oscillates within the pericardial cavity, causing the septum and the left ventricular free wall to move abnormally. The mitral valve moves posteriorly during ventricular systole (*arrow*) (this finding should not be interpreted as mitral prolapse). Again the effusion is not observed behind the left atrium (*LA*). *RVOT* = right ventricular outflow tract; *Sept.* = ventricular septum.

Treatment

Immediate recognition and treatment of acute hemopericardium during cardiac catheterization or associated with noniatrogenic trauma may be lifesaving. If a pericardial effusion is present in a patient with bacterial infection (including tuberculosis), diagnostic pericardiocentesis is indicated, and surgical drainage may be required in addition to medical treatment. Identification of a tumor mass associated with pericardial effusion should lead to surgical exploration for identification of the lesion and appropriate treatment. Other forms of pericardial effusion do not require drainage unless tamponade is present. Treatment of the underlying disease process is initiated during observation for clinical findings of tamponade. On occasion a persistent effusion or recurrent tamponade requires a pericardial window or pericardial resection so that the excess fluid will be absorbed by the pleura. In the presence of cardiac tamponade, needle aspiration or surgical drainage relieves symptoms and provides fluid for diagnostic studies. Needle aspiration may be guided by ultrasound or by electrocardiography. If the needle is attached to the chest lead of the cardiogram, an electrical current of injury or premature ventricular contraction is evidence of contact with the heart. If guidance is by ultrasound the location of the needle is usually easily identified. Injection of saline will opacify the pericardial space if the needle is positioned properly. If the needle has entered a heart chamber, instillation of saline will opacify that chamber instead of the pericardial space.

Relief of tamponade is accomplished by removal of only 50–100 cc of fluid; thus there is no need to completely evacuate the pericardial cavity. Recurrence of tamponade requires another pericardiocentesis or surgical drainage.

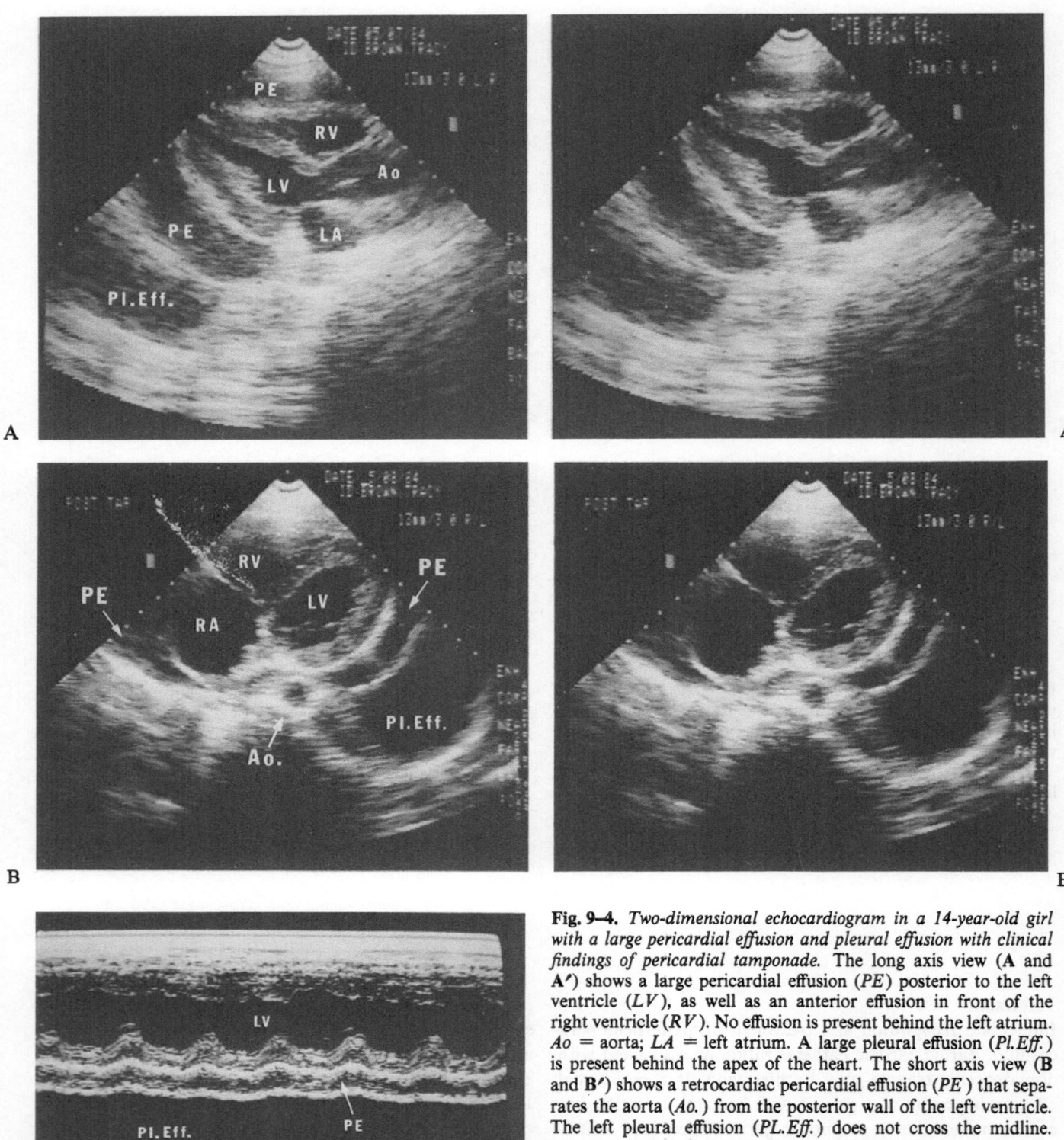

Fig. 9–4. *Two-dimensional echocardiogram in a 14-year-old girl with a large pericardial effusion and pleural effusion with clinical findings of pericardial tamponade.* The long axis view (**A** and **A′**) shows a large pericardial effusion (*PE*) posterior to the left ventricle (*LV*), as well as an anterior effusion in front of the right ventricle (*RV*). No effusion is present behind the left atrium. *Ao* = aorta; *LA* = left atrium. A large pleural effusion (*Pl.Eff.*) is present behind the apex of the heart. The short axis view (**B** and **B′**) shows a retrocardiac pericardial effusion (*PE*) that separates the aorta (*Ao.*) from the posterior wall of the left ventricle. The left pleural effusion (*PL.Eff.*) does not cross the midline. The pericardial effusion is present behind the right atrium (*RA*). On M-mode (**C**) the pericardial and pleural effusions are separated by the parietal pericardium. The right ventricular cavity and the anterior pericardial effusion are not visualized in this view.

Fig. 9–5. *The classic water-bottle appearance of the cardiac silhouette in pericardial effusion.* The pulmonary vasculature is normal. The base of the heart is normal, but the lower portion of the heart is enlarged symmetrically with sharp angulations at the costophrenic angles.

On the lateral projection the retrosternal clear space is obliterated—a finding especially significant since the patient had no signs of right ventricular hypertrophy on the electrocardiogram. Marked cardiomegaly without signs of congestive heart failure is suggestive of pericardial effusion without cardiac tamponade.

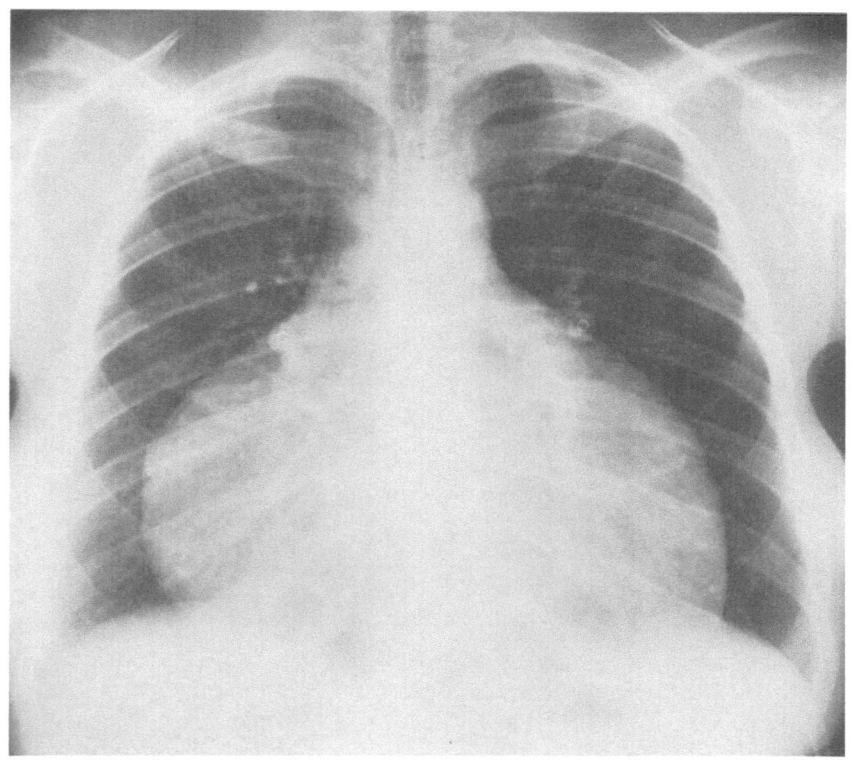

A

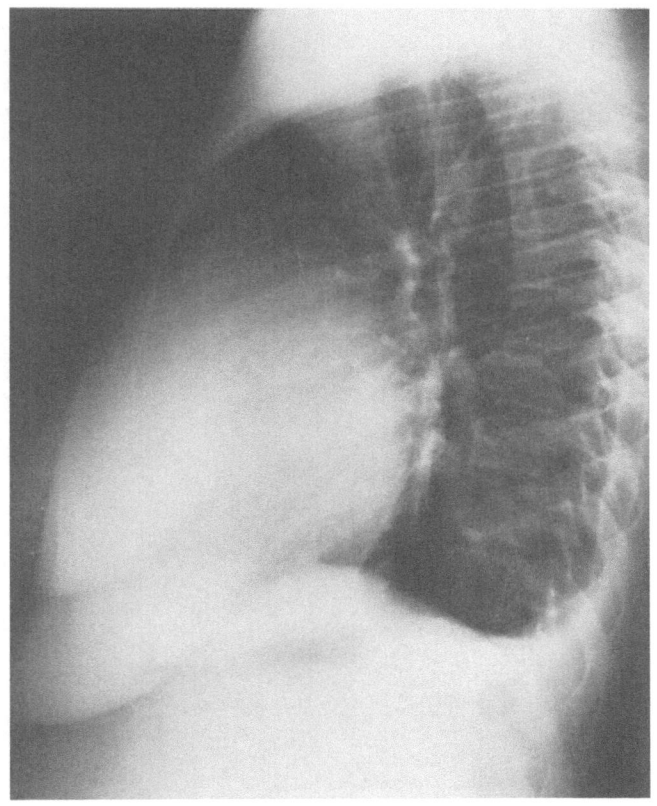

B

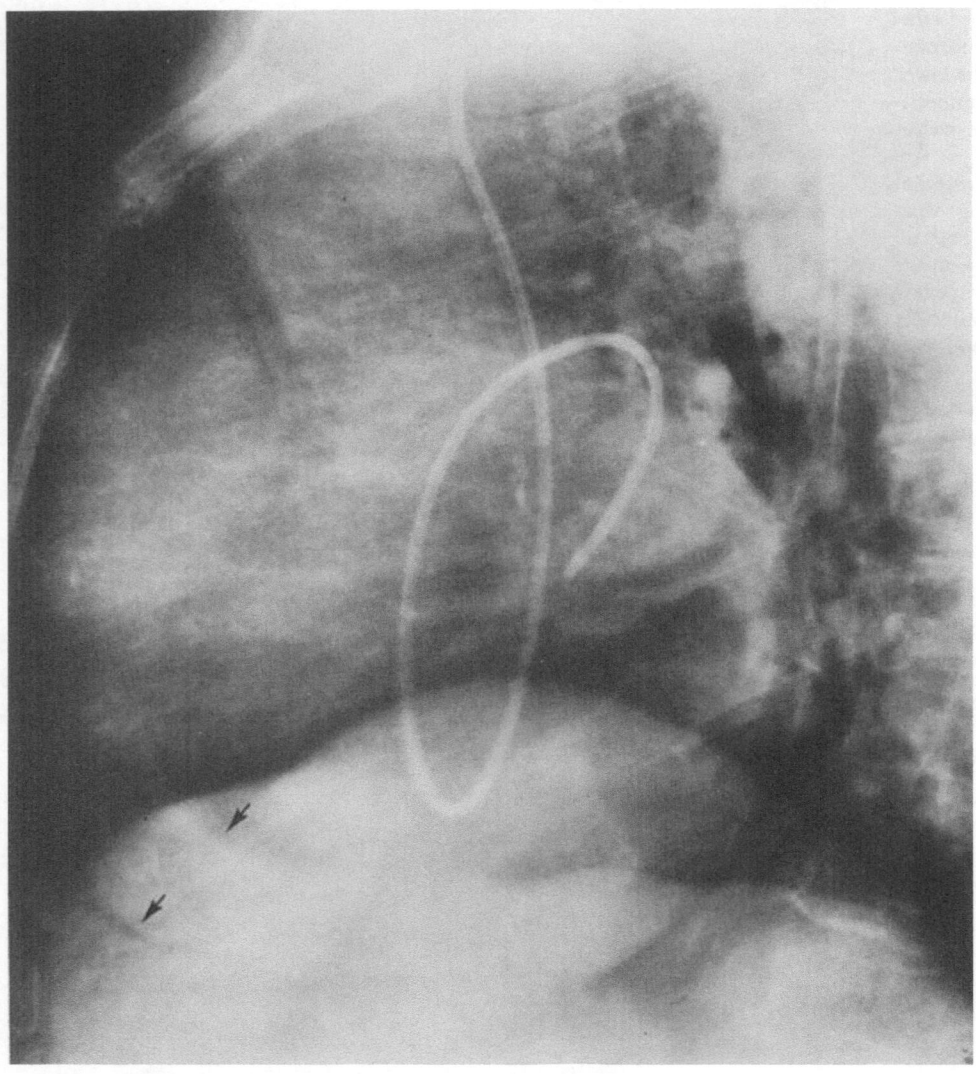

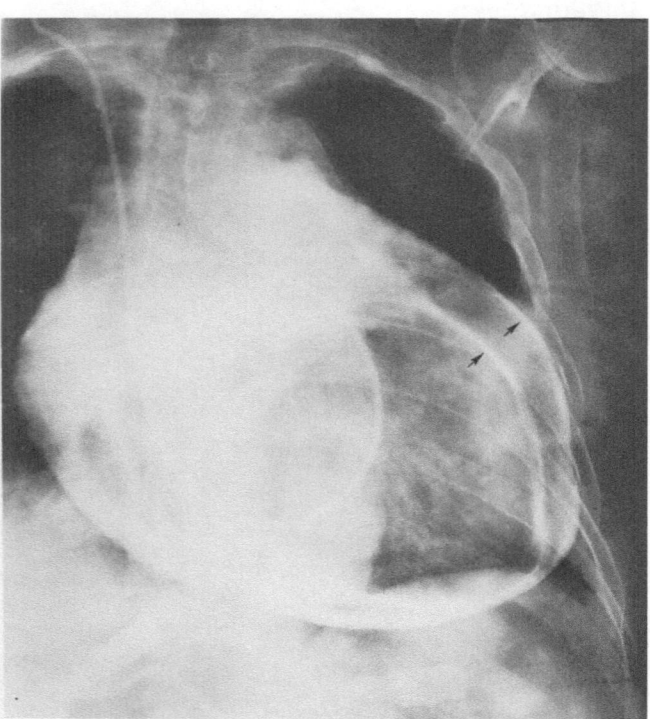

Fig. 9–6. *Large pericardial effusion with cardiac tamponade, secondary to hemopericardium.* In the lateral chest roentgenogram **(A)** the broad radiolucent band represents subepicardial fat that outlines the epicardium (*inner arrow*). The epicardium is widely separated from the mediastinal fat (*outer arrow*) by pericardial fluid. Evacuation of the pericardial cavity was difficult so that contrast material was instilled **(B)**. The arrows in **B** point toward the visceral and parietal pericardium. Since the contrast medium is displaced by clotted blood it does not fill the entire pericardial cavity.

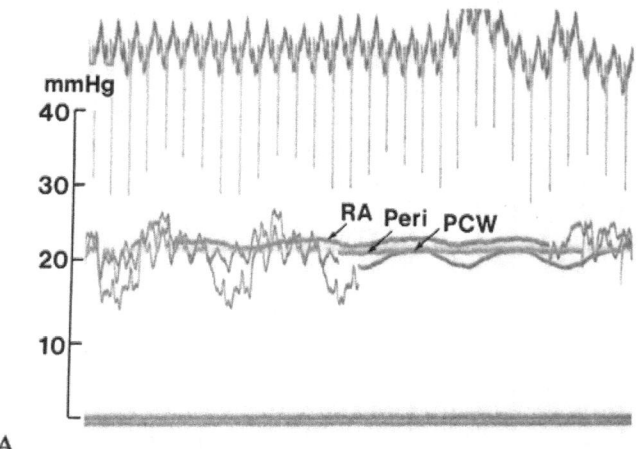

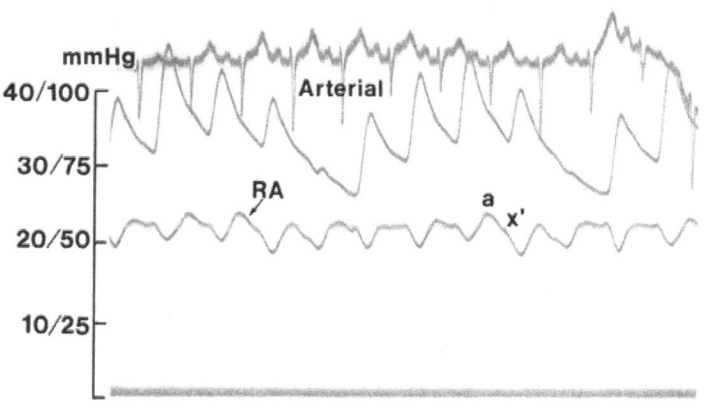

A

B

Fig. 9–7. *Pressure tracings in cardiac tamponade secondary to pericardial effusion.* **A** simultaneous pressure tracings in the right atrium (*RA*), pulmonary capillary wedge (*PCW*) and pericardial cavity (*Peri*). The pericardial cavity was reached by a transthoracic cannula. The pressures are all equal and elevated (mean pressure = 20 mm Hg). The diastolic pressures in the ventricles (not shown) are the same as the pressure in the pericardium and in the atria because all the cardiac chambers are compressed equally by pericardial fluid. **B** simultaneous pressure in the right atrium (*RA*) and brachial artery (*Arterial*). The right atrial pressure has an *a* wave and an *x* descent, but the *y* descent is inconspicuous. The arterial pressure falls dramatically during inspiration, indicating pulsus paradoxus.

Constrictive Pericarditis versus Restrictive Cardiomyopathy

Constrictive pericarditis occurs after recovery from any type of pericardial effusion, including those associated with blunt or penetrating chest trauma; it may occur within 2–3 months or may be delayed for many years.

Restrictive cardiomyopathy is caused by amyloid, sarcoid, hemochromatosis, endomyocardial fibrosis, and neoplastic processes such as metastasis or by direct invasion by carcinoma of the breast and lung, lymphoma, leukemia and melanoma. Ischemic cardiomyopathy may also occur with signs of restrictive cardiomyopathy. Symptoms and clinical findings in both constrictive pericarditis and restrictive cardiomyopathy are caused by increased venous pressure and decreased cardiac output. The clinical presentation of constrictive pericarditis and that of the restrictive cardiomyopathies are therefore very similar; however, treatment is different. Separation of the two groups of entities may, on occasion, be aided by subtle differences in echocardiographic and hemodynamic findings. Table 9–2 compares the findings in constrictive pericarditis and in restrictive cardiomyopathy.

In constrictive pericarditis distention of the neck veins is present with prominent x and y descents recognized as collapsing venous pulses. A pericardial knock may be heard during early diastole. The electrocardiogram may show nonspecific ST and T wave changes. The echocardiogram shows thickening of the pericardium and may demonstrate restricted motion (flattening) of the LV free wall during diastole secondary to limitation of cardiac filling by the noncompliant pericardium. The myocardium is of normal thickness in constrictive pericarditis. Septal motion may be normal or abnormal. Computerized analysis of high–speed M-mode echocardiograms in constrictive pericarditis demonstrates an increase in peak rate of filling and a shortened major filling period as compared to normal. These changes may be due to high venous pressure forcing blood rapidly into the normally compliant ventricle until expansion is halted by the pericardium. On roentgenograms of the chest, pericardial calcification, if present, is highly suggestive of constrictive pericarditis. If pericardial calcification is not present, then the roentgenogram of the chest is not helpful in distinguishing constrictive pericarditis from restrictive cardiomyopathy. Pulmonary venous hypertension and dilatation of the superior and inferior venae cavae may occur with both entities.

Hemodynamically, equal diastolic pressures in all cardiac chambers are characteristic of pericardial disease. A rapid x and y descent of the atrial traces, an early diastolic dip and a late diastolic plateau of the ventricular pressure curves (square root sign; Fig. 9–8) are encountered in restrictive cardiomyopathy as well as in constrictive pericarditis. In patients with constrictive pericarditis, exercise or a diagnostic fluid overload cause the diastolic pressures in all chambers to rise equally. In contrast, in patients with restrictive cardiomyopathy, the diastolic pressure may rise more in the LV than in the RV. On ventriculography in constrictive pericarditis, early ventricular filling is more rapid than normal, but filling ceases midway through diastole. The coronary arteries show abrupt cessation of diastolic motion because the myocardium is limited in its

Table 9–2. Distinguishing Features in Constrictive Pericarditis and in Restrictive Cardiomyopathy

	Constrictive pericarditis	Restrictive cardiomyopathy
Clinical Features	Previous pericarditis, pericardial effusion, etc.; pericardial knock	Clinical features of sarcoid, amyloid, etc. (including neoplastic process)
M-Mode Echocardiography	Rapid early filling, shortened LV filling; flat LV wall during diastole; normal thickness of LV wall; thick pericardium	Thickened wall of LV; slow E–F slope; slow LV filling; prolonged LV filling; ± abnormal ejection phase indices (abnormalities of contractility)
2-D Echocardiography	Confirms M-mode findings	Speckling (sarcoid, amyloid); mass in apex (endomyocardial fibrosis)
Radiological Features	Calcified pericardium (highly suggestive if present)	
Hemodynamic Features	Equal RV and LV diastolic pressures at rest and during fluid challenge	Unequal RV and LV diastolic pressures either at rest or during fluid challenge

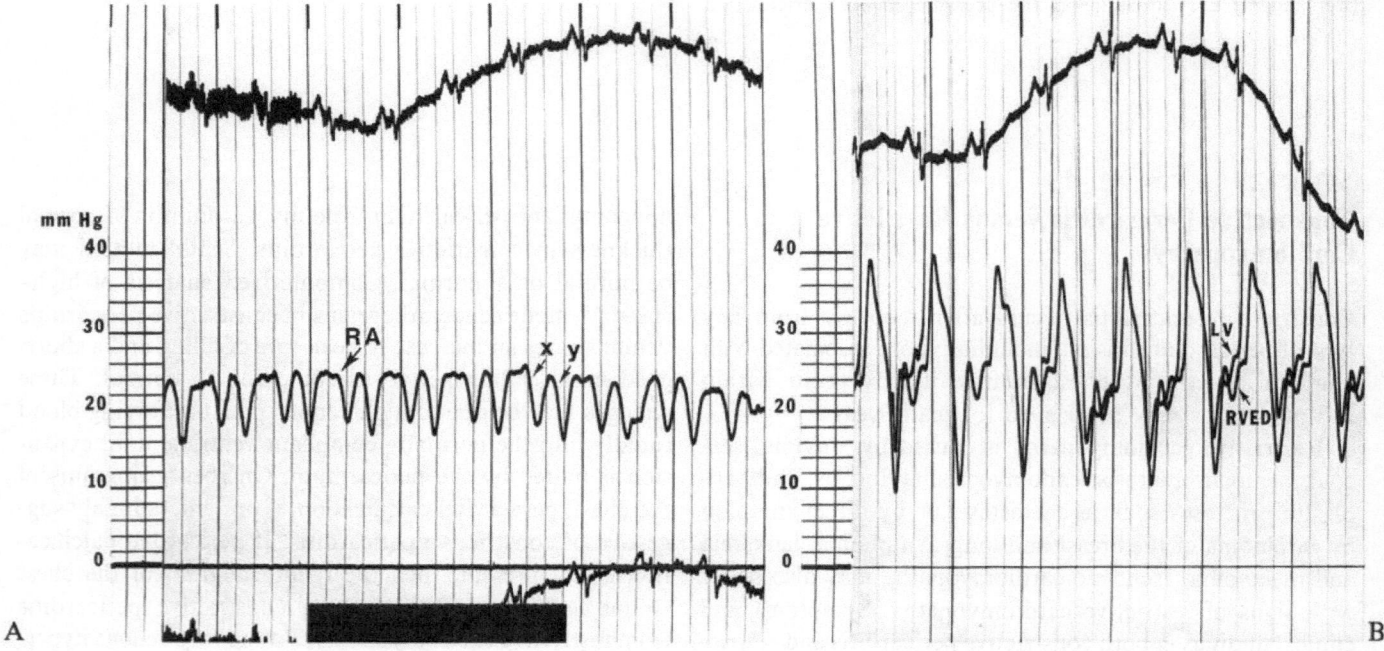

A

B

Fig. 9–8. *Pressure tracings in constrictive pericarditis.* Pressure tracings are similar for constrictive pericarditis and restrictive cardiomyopathy.

A pressure tracing in the right atrium (*RA*), showing elevation of the right atrial pressure (mean pressure = 20 mm Hg), and prominent *x* and *y* descents. The tracing has the shape of a W. **B** simultaneous pressure tracings from the right and left ventricles, showing elevation of both diastolic pressures with an early diastolic dip (the square root sign). In patients with constrictive peri-

carditis the diastolic pressures in the ventricles are equal at rest, and they remain equal during exercise or fluid challenge. In patients with restrictive cardiomyopathy the diastolic pressures are not always equal at rest, and during exercise the diastolic pressure in the left ventricle characteristically rises more than that in the right ventricle. *LV* = left ventricular diastolic pressure; *RVED* = right ventricular diastolic pressure. Courtesy of Richard Grose, M.D.

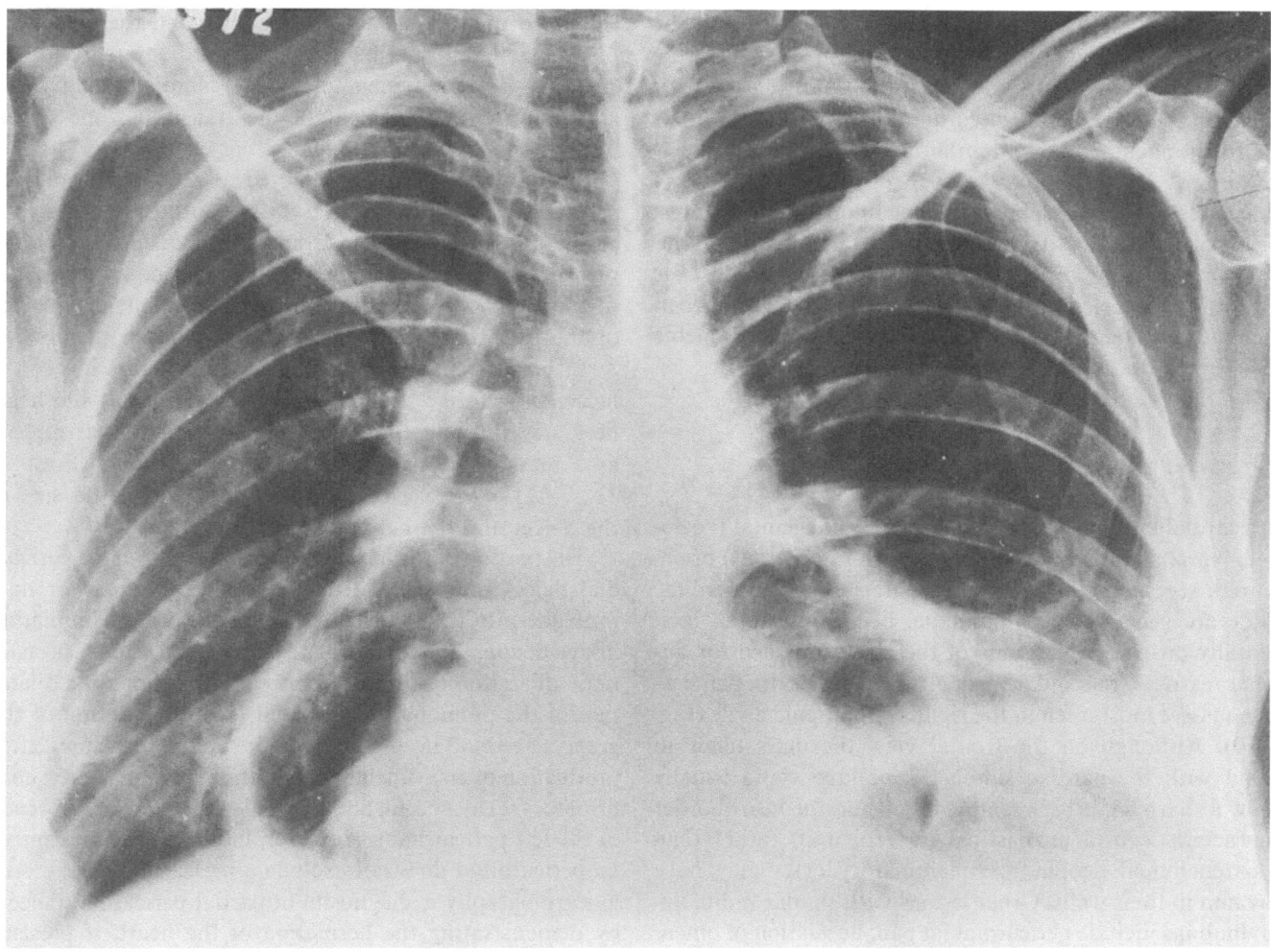

Fig. 9–9. *Pneumopericardium secondary to rupture of an amebic abscess into the pericardium.*

motion by the noncompliant pericardium. In restrictive cardiomyopathy the diastolic motion does not cease as abruptly.

In restrictive cardiomyopathy, as in constrictive pericarditis, the neck veins are distended, and the x and y descent may be easily recognized. A pericardial knock is not present; however, a third or fourth heart sound may be heard. On echocardiography the walls may be thickened and the E–F slope of the mitral valve is slowed. Computer analysis of the M-mode echocardiogram demonstrates a prolonged major filling period, a prolonged period of diastolic thinning of the septum and LV free wall and slow filling of the LV. The pericardium, of course, is not thickened. Amyloid deposits in the myocardium produce a characteristic speckled appearance on 2-D echocardiography (see Fig. 6–28). Mass lesions in the apices of the ventricles, with or without intraventricular calcifications, are evidence for endomyocardial fibrosis. On cardiac catheterization in restrictive cardiomyopathy the diastolic pressures of the ventricles may be different at rest, or the diastolic pressure in the LV may rise more than that in the RV during exercise or after an infusion of fluids. On angiography the presence

of prolonged, slow filling of the ventricles and slow diastolic opening motion of the mitral valve is confirmed. The coronary arteries do not show the abrupt cessation of diastolic motion occurring in constrictive pericarditis. In addition, abnormalities of contractile function may be present. On occasion the distinction between restrictive cardiomyopathy and constrictive pericarditis is not possible even with the application of all parameters described in the foregoing, and surgical exploration is required.

Constrictive pericarditis is treated by surgical resection of the pericardium. Recovery may be slow and incomplete because of an underlying abnormality of the heart muscle or because of residual fibrosis of the epicardium.

Pneumopericardium

Pneumopericardium (Fig. 9–9) may be due to blunt or penetrating trauma to the chest or perforation of a neighboring air-containing structure into the pericardium (e.g., abscess, pneumatocele). Pneumopericardium may be caused intentionally by introduction of gas for diagnostic purposes or unintentionally by a respirator used in severe lung disease or by gas-producing bacilli infecting the pericardium. Often pneumopericardium is combined with pus (purulent pneumopericardium) or blood (hemopneumopericardium). The symptoms in such instances are those of the underlying process; however, pneumopericardium must be recognized since its presence often mandates a major change in therapy. Films of the chest readily demonstrate air inside the pericardium or air-fluid levels or both. Treatment depends on the causative process (e.g., hepatic amebic abscess perforating into the pericardium; Fig. 9–9).

Pericardial Cysts and Diverticula

Pericardial cysts and diverticula may be congenital (coelomic, lymphangiomatous, bronchial or teratomatous) or acquired, secondary to hematoma, parasites or pericarditis. They are generally asymptomatic, being discovered incidentally on roentgenograms of the chest obtained for another reason. Cysts and diverticula are nondescript paracardiac masses most often in the right costophrenic angle (Fig. 9–10). Although on the frontal view the mass tends to blend with the cardiac silhouette, oblique views usually show a sharp angle between the lesion and the heart border characteristic of a mediastinal (extrapleural) rather than a parenchymal neoplasm. Inflammatory cysts may have calcium in their walls. Other lesions with similar radiological findings include pericardial fat pad, herniation of omentum or liver through the foramen of Morgagni and hiatal hernia. Computerized axial tomography is the most specific diagnostic tool to establish the diagnosis. Nevertheless, surgical exploration may be necessary to exclude a neoplasm.

Congenital Absence of the Pericardium

Congenital pericardial deficiency is an uncommon anomaly occurring more often in males than in females in a proportion of 3:1. Partial pericardial defect is more common than complete absence of the pericardium. Partial and complete (unilateral) pericardial defects occur most frequently on the left side. Total absence of the pericardium and defects of the right side of the pericardium are rare.

In patients with a partial defect, herniation of a portion of the heart (usually the left atrial appendage) may occur. Incarceration and strangulation of the herniated segment of the heart have resulted in syncope and sudden death. Intracardiac defects are not infrequently present, including atrial septal defect, patent ductus arteriosus, tetralogy of Fallot and bicuspid aortic valve.

Complete absence of the pericardium generally causes no serious disturbance; however, heart murmurs and discomfort related to the chest have been reported. Pain in the chest may be greatly modified by changes in posture. In patients with complete absence of the left pericardium, the precordium is usually hyperactive, and the apical impulse is shifted to the left. The electrocardiogram may show right axis deviation, incomplete right bundle-branch block, and leftward displacement of the transition zone of the QRS in the precordial leads.

Several theories have attempted to explain the embryogenesis of pericardial defects. Most authors agree that a pericardial defect results from failure of closure of the pleural pericardial foramen, probably secondary to premature atrophy of the left duct of Cuvier, causing insufficiency of the blood supply to the pleuropericardial membrane.

In partial pericardial defects without herniation of the heart, the cardiac silhouette appears normal. If the heart herniates through the defect the herniated part appears as a mass projecting from the cardiac border (Figs. 9–11, 9–12). The size of the mass depends on the size of the defect and the herniated part.

The portion of the heart that herniates through a pericardial defect may straighten the left heart border or may protrude into the left side of the mediastinum, simulating hilar adenopathy, persistent thymus, lung tumor, poststenotic dilatation of the pulmonary artery, idiopathic dilatation of the pulmonary artery and levotransposition of the great arteries. The presence of pneumopericardium after production of an artificial pneumothorax is considered confirmatory evidence in both partial and complete absence of the left pericardium. However, failure to produce pneumopericardium does not exclude a pericardial defect. Angiocardiography is diagnostic in partial pericardial defects by demonstrating the herniation of the heart, if present. Associated cardiac defects may also be demonstrated.

In complete left-sided pericardial defect (Fig. 9–13) the frontal chest roentgenogram shows displacement of the heart to the left, without tracheal shift, and an unusual cardiac configuration (elongated), prominence of the pulmonary artery segment and interposition of lung between the pulmonary artery and the aortic arch and between the left hemidiaphragm and the inferior border of the heart. On the lateral roentgenogram the pulmonary trunk is sharply outlined.

The cardiac silhouette may be normal in size or enlarged. Unusual mobility of the heart may be detected by fluoroscopy or on plain roentgenograms by changing the patient's posture. Echocardiography shows RV and LV dilatation and paradoxical motion of the interventricular septum. The amplitude of motion of the posterior LV wall is increased. The echocardiographic findings are reminiscent of RV volume overload. Radionuclide imaging of the lung demonstrates presence of lung between the heart and the left hemidiaphragm. Normally, lung is excluded from this location by the attachments of the pericardium.

Ectopia Cordis

This usually fatal anomaly is included here because a defect in the pericardium is part of the entity. Ectopia cordis

Fig. 9–10. *Pericardial cyst in a 58-year-old woman.* The frontal film of the chest demonstrates a mass in the right cardiophrenic angle. In all projections the mass blended into the lower right heart border, simulating right atrial enlargement. Computerized tomography **(B)** showed a paracardiac mass completely separate from the heart and pericardium; the density was 15 EMI units, indicating fluid. The anterior blood pool scan **(C)** showed an avascular mass. At surgery a *pericardial diverticulum* was identified containing inspissated mucinous material.

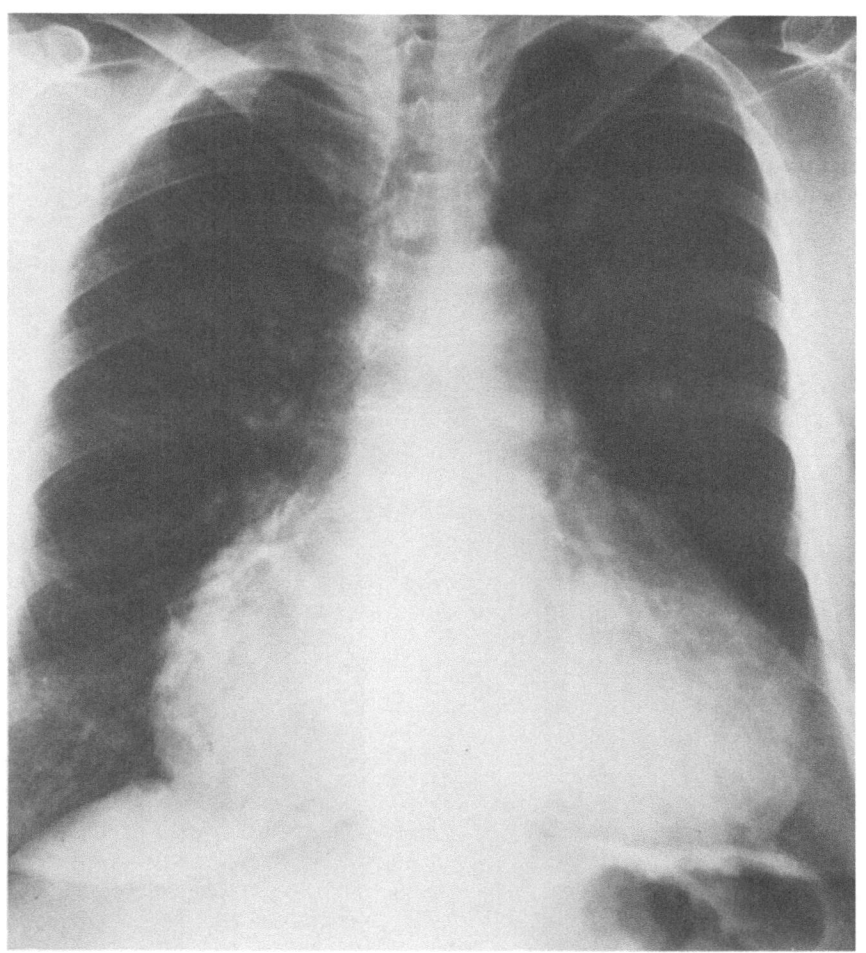

A

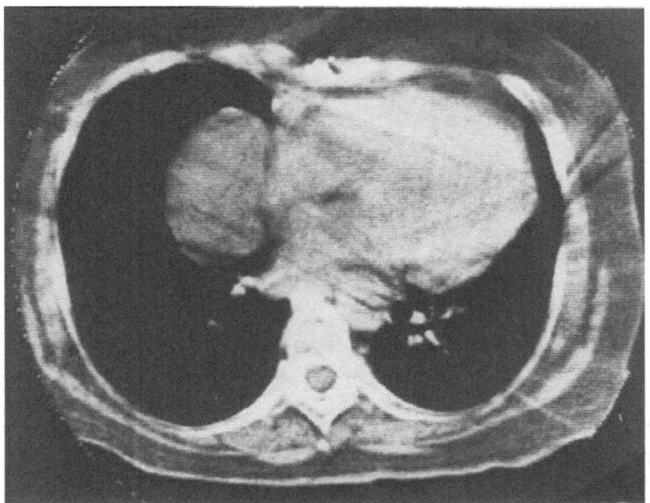

B

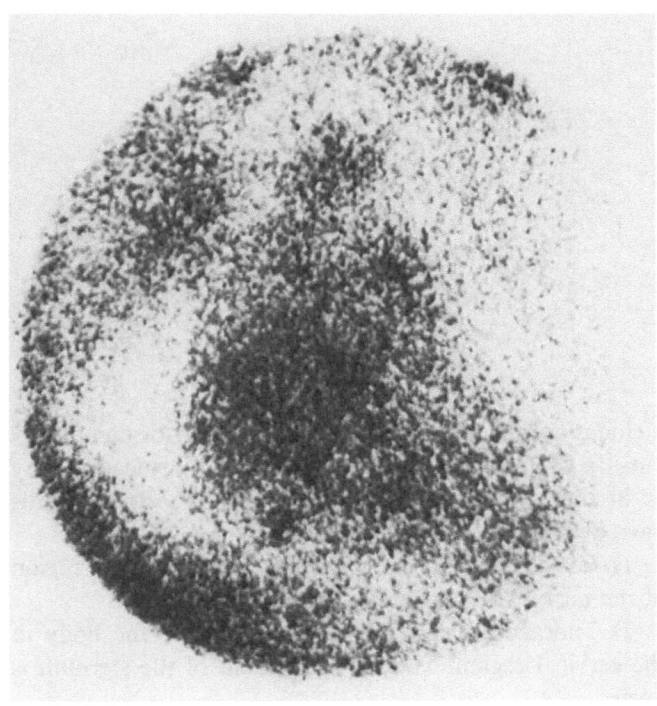

C

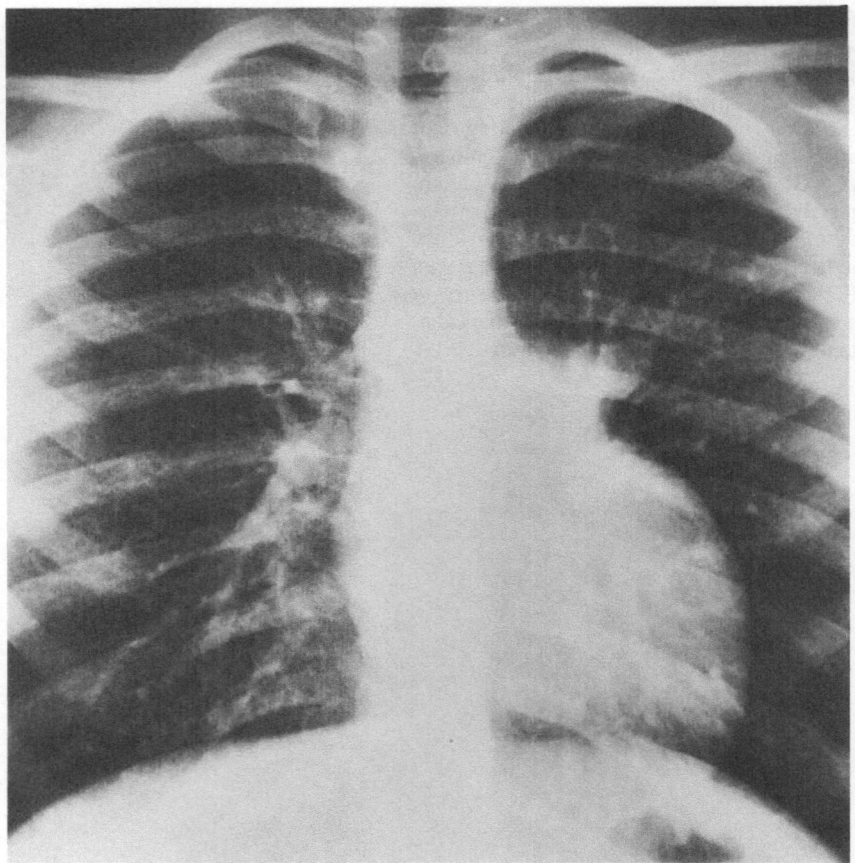

A

includes defects in which the heart is partly or completely outside the chest cavity, actually lying outside the body or in the abdominal cavity. Five types of ectopia cordis have been recognized:

1) Cervical: The heart is outside the body in the region of the neck. The sternum is intact.

2) Thoracocervical: The heart is outside the body in the cervical region. The upper segment of the sternum is open.

3) Thoracic: The sternum is defective. The heart lies outside the thorax.

4) Thoracoabdominal: The sternum is cleft, and a defect is present in the diaphragm, accompanied by a midline abdominal defect such as an omphalocele or diastasis recti.

The heart and abdominal organs protrude partly or completely through the defect.

5) Abdominal: A defect is present in the diaphragm. The heart may be inside the body, lying partly or completely in the abdominal cavity.

A diverticulum of the apex of the LV, extending through a defect in the diaphragm into the abdominal cavity, is considered by some authors as a forme fruste of ectopia cordis. A cleft sternum may also represent a partial form of this anomaly.

Intracardiac defects are virtually always present. Ventricular septal defects are the most common, and are usually part of tetralogy of Fallot or pulmonary atresia. Other defects that may be encountered are single ventricle, trans-

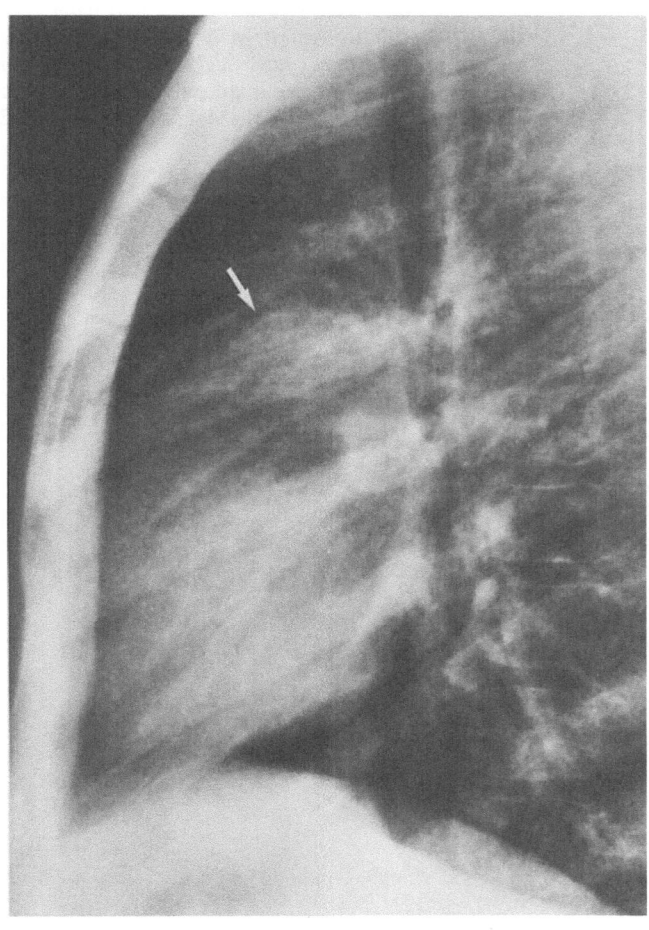

B

position of the great arteries, coarctation of the aorta, truncus arteriosus, double-outlet right ventricle, tricuspid atresis, total anomalous pulmonary venous return and common atrium. Many patients with ectopia cordis have a diverticulum of the LV that projects from the apex anteriorly if the heart lies outside the body or inferiorly if the heart lies partly or completely in the abdomen. These diverticula tend to rupture.

Associated extracardiac anomalies include midline defects of the brain and skull, cleft palate and meningomyelocele. Diagnosis can be made in utero by 2-D echocardiography. At delivery of the infant, physical examination demonstrates the location of the heart outside the body in cervical, thoracic or thoracoabdominal locations. If the heart is in the abdomen it will be a pulsatile mass inside a ventral hernia.

The roentgenogram of the chest in ectopia cordis (Fig. 9–14) shows absence of the heart in its normal position and an extrathoracic cardiac silhouette. A sternal defect is often present (e.g., bifid sternum or absence of sternum). Additional findings are wide separation of the sternal ends of the clavicles and widening of the superior mediastinum.

Surgical treatment has been successful in a few patients with relatively uncomplicated defects. One of the earliest was in a patient with abdominal ectopia cordis. The diverticulum should be amputated and oversewn because of its tendency to rupture.

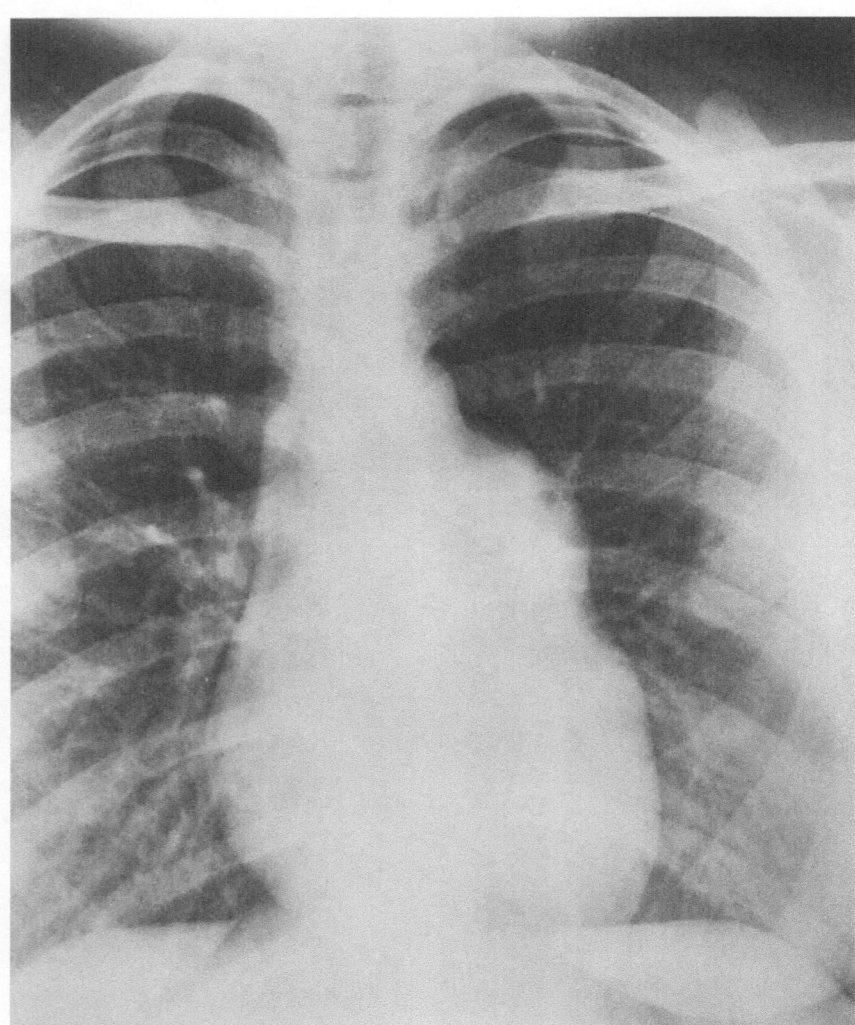

Fig. 9–12. *A partial pericardial defect in an adult who underwent surgery to exclude a mediastinal mass suggested on tomograms.* At surgery the main pulmonary artery protruded through the defect. Courtesy of Edward Burack, M.D.

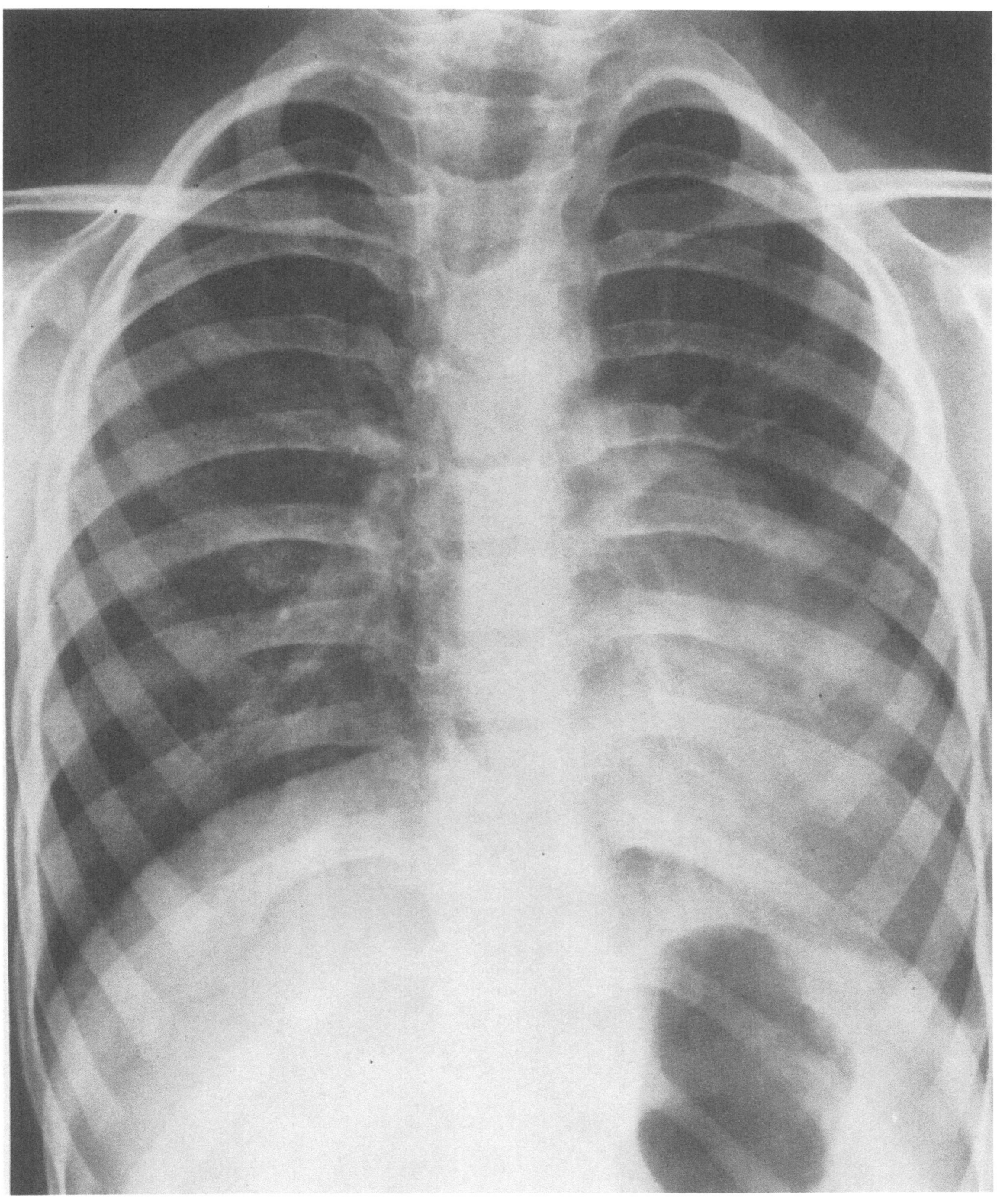

Fig. 9–13. *Absence of the left pericardium in a 3-year-old boy with a systolic ejection murmur.* The cardiac silhouette is elongated and displaced to the left without tracheal shift. On the frontal projection the lucent area below the apex of the heart represents lung interposed between the left hemidiaphragm and the inferior border of the heart. Lung would normally be excluded from this location by the attachments of the pericardium. Lung also herniates between the pulmonary artery and the aortic arch when the left pericardium is absent.

Fig. 9–14. *Thoracic ectopia cordis in a 1-day-old boy.* The frontal view (**A**) shows the cardiac density overlying the right hemithorax. The clavicles are widely separated. These findings are consistent with ectopia cordis. The lateral projection (**B**) confirms the extrathoracic location of the heart. The lungs are not aerated. At autopsy no diaphragmatic hernia was present. Cardiovascular anomalies included hypoplastic left ventricle, ventricular septal defect, atrial septal defect, patent ductus arteriosus and persistent left superior vena cava entering the left atrium.

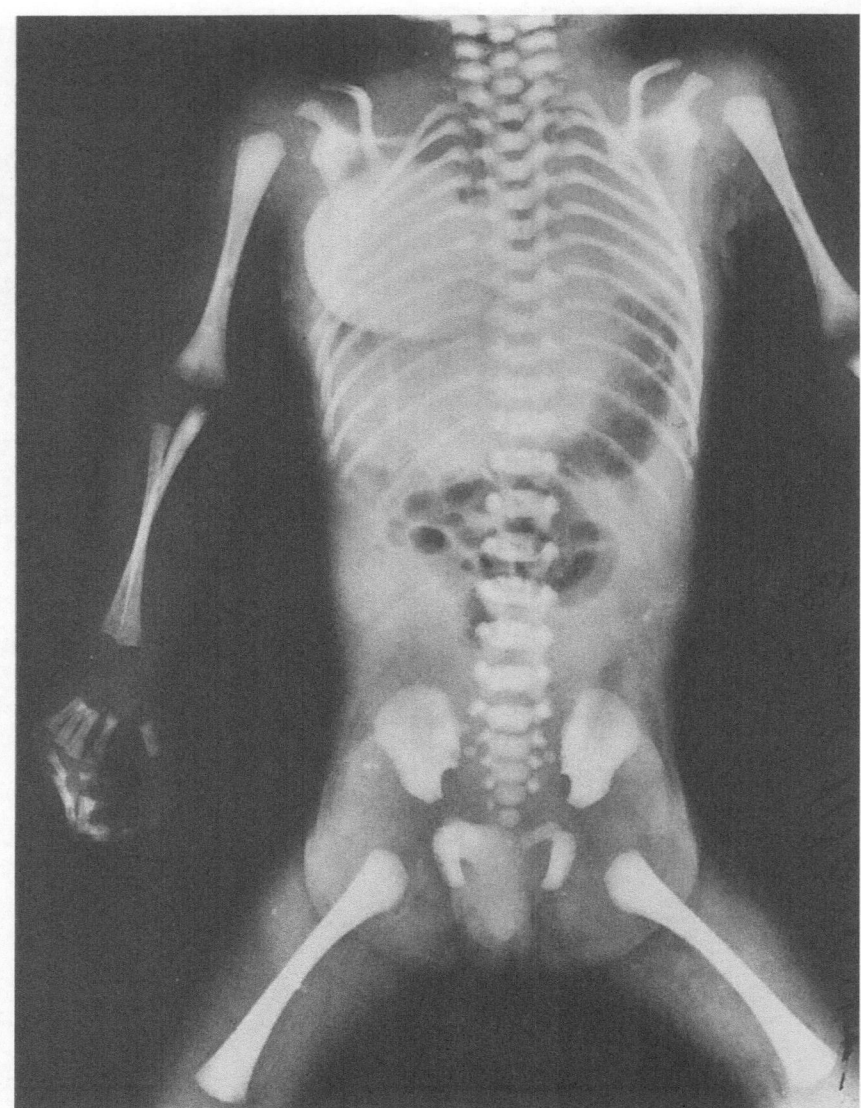

A

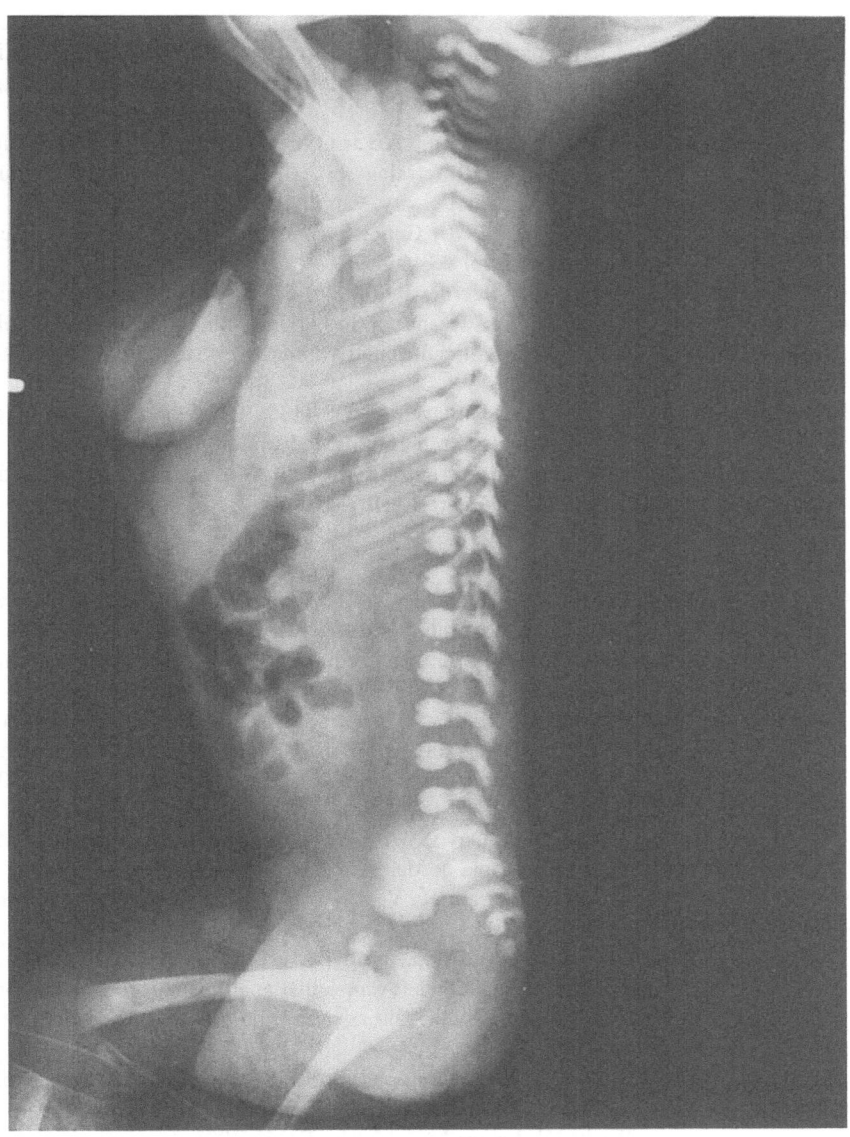

B

Bibliography

Diseases of the Pericardium, Pericardial Effusion and Cardiac Tamponade, Constrictive Pericarditis versus Restrictive Cardiomyopathy

Benotti JR, Grossman W, Cohn PF (1980) Clinical profile of restrictive cardiomyopathy. Circulation 61:1206–1212

Bishop LH Jr, Estes EH Jr, McIntosh HD (1956) The electrocardiogram as a safeguard in pericardiocentesis. JAMA 162:264–265

Carsky EW, Mauceri RA, Azimi F (1980) The epicardial fat pad sign. Radiology 137:303–308

Engle MA, Zabriskie JB, Sentefit LB, Ebert PA (1975) Postpericardiotomy syndrome. A new look at an old condition. Mod Concepts Cardiovasc Dis 44:59–64

Friedman MJ, Sahn DJ, Haber K (1979) Two-dimensional echocardiography and B-mode ultrasonography for the diagnosis of loculated pericardial effusion. Circulation 60:1644–1649

Gaasch WH, Andrias CW, Levine HJ (1978) Chronic aortic regurgitation: The effect of aortic valve replacement on left ventricular volume, mass and function. Circulation 58:825–836

Goldberg BB, Ostrum BJ, Isard HJ (1967) Ultrasonic determination of pericardial effusion. JAMA 202:103–106

Golinko RJ, Kaplan N, Rudolph AM (1963) The mechanism of pulsus paradoxus during acute pericardial tamponade. J Clin Invest 42:249–257

Hawthorne W, Williams C, Bland E (1964) Post-pericardiotomy syndrome and related syndromes. Proceedings of the Second National Conference on Cardiovascular Disease (Federation of American Societies for Experimental Biology), pp 513

Janos GG, Arjunan K, Meyer RA, Engel P, Kaplan S (1983) Differentiation of constrictive pericarditis and restrictive cardiomyopathy using digitized echocardiography. J Am Coll Cardiol 1:541–549

Kremens V (1955) Demonstration of the pericardial shadow on the routine chest roentgenogram: A new roentgen finding. Preliminary report. Radiology 64:72–80

Kronzon I, Cohen ML, Winer HE (1983) Diastolic atrial compression: A sensitive echocardiographic sign of cardiac tamponade. J Am Coll Cardiol 2:770–775

Martin RP, Rakowski H, French JW, Popp RL (1978) Localization of pericardial effusion with wide-angle phased array echocardiography. Am J Cardiol 42:904–912

Meaney E, Shearer M, Weidner C, Mangiardi LM, Smalling R, Peterson K (1976) Cardiac amyloidosis, constrictive pericarditis and restrictive cardiomyopathy. Am J Cardiol 38:547–556

Murphy DJ Jr, Kaplan S (1983) Differentiation of constrictive pericarditis and restrictive cardiomyopathy. Internal Med for the Specialist 4:131–151

Perheentupa J, Autio S, Leisti S, Roitta C, Tunteri L (1973) Mulibrey nanism, an autosomal recessive syndrome with pericardial constriction. Lancet 2:351–355

Peter R, Whalen R, Orgain E, McIntosh H (1966) Post-pericardiotomy syndrome as a complication of percutaneous left ventricular puncture. Am J Cardiol 17: 86–90

St John Sutton MG, Reichek N, Kastor JA, Giucliani ER (1982) Computerized m-mode echocardiographic analysis of left ventricular dysfunction in cardiac amyloid. Circulation 66:790–799

Usher BW, Popp RL (1972) Electrical alternans: Mechanism in pericardial effusion. Am Heart J 83:459–463

Voorhess ML, Husson GS, Blackman MS (1976) Growth failure with pericardial constriction. Am J Dis Child 130:1146–1148

Wong BYS, Lee KR, MacArthur RI (1982) Diagnosis of pericardial effusion by computed tomography. Chest 81:177–181

Congenital Absence of the Pericardium

Boxall R (1887) Incomplete pericardial sac, escape of heart into left pleural cavity. Tr Obstet Soc Lond 28:209–210

Chang CHJ, Leigh TF (1961) Congenital partial defect of the pericardium associated with herniation of the left atrial appendage. Am J Roentgenol 86:517–522

D'Altoria RA, Cano JY (1977) Congenital absence of the left pericardium detected by imaging of the lungs: Case report. J Nucl Med 18:267–268

Ellis K, Leeds NE, Himmelstein A (1959) Congenital deficiencies in the parietal pericardium. A review with 2 new cases including successful diagnosis by plain roentgenography. Am J Roentgenol 82:125–137

Hipona FA, Crummy AB Jr (1964) Congenital pericardial defect associated with tetralogy of Fallot: Herniation of normal lung into pericardial cavity. Circulation 29:132–135

Nasser WK (1970) Congenital absence of the left pericardium. Am J Cardiol 26:466–470

Payvandi M, Kerber RE (1976) Echocardiography in congenital and acquired absence of the pericardium. An echocardiographic mimic of right ventricular volume overload. Circulation 53:86–92

Southworth H, Stevenson CS (1938) Congenital defects of the pericardium. Arch Intern Med 61:223–240

Sunderland S, Wright-Smith RJ (1944) Congenital pericardial defects. Br Heart J 6:167–175

Ectopia Cordis

Blatt ML, Zeldes M (1942) Ectopia Cordis. Report of a case and review of the literature. Am J Dis Child 63:515–529

Byron F (1948) Ectopia cordis. Report of a case with attempted operative correction. J Thorac Surg 17:717–722

Cantrell JR, Haller A, Ravitch MM (1958) A syndrome of congenital defects involving the abdominal wall, sternum, diaphragm, pericardium, and heart. Surg Gynecol Obstet 107:602–614

Chang CHJ, Davis WC (1961) Congenital bifid sternum with partial ectopia cordis. Am J Roentgenol 86:513–516

Kanagasuntheram R, Verzin JA (1962) Ectopia cordis in man. Thorax 17:159–167

Knight L, Neal WA, Williams HJ, Huseby TL, Edwards JE (1976) Congenital left ventricular aneurysm. Part of a syndrome of cardiac abnormalities and midline defects. Minn Med 59:372–375

Scott GW (1955) Ectopia cordis: Report of a case successfully treated by operation. Guys Hosp Rep 104:55–66

Wicks JD, Levine MD, Mettler FA Jr (1981) Juxta-uterine sonography of thoracic ectopia cordis. Am J Roentgenol 137:619–621

10 Magnetic Resonance Imaging of the Heart

Charles B. Higgins

Magnetic resonance imaging (MRI) is a new technique for noninvasive imaging of the heart.[1-5] It involves no ionizing radiation, and for imaging of the cardiovascular system does not require any contrast medium.

MRI depends upon the interaction of nuclei with a strong magnetic field and the intermittently applied radiofrequency pulses to generate tomographic images of the heart. While any atom with an odd number of protons or neutrons may be utilized for MRI, hydrogen is so naturally abundant and efficient (maximum number of nuclei per atomic number) that it is the most ideal nucleus for imaging. Most imaging at the current time employs hydrogen resonance and is referred to as hydrogen or proton MRI.

Localization within an imaged plane is attained by intermittent application of a magnetic field gradient. The magnetic field gradient causes hydrogen nuclei at different sites across the imaged plane to have a resonance frequency that is specific for that site and slightly different from other sites across the plane. By this means, position is encoded for MRI. The signal from any site (voxel) in the image is chiefly dependent upon the concentration of hydrogen nuclei resonating at the frequency specific for that site. The signal received during the MRI process is complex. It is a multiple frequency signal dependent upon the position of each signal within the varying magnetic field. The raw time domain signal undergoes Fourier transformation. Fourier transformation reduces the raw signal into its basic frequency components. The position of the signal depends upon its specific frequency, and the amplitude of the signal depends chiefly upon the concentration of mobile hydrogen nuclei at that site. Depending upon the imaging technique utilized, the T1 (spin-lattice) and T2 (spin-spin) relaxation times also contribute to local signal intensity.

Cardiac imaging requires some form of physiological gating of the imaging sequence. Acquisition of magnetic resonance imaging signals of the thorax without gating results in poor cardiac images because of loss of signal from moving structures and the variable position of cardiac structure relative to imaging pixels when data are acquired indiscriminately throughout the cardiac cycle (Fig. 10–1). An electronically isolated electrocardiographic signal has been used to synchronize the MR data acquisition to a fixed portion of the cardiac cycle.[6] With this technique, anatomically precise images of the central cardiovascular structures have been attained (Fig. 10–1).

When using electrocardiographic gating the MR repetition rate (TR) is defined by the RR interval of the electrocardiogram. With a heart rate of 60/min, the TR is 1.0 second. If the acquisition sequence utilizes every second R wave, then the TR is 2.0 seconds and so forth. The time to acquire sufficient MR signal to generate an image at any tomographic level is approximately 6 to 10 minutes (depending upon the RR interval). Fortunately data can be acquired from five to ten levels during this time. With use of this multisection technique it is possible to obtain a series of tomographic images encompassing nearly the entire heart from base to apex. Direct imaging can be performed in the coronal and parasagittal as well as the transverse planes. Techniques have also been devised for isotropic three-dimensional imaging and for producing images in planes other than the orthogonal planes.

Normal Cardiac Morphology

The transaxial (cross-sectional) imaging format is the one generally used for cardiac MRI studies; it displays cardiac anatomy in a form similar to computerized tomography and sector scan echocardiography. In contradistinction to computerized tomography but similar to echocardiography, the walls of the heart and vascular structures are clearly distinguished without the need for contrast medium.[1-5,7]

Gated MR images of the heart have displayed the internal architecture of the heart (Figs. 10–1 to 10–3). The

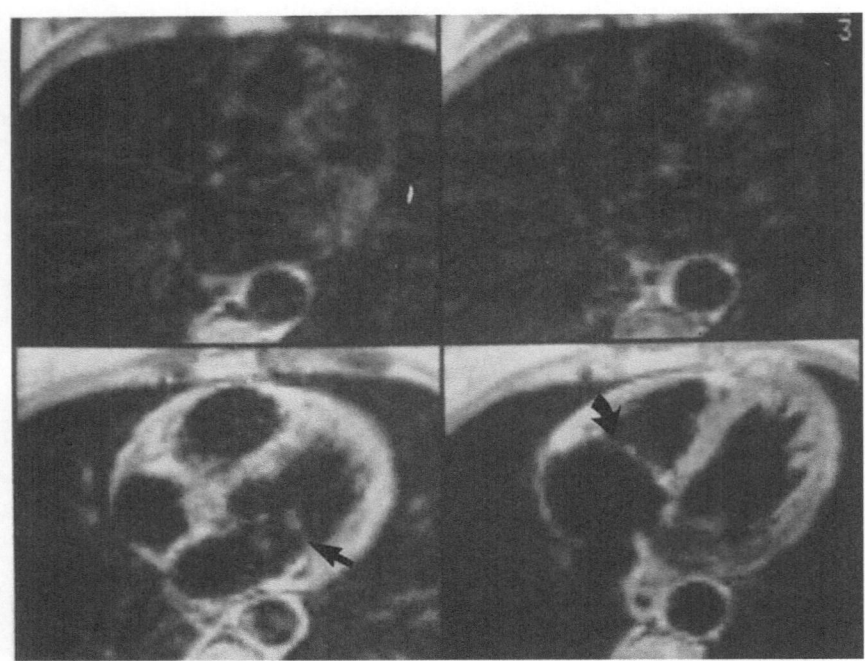

Fig. 10–1. *Nongated* (upper panels) *and ECG gated* (lower panels) *transverse images at two different levels near the middle of the left ventricle.* Note the mitral (*arrow*) and tricuspid (*curved arrow*) valves. Higgins CB, Stark D, McNamara M, Lanzer P, Crooks LE, Kaufman L (1984) Multiplane magnetic resonance imaging of the heart and major vessels: Studies in normal volunteers. *Am J Roentgenol* 142:661–668. Reproduced with permission.

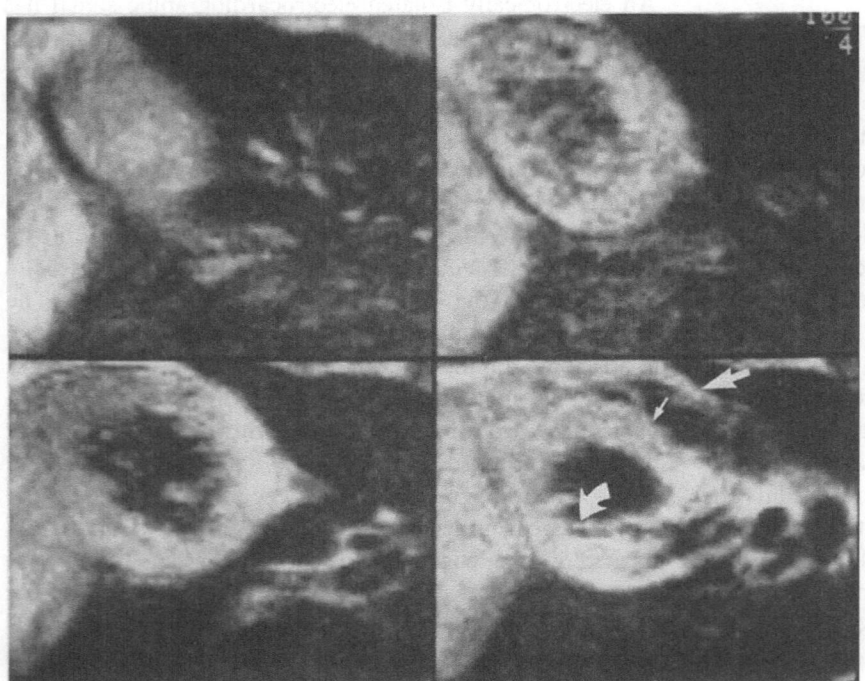

Fig. 10–2. *Gated sagittal images of the left ventricle extending from left* (left upper panel) *to right* (right lower panel). The most medial image cuts through the left and right ventricles. Note in this image the clear delineation of the septal (*small arrow*), posterior (*curved arrow*) and diaphragmatic wall of the left ventricle. The free wall of the right ventricle (*arrow*) is also seen. Higgins CB, Stark D, McNamara M, Lanzer P, Crooks LE, Kaufman L (1984) Multiplane magnetic resonance imaging of the heart and major vessels: Studies in normal volunteers. *Am J Roentgenol* 142:661–668. Reproduced with permission.

natural sharp interface in contrast between moving blood in the cardiac chamber and the cardiac walls results in clear discrimination of the ventricular and atrial septa. Consequently it should be possible to measure wall thickness at all sites within the ventricles. Even at this early time in the development of MRI, the spatial resolution of the imager coupled with the current gating system has permitted visualization of the proximal portions of the left and right coronary arteries (Fig. 10–4); this has been achieved without the injection of any contrast medium. Resolution of the internal morphology of the ventricles

has been sufficient to depict the moderator band of the right ventricle (RV) (Fig. 10–1), the papillary muscles (Fig. 10–5), leaflets of the atrioventricular valves (Fig. 10–1) and cusps of the aortic valve (Fig. 10–4B).

Direct images of the heart in the sagittal and coronal planes are also useful for evaluating certain regions of the cardiac chambers and, together with transaxial images, depict all regions of the myocardium of the left ventricle (LV) (Figs. 10–2, 10–3). The sagittal plane demonstrates the thickness of the anteroseptal and posterior walls of the LV (Fig. 10–2). The coronal plane demonstrates an-

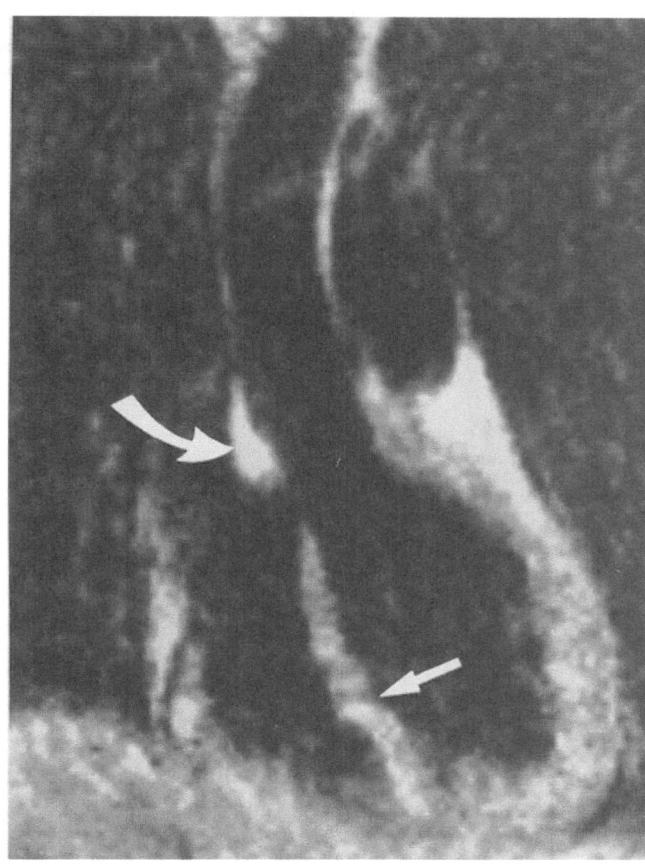

Fig. 10–3. *Gated coronal image through the two ventricles shows the sinus of Valsalva of the aorta* (curved arrow) *and the ventricular septum* (arrow) *of the right and left ventricles.* Higgins CB, Stark D, McNamara M, Lanzer P, Crooks LE, Kaufman L (1984) Multiplane magnetic resonance imaging of the heart and major vessels: Studies in normal volunteers. *Am J Roentgenol* 142:661–668. Reproduced with permission.

other region of the septum as well as the diaphragmatic and lateral walls of the LV (Fig. 10–3).

Chronic Ischemic Heart Disease

Old myocardial infarctions have been demonstrated as regions of wall thinning on MR images[8] (Figs. 10–6, 10–7). The transition between normal myocardial wall thickness and wall thinning has been sharply defined; this has provided an estimate of the extent of the LV involved by the previous infarction. The MRI findings have been correlated with the corroborative LV angiogram or sector scan echocardiogram or both.[8] Gated MR images have displayed regions of extreme wall thinning and bulging of segments of the LV in patients with aneurysms demonstrated on left ventriculography or echocardiography (Fig. 10–8). Posterior aneurysms and infarctions have been depicted, as well as those involving the anterior and septal regions.

LV thrombus was demonstrated on MR images in several patients shown to have this abnormality on either sector scan echocardiography or computerized tomographic

Fig. 10–4. *Gated images in the left ventricular outflow tract beneath the aortic valve* (**A**) *and at level of aortic valve* (**B**). Note the origin of the right coronary artery (*arrowhead*) from the right sinus of Valsalva, and its course in the right atrioventricular groove (*arrow*). Higgins CB, Lanzer P, Stark D, Botvinick E, Schiller NB, Crooks L, Kaufman L, Lipton MJ (1984) Nuclear magnetic resonance imaging in chronic ischemic heart disease in man. Circulation (In press). Reproduced with permission of American Heart Association.

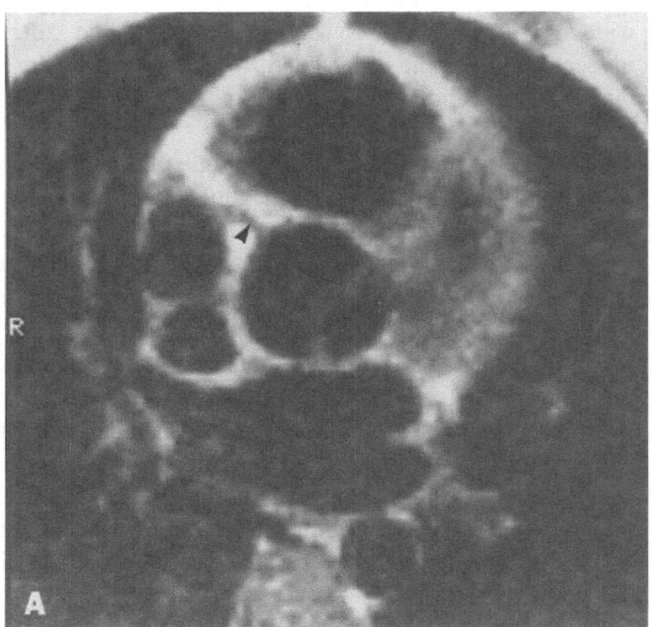

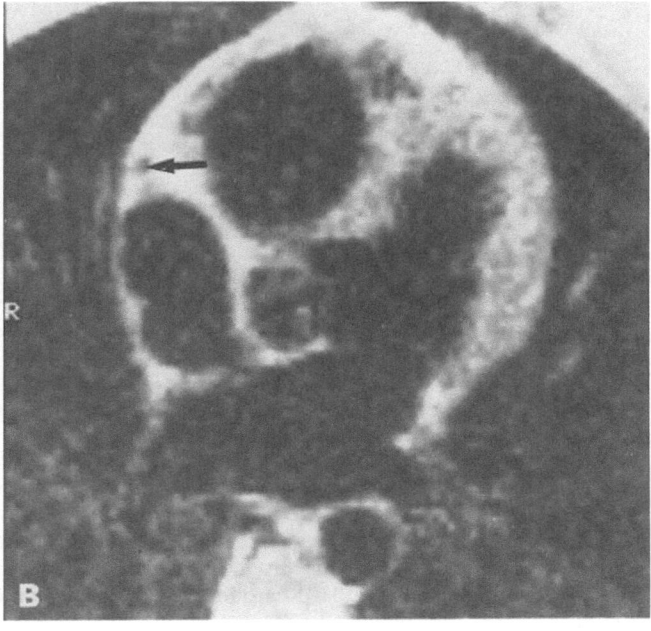

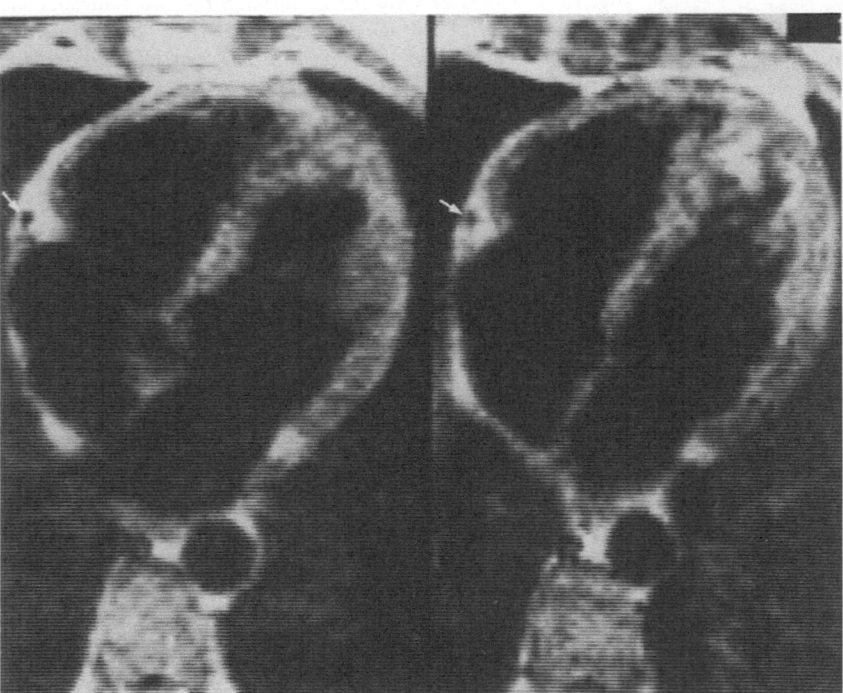

Fig. 10–5. *First echo (TE = 28 msec)* **(A)** *and second echo (TE = 56 msec)* **(B)** images through the middle of the ventricles. Note the papillary muscle in the left ventricle and the right coronary artery (*small arrow*).

A   B

scans. Mural thrombus was noted on MRI as structures of medium signal intensity projecting into the signal void of the LV chamber. Stasis of blood in akinetic and dyskinetic regions of the LV can also produce intracavitary signal. The patterns of the regional intensity of thrombus and stasis are usually different on the first [TE (echo delay time) = 28 msec] and second (TE = 56 msec) spin echo images. Thrombus shows a relative decrease in signal from the first to the second spin echo image. On the other hand,

stasis of blood results in a relatively greater intracavitary signal on the second spin echo image (Fig. 10–8).

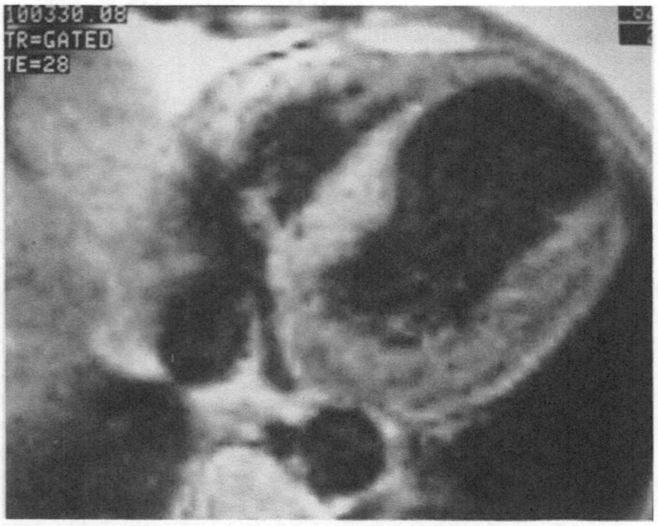

Acute Myocardial Infarction

A recent study in our laboratory[9] used the spin echo technique to image excised canine hearts with 24-hour-old myocardial infarcts within 1 hour after death. In each heart the area of infarction had increased signal intensity compared to normal myocardium. When the animals with experimental myocardial infarctions are considered as a group, the mean value for T1 relaxation times of infarcted myocardium (728 ± 94.8 msec) was higher than the value for normal myocardium (650 ± 87.4 msec). There was a wide range of T1 values between infarcted and normal myocardium. On the other hand, the T1 values of the infarcted myocardium were higher than those of normal myocardium for each individual animal.

The mean value for T2 relaxation time of infarcted myocardium (48.4 ± 2.4 msec) was significantly greater ($p <$ 0.01) than that for normal myocardium (42.1 ± 1.2 msec). There was a narrow range of T2 values for normal myocardium (40.2 − 43.5 msec), and no overlap of individual values between the infarcted and normal groups.

Recently, gated MR images obtained in vivo in intact dogs and patients with 1- to 7-day old myocardial infarctions have also shown that the infarcted myocardium can be distinguished from normal myocardium without the use of contrast medium.[10] Compared to normal myocardium the infarcted myocardium had high signal intensity on MR images produced with the spin echo technique (Fig. 10–9).

Although contrast medium is not needed to delineate

Fig. 10–6. *Gated image in a patient with prior anterior myocardial infarction showing thinning of the anterior septum and anterior wall of the left ventricle.* Higgins CB, Lanzer P, Stark D, Botvinick E, Schiller NB, Crooks L, Kaufman L, Lipton MJ (1984) Nuclear magnetic resonance imaging in chronic ischemic heart disease in man. Circulation 69:523–531. Reproduced with permission of American Heart Association.

Fig. 10–7. *Gated transverse image in a patient with normal pericardium.* Pericardium is represented by a rim of low signal intensity (*arrows*) separating the subepicardial fat (high signal intensity) and pericardial fat. The image also shows thinning of the posterior myocardial wall in this patient with a prior myocardial infarction.

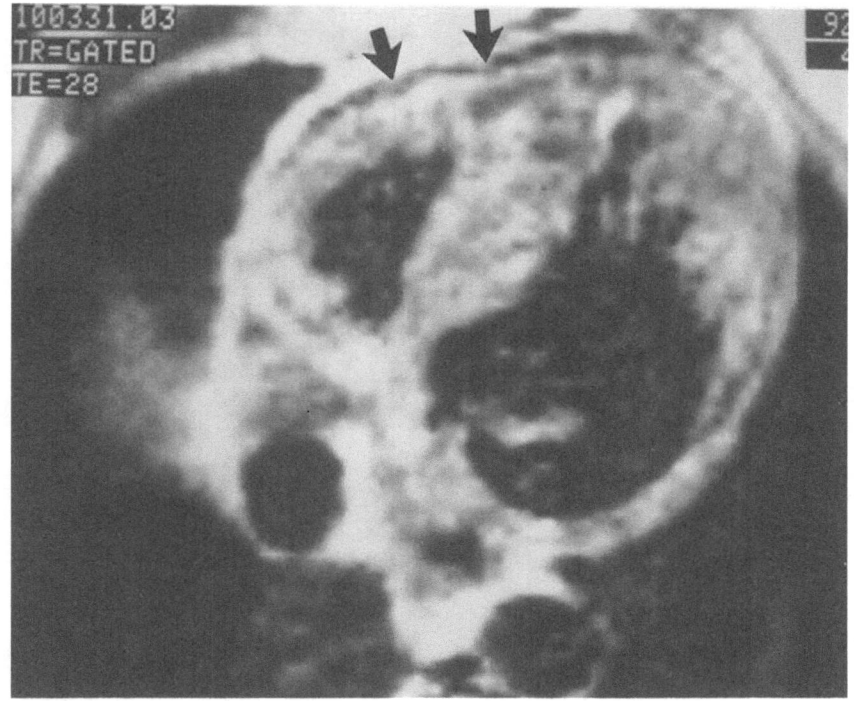

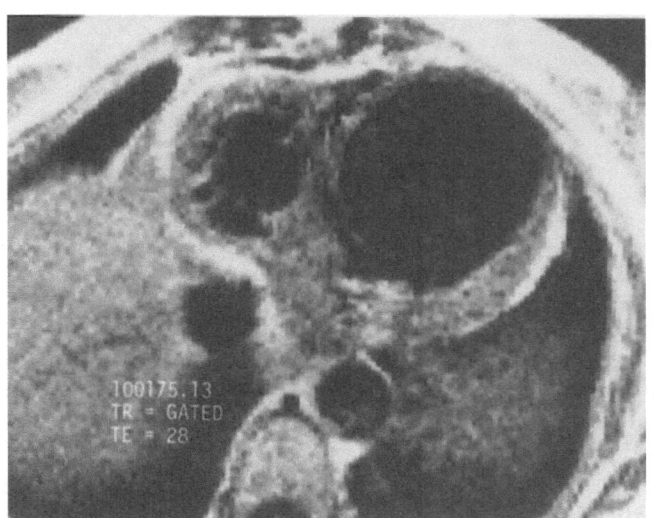

A

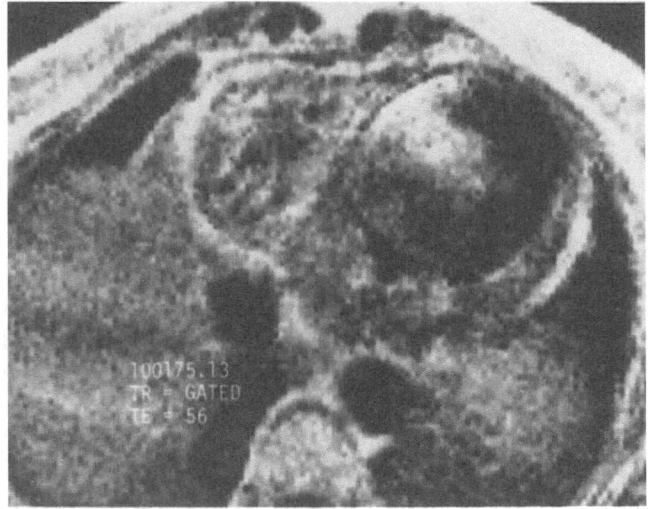

B

Fig. 10–8. *Gated transverse images near the apex of the left ventricle.* First (TE = 28 msec) (**A**) and second (TE = 56 msec) (**B**) spin echo image of a patient with a remote transmural infarction. There is prominent signal intensity in the chamber, presumably due to blood stasis in a region of dyskinesia shown on the second echo image. Higgins CB, Lanzer P, Stark D, Botvinick E, Schiller NB, Crooks L, Kaufman L, Lipton MJ (1984) Nuclear magnetic resonance imaging in chronic ischemic heart disease in man. Circulation 69:523–531. Reproduced with permission of American Heart Association.

Fig. 10–9. *Series of gated spin echo images in a dog with an anterior myocardial infarction.* Images extend from the midventricular level to the apex. Images were obtained within the first week after occlusion of the left anterior descending coronary artery. Infarct has high signal intensity (*arrows*) compared to normal myocardium.

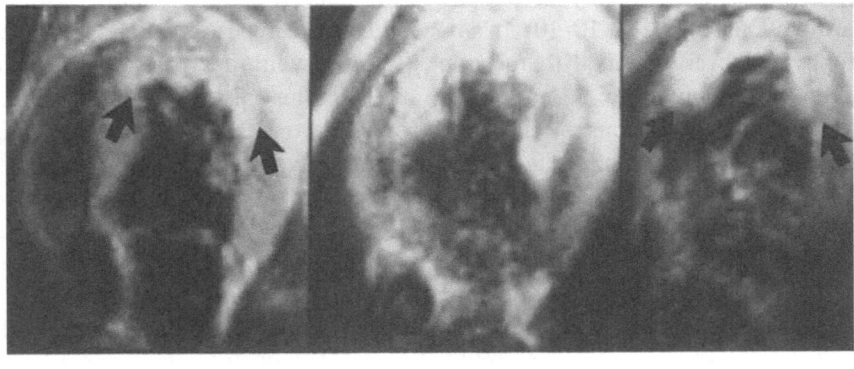

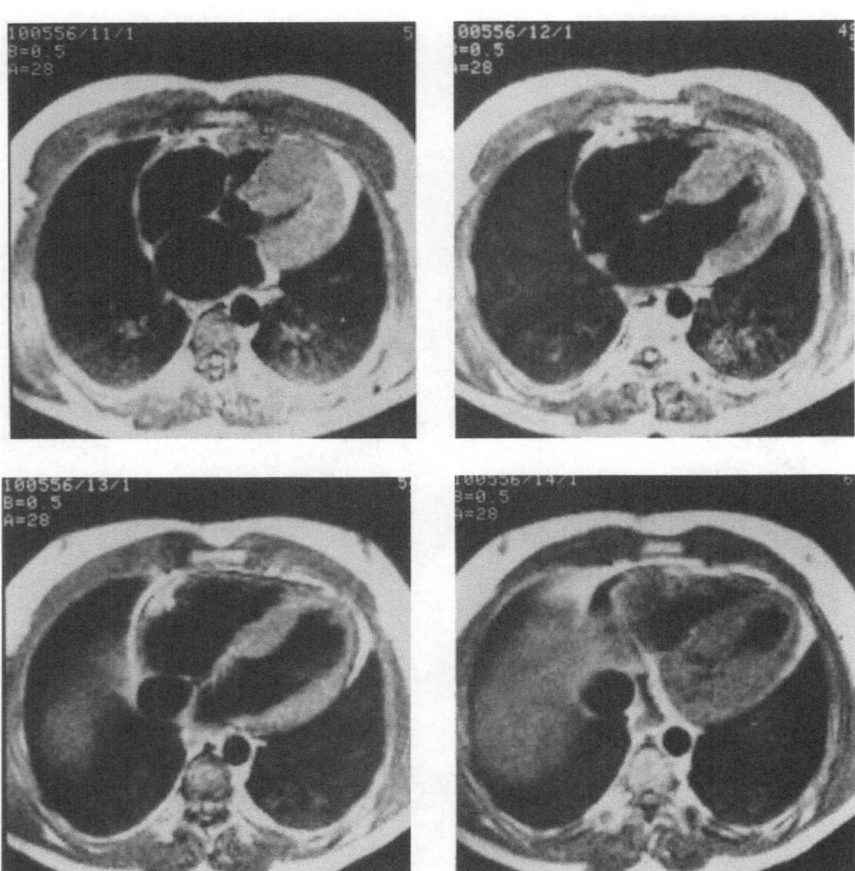

Fig. 10–10. *Series of gated images extending from the base* (left upper panel) *to near the apex* (right lower panel) of the left ventricle in a patient with hypertrophic cardiomyopathy. Note the hypertrophy of the septal and lateral wall of the outflow regions and hypertrophy confined to the septum in the body of the left ventricle.

the blood-tissue interface of the cardiovascular system, it may prove useful as a myocardial perfusion marker. It has not been determined if myocardial ischemia without infarction can be detected by gated proton MRI. In this regard, paramagnetic contrast media have been used to differentiate normally perfused myocardium from jeopardized myocardium after coronary occlusion in canine experimental models.[11]

Cardiomyopathies

Gated MRI has defined the presence, site, extent and severity of septal hypertrophy in patients with hypertrophic cardiomyopathy[12] (Fig. 10–10). In some patients the hypertrophy has been confined to the upper septum, while in others it has involved the entire septum. MRI has also demonstrated extensions of the hypertrophy beyond the septum. The definition of hypertrophic cardiomyopathy shown by gated MRI has correlated closely with that depicted by 2-D echocardiography.

Gated MRI studies in a number of patients with congestive cardiomyopathy have demonstrated the degree of LV and RV enlargement. The sharp depiction of chamber dimensions and wall thickness provided by MRI indicates

that this technique should provide the measurements necessary for accurate calculations of myocardial wall stress. Idiopathic congestive cardiomyopathy reveals uniform thickness of various regions of the LV, while ischemic cardiomyopathy generally shows uniform (regional) wall thinning at sites of previous infarctions. Surprisingly, some patients with idiopathic congestive cardiomyopathy have disproportionate thinning of the septal segment.

Acquisition of images at two different interpulse delays (repetition rate, TR) can be achieved by imaging with the gating interval set to every R wave of the electrocardiogram for one run (TR = RR interval) and to every second R wave for the second run (TR = 2 × RR interval). Data acquired with two different TR intervals permits the calculation of T1 relaxation times of the myocardium. Using the spin echo technique with two different echo delays (TE = 28 msec and 56 msec), the T2 relaxation time can also be determined. This permits the generation of calculated T1 and T2 images; these are essentially maps of the T1 and T2 times of the entire myocardium. They permit visual assessment of the uniformity of relaxation time throughout the myocardium (Fig. 10–11). It will be of interest to determine if relaxation times are altered in hypertrophic cardiomyopathy and the various types of congestive cardiomyopathy.

Fig. 10–11. *Hypertrophic cardiomyopathy.* Images gated to every beat (*left upper panel*) and every other beat (*right upper panel*). Calculated T1 (*left lower panel*) and calculated T2 (*right lower panel*) images demonstrate variations in T1 and T2 relaxation times of the septal and lateral walls. For the T1 and T2 images pixel brightness is directly proportional to the duration of the relaxation times.

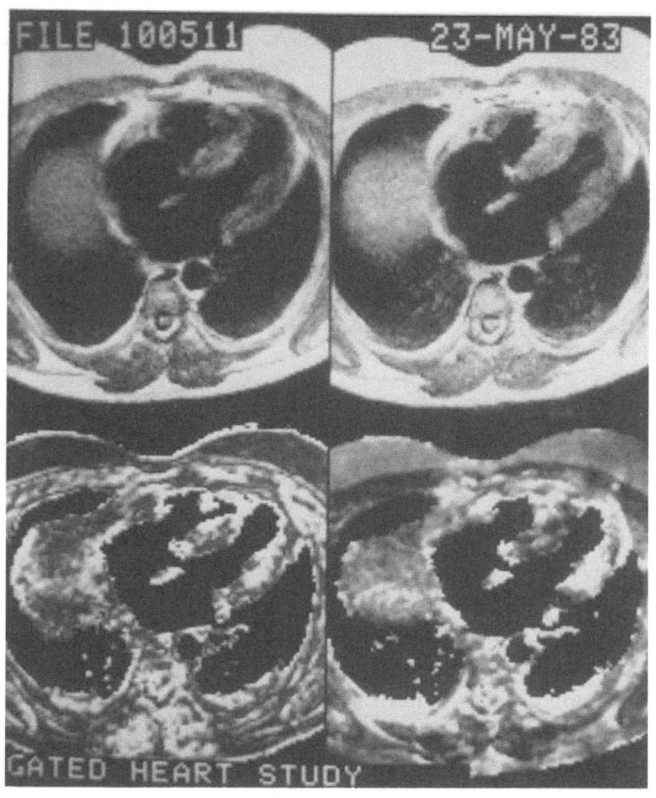

Congenital Heart Disease

MRI has recently been used to define congenital cardiovascular anomalies in our own and other MRI laboratories.[13] Atrial and ventricular septal defects have been demonstrated by gated MRI (Fig. 10–12). Visceroatrial situs and the type of bulboventricular loop can be clearly defined by transverse MR images. Likewise the relationship of the great vessels is demonstrated; the transverse images show the anterior position of the aorta in transposition (Fig. 10–13).

Abnormalities of the tricuspid valve have been well defined on axial and coronal MR images. The axial and coronal images have demonstrated the displacement of the tricuspid valve into the RV in Ebstein anomaly. MRI clearly shows the thickness of the wall of the RV; this is

Fig. 10–12. *Gated images near the base of the heart* (left) *and middle of the ventricles* (right). Note the atrial and ventricular septal defects. The myocardium (*arrows*) in the outflow region and body of the right ventricle is markedly hypertrophied.

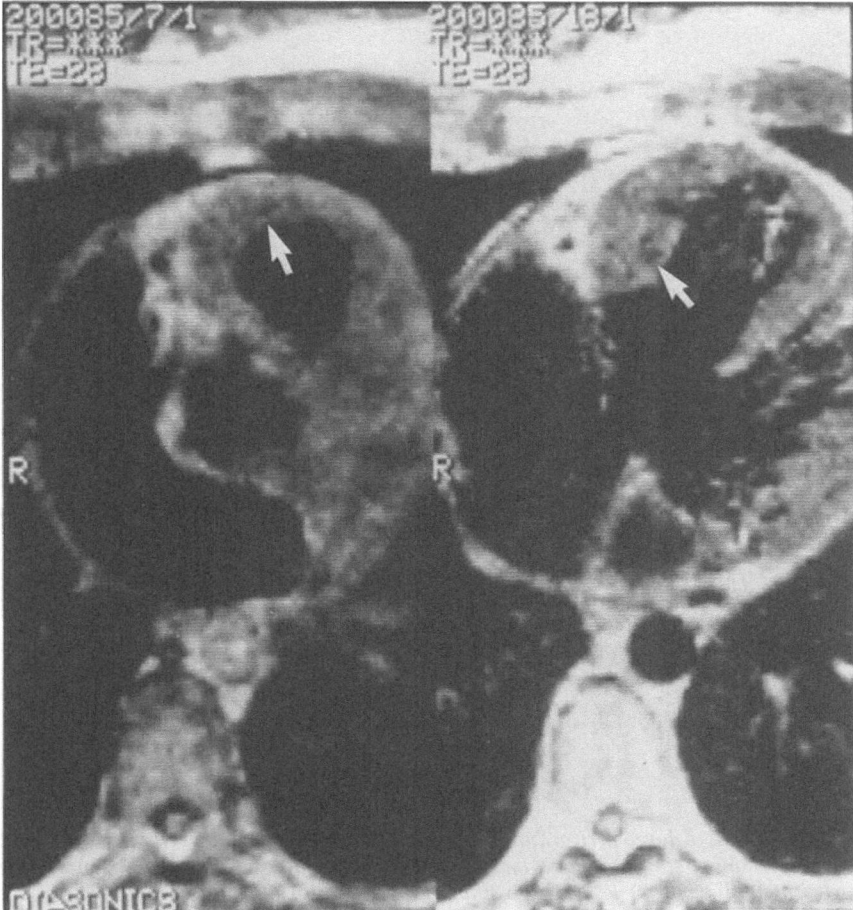

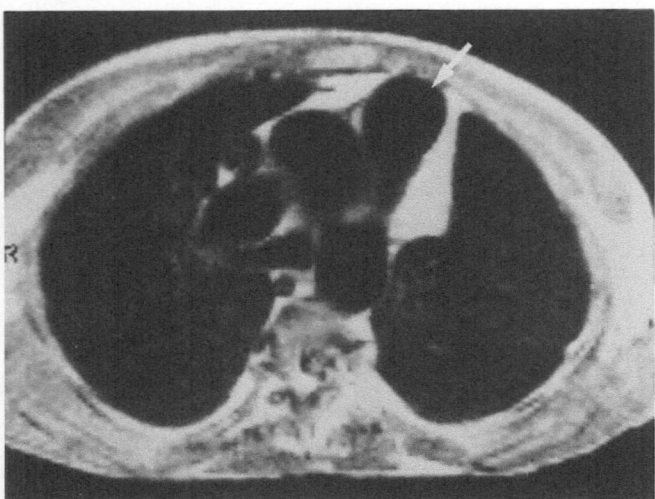

Fig. 10–13. *Transverse image at level of great vessels shows the aorta* (arrow) *positioned anterior and leftward from the pulmonary artery, indicating levotransposition of the great vessels.*

useful for documenting the degree of atrialization of the RV in this anomaly. Gated MRI reveals the size of the functioning RV. This can be important in preoperative assessment of tricuspid valve abnormalities.

MRI is perhaps the most accurate mode for defining wall thickness. In several patients with Eisenmenger syndrome the RV myocardium has been shown to be equivalent to or to exceed the thickness of the LV (Fig. 10–12). Likewise, MRI has shown substantial wall thickening in patients with obstruction of the RV outflow tract.

Pericardial Diseases

The normal pericardium is only 1 to 2 mm in thickness, and the visceral and parietal layers are closely applied to each other. The normal pericardium is composed primarily of fibrous tissue, which produces little MRI signal. Both epicardial and subepicardial fat produce an area of high MRI signal intensity at the external margin of the heart; consequently there is high contrast between the pericardium and adjacent fat. The normal pericardium itself is recognized as a thin lucent line surrounding portions of the circumference of the heart where it is highlighted by adjacent fat (Fig. 10–7). In most normal patients the pericardium is visualized only over the right anterior aspect of the heart. Since pure fluid also produces little or no MRI signal, it is possible that the lucent line is composed of some pericardial fluid adherent to the pericardial layers. Increase in thickness of the dark rim around the myocardium has been observed in the presence of thickened pericardium in patients with constrictive pericarditis.[14] The low signal intensity of the thickened pericardium suggests that it is composed mostly of fibrous tissue, as would be expected in chronic constrictive pericarditis. Recent experience has shown that gated MRI provides clear depiction of a number of pericardial abnormalities, including pericardial effusion, pericardial cysts and pericardial inflammation.[14] The anatomical demonstration of pericardial diseases is similar to that shown by computerized tomography.[15]

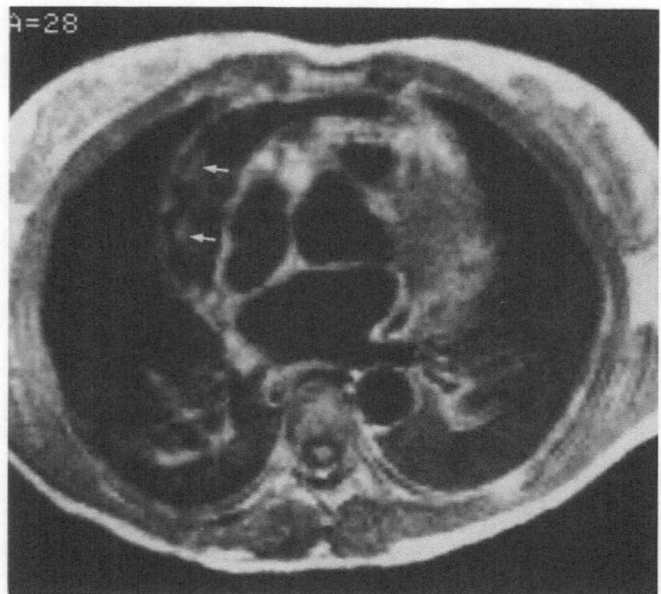

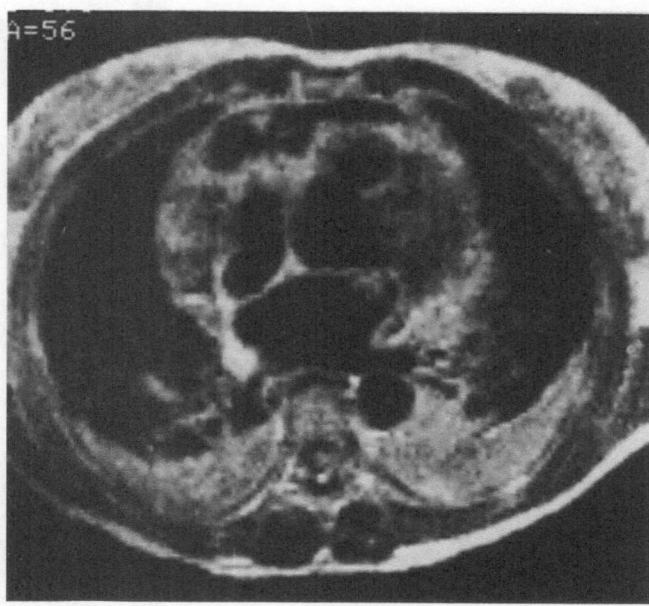

Fig. 10–14. A. *A large pericardial effusion is evident on the gated transaxial magnetic resonance image at TE = 28 msec. Solid debris (small arrows) is evident within the pericardial effusion. The right ventricle is normal in size in this patient with uremic* pericarditis. **B** Magnetic resonance image with TE = 56 msec shows increase in signal intensity of the effusion over the magnetic resonance image at TE = 28 msec, which suggests an inflammatory effusion.

A potential advantage of MRI is that it provides insight into the pathological process involved in the pericardial disease. In the few clinical cases examined to date, gated MRI has defined several inflammatory pericardial processes. In patients with uremic pericarditis the MR images demonstrated pericardial effusion and abundant inflammatory exudate on the pericardium (Fig. 10–14). In contradistinction to the normal pericardium the inflamed pericardium produced strong MRI signal intensity, as did adhesions between the visceral and parietal pericardium (Fig. 10–14). Moreover, the signal intensity of the pericardium was greater on the image with a longer delay time (TE = 28 msec versus TE = 56 msec), which is consistent with a long T2 relaxation time observed with other edematous tissues (increased water content).

Potential of MRI in Cardiac Diagnosis

There is currently too little clinical experience with MRI to predict with any reliance the eventual role of this technique in cardiovascular diagnosis. Cardiovascular MRI offers three intriguing insights into the assessment of cardiovascular disease processes and their response to therapeutic interventions: direct tissue characterization, noninvasive regional blood flow measurements, chemical and metabolic imaging. It is clear that an understanding of MRI for medical diagnosis is still primitive at this early period in its development. Much investigative work lies ahead before full cognizance of the potential of this new method is attained.

References

1. Herfkens RJ, Higgins CB, Hricak H, et al. (1983) Nuclear magnetic resonance imaging of the cardiovascular system; normal and pathological findings. Radiology 147:749–759
2. Kaufman L, Crooks L, Sheldon P, Hricak H, Herfkens R, Bank W (1983) The potential impact of nuclear magnetic resonance imaging on cardiovascular diagnosis. Circulation 67:251–257
3. Hawkes RC, Holland GN, Moore WS, Roebuck EJ, Worthington BS (1981) Nuclear magnetic resonance (NMR) tomography of the normal heart. J Comput Assist Tomogr 5:605–612
4. Crooks LE, Sheldon PE, Kaufman L, Rowan W (1982) Quantification of obstructions in vessels by nuclear magnetic resonance (NMR). IEEE Trans Nucl Sci NS-29:1181–1185
5. Kaufman L, Crooks LE, Sheldon PE, Rowan W, Miller T (1982) Evaluation of NMR imaging for detection and quantification of obstruction in vessels. Invest Radiol 17:554–560
6. Lanzer P, Lorenz V, Schiller NB, Crooks L, Arakawa M, Kaufman L, Davis PL, Herfkens R, Lipton MJ, Higgins CB (1984) Cardiac imaging using gated nuclear magnetic resonance. Radiology 150:121–127
7. Higgins CB, Stark D, McNamara M, Lanzer P, Crooks LE, Kaufman L (1984) Multiplane magnetic resonance imaging of the heart and major vessels: Studies in normal volunteers. Am J Roentgenol 142:661–668
8. Higgins CB, Lanzer P, Stark D, Botvinick E, Schiller NB, Crooks L, Kaufman L, Lipton MJ (1984) Nuclear magnetic resonance imaging in chronic ischemic heart disease in man. Circulation 69:523–531
9. Higgins CB, Herfkens R, Lipton MJ, Sievers R, Sheldon P, Kaufman L, Crooks LE (1983) Nuclear magnetic resonance imaging of acute myocardial infarctions in dogs: Alteration in magnetic relaxation times. Am J Cardiol 52:184–188
10. Wesbey G, Higgins CB, Lanzer P, Botvinick E, Lipton MJ (1984) In vivo imaging and characterization of acute myocardial infarction using gated nuclear magnetic resonance. Circulation 69:125–130
11. McNamara MT, Higgins CB, Ehman RL, Revel D, Sievers R, Brasch RC (1984) MRI contrast-enhancement of acute myocardial ischemia using the paramagnetic pharmaceutical complex gadolinium-DTPA. Radiology (In press)
12. Higgins CB, Byrd BF, Stark D, et al. (1984) Magnetic resonance imaging of hypertrophic cardiomyopathy. Am J Cardiol (In press)
13. Fletcher BD, Jacobstein MD, Nelson AD, Riemenschneider TA, Alfidi RJ (1984) Gated magnetic resonance imaging of congenital cardiac malformations. Radiology 150:137–140
14. Stark DD, Higgins CB, Lanzer P, Lipton MF, Schiller N, Crooks L, Botvinick E, Kaufman L (1984) Nuclear magnetic resonance imaging of the pericardium: Normal and pathologic findings. Radiology 150:469–474
15. Moncada R, Baker M, Salinas M, et al. (1982) Diagnostic role of computed tomography in pericardial heart disease. Congenital defects, thickening, neoplasms and effusions. Am Heart J 103:263–282

Index